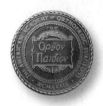
American Academy of Orthopaedic Surgeons

D1418559

OKU
Orthopaedic Knowledge Update:

Home Study
Syllabus

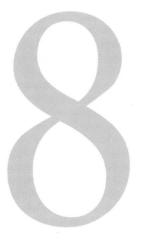

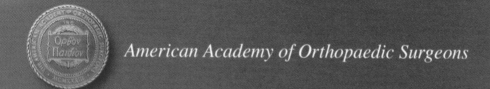
American Academy of Orthopaedic Surgeons

Orthopaedic Knowledge Update:

8

Home Study
Syllabus

Edited by
Alexander R. Vaccaro, MD, FACS
Professor
Co-Chief, Spine Surgery
Co-Chief, Spine Fellowship Program
Co-Director, Delaware Valley Regional Spinal Cord Center
Thomas Jefferson University and the Rothman Institute
Philadelphia, Pennsylvania

Published 2005 by the
American Academy of Orthopaedic Surgeons
6300 North River Road
Rosemont, IL 60018
1-800-626-6726

ISBN 0-89203-338-X
Printed in the USA
Library of Congress Cataloging-in-Publication Data

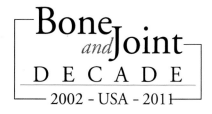

Acknowledgments

Editorial Board, OKU 8

D. Greg Anderson, MD
Associate Professor (Pending)
Department of Orthopaedics
Thomas Jefferson University
Rothman Institute
Philadelphia, Pennsylvania

Daniel J. Berry, MD
Professor of Orthopedics
Mayo Clinic College of Medicine
Department of Orthopedic Surgery
Mayo Clinic
Rochester, Minnesota

Kristen L. Carroll, MD
Associate Professor of Orthopaedics
University of Utah
Department of Orthopaedic Surgery
Shriners Hospital for Children –
  Intermountain
Salt Lake City, Utah

Jeffrey S. Fischgrund, MD
Department of Orthopaedic Surgery
William Beaumont Hospital
Royal Oak, Michigan

Mitchell Freedman, DO
Director of Physical Medicine and
  Rehabilitation at the Rothman Institute
Orthopaedic Department
Thomas Jefferson University Hospital
Philadelphia, Pennsylvania

Gary E. Friedlaender, MD
Wayne O. Southwick Professor and Chair
Department of Orthopaedics and
  Rehabilitation
Yale University School of Medicine
New Haven, Connecticut

Jonathan N. Grauer, MD
Assistant Professor
Yale University School of Medicine
New Haven, Connecticut

Timothy R. Kuklo, MD, JD
Program Director, Orthopaedic Surgery
Director, Spine Surgery
Associate Professor of Surgery
Department of Orthopaedics and
  Rehabilitation
Walter Reed Army Medical Center
Washington, DC

Brian K. Kwon, MD, FRCSC
Assistant Professor
Department of Orthopaedics
University of British Columbia
Vancouver, British Columbia, Canada

Mark D. Lazarus, MD
Associate Professor
Department of Orthopaedic Surgery
Rothman Institute
Thomas Jefferson University
Philadelphia, Pennsylvania

Randall T. Loder, MD
Garcean Professor of Pediatric Orthopaedics
Riley Children's Hospital
Department of Orthopaedic Surgery
Indiana University
Indianapolis, Indiana

Tom G. Mayer, MD
Clinical Professor
Department of Orthopaedic Surgery
University of Texas Southwestern Medical
  Center
Dallas, Texas

Steven M. Raikin, MD
Director, Foot and Ankle Service
Rothman Institute
Assistant Clinical Professor of Orthopaedic
  Surgery
Thomas Jefferson University
Philadelphia, Pennsylvania

Joseph F. Slade III, MD
Associate Professor and Director of Hand
  and Upper Extremity Center
Department of Orthopaedics
Yale University School of Medicine
New Haven, Connecticut

Contributors

William A. Abdu, MD, MS
Associate Professor of Orthopaedic
  Surgery
Medical Director, The Spine Center
Department of Orthopaedic Surgery
Dartmouth-Hitchcock Medical Center
Lebanon, New Hampshire

Robert H. Ablove, MD
Assistant Professor of Orthopaedic
  Surgery
Chief, Hand Surgery Service
University of Wisconsin Medical School
Madison, Wisconsin

Todd J. Albert, MD
Professor and Vice Chairman
Department of Orthopaedic Surgery
Thomas Jefferson University Medical
  College
Philadelphia, Pennsylvania

Arash Aminian, MD
Department of Orthopaedics
Northwestern University
Chicago, Illinois

Michael T. Archdeacon, MD, MSE
Director, Division of Orthopaedic
  Surgery
University of Cincinnati
Cincinnati, Ohio

Gregory J. Argyros, MD
Assistant Chief of Medicine
Program Director, Internal Medicine
  Residency
Department of Medicine
Walter Reed Army Medical Center
Washington, DC

R. Tracy Ballock, MD
Head, Section of Pediatric Orthopaedics
Department of Orthopaedic Surgery
  and Biomedical Engineering
The Cleveland Clinic Foundation
Cleveland, Ohio

Reed L. Bartz, MD
Assistant Professor
Department of Orthopedics
Division of Sports Medicine and
  Shoulder Surgery
University of Colorado School of
  Medicine
Denver, Colorado

John M. Beiner, MD
Clinical Instructor
Yale School of Medicine
Department of Orthopaedics
Connecticut Orthopaedic Specialists
New Haven, Connecticut

Sally Cary Booker, BA
Patient Representative
Medical Center Operations
University of Virginia Health System
Charlottesville, Virginia

Mathias Bostrom, MD
Associate Professor
Weill Medical College of Cornell
  University
New York, New York

Barbara J. Browne, MD
Medical Director, Stroke Rehabilitation
Magee Rehabilitation Hospital
Philadelphia, Pennsylvania

Joseph A. Buckwalter, MD
Professor and Chairman
Department of Orthopaedic Surgery
University of Iowa
Iowa City, Iowa

Susan V. Bukata, MD
Assistant Professor
Department of Orthopaedics
University of Rochester
Rochester, New York

Michael T. Busch, MD
Surgical Director of Sports Medicine
Hemophilia Clinic Consultant
Children's Orthopaedics of Atlanta
Children's Healthcare of Atlanta
Atlanta, Georgia

John A. Carrino, MD, MPH
Co-Director, Spine Intervention Service
Clinical Director, Magnetic Resonance
  Therapy
Department of Radiology
Harvard Medical School/Brigham and
  Women's Hospital
Boston, Massachusetts

Kristen L. Carroll, MD
Associate Professor of Orthopaedics
University of Utah
Department of Orthopaedic Surgery
Shriners Hospital for Children -
  Intermountain
Salt Lake City, Utah

Nena Clark, MPA
Medical Center Manager
Clinics (Orthopaedics, Pain
  Management Clinic, Rheumatology,
  PM & R)
UVA Health System
Charlottesville, Virginia

Brian S. Cohen, MD
Center for Advanced Orthopaedics
Adena Regional Medical Center
Chillicothe, Ohio

Frank A. Cordasco, MD, MS
Associate Professor
Department of Orthopaedic Surgery
Cornell University, Weill Medical
  College
The Sports Medicine and Shoulder
  Service
Hospital for Special Surgery
New York, New York

Roger Cornwall, MD
Attending Hand Surgeon
Department of Orthopaedic Surgery
Children's Hospital of Philadelphia
Philadelphia, Pennsylvania

Jacques L. D'Astous, MD, FRCSC
Associate Professor of Orthopaedics
University of Utah
Department of Orthopaedic Surgery
Shriners Hospital for Children -
  Intermountain
Salt Lake City, Utah

Kenny S. David, MD
Fellow
Department of Orthopedic Surgery
Medical College of Wisconsin
Milwaukee, Wisconsin

Jon R. Davids, MD
Assistant Chief of Staff
Director, Motion Analysis Laboratory
Shriners Hospital for Children
Greenville, South Carolina

Guvinder S. Deol, MD
Orthopaedic Spine Surgeon
Orthopaedic Specialists of North
  Carolina (Private Practice)
Wake Forest, North Carolina

Hargovind DeWal, MD
Fellow, Spinal Surgery
Department of Orthopaedic Surgery
Department of Neurological Surgery
Cleveland Clinic Foundation
Cleveland, Ohio

Christopher J. DeWald, MD
Assistant Professor, Department of
    Orthopedics
Rush University
Orthopaedics and Scoliosis, LLC
Rush University Medical Center
Chicago, Illinois

Edward Diao, MD
Professor of Orthopaedic Surgery and
    Neurosurgery
Chief, Division of Hand, Upper
    Extremity, and Microvascular
    Surgery
Director, UCSF/Mt. Zion Orthopaedic
    Faculty Practice
Director, UCFS Combined Hand
    Surgery Fellowship
Director, Hand Microvascular Lab
Department of Orthopaedic Surgery
University of California, San Francisco
San Francisco, California

Jeanne G. Doherty, MD
Director of NJ Outpatient
    Rehabilitation
Clinical Instructor
Magee Rehabilitation Hospital
Philadelphia, Pennsylvania

Mark Anthony Duca, MD
Clinical Assistant Professor of Medicine
University of Pittsburgh School of
    Medicine
Associate Team Physician
Pittsburgh Steelers Football Club
Pittsburgh, Pennsylvania

Marcel Dvorak, MD, FRCSC
Associate Professor
Head, Division of Spine
Department of Orthopaedics
University of British Columbia
Vancouver, British Columbia, Canada

Mark E. Easley, MD
Ankle and Foot Reconstruction
Department of Surgery/Division of
    Orthopaedic Surgery
Duke University Medical Center
Durham, North Carolina

John M. Esdaile, MD, MPH
Professor and Head
Division of Rheumatology
Department of Medicine
University of Rheumatology
Vancouver, British Columbia, Canada

Alberto Esquenazi, MD
Chair Department of PMTR
Moss Rehabilitation Hospital
Albert Einstein Medical Center
Philadelphia, Pennsylvania

Charles G. Fisher, MD, MHSc, FRCSC
Assistant Professor
Combined Neurosurgical and
    Orthopaedic Spine Program
Department of Orthopaedics
University of British Columbia
Vancouver, British Columbia, Canada

John M. Flynn, MD
Assistant Professor of Orthopaedic
    Surgery
Attending Surgeon
Division of Orthopaedic Surgery
The Children's Hospital of Philadelphia
Philadelphia, Pennsylvania

Guy W. Fried, MD
Director of Outpatient Services
Magee Rehabilitation Hospital
Philadelphia, Pennsylvania

Mark I. Froimson, MD, MBA
Department of Orthopaedic Surgery
Cleveland Clinic Foundation
Cleveland, Ohio

Freddie H. Fu, MD
David Silver Professor and Chairman
Department of Orthopaedic Surgery
University of Pittsburgh School of
    Medicine
Pittsburgh, Pennsylvania

Keith R. Gabriel, MD
Associate Professor
Division of Orthopaedics and
    Rehabilitation
Southern Illinois University School of
    Medicine
Springfield, Illinois

Gary F. Galang, MD
Department of Physical Medicine and
    Rehabilitation
University of Pittsburgh School of
    Medicine
Pittsburgh, Pennsylvania

Leesa M. Galatz, MD
Assistant Professor of Orthopaedic
    Surgery
Shoulder and Elbow Service
Department of Orthopaedic Surgery
Washington University School of
    Medicine
Barnes-Jewish Hospital
St. Louis, Missouri

William B. Geissler, MD
Professor and Chief
Arthroscopic Surgery and Sports
    Medicine
Professor, Division of Hand and Upper
    Extremity
Department of Orthopaedic Surgery
University of Mississippi Medical
    Center
Jackson, Mississippi

Michael Gilbart, MD
Shoulder and Elbow Surgery
Sports Medicine
Allan McGavin Sports Medicine Center
Vancouver, British Colombia

Vijay K. Goel, PhD
Professor and Chair
Co-Director, Spine Research Center
Bioengineering, College of Engineering
University of Toledo
Toledo, Ohio

Jonathan N. Grauer, MD
Assistant Professor
Yale University School of Medicine
New Haven, Connecticut

Nelson Greidanus, MD, MPH, FRCSC
Assistant Professor
Department of Orthopaedic Surgery
University of British Columbia
Vancouver, British Columbia, Canada

Diederick E. Grobbee, MD, PhD
Julius Center for Health Sciences and
    Primary Care
UMC Utrecht
Utrecht, The Netherlands

George J. Haidukewych, MD
Orthopedic Traumatologist
Florida Orthopedic Institute
Tampa General Hospital
Tampa, Florida

Mitchel B. Harris, MD
Associate Professor
Department of Orthopaedics
Chief, Orthopaedic Trauma
Brigham and Women's Hospital
Harvard Medical School
Boston, Massachusetts

Emily A. Hattwick, MD, MPH
Fellow, Hand Surgery
Department of Orthopaedic Surgery
University of California, San Francisco
San Francisco, California

Rex Haydon, MD, PhD
Assistant Professor of Surgery
Department of Surgery/Orthopaedics
University of Chicago
Chicago, Illinois

William Hennrikus, MD
Clinical Associate Professor: UCSF
Department of Orthopaedics
Children's Hospital Central California
Madera, California

Alan S. Hilibrand, MD
Associate Professor of Orthopaedic
    Surgery
Director of Medical Education
The Rothman Institute
Jefferson Medical College
Philadelphia, Pennsylvania

David J. Jacofsky, MD
Instructor in Orthopedic Surgery
Mayo Clinic
Rochester, Minnesota

Jesse B. Jupiter, MD
Hansjorg WYSS/AO Professor of
    Orthopaedic Surgery - Hand Surgery
Department of Orthopaedic Surgery-
    Hand Surgery
Massachusetts General Hospital
Boston, Massachusetts

Lori A. Karol, MD
Associate Professor
University of Texas - Southwestern
Department of Orthopaedic Surgery
Texas Scottish Rite Hospital
Dallas, Texas

Kosmas J. Kayes, MD
Assistant Clinical Professor
Department of Pediatric Orthopaedics
Indiana University School of Medicine
Indianapolis, Indiana

Ashutosh Khandha, MS
Bioengineering, College of Engineering
University of Toledo
Toledo, Ohio

David H. Kim, MD
The Boston Spine Group
Department of Orthopaedic Surgery
New England Baptist Hospital
Boston, Massachusetts

Richard D. Lackman, MD
Paul B. Magnuson Associate Professor
    and Chair
Department of Orthopaedic Surgery
University of Pennsylvania
Philadelphia, Pennsylvania

Joseph M. Lane, MD
Professor of Orthopaedic Surgery
Weill Medical College of Cornell
    University
New York, New York

Mark D. Lazarus, MD
Associate Professor
Department of Orthopaedic Surgery
Rothman Institute
Thomas Jefferson University
Philadelphia, Pennsylvania

Gary M. Lourie, MD
Clinical Assistant Professor,
    Department of Orthopaedics
Emory University School of Medicine
Hand and Upper Extremity Center of
    Georgia
Children's Healthcare of Atlanta at
    Scottish Rite
Atlanta, Georgia

Robert P. Lyons, MD
Shoulder and Elbow Surgeon
OrthoCarolina Orthopaedic and Sports
    Medicine
Presbyterian Orthopaedic Hospital
Charlotte, North Carolina

William G. Mackenzie, MD
Pediatric Orthopaedic Surgeon
Department of Orthopaedics
A.I. duPont Hospital for Children
Wilmington, Delaware

Richard M. Marks, MD, FACS
Associate Professor
Director, Division of Foot and Ankle
    Surgery
Department of Orthopaedic Surgery
Medical College of Wisconsin
Milwaukee, Wisconsin

Eric K. Mayer, MD
Clinical Fellow
Physical Medicine and Rehabilitation
Harvard Medical School, Spaulding
    Rehabilitation Hospital
Boston, Massachusetts

Tom G. Mayer, MD
Clinical Professor
Department of Orthopaedic Surgery
University of Texas Southwestern
    Medical Center
Dallas, Texas

Eric C. McCarty, MD
Associate Professor
Chief of Sports Medicine and Shoulder
    Surgery
Head Team Physician
University of Colorado
Department of Orthopaedic Surgery
Division of Sports Medicine and
    Shoulder Surgery
University of Colorado School of
    Medicine
Denver, Colorado

Robert F. McLain, MD
Member, Surgical Staff
Fellowship Director
Department of Orthopaedic Surgery
Cleveland Clinic Spine Institute
The Cleveland Clinic Foundation
Cleveland, Ohio

Patrick J. McMahon, MD
Shoulder and Elbow Surgery
Sports Medicine
University of Pittsburgh
Pittsburgh, Pennsylvania

Gregory A. Mencio, MD
Associate Professor
Department of Orthopaedics and
    Rehabilitation
Vanderbilt University Medical Center
Nashville, Tennessee

Alexander D. Mih, MD
Associate Professor
Department of Orthopaedic Surgery
Indiana University School of Medicine
Indianapolis, Indiana

Karel G. M. Moons, PhD
Julius Center for Health Sciences and
    Primary UMC Utrecht
Utrecht, The Netherlands

William B. Morrison, MD
Director, Division of Musculoskeletal
    and General Diagnostic Imaging
Department of Radiology
Thomas Jefferson University Hospital
Philadelphia, Pennsylvania

Vincent S. Mosca, MD
Associate Professor of Orthopaedics
Department of Orthopaedics and Sports
    Medicine
University of Washington School of
    Medicine
Seattle, Washington

Owen J. Moy, MD
Clinical Professor of Orthopaedic
    Surgery
SUNY at Buffalo School of Biomedical
    Sciences
Hand Center of Western New York
Buffalo, New York

Michael C. Munin, MD
Associate Professor
Physical Medicine and Rehabilitation
University of Pittsburgh School of
    Medicine
Pittsburgh, Pennsylvania

Mary A. Murray, MD
Associate Professor
Chief, Division of Pediatric
    Endocrinology
University of Utah School of Medicine
Pediatric Endocrinology
University of Utah School of Medicine
Salt Lake City, Utah

George F. Muschler, MD
Full Staff
Department of Orthopaedic Surgery
    and Biomedical Engineering
The Cleveland Clinic Foundation (AYI)
Cleveland, Ohio

Chizu Nakamoto, MD, PhD
Project Staff
Department of Biomedical Engineering
The Cleveland Clinic Foundation
Cleveland, Ohio

Kevin C. O'Connor, MD
Medical Director, Spinal Cord Injury
Assistant Professor
Department of Physical Medicine and
    Rehabilitation
Spaulding Rehabilitation Hospital
Boston, Massachusetts

Debra M. Parisi, MD
Clinical Assistant Professor
Hand and Orthopaedic Surgery
Beth Israel Orthopaedics
Beth Israel Medical Center
New York, New York

Javad Parvizi, MD, FRCS
Assistant Professor
Department of Orthopaedic Surgery
Rothman Institute at Jefferson
    University
Philadelphia, Pennsylvania

Chetan K. Patel, MD
Attending Surgeon
Orthopaedic Spine Center
Douglas, Georgia

Tushar C. Patel, MD
Commonwealth Orthopaedics
Fairfax, Virginia

Michael J. Patzakis, MD
Professor and Chairman
The Vincent and Julia Meyer Chair
Chief of Orthopaedic Surgery Service
Department of Orthopaedic Surgery
Keck School of Medicine of the
    University of Southern California
Los Angeles, California

Andrew D. Pearle
Sports Medicine and Shoulder Service
Hospital for Special Surgery
New York, New York

Frank M. Phillips, MD
Professor of Orthopaedic Surgery
Rush University Medical Center
Chicago, Illinois

Kornelis A. Poelstra, MD, PhD
Physician
University of Virginia
Department of Orthopaedic Surgery
Charlottesville, Virginia
Joel M. Press, MD
Medical Director
Spine and Sports Rehabilitation Center
Rehabilitation Institute of Chicago
Assistant Professor, Physical Medicine
    and Rehabilitation
Northwestern/Feinberg School of
    Medicine
Chicago, Illinois

James J. Purtill, MD
Assistant Professor
Rothman Institute
Thomas Jefferson University
Philadelphia, Pennsylvania

Thomas J. Puschak, MD
Indiana Spine Surgery
Orthopaedic Spine Surgery
Indianapolis, Indiana

Raj D. Rao, MD
Associate Professor
Director of Spine Surgery
Department of Orthopaedic Surgery
Medical College of Wisconsin
Milwaukee, Wisconsin

Mark Cameron Reilly, MD
Assistant Professor, Orthopaedics
Co-Chief Professor, Orthopaedic
    Trauma Service
Department of Orthopaedic Surgery
New Jersey Medical School
Newark, New Jersey

Angelique M. Reitsma, MD, MA
Research Associate
Center for Biomedical Ethics
University of Virginia
Charlottesville, Virginia

William M. Ricci, MD
Associate Professor
Department of Orthopaedic Surgery
Washington University School of
    Medicine
St. Louis, Missouri

B. Stephens Richards III, MD
Professor, Department of Orthopaedic
    Surgery
University of Texas-Southwestern
    Medical Center
Assistant Chief of Staff
Texas Scottish Rite Hospital for
    Children
Dallas, Texas

David Ring, MD
Orthopaedic Hand and Upper
    Extremity Service
Massachusetts General Hospital
Boston, Massachusetts

Anthony A. Romeo, MD
Director, Shoulder Service
Section of Sports Medicine
Associate Professor
Department of Orthopaedic Surgery
Rush University Medical Center
Chicago, Illinois

Mark J. Romness, MD
Commonwealth Orthopaedics
Fairfax, Virginia

Dino Samartzis, BS, PGCEBHC
Faculty of Arts and Sciences Graduate
    Division
Harvard University
Cambridge, Massachusetts
Division of Health Sciences
University of Oxford
Oxford, England

John F. Sarwark, MD
Professor
Department of Orthopaedic Surgery
Northwestern University
Chicago, Illinois

Rick C. Sasso, MD
Indiana Spine Group
Assistant Professor
Clinical Orthopaedic Surgery
Indiana University School of Medicine
Indianapolis, Indiana

Tim Schrader, MD
Children's Orthopaedics of Atlanta
Children's Healthcare of Atlanta-
    Scottish Rite
Atlanta, Georgia

Francis H. Shen, MD, FACS
Assistant Professor
Department of Orthopaedic Surgery
Division of Spine Surgery
University of Virginia
Charlottesville, Virginia

Kam Shojania, MD, FRCPC
Clinical Associate Professor
Division of Rheumatology
Department of Medicine
University of British Columbia
Vancouver, British Columbia, Canada

David Andrew Spiegel, MD
Department of Orthopaedic Surgery
Children's Hospital of Philadelphia
Philadelphia, Pennsylvania
Assistant Professor of Orthopaedic
    Surgery
The University of Pennsylvania School
    of Medicine
Philadelphia, Pennsylvania

Kurt P. Spindler, MD
Professor, Orthopaedics and
    Rehabilitation
Vanderbilt University Medical Center
Nashville, Tennessee

Scott P. Steinmann, MD
Department of Orthopaedic Surgery
Mayo Clinic
Rochester, Minnesota

Daniel J. Sucato, MD, MS
Assistant Professor
Department of Orthopaedic Surgery
University of Texas at Southwestern
    Medical Center
Texas Scottish Rite Hospital for
    Children
Dallas, Texas

Bobby K-B Tay, MD
Assistant Professor of Orthopaedic
    Surgery
Department of Orthopaedic Surgery
University of California, San Francisco
San Francisco, California

Thomas E. Trumble, MD
Professor and Chief
Hand and Microvascular Surgery
Department of Orthopaedics
University of Washington
Seattle, Washington

Eeric Truumees, MD
Attending Spine Surgeon
Orthopaedic Director, Gehring
    Biomechanics Laboratory
William Beaumont Hospital
Royal Oak, Michigan

Sasidhar Vadapalli, MS
Bioengineering, College of Engineering
University of Toledo
Toledo, Ohio

Ann Van Heest, MD
Associate Professor
Department of Orthopaedic Surgery
University of Minnesota
Minneapolis, Minnesota

Eric J. Wall, MD
Director, Sports Medicine
Department of Orthopaedics
Cincinnati Children's Hospital
Cincinnati, Ohio

Jeffrey C. Wang, MD
Chief, Spine Service
Associate Professor of Orthopaedic
    Surgery
Department of Orthopaedic Surgery
University of California, Los Angeles,
    School of Medicine
Los Angeles, California

William C. Warner, Jr, MD
Associate Professor
Department of Orthopaedic Surgery
University of Tennessee-Campbell
    Clinic
Memphis, Tennessee

Peter M. Waters, MD
Director of Hand and Upper Extremity
    Surgery
Department of Orthopaedic Surgery
Children's Hospital
Boston, Massachusetts

Robin Vereeke West, MD
Assistant Professor
Department of Orthopaedics
University of Pittsburgh Medical Center
Pittsburgh, Pennsylvania

David E. Westberry, MD
Assistant Director
Orthopaedic Surgery Education
Greenville Hospital System
Greenville, South Carolina

Eric S. Wieser, MD
Spinal Surgery Specialist
Arlington Orthopedic Associates, PA
Arlington, Texas

Timothy M. Wright, PhD
Senior Member, Research Division
Biomechanics Laboratory
Hospital for Special Surgery
New York, New York

John S. Xenos, MD
Director, Adult Reconstruction
Orthopaedic Surgery Service
Department of Orthopaedic Surgery
    and Rehabilitation
Walter Reed Army Medical Center
Washington, District of Columbia

Andrew Yun, MD
Medical Doctor
Department of Orthopaedic Surgery
The Arthritis Institute
Inglewood, California

Charalampos Zalavras, MD
Assistant Professor
Department of Orthopaedic Surgery
LAC and USC Medical Center
Keck School of Medicine
University of Southern California
Los Angeles, California

Steven Zeiller, MD
Spine Fellow
Department of Orthopaedics
Thomas Jefferson University
Philadelphia, Pennsylvania

Table of Contents

Section 3 Systemic Disorders

Section 4 Upper Extremity

Section 5 Lower Extremity

Section Editors

Daniel J. Berry, MD
Steven M. Raikin, MD

Section 6 Spine

Section Editor

Jeffrey S. Fischgrund, MD

Preface

As trusted and caring orthopaedic physicians, we have a duty to possess, maintain, and gain as much knowledge as we can about our field of medicine. Orthopaedic surgery is dedicated to the management of musculoskeletal disorders. This exciting discipline is constantly developing in terms of its knowledge foundation and ability to improve the quality of our patients' lives. To be productive participants in this evolving field, it is our responsibility to continuously update our understanding of current practices and advances. We accomplish these goals in many ways, including subscribing to medical journals, attending conferences, actively treating patients, and through our own research. It is hoped that this latest edition of Orthopaedic Knowledge Update (OKU 8) will serve as a vital learning aid so that every orthopaedic surgeon can review the most up-to-date information in the field as assembled by many of our respected colleagues.

The 8th volume of OKU includes a comprehensive review of current knowledge as well as of recent advances in musculoskeletal care. It is also intended to function as a bridge between the findings of the past and present to those of the future. The primary purpose of this text is to serve as a user-friendly reference guide for all levels of learning so students, residents, fellows, and practitioners can confidently care for patients with orthopaedic problems in a safe and effective manner. The Orthopadeic Knowledge Update series is, and always will be, the official reference book for information necessary to prepare for in-service or board examinations. The knowledge within this text will undoubtedly become partially obsolete over the ensuing years in time for subsequent editions of Orthopaedic Knowledge Update.

Great thanks is given to the over 100 authors who collaborated to impart their expertise in their contributed chapters. A tremendous amount of sacrificed time and energy was needed to prepare an evidence-based synopsis of their assigned chapters. Their dedication to the field of orthopaedics as well as to their patients is commendable. The table of contents and organization is largely a reflection of the oversight of 14 section editors who have worked countless hours selecting the optimal authors and topics, and ensuring the lack of repetition or duplication of work throughout the book. I would like to express my deepest gratitude to the Academy Publications staff, headed by Marilyn Fox, PhD, and specifically Lisa Claxton Moore and Kathleen Anderson, as well as my assistants, Arjun Saxena and Thomas Day, for their tireless work throughout this enormous project. The Academy staff and assistants have spent innumerable hours coordinating manuscripts and illustrations, organizing meetings, and bringing to reality the final version of OKU 8. I hope you enjoy this most recent edition of Orthopaedic Knowledge Update as much as we did throughout its preparation.

Alexander R. Vaccaro, MD
Editor

Section 1

Basic Science

Section Editors:
Jonathan N. Grauer, MD
Gary E. Friedlaender, MD

Chapter 1

Orthopaedic Research: What An Orthopaedic Surgeon Needs to Know

Charles Fisher, MD, MHSc, FRCSC

Marcel Dvorak, MD, FRCSC

Introduction

Although statistics and clinical epidemiology have been part of the core curriculum for medical schools and some residency programs, most clinicians have only limited knowledge in these areas. This is not from a lack of training or interest, but more because statistical and epidemiologic proficiency requires frequent application and interpretation. Lack of familiarity in these areas may lead the clinician to feel intimidated or to avoid statistics and other methodologic aspects of clinical studies.

Therefore, it is important to be familiar with some of the essential statistical and epidemiologic concepts and study design principles necessary to properly conduct and evaluate clinical research. Although it is impossible to comprehensively derive or explain these concepts within the scope of this chapter, hopefully their practicality will stimulate further application within clinical and academic practice. Surprisingly, many of the errors or flaws found in clinical research are not complex statistical or methodologic issues but more the neglect of fundamental principles that are often forgotten.

It's All in the Question

Although biostatistics plays a prominent role, especially in research, its significance is often overemphasized, particularly relative to issues of study design and methodology. In any research study, the clinician scientist must first develop a question. On the surface this may seem simple, but clearly defining the primary study question is indeed difficult. For example: What are the outcomes of patients with sciatica treated surgically and nonsurgically? This question may appear adequate, but on further inspection what is meant by outcome? Is the outcome pain, function, or return to work? Studies can usually only be designed to answer one question precisely and provide probable or possible answers to other secondary questions. So a better question for this example might be: For patients with sciatica secondary to lumbar disk herniation treated with either surgery or nonsurgical treatment, what is the change in neurologic symptom score from initial assessment to 1 year after treatment? Once a researcher has a clearly defined question the research protocol usually is easy to write. The inclusion criteria, sample size calculation, blinding, random allocation, follow-up schedule, objective outcome measure, and statistical analysis all become much easier with a well-defined question.

Once the study question is clearly identified, then biostatistics becomes fundamental to the understanding and conduct of medical research. Not only do statistics enable physicians to compare treatment strategies in clinical trials, but also in analytical epidemiology the relationship or association between variables can be studied. The classic association of environmental, lifestyle, or biologic factors to the development of disease has been analyzed. The relationship of lung cancer and smoking is probably the most famous example. In clinical research these same statistical tools can be used to examine the relationship between various baseline and demographic variables to an outcome variable of choice. For example, the association of age, surgery, and disease severity on the primary outcome of interest ("pain") can be determined. Ultimately through this analysis the true effect or causation is determined; however, before this can be concluded other possible explanations (bias, confounding, chance, reverse causation) for the associations must be ruled out, such that causation is a diagnosis of exclusion.

The conclusions that can be reached from a data set are limited by the question asked and the design of the study to answer it. Although statistics allow for the summation of data, hypothesis testing, the avoidance or reduction of nonsystematic error, and adjustment for confounding factors, they are not the panacea for a poorly designed study.

Study Design

In general there are two types of clinical studies—those that analyze primary data and those that analyze secondary data. Studies that collect and analyze primary data include case reports and series, case control, cross sectional, cohort (both prospective and retrospective) and randomized controlled trials (RCTs). Analysis of secondary data occurs in systematic reviews or meta-analysis for the purpose of pooling or synthesizing data to answer a question that is perhaps not practical or answerable with an individual study. Another way to broadly characterize studies is as experimental, where an intervention is introduced to subjects, or observational, in which no active treatment is introduced to subjects. The methodologic hierarchy or rating of scientific studies is well summarized in the literature.

Case Reports

Case reports are valuable in rare conditions or if they provide compelling findings that can be hypothesis-generating for further studies. Case reports are limited by small sample size, the lack of a control group, and nonobjective outcome measures. The natural extension of a case report is a case series, which allows for a more valid assessment of a clinical course or response to an intervention. Few conclusions can be made because of the selection bias, subjective assessment, a small, often ill-defined number of subjects (n), and lack of a comparison group. Case series can be improved by addressing some of these limitations such as using objective outcome measures and clearly defining their inclusion criteria, which makes them very similar to cohort studies.

Prevalence Studies

Cross sectional or prevalence studies are common in public health but are rare in the surgical realm. They provide a snapshot of the health experience of a population at a specified period of time. These studies can provide a relatively quick assessment of health status or health needs. They can be hypothesis-generating for ill-defined diseases and are a good design for common diseases of long duration such as osteoarthritis. Unfortunately, they cannot establish temporality, so these studies are prone to reverse causality or protopathic bias. A cross-sectional analysis can be blended with a retrospective cohort study and be quite effective. An example would be to retrospectively define a patient cohort such as cervical burst fractures and then do a cross-sectional outcome analysis on function or quality of life. The follow-up will occur at various times relative to when the patient was injured but can still provide valuable objective long-term outcome information.

Case Control Studies

Case control studies usually involve a cross-sectional analysis on similar subjects and classically compare certain patient groups (cases) with control patients for the presence of risk factors. This design is ideal for assessing etiologic or risk factors for rare diseases and is useful in studies of prognosis. Although these studies are efficient

from a time and cost perspective, there are limitations. Finding appropriately matched controls and defining inclusion and exclusion criteria that are similar for both cases and control patients are steps taken to control for confounding variables. Because both the exposure and disease have already occurred and there is different recall bias between cases and control patients, proving causation is difficult. An example of a surgical case control study would be comparing patients who have had anterior cruciate ligament reconstruction and developed the complication of a stiff knee (cases), to patients without postoperative knee stiffness (controls). The results may allow the identification of risk factors for knee stiffness. Ideally the control:case ratio should be 1:1 up to a maximum of 4:1.

Cohort Studies

Cohort studies can be retrospective or prospective, with prospective studies providing better scientific evidence. Cohort studies are similar to case series, but more tightly controlled. They require a time zero, strict inclusion/exclusion criteria, standardized follow-up at regular time intervals, and efforts to optimize follow-up and reduce dropouts. For these reasons prospective cohort studies are expensive and time-consuming. Cohort designs are ideal for identifying risk factors for disease, determining the outcome of an intervention, and examining the natural history of a disease. The Framingham cohort study examining cardiovascular disease is one of the more famous cohort studies. Prospective cohorts can be compared with historical controls but problems with data quality, selection bias, outcome parameters, and temporal trends make this less desirable than a nonrandomized prospective outcomes study.

Retrospective studies have the advantage of being less expensive and time consuming. The records (usually charts) are made out without knowledge of exposure or disease and therefore recall bias is not an issue. However, because the records used for data are collected for other reasons and in a nonstandardized manner, critical information such as confounders is almost always missing. The incorporation of a cross-sectional outcome analysis to a retrospective cohort study provides a standardized outcome, but many subjects may be deceased or lost to follow-up, leading to poor response rates.

Randomized Controlled Trials

RCTs are justifiably recognized as the gold standard in obtaining clinical evidence; however, they have well recognized disadvantages including high costs, administrative complexity, prolonged time to completion, and difficulty ensuring methodologic vision. Furthermore, RCTs in surgery are complicated by difficulties in blinding, randomization, technique standardization, and generalizability. Nevertheless, the ability to control for known and unknown bias outweighs these disadvantages. Randomization is unrivaled in ensuring the balancing of the experimental and control groups for unknown confounders. Known confounders are also well balanced if the group sizes are large enough; however, if the sample sizes are small the balancing of known confounders can easily be performed through stratification. Blinding is designed to induce comparability in the handling and evaluation of the participants, it preserves the integrity of the randomization, and allows for objective collection and analysis of data. Surgical RCTs are difficult to perform; hence, there is a paucity of information about them in the orthopaedic literature. Practical and ethical issues limit their use in surgery, but above all they are extremely difficult, time consuming and expensive to perform. These factors should not deter clinical scientists from pursuing this study design so that needed answers to important questions can be obtained.

Systematic Reviews

A systematic review provides a rational synopsis of the available literature. By summarizing all relevant literature on a particular topic, the systematic review tends to be a tremendous asset to the busy clinician. A systematic review attempts to overcome the bias that is associated with the majority of "traditional" reviews or more appropriately termed "narrative" reviews. Through the application of rigorous methodology, potential bias is minimized. A properly conducted systematic review will ensure all published and unpublished literature is considered, will evaluate each study for its relevance and quality through independent assessment, and then synthesize the remaining studies in a fair and unbiased manner. A good systematic review is transparent. Transparency implies openness by the authors so that the reader can determine the validity of the conclusions for themselves. A properly conducted systematic review should allow a second group of authors using the same methodology to arrive at the same conclusion(s).

Component studies of a systematic review may be combined qualitatively, or quantitatively with RCTs. When a quantitative synthesis is performed it is termed a meta-analysis. Meta-analysis refers to the statistical technique used for combining independent studies. A meta-analysis is particularly useful when combining several small studies whose results may be inconclusive because of low power. Meta-analyses have a greater ability to detect uncommon but clinically relevant end points such as mortality.

After determining the question being asked in a study, and having an overview of the types of studies used in clinical research, the next step is to look at data analysis, which validates the answer to the question.

Basic Terms and Concepts in Biostatistics
Population and Sample

A population is a complete set of homogenous individuals with a specified set of characteristics. A sample is a subset of a population. The population and sample represent the starting point for all analysis. Total populations are very difficult if not impossible to study. The majority of studies are based on subpopulations or samples of the population of interest. It is the parameters (measurements) of the sample that are used not only to accurately describe the larger population of interest, but also to help answer scientific questions about whether interventions affect these measurements. For instance, the variable might be age and the parameter average age. The parameters used describe the location and variability among the members of a population and are discussed in the following paragraphs.

Mean and Median

A simple figure that provides a measure of central tendency or an average of variability for symmetric or normative data is the mean, which is defined as the sum of all the observations in a sample divided by the number of observations. For nonsymmetric data, a better measure of central tendency or average is the median. The median is the point that divides the distribution of observations in half, if the observations are arranged in increasing or decreasing order. This is relevant because statistical procedures vary depending on the distribution of the population. In other words, certain tests assume a normal distribution, and if the data distribution is not normal, alternative statistical tests must be used to ensure accurate results.

Standard Deviation

The standard deviation (SD) is one of several indices of variability used to characterize the distribution of values in a sample for symmetric data. Numerically, the SD is the square root of the variance. The SD is conceptually easier to use than the variance, which is defined as the average squared deviation from the mean. Degrees of freedom are used in the calculation of SD and are often misunderstood or confusing. They are used in the mathematical formulas that construct tables to determine levels of significance. Specifically, they represent the number of samples and sample size, which are factors in determining significance.

If there were a greater range (maximum to minimum) in the measured variable, then the SD would be larger. Assuming a normal distribution, about 95% of the population falls within 2 SDs of the mean. Therefore, the mean and SD provide a concise summary of a particular variable within a symmetrically distributed population. If a population does not follow a normal distribution then it would be more appropriate to report the median and percentiles.

Another term of variability worth mentioning that is often reported in the literature is standard error of the mean (SEM). SEM estimates the accuracy of the mean computed from the sample compared with mean of the actual population from which the sample was taken. It quantifies the uncertainty in the estimate of the mean; however, it says nothing about the variability of the population itself. The SD measures the variability of the population and is always larger then the SEM, and thus makes the data less statistically appealing.

Randomization

Randomization is a process that arbitrarily assigns subjects to two or more groups by some chance mechanism, rather than by choice. It ensures that each subject has a fair and equal opportunity to be assigned to each group. Randomization is necessary to avoid systematic error (bias) that may produce unequal groups with respect to general characteristics, such as gender, age, ethnicity, and other key factors that may affect the probable course of the disease or treatment. Depending on the distribution of the data and the size of the sample there is a chance that the sample will not be representative just by chance alone.

Variables and Types of Variables

Any division of measurement or classification on which individual observations are made is called a variable. In general, there are two types of variables, qualitative and quantitative. A qualitative variable is subdivided into nominal and ordinal variables. With ordinal variables, the categories have an obvious rank order, such as the stages of bowel cancer. Nominal variables allow for only qualitative classification; for example, gender or occupation. Quantitative variables are either discrete (length of hospital stay) or continuous (age). Continuous variables allow not only ranking of the order of observations that are measured, but also quantification and comparison of the size of differences between observations.

Hypothesis

A hypothesis is a supposition made as a basis for reasoning, without assumption of its truth, or as a starting point for further investigation. In statistics there are two kinds of hypotheses. The null hypothesis (H_o) assumes no effect or differences, whereas the alternate hypothesis (H_a) postulates there is an effect or difference. Statistics are designed to test for the H_o. When the probability of the observed data patterns cannot support H_o, a researcher would reject H_o in favor of H_a. This does not mean that H_o is absolutely incorrect, only that the data at hand cannot support it.

Hypothesis and Significance Testing: P Value

These terms are best explained by an example. A researcher wants to test a new drug for postoperative pain control. The population will be patients undergoing lumbar fusion. Two samples will be randomly chosen from the population, with one getting the standard drug (control) and the other getting the new drug (experimental). The two groups will then rate their pain and the mean and SD pain score for each group will be calculated. Is the observed difference in mean pain scores caused by the drug or by random assignment to the two study samples? This question is answered by quantifying the difference by means of a test statistic. The actual specific statistical test the researcher uses will vary depending on the question and population, but one number will be calculated. The greater the difference between the two means the greater the test statistic number; however, what is the cutoff value for this number between true and random difference?

To obtain the distribution of the test statistic, the researcher will assume the drug has no effect (null hypothesis) and in "theory" run the same experiment a multitude of times using all possible samples from the population. Most test statistic numbers will be small because there is no difference; by chance alone some of these experiments will demonstrate a large test statistic. Say 5% of them will be above this cutoff point even if the H_o is correct.

Having established the cutoff for the test statistic, the experiment is redone with a drug that the researcher hypothesizes will improve pain. If the calculated test statistic is larger than the 5% cutoff point that was determined above, then the chance of the observed difference in pain scores used to calculate this big test statistic number being due to chance alone is 5%. Therefore the experimenter would reject the H_o and accept the H_a at a significance level of 5%. It should be noted that there is still a 5% chance of a false-positive result. The p value is the probability of reporting a difference when one does not exist. The p value should not be regarded as rigid and can be adjusted depending on the question being asked and the clinical implications of the H_o being falsely rejected. The researcher should specify the p value before the study is commenced.

Type I (α) and Type II (β) Error

A type I error occurs in a comparative study when a statistically significant finding occurs by chance alone. In other words, a study's H_o is rejected when it is true and a false-positive result occurs. The probability of a type I error is represented by α, and is widely accepted at 5%.

Not as well recognized is the type II error or false-negative finding of a study. In this situation no difference is identified between experimental and control groups, when in fact there is a difference between the

Table 1 | Influence of the Magnitude of Sample Size Determinants on Sample Size Required

Determinants	Sample Size	
Variability	Increase	Decrease
Effect change	Decrease	Increase
α	Decrease	Increase
β	Decrease	Increase

groups. In medicine, a type II error occurs when a study is "underpowered"; the study has failed to include enough patients to detect a predetermined magnitude of difference between treatments. The chance of making a type II error, represented by β, is commonly accepted to be 20%. The chance of detecting a true positive result is the power of the study $(1-\beta)$ and would be 80%. Unfortunately, it is common for RCTs published in peer-reviewed journals to neglect the power of the study by not reporting a sample size calculation a priori. When a study reveals no difference between groups but does not report the power, the chance of making a type II error is essentially unknown. This significantly limits the validity of a study's findings.

Sample Size or Power Calculation

A power calculation determines the number of patients or experimental units required for the study to detect a difference, if one is present. Too large a sample results in a waste of time and money; conversely, too small a sample leads to a lack of precision in the results (type II error). Formulas are available to determine sample size and vary depending on the statistical analysis being done. The determinants of sample size are α, power $(1-\beta)$, effect change, and variability (Table 1).

One final consideration is a one- or two-tailed significance test. Convention would suggest that all comparative studies be two-tailed such that A analyzed to be better than B and vice versa. However, if it is important to know that A is better than B, a one-tailed test can be done and sample size reduced because α is theoretically larger. An example where a one-tailed test is useful would be a study of a new intervention that is more expensive and the only way it will replace the control is if it is superior to it; equivalence or worse is not of interest.

Statistical Versus Clinical Significance

As discussed, many factors affect statistical significance, such as the magnitude of the effect (effect change), the sample size, the reliability of the effect, and the reliability of the measurement instrument. A clinically significant difference varies depending on factors associated with the intervention and variable of interest. The ge-

neric definition of clinical significance that permits its application to numerous studies is a difference large enough for the clinician to want to choose one treatment over the other, after considering all factors (such as cost or side effects). Determining a clinically significant difference is often difficult, especially if it involves an outcome such as health-related quality of life. It is an important decision because it is an integral component of the sample size calculation.

Confidence Interval

A confidence interval (CI) gives an estimated range of values that are likely to include the unknown population parameter being sought. The CI is usually calculated at 95%, but 99% CIs are also used. The interval describes the confidence with which the true difference in mean values from each group or intervention is within the CI. The CI then describes both the size of the treatment effect and the certainty of the estimation of the treatment effect. The CI can be used for hypothesis testing for if the interval contains zero, then the H_o cannot be rejected. If the interval is 95% confidence this would be analogous to a p value of 0.05. The advantage of using the CI for hypothesis testing is that it provides information about the size of the effect. For example, something might be statistically significant because of a large sample size, but when one sees the quantitative effect it may be clinically insignificant.

Statistical Analysis

The goal of this section is to create familiarity with some of the common statistical methods used in clinical research. Most of these methods are used for hypothesis testing.

t Test (Student's t test) and the Signed-Rank Sum Test

The t test procedure is used to test the H_o where the mean of a single variable of the population from which the sample was drawn is equal to a specified value. The t test is applied if the sample values are independent and normally distributed. If not, a nonparametric method is used, commonly the signed rank sum test. Researchers want to test whether the average score of the Short Form-36 (SF-36) at 1 year postoperative for 10 patients (mean = 39.8, SD = 10.3) differs from published normative population data (mean = 52.0; SD = 8.0) (H_a). Or, if it is likely that the mean score at 1-year follow-up is equal to the normative data (H_o). From a computer statistical package or tables, the exact p value based on a two-sided test is 0.005. This is a significant difference at the 5% level and suggests that the decrease of the SF-36 score in patients at 1-year follow-up is unlikely due to chance and H_o is rejected.

The Paired t Test and Wilcoxon Two-Sample Test

The paired *t* test is generally used when measurements are taken from the same subject or related subject over time or in different circumstances. This implies that the data are from within the same sample and that measurements are related to each other. For example, a paired *t* test can be used to determine the difference in blood pressure before and after treatment. The paired *t* test assesses the average change that an intervention produces. For the paired *t* test, the observed data are from the same subject or from a matched subject and are drawn from a population with a normal distribution. If these assumptions are not met, then one of the nonparametric alternative tests should be applied, for example, the Wilcoxon two-sample test.

Comparisons of Two Means (t Test and the Mann-Whitney U Test)

The *t* test and the Mann-Whitney U test are appropriate where the data have been obtained from two independent samples. The two-sample *t* test determines whether two samples are likely to be from the same population. In addition, the two different samples are assumed to come from populations with the same variance. The *t* test would be commonly used in RCTs comparing the mean score from each of two groups. If the assumption of normality or equality of variance is not met, a distribution-free test that is an alternative to the independent sample *t* test is used. This is called the Mann-Whitney U test and uses ranked scores.

One of the common problems that arise with *t* tests is that of multiple comparisons. The issue of multiple comparisons actually goes beyond *t* tests into issues of subgroup analysis and hypothesis testing versus hypothesis generating analysis. From the explanation of the p value earlier in the chapter, the chance of obtaining a false-positive result is 5%. If a researcher has three groups to compare and does a *t* test for A versus B, B versus C, and A versus C, then the chance for a type I error is greater. For three tests it is 5% + 5% + 5% so it becomes 15%; if it were four groups it would be 30%. In other words the chances of the researcher obtaining a highly coveted significant difference are increased, and the problem is that it may not be a true difference. To avoid this problem there are two approaches. One is to use multiple comparison procedures such as the Bonferroni or Holm *t* test that use appropriate correction factors to address the changing p value. The simplest and initial approach, however, should be to use the analysis of variance (ANOVA) when the experimental design involves multiple groups.

Analysis of Variance

The ANOVA takes the *t* test from two groups to three or more groups. It accomplishes this by replacing multiple *t* tests with the F test. The F test assumes all the underlying group population means are equal. Therefore, if the groups have a common population mean, then the group or sample means should all lie near the population mean. If the group means are sufficiently different, then the F statistic will be large, and it can be concluded that at least one of the population means for the group varies from the others. The ANOVA does not differentiate which group differs from the others. To make that determination, multiple comparison techniques must be used. Beyond the analysis of studies with more than two groups and one factor of interest, ANOVA is valuable for testing whether treatment groups have comparable population means for variables that may influence treatment, but are not the primary variable of interest. Classic examples are age, gender, or comorbidities. In well-designed RCTs this type of analysis will be done to ensure comparable treatment groups.

Rates and Proportions

The tests and examples given above have been concerned with quantitative data made up of continuous or discrete data. Many scientific studies use data that are measured on a nominal scale. These variables are easily described as proportions and are analyzed by a distinct set of statistical tools. Analogous to the *t* test for proportions is the z statistic. The z statistic is derived along the same lines as a *t* test and is only adequate for hypothesis testing when there are two outcomes of interest. The more commonly used test is the chi square test, which is the proportion equivalent of the ANOVA, but is also used when there are only two outcomes of interest.

Comparisons of Two Proportions (Chi-Square Test and the Exact Test)

In a study assessing neurologic outcome in spinal cord injuries, a total of 123 patients were eligible but only 71 consented. Because there were a large number of patients who refused, the researchers wanted to ensure there was no bias introduced based on the subjects who did and did not consent. They wanted to check if there was an association between gender distribution and participation.

The chi square test summarizes the differences between the expected and observed frequencies. The expected frequencies are the number of subjects that would be expected in each group subdivision (consenting/nonconsenting males, consenting/nonconsenting females) if the treatment had no effect, or in this case if there was no relationship between gender and participation. The H_o is that there is no relationship between the two categorical variables, gender and participation. The chi square test is used to test this hypothesis.

For the chi square test to be accurate, all the expected frequencies for each subgroup or cell should exceed 5. If the study is small and expected frequencies are less than 5, two methods of improvement are widely used: the application of continuity correction; and the calculation of Fisher's exact probability. When the expected frequencies are particularly small, say, less than 1, the Fisher's exact test should be applied.

Relative Risk and Odds Ratio in a Cohort and Case-Control Study

A classic cohort study usually makes comparisons between a group of individuals exposed to some factor and a group not exposed. The relative risk (RR) is the probability of the disease in the exposed group divided by the probability of the disease in the unexposed (control) group. RR measures the increased risk (if any) of incurring a particular disease in the exposed individuals compared with the unexposed individuals. For example, the association of lung cancer with smoking is a RR of 10, which would mean that smokers are 10 times more likely to develop lung cancer. If the RR is 1, the risks are equal and if less than 1, then the risk in the exposed group is lower.

In a cohort study, the result of the study can be summarized as a 2 × 2 contingency table illustrated by the generic form shown in Table 2.

The RR of a specific disease for individuals exposed as compared with those not exposed is given by

$$RR = \frac{a/(a + b)}{c/(c + d)}$$

The 95% CI for RR can also be calculated.

Case-control studies are retrospective; therefore, disease rates in the exposed sample and the nonexposed sample cannot be estimated, thus RR cannot be calculated. The data can again be summarized in a 2 × 2 table. In such a case, if the disease in both exposed and nonexposed groups is rare, or *a* and *c* are small in comparison with *b* and *d*, respectively, the odds ratio (OR) will be used to estimate the relative risk.

$$OR = \frac{a/b}{c/d} = \frac{ad}{bc}$$

The OR is the probability of an event occurring, divided by the probability of an event not occurring. The OR is the ratio of the odds of disease for the experimental group relative to the odds of disease in the control group. Similar to the RR, an OR above 1 implies that exposure to the factor under investigation increases the risk of disease, while a value below 1 means the factor reduces the risk of disease.

Statistical Modeling (Regression Analysis)

A statistical model is a detailed mathematical specification of a hypothesis. Modeling helps in examining the relationship or association between variables. For example, do age and weight affect function after total hip re-

| Table 2 | Presentation of Data From a Cohort Study |

Disease Status

Characteristic	Disease	No disease	Total
Exposed	a	b	a + b
Nonexposed	c	d	c + d
	a + c	b + d	n

placement? Ultimately, causation is the factor of interest, but before causation can be determined association must be studied in more detail. Specifically, there are five possible explanations for an association between two variables (A and B). (1) Chance: luck has resulted in the sample that was chosen not accurately reflecting the situation in the true population. (2) Bias: structured or systematic error in design analysis or conduct resulting in an alternative explanation for an observed relationship. There are numerous types of bias. Some of the more common ones include recall, reporting, and selection bias. (3) Confounding: a relationship between A and B reflects the effect of a third variable that is more exactly related to both A and B. For example, a medication (A) designed to decrease postoperative pain (B) in surgical patients, some of whom have narcotic dependence (C). C affects both A and B and therefore would be a confounder in the evaluation of postsurgical pain control. Age and gender are classic confounders as they influence many health variables. (4) Causation: A is a cause of B. (5) Reverse causation: B is a cause of A. For example, the statement that drinking tea causes people to live longer could be attributed to the result of older people drinking more tea rather than tea affecting life expectancy.

It is prudent to think of causation as a diagnosis of exclusion. Once chance has been minimized, confounders have been controlled, and there is appropriate timing with cause preceding effect, then causation is supported. Statistical modeling facilitates this process, but cannot compensate for bias, which is more a product of study design.

One final issue that statistical modeling can detect and deal with is interaction. Interaction is where A's influence on B can change in the presence of a second variable; a hypothetical example is that continuous passive motion and an epidural anesthetic may increase postsurgical knee range of motion more than either intervention alone.

The variables described earlier in the chapter form a hierarchy from continuous to binary. Higher, more descriptive variables can be converted to a lower variable; for example, grouping a continuous variable such as age

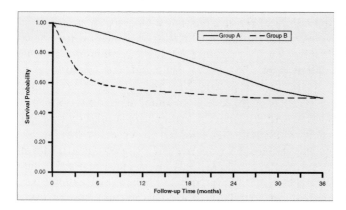

Figure 1 Hypothetical survival probability for medical versus surgical trial. Group A = medical treatment. Group B = surgical treatment.

into 5-year intervals. This will result in loss of detail but can facilitate data analysis.

In the analysis of variables it is important to characterize them into one of two groups depending on the role they play in the evaluation. The dependent or outcome variable is the quantity of interest whose variation in a population is being explained. The independent or explanatory variables are the ones being analyzed to determine if they influence the dependent variable. Independent variables are also referred to as covariates. The researcher determines the status of each variable; it is not an intrinsic property of the variable itself. A dependent variable in one evaluation could be independent in another.

Regression modeling is any statistical model that involves independent or explanatory variables. Regression statistics essentially allow the relationship between the dependent variable and the independent variables in a population to be uncovered, despite the presence of other factors affecting outcome. These principles are needed primarily in observational studies to control for confounders, but regression statistics can be equally valuable in RCTs to adjust for imbalances in treatment groups and known confounders.

Simple linear regression involves one dependent and one independent variable, such as trying to predict the weight of a child by height. Multiple linear regression implies that there are at least two independent variables. For example, is neurologic recovery in spinal cord injury (dependent variable) is associated with surgery, age, gender, and energy of injury (independent variables)? In linear regression the dependent variables are continuous; however, when a dichotomous dependent outcome is selected, then a logistic regression analysis must be done.

Details of regression modeling are beyond the scope of this chapter, but regression or statistical modeling is a very powerful tool that can be used both in observational or cohort studies as well as in RCTs. From a power perspective the basic rule is that 5 to 10 subjects are needed for each independent variable being assessed.

Survival Analysis (Kaplan-Meier Method)

Many clinical trials accrue patients over time, and in certain situations patients are followed for varying lengths of time. Often, event rates such as mortality or frequency of aseptic loosening of a total joint arthroplasty are selected as primary response variables. Analyzing two groups for event rates such as these could be done with chi-square or the equivalent "normal" statistic for comparing two proportions, but because the length of observation for each subject is variable, estimating an event rate is complicated. Moreover, a basic comparison of event rates may be misleading. For example, Figure 1 shows the survival pattern for two different groups. Although their mortality rate at 5 years is nearly identical, the mortality pattern is quite different. This could represent a medical versus surgical trial where surgery might carry a high initial mortality secondary to perioperative and intraoperative risks.

Kaplan-Meier or survival analysis is a nonparametric method to examine and compare the distribution of times between two events. These techniques can provide three main functions. The first is to estimate the cumulative risk of an event (usually adverse) over time. This is plotted as a cumulative proportion of subjects remaining event free and is termed the survival curve. The pattern of this curve becomes smoother and more accurate with increasing numbers of subjects. Second, it can compare the position of two survival curves using proper statistical hypothesis testing. For example, a study to compare the survival patterns between two types of total knee arthroplasties would use the Mantel-Haenszel (log rank) Statistic. Finally, survival analysis techniques can study the influence of various baseline variables on the underlying risk of the event. This can be done in the setting of a natural history study or to adjust for imbalances in prognostic variables (confounders) between two treatment groups. The Cox proportional hazards model allows for adjustment for these imbalances.

Outcomes

Outcomes research and other epidemiologic issues historically have been of little interest to the clinician, but as pressure builds for therapeutic accountability clinicians find themselves in the unfamiliar territory of health-related quality of life (HRQOL), cost effectiveness and other patient based outcomes. Use of these patient-based measures will continue to grow as patients, administrators, policy makers, and professional organizations demand evidence-based medicine.

HRQOL focuses on many different dimensions of health including physical, mental, pain, function, and sat-

Table 3 | Interobserver Variability in Clinical Assessment

Lumbar Spine Interpretation by Musculoskeletal Radiologists		Self-Administered Patient Questionnaires	
Reading	*Kappa**	*Questionnaire*	*Kappa**
Any abnormality	0.51	Sickness impact	0.87
Facet joint sclerosis	0.33	Medical history	0.79
Any narrowed disks	0.49		

*Kappa statistic or intraclass correlation coefficient ranges from 0 to 1, with 1 representing perfect agreement and 0 representing random agreement

isfaction. Despite this specificity, clinicians, especially surgeons, often regarded HRQOL outcomes as soft measures that don't provide the hard distinct data surgeons covet, but patients or society have little interest in. They are perceived as subjective and easily influenced by a patient who exaggerates symptoms or disability. These patient influences are not limited to questionnaires, because mood, motivation and other psychosocial issues can prejudice physiologic measures such as range of motion, strength, and ability to perform functional tasks. Outcomes instruments are developed through a collaborative effort of clinicians and social scientists using vigorous psychometric principles. Even the so-called objective tests such as radiographs that take patient factors out of the equation can be outperformed by the so-called softer questionnaires (Table 3).

In the mid 1980s several articles pointed out the glaring deficiencies in the orthopaedic literature and the somewhat shaky foundation on which treatment decisions are based. The majority of orthopaedic studies were retrospective cohort or case control studies with flawed outcome measures and uncontrolled bias. A 1985 study brought to light the tremendous variability in outcome that could occur if various traditional surgical measures were used on the same patient group. Terms such as excellent, good, or satisfactory were not precise in their definitions and varied depending on the context in which they were used (ie, pain, function, return to work). By combining multiple dimensions of outcome with subjective and unclear questions it was difficult to determine whether surgery was successful or not, nor could results between studies be compared. Furthermore, the importance of a qualified independent patient evaluator was made clear; patients report better results when the surgeon or his/her delegate asks the questions.

There are three general psychometric criteria that should be established in HRQOL measures before they are endorsed. Reliability is the ability of the tool to be reproducible and internally consistent over time. Validity ensures that the instrument is accurately measuring what it is supposed to be measuring. Responsiveness is the ability of the questionnaire to detect clinically relevant change or differences. Responsiveness will vary depending on the type of HRQOL questionnaire and the patient population being evaluated. For example, if an outcome tool is designed for the functional assessment of patients with severe rheumatoid arthritis, and the outcome tool is given to patients with mild osteoarthritis, it would probably produce all perfect scores, the so-called "ceiling effect." Likewise, a questionnaire developed for the general population would not discriminate among severely impaired patients in a rehabilitation setting, because all patients would end up with the worst possible score ("floor effect").

HRQOL questionnaires may only involve one or two questions, but generally consist of several items or questions, organized into domains or dimensions. A domain is an area or experience the questionnaire is trying to measure. Examples would include pain, disability, well-being, and mood. There are two basic types of questionnaires, generic and disease-specific.

Generic instruments attempt to evaluate overall health status. The SF-36 is probably the most well known of the generic tools and is made up of eight domains that can blend to form a physical and mental component score interpreted as the "physical" and "mental" dimensions of health status. The major advantage of generic instruments is that they deal with a variety of areas in any population regardless of the underlying disease. This allows for broad comparisons across various disease states, enabling an assessment of the impact of health care programs. They can also be very useful in assessing the overall HRQOL after a very specific intervention, such as surgery. One final advantage of some of the more frequently used questionnaires is the availability of normative data. This can be very helpful when trying to evaluate patients who do not have a baseline HRQOL score to compare with the postintervention score. For example, in the trauma patient, it is the surgeon's goal to try to return the patient to "normal."

One other generic measure of note is utility measurement. These measurements are somewhat more complicated as they evolved from decision and economic theory. They reflect the patient's preferences for various treatment options and potential outcomes. The primary value of utility measures is in economic analysis; therefore their use will grow exponentially in the coming years.

Disease-specific measures are the other major category of HRQOL outcome tools. These questionnaires concentrate on a region of primary interest that is generally relevant to the patient and physician. As a result of this focus on a region or disease state, the likelihood of increased responsiveness is higher. These instruments can be specific in various ways. Some examples of the primary focus of these instruments include populations (rheumatoid arthritis), symptoms (back pain), and function (activities of daily living). The disadvantage of a disease-specific outcome is that general information is lost, and therefore, it is generally recommended that when evaluating patients, both a disease-specific and generic outcome measure should be used.

How are HRQOL outcome tools used? First, an instrument must be selected. Assuming it has passed psychometric scrutiny, the major determinants are the question or the purpose of the study and the feasibility of applying the instrument. Is the question evaluative or discriminative? What is the domain of interest, the population being studied? Is function important? For example, in a study population of spinal cord injured patients the Functional Independence Measure is a much better choice than the Roland Morris Disability Questionnaire because the former is designed for neurologically impaired patients and any floor effects will be avoided. In most studies after addressing the primary question the physician should be as comprehensive as possible; therefore, the use of both a generic and disease-specific outcome measure is ideal. From a feasibility perspective, patient and investigator burden must be considered. Time to complete, patient comprehension, cost to administer, analyze, store and retrieve data, and interpretability of results are only a few of the issues that must be considered. A concise guide to the appropriate outcome instrument for the anatomic region or disease process being studied is provided on the American Academy of Orthopaedic Surgeons website.

For all the attributes of HRQOL questionnaires there are numerous problems, such as compliance, cost, and collection of "too much" data. Caution must also be exercised not to alter questionnaires or develop creative scoring systems, as these threaten the validity of the instrument, the ability to compare across studies, and ultimately the results of the study. Multiple comparisons are another danger with HRQOL outcomes. Because of the wealth of information they provide in numerous domains, it is tempting for the researcher to go off on a fishing expedition looking for the elusive variable that will result in statistical significance.

One of the most difficult challenges is to determine what magnitude of change in "score" represents a clinically significant change when evaluating a particular intervention. Some outcome measures such as the American Academy of Orthopaedic Surgeons/North American Spine Society Low Back Instrument suggests that a 20% difference is clinically significant. Other questionnaires provide no guidelines and it is left up to the clinical researcher to decide. This issue is not only relevant from an evaluative perspective but is also germane to the power calculation of a study. A 10% to 20% effect change would generally be considered appropriate.

Evidence-Based Medicine

In the current era of increasing accountability for health care services, the issues of quality and access to health care are of overriding importance. A major focus to date has been on efficiency of care, with a view to maximizing productivity and optimizing resource utilization. Recently, the National Academy of Science Institute of Medicine has defined quality of health care as "the degree to which health services for individuals and populations increase the likelihood of desired health outcomes and are consistent with current professional knowledge." Thus, improvements in accountability must clearly include indicators of efficiency. Accountability requires that increased emphasis be placed on bringing patterns of clinical practice in line with current scientific evidence and that the effectiveness of current health services at producing desirable health outcomes be determined.

As pressure grows for increasing accountability in the use of medical resources, the clinician must play a greater role in leading the design of the studies that evaluate care. It is by ensuring that the care is based on sound evidence, that clinicians will be able to remain ethical advocates of effective patient care.

Annotated Bibliography

American Academy of Orthopaedic Surgeons Website. AAOS Normative Data Study and Outcomes Instruments, Table of Contents. Available at: http://www3.aaos.org/research/normstdy/main.cfm/. Accessed January 26, 2004.

Eleven functional outcomes instruments related to the musculoskeletal system are presented. Seven of the instruments contain the generic outcomes instrument, the SF-36. Not only are the instruments available to assess baseline levels and responsiveness to treatment, normative data from the general population are provided to serve as a point of reference.

Atlas SJ, Keller RB, Chang Y, Deyo RA, Singer N: Surgical and non-surgical management of sciatica secondary to lumbar disc herniation: Five year outcomes from the main lumbar spine study. *Spine* 2001;26:1179-1187.

A well designed prospective outcome study comparing the results of the two recognized treatment approaches for lumbar disk herniation is presented. Validated outcome instruments are used along with appropriate statistical analysis to show surgical intervention to be superior. The influence of various baseline variables on these outcomes is also analyzed.

Bailey CF, Fisher CG, Dvorak MF: Type II error in the spine surgical literature. *Spine* 2004;29:1723-1730.

The primary purpose of this study was to determine the frequency of potential type II errors published in the surgical spine literature. The article clearly defines type I and type II errors and emphasizes their importance, along with the significance of identifying one primary research question. Only 17% of the randomized trials had adequate power to determine an appropriate difference and merely 27% had identified a primary question. The results support appropriate scrutiny of RCTs before implementing their results.

Fisher CG, Dvorak MF, Leif J, Wing P: Comparison of outcomes for unstable cervical flexion teardrop fractures managed with halo thoracic vest vs. anterior corpectomy and plating. *Spine* 2002;27:160-166.

This study uses a retrospective cohort design with a cross sectional outcome analysis to assess the radiographic and clinical outcomes of two treatment methods. This design eliminates some of the inherent biases of a retrospective study by obtaining objective long term validated and reliable outcome measures. Although the study demonstrates improved radiographic measurements with surgery, this does not necessarily correlate with clinical outcome.

Glantz SA: *Primer of Biostatistics*, ed 5. New York, NY, McGraw-Hill, 2001, pp 6-7.

This book provides a superb overview of biostatistics and is a great reference for both the novice and the part-time researcher. All the essential aspects of statistics are covered in an easy to read and stimulating way and reinforced with relevant examples. Summary tables provide quick check references for the appropriateness of commonly used statistical methods.

Institute for Clinical Evaluative Sciences Website. Practice Atlas Series, 2000, Toronto, Ontario. Available at: http://www.ices.on.ca. Accessed January 26, 2004.

This is a reference for nonbiased evidence-based research in the areas of health care delivery, service utilization, health technologies, treatment modalities, and drug therapies. The major objective of the Institute for Clinical Evaluative Sciences is to perform population-based health delivery research that is germane to the clinician and the makers of health policy.

Journal of Bone and Joint Surgery Website. Levels of evidence for primary questions. Available at: http://www.ejbjs.org/misc/public/instrux.shtml. Accessed January 26, 2004.

A concise table outlining the hierarchy and spectrum of the various study designs for clinical research is presented. The table serves as a guide as to the strength of evidence of a particular study, with level 1 being the gold standard.

National Heart: Lung and Blood Institute Website. Framingham Heart Study. Available at: http://www.nhlbi.nih.gov/about/framingham/. Accessed January 27, 2004.

A comprehensive review and current status of the landmark cohort study assessing variables that influence cardiovascular disease is presented. Design, objectives, results, and ancillary studies are discussed.

Classic Bibliography

Begg C, Cho M, Eastwood S, et al: Improving the quality of reporting of randomized controlled trials: The CONSORT statement. *JAMA* 1996;276:637-639.

Bombardier C, Kerr M, Shannon H, Frank J: A guide to interpreting epidemiologic studies on the etiology of back pain. *Spine* 1994;19(suppl 18):2047S-2056S.

Deyo RA, Andersson G, Bombardier C, et al: Outcome measures for studying patients with low back pain. *Spine* 1994;19(suppl 18):2032S-2036S.

Gartland JJ: Orthopaedic clinical research: Deficiencies in experimental design and determinations of outcome. *J Bone Joint Surg Am* 1988;70:1357-1364.

Howe J, Frymoyer J: Effects of questionnaire design on determination of end results in lumbar spine surgeries. *Spine* 1985;10:804-805.

Lieber RL: Statistical significance and statistical power in hypothesis testing. *J Orthop Res* 1990;8:304-309.

Markel MD: The power of a statistical test. What does insignificance mean? *Vet Surg* 1991;20:209-214.

Sledge CB: Crisis, challenge, and credibility. *J Bone Joint Surg Am* 1985;67:658-662.

Chapter 2

Soft-Tissue Physiology and Repair

Robin Vereeke West, MD

Freddie H. Fu, MD

Introduction

Progressive advances including research on stem cells, growth factors, and tissue engineering continue to be made in the treatment of soft-tissue diseases and injuries. Although cells have been cultured in the laboratory for many years, the replication of the function and the structure of complex human tissues is a relatively recent development. There are currently many advances being made regarding tissue engineering. Continuing progress also is being made in the understanding of the genetic basis of diseases such as degenerative joint disease, and the biologic response to soft-tissue injury.

Articular Cartilage

Structure and Function

Articular cartilage is a highly organized viscoelastic material composed of chondrocytes, water, and an extracellular matrix (ECM) and is devoid of blood vessels, lymphatics, and nerves. Complex interactions between the chondrocytes and the ECM actively maintain tissue balance.

Chondrocytes from different cartilage zones vary in size, shape, and metabolic activity. All chondrocytes are active in the homeostasis of their surrounding matrix and derive nutrition from the synovial fluid. The chondrocytes sense mechanical changes in their surrounding matrix through intracytoplasmic filaments and short cilia on the surface of the cells.

The ECM consists primarily of water (65% to 80% of its total wet weight), proteoglycans, and collagen. The predominant collagen is type II (95%), but smaller amounts of other collagens (types IV, VI, IX, X, XI) have also been identified. The exact function of the other collagens is unknown, but they may be important in matrix attachment and stabilization of the type II collagen fibers.

The collagen forms a three-dimensional network that encases proteoglycan molecules, predominantly chondroitin and keratan sulfates. This lattice framework is responsible for the structural properties of articular cartilage, including tensile strength and resiliency. The proteoglycans are negatively charged and attract water along with cations. These sulfated proteoglycans are linked to hyaluronate and are responsible for the high water content of the ECM. The rate of deformation of articular cartilage is directly correlated with how quickly water is discharged, and therefore is affected by the structural integrity of the collagen.

The normal thickness of articular cartilage is determined by the contact pressures across the joint. The higher the peak pressures, the thicker the cartilage. The patella has the thickest articular cartilage in the body.

Articular cartilage can be divided into four distinct layers: superficial, middle, deep, and calcified (Figure 1). These layers differ in cellular morphology, biomechanical composition, and structural properties. In the superficial layer, the collagen orientation is parallel to the surface. It changes to a more random, less densely packed array in the middle zone. The collagen bundles are perpendicular to the joint surface and subchondral bone in the deep and calcified layers. The deep zone has the largest collagen fibers, the highest concentration of proteoglycans, and the lowest concentration of water.

The morphology and arrangement of the chondrocytes differ in each zone. In the calcified zone, the chondrocytes are small and randomly arranged. The chondrocytes transition to a columnar arrangement and spherical shape in the deep zone, to a more random array of cells in the middle zone, and to a flat, parallel array of cells in the superficial zone (Figure 2). The tidemark, a thin, basophilic line that is seen on light microscopy sections of articular cartilage, represents the boundary between the calcified and uncalcified cartilage.

Injury and Repair

Injuries to articular cartilage can be divided into three distinct types: type 1 injuries involve microscopic damage to the chondrocytes and ECM (cell injury) and type 2 injuries involve macroscopic disruption of the articular cartilage surface (chondral fractures or fissuring). These two injury types have an extremely poor healing

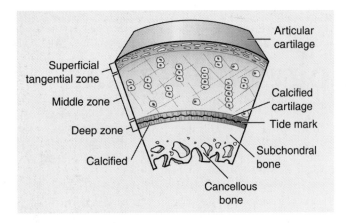

Figure 1 Articular cartilage layers.

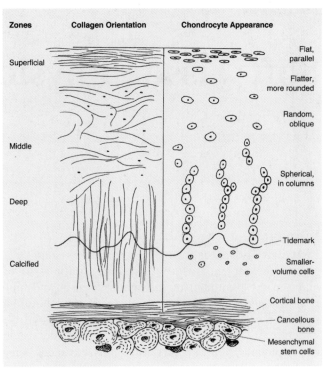

Figure 2 Basic structural anatomy of articular cartilage. *(Reproduced from Browne JE, Branch TP: Surgical alternatives for treatment of articular cartilage lesions.* J Am Acad Orthop Surg *2000;8:180-189.)*

potential because they do not penetrate the subchondral bone and therefore do not bring forth an inflammatory response. Type 3 injuries involve disruption of the articular cartilage with penetration into the subchondral bone (osteochondral fracture). Type 3 injuries produce a significant inflammatory process. A fibrin clot is formed, and mesenchymal undifferentiated cells produce a reparative tissue, which is not normal articular cartilage but fibrocartilage that consists primarily of type I collagen and has a tendency to undergo early degenerative changes.

Articular cartilage injuries have frequently been observed in conjunction with anterior cruciate ligament (ACL) injuries. An occult osteochondral lesion or bone bruise may be detected with MRI in up to 80% of patients. The most common locations of these lesions are within the lateral compartment of the knee, on the lateral femoral condyle at the sulcus terminalis, and at the posterolateral tibial plateau (Figure 3). Although the area may appear normal during arthroscopic evaluation, in vivo histologic studies have shown significant disruption of the articular cartilage. Current data strongly indicate that chondrocyte apoptosis can be stimulated by the application of a single, rapid impact load and that the extent of apoptosis is related to the amount of load applied.

Treatment

Surgical treatment options for full-thickness cartilage defects are simple arthroscopic débridement, abrasion arthroplasty, microfracture, autologous chondrocyte cell implantation, and mosaicplasty with either autologous tissue or fresh allograft. In a recent study of autologous osteochondral mosaicplasty in the treatment of full-thickness cartilage defects, good to excellent results were achieved over a 10-year period.

Actual regeneration of articular cartilage is accomplished when the present cells become mature chondrocytes that are capable of restoring the biomechanical and structural integrity of the articular surface. Current research is focused on inducing the newly attracted or transplanted cells to become mature chondrocytes using growth factors (polypeptides that bind to cell surface receptors). These growth factors act in a paracrine manner and have a variety of regulatory effects on cells. Bone morphogenetic proteins (BMPs) are members of the transforming growth factor superfamily (except BMP-1) and have a regulatory role in the differentiation of cartilage-forming and bone-forming cells from pluripotent mesenchymal stem cells. More than a dozen BMPs have been discovered.

Acceleration of cartilage healing has been shown in vivo with the implantation of genetically modified chondrocytes, expressing BMP-7. Large articular cartilage defects in the patellofemoral joints of 10 horses were implanted with either controls or the genetically modified chondrocytes. The lesions that were treated with the BMP-7 chondrocytes showed an accelerated healing response at the 4-week biopsy. The 8-month biopsy revealed a similar healing response in both the control and the study groups. A recent study was performed to evaluate the clinical outcomes and histologic results of isolated femoral articular cartilage defects treated with either a microfracture or an autologous chondrocyte implantation. No significant differences were found between the two groups regarding the clinical and biologic outcomes.

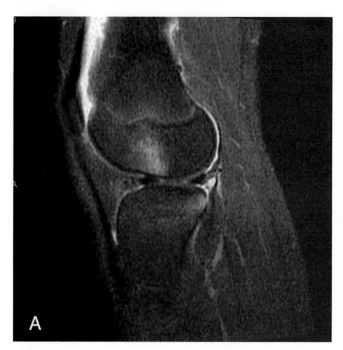
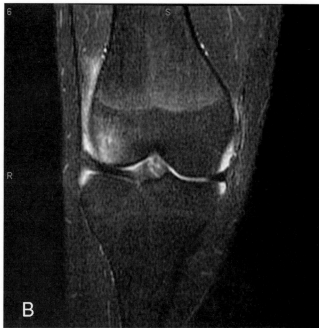

Figure 3 MRI of common occult bone bruises associated with ACL injuries in the sulcus terminalis of the lateral femoral condyle **(A)** and the posterolateral tibial plateau **(B)**.

Alternatives to surgery are also being promoted in the treatment of arthritis. Viscosupplementation, or intra-articular injections of hyaluronic acid, has been used to treat osteoarthritis. The proposed mechanisms of action result from the physical properties of the hyaluronic acid, as well as the anti-inflammatory, anabolic, local analgesic, and chondroprotective effects. Hyaluronic acid has both viscous and elastic properties. At high shear forces, the molecules exhibit increased elastic properties and reduced viscosity. At low shear forces, the opposite effects are seen. The anti-inflammatory effects of hyaluronic acid include inhibition of phagocytosis, adherence, and mitogen-induced stimulation. The anabolic effects have been demonstrated in vivo with studies showing that intra-articular injections of hyaluronic acid may stimulate fibroblasts. The anti-inflammatory effects may explain the analgesic effect. Although hyaluronic acid has been shown to stimulate cartilage matrix production, the chondroprotective effects have not been confirmed. Several studies have failed to show a statistically significant benefit for hyaluronic acid injections when compared with a placebo. Furthermore, viscosupplementation is relatively expensive, with the cost of a series of injections at more than $500 per knee.

Numerous studies have investigated other potential chondroprotective agents (substances that are capable of increasing the anabolic activity of chondrocytes while suppressing the degradative effects of cytokine mediators) on cartilage. These agents include chondroitin sulfate, glucosamine sulfate, piroxicam, tetracylines, corticosteroids, and heparinoids. Glucosamine serves as a substrate for the biosynthesis of chondroitin sulfate, hyaluronic acid, and other macromolecules located in the cartilage matrix. Chondroitin sulfate, which is covalently bound to the proteins as proteoglycans, is secreted into the ECM. The load-bearing properties of the cartilage are attributable to the compressive resilience and affinity for water that the proteoglycans possess. Studies have supported the effectiveness of glucosamine and chondroitin sulfate for the relief of symptoms of osteoarthritis based on clinical trials and short-term follow-up. These studies have shown a progressive and gradual decline of joint pain and tenderness and improved motion; few side effects have been reported. However, many questions surround the long-term effects, the most effective dosage and delivery route, and the purity of glucosamine and chondroitin sulfate products. Prospective studies that use validated outcome measures for pretreatment and posttreatment and that stratify major confounding variables are needed.

Meniscus
Structure and Function
The meniscus is a specialized viscoelastic fibrocartilaginous structure capable of load transmission, shock absorption, stability, articular cartilage lubrication, and proprioception. The meniscus is more elastic and less permeable than articular cartilage and is composed of a complex three-dimensional interlacing network of collagen fibers, proteoglycan, glycoproteins, and fibrochondrocytes that are responsible for the synthesis and maintenance of the ECM. The meniscus is composed of 75%

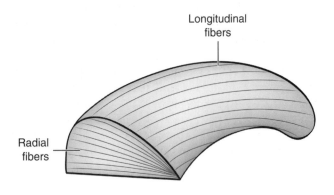

Figure 4 Collagen fiber ultrastructure with longitudinally and radially oriented fibers.

collagen, 8% to 13% noncollagenous protein, and 1% hexosamine. Type I collagen is predominant (90%); small amounts of types II, III, V, and VI are present.

The collagen fiber ultrastructure influences the load-bearing role of the meniscus. Radial collagen bundles run from the periphery to the center of the meniscus and large collagen fibers have a predominately circumferential arrangement (Figure 4). Collagen bundles on the superficial surfaces of the meniscus have no organization. The rate of fluid exudation from the meniscal tissue determines the rate of creep. The collagen proteoglycan matrix and the applied load affect the deformation of the meniscus.

The peripheral meniscus obtains its blood supply from a circumferentially arranged perimeniscal capillary plexus from the superior and inferior geniculate arteries. This capillary plexus penetrates up to 30% of the medial and 25% of the lateral meniscus. The inner two thirds of the meniscus are essentially avascular and receive nutrition from the synovial fluid. Free nerve endings and corpuscular mechanoreceptors have been found in meniscal tissue, concentrated at the root insertion sites and the periphery.

Kinematic analysis has shown that the meniscus is a dynamic structure, moving anterior with knee extension and posterior with knee flexion. Because the peripheral attachments of the lateral meniscus are interrupted by the popliteus, it has greater mobility than the medial meniscus.

Through its shape and structure, the meniscus provides several important functions in the knee joint. The shape of the meniscus improves the congruency of the articulating surfaces and increases the surface area, thus aiding in load transmission across the joint. The meniscus is responsible for transmitting 50% of the joint force in knee extension and 90% of the joint force in deeper flexion.

Meniscal Tears and Repairs

The detrimental effects of partial and complete meniscectomy have been shown in numerous studies. Partial and complete meniscectomies have been shown to in-

crease contact pressure by as much as 65% and 200%, respectively. Meniscal loss leads to alterations in load transmission and accelerated rates of articular cartilage degeneration. The healing potential of meniscal tears varies according to patient age and the location/chronicity of the tear.

The success of meniscal repairs depends on multiple factors, including vascular supply, tissue stability, tear pattern, associated injuries, and chronicity of the tear. The types of tears that can be repaired include acute, peripheral, and unstable tears in the vascular zone of the meniscus. Complex, radial, or flap tears are not usually appropriate for repair because excision is often necessary. Partial-thickness or stable tears usually do not require repair.

The poor healing potential of central meniscal tears has led to the investigation of methods to provide blood supply to the injured area. These methods include the use of fibrin clot, fibrin glue, endothelial cell growth factor, vascular access channels, and synovial pedicle flaps. Studies support the use of exogenous fibrin clots to promote healing of meniscal tears in the avascular zone. The clot provides chemotactic and mitogenic factors, such as platelet-derived growth factor and fibronectin, which stimulate the cells involved in wound repair. The clot also provides a scaffold for the support of the reparative process.

A stable knee is important for successful meniscal repair and healing. Meniscal repairs have a success rate of as high as 90% to 100% when associated with a concomitant ACL reconstruction. In contrast, the success rate drops to 30% to 70% when the repair is performed in an unstable knee. Healing rates of meniscal repairs are lower in ACL-intact knees when compared with healing rates in ACL-reconstructed knees, but are higher than in ACL-deficient knees. The increased rates of healing in ACL-reconstructed knees is possibly a result of drilling, which provides an exogenous source of blood to promote healing of the repair.

Meniscal Replacement

Although autografts, biocompatible prostheses, bioabsorbable collagen scaffold, and synthetic materials have been used as meniscal replacements, the only currently available method to replace the entire meniscus is meniscal allograft transplantation. The ideal candidate for a meniscal transplant is a symptomatic patient with a prior meniscectomy, persistent pain in the involved compartment, intact articular cartilage (less than grade III changes), normal alignment, and a stable joint. Localized chondral defects should be treated concomitantly. Osteotomies or ligament reconstruction can be performed as a staged procedure or concurrently. Additional contraindications include inflammatory arthritis, obesity, and previous infection.

Other factors that should be considered before performing the transplantation include antigenicity, sterilization techniques, and remodeling capabilities of the allograft. Class I and II histocompatibility antigens are expressed on the cells of the meniscal allograft, indicating the potential for an immune response. However, there is only one report of frank immunologic rejection of a cryopreserved, non–tissue-matched meniscal allograft. Immunoreactive cells (B lymphocytes and T-cytotoxic cells) have been identified in recipients of fresh-frozen allografts. The effect of the immune response is unknown, but the reaction may stimulate healing, incorporation, and revascularization.

The American Association of Tissue Banks has defined the recommended testing protocol for allograft screening. Serologic screening is performed for human immunodeficiency virus (HIV) p24 antigen, HIV-1/HIV-2 antibodies, human T cell lymphoma/leukemia virus-1 and -2, hepatitis B surface antigen and core antibody, hepatitis C antibody, and syphilis. Many tissue banks perform polymerase chain reaction testing, which can detect 1 in 10 HIV-infected cells. Cultures for aerobic and anaerobic bacteria also are performed. Following the harvest, the tissue can be preserved by one of four methods: fresh, cryopreserved, fresh-frozen, or lyophilized. Only fresh and cryopreserved allografts contain viable cells at the time of transplantation. However, it is not known if these cells survive after the transplantation. Several studies have shown that the donor cells are replaced by the host-derived cells. Additional sterilization with ethylene oxide, gamma irradiation, or chemical methods has been shown to have deleterious effects on the graft tissue. The amount of gamma radiation required to eliminate viral DNA (at least 3.0 Mrad) may adversely affect the material properties of the allograft. Ethylene oxide produces by-products that may cause synovitis.

Meniscal allografts are repopulated by host-derived cells that appear to originate from the synovial membrane. The repopulation occurs from the peripheral zone to the central core. Active collagen remodeling by the host cells has been shown, but the long-term ability of these cells to synthesize appropriate matrix proteins and maintain the ECM is unknown. The transplanted menisci also undergo a gradual, incomplete revascularization, with new capillaries derived from the capsular and synovial attachments.

Intervertebral Disk

The intervertebral disk forms the primary articulation between the vertebral bodies and is the major constraint to motion of the functional spinal unit. The disk is composed of two morphologically separate parts, the outer and the inner part. The outer part, the anulus fibrosus, is made up of fibrocartilage and type I collagen. At the periphery, the collagen fibers are oriented vertically. They become more oblique with each underlying layer, with the fibers in each adjacent sheet running at about 30° angles to each other. Lamination of these layers strengthens the anulus fibrosus. Some peripheral fibers extend past the cartilage end plate to insert onto the vertebral bodies as Sharpey's fibers. Neural fibers are found in the outer rings of the anulus fibrosus. The nerve fibers are dorsal branches of the sinu vertebral nerve; the ventral branches arise from the sympathetic chain that courses anterolaterally over the vertebral bodies.

The inner part of the intervertebral disk is the nucleus pulposus. In young people, the nucleus pulposus is composed of 90% water. The other components are type II collagen and proteoglycans, which bind water. With the gradual loss of proteoglycans, the water content of the nucleus pulposus declines with advancing age. After the third decade of life, there is a gradual fluid loss and concomitant replacement of the nucleus pulposus with fibrous tissue. By the sixth or seventh decade of life, the entire nucleus pulposus is replaced by fibrocartilage.

The disk is separated from the vertebral bodies by hyaline cartilage end plates. Because the intervertebral disk is avascular, nutrients and fluid enter the disk by diffusion through the end plates or the anulus fibrosus. Glucose diffuses through the end plates and sulfate ions diffuse mainly through the anulus. The diffusion is influenced by mechanical and biologic factors. An outflow of fluid occurs with increased load, and a fluid influx occurs with decreasing load. End plate permeability is reduced by patient factors such as smoking and exposure to vibration and is enhanced with dynamic exercise.

The nucleus pulposus functions to resist compressive loads. In axial compression, the increased intradiskal pressure is counteracted by annular fiber tension and disk bulge. Asymmetric and cyclic loading with combined lateral bend, compression, and flexion is a risk factor for disk herniation. The lumbar motion segment can resist a combination of a bending moment and a shear force of 156 Nm and 620 N, respectively, before complete disruption occurs. These numbers are much lower than the failure load in compression. About 35% of the torque resistance is provided by the disk, whereas the remainder of the resistance is provided by the posterior elements and ligaments. Therefore, any injury to the posterior elements may increase the risk for disk failure.

Viscoelastic intervertebral disk changes have been shown both in vivo and in vitro. Disk height increases with decreasing compressive loads because the decreased intradiskal osmotic pressure allows water to flow into the disk. Reported diurnal changes in the overall height of individuals range from 6.3 mm to 19.3 mm, with an average of 15.7 mm. The average person is 1% shorter in the evening than in the morning.

Information on disk degeneration, herniation, traumatic injury, and treatment can be found in section 6. The effects of aging on intervertebral disks are discussed in chapter 6.

Ligament

Structure and Function

Ligaments are dense connective tissues that link bone to bone. The gross structure of the ligaments varies with their location (intra-articular or extra-articular, capsular) and function. Some ligaments (ACL, posterior cruciate ligament, and inferior glenohumeral ligaments) have geometric variations between their bundles.

Ligaments are composed primarily of water. Collagen makes up most of the dry weight of ligaments, with type I collagen the predominant protein at 90% and type III accounting for the remainder of the collagen. Type III collagen is often found in injured ligaments. Elastin accounts for about 1% of the dry weight of ligaments, but is even more prevalent in spine ligaments.

Microscopically, the collagen fibers are relatively parallel and aligned along the axis of tension. Fibroblasts are located between the rows of fibers and are responsible for producing and maintaining the ECM. Strength is enhanced by the cross-linked structure of the collagen fibers. Proteoglycans in the ECM store water and affect the viscoelastic properties; the rate of deformation is directly related to the amount of stored water.

The direct insertion (for example, the medial collateral ligament [MCL] attachment) is the most common type of insertion site and attaches the ligament to the bone through four distinct zones. Zone 1 is made up of collagen with ECM and fibroblasts. Zone 2 is composed of fibrocartilage with cellular changes, whereas mineralized cartilage is found in zone 3. Zone 4 is characterized by an abrupt transition to bone. In indirect insertions (for example, the tibial attachment to the MCL), the superficial layer connects directly to the periosteum, whereas the deep layer anchors to bone by Sharpey's fibers.

Ligament Properties

The structural properties of ligaments, expressed by the load-elongation curve, reflect the behavior of the entire bone-ligament-bone complex, including its geometry, insertion sites, and material characteristics. The mechanical properties of ligaments, characterized by the stress-strain curve, depend on the ligament substance, molecular bonds, and composition. Over an extended period of time, ligaments respond to loading with an overall increase in mass, stiffness, and load to failure. In addition to these structural changes, the material properties show an increase in ultimate stress and strain at failure.

Stress is defined as force per unit area, and strain describes the change in length relative to the original length. Under tension, a ligament deforms in a nonlinear fashion. In the initial phases of applied tension, the coiled nature of collagen and the crimping become more aligned along the axis of tension; the collagen fibers then become taut and stretch with continued tension. The slope of the linear-elongation curve describes the tissue stiffness, and the slope of the stress-strain curve denotes the tensile modulus. The point at which overload occurs and the tissue fails is the yield point. The ultimate load and elongation are defined as this overload point for structural properties, and the ultimate tensile stress and strain are defined as this yield point for mechanical properties. Besides the nonlinear nature of these curves, ligaments and tendons also show a time-dependent viscoelastic behavior. More information on the biomechanics of ligaments can be found in chapter 4.

Other Influences

An increased prevalence of ACL injuries in females and gender-specific muscle response to sport-specific maneuvers have been discussed in the literature. Anatomic features (smaller intercondylar notch, higher Q angle, low hamstring/quadriceps force ratio), intrinsic factors (estrogen/relaxin receptors within the ACL), and landing techniques (straight-knee landing, one-step stop landing with the knee hyperextended) have been suggested as contributing factors to the increased incidence. Estrogen, progesterone, and relaxin receptors have been identified in the human ACL. In vitro fibroblast proliferation and collagen synthesis have been shown to directly correspond to estrogen levels. Increasing estrogen levels lead to a decrease in cellular proliferation and collagen synthesis of fibroblasts.

Skeletal maturity and age also have been shown to affect the mechanical and structural properties of ligaments. The load at failure from specimens of older human ACL has been found to be 33% to 50% of that in younger bone-ligament-bone specimens.

Effects of Disuse and Immobilization

Immobilization and disuse dramatically compromise the structural and material properties of ligaments. In a 2003 study, immobilization led to a significant decrease in the ability of scars to resist strain. According to another study, after 12 weeks of immobilization, the ACL-bone unit showed a significant decrease in maximum load to failure, energy absorbed to failure, and stiffness (increased compliance). At 5 months after remobilization, a decrease in ligament strength was still apparent (stiffness and compliance parameters had returned to baseline levels). At 12 months, ligament strength had returned to a near-normal level.

The effect of immobilization on the ligament units depends on the histologic characteristics of the attachment site. The ACL attachment site, through zones of fibrocartilage, was slightly affected after immobilization; however, the direct tibial insertion of the superficial MCL was significantly disrupted. This disruption was caused by cortical and subchondral bone resorption after the period of immobilization. Collagen degradation increases and collagen synthesis decreases with longer periods of immobilization.

Injury and Repair

The healing process of extra-articular ligaments can be divided into four phases: the inflammatory response, cell proliferation and fibrin clot organization, remodeling, and scar maturation. The ratio of type I to type III collagen normalizes during these final phases. The tensile strength gradually increases. As a result of matrix changes involving collagen reorganization and cross-linking, there is a gradual increase in tensile strength; however, the injured ligament is never as strong as the uninjured ligament. Ligament scarring is dominated by small-diameter collagen fibers and decreased cross-link density.

An intrinsic healing response has not been observed in intra-articular ligaments such as the ACL, because intra-articular ligaments have a limited blood supply and the synovial fluid may not allow an inflammatory response. Fibroblast adhesion and migration is different between the MCL and ACL in an inflammatory environment. Platelet-derived growth factor and transforming growth factor-beta are increased during MCL healing, whereas the opposite effect is found in the healing ACL animal model. Low-intensity pulsed ultrasound has been shown to enhance early healing of transected MCLs in rats. Superior mechanical properties were found 12 days after the injury when compared with a placebo group. At 21 days after injury, the mechanical properties were similar between the placebo and ultrasound groups.

Ibuprofen has been shown to have no significant effect on early MCL healing. Studies have shown no significant differences between the mechanical properties of placebo-treated and ibuprofen-treated rats after MCL transection. However, cyclooxygenase-2 specific inhibitors have been shown to impair ligament healing in rats. When compared with a placebo-treated group, the rats treated with celecoxib for 6 days after an MCL transection had 32% lower load to failure.

Tendon

Structure and Function

Tendons function to transmit high tensile loads from muscle to bone. Tendons are made up of densely packed parallel-oriented bundles of collagen, composed mainly of type I and III collagen by dry weight (86% and 5%

respectively). Three collagen chains comprise one collagen molecule, which is then organized into microfibrils and fibrils. Proteoglycans (which influence the viscoelastic properties of tendons), glycoproteins, and water combine with fibrils into a matrix to form fascicles. The fascicles come together to form bundles, which are surrounded by endotenon. The vascular supply, lymphatics, and nerves are supported by the endotenon. Surrounding the collagen bundles are the epitenon and paratenon.

The composition and organization of tendons make them ideal to resist high tensile forces. Tendons deform less than ligaments under an applied load and are able to transmit the load from muscle to bone.

The toe region on the load-elongation curve, which represents the structural properties of the bone-tendon-muscle unit, shows the initial stretch of the tendon, which results from straightening of the cramped fibrils and orientation of the longitudinal collagen fibers. Because tendons have more parallel collagen fibers than ligaments and less realignment occurs during initial loading, the toe region of the curve is smaller in tendons than in ligaments. In addition, as the amount of crimp decreases with age, the toe region becomes smaller.

The elastic modulus of the tendon is represented by a linear region on the load-elongation curve that follows the toe region. Tendon failure occurs in a downward curve, representing permanent structural changes. Shortening of the muscle occurs when, during isometric contractions, the length of the muscle-tendon unit remains constant but elongation of the tendon occurs secondary to creep. Creep improves muscle function during isometric contractions.

Tendons surrounded by a paratenon receive their blood supply from the periphery and a longitudinal system of capillaries. The perimysium and osseous insertions also provide a vascular supply to these tendons. The perimysium, the periosteal insertion, and the long and short vincula from the proximal mesotendon provide the blood supply for tendons within a sheath.

Factors Affecting Tendon Properties

Tendons become weaker, stiffer, and less yielding as a result of the vascular, cellular, and collagen-related alterations that occur with aging. Aging causes many changes in the properties of collagen, including a reduction in collagen turnover and a decrease in water and proteoglycan content.

Studies have shown that exercise has positive effects on the mechanical and structural properties of tendons, whereas immobilization adversely affects their biomechanical properties, resulting in decreased tensile strength, increased stiffness, and a reduction in total weight. Therefore, early mobilization should be initiated whenever possible.

Table 1 | Muscle Contractions

Type	Characteristics
Isometric	Fixed load with no joint motion
Concentric	Joint moves with a load and the muscle contracts
Eccentric	Results in muscle lengthening while controlling a load during joint motion
Isokinetic	Variable load with constant velocity

(Reproduced with permission from Woo SL-Y, Debski RE, Withrow JD, Janqueshek MA: Biomechanics of knee ligaments. Am J Sports Med 1999;27:533-543.)

Injury and Repair

There are three types of tendon injuries: direct trauma with transection of the tendon; indirect injury with avulsion of the tendon from the bone, and indirect intrasubstance injury stemming from intrinsic or extrinsic factors. Transections or partial lacerations are associated with trauma and are most common in the flexor tendons of the hand. Bone avulsions can occur after overwhelming tensile loads. Degenerative changes within a tendon can occur from submaximal overload (Achilles tendinitis) or from repetitive pressure against a bony surface.

Tendon healing after an acute injury follows a similar pattern as other soft-tissue healing. The inflammatory response provides an extrinsic source of cells to begin the reparative process. Proliferation of the cells and increased vascularity follows, whereas collagen synthesis increases and the tissue matures.

Successful tendon-to-bone healing is necessary for good outcomes in many reconstructive procedures. As the tendon heals within a bony tunnel, fibrovascular interface forms and bony ingrowth is started. An indirect insertion of the tendon collagen fibers then occurs. Based on the results of animal models, it has been shown that there is no advantage in repairing a tendon to a cancellous bone trough compared with direct repair to cortical bone. In MCL reconstruction in rabbits, the initial maximum failure load was higher in the tendons repaired to cortical bone when compared with those repaired to cancellous bone. By 8 weeks after the reconstruction, the tendon attachments in both groups had matured to almost baseline.

Suture material, type of repair, suture knots, quality of the tissue, continuous passive motion, gap formation, and load experienced by the tendon are all factors that can affect tendon repair. Aggressive early active motion along with weight bearing has been shown to increase the rate of tendon re-rupture and gap formation. However, controlled passive motion improves the repair strength in the early period after repair and decreases adhesions. An optimum level of stress and motion exists that promotes healing without resulting in damage to the repaired tendon.

Growth factors are cell-secreted proteins that regulate cellular functions and are involved in cell differentiation and growth, including the normal processes of development and tissue repair. Several growth factors, recently identified as playing a role in tendon healing, include vascular endothelial growth factor, insulin-like growth factor, platelet-derived growth factor, basic fibroblast growth factor, and transforming growth factor beta. In addition, the transcription factor NF-kappaB has been implicated in the signaling pathways of these growth factors. The type and timing of cytokine delivery to facilitate the most rapid and quality repair has yet to be determined.

Muscle

Structure and Function

Skeletal muscle constitutes the largest tissue mass in the body, making up 40% to 45% of total body weight. Skeletal muscle originates from bone and adjacent connective tissue and inserts into bone via tendon.

The microscopic and macroscopic anatomy of muscle includes the motor unit, the muscle fiber bundles, individual fibers, myofibrils within the fibers, and the myofibril contractile unit (sarcomere). Muscle contraction occurs in response to input via nerve fibers through the neuromuscular junction. The force of the muscle contraction depends on the number of motor units firing. The size of the motor unit depends on the number of muscle fibers that are innervated by the nerve fiber. Muscle contractions can either be isometric, concentric, eccentric, or isokinetic (Table 1).

The three basic muscle types are I, IIA, and IIB. Types I and II are determined by the speed of the contraction. Type I, or slow-twitch oxidative fibers, predominate in postural muscles and are well suited for endurance by aerobic metabolism. They have an ability to sustain tension, relative fatigue resistance, and have high amounts of mitochondria and myoglobin. In addition to a slow contraction rate, type I fibers have a relatively low strength of contraction. Type II muscle fibers are fast-twitch, have a fast rate of contraction, and a relatively high strength of contraction. Type II fibers are either A or B, depending on their mode of energy utilization. Type IIA fibers have an intermediate aerobic capacity, whereas type IIB fibers are primarily anaerobic. Type IIB fibers are common in muscles that require a rapid generation of power, but they are less capable of sustaining activity for a prolonged period because of lactic acid buildup (Table 2).

Factors Affecting Muscle Properties

Like other tissues in the body, skeletal muscle undergoes changes with aging. Muscle mass decreases, the number and diameter of muscle fibers decrease, stiffness

Table 2 | Characteristics of Human Skeletal Muscle Fibers

	Type I	Type IIA	Type IIB
Other names	Red, slow-twitch Slow, oxidative	White, fast-twitch Fast, oxidative, glycolytic	Fast, glycolytic
Speed of contraction	Slow	Fast	Fast
Strength of contraction	Low	High	High
Fatigability	Fatigue-resistant	Fatigable	Most fatigable
Aerobic capacity	High	Medium	Low
Anaerobic capacity	Low	Medium	High
Motor unit size	Small	Larger	Largest
Capillary density	High	High	Low

(Reproduced from Garrett WE Fr, Best TM: Anatomy, physiology, and mechanics of skeletal muscle, in Simon SR (ed): Orthopaedic Basic Science. Rosemont, IL, American Academy of Orthopaedic Surgeons, 1994, pp 89-125.)

increases, and collagen content increases with aging. The loss of muscle size and strength can be diminished with strength training.

Muscle loses contractile strength and mass with disuse or immobilization. As the muscle atrophies, both macroscopic and microscopic changes occur, with decreasing fiber size and number, as well as changes in the sarcomere length-tension relationship.

Changes that accompany immobilization of the muscle are related to the length at which muscles are immobilized. Atrophy and loss of strength are much more prominent in muscles immobilized under no tension than muscles placed under some stretch during immobilization. This greater tension induces a physiologic response to load, making the immobilization of muscles in a lengthened position less deleterious. The profound strength and mass reduction in inactive muscles can be reversed quite quickly because of the excellent vascular supply.

Muscle tissue is capable of significant adaptions. Muscle training can involve exercises aimed at increasing strength, endurance, and anaerobic fitness. Strength training (high force, low repetition) leads to an increase in muscle strength, which is proportional to the cross-sectional area of the muscle fibers. The increased muscle fiber size results in an increased amount of contractile proteins. There is also a strong neurologic component to strength training. A poorly conditioned muscle has only about 60% of the fibers firing simultaneously, whereas a well-conditioned muscle has over 90% active fibers.

Endurance training, with low tension and high repetition, increases capillary density and mitochondria con-

centration, resulting in an increased Vo_{2max} and improved fatigue resistance. Improvements in endurance result from changes in both central and peripheral circulation and muscle metabolism. The muscle adapts to use energy more efficiently.

Anaerobic (sprint) training is high-intensity exercise that lasts for a few seconds up to 2 minutes. These exercises rely primarily on adenosine triphosphate in the form of phosphagens and on the anaerobic pathways.

Injury and Mechanisms of Repair

Muscle injury can result from an indirect injury that overpowers the muscle's ability to respond normally, or from a direct injury, such as a contusion or laceration. The indirect mechanism of injury includes muscle strains and delayed-onset muscle soreness (DOMS). Muscle strains usually result during eccentric contractions, when the muscle is unable to accommodate the stretch during the contraction. Muscles that cross two joints, such as hamstrings, are more prone to strain injury. Muscle injuries most commonly occur at the myotendinous junction, and fatigue has also been associated with increased rates of strain injury.

The severity of muscle injury varies from microscopic damage, to partial tears, to complete tears. The healing process is initiated with an inflammatory phase. Fibroblast proliferation and collagen production lead to scar formation, with muscle regeneration resulting from myoblasts stemming from satellite cells. Motion during healing has been shown to reduce scar size, but healing muscles are at increased risk for reinjury. Therefore, return to strenuous activity should be delayed until satisfactory healing has occurred.

DOMS is defined as muscle pain that generally occurs 24 to 72 hours after intense exercise. Muscle swelling and pain typically reach maximum levels after 1 to 3 days. Several treatment strategies have been introduced to help alleviate the severity of DOMS and to restore the maximal function of muscles as rapidly as possible. Nonsteroidal anti-inflammatory drugs have shown dose-dependent effects that may also be influenced by the time of administration. Massage has shown varying results that may be attributed to the time of application and the type of technique used. Cryotherapy, stretching, homeotherapy, ultrasound, and electric current modalities have demonstrated no effect on the alleviation of muscle soreness or other DOMS symptoms.

Myositis ossificans (MO) is a benign aberrant reparative process that results in heterotopic ossification in soft tissues. Myositis ossificans is a misnomer because the condition does not involve muscle inflammation, and the process is not limited to muscle. MO circumscripta results from soft-tissue trauma, whereas MO progressiva is an autosomal dominant genetic disorder. About 80% of MO occurs in the thigh or arm. Ossification occurs in three zones: the central zone is undifferentiated matrix, the surrounding area is composed of immature osteoid, and the most peripheral zone is made of mature bone. Treatment consists of immobilization and the administration of anti-inflammatory drugs. Surgical intervention should only be considered when the MO is completely mature (6 to 24 months) and is recommended when joint motion is compromised or neurologic impingement occurs.

Nerve

Structure and Function

The axon (conducts information by propagating electrical signals), dendrites (branches from the cell body that receive signals from other nerve cells), presynaptic terminal (transmits information to cell bodies or dendrites of other neurons), and the cell body (the metabolic center of the neuron containing the nucleus and organelles for protein and RNA synthesis) are the main components of the neuron, or nerve cell. The action potential that originates at the axon hillock is an all-or-none phenomenon. Proteins that support the structure and function of the axon are synthesized in the cell body and travel along the axon via slow and fast antegrade transport systems. Axons with a myelin sheath that is produced by Schwann cells have a higher conduction velocity than noninsulated axons.

The axon and myelin sheath make up the nerve fiber. The fiber is enclosed with a basement membrane and connective tissue layer, the endoneurium. The fibers are further grouped into a bundle, called a fascicle, which is surrounded by the perineurium. Several fascicles make up the peripheral nerve, which is encased by the epineurium. The vascular supply of the peripheral nerves has an intrinsic and extrinsic component. A vascular plexus within the endoneurium, perineurium, and epineurium comprises the intrinsic component. The extrinsic component is made up of regional blood vessels that enter the axon at various sites and travel along the epineurium. The blood-nerve barrier, like the blood-brain barrier, protects and maintains an appropriate endoneurial environment.

Peripheral nerves demonstrate similar viscoelastic properties typical of other connective tissues. Their stress-strain curve shows a linear region at higher stress and follows a compliant, low-strained toe region. During normal physiologic function, the peripheral nerves work in the toe region of the curve. However, low levels of strain can result in alterations in peripheral nerve conduction and blood flow impairment. Ischemic permanent changes are noted at strain rates as low as 15%. Nerve repairs can place excess tension on the nerve at the repair site, and joints at or near the repair site are frequently immobilized to protect the repair.

Injury, Degeneration, and Regeneration

Peripheral nerve injuries can be categorized as (1) having no axonal discontinuity with only temporary loss of nerve conduction, or as (2) having axonal damage with proximal and distal degeneration of the axon. The reaction after the second category of injury occurs in two phases. In the first phase, the axon and myelin sheath disintegrate along the entire distance distal to the injury and for some distance proximal to the injury. These changes are termed wallerian degeneration and result in denervation. Depending on the severity and location of the injury, the cell body either regenerates the axon or autodegenerates (resulting in cell death). Degeneration of the myelin sheath results in loss of nerve conduction.

Neurapraxia is usually a result of compression and involves loss of conduction across the injured site without wallerian degeneration. Because the axon is not injured, recovery is complete. Axonotmesis involves disruption of the axon with some preservation of the nerve connective tissue. Wallerian degeneration occurs with axonotmesis, but the endoneurial sheath remains intact and serves to guide the regenerating axon during recovery. Neurotmesis is physiologic discontinuity of the nerve and is divided into varying degrees of severity. The likelihood of recovery decreases with each degree of severity.

The Schwann cells of normal intact myelinated fibers do not divide. However, within 24 hours of nerve transection, the Schwann cells throughout the distal segment undergo a series of mitosis. Schwann cells maintain cytoplasmic tubes, called bands of Büngner, which guide the process of regeneration. These cells also produce nerve growth factor and nerve growth receptors. Macrophages and Schwann cells are responsible for the phagocytosis of debris.

Factors applied locally or systemically that enhance regeneration include hormones, proteins, and growth factors. Patient outcome after peripheral nerve injuries is quite variable. Factors affecting the outcome of nerve repair include patient age, the type of nerve injured, length of the injury zone, timing of the repair, status of the target organ at the time of repair, and technical skill of the surgeon.

Nerve Repair

Peripheral nerve repair is used to establish the continuity of the nerve. The best results are achieved when the repair is done soon after transection in a tension-free environment. A primary repair requires adequate soft-tissue coverage, skeletal stability with low nerve tension, and a good blood supply. However, nerve grafting may be required with an extensive crush injury, or when excessive gap or tension is present. Mobilization of the stump during repair should be limited because ischemia and diminished profusion can result. Better results are typically seen in patients younger than age 50 years, and in patients with more distal injuries.

There are two types of peripheral nerve repair: grouped fascicular repair and simple epineurial repair. Fascicular repair theoretically is preferred over epineurial repair because axon realignment can be more accurate. However, fascicular repair may require additional dissection, which may result in increased scarring and decreased vascular supply. A prospective study comparing epineurial to fascicular repair showed no difference between the two groups.

Nerve Grafting

Nerve grafting is considered in injuries that have a large gap that may result in undue tension after repair. Autogenous tissue (the sural nerve or the medial and lateral antebrachial cutaneous nerves) is the most common source used for nerve grafting. When possible, the fascicular groups on the injured nerve are matched to the autogenous graft. A single segment is typically used for grafting smaller nerves, whereas a few segments of graft may be used with larger nerves. Alternatives to the autograft, including biologic or artificial conduits (such as arteries, veins, muscle, collagen, or silicone tubes) and allografts, which avoid donor-site morbidity and nerve loss. The main complication with the use of allografts has been the immunogenic host response. The rate of axonal elongation has been shown to increase if the silicone tubes are filled with extracellular matrix proteins such as collagen, laminin, and fibronectin.

Annotated Bibliography

Articular Cartilage

Borrelli J Jr, Tinsley K, Ricci WM, Burns M, Karl IE, Hotchkiss R: Induction of chondrocyte apoptosis following impact load. *J Orthop Trauma* 2003;17:635-641.

The presence and extent of chondrocyte apoptosis following an impact load to articular cartilage was studied in an in vivo model. The data suggested that there is a relationship between apoptosis and a single, rapid impact load and that the extent of the apoptosis is related to the amount of load applied.

Hangody L, Fules P: Autologous osteochondral mosaicplasty for the treatment of full thickness defects of weight-bearing joints: Ten years of experimental and clinical experience. *J Bone Joint Surg Am* 2003;85(suppl 2):25-32.

Outcomes of 831 patients who underwent mosaicplasty were evaluated with clinical scores, imaging techniques, and biopsy samples. Good-to-excellent results were achieved in 92% of patients treated with femoral defects, 87% of those with tibial defects, 79% of those with trochlear and patellar mosaicplasties, and 94% of those treated for talar defects.

Hidaka C, Goodrich LR, Chen CT, Warren RF, Crystal RG, Nixon AJ: Acceleration of cartilage repair by genetically modified chondrocytes over expressing bone morphogenetic protein-7. *J Orthop Res* 2003;21:573-583.

Large articular cartilage defects in the patellofemoral joint of 10 horses were implanted with either genetically modified chondrocytes, expressing BMP-7, or a control group of chondrocytes. The study group showed accelerated healing at 4 weeks and similar healing at 8 months when compared with the control group.

Knutsen G, Engebretsen L, Ludvigsen T, et al: Autologous chondrocyte implanation compared with microfracture in the knee: A randomized trial. *J Bone Joint Surg* 2004;86:455-464.

Autologous chondrocyte implantation was compared with microfracture in a randomized trial. Short-term clinical results were acceptable for both methods.

Leopold SS, Redd BB, Warme WJ, Wehrle PA, Pettis PD, Shott S: Corticosteroid compared with hyaluronic acid injections for the treatment of osteoarthritis of the knee: A prospective, randomized trial. *J Bone Joint Surg Am* 2003;85:1197-1203.

No significant differences in pain relief or function were found in patients treated with corticosteroid compared with hyaluronic acid injection.

Steadman JR, Briggs KK, Rodrigo JJ, Kocher MS, Gill TJ, Rodkey W: Outcomes of microfracture for traumatic chondral defects of the knee: Average 11-year follow-up. *Arthroscopy* 2003;19:477-484.

Functional outcomes of 72 patients who were treated arthroscopically with microfracture for full-thickness traumatic defects of the knee were evaluated. Patients under the age of 45 years who underwent this procedure, without associated meniscus or ligament pathology, showed significant improvement in function.

Meniscus

Cole BJ, Carter TR, Rodeo SA: Allograft meniscal transplantation: Background, techniques, and results. *Instr Course Lect* 2003;52:383-396.

Meniscal allograft transplantation can be effective in symptomatic meniscectomized patients, alleviating pain and providing improved function.

Vangsness CT Jr, Garcia IA, Mills CR, Kainer MA, Roberts MR, Moo TM: Allograft transplantation in the knee: Tissue regulation, procurement, processing, and sterilization. *Am J Sports Med* 2003;31:474-481.

This article is a review of the present issues that surround the allograft industry, including regulation of tissues and tissue banks, procurement, sterilization, and storage of allografts.

Yoldas EA, Sekiya JK, Irrgang JJ, Fu FH, Harner CD: Arthroscopically assisted meniscal allograft transplantation with and without combined anterior cruciate ligament reconstruction. *Knee Surg Sports Traumatol Arthros* 2003;11:173-182.

Clinical and subjective outcomes of 31 patients (34 meniscal transplants) who either underwent an isolated meniscal transplantation or a combined transplantation and ACL reconstruction were reviewed. Relief of symptoms was provided in carefully selected patients with joint line pain and instability.

Ligament

Bogatov VB, Weinhold P, Dahners LE: The influence of a cyclooxygenase-1 inhibitor on injured and uninjured ligaments in the rat. *Am J Sports Med* 2003;31:574-576.

The cyclooxygenase-1 inhibitor was found to improve the strength of the uninjured ligament, but was not found to improve the strength of ligament healing.

Takakura Y, Matsui N, Yoshiya S, et al: Low-intensity pulsed ultrasound enhances early healing of medial collateral ligament injuries in rats. *J Ultrasound Med* 2002; 21:283-288.

The effect of low-intensity pulsed ultrasound on the healing of medial collateral ligament injuries was studied. This method was shown to be effective in enhancing early healing.

Thornton GM, Shrive NG, Frank CB: Healing ligaments have decreased cyclic modulus compared to normal ligaments and immobilization further compromises healing ligament response to cyclic loading. *J Orthop Res* 2003; 21:716-722.

The cyclic stress-strain response of normal and healing ligaments to repetitive low loads was examined. Immobilization significantly decreased the ability of scars to resist strain, with the majority of immobilized scars failing during repetitive loading.

Tendon

Oguma H, Murakami G, Takahashi-Iwanaga H, Aoki M, Ishii S: Early anchoring collagen fibers at the bone-tendon interface and conducted by woven bone formation: Light microscope and scanning electron microscope observation using a canine model. *J Orthop Res* 2001;19:873-880.

Light microscopy and scanning electron microscopy was used to examine the process of anchoring of collagen fibers to bone in a canine model. The formation of woven bone was important during the early recovery of the tendon-bone interface before the completion of fibrocartilage-mediated insertion.

Soda Y, Sumen Y, Murakami Y, Ikuta Y, Ochi M: Attachment of autogenous tendon graft to cortical bone is better than to cancellous bone: A mechanical and histological study of MCL reconstruction in rabbits. *Acta Orthop Scand* 2003;74:322-326.

The MCL of 33 rabbits was reconstructed using autogenous tendon graft to cortical or cancellous bone. At 8-week follow-up, the cortical bone group showed a tendency to an increase in maximum failure load. With time, the tendons in both groups matured.

Muscle

Babul S, Rhodes EC, Taunton JE, Lepawsky M: Effects of intermittent exposure to hyperbaric oxygen for the treatment of an acute soft tissue injury. *Clin J Sport Med* 2003;13:138-147.

Sixteen sedentary female university students were subjected to 300 maximal voluntary eccentric contractions. One group was treated with 100% oxygen at 2 atmospheres and the other was treated with 21% oxygen at 1.2 atmospheres absolute. No significant difference was found between the two groups for pain, strength, or quadriceps circumference.

Cheung K, Hume P, Maxwell L: Delayed onset muscle soreness: Treatment strategies and performance factors. *Sports Med* 2003;33:145-164.

This review article on delayed onset muscle soreness examines the mechanisms of injury and treatment strategies.

Deal DN, Tipton J, Rosencrance E, Curl WW, Smith TL: Ice reduces edema: A study of microvascular permeability in rats. *J Bone Joint Surg Am* 2002;84:1573-1578.

This study investigated the relationship between cryotherapy and edema by determining the microvascular permeability before and after contusion in rats. The application of ice significantly decreased the microvascular permeability after striated muscle contusion.

Nerve

Midha R, Munro CA, Dalton PD, Tator CH, Shoichet MS: Growth factor enhancement of peripheral nerve regeneration through a novel synthetic hydrogel tube. *J Neurosurg* 2003;99:555-565.

A synthetic hydrogel tube was used to repair surgically created 10-mm gaps in the rat sciatic nerve. The tubes supported nerve regeneration in 90% of cases, and fibroblast growth factor-1 enhanced tubes showed significantly better regeneration.

Wang S, Cai Q, Hou J, et al: Acceleration effect of basic fibroblastic growth factor on the regeneration of peripheral nerve through a 15-mm gap. *J Biomed Mater Res* 2003;66A:522-531.

Nerve guides embedded with basic fibroblast growth factor were used in the repair of transected sciatic nerves (15-mm gaps). The recovery and function of the regenerated nerves was significantly accelerated by basic fibroblast growth factor, as indicated by an electrostimulation test and histologic assays.

Classic Bibliography

Arnoczky SP, Warren RF: Microvasculature of the human meniscus. *Am J Sports Med* 1982;10:90-95.

Arnoczky SP, Warren RF, Spivak JM: Meniscal repair using an exogenous fibrin clot: An experimental study in dogs. *J Bone Joint Surg Am* 1988;70:1209-1217.

Buckwalter JA, Mankin HJ: Articular cartilage: Degeneration and osteoarthritis, repair, regeneration, and transplantation. *Instr Course Lect* 1998;47:487-504.

Fu FH, Harner CD, Johnson DL, Miller MD, Woo SL: Biomechanics of knee ligaments: Basic concepts and clinical application. *Instr Course Lect* 1994;43:137-148.

Gelberman RH, Manske PR, Akeson WH, Woo SL, Lundborg G, Amiel D: Flexor tendon repair. *J Orthop Res* 1986;4:119-128.

Inaba H: Biomechanical study on contact pressure in the femoral-tibial joint. *Nippon Seikeigeka Gakkai Zasshi* 1987;61:1073-1080.

Jackson DW, McDevitt CA, Simon TM, Arnoczky SP, Atwell EA, Silvino NJ: Meniscal transplantation using fresh and cryopreserved allografts: An experimental study in goats. *Am J Sports Med* 1992;20:644-656.

Kline DG, Hudson AR, Bratton BR: Experimental study of fascicular nerve repair with and without epineurial closure. *J Neurosurg* 1981;54:513-520.

Walker PS, Erkman MJ: The role of the menisci in force transmission across the knee. *Clin Orthop* 1975;109:184-192.

Woo SL, Hollis JM, Adams DJ, Lyon RM, Takai S: Tensile properties of the human femur-anterior cruciate ligament-tibia complex: The effects of specimen age and orientation. *Am J Sports Med* 1991;19:217-225.

Chapter 3

Bone Healing and Grafting

George F. Muschler, MD

Chizu Nakamoto, MD, PhD

Jonathan N. Grauer, MD

Introduction

An understanding of the principles of bone healing and grafting is needed for the treatment of acute fractures, repair of nonunions, filling of bone voids, healing of osteotomies, correction of angulatory or length deformities, and arthrodeses of the spine and extremities. The effective use of a broad range of methods and strategies is required to optimize outcome for each patient.

The formation of bone relies on three crucial processes. Osteogenesis is the ability of grafted cells to form bone via osteoblastic stem cells and/or progenitor cells. Osteoinductivity is the ability to modulate the differentiation of stem cells and progenitor cells along an osteoblastic pathway. Osteoconductivity is the ability to provide the scaffold on which new bone can be formed.

The many molecular, cellular, local, mechanical, and systemic variables affecting bone healing must be effectively aligned for the bone healing response to be successful. The surgeon must identify settings in which these conditions are deficient, and use appropriate methods to optimize conditions. Bone tissue engineering has evolved rapidly in the past decade, translating fundamental knowledge and developments in physics, chemistry, and biology to achieve practical clinical benefits in the form of a variety of new materials, devices, systems, and strategies.

Variables Affecting Bone Healing

The many variables that are crucial to bone formation must be considered in the formulation of a treatment plan for a fracture, the decision to proceed with an elective procedure, and the assembly of a construct during surgery. Some variables are beyond the control of the surgeon. However, other variables can be manipulated to better achieve the desired orthopaedic goal.

Patient characteristics directly affect bone formation. The nutritional status of the patient must be maximized to withstand anabolic events and to limit complications such as infection. Patient use of substances such as nicotine and nonsteroidal anti-inflammatory medications has been linked to decreased bone formation, whereas other factors, such as parathyroid hormone, have been suggested as having beneficial effects.

Local factors also alter the bone healing responses, justifying an increased emphasis on careful handling of soft tissue; specifically, limiting local physical, thermal, and chemical trauma and preserving local blood supply. Fracture treatment with limited exposure using intramedullary rods or sliding of plates across an injury zone with minimal direction has been developed to better achieve this goal. The value of soft-tissue coverage (possibly including skin/muscle flaps) has become more apparent, particularly in patients with open tibia fractures, where the risk of nonunion is increased.

Mechanical factors must also be considered. Appropriate compressive forces across the site of potential bone formation have been found to maximize the healing response. During fracture healing and with osteotomies, mechanical alignment must be restored. For example, in spinal fractures, the anterior column, which is primarily under compression, generally heals more efficiently than the posterior column, which is under tension. Instrumentation and immobilization are effective methods of holding desired alignment and favorably modifying mechanical forces.

Phases of Bone Healing

The process of bone formation follows an orderly cascade of events. Initially, the tissue volume in which new bone is to be formed is filled with a matrix, generally including a blood clot or hematoma. At this hematoma stage, the matrix within the site is bordered by local tissues, which also are often traumatized resulting in focal necrosis and reduced blood flow. An effective bone healing response will include an initial inflammatory phase, characterized by an increase in regional blood flow, invasion of neutrophils and monocytes, removal of cell debris, and degradation of the local fibrin clot.

These phases blend into a revascularization phase that is associated with the invasion of new blood vessels formed by endothelial progenitor cells, and subsequently a cell proliferation phase during which there is multiplication of a highly proliferative population of connective tissue progenitor cells (derived from regional or circulating precursor cells). These progenitor cells are capable of forming bone, but also may form fibrous tissue, cartilage, and possibly other tissues, depending on local conditions at the site. A subsequent matrix synthesis phase coincides with the initial differentiation of these progenitor cells.

Differentiation is strongly influenced by the local oxygen tension and mechanical environment, as well as by signals from local growth factors. Regions of high strain tend to promote fibrous tissue formation. Regions of low strain and high oxygen tension are associated with direct formation of woven bone (intramembranous bone formation) whereas regions of intermediate strain and low oxygen tension are associated with cartilage formation. In many instances, cartilage formation may add to the mechanical stability of the site, improving strain conditions for regional bone formation, and may subsequently be remodeled into bone tissue (endochondral bone formation).

Remodeling is the final phase of bone formation. It is characterized by the systematic removal of the initial matrix and tissues that formed in the site, primarily through osteoclastic and chondroclastic resorption, and their replacement with more organized lamellar bone aligned in response to the local loading environment.

The basic biologic processes and mechanisms associated with these phases of bone repair are similar in closed fractures, bone graft sites, and sites of distraction osteogenesis; however, the spatial and temporal relationship between these events may vary significantly depending on the setting. For example, in distraction osteogenesis, the initial inflammatory response is limited to a relatively small tissue volume at the site of the corticotomy. Revascularization is rapid in the osteotomy site. Distraction is begun after revascularization and during the early proliferative phase. Through distraction, the proliferative phase of wound healing is prolonged in the central region of the regenerate, providing a continuous source of progenitor cells that enter into matrix synthesis and remodeling processes adjacent to the distraction zone. Similarly, distraction osteogenesis is associated with little or no cartilage formation. Angiogenesis at the site is generally rapid enough to prevent regions of low oxygen tension, and strain at the site is controlled.

The cascade of bone formation is also altered by varying degrees of instrumentation and immobilization. Rigid fixation and a low strain environment (500 to 2000 microstrain) tends to promote osteoblastic differentiation without formation of intermediary cartilage. In contrast, regions of motion that produce hydrostatic loading within a healing bone site tend to promote cartilaginous differentiation. Regions of tensile loading promote signaling that leads to fibroblastic differentiation.

Mass Transport and Metabolic Demand in Bone Healing

Access to substrate molecules (oxygen, glucose, amino acids) and clearance of metabolic products (CO_2, lactate, urea) are of critical importance to cell survival. The processes by which molecules are moved in and out of a fracture or graft site are collectively referred to as mass transport. This process may be mediated by fluid flow (convection) or by diffusion of molecules along concentration gradients or in response to electromagnetic forces. Fluid flow in the circulatory system, as well as flow induced by muscle contraction, gravitational pooling, and pulsation of arterial structures all are examples of convection, and, most importantly, passive diffusion along concentration gradients.

In native bone marrow tissues, the distance between a cell and a capillary lumen is generally less than 40 μm; however in osteocytes this distance can be up to 200 μm and represents the distance over which extravascular convection and diffusion must occur. At distances greater than 200 μm, the transport of oxygen and other nutrients rapidly becomes a limiting factor for cell survival.

In nondisplaced fractures or corticotomies, the distance between osteogenic cells and a local blood supply may be small, providing an effective mass transport system for much of the fracture hematoma. However, this situation does not exist in displaced fractures or at most sites of bone grafting. In these settings, the osteogenic cells of the fracture hematoma or cells that are transplanted into a graft are subject to significant metabolic challenges. These challenges are imposed by the imbalance between the rate at which oxygen and other nutrients (such as glucose) diffuse into the site, and the rate of consumption of oxygen and other nutrients by other cells that are present in the site (metabolic demand).

The transport of oxygen into the center of most clinical graft sites must occur over relatively vast distances (a minimum of 5 mm in most bone grafts, which is approximately 50 times the diffusion distance in normal tissues). Because of this limitation, transplanted cells are not likely to survive if they are more than 0.5 to 1.0 mm from the surface of the graft. The depth of cells that survive is expected to be slightly better with less cellular grafts, such as bone marrow aspirates; however, even in these grafts the concentration of transplanted cells limits the predicted cell survival to a maximum depth of approximately 3 mm. As a general rule, there is an inverse square relationship between cell concentration and the depth of cell survival, such that fourfold reductions in the concentration of implanted cells will double the depth of their survival within an implant.

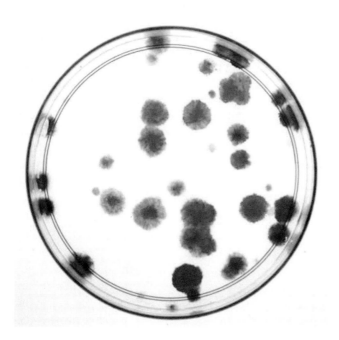

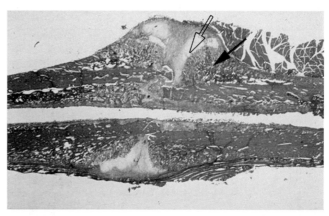

Figure 2 Fracture healing in a rat femur immobilized with an intramedullary rod. Bone formation, mediated by osteogenic cells, progresses at different rates and through different pathways of differentiation and remodeling depending on local signals, vascularity, and mechanical forces. Enchondral ossification forms in regions of higher strain and lower oxygen tension (open arrow). Direct intramembranous bone formation occurs in regions of lower strain and higher oxygen tension (black arrow). *(Reproduced with permission from Einhorn T: The cell and molecular biology of fracture healing.* Clin Orthop *1998;355 (suppl):S7-S21.)*

Figure 1 This image of a 10-cm diameter tissue culture dish illustrates colony formation by cells derived from human bone marrow harvested by aspiration. These colonies were allowed to grow for 9 days before being stained to label those colonies expressing alkaline phosphatase, a marker of early osteoblastic differentiation. The colonies vary in size, illustrating the variation in biologic potential between individual progenitor cells. The prevalence of osteoblastic colonies shown here is about average, approximately 50 colonies per million bone marrow derived nucleated cells, or 1 in 20,000. *(Reproduced with permission from Muschler GF, Nakamoto C, Griffith LG: Engineering principles of clinical cell-based tissue engineering.* J Bone Joint Surg Am *2004;86: 1541-1548.)*

Osteogenesis
Biology
Stem cells are distinguished from progenitor cells by their capacity to avoid being consumed or used up. This characteristic is the result of activation through a process of self renewal, which is accomplished by a process of asymmetric cell division that produces two daughter cells. One daughter cell is identical to the original stem cell and remains available to be activated again by an appropriate signal. A second daughter cell continues to divide and produces many additional progenitor cells that ultimately give rise to new tissues. In contrast to the stem cell, progenitor cells (also called transit cells) eventually develop into terminally differentiated cells.

Many adult musculoskeletal tissues contain stem and progenitor cells that are capable of differentiation into one or more mature cell phenotypes, including bone, cartilage, tendon, ligament, fat, muscle, or nerve. These cells are particularly concentrated in bone marrow, periosteum, vascular pericytes, and peritrabecular tissues and are best characterized in bone marrow aspirates, where they comprise approximately 1 in 20,000 of the nucleated cells. Cellularity and the prevalence of precursor cells greatly varies between different individuals and

anatomic sites. Aging and gender are factors that have been shown to account for only a small portion of this variation (Figure 1).

Repair Mechanisms
The contribution of individual stem and progenitor cells to new tissue formation is dependent on their activation, proliferation, migration, differentiation, and the survival of their progeny. These cell functions are modulated in three-dimensional space by chemical and physical signals, including receptor-mediated signaling through contact with ligands on other cells or through ligands presented in the extracellular matrix (Figure 2). However, repair of bone is also dependent on the number of stem and progenitor cells that are available to participate in new tissue formation at a given site. Local bone repair can be limited by a deficiency in the number of osteogenic stem or progenitor cells. This deficiency can be improved by transplantation of autogenous osteogenic cells from other sites, via grafts from autogenous cancellous bone, bone marrow, periosteum, or vascularized bone (such as fibula grafts).

Treatment Alternatives
Bone from the ilium is the most commonly used source of progenitor cells. Grafts from the tibia and rib also are used, although the number of progenitor cells from these sources is less characterized than bone and marrow from the iliac crest. Autograft bone also provides osteoinductive and osteoconductive properties; however, these desirable features are offset significantly by the morbidity that is associated with the harvest of such grafts.

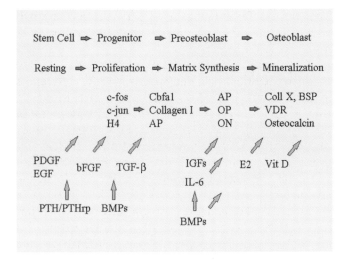

Figure 3 Individual growth factors often promote osteoblastic differentiation at specific stages. The characteristic genes expressed at each stage are listed and the approximate stage of the principal action of the most active osteotropic growth factors and hormones are shown. H4 = histone; AP = alkaline phosphatase; OP = osteopontin; ON = osteonectin; BSP = bone sialoprotein; VDR = vitamin D receptor; PDGF = platelet-derived growth factor; EGF = epithelial growth factor; bFGF = basic fibroblast growth factor; BMPs = bone morphogenetic protein family members; TGF-β = transforming growth factor-beta; IGFs = insulin-like growth factors I and II; IL-6 = interleukin-6; E2 = estradiol; Vit D = vitamin D$_3$; PTH = parathyroid hormone; PTHrP = parathyroid hormone-related peptide; Cbfa1 = transcription core binding factor-alpha 1; Coll X = collagen type X. *(Reproduced with permission from Fleming JE, Cornell CN, Muschler GF: Bone cells and matrices in orthopedic tissue engineering.* Orthop Clin North Am *200;31: 357-374.)*

Bone marrow aspirates have recently become much more widely used as a safer and less costly alternative source of transplantable osteogenic cells. Anticoagulated bone marrow can be further manipulated to selectively concentrate osteogenic cells and remove cells that are unlikely to contribute to a bone healing response (such as red blood cells and most lymphocytes). Simple centrifugation and buffy coat isolation can increase the concentration of marrow-derived nucleated cells by as much as fourfold. Selective adherence and retention on some implantable matrices (such as Cellect, DePuy, Warsaw, IN) can also improve local bone repair by increasing the concentration of target cells and potentially improving their survival by reducing the number of nonosteogenic cells, which then reduces competition for oxygen and other substrates.

Future sources of osteogenic cells for transplantation may include cells that are harvested from fat, muscle, or marrow, and then expanded in tissue culture. This technique can be used to increase the number of cells available for transplantation. In vitro expansion also may provide an opportunity to modify osteogenic potential by the selection of optimal subpopulations, selective differentiation, or by genetic engineering techniques. However, these techniques and their potential to improve efficacy will need to be balanced against their cost and their potential to generate undesirable cell behavior.

Osteoinductivity
Biology
Osteoinductive materials include a variety of soluble growth factors that can be used to modulate the behavior of the osteogenic cells to become activated, to proliferate, and to differentiate into cells that make new bone tissue rather than into cells that remain quiescent or differentiate into other tissues. This multistep process involves biologic signals expressed in a spatially and temporally regulated manner during the fracture healing and bone repair processes. Individual signals can have specific effects on the recruitment, proliferation, differentiation, and survival of osteoblastic progenitors (Figure 3).

The ability of proteins extracted from demineralized bone matrix to induce bone formation was first described by Urist in the 1960s. These observations led to the discovery of a family of signaling proteins now known as bone morphogenetic proteins (BMPs) that are part of the larger transforming growth factor-beta (TGF-β) superfamily. Fourteen BMPs are now recognized (BMP-2 through BMP-15). These proteins are secreted as homodimers or heterodimers of 110 to 140 amino acid peptides linked by one disulfide bond (molecular weight of approximately 30 kd).

Other growth factors also can contribute to osteoinduction. Both epidermal growth factor and platelet-derived growth factor are capable of inducing colony formation by osteoblastic stem and progenitor cells. Vascular endothelial growth factors also play several important roles in angiogenesis, osteoclast migration, and osteoblastic activity. Although vascular endothelial growth factors and TGF-β do not induce bone formation directly, they have been shown to act synergistically to enhance BMP activity in fracture healing and during distraction osteogenesis.

Repair Mechanisms
In vivo, these growth factors have autocrine and paracrine effects as soluble factors. Many growth factors are also embedded in bone matrix where they are believed to play a role in bone remodeling and the coupling of osteoclastic and osteoblastic activity. TGF-β is most abundant and is found in bone matrix at a concentration of approximately 1 mg/kg. The effects of these growth factors can only be mediated on cells expressing specific cell surface receptors. For example, cells must express both a type I and a type II BMP receptor (serine/threonine kinases) to be responsive to BMPs. To date, three type I and three type II BMP receptors have been identified. Each BMP shows a unique binding pattern for the individual receptors, some of which are also responsive to other TGF-β family members. Receptor activation by both TGF-β and BMPs results in activation of an intracellular signaling cascade involving SMAD pathway leading to changes in gene expression.

In vitro, BMPs influence differentiation and other cell functions in a dosage range from 1 to 100 ng/mL. Wheras BMPs often appear to share similar functions and act through a limited set of receptors, each is independently regulated in both space and time during embryonic development and fracture healing. The activity of BMPs is also modulated by specific inhibitors (such as noggin, chordin, gremlin, and follistatin).

Treatment Alternatives

Demineralized bone matrix preparations are widely available for clinical use. Because of their mild osteoinductive potential and desirable osteoconductive properties, they are frequently used as bone graft supplements or secondary extenders, or as a means for transplanting bone marrow derived cells. Nonetheless, different demineralized bone matrix preparations appear to vary in biologic activity, depending on the quality of the donor bone and on the bone processing method. Currently, there is no generally accepted method for proving or screening for biologic activity, though several in vitro and in vivo assays are available. In this regard, demineralized bone matrix preparations lag behind the regulatory standards that have been applied to the purified recombinantly manufactured human osteoinductive growth factors (such as BMPs) that are becoming available for clinical use.

Available data clearly show that BMPs will provide valuable tools for enhancing bone healing in some settings. Among the individual recombinant human BMPs (rhBMPs), BMP-2 and BMP-7 (known as osteogenic protein-1 or OP-1) have both been developed and are now approved by the Food and Drug Administration for use in a limited set of clinical applications. BMP-14 (known as MP52 and growth and differentiation factor-5 or GDF-5) is also under development. BMP-2 in a collagen carrier called InFuse (Medtronic, Minneapolis, MN) has been evaluated and approved for use in the setting of anterior interbody fusion using specific metallic and allograft devices. The OP-1 Device (Stryker Biotech, Hopkinton, MA) has been approved under a humanitarian device exemption for use in tibial nonunions where conventional treatment has failed. Clinical trials of these and other BMP preparations are ongoing.

One of the principal requirements for optimal performance of BMPs or other growth factors is the presence of a local population of target precursor cells that express appropriate receptors. For a BMP to be optimally effective, these target cells must be activated in sufficient numbers to produce the desired result. If an optimal number of responsive cells are not present, the biologic response to the protein will be reduced and implantation of a BMP may be ineffective. Very high concentrations of BMP are required to induce a clinically useful volume of bone in higher animals and humans.

The current formulations of BMPs deliver approximately 50 times the total amount of BMP that is present in the human skeleton.

These massive doses of BMPs are currently required for many reasons, including species-specific differences in dose response to BMPs, the lower concentration of osteogenic cells in higher order animals, the decrease in the concentration of osteogenic cells in human tissues that occurs with advancing age, and other clinical factors. It is also related to the inefficiency of delivery associated with a declining surface to volume ratio as the size of graft sites increases. As graft sites increase in size, more of the implanted growth factor is placed farther away from tissue surfaces where target cells are located. As a result, overdose molecules of BMP become less likely to interact with a responding cell. This situation results in a progressive decrease in surface-to-volume ratio in larger graft sites. Assuming penetration of the BMP to the same depth within tissue, increases in graft volume result in activation of proportionately fewer target cells per unit volume. Increasing the dose (BMP concentration in the defect) may increase the depth penetration of the signal, partly offsetting this limitation. The concentration or biologic potential of target cell populations vary in individual patients, which presents another challenge. Also, the concentration and prevalence of targeted stem and progenitor cells and their biologic performance varies significantly from tissue to tissue (bone, bone marrow, periosteum, muscle, fat) and site because of local or systemic disease. Increasing the BMP dosage may compensate for some of this variation.

Other opportunities for further advancement and refinement of the use of BMPs and other growth factors include modification of their molecular structure, dosage, carrier, formulation, delivery kinetics, and on-site retention.

Osteoconductivity

Three-dimensional porous scaffolds are used extensively in bone grafting and skeletal reconstruction. The principal function of these implants is to provide a surface and structure that facilitates the attachment, migration, proliferation, differentiation, and survival of osteogenic stem and progenitor cells throughout the implant site. Scaffolds also may serve as a space holder to prevent other tissues from occupying the space where new tissue is desired, improve local mechanical stability (as a supportive block, stent, or strut), and facilitate revascularization.

Structural properties refer to the spatial distribution of bulk material of the scaffold (the scaffold architecture). These features can be at nanoscale, microscale, and macroscale (the molecular, cellular, and tissue levels, respectively). Macroporous features of the scaffold

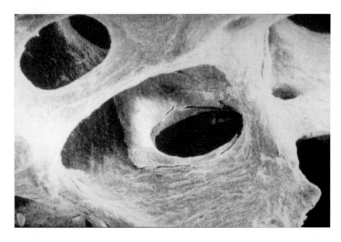

Figure 4 This image shows the macroporous architecture of allograft cancellous bone, which provides a large interconnected void volume for fluid flow and revascularization and progenitor cell attachment migration, proliferation, and differentiation. The microporous texture on the surface of the allograft matrix is also shown. Nanostructural features and porosity are too small to be seen in this image. *(Reproduced with permission from Bullough PG, Vigorita VJ: Slide Atlas of Orthopaedic Pathology. New York, NY, Gower Medical Publishing, 1984.)*

define the initial void space that is available for cell migration and ingrowth of new blood vessels. In most settings, where bone ingrowth is needed to depths of 3 to 5 mm, a macropore size between 150 and 1,000 μm is optimal. Microstructural features define the surface texture that cells encounter, which can have important biologic effects on cell functions. Features at all levels may influence fluid flow and diffusion of oxygen and other nutrients through the scaffold (Figure 4).

The mechanical properties (such as strength, modulus, toughness, ductility) of available scaffolds vary widely, and are determined by the mechanical properties of the bulk material (material properties) and the structural properties of the implant. Mechanical properties of a scaffold must be matched to the graft environment and demands. For example, the ability to accommodate early loading may be crucial in some situations (interbody spinal struts) but not necessary in others (posterolateral lumbar fusions).

Repair Mechanisms
General Concepts
The conditions at the host-implant interface are defined by the chemical properties of the implant and by the local response of the host cells and tissues. Biomolecules derived from the host fluids and tissues are rapidly adsorbed and become the principal mediators of the cellular response to the material, modulating cellular attachment, migration, proliferation, and differentiation events.

The resorbability of plasticizing agents often has important early effects. Low molecular weight soluble compounds (such as glycerol and calcium sulfate) create a hyperosmotic environment that will prevent early cell survival in or adjacent to the implant. Dissolution or degradation may also release acidic by-products (for example, sulfate or carbonate), creating a nonphysiologic pH in the region in and around the implant. These conditions preclude the use of some materials as a vehicle for transplantation of viable cells.

Scaffolds that do not degrade (for example, metals and some ceramics) avoid complications associated with early solubility or later degradation and can have excellent and durable function when integrated with tissues. However, these same materials also can compromise later function in some settings by disrupting tissue remodeling in a way that compromises long-term mechanical function. Stress shielding or stress concentration around these implants can result in local bone loss or in increased risk of mechanical failure. Durable materials also may physically obstruct or complicate future intervention (such as revision surgery). These considerations have led to interest in biologically resorbable scaffolds whenever feasible. One example is the use of impaction grafting for reconstruction of contained and protected periprosthetic defects. Another example is the recent shift in bone void fillers from very slowly degradable ceramics (such as hydroxyapatite) to more rapidly resorbed materials (such as tricalcium phosphate, calcium sulfate, or calcium carbonate).

During the process of degradation of a resorbable implant, the biologic environment adjacent to the implant will be defined by the degradation products that are produced and the biologic effects these products have on local cells. The concentration of degradation products is determined by the balance between their rate of release into the graft site and their rate of clearance from the site. Polyesters, such as polylactides and polyglycolides, are the most commonly used synthetic degradable surgical materials (surgical meshes, suture anchors, and screws). However, the release profile of these materials remains imperfect, despite the fact that degradation can be extended over a range of weeks to years because these materials are degraded by hydrolysis. Early degradation of these materials is characterized by random hydrolysis of long polymeric chains resulting in a progressive reduction of the molecular weight of the bulk material and reduction of its material properties. However, the total mass of the polymer remains in the site until the molecular weight of the fragments that are created is small enough to make them soluble. When this occurs, soluble material can be generated rapidly, liberating the bulk polymer into solution but creating a profound local decrease in pH. This process is the origin of late local osteolysis and the formation of sterile cysts in bone and soft tissue that have been observed after implantation of these materials. These limitations are beginning to be addressed by the development of new materials that are degraded by gradual surface erosion (often cell mediated) without the risk of accelerated release of degradation products.

Treatment Alternatives

The most commonly used scaffold materials are derived from allograft bone and are available in a broad range of physical forms including structural blocks, wedges, rings, dowels, and nonstructural chips, fibers, and powders. Nonstructural allograft preparations have been combined with plasticizing agents, such as carboxymethylcellulose, hyaluronan, and glycerol, to improve handling properties. Nonbone tissue-derived scaffolds have been introduced, including allograft and xenograft skin matrix, and xenograft intestinal submucosa. Biologic polymers (for example, collagen, hyaluronan, chitin, or fibrin), ceramic or mineral-based matrices (for example, tricalcium phosphate, hydroxyapatite, or calcium sulfate), metals (for example, titanium, tantalum, or cobalt-chromium-molybdenum alloy), and composites of two or more of these materials are also widely used as scaffold materials for tissue ingrowth and regeneration. Synthetic polymer materials (for example, polylactide, polyglycolide, polytyrosine carbonates, polycaprolactone) varying copolymers, and synthetic gel-like polymers (polyethylene oxide-based) are also being adapted from other surgical uses or developed de novo to improve properties of mechanical performance, degradation, and cell interaction. Other scaffold materials include hybrids of biologically-derived polymers such as alginate or fibrin that are chemically modified with cell adhesion peptides or growth factors. Some of these new scaffold materials are in advanced stages of development in animal studies.

Options for the structural distribution of scaffolds are almost infinite. The macro structures include regular geometric shapes (blocks, pellets, and dowels), amorphous structures (randomly packed chips, granules, or fibers), randomly integrated structures (foams or freeze dried materials), and formally designed regular structures (machined, printed, woven, or assembled structures). Gel or putty preparations can also be made from powders or fibers by mixing them with plasticizing agents (such as glycerol, methylcellulose, and hyaluronan).

In some instances, a desirable structure or porosity can be derived from nature. Allograft bone matrix can vary significantly according to sample and donor; however, through selective processing (machining, size and density selection, washing, demineralization), a variety of relatively uniform and optimized allograft materials can be made for specialized clinical settings (for example, chips, powders, struts, dowels, rings, wedges, screws). During the past decade, significant advances have been made in methods for producing more precise hierarchical microstructures from a variety of materials (tantalum, titanium, collagen, synthetic polymers, ceramics), which are now being applied to the creation of devices with strategically oriented channels and pores.

Many new types of scaffolds also are being developed to optimize bulk characteristics, three-dimensional architecture and porosity, mechanical properties, surface chemistry, initial scaffold environment (osmolarity, pH) and late scaffold environment (degradation characteristics). Each property has important implications in the biologic response to a scaffold and its usefulness in supporting the transplantation, homing, or biologic activity of local stem cells and progenitor cells.

The Evolving Science Leading to Optimized Bone Healing

Bone healing is an intricate process with many contributing variables. Tools for understanding and manipulating the bone healing process and for optimizing successful bone grafting are becoming increasingly available in the clinical setting. As a result, autogenous bone grafting is slowly being replaced as the gold standard against which all other bone graft alternatives are compared. Although no material is clinically more effective than autograft, the significant morbidity involved in harvesting these grafts creates the need for alternative materials that can provide comparable efficacy.

The translation of new materials and strategies into clinical practice requires significant basic benchtop science, preclinical assessment in animal models, and clinical assessment in either targeted cohort studies or prospective randomized trials. This stepwise approach is necessary to provide the burden of proof that is needed to support wide adoption of these new methods.

In addition to implantable or injectable bone graft substitutes, additional methods of facilitating bone healing and fusion remain equally important. Other methods for promoting bone healing include optimizing patient nutrition, patient cessation of tobacco use, and application of graded mechanical loading (for example, progressive weight bearing or dynamization of internal or external fixation). Biophysical stimulation using electromagnetic field stimulation or ultrasound also may be effective in reducing healing time and increasing the rate of union in selected settings.

It is important to make clinical decisions based on sound biologic and mechanical principles and objective data. To ensure the most predictable outcome and rapid patient recovery, attention to clinically proven guidelines, careful patient assessment, monitoring, and the reporting of clinical outcomes are required.

Annotated Bibliography

Mass Transport and Metabolic Demand in Bone Healing

Muschler GF, Nakamoto C, Griffith LG: Engineering principles of clinical cell-based tissue engineering. *J Bone Joint Surg Am* 2004;86-A:1541-1548.

This article reviews the current state of cell-based tissue engineering, the central engineering principles and strategies involved in the design and use of cell-based tools and strategies, and examines the challenges of mass transport.

Osteogenesis

Muschler GF, Midura RJ, Nakamoto C: Practical modeling concepts for connective tissue stem cell and progenitor compartment kinetics. *J Biomed Biotechnol* 2003; 2003:170-193.

Current concepts in stem cell biology, progenitor cell growth, and differentiation kinetics are reviewed in the context of bone formation. A cell-based modeling strategy is developed and offered as a tool for conceptual and quantitative exploration of the key kinetic variables and organizational hierarchies in bone tissue development and remodeling and in tissue engineering strategies for bone repair.

Osteoinductivity

Burkus JK, Gornet MF, Dickman CA, et al: Anterior lumbar interbody fusion using rhBMP-2 with tapered interbody cages. *J Spinal Disord Tech* 2002;15:337-349.

The findings of a multicenter, prospective, randomized, nonblinded study of patients with degenerative lumbar disk disease who underwent interbody fusion using two tapered threaded fusion cages is presented. The investigational group (143 patients) received rhBMP-2 on an absorbable collagen sponge. A control group (136 patients) received autogenous iliac crest bone graft. At 24-month follow-up, patients in the BMP-2 group showed a fusion rate of 94.5%. The patients in the autograft group showed a fusion rate of 88.7%.

Cheng H, Jiang W, Phillips FM, et al: Osteogenic activity of the fourteen types of human bone morphogenetic proteins (BMPs). *J Bone Joint Surg Am* 2003;85-A:1544-1552.

A comprehensive analysis of the osteogenic activity of 14 types of BMPs in osteoblastic progenitor cells is presented. BMP-2, BMP-6, and BMP-9 may play an important role in inducing osteoblast differentiation of mesenchymal stem cells. Most BMPs are able to stimulate osteogenesis in mature osteoblasts.

Einhorn TA: Clinical applications of recombinant human BMPs: Early experience and future development. *J Bone Joint Surg Am* 2003;85-A(suppl 3):82-88.

A review of BMPs and their clinical application is presented.

Friedlaender GE, Perry CR, Cole JD, et al: Osteogenic protein-1 (bone morphogenetic protein-7) in the treatment of tibial nonunions. *J Bone Joint Surg Am* 2001;83 (suppl 1):S151-S158.

A multicenter, prospective, randomized study of patients with established tibial nonunions who underwent treatment with bone grafting and intramedullary rod fixation is presented. Patients in the investigational group (63 fractures) received rhOP-1 on a type I collagen carrier. Patients in the control group (61 fractures) received an autogenous iliac crest bone graft. At 9 months, 75% of the fractures treated with OP-1 had healed compared with 84% of the fractures treated with autograft. The rhOP-1 group had a significantly lower incidence of postoperative infection and no donor site pain.

Govender S, Csimma C, Genant HK, et al: Recombinant human bone morphogenetic protein-2 for treatment of open tibial fractures: A prospective, controlled, randomized study of four hundred and fifty patients. *J Bone Joint Surg Am* 2002;84-A:2123-2134.

This article presents the findings of a prospective, randomized, single-blind study of patients treated for open tibial fractures using intramedullary nail fixation. In the study group, patients were treated with an rhBMP implant (doses of 6 mg or 12 mg in an 8 mL collagen carrier) at the time of wound closure. The control group did not receive an implant. Patients receiving the 12 mg dose of rhBMP had significantly fewer subsequent procedures, more rapid union, fewer hardware failures, fewer infections, and faster wound healing when compared with the control group or the group who received the 6-mg dose of rhBMP.

Muschler GF, Nitto H, Matsukura Y, et al: Spine fusion using cell matrix composites enriched in bone marrow-derived cells. *Clin Orthop* 2003;407:102-118.

Posterior spinal fusion model and cancellous bone matrix was used to compare an enriched cellular composite bone graft alone, bone matrix plus bone marrow clot, and an enriched bone matrix composite graft plus bone marrow clot. The union score, fusion volume, and fusion area for the enriched bone matrix plus bone marrow clot composite were superior to the enriched bone matrix alone and the bone matrix plus bone marrow clot. The addition of a bone marrow clot to an enriched cell-matrix composite graft results in significant improvement in graft performance.

The Evolving Science Leading to Optimized Bone Healing

Hodges SD, Eck JC, Humphreys SC: Use of electrical bone stimulation in spinal fusion. *J Am Acad Orthop Surg* 2003;11:81-88.

A review of the effect of three types of electrical stimulation (direct current electrical stimulation, pulsed electromagnetic fields, and capacitively coupled electrical stimulation) on spinal fusion is presented. Direct current electrical stimulation showed positive effects although there was difficulty in determining the end point of fusion and incorporating the effect of patient parameters.

Rubin C, Bolander M, Ryaby JP, Hadjiargyrou M: The use of low-intensity ultrasound to accelerate the healing of fractures. *J Bone Joint Surg Am* 2001;83-A:259-270.

A review of the efficacy of low-intensity ultrasound in fracture management is presented.

Classic Bibliography

Aronson J: Limb-lengthening, skeletal reconstruction, and bone transport with the Ilizarov method. *J Bone Joint Surg Am* 1997;79:1243-1258.

Bauer TW, Muschler GF: Bone graft materials: An overview of the basic science. *Clin Orthop* 2000;371:10-27.

Boden SD, Zdeblick TA, Sandhu HS, et al: The use of rhBMP-2 in interbody fusion cages: Definitive evidence of osteoinduction in humans. A preliminary report. *Spine* 2000;25:376-381.

Connolly JF: Clinical use of marrow osteoprogenitor cells to stimulate osteogenesis. *Clin Orthop* 1998; 355(suppl):S257-S266.

Green SA: Ilizarov method. *Clin Orthop* 1992;280:2-6.

Muschler GF, Boehm C, Easley K: Aspiration to obtain osteoblast progenitor cells from human bone marrow: The influence of aspiration volume. *J Bone Joint Surg Am* 1997;79:1699-1709.

Rhinelander FW: Tibial blood supply in relation to fracture healing. *Clin Orthop* 1974;105:34-81.

Stevenson S: Biology of bone grafts. *Orthop Clin North Am* 1999;30:543-552.

Urist MR: Bone: Formation by autoinduction. *Science* 1965;150:893-899.

Wiss DA, Stetson WB: Tibial nonunion: Treatment alternatives. *J Am Acad Orthop Surg* 1996;4:249-257.

Wozney JM, Rosen V, Celeste AJ, et al: Novel regulators of bone formation: Molecular clones and activities. *Science* 1988;242:1528-1534.

Chapter 4

Musculoskeletal Biomechanics

Vijay K. Goel, PhD

Ashutosh Khandha, MS

Sasidhar Vadapalli, MS

Introduction

Biomechanics involves the use of the tools of mechanics (the branch of physics that analyzes the actions of forces) in the study of anatomic and functional aspects of living organisms. The musculoskeletal interactions are a good example of a mechanical system. The primary functions of the musculoskeletal system are to transmit forces from one part of the body to another and to protect certain organs (such as the brain) from mechanical forces that could result in damage. Therefore, the principal biologic role of skeletal tissues is to bear loads with limited deformation. To appreciate the mechanical functions that these tissues must perform, it is necessary to understand the forces that whole bones normally carry. In most cases, these forces result from loads being passed from the part of the body in contact with a more or less rigid environmental surface (such as the heel and the ground surface during walking) through one or more bones to the applied or supported load (such as the torso). In addition to the forces transmitted through bone-to-bone contact, large and important forces exerted by the muscles and ligaments act on the bones. Most muscle, ligament, and bone-to-bone contact forces act in or near the body's major diarthrodial joints. Basic engineering concepts used in the conventional analysis of mechanical systems and their principles can be applied to the musculoskeletal system.

Concepts and Terminology of Mechanics

Scalars, Vectors, and Tensors

In mechanics, two basic quantities are defined. Scalar quantities (such as mass, temperature, work, and energy) have magnitude. A vector quantity (such as force, velocity, and acceleration) has both magnitude and direction. Unlike scalars, vector quantities add in a tip to tail fashion.

Consider two force vectors, $\overline{A}$ and $\overline{B}$. The length of the vectors represents the magnitude and arrows point in the direction of the forces. To replace these two vectors with a single vector that has the same effect on the body, the two vectors are drawn tail to tail. Next, lines are drawn parallel to each vector to create a parallelogram. The resultant force (or the force that can replace the two vectors and still have the same effect on the body as the two original vectors) is the diagonal of the parallelogram ($\overline{R}$).

An example of vector resolution to predict contact force at the knee joint is shown in Figure 1. If the direction and magnitude of the muscle and tendon forces are as shown in the figure, the resultant joint contact force can be found by using the parallelogram law. The resultant joint contact force is at a 45° angle to the line of action of the tendon force and its magnitude is given by the vector addition (the square root of the squares of the two forces), which is 71 lb.

Tensors, defined mathematically, are simply arrays of numbers, or functions, which transform according to certain rules, under a change of coordinates. In physics, tensors characterize the properties of a physical system. A tensor consisting of a single number is referred to as a tensor of order zero, or simply, a scalar. A tensor of order one, known as a vector, is a single row or a single column of numbers. Tensors can be defined to all orders. The next order above a vector are tensors of order two, which are often referred to as matrices. Second order components are not only associated with magnitude and direction, but they are also dependent on the plane over which they are determined. The components of a second order tensor can be written as a two-dimensional array consisting of rows and columns as shown below:

$$\begin{vmatrix} \sigma_{xx} & \sigma_{xy} & \sigma_{xz} \\ \sigma_{yx} & \sigma_{yy} & \sigma_{yz} \\ \sigma_{zx} & \sigma_{zy} & \sigma_{zz} \end{vmatrix}$$

Just as vectors represent physical properties more complex than scalars, matrices represent physical properties more complex than can be described by vectors.

Force, Mass, and Weight

Force may be defined as mechanical disturbance or load and is associated with the result of muscle activity.

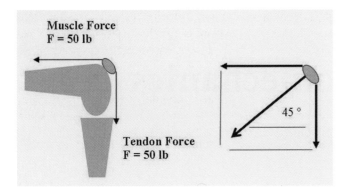

Figure 1 Vector resolution to calculate joint contact force at the knee.

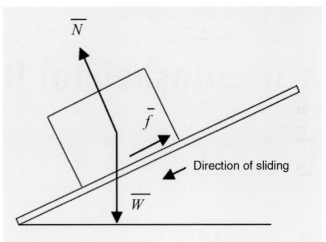

Figure 2 Normal and tangential forces when a block slides.

When an object is pulled or pushed, force is applied to the object. Force is also exerted when a ball is thrown or kicked. Force acting on an object can deform the object and/or change its state of motion. Force is also defined as a vector quantity and is equal to mass multiplied by the acceleration. The unit of force is the newton.

A force may be broadly classified as external or internal. When a nail is hit with a hammer, an external force is applied to the nail. Internal forces are those that hold a body together when the body is under the effect of externally applied forces. If the human body is considered as a whole, then the forces generated by muscle contractions are the internal forces.

A normal force acts in a direction perpendicular to a particular surface. A tangential force acts in a direction parallel to the surface. In Figure 2 the weight ($\overline{W}$) of the sliding block acts on the floor as shown. The floor applies a counteracting normal force ($\overline{N}$) on the block. The frictional force ($\overline{f}$), which develops between the block and the floor, is an example of a tangential force.

A compressive force tends to shrink the body in the direction of the applied force, whereas a tensile force tends to stretch or elongate the body in the direction of the applied force. Muscles contract to produce tensile forces that pull together the bones to which they are attached. Muscles cannot produce compressive forces.

Mass and weight are terms that are often confused. Mass is the amount of matter present in a body and is an intrinsic property of the body; the mass of an object always remains the same. Weight, however, is the force that a given mass feels because of the gravity at its place. Mass is measured in kilograms, whereas weight is measured in units of force such as the newton.

Moment and Torque Vectors

In general, torque is associated with the rotational and twisting action of applied forces, whereas moment is related to its bending effect. A torque is said to be applied to a structure when the plane in which force acts is perpendicular to the long axis of the structure. Examples of torque are forces applied on a screwdriver and the

steering wheel of a car. A bending moment is said to be applied to a structure when the force plane is parallel to the long axis of the structure. An example of a bending moment is the bending of a diving board caused by the weight of a diver. However, the mathematical definition of moment and torque is the same.

The magnitude of the moment of a force about a point is equal to the magnitude of the force times the length of the shortest distance between the point and the line of the action of the force, which is known as the lever or moment arm. Figure 3 shows how the moment caused by a force acting on the wrist is calculated about a point on the elbow. The direction of moment is per-

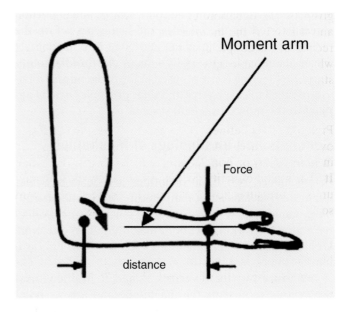

Figure 3 Moment of force acting on the wrist about a point on the elbow. *(Reproduced with permission from Mow VC, Hayes WC: Analysis of muscle and joint loads, in Basic Orthopaedic Biomechanics, ed 2. Philadelphia, PA, Lippincott-Raven, 1997, p 3.)*

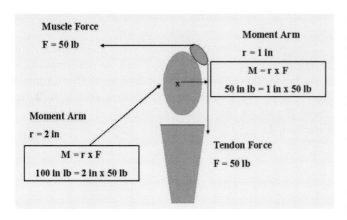

Figure 4 Change in moment arm changes the value of moment.

pendicular to the plane on which the point and force lie, and is found by the right hand rule. The right hand rule states, "When the fingers of the right hand curl in the direction that the applied force tends to rotate the body about a point, the right thumb points in the direction of the moment vector."

Figure 4 shows how a change in the moment arm changes the moment. When the moment is calculated about "x," the muscle force has a moment arm of 2 inches and therefore, the moment is 100 in-lb. However, when the force has a moment arm of 1 inch, the moment reduces to 50 in-lb. The change in moment arm can be the result of surgery.

A couple or pure moment is a system of forces whose resultant force is zero. The system typically consists of two parallel coplanar forces of equal magnitude and opposite directions. The magnitude of the couple is given by the equation: C = F × r, where F is the force and where r is the moment arm. The magnitude and direction of the couple does not change as the point about which the couple changes, because the moment arm stays the same.

Pressure

Pressure (P) is defined as the amount of force (F) acting over a given area (A). Pressure is commonly measured in Pascal (Pa) or pounds per square inch (psi or lb/in^2). It is a scalar quantity. Stress is measured in the same units as pressure; however, stress is a second order tensor.

Displacement, Velocity, and Acceleration

Displacement is a vector measure of the interval between two locations measured along the path connecting them.

Velocity is defined as the rate of change of position of a point or rigid body with respect to a coordinate system or another body. If the motion is translational, then it is termed as linear velocity. If the motion is rotational,

it is termed as angular velocity. Velocity is similar to speed, except that speed is a scalar quantity, whereas velocity is a vector because it has direction in addition to its magnitude.

Acceleration is defined as the rate of change of velocity and can be linear or angular. An example of linear acceleration is a driver pressing the accelerator of a car. Angular acceleration is the rate of change of angular velocity.

Statics and Dynamics

Statics and dynamics are two major subbranches of mechanics. Statics is an area within the field of applied mechanics dealing with the analysis of rigid bodies in equilibrium. The term equilibrium implies that the body of concern is either at rest or moving with a constant velocity. Dynamics is the study of systems in which acceleration is present.

Newton's Laws of Mechanics

Newton's first law states that a body that is originally at rest will remain at rest, or a body moving with a constant velocity in a straight line will maintain its motion unless an external force acts on the body.

Newton's second law states that if the net force acting on a body is not zero, then the body will accelerate in the direction of the resultant force. Furthermore, the magnitude of the acceleration of the body will be directly proportional to the magnitude of the net force acting on the body and inversely proportional to its mass. Newton's second law can be formulated as:
Equation 1:

$$\overline{F} = m \cdot \overline{a}$$

where $\overline{F}$ is the net force acting on the body, m is the mass of the body, and $\overline{a}$ is its acceleration. This is also known as the equation of motion.

Newton's third law states "to every action, there is an equal and opposite reaction." This law is particularly useful in analyzing complex problems in biomechanics in which there are several interacting bodies.

Conditions for Equilibrium

If the net force and the net moment acting on a body are zero, then acceleration (linear and angular) of the body is zero, and consequently, the velocity (linear and angular) of the body is either constant or zero. Therefore, two conditions need to be satisfied for equilibrium. The body is said to be in translational equilibrium if the net force (vector sum of all forces) acting on it is zero.
Equation 2:

$$\sum \overline{F} = 0$$

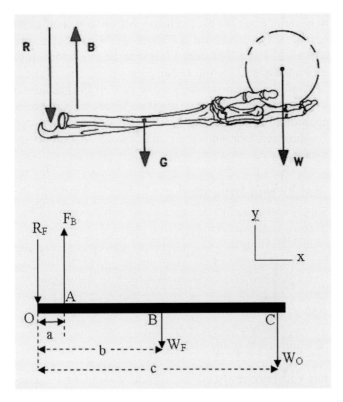

Figure 5 Free-body diagram showing the forces acting on the lower arm while holding a weight with the arm flexed to 90°. *(Reproduced with permission from Mow VC, Hayes WC: Analysis of muscle and joint loads, in* Basic Orthopaedic Biomechanics, *ed 2. Philadelphia, PA, Lippincott-Raven, 1997, p 6.)*

The body is in rotational equilibrium if the net moment (vector sum of all moments) acting on it is zero.
Equation 3:

$$\sum \overline{M} = 0$$

Free-Body Diagrams

Free-body diagrams (FBDs) are constructed to help identify the forces and moments acting on individual parts of a system and to ensure the correct use of the equations of equilibrium. For this purpose, the system is isolated from its surroundings and proper forces and moments replace the effects of the surroundings. For example, Figure 5 shows the forearm holding a weight. Point O is designated the axis of rotation of the elbow joint, which is assumed to be fixed for practical purposes. Point A is the attachment of the biceps muscle with the radius, B is the center of gravity of the forearm, and C is a point on the forearm that lies along the vertical line passing through the center of gravity of the weight in the hand. The distances between O and A, O and B, and O and C are measured as a, b, c, respectively. W_O is the weight of the object held in the hand and W_F is the total weight of the forearm. F_B is the magnitude of the force exerted by the biceps on the radius, and R_F is the reaction force at the elbow joint. The line of ac-

tion of the muscle force is assumed to be vertical. The gravitational forces are vertical as well.

The magnitudes of the muscle tension (F_B) and joint reaction force at the elbow (R_F) can be determined by considering the equilibrium conditions at the forearm. Considering the rotational equilibrium of the forearm about the elbow joint (point O) will yield:
Equation 4a:

$$\sum M_o = 0 :$$

$$F_B \times a - W_F \times b - W_O \times c = 0$$

$$F_B = \frac{1}{a}(bW_F + cW_O)$$

Considering the translational equilibrium of the forearm along the y direction:
Equation 4b:

$$\sum F_y = 0 :$$

$$R_F - F_B + W_F + W_O = 0$$

$$R_F = F_B - W_F - W_O$$

Equations 4a and 4b can be solved for F_B and R_F for a given set of geometric parameters of a, b, c and weights W_O and W_F. For example, assume a = 4 cm, b = 15 cm, c = 35 cm, W_O = 80 N, and W_F = 20 N. Then from equations 4a and 4b:

$$F_B = \frac{1}{0.04}[(0.15)(20)+(0.35)(80)] = 775N \ (+y)$$
$$R_F = 775 - 20 - 80 = 675N \ (-y)$$

FBDs can also be used to calculate external intersegmental forces and moments at different joints during human locomotion, as shown in Figure 6. In Figure 6, *A*, the subscripts "*f*," "*s*" and "*t*" stand for foot, shank, and thigh, respectively. The letter "*I*" represents the moment of inertia, "a" represents the angular acceleration, "g" represents the gravitational acceleration, "*m*" represents the mass of the segment concentrated at the centroid, and "*a*" represents the linear acceleration. In Figure 6, *B*, the subscripts "*g*," "*a*," "*k*," and "*h*" stand for ground, ankle, knee, and hip, respectively. "*F*" stands for the force and "*T*" is the resultant torque.

After an FBD is drawn, equilibrium equations are used to calculate the unknown proximal forces. Calculations proceed from the distal to proximal end and start at the foot. With the help of equilibrium equations, the force and torque at the ankle are calculated. The force and torque at the distal end of the shank are equal and opposite to the force and torque at the ankle. With the distal force and torque of the shank known, the proximal end force and torque are then calculated. In most cases, however, the number of equations available for the solution of such problems are fewer than the number of unknowns. Therefore, additional assumptions

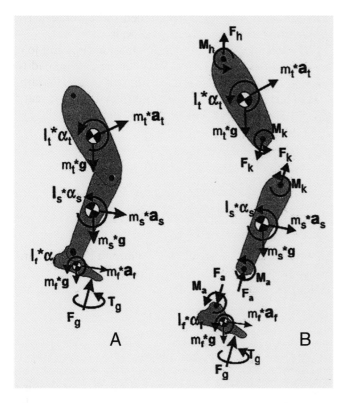

Figure 6 A and **B**, model of the lower extremity and the corresponding free-body diagrams. See text for details. *(Reproduced with permission from Mow VC, Hayes WC: Musculoskeletal dynamics, locomotion, and clinical applications, in Basic Orthopaedic Biomechanics, ed 2. Philadelphia, PA, Lippincott-Raven,1997, p 44.)*

need to be made to obtain a solution. A common method for solving an indeterminate problem is to seek an optimum solution (a solution that maximizes or minimizes some process or action).

Kinematics and Kinetics

The general field of dynamics consists of two major areas: kinematics and kinetics. The field of kinematics addresses the description of geometric and time-dependent aspects of motion without dealing with the forces causing the motion. Kinematic analyses are based on the relationships between position, velocity, and acceleration vectors. These relationships appear in the form of differential and integral equations.

The field of kinetics is based on kinematics and includes the effects of forces and torques that cause the motion in the analyses. There are several different approaches to the solutions of problems in kinetics. Different methods may be applied to different situations, depending on the parameter that needs to be determined. For example, the equation of motion is used for problems requiring the analysis of acceleration, whereas the analysis of forces related to changes in velocity uses a different method known as the energy method.

It is a common practice in the study of kinematics and kinetics to categorize motion as translational, rotational,

or general. Translational or linear motion occurs if all parts of the body move the same distance at the same time and in the same direction. An example of a translational motion is the vertical motion of an elevator in a shaft. Linear motion also may be thought of as motion along a line. If the line is straight, the motion is rectilinear. If the line is curved, the motion is curvilinear.

Rotational or angular motion occurs when a body moves in a circular path such that all parts of the body move through the same angle at the same time. The angular motion occurs about a central line known as the axis of rotation, which lies perpendicular to the plane of motion.

General motion occurs when a body undergoes both translational and rotational motions simultaneously; it is more complex to analyze motions composed of both translation and rotation. Most human body segmental motions are of the general type. For example, while walking, the lower extremities both translate and rotate.

Degree of freedom is an expression that describes the ability of an object to move in space. A completely unrestrained object, such as a ball, has six degrees of freedom (three related to translational motion along three mutually perpendicular axes, and three related to rotational motion about the same axes).

Stress and Strain

In addition to tensile and compressive forces, there is a third important category of force, termed shear. Whereas compressive and tensile forces act along the longitudinal axis of a bone or other body to which they are applied, shear force acts parallel or tangent to a surface. Shear force tends to cause a portion of the object to slide, displace, or shear with respect to another portion of the object. For example, a force acting at the knee joint in a direction parallel to the tibial plateau is a shearing force at the knee. During the performance of a squat exercise, joint shear at the knee is greatest at full squat position, which places a large amount of stress on the ligaments and muscle tendons that prevent the femur from sliding off the tibial plateau.

The area moment of inertia is a measure of the distribution of the material in the cross section of a structure characterizing its bending stiffness and strength. The cross section of a bone, shown in Figure 7, is divided into many small elements of area (ΔA).

The area moment of inertia about the X and Y axes are given by:

Equation 5a:

$$I_x = \Sigma \, y^2 \cdot \Delta A$$

Equation 5b:

$$I_y = \Sigma \, x^2 \cdot \Delta A$$

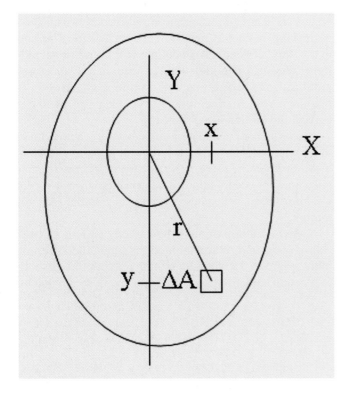

Figure 7 Area and polar moment of inertia defined for a cross section of bone.

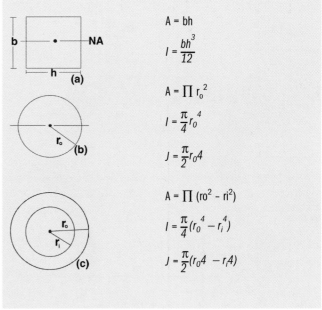

Figure 8 Area moment of inertia and polar moment for three geometries: rectangle (a), solid cylinder (b), and hollow cylinder (c). A = Area ; I = area moment of inertia; J = polar moment of inertia; NA = neutral axis. *(Reproduced with permission from Ozkaya N, Nordin M:* Fundamentals of Biomechanics, *ed 2. New York, NY, Springer-Verlag, 1998.)*

The polar moment of inertia is a measure of the distribution of material in the cross section of a structure characterizing its torsional stiffness and strength. The mathematical expression for the polar moment of inertia (J) about the centroid of the cross section is as follows:

Equation 6:

$$J = \Sigma \ r^2 \cdot \Delta A$$

Material distribution in a structure has an impact on strength and bending (Figure 8). A solid cylindrical rod of 5 mm radius has an area moment of inertia of 491 mm^4. Redistributing the same material into a hollow tube of 1-mm thickness results in an outer radius of 13 mm and an area of moment of inertia of 6,146 mm^4. The bending strength (the area of moment of inertia divided by the radius) of the two different geometries now can be calculated. It is found that the 13-mm tube is 4.8 times as strong as the 5-mm rod. Human bone is an excellent example of this type of construction. Bones are hollow and cancellous on the inside and hard and cortical on the outside. This construction provides maximum strength to the bone.

Stress

An important factor affecting the outcome of the action of forces on the human body is the manner in which the force is distributed. Whereas pressure represents the distribution of force external to a solid body, stress represents the resulting force distribution inside a solid body when an external force acts. Stress (σ) is quantified in the same way as pressure. Stress = force (F) per unit area (A) over which the force acts.

Equation 7:

$$\sigma = \frac{F}{A}$$

A given force acting on a small surface produces greater stress than the same force acting over a larger surface. When a blow is sustained by the human body, the likelihood of injury to body tissue is related to the magnitude and direction of the stress created by the blow. Compressive stress, tensile stress, and shear stress are terms that indicate the direction of the acting stress.

From a mechanical perspective, long bones can be compared to structural beams. A bone's ability to resist a shear force is more important than its ability to resist an axial force. A bone can be subjected to three-point bending and four-point bending as shown in Figure 9. When a bone is bent, it is subjected to stresses occurring in the longitudinal direction or in a direction normal to the cross section of the bone. Based on the loading configuration shown in Figure 9 *A*, the distribution of these normal stresses over the cross section of the bone is such that it is zero on the neutral axis (NA), negative (compression) above the neutral axis, and positive (tensile) below the neutral axis.

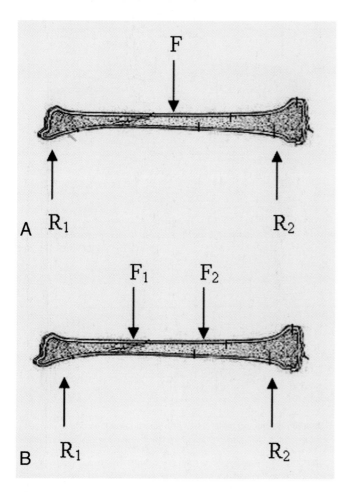

Figure 9 Types of bending. **A,** three-point and **B,** four-point.

For a bone subjected to pure bending, the stress σ_x is given by the following equation known as the flexural formula.

Equation 8:

$$\sigma_x = \frac{(M) \cdot (y)}{(I)}$$

M is the bending moment, y is the vertical distance between the neutral axis and the point at which the stress is sought, and I is the area moment of inertia of the cross section of the beam about the neutral axis.

For example, if the bending moment has a value of 10,000 N-mm^4, the distance from the neutral axis at which stress is to be calculated is 10 mm, and the area moment of inertia of the cross section is 200,000 mm, the stress is calculated as:

$$\sigma_x = 10000 \times 10/200,000$$

$$= 0.5 \text{ N/mm}^2 = 0.5 \text{ MPa}$$

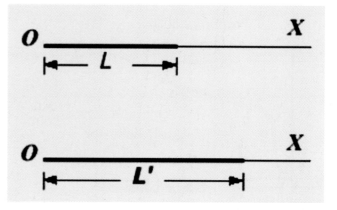

Figure 10 Uniaxial strain for a rod in elongation.

Strain

Strain, which is also known as unit deformation, is a measurement of the degree or intensity of deformation. Consider a rod with initial length L which is stretched to a length L' (Figure 10). The strain measure ε, a dimensionless ratio, is defined as the ratio of elongation with respect to the original length.

Equation 9:

$$\varepsilon = \frac{L' - L}{L}$$

A common term encountered in biomechanics is strain rate (the rate at which strain occurs). Mathematically, it is obtained by dividing strain (dimensionless) by the time (seconds) of application of load, thus imparting the unit of measurement as second^{-1} (s^{-1}).

Stress-Strain Diagram

When any stress is plotted on a graph against the resulting strain for a material, the resulting stress-strain diagram has several different shapes, depending on the kind of material involved. As an example of a stress-strain diagram, Figure 11 illustrates the behavior of a particular metal when subjected to increasing tensile (stretching) stress. On the first portion of the curve (up to a strain of less than 1%, 0a), the stress and strain are proportional. This condition holds until the point "a", the proportional limit, is reached. It is known that stress and strain are proportional because this segment of the line is straight (Hooke's Law). Young's modulus is essentially the slope of the straight line on the stress-strain diagram. Every material has a unique Young's modulus value. The larger the Young's modulus for a material, the greater stress needed for a given strain. The greater the Young's modulus for a material, the better it can withstand greater forces.

From points "a" to "b" on the diagram, stress and strain are not proportional; however, if the stress is removed at any point between "a" and "b," the curve will

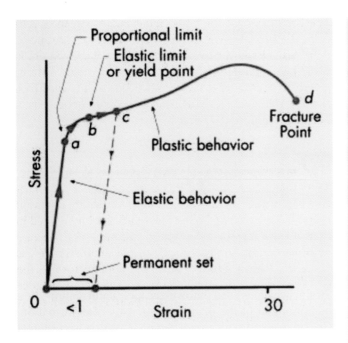

Figure 11 Stress-strain diagram. (Adapted from Examining the effects of space flight on the skeletal system, Houston, Texas, National Space Biomedical Research Institute.)

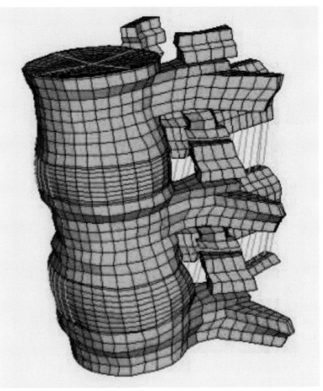

Figure 13 Finite element model of the L3-L5 lumbar segment.

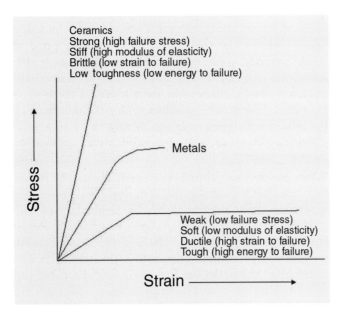

Figure 12 Stress-strain behavior of different materials.

be retraced in the opposite direction and the material will return to its original shape and length. In the region "*ab*," the material is said to be elastic or to exhibit elastic behavior and the point "b" is called the elastic limit.

If the material is stressed further, the strain increases rapidly, but when the stress is removed at some point beyond "b," say point "c," the material does not revert to its original shape or length but returns along a different path to a different point. Further increase of stress beyond "c" produces a large increase in strain until point "d" is reached and fracture occurs. From points "b" to "d," the metal is said to undergo plastic deformation. If the plastic deformation that takes place between the elastic limit and the fracture point is large, the metal is said to be ductile. Such materials are capable of being drawn out like a wire or hammered thin like gold leaf. If, however, fracture occurs soon after the elastic limit is passed, the metal is said to be brittle. Figure 12 compares the stress-strain behavior of different types of materials and includes characteristic mechanical properties.

It is often necessary to compute stresses and displacements in different regions of biologic structures that have complex geometries. Usually, it is not feasible to make in vitro or in vivo measurements of these parameters. A technique called finite element modeling is useful in such cases. As the name suggests, this technique involves constructing a complex geometric model using a finite number of elements of different shapes, sizes, and properties, and then analyzing the structure. Mathematically, it is defined as a procedure to obtain approximate numerical solutions to equations that express the fundamental laws of physics (such as equilibrium and balance of mass and energy). Figure 13 shows a validated finite element model of the L3-L5 ligamentous spinal lumbar segment.

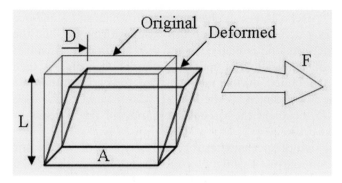

Figure 14 Shear force (F) deforms a cube into a parallelepiped.

Young's Modulus, Shear Modulus, and Poisson's Ratio

The modulus of elasticity in tension, also known as Young's modulus (E), is the ratio of stress to strain on the "loading plane" along the "loading direction" when the material is in the elastic limit.
Equation 10:

$$E = \frac{\sigma_{xx}}{\varepsilon_{xx}}$$

Common sense (and the second law of thermodynamics) indicates that a material under uniaxial tension must elongate in length. Therefore, the Young's modulus *(E)* is required to be nonnegative for all materials *(E > 0)*.

A similar property known as shear modulus is used to define material stiffness. Shear modulus is the ratio of shear stress to shear strain of a material. Shear modulus (G) is measured in Pa or newton per square meter (N/m^2). In the cube shown in Figure 14, application of a shear force (F) deforms the cube into a parallelepiped (a solid with parallel sides that are not perpendicular to each other). This results in shear stress, τ (F/A) and shear strain, γ (D/L).
Equation 11:

$$\text{Shear modulus, } (G) = \frac{(F/A)}{(D/L)} = \tau/\gamma$$

Also, a rod-like specimen subjected to uniaxial tension will exhibit some shrinkage in the lateral direction for most materials. The opposite is true for the compression force. The ratio of lateral strain and axial strain is defined as Poisson's ratio (v).
Equation 12:

$$v = -\frac{\varepsilon_{yy}}{\varepsilon_{xx}}$$

The Poisson's ratio for most materials will fall in the range,

$$0 \leq v \leq \frac{1}{2}$$

The Poisson's ratio for most metals falls between 0.25 to 0.35. Rubber has a Poisson's ratio close to 0.5 and is therefore almost incompressible. Theoretical materials with a Poisson's ratio of exactly 0.5 are truly incompressible, because the sum of all their strains leads to a zero volume change. Cork, on the other hand, has a Poisson's ratio close to zero.

Torsion

Torsion occurs when a structure is caused to twist about its longitudinal axis, typically when one end of the structure is fixed. Torsional fractures of the tibia are common in football and skiing injuries in which the foot is held in a fixed position while the rest of the body undergoes a twisting motion. The magnitude of the shear stress (τ) is related to the magnitude M of the applied torque, the cross-sectional area of the shaft, and the radial distance (r) between the center line and the point at which shear stress is to be determined.
Equation 13:

$$\frac{\tau = (M) \cdot (r)}{(J)}$$

Mechanical Properties of Tissues

Biomechanical principles guide the manner in which components of the musculoskeletal system respond to trauma, stresses, and loads and therefore determine the success of this system to withstand external forces that may threaten the more vulnerable organs. These principles also apply to body motions such as bending, lifting, and fine manipulation. It also is important to realize that the behavior of the muscles and tissues depends on intrinsic material properties. In general, materials respond differently to different loading configurations. For a given material, there may be different mechanical properties that must be considered in analyzing its response to, for example, tensile loading as compared with loading that may cause bending or torsion. To apply biomechanical principles to the musculoskeletal system, it is essential to understand the mechanical properties of tissues.

Extensibility and Elasticity

The properties of extensibility and elasticity are common to many biologic tissues. Extensibility is the ability to be stretched and elasticity is the ability to return to normal length after extension or contraction.

The elastic behavior of muscle consists of two major conceptual components. As shown in Figure 15, the muscle membranes represent the parallel elastic component, which provides resistive tension when a muscle is passively stretched. The tendons represent the series elastic component, which acts as a spring to store elastic energy when an active muscle is stretched. These com-

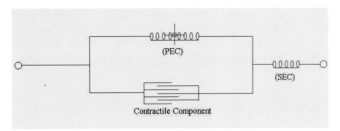

Figure 15 Conceptual components to explain muscle elasticity. PEC = parallel elastic component; SEC = series elastic component. *(Reproduced with permission from Hall SJ: The biomechanics of human skeletal muscle, in* Basic Biomechanics, *ed 3. New York, NY, McGrawHill, 1999.)*

ponents of muscle elasticity are so named because the membranes and tendons are respectively parallel to and in series with the muscle fibers, which provide the contractile component. The elasticity of human skeletal muscle is believed to result primarily from the series elastic component.

Irritability and the Ability to Develop Tension

Another characteristic property of muscle is irritability, which is the ability to respond to a stimulus. Muscles are affected by either electrochemical stimuli (such as an action potential from the nerve) or mechanical stimuli (such as an external blow to a portion of a muscle). If the stimulus is of sufficient magnitude, the muscle responds by developing tension.

Viscoelasticity

Viscoelasticity is the time-dependent mechanical property of a material. As the name suggests, two basic components of viscoelasticity are viscosity and elasticity. Viscosity is a fluid property and is a measure of resistance to flow. Elasticity is a solid material property. A viscoelastic material is one that possesses both fluid and solid properties. It has been experimentally determined that most biologic materials, such as bone, ligaments, tendons, and passive muscles exhibit viscoelasticity.

Creep and relaxation are two characteristics of viscoelastic materials that are used to document their behavior quantitatively. Creep is a phenomenon in which a material or a structure deforms as a function of time under the action of a constant load. A creep test involves the application of a sudden load, which is then maintained at constant magnitude. Measurements of deformation are recorded as a function of time. When an individual's height is measured in the morning and again at night after weight bearing throughout the day, the nighttime measurement is less than the morning measurement. This change in height (deformation) is not caused by any additional weight the person might have gained during the day, but rather by creep of the intervertebral disks, and to a lesser extent by the effects of compression of the cartilage of load-bearing joints.

Relaxation is a phenomenon in which stress or force in a deformed structure decreases with time, while the deformation is held constant. A relaxation test involves the application of sudden deformation, which is then maintained during the test. The force- or stress-time curve obtained is called the relaxation curve and is used to document the viscoelastic nature of the material or structure.

Another characteristic that is typical of viscoelastic materials is sensitivity to the rate of loading. The stress-strain curve of a viscoelastic material is dependent on the rate of loading. A higher rate of loading generally results in a steeper curve. For example, a slow pull on a material such as Silly Putty can produce a deformation of as much as several thousand percent before failure. The behavior of this material is classified as ductile. A fast pull, however, will break the putty at less than 5% deformation, and will require a relatively large force. The material property may now be called brittle. The literature of biomechanics has established that bone, ligaments, tendons, and passive muscles are sensitive to the rate of loading.

The other major characteristic of a viscoelastic material is hysteresis or energy dissipation. This property means that if a viscoelastic material is loaded and unloaded, the unloading curve will not follow the loading curve. The difference between the two curves represents the amount of energy that is dissipated or lost during loading.

Anisotropy of Materials

A material is called anisotropic if its mechanical properties (such as strength and modulus of elasticity) are different in different directions. Experiments have shown that bone is highly anisotropic. For example, strength of bone in the mid-diaphysis of a long bone varies in different directions. Generally, the axial strength for bone is the greatest, followed by radial strength, and then the circumferential strength.

Biomechanical Evaluation of Human Tissues

Most biologic tissues are composite materials (consisting of materials with different properties) with nonhomogeneous and anisotropic properties. The mechanical properties of living tissues may vary from point to point within the tissue, and their response to forces applied in different directions may be different. Among the common components of biologic tissues, collagen and elastin fibers have the most important mechanical properties affecting the overall mechanical behavior of the tissue in which they are present.

Collagen is a protein made of crimped fibrils that aggregate into fibers. The mechanical properties of collagen fibrils are such that each fibril can be considered a mechanical spring and each fiber as an assemblage of

Table 1	Ultimate Strength for Human Femoral Cortical Bone	
Loading Mode	**Ultimate Strength**
Longitudinal	
Tension	133 MPa
Compression	193 MPa
Shear	68 MPa
Transverse	
Tension	51 MPa
Compression	133 MPa

$(1 \text{ MPa} = 10^6 \text{ Pa}; 1 \text{ GPa} = 10^9 \text{ Pa})$

(Reproduced with permission from Mow VC, Hayes WC: Biomechanics of cortical and trabecular bone, in Mow VC, Hayes WC (eds): Basic Orthopaedic Biomechanics, ed 2. New York, NY, Raven Press, 1997, p 85.)

Table 2	Elastic and Shear Moduli for Human Femoral Cortical Bone	
Young's Moduli/ Elastic Moduli, E	
Longitudinal	17.0 GPa
Transverse	11.5 GPa
Shear Modulus, G	3.3 GPa

$(1 \text{ MPa} = 10^6 \text{ Pa}, 1 \text{ GPa} = 10^9 \text{ Pa})$

(Reproduced with permission from Mow VC, Hayes WC: Biomechanics of Cortical and trabecular bone, in Mow VC, Hayes WC (eds): Basic Orthopaedic Biomechanics, ed 2. New York, NY, Raven Press, 1997, p 85.)

springs. The primary mechanical function of collagen fibers is to withstand axial tension. Because of their high length-to-diameter ratios (aspect ratio), collagen fibers are not effective under compression. Whenever a fiber is pulled, its crimp straightens and its length increases. Like a mechanical spring, the energy supplied to stretch the fiber is stored, and it is the release of this energy that returns the fiber to its unstretched configuration when the applied load is removed. Collagen fibers exhibit viscoelastic behavior and possess relatively high tensile strength.

Among the noncollagenous tissue components, elastin is another fibrous protein with material properties that resemble the material properties of rubber. Fibers containing elastin are highly extensible, and their extension is reversible even at high strains. Elastin fibers behave elastically with low stiffness.

Biomechanics of Bone

Bone is the primary structural element of the human body that protects internal organs, provides kinematic links, provides muscle attachment sites, and facilitates muscle actions and body movements. Bone is also unique in that it is self-repairing. Bone also can alter its shape, mechanical behavior, and mechanical properties to adapt to the changes in mechanical demand. The major factors influencing the mechanical behavior of bone are the mechanical properties of tissues comprising the bone; the size and the geometry of the bone; and the direction, magnitude, and rate of applied loads.

At the macroscopic level, all bones consist of two types of tissues. The cortical or compact bone tissue is a dense material forming the outer shell (cortex) of bones and the diaphysial region of long bones. The cancellous, trabecular, or spongy bone tissue consists of thin rods and plates (trabeculae) in a lattice-like structure that is enclosed by the cortical bone.

The mechanical response of bone can be observed by subjecting it to tension, compression, bending, and torsion. Various tests to implement these conditions are performed using uniform bone specimens or whole bones. Results from these tests indicate that the compressive strength of bone is greater than its tensile strength. Also, bone is much better at resisting rapidly applied loads than at resisting slowly applied loads. Bone is stiffer and stronger at higher strain rates. The energy absorbed by bone tissue, which is proportional to the area under the stress-strain curve, increases with an increasing strain rate. It should be noted that during normal daily activities, bone tissues are subjected to a strain rate of about 0.01 s^{-1}.

The stress-strain behavior of bone is also dependent on the orientation of bone with respect to the direction of loading. Cortical bone has a larger ultimate strength (indicating that it is stronger) and a larger Young's modulus or elastic modulus (indicating that it is stiffer) in the longitudinal direction than the transverse direction. Bone specimens loaded in the transverse direction fail in a more brittle manner (without showing considerable yielding) compared with bone specimens loaded in the longitudinal direction. The ultimate strength values for adult femoral cortical bone under various modes of loading and its elastic and shear moduli are listed in Tables 1 and 2.

Long bones have a tubular structure in the diaphyseal region, which provides considerable mechanical advantage over solid circular structures of the same mass. Tubular structures are more resistant to torsional and bending loads when compared with solid cylindrical structures. Furthermore, a tubular structure can distribute the internal forces more evenly over its cross section compared with a solid cylindrical structure of the same cross-sectional area.

Bone will fracture when the stresses generated in any region of bone are larger than the ultimate strength of bone. Fractures caused by pure tensile forces are seen in bones with a large proportion of cancellous bone tissue. Fractures caused by compressive loads are com-

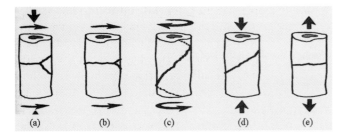

Figure 16 Lines of fracture vary depending on whether the load is a combination of compressive and bending forces **(a)**, bending force **(b)**, torsional force **(c)**, compressive force **(d)**, and tensile force **(e)**.

Table 3 | Stresses in Tendon During Various Activities

Stress (MPa)	Tendon	Activity
23	Goat patellar tendon	Walking
29	Goat patellar tendon	Trotting
59	Human Achilles tendon	Walking
110	Human Achilles tendon	Running

(Reproduced with permission from An Kn: In vivo force and strain of tendon, ligament, and capsule, in Guilak F, Butler DL, Goldstein SA, Mooney DJ (eds): Functional Tissue Engineering. New York, NY, Springer, 2003.)

monly encountered in the vertebrae of elderly patients, whose bones are weakened as a result of aging. Clinically, most bone fractures occur as a result of complex combined loading situations rather than simple loading mechanisms. Figure 16 shows the differing lines along which fractures in bone occur depending on the type of load encountered.

Biomechanics of Tendons and Ligaments

Tendons and ligaments are fibrous connective tissues. Tendons help execute joint motion by transmitting tension from muscles to bones. Ligaments join bones and provide stability to the joints. Unlike muscles, which are active tissues and can produce mechanical forces, tendons and ligaments are passive tissues and cannot actively contract to generate forces. Tendons and ligaments do not rupture easily. Damage to tendons and ligaments usually occurs at their junctions with bones.

Compared with skeletal muscles, tendons are stiffer, have higher tensile strengths, and can endure larger stresses. The relatively low ultimate strength of muscles would require that they have relatively large cross-sectional areas to transmit sufficiently high forces to bones without tearing. Tendons are better designed to perform this function. Therefore, around the joints where the space is limited, muscle attachments to bones are made by tendons. Tendons are capable of supporting very large loads with very small deformations.

Tendons are believed to function in the body at strains of up to about 0.04, which is believed to be their yield strain. Tendons rupture at strains of about 0.1 (ultimate strain), or stresses of about 60 MPa (ultimate stress). The magnitude of tendon tension has been estimated by various analytical methods, and also by combined experimental and analytical methods. Direct measurements also have been attempted. The most commonly studied tendons include the patellar tendon of the knee, the flexor tendons of the finger (the flexor digitorum superficialis and flexor digitorum profundus), and the Achilles tendon. Tendon stresses and forces reported in the literature are listed in Table 3 and Table 4 respectively.

Compared with tendons, ligaments often contain a greater proportion of elastic fibers that account for their high extensibility but lower strength and stiffness. Like tendons, they are viscoelastic and exhibit hysteresis, but deform elastically up to strains of about 0.25 (yield strain), which is about five times as much as the yield strain of tendons.

Biomechanics of Articular Cartilage

Cartilage covers the articulating surfaces of bones within the diarthrodial (synovial) joints. The primary function of cartilage is to facilitate the relative movement of articulating bones. Cartilage reduces stresses

Table 4 | Tendon Forces During Various Activities

Tension (N)	Tendon	Activity
207	Goat patellar tendon	Standing
801	Goat patellar tendon	Walking
999	Goat patellar tendon	Trotting
13	Rabbit flexor digitorum profundus	Standing
50	Rabbit flexor digitorum profundus	Level hopping
82	Rabbit flexor digitorum profundus	Inclinal hopping
2,600	Human Achilles tendon	Walking
9,000	Human Achilles tendon	Running
4,000	Human Achilles tendon	Running
480-661	Human Achilles tendon	Cycling
1,895-2,233	Human Achilles tendon	Squat jump
3,786	Human Achilles tendon	Hopping
1-9	Human flexor digitorum profundus	Passive motion
35	Human flexor digitorum profundus	Active motion
120	Human flexor digitorum profundus	Pinch
8-16	Human flexor digitorum superficialis	Keystroke

(Reproduced with permission from An Kn: In vivo force and strain of tendon, ligament, and capsule, in Guilak F, Butler DL, Goldstein SA, Mooney DJ (eds): Functional Tissue Engineering. New York, NY, Springer, 2003.)

applied to bones by increasing the area of contact between the articulating surfaces and reduces bone wear by reducing the effects of friction. From an engineering perspective, the mechanical behavior of cartilage is considered to be remarkable.

During daily activities, the articular cartilage is subjected to tension and shear stresses as well as compressive stresses. Under tension, cartilage responds by realigning the collagen fibers that carry the tensile load applied to the tissue. The higher the collagen content, the higher the tensile strength of cartilage. Shear stresses on the articular cartilage are caused by frictional forces between the relative movements of articulating surfaces. The importance of cartilage to bear load and to maintain its mechanical integrity becomes clear when the magnitude of the forces involved at the human hip joint are considered. The hip bears a load of about five times the body weight during ordinary walking; the load is much higher during running and jumping.

An essential step toward a better understanding of the mechanics of articular cartilage is the development of appropriate constitutive models for this tissue that relate the state of stress to the state of strain, and fluid and solute fluxes to electrochemical gradients. These mathematical models, when validated through experiments, can provide valuable insight into the functioning of this tissue.

Joint Lubrication

The design and lubrication of human joints are major factors in the capacity for swift and prolonged mobility. The loads on many joints are as great as two to four times body weight during ordinary activities. These loads increase to even higher multiples in other activities. One of the most critical biomechanical characteristics of human joints, which allows them to function for 70 to 80 years, is their system of lubrication. Several attempts have been made to explain the underlying mechanisms.

Basic Concepts and Definitions

When a joint in the body is subjected to external forces, in the form of external loads and muscle forces, the internal reaction forces acting at the contact surfaces are called the joint reaction forces. For example, the contact surface of the metacarpal portion of a metacarpophalangeal joint has two components of joint reaction forces acting on it. One is perpendicular to the contact surface and is called the normal joint reaction force. The other force is parallel to the surface and is called the tangential joint reaction force or the frictional force. The normal component is always compressive and is generally large. The tangential component is generally small. The ratio of the two components (tangential to normal) is called the coefficient of friction.

For example, a skater can glide effortlessly on ice because the ratio of effort (the tangential or frictional force) to body weight (the normal compressive force) is very small. This interbody action has a rather low coefficient of friction. Typical values range from 0.01 (such as a bearing with lubrication) to 0.75 (such as a stone on the ground).

Another important joint parameter is the contact area, which is the area of contact between the two joint surfaces. In general, the greater the contact area the smaller the contact stress or the stress at the contacting surface. An injury, joint misalignment, or disease process may lead to a decrease in the contact area and, therefore, to an increase in contact stresses and wear of the joint surfaces. The contact area depends on the congruency of the mating surfaces, physical properties of cartilage and supporting bone, and the forces that press the two surfaces together. The contact area also increases when either the contacting surfaces decrease in stiffness or the joint forces increase. In the hip joint, the diameter of the femoral head is slightly larger than that of the acetabulum resulting in contact that begins around the periphery. As the load is increased, the contact area of the femoral head extends toward the center. With such a design, the contact area increases with increasing load, thus keeping the contact stresses relatively constant. This factor is especially important when the load reaches its maximum value. At that time, the load is spread all the way to the periphery, thus reducing the peak stress in the central regions of the head.

In a lubricant, viscosity is essential for providing lubrication between two loaded joint surfaces and is defined as the property of a material to resist shear load. The lubricant is sheared by the sliding action of one surface against the other. Experiments showed that the friction in an animal joint increased dramatically when the synovial fluid was replaced by water, which is relatively less viscous. The coefficient of viscosity is a measure of the viscosity of a fluid. A more viscous fluid has a higher coefficient of viscosity. Water, for example, has a low coefficient of viscosity and motor oil has a high coefficient of viscosity. The coefficient of viscosity may be constant or it may vary with the speed of shearing. Fluids that have constant viscosity coefficients are called newtonian fluids and include water and glycerin. Fluids that decrease in viscosity at higher shearing rates are called thixotropic and include synovial fluid.

Hydrodynamic Lubrication

Hydrodynamic lubrication is a mechanism that decreases the friction between two sliding surfaces by maintaining a fluid film caused by the sliding motion between the surfaces. Consider a circular metal shaft placed in a slightly larger hole in a metal block or bearing. As shown in Figure 17, *A*, when the shaft is stationary and carries an ex-

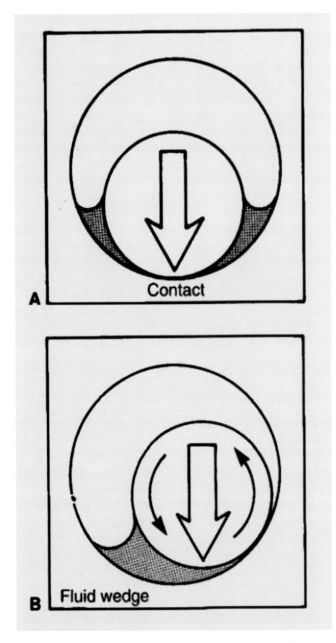

Figure 17 Hydrodynamic lubrication. *(Reproduced with permission from Panjabi MM, White AA III: Joint friction, wear, and lubrication, in Biomechanics of the Musculoskeletal System. New York, NY, Churchill Livingstone, 2001.)*

Elastohydrodynamic Lubrication

Elastohydrodynamic lubrication is a mechanism that decreases friction between two sliding surfaces by maintaining a fluid film between the surfaces caused by both the sliding motion and the elastic deformation of the surfaces.

In some machine parts, the loads are too high and the geometry of the bearing surfaces is not ideal for producing a dynamic wedge of fluid film. An example of this situation is the gear teeth in an automotive gear box in which both the surfaces are convex, making it difficult to produce a wedge film. However, the measured friction in the gear teeth is low, which can be explained by the effects of elastohydrodynamic lubrication. The basic idea is that the high loads carried by the two convex surfaces deform the surfaces significantly on a microscopic scale to produce a geometry of the mating surfaces that is suitable for the development of a fluid film. Human cartilage can deform elastically under load and thus provides the potential for elastohydrodynamic lubrication.

Weeping Lubrication

Weeping lubrication is a mechanism by which the joint load is borne by the hydrostatic pressure created by the water phase of the synovial fluid escaping from the cartilage. Because cartilage is permeable, the water phase of the synovial fluid can move in and out of it. Under the application of load, the water phase of the synovial fluid is released from cartilage. As the fluid is pushed into the joint cavity, it separates the two cartilage surfaces because of its hydrostatic pressure and, thus, decreases the friction. The reverse happens when the joint is unloaded and the water phase of the synovial fluid is sucked into the cartilage, thus completing the cycle. This squeeze-out/suck-in occurrence provides a self pressurizing and load-bearing mechanism that is not dependent on the speed of sliding. This theory is based on some experimental studies of animal joint lubrication.

Squeeze Film Lubrication

Squeeze film lubrication is a mechanism by which the joint load is carried by the fluid pressure developed between the two surfaces as a result of the relative movement of the approaching surfaces. As the two surfaces approach each other, the fluid trapped between the cavities of the cartilage is squeezed out, thus creating a cushion and providing a load-bearing capacity for the joint. When the surfaces touch, there is no longer a squeeze film. Thus, this mechanism cannot explain the joint lubrication under normal physiologic conditions. However, in situations where a joint is suddenly loaded, such as landing on the ground after a jump, the squeeze film mechanism may be responsible for reducing shock and injury to the cartilage.

ternal load, the lubricant is squeezed out and there is direct contact between the shaft and its bearing. However, when the shaft starts rotating, the fluid is brought in between the shaft and the bearing, creating a fluid wedge (Figure 17, *B*). This action has the effect of lifting the shaft above the bearing and thus decreasing friction and wear. Although this lubrication mechanism explains the low friction found in high speed and highly loaded machinery (for example, the bearings of the automotive crankshaft), it does not explain the lubrication of a body joint, which has a sliding velocity that is too slow to generate any significant wedge of fluid film.

Simultaneous Fluid Exudation and Imbibition

Although the weeping and squeeze film theories provide explanations of some aspects of animal and human joint lubrication, they do not give a detailed description of the actual interaction between the cartilage and synovial fluid during joint motion under load. Backed by mathematical description and experimental evidence, some recent work has attempted to describe the actual fluid flow in the cartilage, an essential step toward understanding joint lubrication.

Consider a sheet of sponge soaked with water. When a finger is pressed into the sponge, water exudes out from the region around the finger (Figure 18, *A*). Accompanying this wet region, surrounding the finger, is a drier region under the finger. Pressing the finger into the sponge simply displaces the water from under the finger to its surroundings. By lifting the finger, the water is reabsorbed by the sponge, thus restoring the original condition. If motion is added to the above experiment (Figure 18, *B*), it is found that the wet region that is ahead of the finger motion is wetter, and the wet region that is behind the finger is now drier. The motion of the finger produces a flow of the fluid from behind to in front of the finger. The reverse will occur if the direction of motion is reversed. Researchers have provided a mathematical model for this process. A diagrammatic representation of the concept as it applies to the cartilage is shown in Figure 18, *C*. As one cartilage-covered bone moves over another, the water phase of the synovial fluid is squeezed out (exudation) and pushed ahead of the moving contact area. At the same time, the water phase of the synovial fluid is sucked in (imbibition) behind the contact area. Because the permeability of the cartilage is significantly reduced under load in the contact area, there is enhancement of the fluid film to carry the load.

The interpretation of experimental results requires the proper formulation of a lubrication theory for cartilage. Any such formulation must be able to predict a variety of experimental outcomes using physically and mathematically consistent equations. The formulation of such a theory is a great challenge in the field of biotribology; research is still needed to fully understand the physiologic lubrication processes in vivo.

New Approaches and Future Perspectives

Over the past few years, substantial progress has occurred not only in measurement techniques of biomechanical parameters, but also in the techniques used to aid healing of injured tissue.

Imaging Techniques

To better document the load environment in various components of the musculoskeletal system, more direct in vivo measurements are essential. Newer techniques

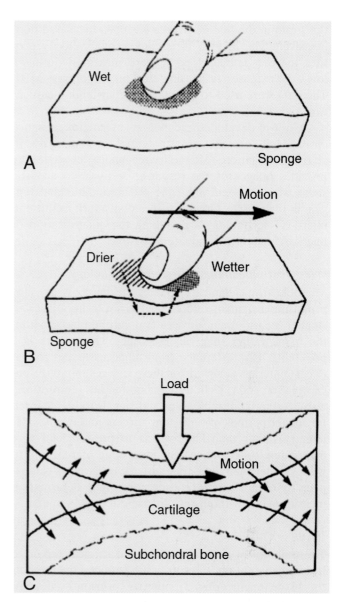

Figure 18 Diagrammatic representation of a new concept to describe fluid flow in cartilage. *(Reproduced with permission from Panjabi MM, White AA III: Joint friction, wear, and lubrication, in Biomechanics of the Musculoskeletal System. New York, NY, Churchill Livingstone, 2001.)*

should enable in vivo signals to be measured less invasively than with conventional strain gauges and transducers. Noninvasive techniques based on image analysis are useful tools for such measurements.

A technique for quantifying two-dimensional strain using MRI has been developed. Images are collected on a 1.5 Tesla scanner using a two-dimensional spin-echo technique, which uses a pattern-matching algorithm to quantify tissue deformation from the "unstrained" and "strained" images. No markers are placed on or within the tissue as had been done using traditional methods. Instead, this approach uses patterns naturally inherent to the tissue, treating small rectangular regions of the image as discrete, unique markers. Using this technique, the strain in the human patella has been measured noninvasively. The in vivo three-dimensional velocity profiles for the patellar tendon were measured during a low-load extensor task using cine phase contrast MRI. The data were used to calculate patellar tendon elongation and strain.

A newly developed technology, magnetic resonance elastography, provides great potential for noninvasive in vivo investigation. Magnetic resonance elastography provides images of the response of tissue to acoustic shear waves to determine the shear modulus and tension in the muscle. Other advancements, such as those in micro-CT technology are making the quantification of microarchitectural parameters possible.

Microelectromechanical Systems Technology

Microelectromechanical systems technology is also promising. Scientists and engineers are trying to design smaller measurement devices that can be placed within the tissue rather than on its surface where there is a possibility of interference from adjacent tissues. Transducer materials selected for these devices minimize encapsulation and rejection by the body. These transducers also need to be durable to permit signals to be recorded for longer periods of time after surgery and may use telemetry rather than hard wiring to prevent lead wire and connector damage. By measuring signals up to weeks rather than days after surgery, researchers can expect to obtain more realistic force and deformation measurements without the adverse effects of surgery.

Tissue Engineering

The inability of natural healing and surgical repair to truly regenerate normal soft tissue has been the impetus for tissue engineering. Combining principles of engineering and biology, tissue engineering endeavors to fabricate new tissues in the laboratory that are designed to rapidly restore tissue form (three-dimensional architecture and composition of normal tissue) and function (normal structural and material properties). The tissue engineering process typically involves introducing living cells and a "carrier" into a wound site or mixing these cells and a carrier with a natural or man-made scaffold material. Collagen gels often serve as carriers for these cells; in the past, scaffolds have included carbon fibers, collagen fibers, polylactic acid, polyglycolic acid, and Dacron sutures. Biologic scaffolding materials, such as small intestine mucosa obtained from porcine small intestines, are gaining wide acceptance. When these constituents are combined, cellular recruitment and tissue ingrowth are encouraged in the implants. The stiffer scaffold material protects the cells and newly forming repair tissue from high forces during the early phases of repair. To avoid stress shielding, however, the scaffold should degrade at the same rate as the rate of increase in the capability of the newly formed tissue to bear significant load. The degrading scaffold should pose no threat of rejection.

Functional Tissue Engineering

Functional tissue engineering extends the goals of tissue engineering by taking into consideration the actual functional demands placed on the implants that are intended to repair the damaged tissue. Tissue engineers then incorporate these requirements into meaningful parameters that are designed into the constructs before surgery. Presuming that tissue-engineered implants alone will not possess sufficient strength and stiffness, biomaterials experts and tissue engineers should work together to formulate scaffolds with the correct mechanical integrity, degradation characteristics, and biocompatibility to facilitate an aligned extracellular matrix of the correct composition. Novel biologic and bioengineering techniques, including application of growth factors, gene transfer, and cell therapy offer the potential to improve the quality of healing tissues.

Growth factors are small proteins that are known to induce a variety of cellular responses, including cell proliferation and matrix synthesis. The induction of these biologic effects is mediated by binding of growth factors to their specific receptors on cell surfaces. In vivo studies have shown that treatment of platelet-derived growth factor-BB affects the biomechanical properties of the rabbit femur-medial collateral ligament complex. Specifically, this growth factor increased the ultimate load, energy absorbed to failure, and ultimate elongation of the rabbit femur-medial collateral ligament complex.

Recent advances in genetic engineering are providing excellent advantages for recreating and investigating various human skeletal disease states in transgenic (organisms whose genome has been altered by the transfer of a gene or genes from another species or breed) mice animal models. Various studies have shown the profound effect of several noncollagenous proteins through the alteration of the normal mineralization process or collagen fibrillogenesis. Transgenic mouse models also make it possible to investigate the effect of genetic disease, such as osteogenesis imperfecta, on the mechanical function of bone. Using gene transfer technology, it is possible to increase cellular production of specific proteins (such as growth factors) that are functionally important for tissue healing. Two approaches, ex vivo and in vivo, are often used for gene transfer. With the ex vivo approach, genes are placed into cells in culture and the cells are later transferred back to the host tissues of interest. With an in vivo approach, genes are transferred to cells in host tissues by direct injection of a carrier into the host tissues.

It has been established that mesenchymal progenitor cells (MPCs) from both humans and animals can differentiate into a variety of cell types, including fibroblasts, osteoblasts, and endothelial cells. These cells are responsible for tissue wound healing. Bone marrow, blood, muscle, or adipose tissue are potential sources of MPCs for cell therapy. For cell therapy, MPCs are isolated from the bone marrow, cultured, and finally transplanted into host tissues. MPCs appear to retain their developmental potential even after extensive subculturing. Implantation of MPCs into an injured tendon significantly improves its mechanical properties.

The basis for future treatments eventually may use a combination of approaches to treat injuries that include seeding cells on a scaffold that is conditioned with the right combination of mechanical stimuli, growth factors, and gene therapy. Because these experiments will require a combination of techniques that simultaneously address the structure, biochemistry, and biology of a tissue to enhance healing, a significant effort must be made to encourage collaboration among investigators from different disciplines. By combining appropriate engineering mechanics with other basic sciences, improved outcomes can be achieved.

Annotated Bibliography

An KN: In vivo force and strain of tendon, ligament and capsule, in Guilak F, Butler DL, Goldstein SA, Mooney DJ (eds): *Functional Tissue Engineering*. New York, NY, Springer, 2003, pp 96-105.

In vivo force and strain measurements in soft tissue were presented in six groups: tendon tension, ligament deformation, capsular pressure, tendon surface friction, soft-tissue stress, and soft-tissue strain.

Ateshian GA, Hung CT: Functional properties of native articular cartilage, in Guilak F, Butler DL, Goldstein SA, Mooney DJ (eds): *Functional Tissue Engineering*. New York, NY, Springer, 2003, pp 46-68.

Important mechanical properties of the cartilage including viscoelasticity, anisotropy, tension-compression nonlinearity, and inhomogeneity were assessed. Valuable measures of the functionality of the tissue-engineered constructs were included.

Butler DL, Dressler M, Awad H: Functional tissue engineering: Assessment of function in tendon and ligament, in Guilak F, Butler DL, Goldstein SA, Mooney DJ (eds): *Functional Tissue Engineering*. New York, NY, Springer, 2003, pp 213-226.

This chapter discusses the issues that confront researchers in fabricating structures from cells. State-of-the-art applications of biologic-microelectromechanical systems, imaging, and other technologies are described.

Efunda: Engineering Fundamental Website. Available at: http://www.efunda.com. Accessed June, 2004.

This website provides information that is helpful in the understanding of biomechanics. Information includes formulas for beam deflection, bending, and twisting and on stress and strain parameters for materials.

Keaveny TM, Yeh OC: Architecture and trabecular bone: Toward an improved understanding of the biomechanical effects of age, sex and osteoporosis. *J Musculoskeletal Neuronal Interactions* 2002;2:205-208.

This study reviews what is known about architectural changes in trabecular bone associated with age, gender, and osteoporosis and the role of these changes in the mechanical properties of tissue. Recent developments in three-dimensional high-resolution imaging technologies have provided more accurate measures of quantitative metrics of architecture, thereby providing new data and raising questions about earlier conclusions.

NSBRI: National Space Biomedical Research Institute Website. Available at: http://www.nsbri.org. Accessed June, 2004.

This website provides a description of areas of research such as bone loss, muscle atrophy, and other current research projects.

Panjabi MM, White AA III: *Biomechanics of the Musculoskeletal System*. New York, NY, Churchill Livingstone, 2001.

This book describes the principles of biomechanics in a simple manner and is suitable for orthopaedic residents and fellows.

Puska MA, Kokkari AK, Närhi TO, Vallittu PK: Mechanical properties of oligomer-modified acrylic bone cement. *Biomaterials* 2003;24:417-425.

Mechanical properties of oligomer-modified acrylic bone cement with glass fibers were studied. The three-point bending test was used to measure the flexural strength and modulus of the acrylic bone cement composites using analysis of variance between groups. A scanning electron microscope was used to examine the surface structure of the acrylic bone cement composites.

Woo SL, Abramowitch SD, Loh JC, Musahl V, Wang JH: Ligament healing: Present status and the future of functional tissue engineering, in Guilak F, Butler DL, Goldstein SA, Mooney DJ (eds): *Functional Tissue Engineering*. New York, NY, Springer, 2003, pp 17-34.

Properties of normal ligaments, including their anatomic, biologic, biochemical, and mechanical properties, and changes that occur after injury, were described. Functional tissue engineering methods and preliminary findings were presented.

Classic Bibliography

Burstein AH, Reilly DT, Martens M: Aging of bone tissue: Mechanical properties. *J Bone Joint Surg Am* 1976; 58:82-86.

Ding M, Dalstra M: Danielsen CC, Kabel J, Hvid J, Linde F: Age variations in the properties of human tibial trabecular bone. *J Bone Joint Surg Br* 1997;79:995-1002.

Hall SJ: *Basic Biomechanics,* ed 3. New York, NY, McGrawHill, 1999.

Martin BR, Burr DC, Sharkey NA: *Skeletal Tissue Mechanics*. New York, NY, Springer, 1998.

Mow VC, Ateshian GA: Lubrication and wear of diarthrodial joints, in Mow VC, Hayes WC (eds): *Basic Orthopaedic Biomechanics,* ed 2. New York, NY, Raven Press, 1997, pp 275-316.

Ozkaya N, Nordin M: *Fundamentals of Biomechanics,* ed 2. New York, NY, Springer-Verlag, 1998.

Chapter 5

Biomaterials and Bearing Surfaces in Total Joint Arthroplasty

Timothy M. Wright, PhD

Introduction

Synthetic materials play a prominent role in orthopaedic surgery because of the continuing need to replace, stabilize, or augment damaged musculoskeletal tissues. Materials used for orthopaedic devices must be safe and effective; therefore they must be biocompatible, resistant to corrosion and degradation, possess superior mechanical and wear properties, and meet high quality standards—all at a reasonable cost. The interplay between synthetic materials and the surrounding environment is an important factor to consider when using such materials to temporarily stabilize a fracture or to permanently replace a structure such as the hip joint.

Implant wear is the major complication that limits the longevity of total joint arthroplasties. Substantial clinical evidence exists that links the release of large amounts of submicron particulate debris from articular and modular interfaces in implant components to subsequent osteolysis and implant loosening. Bioengineering solutions to the wear problem are based on two approaches: (1) replacing the conventional metal-on-ultrahigh molecular weight polyethylene (UHMWPE) articulation with alternative combinations of bearing materials with improved wear resistance, and (2) using improved designs aimed at lowering contact stresses and sliding distances between moving parts. Only long-term clinical experience will ultimately establish the efficacy of these approaches; however, laboratory results and short-term clinical experience suggest that such approaches are beneficial in reducing implant wear.

Appreciation of the basic science behind these and other uses of biomaterials in orthopaedic surgery requires knowledge of the basic structure and composition of these materials and an understanding of how a material's structure and composition determine its ability to meet necessary performance criteria essential to its clinical efficacy. For many applications of biomaterials in orthopaedics, the failure criteria for the material can be measured and directly compared with the expected mechanical burden the material will be subjected to for use in vivo. For many other applications, however, the situation is not as straightforward.

The goal of improving implant wear resistance is a difficult task. The introduction of new forms of existing materials or alternative bearing materials is hampered by the lack of strong scientifically based relationships between specific material properties (measured using standardized laboratory tests) and in vivo wear behavior. Knowledge has been gained by analyzing the stresses that occur in bearing materials under realistic geometries and loading conditions; however, the link between specific wear mechanisms and the controlling material properties remains circumstantial. Thus, material selection cannot be made on the simple basis of specifications such as elastic modulus, fracture toughness, or yield stress. Similarly, standard laboratory experiments on simple geometries, such as pin-on-disk tests, do not adequately recreate the mechanical stresses that the material will experience in vivo.

Because of these limitations, screening tests using hip and knee joint simulators have become the accepted approach for providing preclinical test data on wear performance. Wear is measured gravimetrically on the basis of periodic measurements of the small amount of weight that is lost as material is worn from the articular surface during the simulator test. Joint simulators are validated in the sense that, under certain kinematics and loading conditions, they produce worn polyethylene surfaces and generate wear particle sizes and shapes similar to those observed on retrieved implants. Hip simulators also produce wear rates over the course of the test that generally agree with clinical wear rates determined from component thickness changes observed on serial radiographs (assuming one million cycles of test equals 1 year of clinical use).

The reliance on joint simulator tests is especially important because the clinical ramifications of improved wear are not known until many years after the introduction of a new material. If a bearing material is intended to produce a meaningful reduction in wear, its effectiveness can only be shown through long-term studies; however, this requirement makes it difficult for both indus-

Table 1 | Benefits and Disadvantages of Bearing Material Combinations

Bearing Combination	Benefits	Disadvantages
Metal-on-polyethylene	Long-term clinical results Design effects well known Long-term clinical results Low wear Excellent resistance to degradation	Osteolysis May be unsuitable for young patients Limited shelf life before implantation Wear rates not as low as elevated cross-linked polyethylene
Ethylene oxide or gas plasma sterilized polyethylene-on-metal or ceramic	Excellent resistance to degradation	Wear rates not as low as elevated cross-linked polyethylene
Polyethylene sterilized in low oxygen/inert environment	Excellent resistance to degradation Low wear	Wear rates not as low as elevated cross-linked polyethylene Possible residual free radicals
Elevated cross-linked polyethylene-on-metal or ceramic	Excellent wear resistance Excellent resistance to degradation	Short-term clinical use Reduced toughness could be problematic High cost
Metal-on-metal	Usually low wear Possible lubrication film	Sometimes high wear Local and systemic accumulation of metallic debris and ions
Ceramic-on-polyethylene	Low wear Good resistance to third body wear	Component fracture/difficult revision High cost
Alumina-on-alumina	Usually low wear Excellent biocompatibility Possible lubrication film	Sometimes high wear Component fracture High cost

(Adapted from McKellop HA: Bearing surfaces in total hip replacements: State of the art and future developments. Instr Course Lect *2001;50:174.)*

try and the Food and Drug Administration (FDA) to bring improved technologies to the marketplace safely and expeditiously. Current evaluation of the performance of new bearing materials must be centered on their intended benefits and disadvantages (Table 1) and the results of laboratory and short-term clinical tests.

Metallic Materials

Stainless steels, cobalt alloys, and titanium alloys have been used in orthopaedic devices for decades. They are generally corrosion resistant and biocompatible and possess mechanical properties sufficient for use as structural load-bearing implants. These materials are fabricated using a wide variety of techniques (including casting, forging, extrusion, and hot isostatic pressing) which lend flexibility in terms of both mechanical properties and shape.

Stainless steels are predominantly iron-carbon alloys. Carbon is added to allow the formation of metallic carbides within the microstructure. Carbides are much harder than the surrounding material, and a uniform distribution of carbides provides strength. Additions of other alloying elements, such as molybdenum, stabilize the carbides. Chromium provides the stainless quality to stainless steel. It forms a strongly adherent surface ox-

ide, which serves as a protective passive layer between the corrosive body environment and the bulk steel.

Cobalt alloys are composed primarily of cobalt, chromium, and molybdenum. Chromium is added for increased hardness and corrosion resistance. As is the case with stainless steel, the chromium forms a strongly adherent passive oxide film. Molybdenum is added to provide high strength. Standard cobalt alloy contains significant amounts of carbon that allows for the formation of hard carbides, which strengthen the alloy and improve its wear resistance. The addition of nickel forms an alloy suitable for forging, which further enhances the material's strength.

The most commonly used titanium alloy for orthopaedic applications is titanium-aluminum-vanadium alloy, often referred to as Ti-6Al-4V because the primary alloying elements, aluminum and vanadium, comprise about 6% and 4%, respectively, of the alloy. Titanium has the ability to self passivate, forming its own oxide that imparts a high degree of corrosion resistance. Oxygen concentration is kept very low to maximize strength and ductility. Despite long-term clinical evidence of excellent biocompatibility, concern that the release of vanadium (a cytotoxic element) could cause local and systemic complications has led to the introduction of other titanium alloys in which vanadium is replaced by more inert elements such as niobium.

Stainless steel is the material that is most susceptible to both galvanic and crevice corrosion. The area between the screw heads and countersunk holes in stainless steel bone plates is a common location for crevice corrosion. Continual removal of the passive layer can be caused by fretting and can lead to the corrosion of all three metallic alloys. Modular metallic devices, including femoral components for total hip replacement and stemmed components for revision knee replacement, provide both the micromotion that causes fretting and the enclosed environment needed for crevice corrosion. Damage caused by corrosion and fretting often is found on retrieved modular components, and is associated with local and systemic accumulations of alloy elements such as titanium and chromium.

Corrosion and strength concerns have largely relegated the use of stainless steel components to temporary implant devices, such as fracture plates, screws, and hip nails; however, with appropriate designs, stainless steel is still used in permanent implants such as Charnley style femoral components for hip replacement. Cobalt alloys, because of their high strength and their ability to be polished to a very smooth surface finish, are the most common materials used for metallic total joint arthroplasty components.

Titanium alloys possess roughly one half of the elastic modulus of stainless steel or cobalt alloy materials; therefore, for the same component design, a titanium version will have one half the structural stiffness (whether subjected to axial, bending, or torsion loads). This property makes titanium alloys attractive in situations in which more load is to be shared with the surrounding bone. The low modulus and excellent strength of these alloys make them useful in a host of devices for trauma, spinal fixation, and arthroplasty. The latter application, however, no longer extends to articular surfaces because significant scratching and wear of titanium alloy femoral heads has been observed, particularly in the presence of third body wear.

Metal-on-Metal Bearings

The problems of wear and osteolysis in total joint arthroplasties have led to a resurgence of interest in metal-on-metal bearing surfaces. Metal-on-metal articulations were among the first to be used in total hip arthroplasty and had clinical success in the 1960s and 1970s in designs such as the McKee-Farrar (Howmedica, Limerick, Ireland) hip replacement. Recent studies suggest that many of these early implants have performed well, even after implantation intervals approaching 30 years.

Metal-on-metal hip joint replacements fell from favor when the clinical results of polyethylene-on-metal

joints proved superior and as carcinogenic concerns over local and systemic accumulation of particulate and ionic metallic debris grew. These early failures were partly the result of poor metallurgy and less than optimum implant design. Casting of metallic alloys often resulted in microstructures with large grains and poorly distributed carbides, resulting in inhomogeneity in surface hardness. Early metal-on-metal designs often had small head to neck ratios; therefore, impingement between the neck of the femoral component and the rim of the acetabular components was a common occurrence.

More recently, improved metallurgy and manufacturing techniques have led to the reintroduction of metal-on-metal bearings for hip replacement. Cobalt-chromium alloys with well-controlled grain sizes and finely distributed carbides provide superior hardness and wear resistance compared with earlier versions of the alloy and to implants made of stainless steel and titanium alloy. Laboratory evidence from hip joint simulator studies has confirmed that these improved bearing surfaces can provide low friction and low wear articulations. Clearance and conformity between the mating surfaces are now recognized as important parameters that must be controlled as part of the design and manufacturing processes.

The strength of cobalt-chromium alloys (compared with polyethylene) and their increased toughness over ceramics provides additional benefits from the standpoint of hip implant design. For example, the wall thickness of solid metallic acetabular components can be smaller than modular polyethylene and metal or ceramic and metal implants, so larger head sizes can be incorporated, providing an advantage for patients where joint stability is a concern. Similarly, the ability to manufacture large metallic shells allows for surface replacement of the hip joint, which is a bone-conserving operation with particular indications for young, active patients with good bone stock in the femoral head and neck.

Laboratory and analytical evidence suggest that wear rates of metal-on-metal bearings can be markedly affected by head size. Unlike metal-on-polyethylene bearings, in which larger head sizes tend to increase wear because of increased sliding distances between the articulating surfaces, wear decreases significantly in metal-on-metal bearings with larger heads. Large femoral head-acetabular component combinations seem to form a protective lubricating film that separates the surfaces. Smaller head sizes (≤ 28 mm) have much less or no separation and therefore increase the propensity for adhesive and abrasive wear.

Corroborating clinical evidence of the effect of head size on wear rates in metal-on-metal hip replacements does not yet exist. With most modern versions of alternative bearings, clinical results are available only for short- to intermediate-term usage. To date, few serious wear-related problems such as osteolysis have been found. Nonetheless, serum concentrations of metallic elements including chromium, cobalt, and molybdenum are found in increased levels in patients receiving metal-on-metal hip replacements compared with control groups and patients receiving metal-on-polyethylene joint implants. The same cytokines found in abundance around failed metal-on-polyethylene joints have been identified around failed metal-on-metal joints, suggesting that the same biologic pathways for osteolysis exist in these joints. Laboratory evidence also suggests that increased adhesion can occur between metal-on-metal bearing surfaces at the startup of motion after a resting period (common in patients' daily activities); the clinical ramifications remain unknown.

Only longer and more extensive clinical experience will determine if the reduced volumetric wear with metal-on-metal bearings will lower the incidence of osteolysis and wear-related failures. Data will soon become available because metal-on-metal hip joints have received approval by the FDA for commercial distribution in the United States. Surface replacements using metal-on-metal bearings are currently in the investigational stage. An early report (2- to 6-year follow-up) showed a revision rate of 3% because of loosening and femoral neck fracture.

Metal-on-metal bearings have not been used for other joints, such as the knee. Most other joints require very different design concepts and are subject to additional wear mechanisms for which metal-on-metal surfaces have few advantages.

Ultra-High Molecular Weight Polyethylene

Clinical follow-up for polyethylene-on-metal bearings now extends beyond 25 years, which is longer than for some other bearing types. Considerable biologic and clinical evidence shows that polyethylene wear debris elicits a deleterious biologic response culminating in osteolysis. Biomaterial approaches to combat polyethylene wear that do not require the introduction of alternative bearing materials are attractive because they can capitalize on the relatively low cost of manufacturing polyethylene components, the material biocompatibility and toughness in bulk form, and an easier path to regulatory approval. In the past, polyethylene components have been sterilized by exposure to gamma radiation at a higher dose than 25 kGy in an ambient environment. It is now known that this technique causes oxidative degradation. The exposure to radiation energy causes chain scission, chain cross-linking, and the creation of free radicals in the material, resulting in a decrease in molecular weight, an increase in density, and detrimental alterations in mechanical properties that add significantly to the wear problem.

In response to these findings, several alternative sterilization techniques have been introduced with the aim of eliminating degradation. These techniques do not have the same beneficial impact on wear. Sterilization techniques that eliminate irradiation, such as exposure to gas plasma and ethylene oxide, also eliminate the potential benefit of the additional cross-linking produced by irradiation. Hip joint simulator studies have shown a higher rate of wear for components sterilized with gas plasma and ethylene oxide compared with gamma irradiation; however, the long-term clinical relevance of these differences remains unknown. Little is known about the impact of irradiation-free sterilization techniques on the pitting and delamination surface damage that occurs in total knee polyethylene components. Studies of retrieved tibial components originally sterilized in ethylene oxide have shown less evidence of cracking than conventionally sterilized components.

Other sterilization techniques that use irradiation in an inert or low-oxygen environment are more beneficial in improving wear resistance, based on improved wear rates found in hip simulator studies. The improvement in wear behavior is probably the result of the cross-linking of polyethylene chains that occurs with irradiation. However, free radical production is still a detrimental result, and postirradiation thermal treatment is performed to quench free radicals and prevent degradation that could occur with subsequent exposure to an oxygen environment.

The fabrication technique used in manufacturing polyethylene total joint components also affects wear behavior. Direct compression molding in which polyethylene powder is heated and pressed in molds to form a finished product results in polyethylene components resistant to oxidative degradation. In clinical use for more than 20 years, directly molded hip and knee replacement components have shown favorable wear resistance, based on clinical evidence, studies of wear damage in retrieved components, and laboratory wear tests compared with components machined from extruded polyethylene stock. The lower elastic modulus that results from compression molding may be a key factor. Under the same load conditions, a lower modulus polyethylene will have larger contact areas and will experience lower stresses than a higher modulus polyethylene under the same load conditions.

The most significant recent alteration in fabrication techniques for manufacturing polyethylene joint arthroplasty components is the inclusion of elevated levels of radiation to induce even higher levels of cross-linking than occur with the conventional sterilization dose (25 kGy). Advantages of elevated cross-linking include significantly reduced wear (as shown in hip and knee joint simulator test) and, in the case of knee joints, a resistance to pitting and delamination. Wear rates of essentially zero have been shown, for example, in hip simulator tests for elevated cross-linked polyethylenes (Figure 1). Few well-controlled clinical studies in the peer-reviewed literature exist to date on the in vivo wear behavior of these materials. Short-term results suggest an improvement in wear; however, a longer follow-up period is required.

The improved abrasive and adhesive wear resistance that accompanies elevated cross-linking provides other potential benefits. Backside wear in modular implants, for example, is an important complication that could be reduced with the use of elevated cross-linked instead of conventional polyethylene. Increased wear resistance also has renewed interest in the use of larger femoral heads for total hip replacement. The risk of dislocation is markedly reduced with a larger head size. However, because sliding distance between the bearing surfaces and the amount of wear is higher with a larger head, conventional polyethylene-metal bearings usually have a small diameter ($\leq$ 32 mm). Larger head sizes are now available with matching larger diameter, elevated cross-linked polyethylene acetabular components. The wall thicknesses of these components are thin (less than 5 mm in some instances), making the strength and toughness of elevated cross-linked polyethylenes an important consideration.

Changes in mechanical properties that accompany increased cross linking may pose the biggest threat to the clinical efficacy of these materials. Reduced toughness and resistance to fatigue crack propagation have been shown in several laboratory studies using standardized specimens under controlled loading conditions. These findings suggest greater susceptibility to pitting and delamination wear damage, to gross failure should a crack propagate entirely through a component, and to dissociation that could result from the failure of a locking mechanism that relied on the structural integrity of the polyethylene. The clinical relevance of standardized fracture and fatigue test results is difficult to interpret, because the fracture conditions in implant components depend on geometry and loading conditions that differ from those of standard laboratory specimens. Analytical attempts to interpret performance with consideration of

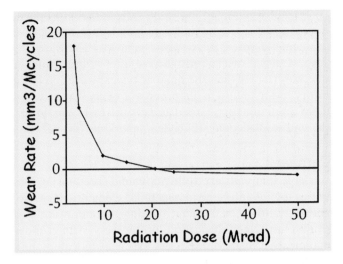

Figure 1 The wear rates of acetabular cups tested in a hip simulator decrease with exposure to higher doses of radiation applied to the components prior to testing. *(Adapted with permission from McKellop H, Shen FW, Lu B, Campbell P, Salovey R: Development of an extremely wear-resistant ultra high molecular weight polyethylene for total hip replacements. J Orthop Res 1999;17:157-67.)*

lowered toughness and crack propagation resistance are hampered by the lack of good nonlinear material models for polyethylene's stress-strain behavior. Close monitoring of data from the clinical experience will be needed to establish the extent of this problem.

Wear tests of knee-like geometries (with nonconforming bearing surfaces) and knee joint simulator studies show that elevated cross-linked materials perform well in comparison with conventional polyethylene. Given their decreased fracture resistance, the hypothesis would be the opposite—wear rates and pitting and delamination damage should be worse for elevated cross-linked materials. Lowering of the elastic modulus that accompanies the post cross-linking thermal treatment used to quench free radicals may explain these positive findings. As in the case of compression-molded polyethylene, the lower modulus creates larger contact areas, lower stresses, and better resistance to wear damage (Figure 2).

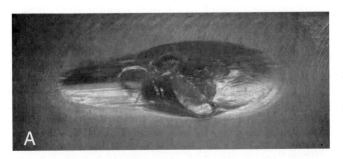
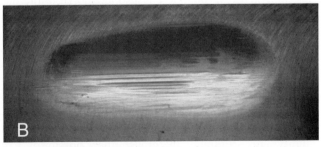

Figure 2 Wear tracks from a conventional polyethylene (1050 resin irradiated at 25 kGy) **(A)** and an elevated cross-linked polyethylene (1050 resin irradiated at 65 kGy) **(B)**, which were tested on a knee-like wear apparatus for 2 million cycles under identical conditions show more severe damage in the conventional material. The elastic moduli were 1.0 GPa for the conventional and 800 MPa for the elevated cross-linked material. *(Reproduced with permission from Furman BD, Maher SA, Morgan T, Wright TM: Elevated crosslinking alone does not explain polyethylene wear resistance, in Kurtz SM, Gsell R, Martell J (eds): Crosslinked and Thermally Treated Ultra-High Molecular Weight Polyethylene for Joint Arthroplasties ASTM STP 1445. West Conshohocken, PA, ASTM International, pp 248-261.)*

Recent findings of increased fatigue crack propagation in elevated cross-linked polyethylenes may prove problematic for in vivo wear behavior. These results suggest that if cracks form in vivo after a large number of cycles (larger than the number typically used in laboratory tests), failure might progress rapidly. Thus, even if crack initiation is retarded because stresses are lower, the end results could still be less favorable.

Ceramics

Ceramic materials are solid, inorganic compounds consisting of metallic and nonmetallic elements. Held together by ionic or covalent bonding, ceramics are stiff (high elastic modulus), hard, brittle, very strong under compressive loads, and possess excellent biocompatibility and exceptional wear resistance. Ceramic materials usually have polygranular microstructures similar to metallic alloys. Their properties depend on factors such as grain size and porosity (for example, strength is inversely proportional to both grain size and porosity).

Fully dense ceramics, such as alumina and zirconia, are used in total joint arthroplasty components specifically because they provide more wear-resistant bearing surfaces; they have few other mechanical advantages for joint arthroplasty. Ceramic-on-polyethylene bearings have been commercially available for some time as alternatives to conventional metal-on-polyethylene. Ceramic-ceramic bearings have only recently received regulatory approval for commercial distribution in the United States. Because of their hardness and strength, ceramics can be polished to a very smooth finish and resist roughening while in use as a bearing surface. They possess good wettability, suggesting that lubricating layers may form between ceramic couplings, thus reducing adhesive forms of wear.

The most significant disadvantage of ceramics is low toughness, which resulted in a significant number of ceramic head fractures during early clinical use in total hip replacement. More recently, however, improvements in ceramic quality, most notably increased chemical purity and reduced grain size, has led to a dramatic reduction in head fractures. Toughness is also a concern in the use of ceramic-on-ceramic acetabular components for hip replacements. Retrieval studies of polyethylene acetabular components suggest that impingement between the neck of the femoral component and the rim of the acetabular component is a common occurrence. With the use of ceramic components, impingement could cause significant damage and eventual fracture. Recent laboratory tests suggest, however, that with the improved quality of ceramic materials the possibility of impingement-related failure is quite low.

Three types of ceramic bearing materials are commercially available. Bulk implant materials made from alumina and zirconia have been used for decades, mainly for femoral heads in total hip arthroplasties. Long-term clinical experience with these materials has been published. More recently, an oxidized zirconium material has been introduced into both hip and knee replacement components for articulation against polyethylene; however, few results are available and clinical experience with this material is short term.

Long-term experience with alumina-on-polyethylene bearings for hip replacement shows reduced wear rates compared with metal-on-polyethylene bearings and an associated decrease in the presence of osteolysis, suggesting that these types of bearings are beneficial in improving clinical performance. Alumina-on-polyethylene bearings for knee replacements have a much more limited use. Mid-term results are excellent; however, the absence of direct comparisons with conventional metal-on-polyethylene bearing surfaces of the same design and the lack of long-term results make it difficult to assess the clinical benefits.

The use of zirconia as a bearing surface against polyethylene has not been proven as clinically successful as alumina-on-polyethylene bearings. High wear rates, which resulted in catastrophic failure as early as 5 years after implantation, have been reported; however, these failures may have resulted from the use of an enhanced form of polyethylene (Hylamer, DePuy-Dupont, Newark, DE) in the acetabular component, that has been prone to rapid wear. More convincing data exist from a direct comparison between alumina-, zirconia-, and metal-on-conventional polyethylene bearings in patients with total hip arthroplasties. Data show the highest wear rate in the zirconia group, which is consistent with an increased monoclinic content on the surface of retrieved zirconia heads from the same series. The propensity for zirconia to transform from a tetragonal crystalline form, which is stable at elevated temperatures, to the less tough monoclinic form is a disadvantage of this material and has led to FDA warnings against autoclave resterilization of zirconia heads. The decrease in toughness makes the material more susceptible to roughening and increased wear. Manufacturing problems led to a high incidence of fracture and prompted a recent voluntary recall of nine batches of zirconia femoral heads, which further undermined confidence in this material.

Ceramic-on-ceramic bearings have been used extensively in total hip arthroplasty in Europe, though hip implants using this bearing combination have only recently received regulatory approval in the United States. Alumina-on-alumina joints have shown very low clinical wear rates; however, the results are design dependent (these bearings can show excessive wear if incorporated into an inferior design). Recent reports also show excellent wear resistance of alumina-on-alumina joints in young patients with no measurable wear and no evidence of osteolysis even at more than 10-year follow-up. Furthermore, head fractures have not been observed in this high-demand patient population, which supports the supposition that alumina-ceramic materials have improved mechanical properties. Zirconia-on-zirconia bearings have not performed well based on laboratory findings of high wear.

The use of ceramic bearings in other joint arthroplasties is more limited in scope. For implant designs dominated by the potential for abrasive and adhesive wear (bearing surfaces that remain conforming throughout the useful ranges of motion of the implant), ceramic bearing surfaces may have all of the potential benefits of ceramic hip replacement components. For joint designs such as conventional knee replacements that require nonconforming articulations to adequately function, the advantages of ceramic materials are less clear. Although knee joint simulator data show substantial decreases in wear rate (for example, an oxidized zirconia surface bearing against polyethylene), the clinical benefit of this decreased wear rate remains uncertain. Osteolysis has not been as significant a complication in knee replacement as in hip replacement surgery; long-term clinical data will be required to substantiate a clear advantage. Fatigue-related pitting and delamination is the main wear problem after knee replacement. This type of wear is caused by the large cyclic stresses generated at and near the polyethylene surface of the tibial component as the more rigid femoral component moves across it. Ceramic materials provide no advantage in such a situation.

Bulk ceramic components for knee replacement have been used primarily in Japan, where both ceramic-on-polyethylene and ceramic-on-ceramic bearings have been used clinically. Evidence of the efficacy of either bearing combination is limited by the length of follow-up (< 9 years), the lack of comparative data for other bearing surfaces with the same design, and patient selection (for example, one study was limited to patients with rheumatoid arthritis). Whereas satisfactory outcomes have resulted with the use of ceramic bearings in total knee arthroplasty, no data yet exist to prove them superior to the more common metal-on-polyethylene articulations.

Cements

Polymethylmethacrylate (PMMA) bone cement has been the polymer of choice as a grouting agent to secure implant components to bone since its introduction by Charnley in the 1970s. The basic principles of the in situ polymerization remain the same. Liquid methylmethacrylate monomer with the addition of hydroquinone (to inhibit premature polymerization) and N,N,-dimethyl-p-toluidine (to accelerate polymerization once mixing commences) is mixed with prepolymerized PMMA, which also contains dibenzoyl peroxide (to initiate the polymerization process) and a radiopaque material (usually barium sulfate or zirconia). Variations on

this basic approach include powders that are a blend of a copolymer (PMMA and polystyrene or PMMA and methacrylic acid) to increase toughness.

The heat given off during polymerization is substantial. The rise in temperature that occurs in the adjoining tissues is dictated by the volume and shape of the cement bulk and the heat transfer properties of the surrounding structures. Bone cement temperatures during in vivo polymerization are usually below that required to denature proteins or kill bone cells. The long-term successful use of such cement in an array of orthopaedic applications shows that the thermal properties do not affect clinical efficacy.

Antibiotics can be added to bone cement to provide prophylaxis or treatment of infection. The elution of antibiotic from the cement is dictated by the preparation technique, chemistry, and surface area of the cement. The elution of gentamycin from commercially available cements varies significantly depending on the brand used. Bone cement properties can be detrimentally altered by the addition of antibiotics during the mixing process, an important clinical concern when antibiotics are added to the cement at surgery. The FDA has recently approved commercially prepared antibiotic cements for use in the United States; this will markedly reduce potential complications.

The performance of cement as a grout for fixation of joint arthroplasty components has been enhanced by improved protocols in cement handling, bone preparation, and cement delivery. For example, vacuum-mixed or low viscosity formulations of cement that are delivered into the bone under pressure using a cement gun have a significantly reduced porosity compared with hand-mixed cement. Reducing the porosity results in more cement in the mantle and increased structural strength, even though the material properties of the cement itself remain unaltered. Although difficult to prove clinically, a reduction in porosity should reduce the chances of cement mantle fracture and subsequent implant loosening.

PMMA cement has often been used solely as a structural component to fill bone defects and as a load-carrying element of the resulting composite. Vertebroplasty and kyphoplasty are gaining acceptance as treatments for painful osteoporotic compression fractures. Vertebroplasty was first used for osteolytic spinal conditions secondary to cancer; injection of cement into the vertebral body can prevent further collapse and relieve pain. Kyphoplasty, an extension of vertebroplasty, uses an inflatable bone tamp to restore the vertebral height while creating a cavity to be filled with bone cement. Short-term clinical results with both procedures are promising; however, several biomechanical questions remain, including the appropriate properties for the cement, the amount of fill, and the effects of vertebra reinforcement on the adjacent spinal motion segments.

Serious complications related to cement leakage, including soft-tissue damage and nerve root pain and compression, have prompted the FDA to issue a public health notification concerning this off-label use of cement.

Interest in using bioactive cements in these types of applications is growing. Cements based on hydroxyapatite and calcium phosphate have been studied to determine their ability to provide strength and stiffness to osteoporotic vertebral bodies compared to that achieved with PMMA. Handling and radiopacity difficulties have hampered the clinical use of these cements in spinal applications. These cements have been found to be effective as augments to standard fixation in several fractures, including those of the distal radius and femoral neck.

Biodegradable Polymers

Biodegradable polymers degrade chemically in a controlled manner over time. Orthopaedic applications for these materials include sutures, screws, anchors, and pins designed to slowly lose their mechanical function as they resorb and the surrounding tissue heals. The tissue assumes its normal mechanical role, while the resorption of the polymer eliminates the need for a second surgical procedure to remove the device. Resorbable polymers also are used for drug delivery, and considerable research is underway to develop biodegradable scaffolds for tissue engineering. This last application is especially challenging because the scaffold must provide a suitable biologic environment for the cells to be delivered within the material and a suitable mechanical environment so that they manufacture extracellular matrix with the appropriate biomechanical properties. Biocompatibility is a very important consideration; the polymer must degrade without adversely affecting the cells or the tissues that replace it.

Common bioresorbable polymers include polylactic acid, polyglycolic acid, polydioxanone, and polycaprolactone. Their mechanical properties span large ranges, depending on polymer type, the addition of copolymers, molecular weight, fabrication technique, and the addition of reinforcing materials such as fibers. Orthopaedic applications are limited by the strengths of these materials, which are insufficient for many load-bearing situations common in the musculoskeletal system. Bioresorbable polymers are most often used in applications involving trauma; such as the fixation of small cancellous bone fractures. The most common use reported in the literature is in association with malleolar fractures.

Hydrogels are a soft, porous-permeable group of polymers that are nontoxic, nonirritating, nonmutagenic, nonallergenic, and biocompatible. They readily absorb water (and thus have high water contents), and have low coefficients of friction and time-dependent mechanical properties that can be varied through altering the material's composition and structure. Hydrogels have been considered for use in a wide range of biomedical and pharmaceutical applications; orthopaedic applications include tissue engineering of cartilage and bone and for drug delivery.

Interfaces

In orthopaedic applications, biomaterials are generally used to fabricate entire structures for specific purposes (for example, a fracture plate or a tibial knee replacement insert). Difficulties in achieving long-term permanent fixation of orthopaedic devices to the skeleton has led to the development of specific materials and technologies intended to enhance biologic fixation. For example, tantalum is a highly biocompatible, corrosion-resistant, osteoconductive material. Recently, porous forms of tantalum deposited on pyrolytic carbon backbones have been suggested as superior structures for bone ingrowth. Orthopaedic applications include coatings for joint arthroplasty components (acetabular cups and tibial trays) and as spinal cages. Experimental work in animal models and randomized trials in humans suggest that this may be a useful material for achieving fixation to bone.

Hydroxyapatite, a ceramic, has been available as a coating on joint arthroplasty implants for some time. Animal studies showed that such coatings increase fixation strength by preferential deposition of new bone at the interface. Despite this in vivo evidence, no clear advantage has been shown in the clinical literature; whereas some reports suggest enhanced fixation, others show no benefit. This disagreement may be the result of several factors, including patient selection, implant design, and the quality and type of hydroxyapatite used.

Summary

A clinical improvement in wear rate is possible with the introduction of alternative bearing materials. In all cases, however, compromises exist; although wear behavior can be improved, other properties are altered in potentially detrimental ways (Table 1). The use of preclinical assessment tools such as joint simulators are vital to establishing efficacy, but the shortcomings of these tools must be considered when interpreting the clinical relevance of test results. Long-term follow-up data from well-controlled studies remain the only real test of efficacy.

Annotated Bibliography

General Reference

McKellop HA: Bearing surfaces in total hip replacements: State of the art and future developments. *Instr Course Lect* 2001;50:165-179.

This review article discusses the advantages and disadvantages of bearing surfaces including the new polyethylenes, modern metal-metal, and ceramic-ceramic bearings. The goal of this review is to provide surgeons with the information needed to assess the risk-benefit ratios of each of the new bearing combinations.

Santavirta S, Bohler M, Harris WH, et al: Alternative materials to improve total hip replacement tribology. *Acta Orthop Scand* 2003;74:380-388.

This review article examines proposed improvements in tribology of bearing surfaces for total hip replacement. The three approaches examined were highly cross-linked UHMWPE, aluminum oxide, and metal-on-metal. The findings in support of their efficacy were emphasized.

Wright TM, Goodman SB (eds): *Implant Wear in Total Joint Replacement: Clinical and Biologic Issues, Materials and Design Considerations*. Rosemont, IL, American Academy of Orthopaedic Surgeons, 2001.

This monograph provides answers to important clinical, biologic, and bioengineering questions concerning the complications caused by wear in total joint arthroplasties. The answers were drafted by invited attendees at a workshop sponsored by the National Institutes of Health and the American Academy of Orthopaedic Surgeons and are supported by a comprehensive bibliography.

Metal-on-Metal Bearings

Amstutz HC, Beaule PE, Dorey FJ, Le Duff MJ, Campbell PA, Gruen TA: Metal-on-metal hybrid surface arthroplasty: Two to six-year follow-up study. *J Bone Joint Surg Am* 2004;86:28-39.

Encouraging results were found in this follow-up study (average follow-up 3.5 years) of 400 hips treated with metal-on-metal surface arthroplasties. Survival rates of the arthroplasties at 4 years were 94.4%; however, a 3% revision rate for loosening of the femoral component and femoral neck fracture were also found.

Goldberg JR, Gilbert JL, Jacobs JJ, Bauer TW, Paprosky W, Leurgans S: Links: A multicenter retrieval study of the taper interfaces of modular hip prostheses. *Clin Orthop* 2002;401:149-161.

This study found that corrosion and fretting of modular taper surfaces was significantly worse for mixed alloy couples compared with similar alloy couples and were also dependant on implantation time and flexural rigidity of the neck. The results suggest that this damage was attributable to a mechanically assisted, crevice corrosion process.

Smith SL, Dowson D, Goldsmith AA: The effect of femoral head diameter upon lubrication and wear of metal-on-metal total hip replacements. *Proc Inst Mech Eng [H]* 2001;215:161-170.

A hip joint simulator study of metal-on-metal joints with different head diameters showed no surface separation with smaller heads and significantly higher wear rates compared with those found with larger diameter heads. In the larger heads, surface separation occurred, suggesting the formation of a protective lubricating film.

Ultra-High Molecular Weight Polyethylene

Burroughs BR, Rubash HE, Harris WH: Femoral head sizes larger than 32 mm against highly cross-linked polyethylene. *Clin Orthop* 2002;405:150-157.

In vitro wear testing and anatomic studies, together with prior clinical studies in which large femoral heads were used, support the hypothesis that highly cross-linked UHMWPE allows the use of femoral heads larger than 32 mm.

Collier JP, Currier BH, Kennedy FE, et al: Comparison of cross-linked polyethylene materials for orthopaedic applications. *Clin Orthop* 2003;414:289-304.

Physical and mechanical properties of six commercially available cross-linked polyethylene materials were obtained from tests in a single laboratory and reported along with wear data and summary descriptions of the materials by the manufacturers.

Digas G, Karrholm J, Thanner J, Malchau H, Herberts P: Highly cross-linked polyethylene in cemented THA: Randomized study of 61 hips. *Clin Orthop* 2003;417:126-138.

Highly cross-linked polyethylene components (irradiated to 95 kGy) were compared with conventional polyethylene components in a randomized study of cemented hip replacements. At 2-year follow-up, the highly cross-linked cups showed 50% reduction of proximal wear based on radiostereometric examinations; however, the follow-up period was short and the results preliminary.

D'Lima DD, Hermida JC, Chen PC, Colwell CW Jr: Polyethylene cross-linking by two different methods reduces acetabular liner wear in a hip joint wear simulator. *J Orthop Res* 2003;21:761-766.

A comparison of wear reduction by two different cross-linking methods, 9.5 Mrad electron beam and 10 Mrad gamma irradiation, showed no clinically significant differences. Both methods were superior to conventional nominally cross-linked (gamma sterilized) polyethylene in wear resistance.

Endo MM, Barbour PS, Barton DC, et al: Comparative wear and wear debris under three different counterface conditions of crosslinked and non-crosslinked ultra high molecular weight polyethylene. *Biomed Mater Eng* 2001;11:23-35.

The wear of grade GUR 1020 cross-linked, GUR 1120 cross-linked, and non–cross-linked GUR 1020 UHMWPE (Ticona, Summit, NJ) was compared in multidirectional wear tests using three different counterface conditions. Better wear resistance was found with cross-linking for smooth counterfaces, but with rough and scratched counterfaces, the GUR

1020 cross-linked material produced significantly higher wear rates than the non–cross-linked material.

Hopper RH Jr, Young AM, Orishimo KF, Engh CA Jr: Effect of terminal sterilization with gas plasma or gamma radiation on wear of polyethylene liners. *J Bone Joint Surg Am* 2003;85:464-468.

Patients who received hip replacements with polyethylene acetabular liners sterilized with gamma radiation (61 hips at mean follow-up of 5.2 years) experienced an average of 50% less wear than patients with non–cross-linked liners sterilized with gas plasma (63 hips at mean follow-up of 3.9 years).

Muratoglu OK, Bragdon CR, O'Connor DO, Perinchief RS, Jasty M, Harris WH: Aggressive wear testing of a cross-linked polyethylene in total knee arthroplasty. *Clin Orthop* 2002;404:89-95.

A knee simulator study comparing elevated cross-linked and conventional tibial inserts showed extensive delamination and cracking as early as 50,000 cycles for conventional polyethylene inserts, whereas the cross-linked polyethylene inserts did not show any subsurface cracking or delamination at 0.5 million cycles.

Ceramics
Allain J, Roudot-Thoraval F, Delecrin J, Anract P, Migaud H, Goutallier D: Revision total hip arthroplasty performed after fracture of a ceramic femoral head: A multicenter survivorship study. *J Bone Joint Surg Am* 2003;85:825-830.

One hundred five surgical revisions to treat a fracture of a ceramic femoral head, performed at 35 institutions, were studied. Although the fractures were potentially serious events, treatment with total synovectomy, cup exchange, and insertion of a cobalt-chromium or new ceramic femoral ball minimized the risk of early loosening and the need for one or more repeat revisions.

Hamadouche M, Boutin P, Daussange J, Bolander ME, Sedel L: Alumina-on-alumina total hip arthroplasty: A minimum 18.5-year follow-up study. *J Bone Joint Surg Am* 2002;84:69-77.

A retrospective long-term study showed a 20-year survival rate of 85% for alumina-on-alumina hip replacements with minimal wear rates and limited osteolysis, provided that the acetabular component remained well-fixed. No alumina head or socket fractures occurred and osteolysis was moderate in about 10% of the patients.

Hernigou P, Bahrami T: Zirconia and alumina ceramics in comparison with stainless-steel heads: Polyethylene wear after a minimum ten-year follow-up. *J Bone Joint Surg Br* 2003;85:504-509.

Comparison of ceramic and metal bearing surfaces showed increased polyethylene wear at 5- to 12-year follow-up for zirconia and metal heads. The group with the zirconia heads had

more severe wear. No change in wear rate occurred in the alumina group, which showed considerably less wear.

Urban JA, Garvin KL, Boese CK, et al: Ceramic-on-polyethylene bearing surfaces in total hip arthroplasty: Seventeen to twenty-one-year results. *J Bone Joint Surg Am* 2001;83:1688-1694.

Findings showed that long-term use of ceramic-on-polyethylene bearings implanted with cement by one surgeon resulted in outstanding long-term clinical and radiographic results and wear rates lower than those previously reported for metal-on-polyethylene bearings. These findings support the use of such bearings in total hip arthroplasty.

Cements
Cassidy C, Jupiter JB, Cohen M, et al: Norian SRS cement compared with conventional fixation in distal radial fractures: A randomized study. *J Bone Joint Surg Am* 2003;85:2127-2137.

A prospective, randomized multicenter study of closed reduction and immobilization with and without the use of calcium phosphate bone cement for the treatment of distal radial fractures, found significant clinical improvement during the first 3 months of treatment with cement augmentation.

Garfin SR, Reilley MA: Minimally invasive treatment of osteoporotic vertebral body compression fractures. *Spine J* 2002;2:76-80.

A literature review with presentation of early results of a national, clinical study showed 95% of patients treated for painful osteoporotic compression fractures had significant improvement in symptoms and function after kyphoplasty or vertebroplasty. Only kyphoplasty improved vertebral height and kyphosis.

Lewis G: Fatigue testing and performance of acrylic bone-cement materials: State-of-the-art review. *J Biomed Mater Res* 2003;66B:457-486.

A literature review of the fatigue behavior of acrylic bone-cement formulations showed that an increase in molecular weight leads to an increase in fatigue life; the effect of vacuum mixing on fatigue life remains controversial.

Biodegradable Polymers
Grande DA, Mason J, Light E, Dines D: Stem cells as platforms for delivery of genes to enhance cartilage repair. *J Bone Joint Surg Am* 2003;85(suppl 2):111-116.

Stem cells transduced with either bone morphogenetic protein-7 or sonic hedgehog gene were delivered to osteochondral defects in rabbits using bioresorbable scaffolds. The addition of either factor enhanced the quality of the repaired tissue, showing the utility of tissue-engineering gene therapy strategies.

Hovis WD, Kaiser BW, Watson JT, Bucholz RW: Treatment of syndesmotic disruptions of the ankle with bioabsorbable screw fixation. *J Bone Joint Surg Am* 2002; 84:26-31.

Syndesmotic disruptions associated with malleolar fractures in which the syndesmosis was fixed with poly-L-lactic acid screws healed without displacement of the syndesmosis or widening of the medial clear space. No episodes of osteolysis or late inflammation secondary to the hydrolyzed polylactide occurred.

Interfaces

Kim YH, Kim JS, Oh SH, Kim JM: Comparison of porous-coated titanium femoral stems with and without hydroxyapatite coating. *J Bone Joint Surg Am* 2003;85: 1682-1688.

At a mean follow-up of 6.6 years postoperatively, the clinical and radiographic results associated with proximally porous-coated femoral prostheses with identical geometries that differed only with regard to the presence or absence of hydroxyapatite coating were found to be similar.

Wigfield C, Robertson J, Gill S, Nelson R: Clinical experience with porous tantalum cervical interbody implants in a prospective randomized controlled trial. *Br J Neurosurg* 2003;17:418-425.

A prospective randomized study of the ability of porous tantalum implants to achieve cervical interbody fusion showed inferior end-plate lucency in four patients raising concerns about delayed or nonfusion. Fusion subsequently occurred in all patients at 12 months after surgery.

Classic Bibliography

Bartel DL, Rawlinson JJ, Burstein AH, Ranawat CS, Flynn WF Jr: Stresses in polyethylene components of contemporary total knee replacements. *Clin Orthop* 1995;317:76-82.

Bobyn JD, Toh KK, Hacking SA, Tanzer M, Krygier JJ: Tissue response to porous tantalum acetabular cups: A canine model. *J Arthroplasty* 1999;14:347-354.

Boehler M, Plenk H Jr, Salzer M: Alumina ceramic bearings for hip endoprostheses: The Austrian experiences. *Clin Orthop* 2000;379:85-93.

Chan FW, Bobyn JD, Medley JB, Krygier JJ, Tanzer M: The Otto Aufranc Award. Wear and lubrication of metal-on-metal hip implants. *Clin Orthop* 1999;369: 10-24.

Dorr LD, Wan Z, Longjohn DB, Dubois B, Murken R: Total hip arthroplasty with use of the Metasul metal-on-metal articulation: Four to seven-year results. *J Bone Joint Surg Am* 2000;82:789-798.

Dorr LD, Wan Z, Song M, Ranawat A: Bilateral total hip arthroplasty comparing hydroxyapatite coating to porous-coated fixation. *J Arthroplasty* 1998;13:729-736.

Fenollosa J, Seminario P, Montijano C: Ceramic hip prostheses in young patients: A retrospective study of 74 patients. *Clin Orthop* 2000;379:55-67.

Jacobs JJ, Skipor AK, Patterson LM, et al: Metal release in patients who have had a primary total hip arthroplasty: A prospective, controlled, longitudinal study. *J Bone Joint Surg Am* 1998;80:1447-1458.

McKellop H, Shen FW, Lu B, Campbell P, Salovey R: Development of an extremely wear-resistant ultra high molecular weight polyethylene for total hip replacements. *J Orthop Res* 1999;17:157-167.

Oonishi H, Kadoya Y: Wear of high-dose gamma-irradiated polyethylene in total hip replacements. *J Orthop Sci* 2000;5:223-228.

Ritter MA: Direct compression molded polyethylene for total hip and knee replacements. *Clin Orthop* 2001; 393:94-100.

Rokkanen PU, Bostman O, Hirvensalo E, et al: Bioabsorbable fixation in orthopaedic surgery and traumatology. *Biomaterials* 2000;21:2607-2613.

Chapter 6

Physiology of Aging

Susan V. Bukata, MD

Mathias Bostrom, MD

Joseph A. Buckwalter, MD

Joseph M. Lane, MD

Introduction

Aging is a complex process that involves changes in many of the physiologic functions of the body; aging also may create changes in social and economic conditions that influence lifestyles and daily routines. The accumulated effects of past diseases, side effects of medications, and environmental factors can change an individual's ability to perform daily activities. Older people often have difficulty sleeping and many experience at least some recent memory loss. The heterogeneity of the aging body also makes patient response to a particular medication or treatment much more variable than in a younger population. To care for the elderly patient and improve quality of life, it is important to understand the changes that occur with aging and to address the special needs that these changes produce. The United States Census Bureau projects that by the year 2010, one quarter of the US population will be age 55 years or older. This projection is based in part on increasing life expectancies for men and women. Health care providers must understand the special needs associated with aging to provide appropriate treatment for this expanding population of patients.

Changes in Neuromuscular Control

The maintenance of a moderate level of neuromuscular control is essential for the continuation of normal daily routines. Many changes that occur with natural aging affect neuromuscular control. These changes affect an individual's ability to perform certain tasks and result in changes in proprioception that affect balance and increase the risk for falling. Changes in proprioception stem from a variety of sources, such as sensory changes that affect vision, hearing, and vestibular function, as well as age-related changes in the central and peripheral nervous systems. All of these changes affect coordination and musculoskeletal function by altering the neural control and stimuli of muscles, which affect mobility.

Many other changes occur in the central and peripheral nervous systems with aging. Brain atrophy of 30% to 40% in the frontal lobe, temporal lobe, and basal ganglia occurs with a decrease in the total number of neurons. A decrease in brain tissue metabolism accompanies a decrease in cerebral blood flow. Processing in both nervous systems slows with increasing age, with nerve conduction velocity decreased 10% to 15%. Autonomic and muscle stretch reflexes become less sensitive and righting reflexes decrease in acuity, resulting in increased body sway that makes it more difficult for elderly people to respond to sudden positional changes. Reaction times in older adults are 20% longer than those in young adults, which partially accounts for the 35% to 40% increase in falls seen in adults older than 60 years.

An age-related decrease in the number of spinal motor neurons probably contributes to these changes. Single peripheral motor neurons innervate groups of skeletal muscle fibers forming a motor unit. Accompanying the loss of spinal motor neurons is a concomitant loss in the total number of motor units in old muscles and remodeling of other motor units. This decrease in total motor units is actually a specific loss of fast motor units and an increase in slow motor units. During normal aging, a reorganization of the motor unit pool for skeletal muscle occurs, which supports the belief that some fast fibers may undergo denervation and others may be reinnervated by sprouting nerves from the slow motor units. Changes also occur at the neuromuscular junction, which affect the recruitment of muscle fibers for coordinated activity. With aging, there is a degeneration of the neuromuscular junction that prevents or slows the transmission of neural stimuli to muscle fibers. All of these changes contribute to slower reaction times.

Many sensory changes also occur with aging that can make it difficult for eldery people to respond to changes in their environment. Increasingly poor vision, macular degeneration, stereopsis, cataracts, and poor night vision commonly occur with aging. Hearing loss with a decrease in high-frequency acuity (affecting the ability to distinguish words from background noise) affects almost 30% of patients older than 70 years and almost 90% of nursing home residents. Impaired vestibular function also affects many older patients and may play a signifi-

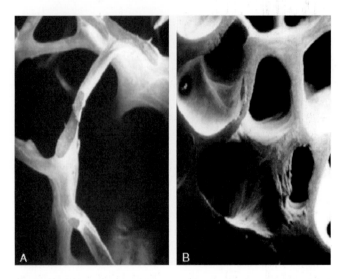

Figure 1 A, Osteoporotic trabecular bone. **B,** Normal trabecular bone. *(Adapted with permission from Dempster DW, Shane E, Horbert W, Lindsay R: A simple method for correlative light and scanning electron microscopy of human iliac crest bone biopsies: Qualitative observations in normal and osteoporotic subjects. J Bone Miner Res 1986; 1:15-21.)*

cant role in balance impairment and falls. Neuropathy secondary to diabetes and nerve injuries can limit sensation in the feet and impair the ability to respond to uneven terrain. Impaired cognition secondary to medications, dementia, depression, or stroke also can impair an older person's ability to respond appropriately to their environment and is a risk factor for appendicular fracture.

Changes in Body Composition and Functional Reserve

Age-related changes occur in body composition that result in decreased bone mass, decreased muscle mass, and an increase in body fat. Sarcopenia, or muscle mass loss, reduces basal metabolism and is the predominant cause of decreased muscle strength seen with aging. This loss of strength can have a profound effect on an elderly person's ability to perform simple tasks such as walking and rising from a chair. Peak muscle mass is attained at approximately 30 years of age. After age 50 years, approximately 15% of muscle mass is lost per decade, increasing up to 30% per decade after age 70 years. Muscle atrophy occurs from both a reduction in fiber size and quantity. The equal loss of type I (fast twitch) and type II (slow twitch) fibers accounts for most of the atrophy associated with aging; however, the type II fibers also decrease in size more than the type I fibers and subsequently compose a smaller percentage of the muscle cross-sectional area. A 26% reduction in the size of type II fibers occurs from age 20 to 80 years and accounts for a large proportion of age-related muscle mass loss. This decrease in fiber size is not seen with normal disuse atrophy. Overall muscle cross-sectional area de-

creases 40% and the total number of fibers declines 39% between the ages of 20 and 80 years. In addition, greater muscle mass is lost in weight-bearing muscles than in non–weight-bearing muscles. These combined changes in muscle mass lead to a prolongation of twitch contraction and a reduction in voluntary strength. Poor quadriceps function has been identified as a key risk factor for falls and hip fracture.

Aging also causes many significant changes in the cardiovascular system, such as changes in functional reserve capacity that affect an individual's ability to respond to physiologic stresses. Increased vascular stiffness, hypertension, and other factors result in a decreased ability to increase cardiac output in response to physiologic stress. Maximal oxygen consumption, a measurement that serves as a good measure of athletic fitness, declines 5% to 15% each decade after age 25 years. Endurance training is able to slow this decline up to 50% until approximately age 70 years. Older patients are able to respond to exercise and to improve muscle strength and tone and cardiovascular response; however, even very fit older adults may have a maximal functional reserve that only is equivalent to that of younger sedentary individuals.

Bone mass also changes as a part of normal aging. Peak bone mineral density is reached between age 25 and 30 years and begins to decline in the fourth and fifth decades of life. Bone mineral density declines 0.3% to 0.5% per year and the rate of loss may increase for women to 2% to 3% per year in the 7- to 10-year period of perimenopause. The rate of bone loss and the associated increase in fracture risk is related to a complex combination of genetics, body mass characteristics, nutritional factors, and diseases. A complex relationship, commonly referred to as coupling, exists between osteoblasts and osteoclasts, which balances bone formation with bone resorption. It is ultimately this relationship between the osteoblasts and osteoclasts that determines the rate of bone mineral density loss. After peak bone mass is attained, the full bone remodeling unit is not completely replaced during the process of normal bone turnover, which results, over time, in decreased bone mass. During the perimenopausal period, the activity of osteoclasts is enhanced and osteoblasts are unable to replace bone at the same pace. Architectural changes eventually occur as bone trabeculae decrease in number and lose continuity. Whereas cortical bone thins, the losses are greater in the trabecular bone mass (Figure 1). More information about bone mineral density and bone remodeling can be found in chapter 18. All of these processes combine to increase the fragility of aging bone. Fracture repair is not delayed or compromised, but fixation failure is more common because of inadequate bone stock. Almost 98% of elderly patients who sustain a hip fracture have some level of bone deficiency. Low-energy hip fractures are associated with a

20% increase in mortality within the first 6 months after injury. Although patients with two or more vertebral fractures have a 25% to 30% increase in mortality compared with peers who do not sustain such fractures, this difference is reflected over the much longer period of 5 years. Because of age-associated bone loss, elderly people are at greater risk for low-energy fractures and related mortality.

Normal aging results in many changes in the endocrine system that affect a variety of body tissues and functions. Changes in glucose metabolism include an increase in peripheral glucose resistance and an increase in postprandial blood glucose and insulin levels. These changes are influenced by diet, exercise, and body fat content, all of which often change with aging. This altered glucose metabolism results in a higher rate of insulin-resistant diabetes (type II diabetes) in the older population. Decreased levels of growth hormone, insulin growth factor, estrogen, and testosterone also occur with aging. Patients have been treated with growth hormone supplementation, but the benefits are not clear. Estrogen supplementation was used for many years as the mainstay of treatment for patients with perimenopausal bone loss; however, global risk including increases in the prevalence of breast cancer, strokes, pulmonary emboli, and blood clots are believed to outweigh the benefits obtained in fracture reduction and decreased bone loss. Estrogen supplementation is no longer recommended as a treatment if its sole purpose is to prevent bone loss.

Age-Related Changes in Articular Cartilage

Most of the cells and extracellular matrix proteins of articular cartilage undergo very little turnover, which results in an accumulation of age-related changes and damage to the tissue over many years. In the world population, almost 25% of people older than 60 years have osteoarthritis, which makes age the greatest risk factor for developing this disease. However, the relationship between age and osteoarthritis is not well understood. The age-related changes in articular cartilage are somewhat different from those seen in osteoarthritis; however, these changes affect the biomechanical, biochemical, and cellular characteristics of the tissue and possibly increase the risk of damage and progression to osteoarthritis. The extent of degenerative changes varies by joint; however, not all degenerative changes are associated with joint pain and loss of motion. All degenerative changes do not progress to osteoarthritis, which further indicates the complex relationship between the two processes. Age-related changes to the synovium, subchondral bone, menisci, ligaments, and the joint capsule may all contribute to the progression of joint symptoms and the establishment of osteoarthritis.

Articular cartilage undergoes age-related changes in thickness, cellular function, matrix tensile properties, ma-trix composition, and molecular organization. Localized, superficial fibrillation of articular surfaces can be first seen in adolescents as they approach skeletal maturity. During skeletal growth, there is a noted decrease in chondrocyte density, an associated decrease in synthetic activity, and a change in the proteoglycan component ratios. With increasing age, there is a decrease in the ratio of chondroitin sulfate to total glycosaminoglycans, an increase in the production of chondroitin 6 sulfate, and a decrease in the production of chondroitin 4 sulfate. There also is a decreased response to growth factors, especially transforming growth factor-β, which exerts almost no influence on chondrocytes once skeletal maturity is reached, but is a strong stimulant to glycosaminoglycan production (particularly chondroitin 4 sulfate). There is an age-associated decrease in the water content of cartilage, in direct contrast to the changes that occur with degenerative arthritis. In osteoarthritis, water content initially increases as a result of a disruption in the architecture of the matrix molecules. Other matrix changes associated with aging include an increase in decorin concentration, collagen cross-linking, collagen fibril diameter, and variability in collagen fibril diameter.

Chondrocyte proliferation and cell density begin to decline from birth, and reach a steady plateau by skeletal maturity. Although cell number may not vary significantly with increasing age, the synthetic capabilities and cell morphology continue to change. Cells accumulate intracytoplasmic filaments and may lose some of their endoplasmic reticulum. Cell culture studies using chondrocyte samples extracted from human articular cartilage show a decrease in absolute chondrocyte yield and in cell proliferation after the age of 30 years. These cell cultures are responsive to platelet-derived growth factor–BB, with a threefold increase in glycosaminoglycan production up to age 40 years; there is minimal response after that age. A recent study showed that human articular cartilage chondrocytes become senescent with increasing patient age, which may account for the decreased capacity of chondrocytes to respond to injury. In addition, oxidative stress to the cartilage tissue may cause premature chondrocyte senescence, making the tissue susceptible to injury for a longer period of time. Chondrocyte cultures maintained in 5% oxygen doubled 60 times before becoming senescent, whereas increasing the oxygen concentration to 21% cut the number of population doublings to 40. Increased oxidative stress occurs after trauma and with inflammation and may explain why injury increases a patient's risk for osteoarthritis.

Mechanical studies have shown significant age-related changes in the tensile properties of articular cartilage including decreases in stiffness, fatigue resistance, and strength. The exact cause of these changes is not known but it is likely that changes in the collagen matrix, the proteoglycans, and the decrease in water content all play a role. The increase in advanced glycosylation end products (AGEs) and their effect on cartilage mechanical properties are of significant interest. AGEs adversely influence cartilage turnover, causing decreases in matrix synthesis and degradation. Their presence is accompanied by increased cartilage stiffness and brittleness, possibly because of increased cross-linking of the collagen molecules by the AGEs. A canine model of anterior cruciate ligament (ACL) transaction showed increased collagen damage, impaired matrix repair, decreased proteoglycan synthesis, and more severe osteoarthritis in the animals treated to have a higher concentration of AGEs in their tissues, similar to that found in older dogs. If there is confirmation that these findings are correlated with the onset of osteoarthritis, reversing or preventing the changes modulated by AGEs may represent a novel approach to preventing the onset of osteoarthritis. Collagen fibrils also become larger in diameter and more variable in size with aging; this change is attributed to a decrease in the type XI collagen component. The larger, more cross-linked fibrils are more rigid and may limit the ability of the articular cartilage surface to deform without cracking.

Age-Related Changes in Intervertebral Disk

Low back pain, which affects a substantial portion of the adult population, is one of the most common reasons for an adult to consult a primary care physician. Although it is difficult to separate age-related changes from degenerative changes to the intervertebral disk, it is clear that substantial changes occur (possibly more than occur to any other musculoskeletal tissue) as a result of aging. There are also substantial individual differences in the rate that these changes occur, which may explain the difficulty in separating the effects of aging from those of degeneration. Several general trends link the blood supply, cellular and matrix proliferation, and tissue hydration to the structural changes observed in the intervertebral disk.

Beginning at birth, the abundant notochordal cells found in the nucleus pulposus begin to disappear, whereas chondrocyte density increases. The cellular density at the disk end plates begins to increase and disorganization of the cartilaginous regions is noted. By the second decade of life, blood vessels within the disk begin to disappear and cleft formation in the nucleus pulposus begins. During adulthood, the number of clefts continues to increase and radial tears develop that extend into the disk periphery and the anulus fibrosus. There is a marked decline in the number of cells within the disk, and the rate of cellular apoptosis increases. Both the volume and shape of the disk change. Mucoid degeneration with an increase in noncollagenous protein content occurs and there is a concomitant decrease in proteoglycan and water content. Collagen content de-

clines and the remaining collagen is composed of fibrils with increased diameter and diameter variability, and decreased pyridinoline crosslinks. In later adulthood, there is increased scar formation within the disk (including the anulus fibrosus), a disruption in the normal lamellar pattern of collagen fibrillar layers within the anulus fibrosus, and a decrease in the functional stretch of these collagen molecules. In elderly people, it becomes difficult to distinguish the anatomic regions of the disk.

Significant alterations in the blood supply to the disk appear to parallel the structural changes. With increasing age, physiologic vessels within the disk disappear. The ossification of the vertebral end plates that occurs with skeletal maturity may significantly affect the nutritional supply and hydration of the adjacent disk. The cells within the disk begin to depend on diffusion of nutrients from the periphery, a process that appears to be hindered as the number of vessels supplying the disk declines and increased intradiskal matrix slows diffusion through the tissues. Decreased hydration of the central nucleus pulposus leads to stiffening of the surrounding anulus fibrosus and changes in spine biomechanics that can affect load sharing between the adjacent facet joints, ligaments, paraspinal muscles, and vertebral bodies. Other diseases and lifestyle habits that affect small vessel proliferation and function, including diabetes and smoking, may accelerate the rate of change in the disk tissues.

Age-Related Changes in Tendon, Ligament, and Joint Capsule

Injuries to ligaments, tendons, and joint capsules are commonly seen in middle-aged and elderly individuals. These injuries can result in significant impairment in strength, range of motion, and stability in the regions where they occur. Significant pain and disability can result from low-energy ruptures of the rotator cuff, quadriceps, patellar, bicep, or posterior tibial tendons, and form ruptures to spinal and wrist ligaments following physical activity or even as a result of the normal activities of daily living.

Although the cellular and mechanical properties that change with aging have not been fully defined in all of these tissues, similarities in structure and composition suggest that the known observations are probably applicable to all of these tissues. Fibroblast cells form a major proportion of ligaments, tendons, and joint capsules. As fibroblasts age, the cells flatten, elongate, and lose most of their protein-producing cell organelles, including the rough endoplasmic reticulum and Golgi apparatus. This finding suggests that the tissues are less biosynthetically active, and may be less able to efficiently respond to injury. Several factors may contribute to the age-related increase in injuries to these tissues. A decreasing blood supply may cause changes in cell activity and matrix composition and organization that lead to tissue degeneration. Although biochemical analysis of these tissues has not identified dramatic changes in the matrix composition, a decrease in collagen cross-links (common in many musculoskeletal tissues with aging) may contribute to the observed age-related decrease in water content. Collagen bundles in these tissues are highly oriented, a property that contributes to the mechanical characteristics of the tissues. Animal studies have suggested that changes in the collagen organization, including fibril alignment and fiber bundle orientation, occur with aging. This change in the organization of the collagen fibers may account for the altered mechanics and changes in the ultimate load-to-failure. One study of human ACLs showed decreasing tensile stiffness and ultimate load-to-failure with increasing age. Another study showed that the ligament-bone complexes in people older than 60 years tolerated only one third the load before failing compared with those of young adults. A recent study of human posterior cruciate ligaments found a decrease in collagen fiber diameter and an increase in collagen fibril concentration with aging.

Nutrition

Many changes occur to the gastrointestinal system as a part of natural aging. Changes in the autonomic nervous system affect colonic motility and can result in constipation, whereas other neurologic changes to the anorectal region can result in fecal incontinence. Past diseases also can have an effect on the gastrointestinal system. Elderly patients with a history of diabetes may have special dietary needs to regulate their blood glucose levels and also may have additional bowel motility needs as a result of neuropathic changes. Patients may have difficulty swallowing (secondary to stroke) and also may have special dietary needs after abdominal surgery for ulcers, diverticulitis, or colon cancer. All of these concerns can make it difficult for elderly patients to obtain adequate nutrition from food intake alone.

Protein is essential for the maintenance of muscle mass and for the formation of some of the extracellular components of bone, especially collagen. Follow-up on age-related bone loss for patients in the Framingham study showed lower levels of bone loss if adequate protein was present in the diet. It is widely recognized that patients with low serum albumin levels have difficulty with wound healing. Survival rates in elderly patients with hip fractures also is well correlated with adequate serum albumin levels. Many elderly patients do not receive adequate protein in their diets because of dietary choices or social or economic concerns; such patients should be encouraged to increase protein intake until serum albumin levels are within normal limits. Some patients also have inadequate caloric intake. If patients are unable to consume adequate calories with their normal meals, supplemental nutrition (such as shakes and puddings) should be added to their daily diet.

Older age is associated with a decrease in gastric acidity, which affects the absorption of calcium and vitamin B12. When prescribing calcium supplementation for elderly patients, it is important to remember that a high percentage of them will be naturally achlorhydric or taking an H_2 blocker and are unable to absorb calcium carbonate supplements. Such patients must take calcium citrate supplements, which can be absorbed in the absence of stomach acid. A dietary goal for calcium intake should be 1,500 mg daily for older individuals, which should be taken in divided doses of 500 mg or less to optimize absorption from each dose.

Although changes occur in the liver that affect the efficiency of drug metabolism, these changes do not seem to be the primary cause of vitamin D deficiency in elderly people. Serum 25-hydroxyvitamin D levels decline with age primarily because of decreased sun exposure and a decrease in the efficiency of vitamin D production in the skin. Changes in the kidney do not seem to affect vitamin D levels, except in patients with renal failure. Supplementation with 400 to 800 IU of vitamin D daily is recommended for all older patients. Those who are vitamin D-deficient (such as patients taking seizure medications, those with sprue, or with irritable bowel syndrome) may require a higher dosage.

Fracture Healing

Fracture healing occurs either through a cartilage callus (endochondral bone formation) when fracture fragments are not in close apposition, directly onto the surface of existing bone (appositional bone formation), or along a collagen matrix that does not contain any cartilage (intramembranous bone formation). These modes of fracture healing occur in people of all ages, but the speed and efficacy of bone healing declines with increasing age. When skeletal maturity is reached, the periosteum gradually thins and the chondrogenic and osteogenic potential of its mesenchymal cells declines with age. A recent study with rabbits showed that the percentage of proliferating mesenchymal chondrocyte precursor cells did not change between young and old animals. However, the same study showed that the absolute number of proliferating cells decreased in the older rabbits because the size and total cell number in the periosteum was decreased. Conflicting evidence has been found concerning the change in the number and the proliferative capacity of osteoprogenitor cells. One study of human bone marrow that was aspirated from the iliac crest showed an age-related gradual decline in precursor colony-forming units. Another study of human iliac crest bone marrow also found no change in precursor cell number or proliferative capacity with advancing age or with the presence of osteoporosis.

Delayed fracture healing has been reported both in humans and in animals with aging. Because most experiments done on fracture healing have involved young or young adult animals, few data exist on fracture healing in older animals. Experiments performed to assess the effect of aging on fracture healing showed no differences in the biochemical parameters of fracture healing. One recent study comparing 6-week-old rats with 1-year-old rats showed no differences in the messenger RNA (mRNA) expression of several cytokines and proteins involved in fracture healing. Despite this similarity in mRNA expression, femur fracture healing was delayed in the older animals. Expression of Indian hedgehog and bone morphogenetic protein-2 was lower in the older animals at the time of fracture callous formation and may have contributed to the delay in healing. This same study found differences in the baseline expression mRNA levels in the young rats even over the short period of the study, suggesting that the age and metabolic status of the animal or patient must be taken into account when interventions are considered to enhance bone repair. In another rat study, fractures in young animals were healed in 40 days and the bones had normal mechanical properties by 4 weeks. In the older animals, fracture healing was delayed to 80 days, and normal mechanical properties were not regained until 12 weeks. The delayed return of mechanical properties may reflect the increased incidence of hardware failure in older patients with fractures. The bone holding the hardware in place actually fails in many older patients, rather that the hardware itself breaking before fracture healing is complete.

The age-related decline in the rate of fracture healing may be explained by several mechanisms. Aging is related to a general functional decline in the homeostatic mechanisms of skeletal tissues. There is a decline in the expression of osteoinductive cytokines and growth factors both at baseline and with injury in older animals, caused in part by a reduction in the inflammatory response to injury. In addition, the bone inductive potential of demineralized bone matrix decreases with aging. The inductive potential of bone matrix appears to be growth hormone-dependent; growth hormone secretion decreases with age.

Exercise and Fall Prevention

More than 300,000 hip fractures occur annually in the United States, and over 90% of these fractures are associated with a fall. Each year, 30% of community dwelling people older than 65 years fall, and nursing home dwellers average 1.5 falls per person per year. A variety of factors increase the risk of a fall, including muscle weakness, abnormalities in gait or balance, poor vision, decreased sensation in the lower extremities and associated changes in proprioception, functional limitations,

cognitive impairments, and the side effects of medications. The risk of falling increases with an increased number of impairments, ranging from 8% in patients with no impairments to 78% in patients with four or more impairments. Abnormal body sway and gait are correlated with falls; several tests can be used to assess these risks in patients. The average osteoporotic 80-year-old patient should be able to perform a single leg stance for at least 12 seconds. An inability to perform this maneuver implies compromised balance. Timed get up and go tests (which evaluate a patient's ability to rise from a chair without using their arms and to transition to beginning gait) and evaluation of heel-toe straight line walking can be used to identify patients at risk for falls.

Several strategies can be used to prevent falls and injuries associated with falls. Identification of a patient's risk factors for falling are an important initial step in choosing preventive strategies. Patients with gait abnormalities and muscle weakness may require an assistive device such as a cane or walker to improve mobility. The removal of throw rugs, the installation of safety rails in the bathroom and on stairs, the use of nightlights, and the use of proper shoe wear can help to reduce the risk of falling posed by home hazards. Other preventive measures may include the withdrawal of medications that are associated with falls (especially psychotropic drugs). Exercise programs such as tai chi and physical therapy can improve balance, muscle strength, and flexibility, reducing falls by 46%. The use of energy-absorbing flooring and hip protectors are indicated for patients who are at high risk for injury from falls. Hip protectors are made of molded polypropylene or polyethylene and worn as a part of an undergarment over normal underwear. The use of hip protectors has been shown to reduce the average patient's overall risk of hip fracture by 60%, and by more than 80% if the hip protector was being worn at the time of the fall. Patient compliance in using this device is often less than 60% because of the bulkiness of the undergarment and the difficulties some patients have donning and removing it.

Exercise has been shown to decrease the rate of decline of many physiologic changes associated with aging by improving cardiac function, strength, balance, and flexibility. Muscle strength reliably increases in older patients who begin resistance exercises, and improvements in muscle mass and flexibility also are seen. Weight-bearing exercises also decrease bone density losses. An exercise program for older patients must take into account their functional limitations and goals, modifying the choice of exercises as well as the frequency and duration of the training to increase compliance with the program. Elderly people can improve their functional independence, increase mobility, and reduce the risk of falling by participating in an exercise program. Elderly patients who maintain a reasonable level of exercise tolerance or who can be rehabilitated to this level of activity with a proper physical conditioning program can reduce the decline in overall function that occurs with advancing age.

Annotated Bibliography

Changes in Body Composition and Functional Reserve

Buckwalter JA, Heckman JD, Petrie DP: An AOA critical issue: Aging of the North American population. New challenges for orthopaedics. *J Bone Joint Surg Am* 2003; 85:748-758.

A comprehensive review of the physiologic changes that occur with aging and the demands these changes create for the health care system is presented. The authors also address the response the health care system may need to make to serve the aging population of North America.

Cummings SR, Melton LJ: Epidemiology and outcomes of osteoporotic fractures. *Lancet* 2002;359:1761-1767.

The rate of osteoporotic fractures is increasing with the aging of the world population. The authors note the need for epidemiologic research to identify those individuals most at risk for fracture (especially hip fracture) and for treatment with medication. Financial resources for treatments could then be allocated to those most at risk for a disabling fracture.

Stenderup K, Justesen J, Eriksen EF, et al: Number and proliferative capacity of osteogenic stem cells are maintained during aging and in patients with osteoporosis. *J Bone Miner Res* 2001;16:1120-1129.

The results of a study that examined the effect of aging and osteoporosis on the mesenchymal stem cell population are presented. Iliac crest bone marrow from 23 younger patients (age range, 22 to 44 years), 15 older patients (age range, 66 to 74 years), and 13 osteoporotic patients (age range, 58 to 83) were cultured in vitro. Total colony-forming units, colony sizes, and cell density per colony were assessed. Results showed no differences for any group in the number and proliferative capacity of osteoprogenitor cells. The results of this study were in contrast with some previous studies and suggest that the defective osteoblast functions seen with aging and osteoporosis are caused by some other factor.

Age-Related Changes in Articular Cartilage

Degroot J, Verzijl N, Wenting-van Wijk MJ, et al: Accumulation of advanced glycation end products as a molecular mechanism for aging as a risk factor in osteoarthritis. *Arthritis Rheum* 2004;50:1207-1215.

This study examined the role of AGEs in the development of osteoarthritis. Using a canine ACL transection model, the affected joints were injected with ribose to mimic the presence of AGE found in older dogs. The development of osteoarthritis and the degree of collagen damage and proteoglycan release was then analyzed. AGEs were associated with more severe osteoarthritis.

Martin JA, Lingelhutz AJ, Moussavi-Harami F, Buckwalter JA: Effects of oxidative damage and telomerase activity on human articular cartilage chondrocyte senescence. *J Gerontol A Biol Sci Med Sci* 2004;59:324-337.

Chondrocyte cell lines were grown at 5% oxygen and at 21% oxygen and analyzed for population doublings. Those grown at 21% oxygen reached senescence at 40 population doublings, whereas those exposed to 5% oxygen concentration reached senescence at 60 population doublings. These findings show that oxidative stress, like that seen in injury and inflammation, can lead to premature chondrocyte senescence. This finding is also an important consideration in establishing the conditions necessary during chondrocyte transplantation.

Ulrich-Vinther M, Maloney M, Schwarz EM, et al: Articular cartilage biology. *J Am Acad Orthop Surg* 2003;11: 421-430.

A comprehensive review is presented of the current information available about the biology of articular cartilage and the effects on this tissue on various injuries and diseases including osteoarthritis, osteochondral fracture, and microscopic damage. This article also summarizes the cytokines and growth factors that are involved in both normal tissue metabolism and response to injury. A discussion of the rationale and evidence of effectiveness of currently available treatments for osteoarthritis precedes a discussion of future strategies for treatment based on new information about articular cartilage biology.

Age-Related Changes in Intervertebral Disk

Boos N, Weissbach S, Rohrbach H, Weiler C, Spratt KF, Nerlich AG: Classification of age-related changes in lumbar intervertebral discs: 2002 Volvo Award in basic science. *Spine* 2002;27:2631-2644.

A thorough analysis of the histologic age-related changes that occur to the human intervertebral disk is presented. One hundred eighty intervertebral disk specimens from a broad age range of individuals (range, fetal to 88 years of age) were analyzed for histologic changes in the cells, matrix, blood supply, and overall structure. The study is the first to provide histologic evidence of the changes in blood supply that occur to the disk and precede the structural and cellular changes that are associated with aging and degeneration of the intervertebral disk.

Age-Related Changes in Tendon, Ligament, and Joint Capsule

Sargon MF, Doral MN, Atay OA: Age-related changes in human PCLs: A light and electron microscopic study. *Knee Surg Sports Traumatol Arthrosc* 2004;12:280-284.

This study of 36 specimens from patients of various ages used light and transmission electron microscopy to analyze ultrastructural differences. Collagen fibers were most variable in diameter in patients age 10 to 19 years. Aging was associated with a decrease in collagen fiber diameter and an increase in collagen fibril concentration with a maximum fibril concentration occurring in patients age 60 to 69 years.

Nutrition

Meydani M: The Boyd Orr lecture: Nutrition interventions in aging and age-associated disease. *Proc Nutr Soc* 2002;61:165-171.

This article presents a review of the physiologic changes that occur with aging and the concomitant socioeconomic factors that influence the dietary regimen of elderly people. Dietary modifications to maximize the nutritional intake and accommodate the normal changes of aging are discussed.

Fracture Healing

Koval KJ, Meek R, Schmitsch E, Liporace F, Strauss E, Zuckerman JD: Geriatric trauma: Young ideas. *J Bone Joint Surg Am* 2003;85:1380-1388.

A review of the special considerations needed when treating trauma injuries in elderly patients is presented. Discussion includes the physiologic changes to bone and soft tissues that occur with aging, as well as patient factors including medical comorbidities and cognitive status issues that are common in this population. The article reviews the current information on the timing of surgery, anesthesia considerations, implant choices, fixation enhancement, and postoperative care for the elderly population.

Meyer RA Jr, Meyer MH, Tenholder M, Wondracek S, Wasserman R, Garges P: Gene expression in older rats with delayed union of femoral fractures. *J Bone Joint Surg Am* 2003;85:1243-1254.

The levels of mRNA gene expression during fracture healing are the same in young rats and older rats, even though a delay in fracture healing is observed in the older rats. Lower levels of Indian hedgehog and bone morphogenetic protein-2 were detected in the fracture callous of the older rats, which may contribute to slower fracture repair.

O'Driscoll SW, Saris DB, Ito Y, Fitzimmons JS: The chondrogenic potential of periosteum decreases with age. *J Orthop Res* 2001;19:95-103.

The chondrogenic potential of the periosteum of rabbits ranging in age from 2 weeks to 2 years decreased with aging. The most notable change occurred in the total number of cells and the thickness of the periosteum. Although the percentage of proliferating cells did not dramatically change with age, the decrease in the total number of proliferating cells correlated with the decline in the chondrogenic potential of the periosteum with aging of the rabbits.

Exercise and Fall Prevention

DeRedeneire N, Visser M, Peila R, et al: Is a fall just a fall? Correlates of falling in healthy older persons: The Health, Aging, and Body Composition Study. *J Am Geriatr Soc* 2003;51:841-846.

This study evaluated 3,075 high-functioning adults (70 to 79 years of age) who were living independently in the community. Frequency of falls over a 1-year period were studied. Results indicated that 24% of women and 18% of men in this study fell at least once during that 1-year period. Factors associated with falling included female gender, Caucasian race, the presence of an increased number of chronic diseases, use of medications, decreased leg strength, poor balance, slower walking rates, and lower muscle mass. The authors recommend that all elderly patients should be assessed for fall risk.

Lin JT, van der Meulen MCH, Myers ER, Lane JM: Fractures: Evaluation and clinical implications, in Favus MJ (ed): *Primer on the Metabolic Bone Diseases and Disorders of Mineral Metabolism*. Washington, DC, American Society for Bone and Mineral Research, 2003, pp 147-151.

This chapter describes the compositional changes that occur to bone with aging and how this affects the ability of bone to absorb loads. Fall prevention strategies and environmental interventions to decrease applied loads at the time of a fall are discussed.

Marks R, Allegrante JP, MacKenzie CR, Lane JM: Hip fractures among the elderly: Causes, consequences, and control. *Ageing Res Rev* 2003;21:57-93.

A comprehensive review of the physiologic changes of aging and the risk factors and treatment options for hip fractures is presented. Comprehensive references for all of the pertinent articles published in the past decade, which define risk factors for hip fracture and physiologic factors related to fracture, are provided.

Tinetti ME: Clinical practice: Preventing falls in elderly persons. *N Engl J Med* 2003;348:42-49.

Case examples are presented to address the potential causes (use of medication, sensory changes, visual disturbances, and cognitive problems) of falls in the elderly population. The author presents recommendations for assessing a patient during an office visit for fall risk and offers interventions that can be used based on the deficits noted.

Classic Bibliography

Bemben MG: Age-related alterations in muscular endurance. *Sports Med* 1998;25:259-269.

Buckwalter JA: Aging and degeneration of the human intervertebral disc. *Spine* 1995;20:1307-1314.

Galea V: Changes in motor unit estimates with aging. *J Clin Neurophysiol* 1996;13:253-260.

Galloway MT, Jokl P: Aging successfully: The importance of physical activity in maintaining health and function. *J Am Acad Orthop Surg* 2000;8:37-44.

Hannan MT, Tucker KL, Sawson-Hughes B, Cupples LA, Felson DT, Kiel DP: Effect of dietary protein on bone loss in elderly men and women: The Framingham Osteoporosis Study. *J Bone Miner Res* 2000;15:2504-2512.

Martin PE, Grabiner MD: Aging, exercise, and the predisposition to falling. *J Appl Biomech* 1999;15:52-55.

Melton LJ: Epidemiology of hip fractures: Implications of the exponential increase with age. *Bone* 1996;18:121S-125S.

Nishida S, Endo N, Yamagiwa H, et al: Number of osteoprogenitor cells in human bone marrow markedly decreases after skeletal maturation. *J Bone Miner Metab* 1999;17:171-177.

Noyes FR, Grood ES: The strength of the anterior cruciate ligament in humans and rhesus monkeys: Age-related and species-related changes. *J Bone Joint Surg Am* 1976;58:1074-1082.

Quarto R, Thomas D, Liang CT: Bone progenitor cell deficits and the age-associated decline in bone repair capacity. *Calcif Tissue Int* 1995;56:123-129.

Sherman S: Human aging at the millennium, in Rosen CJ, Glowacki J, Bilizikian JP (eds): *The Aging Skeleton.* New York, NY, Academic Press, 1999, pp 11-18.

Taafe DR, Marcus R: Musculoskeletal health and the older adult. *J Rehabil Res Dev* 2000;37:245-254.

Woo SL-Y, Hollis JM, Adams DJ, et al: Tensile properties of the human femur-anterior cruciate ligament-tibia complex: The effects of specimen age and orientation. *Am J Sports Med* 1991;19:217-225.

Section 2

2

General Knowledge

Section Editors:
D. Greg Anderson, MD
Timothy R. Kuklo, MD, JD

Chapter 7

Managing Patient Complaints, Patient Rights and Safety

Sally C. Booker, BA

Nena Clark, MPA

Introduction

Equal in importance to the skills and knowledge of the medical practice of orthopaedics are the skills that an orthopaedic surgeon must have or develop to deal effectively with patients from a social and psychological perspective. Experts confirm what may seem obvious, that patients are unlikely to become involved in litigation with physicians whom they like. Also, the overall success of a physician's practice is highly linked to their ability to interact with patients on a social level.

Dealing with the disgruntled patient or family can be difficult. Even the most compassionate and skilled orthopaedic surgeon will encounter unhappy patients. It is important to examine the factors that lead to the problem and develop effective strategies for dealing with the disgruntled patient. New guidelines have been developed by patient advocacy groups, hospitals, and the federal government regarding patient rights and responsibilities, patient safety, and patient privacy and confidentiality.

The Social Side of Patient Care

A successful patient interaction often begins with appearance. A professional, well-groomed physician will foster patient confidence, whereas a disheveled or distracted physician may lead to a sense of distrust. Good manners and time-honored etiquette go a long way toward making a patient feel comfortable. Most importantly, the physician should always treat a patient with respect, dignity, courtesy, graciousness, and compassion.

The patient's interaction with office staff is equally important to the overall success of the medical experience. Patients look for continuity in communication and view office staff as an extension of the physician. Therefore, ensuring that office staff is fostering an environment that is patient-friendly is of paramount importance.

The Disgruntled Patient or Family

Physicians with excellent bedside manners will encounter unhappy patients, although less often than those physicians who are perceived as arrogant or uncaring. An understanding of the many factors that can lead to patient dissatisfaction is important because many situations can be prevented or addressed early, thus minimizing the degree of frustration. Repeated complaints should lead the physician to carefully analyze their approach to patients and make improvements in their practice.

A patient sometimes may be dealing with an array of emotions (sensitivities, embarrassments, fears, shame, anger, and antagonism) when interacting with the physician and staff. In addition, health problems produce psychological stress that can bring out traits the patient would not display in normal situations. Prolonged or painful conditions can lead to frustration and despair that heighten the patient's emotional response.

Remember that a patient's complaint is their perception of events and attitudes or, in other words, is the patient's version of the truth. When dealing with an angry patient, the physician should avoid becoming angry or defensive and remember that the patient's anger may be based in fear, loss of control, the feeling of being disrespected or misunderstood, personal issues unrelated to the medical situation, or an organic or psychiatric disorder.

Several identifiable factors contribute to patient complaints, such as inconsistency in communication, promises that are not kept, lack of sufficient details regarding the diagnosis and treatment plan, perceived rudeness, lack of understanding regarding known procedural/surgical complications, the perception that the physician and staff are too busy to be concerned with the patient's problem, long wait times, and frustration with the inability to "fix" a painful condition.

Complaint Avoidance

Complaint avoidance often begins with a well-run office. Avoiding long waits and working with courteous staff go a long way toward avoiding unhappy patients. The physician's behavior is also paramount in setting the stage for a positive patient interaction. The physi-

Table 1 | Template for Letter of Response to a Patient Complaint

Paragraph One

Acknowledge the complaint. Thank the patient for taking the time to express thoughts or concerns. Assure the patient that a complaint represents an opportunity for the physician to grow. Let the patient know that his/her concerns have been reviewed and discussed.

Paragraph Two

Address the issue. Explain clinical facts in a language the patient can understand. If appropriate, tell the patient what steps have been taken to avoid such an occurrence in the future. If the issue involves potential liability, a Risk Manager should be consulted before responding to the patient. Do not respond to the patient in anger.

Paragraph Three

Thank the patient again. Assure the patient that his or her feedback will or has been used to discuss the concern among staff, that the concern has given you the opportunity to examine your practices, service delivery, and others. Tell the patient that it is through patient feedback that your practice or institution can grow.

cian should be warm and cordial, balancing concern and interest. Generally, it is best for the physician to sit down and speak to the patient at their level.

The physician needs to be an excellent listener and if he/she senses a problem, it is generally best to address it immediately. A prompt response and action may solve the problem immediately and prevent the issue from deteriorating to a frustrating situation.

How to Manage a Patient Complaint

When a complaint cannot be avoided or diffused, it is important to know how to manage a formal complaint. The first thing to remember is that all complaints must be taken seriously. The physician is required by law to respond to all formal complaints in writing. Often additional information about the complaint is needed and may be obtained from the patient or an institutional patient representative. It is advisable at this time to provide the patient the phone numbers to the patient representative department and allow the patient to take the initiative to contact the department. The patient should be asked if he/she would like to receive a telephone call or a visit from the patient representative. It is always best to allow the patient to make the decision.

When speaking with dissatisfied patients, always listen attentively to their concern. Avoid the pitfalls of interrupting or becoming defensive. Acknowledge the patient's concerns, even if they are unreasonable. Provide accurate information to help clarify the situation. Be frank and honest. Avoid negative comments about other health care providers.

As with all medical care, documentation is vital when dealing with an unhappy patient. First, the medical assessment should be accurately performed and doc-

umented. Next, the nature of any discussions with the patient and the outcome of the discussion should be recorded. Finally, all serious complaints should be formalized by sending a written response. The Center for Medicare and Medicaid Services specifies as a condition of participation that all complaints be addressed with a written response to the patient in a timely manner. A formal letter provides acknowledgment of the complaint and furthers documents complaint management. When writing a letter, it is important to address the complaint frankly and courteously. In addition to providing the basis of good medical practice, accurate and detailed documentation is vital for cases that result in litigation.

To create a good system for complaint management, all complaints and records regarding their management should be kept in a secure location, and labeled "quality improvement" or "quality assurance". Surveys may be useful tools and provide feedback about issues of concern to patients that may never reach the formal complaint process. Complaints should be viewed as a process of learning or quality improvement for the physician and his/her practice.

Which Complaints Require a Written Response?

A formal written complaint requires a written response to the patient. A formal complaint is one where the patient explicitly asks that a written report be generated. A formal complaint also exists when there is a dispute about charges based on the patient's perception of quality of care. If the patient chooses to file a formal complaint, the patient representative in most health care organizations will record the patient's feelings and perceptions and submit that report to the attending physician in charge of the patient's care, or to the manager of the area where the problem occurred. The physician or his/her designee is then obligated to respond to the patient in writing (Table 1). In a teaching hospital, it is always preferable for the attending physician to respond to the patient rather than the medical or surgical resident.

Health Insurance Portability and Accountability Act of 1996

The Health Insurance Portability and Accountability Act of 1996 (HIPAA), Public Law 104-191 required the Secretary for the US Department of Health and Human Services to implement Sections 261 through 264 of HIPAA. The purpose of these sections, known as the Administrative Simplification provisions, is to improve the efficiency and effectiveness of the health care system by mandating national privacy standards to enable electronic exchange of consumers' health information. The Standards for Privacy of Individually Identifiable Health Information or the Privacy Rule requires cov-

Table 2 | What Privacy Rule Says About Disclosure of Protected Health Information

Uses and Disclosures of Patient Health Information	Situations
Required disclosures	To the individual (or individual's representative) who is the subject of information To Department of Health and Human Services during a compliance review, investigation or enforcement action
Permitted uses and disclosures (without an individual's authorization)	To the individual who is the subject of information For treatment, payment, and health care operations By simply asking for permission from the individual which then give the individual the opportunity to agree or object Use or disclosure of information incident to an already permitted use or disclosure of information as long as the covered entity has adopted reasonable safeguards and the release of information is limited to the minimum amount of protected health information needed to accomplish the pur pose as required by the Privacy Rule Public interest and benefit activities (eg, court order, serious threat to health or safety, essential government functions) Limited dataset for the purposes of research, public health or health care operation
No restriction	De-Identified Health Information (removal of individually identifiable health information)
Not covered under privacy rule	Employment records held or maintained by a covered entity as an employer Education and other records defined in the Family Educational Rights and Privacy Act

ered entities (such as health plans, health care clearinghouses, and health care providers) and its business associates to implement the national standards to protect the security and privacy of all individually identifiable health information. The Privacy Rule also requires covered entities to provide individuals an adequate notice of its privacy practices and a description of their individual rights. Furthermore, covered entities are to make a good faith effort to obtain a written acknowledgment of notice of receipt from the individual (Federal Register, 2002, p. 53182.).

Protected health information includes demographic information such as name, address, birth date, Social Security number, medical record number, and account numbers that relate to: (1) the individual's past, present, or future physical or mental health, or (2) the provisions of health care to the individual, or (3) the past, present, or future payment for the provision of health care to the individual. (Office of Civil Rights [OCR] Privacy Brief, 2003, p. 4). Table 2 presents information about uses and disclosures of Protected health information.

Enforcement of Compliance/Penalties for Noncompliance

Compliance with the Privacy Rule standards is voluntary. The OCR of the Department of Health and Human Services will perform the enforcement of compliance. The OCR will investigate reports of violation and covered entities will be subjected to progressive disciplinary actions to demonstrate compliance. The OCR may impose civil penalties of $100 for each act of noncompliance of the standards and up to $25,000 per year for multiple identical violations. However, for criminal penalties, the Department of Justice will perform the investigation, and may impose a fine depending on the severity of violation from $50,000 to $250,000 and imprisonment of 1 to 5 years (OCR Privacy Brief, 2003, pp 17-18).

Patient Safety Issues

The Joint Commission on Accreditation of Healthcare Organizations (JCAHO) is the major accrediting agency for hospitals. In 1996, JCAHO developed a sentinel-event reporting policy that encouraged an accredited health care organization to voluntarily report sentinel events within 5 days and to submit a root cause analysis within 45 days following discovery. JCAHO expects health care organizations to perform root cause analyses of systems and processes of the organization rather than the performance of individuals. JCAHO defines a sentinel event as "an unexpected occurrence involving death or serious physical or psychological injury or the risk for which a recurrence would carry a significant chance of a serious adverse outcome."

Based on the root cause analyses of sentinel events reported by accredited organizations, JCAHO has identified the need to establish national patient safety goals (Table 3). JCAHO intends to reevaluate the national patient safety goals every year. The goals are to be announced in July of each year and to become effective in January of the following year. In July 2002, JCAHO announced the first National Patient Safety Goals, and in January 1, 2003, all accredited health care organizations were required to comply with the established patient safety goals and its corresponding recommendations. JCAHO will allow accredited organizations to implement alternatives to specific recommendations as long as the alternative is as effective as the original recommendation in achieving a specific patient safety goal. Accredited organizations may submit alternative approaches by completing a "Request for Review of an Alternative Approach to a National Patient Safety Goal Requirement" form available on the JCAHO Website: http://www.jcaho.org/accredited+organizations/patient+safety/04+npsg/04_npsg_altform.htm.

Table 3 | 2005 National Patient Safety Goals

National Patient Safety Goal	Associated Recommendation	Suggestions for Compliance
Improve the accuracy of patient identification	Use at least two patient identifiers (neither to be the patient's room number) when taking blood samples or administering medications or blood products.	Possible identifiers include: Patient's name Patient's birth date Patient's medical record number Patient's Social Security number Patient's address Example: Ask patient to state his or her name and verify identification with the patient's wrist band. Name and identification number on the patient's wrist band should be verified and compared with the name and identification number on the ordered service.
	Prior to start of any surgical or invasive procedure, conduct a final verification process, such as "time-out," to confirm the correct patient, procedure, and site, using active—not passive—communication techniques.	All activities in the operating room should cease in order for all members of the surgical team to participate. The surgeon or the circulating nurse must state aloud the patient's name, type of surgery, and location of surgery, as stated in the patient's informed consent form. All members of the surgical team should respond orally to affirm that the patient's name, procedure, and location of surgery are correct.
Improve the effectiveness of communication among caregivers	Implement a process for taking verbal or telephone orders that require a verification "read-back" of the complete order by the person receiving the order.	Apply to all verbal or telephone orders (not just for medication orders) including all critical test results that are reported verbally or by telephone. Read-back requirements apply to all including physicians. The National Coordinating Council for Medication Error Reporting and Prevention has made recommendations for improving the use of verbal orders, some of which are: Verbal orders should be limited to urgent situations Entire verbal orders should be repeated back to the prescriber. Verbal orders should be documented in the patient's medical record, reviewed, and countersigned by the prescriber as soon as possible
	Standardize the abbreviations, acronyms, symbols not to use.	JCAHO has released a "do not use" list of abbreviations such as: U should be written as "unit" IU should be written as "international unit" Q.D., QOD should be written as "daily" and "every other day" Never write a zero by itself after a decimal point (for example, 1.0 mg). Trailing zero after decimal point can be mistaken as 10 mg if the decimal point is not seen. Always use a zero before a decimal point (for example, 0.5 mg). Lack of leading zero before a decimal dose (for example, 0.5 mg) can be mistaken as 5 mg if the decimal point is not seen. MS, MSO_4, $MgSO_4$ should be written as "morphine sulfate" or "magnesium sulfate" The Institute for Safe Medication Practices has also published a list of dangerous abbreviations and is available on the Website at: http://www.ismp.org/MSAarticles/improve.htm

Table 3 CONTINUED | 2005 National Patient Safety Goals

National Patient Safety Goal	Associated Recommendation	Suggestions for Compliance
Improve the safety of using high-alert medications	Remove concentrated electrolytes (including, but not limited to, potassium chloride, potassium phosphate, sodium chloride > 0.9%) from patient care units. Standardize and limit the number of drug concentrations available in the organization.	Applies to all concentrated electrolytes
Eliminate wrong site, wrong patient, wrong procedure surgery	Create and use a preoperative verification process, such as a checklist, to confirm that appropriate documents are available such as medical records and imaging studies.	Applies to all invasive procedures performed in the operating room or special procedures unit (for example, endoscopy unit, interventional radiology) that exposes patients to more than minimal risk (exception: venipuncture, peripheral intravenous line placement, placement of nasogastric tube or Foley catheter).
	Implement a process to mark the surgical site and involve the patient in the marking process	Marking the site is required for procedures involving right or left distinction and multiple structures (fingers, toes) or levels (spinal procedures). The American Academy of Orthopaedic Surgeons has developed a checklist for safety called the "Sign Your Site" initiative that involves patients to watch and confirm as the surgeon marks the surgical site. The checklist is available on the Website: http://www.aaos.org/wordhtml/papers/advistmt/1015.htm
Improve the safety of using infusion pumps	Ensure free-flow protection on all general-use and patient controlled analgesia intravenous infusion pumps used in the organization.	
Improve the effectiveness of clinical alarm systems	Implement regular preventive maintenance and testing of alarm systems.
Assure that alarms are activated with appropriate settings and are sufficiently audible with respect to distances and competing noise within the unit.	
Reduce the risk of health care-acquired infections	Comply with current Centers for Disease Control and Prevention (CDC) hand hygiene guidelines	Each of the CDC guidelines is categorized on the basis of the strength of evidence supporting the recommendation. All category I must be implemented for accreditation purposes. Examples include:
When hands are visibly dirty or contaminated, wash hands with a nonantimicrobial soap and water or an antimicrobial soap and water.
If hands are not visibly soiled, use an alcohol-based hand rub for routinely decontaminating hands in all other clinical situations.
Decontaminate hands before having direct contact with patients.
Decontaminate hands after contact with a patient's intact skin, nonintact skin, body fluids or excretions, mucous membranes, and wound dressings.
Decontaminate hands after removing gloves.
Before eating and after using a restroom, wash hands with a non-antimicrobial soap and water or with an antimicrobial soap and water.
The full report on the CDC guidelines is available on the Website: http://www.cdc.gov/mmwr/preview/mmwrhtml/rr5116a1.htm
	Manage as sentinel events all identified cases of unanticipated death or major permanent loss of function associated with a health care-acquired infection.	This is already required for any outcomes that resulted in unanticipated death or major permanent loss of function.

Table 4 | Consumer Bill of Rights

General Principles	Consumer Rights
Information disclosure	Consumers have the right to receive accurate and easily understood information about health plan, health care professionals, and health care facilities. Suggestions for health care organizations to ensure this right: Provide reasonable accommodation to meet the needs of patients with language barrier, physical or mental disability. Health care providers educational preparation (eg, education, board certification, recertification) and appropriate experience in performing procedures and services. Performance measures such as consumer satisfaction. Provide complaints and appeals processes.
Choice of providers and plans	Consumers have the right to a choice of health care providers that is sufficient to ensure access to appropriate high-quality health care. Suggestion for health plans to ensure this right: Provide sufficient numbers and types of providers to encompass all covered services.
Access to emergency services	Consumers have the right to access emergency health care services when and where the need arises. Health plans should provide payment when a consumer presents to an emergency department with acute symptoms of sufficient severity - including severe pain - such than a "prudent layperson" could reasonably expect the absence of medical attention to result in placing that consumer's health in serious jeopardy, serious impairment to bodily functions, or serious dysfunction of any bodily organ or part. Suggestions to ensure this right: Health plans to educate their members about availability, location, and appropriate use of emergency and other medical services. Emergency department personnel to contact the patient's primary care provider or health plan as quickly as possible to discuss continuity of care.
Participation in treatment decisions	Consumers have the right and responsibility to fully participate in all decisions related to their health care. Consumers who are unable to fully participate in treatment decisions have the right to be represented by parents, guardians, family members, or other conservators. Suggestions for health care organizations/health care providers to ensure this right: Provide patients with easily understood information and opportunity to decide among treatment options consistent with informed consent. Provide effective communication with health care providers for patients with disabilities. Respect the decisions made by patients and/or representatives consistent with the informed consent process.
Respect and nondiscrimination	Consumers have the right to considerate, respectful care from all members of the health care system at all times and under all circumstances. An environment of mutual respect is essential to maintain a quality health care system. Suggestion for health care organizations to ensure this right: Provide health care services to patients consistent with the benefits covered in their policy or as required by law based on race, ethnicity, national origin, religion, sex, age, mental or physical disability, sexual orientation, genetic information, or source of payment.
Confidentiality of health information	Consumers have the right to communicate with health care providers in confidence and to have the confidentiality of their individually identifiable health care information protected. Consumers also have the right to review and copy their own medical records and request amendments to their records. Suggestion to ensure this right: Compliance with the Privacy Rule standards.
Complaints and appeals	Consumers have the right to a fair and efficient process for resolving differences with their health plans, health care providers, and the institutions that serve them, including a rigorous system of internal review and an independent system of external review. Suggestion to ensure this right: Internal and external appeals systems and procedures should be made available to patients and resolution should be performed in a timely manner and/or consistent as required by Medicare (eg, 72 hours).

Table 4 CONTINUED | Consumer Bill of Rights

General Principles	Consumer Rights
Consumer responsibility	Some of the consumer's responsibilities include: Maximizing health habits, such as exercising, not smoking, and eating a healthy diet Become involved in specific health care decisions Work collaboratively with health care providers in developing and carrying out agreed upon treatment plans Disclose relevant information and clearly communicate wants and needs Use the health plan's internal complaint and appeal processes to address concerns that may arise Avoid knowingly spreading disease Become knowledgeable about his or her health plan coverage and health plan options (when available) including all covered benefits, limitations, and exclusions, rules regarding the use of network providers, coverage and referral rules, appropriate processes to secure additional information, and the process to appeal coverage decisions Show respect for other patients and health workers Make a good-faith effort to meet financial obligations

Patient Rights and Safety

The Advisory Commission on Consumer Protection and Quality in Health Care Industry, appointed by President Clinton in 1997, drafted a "consumer bill of rights." Health care organizations, both public and private, have adopted the general principles as cited in the consumer bill of rights (Table 4).

Annotated Bibliography

Bartlett EE: Physician stress management: A new approach to reducing medical errors and liability risk. *J Health Care Risk Manag* 2002;22:3-6.

This article focuses on the scope and effects of medical stress, conceptual approaches to physician stress control, and stress reduction programs, resources, and research. The author concludes that stress reduction programs can result in better patient relations, improved clinical performance, fewer medical errors, and reduced malpractice risk.

Danner C: Working with angry patients. *Behavioral Medicine Brief, Department of Family Practice and Community Health.* Minneapolis, MN, Family Medicine and Community Health, University of Minnesota, Issue 19, 2001.

This article discusses how anger can influence the physician-patient relationship. A three-step model for physicians for effective physical and mental management of critical and angry patients is outlined. The need for the physician to successfully manage anger in order to avoid a malpractice suit and compromised patient care are also discussed.

Hickson GB, Federspiel CF, Pichert JW, Miller CS, Gauld-Jaeger J, Bost P: Patient complaints and malpractice risk. *JAMA* 2002;287:2951-2957.

The topic of this article is physicians who receive a large number of malpractice claims, resulting in high costs. The

premise that a physician's bedside manner and interpersonal skills can help influence patient satisfaction is discussed.

Joint Commission on Accreditation of Health Care Organizations web site: 2004 National Patient Safety Goals. Available at: http://www.jcaho.org/. Accessed December 18, 2003.

The JCAHO's National Patient Safety Goals are listed, which were developed as a result of lessons learned from sentinel events reported by health care organizations.

National Coordinating Council for Medication Error Reporting and Prevention web site: February 20, 2001. Available at: http://www.nccmerp.org/council/council 2001-02-20.html. Accessed December 18, 2003.

Valuable information and recommendations on how to reduce medication errors related to labeling and packaging of drugs and other related products, verbal orders and prescriptions, dispensing of drugs, and drug administration are presented.

Sage WM: Putting the patient in safety: Linking patient complaints and malpractice risk. *JAMA* 2002;287:3003-3005.

Customer satisfaction is connected to clinical safety. Health care organizations should document information from patients relevant to patient safety and provide that information to health care professionals who manage and provide health care.

US Department of Health and Human Services web site: Office for Civil Rights. OCR Privacy Brief: Summary of the HIPAA Privacy Rule. Washington, DC, GPO, May 2003. Available at: http://www.hhs.gov/ocr/privacysummary.pdf. Accessed August 8, 2003.

A summary of the HIPAA Privacy Rule such as statutory and regulatory background, who is covered by the Privacy Rule, what information is protected, general principles for usage and disclosures, and enforcement and penalties for noncompliance is presented.

US Department of Health and Human Services web site: Office of the Secretary. 45 CFR Parts 160 and 164 Standards for Privacy of Individually Identifiable Health Information; Final Rule. Federal Register. Washington, DC, GPO, August 14, 2002. Available at: http://www.hhs.gov/ocr/hipaa/privrulepd.pdf. Accessed August 8, 2003.

The entire document of the rules and regulations for the Privacy Rule released by the Department of Health and Human Services is presented.

President's Advisory Commission on Consumer Protection and Quality in the Health Care Industry web site: Consumer Bill of Rights and Responsibilities. Executive Summary. Washington, DC, GPO, November 1997. Available at: http://www.hcqualitycommission.gov/cborr/exsumm.html. Accessed August 3, 2003.

A summary of the Consumer Bill of Rights and Responsibilities is presented.

Wang EC: Dealing with the angry patient. *Permanante J* 2003;7:77-78.

Communication skills for physicians faced with an angry patient are discussed, along with insight on what steps might be taken for management of this situation.

Classic Bibliography

Levinson W, Roter DL, Mullooly JP, Dull VT, Frankel RM: Physician-patient communication: The relationship with malpractice claims among primary care physicians and surgeons. *JAMA* 1997;277:553-559.

Rogers C: Communicate, in *The American Academy of Orthopaedic Surgeons, Bulletin.* Rosemont, IL, 2003, vol 48, No 6.

Chapter 8

Selected Ethical Issues in Orthopaedic Surgery

Angelique M. Reitsma, MD, MA

Kornelis A. Poelstra, MD, PhD

Surgical Ethics in the 21st Century

Ethical values that guide surgeons toward concrete actions in the care of patients are provided by ethicists and by the professional surgical societies. The ethical principles of beneficence, nonmalfeasance, respect for autonomy, and justice were first presented in 1979 as part of the framework known as principlism. Attention is given in the literature to virtue as an additional moral value to be considered. This renewed interest in virtue as an ethical requirement is one that is in concert with surgeons' perceptions of what it means to be a moral physician. Professional societies such as the American College of Surgeons (ACS) and the American Academy of Orthopaedic Surgeons (AAOS) have adopted statements referring to an honorable surgeon's character. The AAOS adopted ten Principles of Medical Ethics and Professionalism in Orthopaedic Surgery, first in 1991 and most recently revised in 2002. The principles are considered standards of conduct, not laws, defining the essentials of appropriate behavior.

Perceptions of a moral physician's conduct have shifted somewhat during the past century. For example, paternalism was perfectly acceptable in medical and surgical practice for many years, but since the mid 1960s has been considered a breach of patient autonomy. Major improvements in respecting a patient's autonomy were also made in the area of human subject research. Currently, it would be unthinkable to enroll a patient or a healthy volunteer into a clinical trial without their informed consent, a requirement that was not obvious to early investigators. As will be discussed later, informed consent for some types of surgical research is still not uniform and is an issue for orthopaedic surgeons to consider carefully.

In some areas of medicine the patient is the sole medical decision maker, with the physician as mere counselor, offering a virtual and perhaps overwhelming assortment of available therapies. In surgical situations, this approach is not always feasible, because some of the decision making occurs while the patient is unconscious and incapable of making decisions. As procedures become increasingly complex and consent forms get longer, truly informed consent may seem a distant goal.

Perceptions of what constitutes physical harm have also changed, albeit in many separate and perhaps less obvious ways. Therapies that were once state-of-the-art may now be considered obsolete and perhaps even harmful. As new evidence about outcomes became available, procedures have been reshaped or abandoned. Evidence-based surgery continues to expand. It is no longer sufficient to offer a procedure to a patient merely based on good intentions without some evidence of benefit. Although modern surgery demands scientific evidence, this requirement is not always so easy to comply with. Although drugs can be tested in a randomized controlled trial using a placebo for the control, surgeons must invent more intricate and sometimes more invasive placebos. Although challenging this goal is not impossible, the use of sham surgery is not without controversy. Despite strong criticism of such research designs, it must be conceded that surgical controls are a difficult issue and surgery itself can possibly have quite a strong placebo effect.

Some predicted developments in the future of surgery are dazzling and will pose new moral challenges. One example is the use of computers and robotics to enhance surgical precision and safety. These technologies raise ethical questions about training (Who is qualified to operate such devices, and how much expertise is required?), responsibility (Who is responsible for operating the device, who is legally responsible for breakdowns?), and perhaps even fears of too much dependence on machinery (What if it breaks down? Should the surgeon be skilled to perform the procedure without it? Or will the procedure be abandoned?).

Other advances will challenge conventional thinking. As discussed in a recent article, some of these developments include human cloning, genetic engineering, tissue engineering, limb morphogenesis, intelligent robotics, nanotechnology, suspended animation, regeneration, and species prolongation. The potential of these new technologies to disrupt conventional surgical thinking is huge. Of direct impact on orthopaedics in the 21st century are the ethical issues concerning tissue engineering, regeneration, and intelligent prostheses. Bioartificial skin and blood vessel segments already can be found in laboratories. The anticipated long-term goal is the regeneration of body parts, such as parts of limbs and eventually, complete prostheses. Will the orthopaedic surgeons of the future simply replace a diseased hip joint, intervertebral disk, or leg with a new one? To approach these new technologies, an ethical framework will be required.

Ethical Approaches to a Patient Dilemma

Every day, physicians are faced with different dilemmas in patient care. These vary from simple issues such as ordering diagnostic tests or surgical scheduling to more complex issues involving decisions about terminal illnesses and withdrawal of treatment. Deciding on the morally best course can be challenging. Although it is impossible to provide formulaic answers to every ethical dilemma encountered in clinical practice, ethical theories can guide the orthopaedic surgeon in moral decision making. An actual case is presented to illustrate the prominent ethical theories and to serve as an example of how to work through the nuances of ethical thinking.

The Case

Mr. B is an 87-year-old man who has severe injuries, but no head, severe chest, or abdominal injuries, after a head-on motor vehicle collision. He is transferred to a Level 1 trauma center. However, he has several severe orthopaedic injuries, including bilateral grade IIIB open pilon and segmental tibial shaft fractures, a right closed tibial plateau fracture, a displaced femoral neck fracture, and a left closed supracondylar femur fracture. He also has bilateral comminuted foot fractures and dominant right arm fractures. Prior to the accident he had lived independently, close to his only daughter.

Mr. B undergoes emergent irrigation and débridement and A-frame external fixator placement of both legs. He is then transferred, while intubated and in stable condition, to the surgical intensive care unit for further management. A durable power of attorney had been granted to his daughter. She is contacted to obtain consent for urgent right below-knee amputation, repeat irrigation and débridement of the left ankle with possible amputation, and hemiarthroplasty replacement of the right hip. Despite repeated requests, she strongly refuses to give approval for any further interventions that could prolong her father's life, despite the understanding of the severity of the open fractures and the risk for sepsis or pulmonary complications. She states that she and her father had discussed his wishes many years before, and he had expressed his desire to die at home without any nursing home care or dependency on a ventilator for a prolonged period of time.

The patient is extubated 2 days after the index procedures. Severe tissue necrosis becomes apparent at the open wounds on both legs. He is unable to tolerate elevation of the head of the bed more than 30° because of hip pain. Although he recognized his daughter, the patient remains poorly oriented to place and time and coherent conversations with the patient remain very difficult. The Mini-Mental Status Examination is consistent with early dementia.

Controversy about the management of this case causes moral distress among staff and leads to heated discussions. Therefore, a meeting with the ethics committee is requested. Two designees of the committee, a lawyer from the Department of Risk Management and a psychiatrist not involved in the case, are present. During this meeting, the daughter continues to strongly refuse consent for further treatment, stating that 'those were his wishes'. Although sympathetic to the surgeons' plight, the attorney states that it would be legally inadvisable to continue with the surgical intervention as the patient's earlier wishes were conveyed by the power of attorney, and it is impossible to clearly establish whether he had any decisional capacity to counter this. A surgeon on the committee thought the attorney's advice to be 'outrageous', stating that not treating this patient amounted to 'torturing the patient to death'.

Discussion

The approaches that dominate the ethical literature are deontology and utilitarianism. In addition to these two major moral philosophies, clinical ethics cannot be understood without taking into account the principles of biomedical ethics: self-determination, beneficence, nonmaleficence, and justice. Important ethical principles are listed and defined in Table 1.

The deontologic approach is also called 'duty-based ethics', considering the duties that people have toward one another. In this case, it is reminiscent of the familiar notion that the surgeon has certain special duties toward the care of the patient with whom a therapeutic relationship has been established. From a strictly deontologic point of view, the right approach would be for the orthopaedists to perform the surgeries they believe are indicated, as it is their duty as Mr. B's treating physicians to give him the necessary treatments. This is what the orthopaedic surgeons in this case suggested be done and requested consent for, to no avail, leading to the ethical controversy in the first place.

The utilitarianism approach is the view that actions are to be morally evaluated according to the amount of well being they promote. This approach is consistent with preoccupation with the outcomes or consequences of an intervention, and is why one treatment is recommended over another if it is more likely to provide a desired result. Although this approach has been criticized for its "the ends justify the means" image, utilitarianism must be taken into account in public policy as it strives to emphasize the social consequences of an action. In the case of Mr. B, the utilitarian approach may suggest that the intervention is not warranted if the results cannot be expected to be favorable. Of course, exactly what the outcome of an intervention will be is not always clear, leading to controversy such as in the present case.

Self-determination or respect for autonomy is expressed through an informed consent process. By giving an informed consent, the patient chooses the treatment that they wish according to his or her own values. If a patient is not capable of making or of communicating decisions and if an advance directive is not available, a surrogate must make treatment decisions on behalf of the patient. In this case, Mr. B was considered decisionally incapacitated. His daughter was the indicated surrogate decision maker as having been appointed by the durable power of attorney. Even if she had not been appointed by the patient, the daughter would have probably been the obvious surrogate by legal standards as the closest next of kin. Although in the absence of written advance directives it is not possible to know without a doubt what a patient would have wanted, the durable power of attorney is designed to convey previously uttered (verbal) wishes. In this case, respecting the patient's autonomous decision implies that the request for withholding further surgery should be honored.

If Mr. B's prior wishes were unknown, his daughter could have used the best-interest standard to make decisions on his behalf. The best interest for a patient is calculated by weighing the benefits against the burdens of treatment. From a legal perspective, it is unlikely that Mr. B (or his daughter) would be forced to continue with the surgical treatment against his wishes. If the daughter had wanted to continue aggressive limb salvage treatment despite a limited chance of success it is likely that that decision, too, would have been respected. Increasingly, however, physicians are questioning their responsibilities to patients in situations where they consider the intervention to have no medical benefit.

Beneficence, or the obligation to do good for the patient, is closely related to the traditional Hippocratic obligation to avoid harm, or the principle of nonmaleficence. The discussion of beneficence here will include nonmaleficence. In this case, a beneficent act might constitute the amputation of both lower extremities to prevent pain and possibly reduce the risk for septicemia.

Justice is the point of reference for discussion of access to health care and of distribution of (scarce) resources as a matter of social policy, and will be left out of the discussion in this case.

In the case of Mr. B, it was decided to honor the verbal advance directive given to the daughter. Plans were developed to provide sufficient medication and pallia-

Table 1	Principles of Biomedical Ethics

The four clusters of moral basic principles that guide ethics are:

Respect for autonomy	A norm of respecting the decision-making capacity of autonomous persons. This principle is expressed by the doctrine of informed consent.
Nonmaleficence	A norm of avoiding the causation of harm. This principle requires intentionally refraining from actions that cause harm, and is expressed by: "One ought not to inflict evil or harm."
Beneficence	A group of norms for providing benefits and balancing benefits against risks and costs. This principle is expressed by: "One ought to prevent evil or harm; one ought to remove evil or harm; and one ought to do or promote good."
Justice	A group of norms for distributing benefits, risks, and costs fairly. Applicable to both medical care and biomedical research with human subjects.

Two relevant moral philosophical theories that further guide decision making in biomedical ethics are:

Utilitarianism	A consequence-based moral theory holding that actions are right or wrong according to the balance of their good and bad consequences. The right act in any circumstance is the one that produces the best overall result, as determined from an impersonal perspective.
Deontology	A duty-based moral theory holding that some features of actions other than or in addition to consequences make actions right or wrong.

tion to ensure the patient's comfort during the following days in the hospital.

The Role of the Institutional Review Board in Modern Orthopaedics

According to the Department of Health and Human Services, "research" is defined as any systematic investigation designed to develop and contribute to general knowledge. "Human subject" is defined as a living individual about whom an investigator obtains either (1) data through interaction or intervention (such as surgery), or (2) identifiable private information. Research involving human subjects is socially important but morally perilous because it can expose subjects to risks for the advancement of science. Ethically justifiable research must satisfy several conditions, including (1) a reasonable prospect that the research will generate the knowledge that is sought, (2) the necessity of using human subjects, and (3) a favorable balance of potential benefits over risks to the subjects, and (4) fair selection of subjects. Only after these conditions have been met is it appropriate to ask potential subjects to participate.

Assessing if a proposed study met all the criteria above was initially left to the discretion of the physician-investigator, but the dual roles of research scientist and clinical practitioner pull in different directions and present conflicting obligations and interest, endangering the objectivity of the assessment. Therefore, the responsibility to assess the morality of clinical research was given to outside reviewers. In its 1989 revision of the Declaration of Helsinki, the World Medical Association sets as the international standard for biomedical research involving human subjects this requirement: "Each experimental procedure involving human subjects should be clearly formulated in an experimental protocol which should be transmitted for consideration, comment and guidance to a specially appointed committee independent of the investigator and sponsor."

The purpose of the Institutional Review Board (IRB) is to ensure that research with human volunteers is designed to conform to the relevant ethical standards. These standards concern protecting the rights and welfare of individual research subjects, ensuring voluntary informed consent is obtained before participation in a study, and an evaluation of risks and benefits. Since 1978, an additional moral standard has been added by the National Commission for the Protection of Human Subjects of Biomedical and Behavioral Research (The National Commission). The Commission's "Belmont Report" required IRBs to guarantee equity in the selection and recruitment of human subjects.

Across the United States, IRBs may have local names, such as "Human Investigations Committee" or "Committee for Research Subject Protection," and have a decidedly local character, although they are required to comply with federal regulations when reviewing activities involving Food and Drug Administration-regulated investigational drugs or devices, and when reviewing research supported by federal funds. Furthermore, all institutions that receive federal research grants and contracts are required to file a "statement of assurance" of compliance with federal regulations. In these assurances virtually all institutions voluntarily promise to apply the principles of federal regulations to all research they conduct, regardless of the source of funding.

The IRB system has long been subject to criticism, accused of stifling creativity and impeding progress. In many institutions, there is a paucity of surgeons that sit on IRBs, thus risking that decisions about surgical studies will be made with insufficient surgical knowledge. IRBs have also been accused by bioethicists and patient advocates of providing inadequate protection to prospective research subjects. Even the US federal government criticized the work of several IRBs through its Office of Human Research Protections (OHRP). The OHRP was reconstituted by the Department of Health and Human Services in 2002 and is responsible for improving the system of oversight and enforcing the departments' regulations.

Regardless of the criticism they endure, IRBs are currently the only formal and federal mechanism to safeguard the interests of human research subjects. As such, they are an important line of protection to safeguard human participants of clinical research. Most IRBs have a home page on their institution's Website, on which they provide information and submission forms to download and complete.

Although the regulations for submitting research proposals to an IRB are fairly straightforward, uncertainties remain as to what protocols should and should not be reviewed. This is especially the case among clinicians who do not regularly perform research with human participants. One common false assumption is that retrospective studies do not require IRB review. Retrospective studies whose results are to be published or otherwise professionally shared do need to be reviewed by an IRB. Another common misperception is that a study that is likely to be exempt does not have to be reviewed. Officially, only an IRB can make the determination that a study is exempt from full review, although many IRBs will have an expedited review process for studies that are exempt. The important principle to remember is that all human research should be submitted for IRB review, whether it entails a simple chart review or an extensive intervention.

Another area of debate is the use of innovative or experimental surgery. The introduction of surgical innovations frequently occurs under the header of therapeutic intervention, without protocols or consents. This scenario has the potential to produce an "informal study" without specific study consent, which is currently being examined by the surgical and ethical communities alike. In the future, federal regulations or at least professional standards will likely be developed to address this area of surgery to ensure that new innovations are conducted with appropriate protection of human subjects while promoting research and technical advances within the field. Presently, the issue of what constitutes a significant enough innovation as to require an ethical review or specific consent is left to the discretion of the surgeon.

New Technology in Orthopaedic Surgery

Developing new technologies has been the driving force for improvement in surgery. Innovation is necessary if future gains in patient care are desired. Orthopaedists are among the most innovative surgeons in the United States; therefore, attention needs to be paid to the ethics of innovation in orthopaedic surgery. This seems especially important given the promise of emerging new technologies such as cell therapy or the use of growth factors, for which there currently are no clear federal regulations, nor are there any clear guidelines pertaining to innovative surgical procedures.

On a professional level, some attempts have been made to address the issue. The ACS has adopted self-imposed guidelines for emerging surgical technologies and their application to the care of patients, as formulated by the Committee on Emerging Surgical Technologies and Education. The introduction of new technology to surgeons and the public must be done ethically in accordance with the ACS Statement on Principles. These Principles require prior and continued IRB (or equivalent) review of the protocol, full description of the procedure, and informed consent of the patient.

As major innovators, orthopaedic surgeons should assume an active role in thinking through the issue of new surgical technologies. By doing so, orthopaedists can provide practical guidance for their colleagues as well as take on a leadership role within the entire surgical community. Differing views often exist on how to best introduce surgical innovations in an ethically responsible way. Although there is no uniform policy to date, some truths appear valid and of practical use to the innovative orthopaedic surgeon. First, the innovator should be familiar with existing rules and regulations that govern human subject research, and know if and when an innovation is in fact a research activity. This determination includes the question of whether IRB submission and the patient's informed consent is necessary. When a proposed surgical procedure falls short of being definite research but yet is experimental in a narrower sense, or when expected risks are deemed significant or risks and benefits are largely unknown because of the very novelty of the procedure, additional precautions appear prudent and moral. Reasonable precautions are prior consultation (for example, with peers, surgeon-in-chief, and department chair or division head) and full disclosure of the experimental nature of the procedure to the patient with perhaps a separate consent form. It would also be necessary to carefully monitor the outcome of the new technology, if only to assess if further formal evaluation in a trial would be warranted.

Other Selected Ethical Issues in Orthopaedics

The HIV-Positive or Hepatitis B- or C-Positive Health Care Worker

There still is considerable debate concerning the management of health care workers infected with hepatitis B virus (HBV), hepatitis C virus (HCV), or human immunodeficiency virus (HIV). In 1991, the Centers for Disease Control and Prevention (CDC) issued guidelines for health care workers infected with HBV or HIV. These guidelines set restrictions that still apply today. The CDC's guidelines were established with the premise that the risk for transmission of HBV and HIV to patients is greatest during certain definable "exposure-prone" procedures. Exposure-prone proce-

dures include insertion of a needle tip into a body cavity, or the simultaneous presence of a health care worker's fingers and a needle or other sharp object in a highly confined anatomic site. Health care workers who are positive for HIV or HBV should not perform exposure-prone procedures unless they have obtained expert counsel regarding the circumstances under which they may perform such procedures. Furthermore, health care workers should inform patients of their infection status before conducting exposure-prone procedures. Arguably, there are some limitations to the CDC recommendations. First, they do not specify exposure-prone procedures, leaving such determinations to the "expert counsel," allowing for a diversity of opinions and decisions impacting individual infected surgeons or health care workers. In addition, there are no recommendations that restrict professional activities of health care workers infected with HCV, although five cases of viral transmission from health care workers to patient have been documented to date. Of these cases of viral transmission, three involved surgeons; one gynecologist and two cardiac surgeons. Perhaps the most important shortcoming is that serostatus disclosure as proposed by the CDC does not improve patient safety, while it violates physician privacy.

In addition to the CDC recommendations, other professional societies such as the American Cancer Society, American Medical Association (AMA), and AAOS have issued guidelines. Unfortunately, most guidelines offer no, minimal, or fairly nonspecific guidance as to what constitutes exposure-prone procedures. Also, the issue of disclosure to patients remains controversial. Most organizations do not recognize a need for disclosure; some guidelines still favor either postexposure or preprocedure disclosure and/or identification of the source of infection. It has been argued that the law should not require health care workers to disclose their HIV status (or HBV or HCV status) because this is seen as an invasion of privacy.

Regardless of the ongoing controversy, some relevant experiential information is available to the HIV- or HCV-infected orthopaedic surgeon. The AAOS provides practical guidance for HIV-, HBV-, and HCV-infected orthopaedic surgeons to ensure the maximum safety of the patient. Orthopaedic surgeons infected with HCV should always follow strict aseptic technique and vigorously adhere to universal precautions. In addition, they should seek medical evaluation and treatment to prevent chronic liver disease. Specific recommendations for the prevention of HCV transmission from infected health care workers may be developed as more is learned about the virus and its associated risks. HIV carries a lower risk of transmission than either HBV or HCV. There are only two known cases of HIV transmission occurring from an infected health care worker to a patient, and one instance where transmission is suspected. In 1990, a cluster of six patients was infected by a dentist in Florida. In 1997, an orthopaedic surgeon in France transmitted HIV to one of his patients during a total hip joint arthroplasty. A third case where transmission is suspected concerns an instance of HIV transmission from an infected nurse to a surgical patient in France.

Although current data indicate that the risk of transmitting a blood-borne pathogen in a health care setting is exceedingly low, some risk is still present. The orthopaedic surgeon should therefore be familiar with the established guidelines of the CDC and the AAOS. It is important that all recommendations to prevent the transmission of blood-borne pathogens are consistently followed. In general, the guidelines for preventing transmission from patients to health care workers also apply to preventing transmission from health care workers to patients. Additionally, health care workers are encouraged to know their own HBV, HCV, and HIV infection statuses. Voluntary and confidential testing of health care workers for blood-borne pathogens is recommended. Preventing injuries to health care workers and subsequent blood exposure to patients offers the greatest level of protection. Health care workers who have preexisting conditions, such as exudative lesions or weeping dermatitis, should refrain from direct patient care until the condition is resolved. The affected health care worker should also refrain from handling patient-care equipment and devices used to perform invasive procedures. If a member of a surgical team is injured during a procedure, the instrument responsible should be removed from the surgical field without being reused on the patient until appropriately resterilized. Additionally, any disposable items that come into contact with a health care worker's blood should be removed from the surgical field and discarded into an appropriate biohazard bag or container.

Finally, it is advisable for any orthopaedic surgeon infected with HIV or HCV to seek expert legal counsel in addition to medical treatment. An infected surgeon may encounter problems with malpractice insurability, even while in remission and expected to practice. Also, legal charges have been leveled against seropositive surgeons by former patients, even in the absence of infection, claiming psychological stress.

Care of the Uninsured Patient

The AAOS Opinion on Ethics and Professionalism: Care and Treatment of the Medically Underserved, originally formulated in 1998 and recently revised, discusses the dismal health care insurance situation in the United States, noting that increasing percentages of Americans are uninsured, underinsured, and have inadequate access to medical care. The obligations of society and the medical profession to treat the medically underserved

are also discussed. These recommendations are based on the 1993 AMA Council on Ethical and Judicial Affairs guideline.

Also noted in the document, it is stated that physicians should be encouraged to devote some time to the provision of care for individuals who have no means of paying.

Caring for the uninsured, however, can have a considerable impact on the orthopaedic surgeon's practice. One challenge surgeons encounter when attending to the uninsured or underinsured is how to discuss treatment plans. According to the literature, the economic constraints on the available care are beyond the physician's control, yet they raise specific ethical issues for the physician. The question is whether the physician is obligated to disclose all potentially beneficial medical treatment, even the ones that exceed ordinary standards of care, and which probably will be unaffordable or unavailable.

Another more pressing problem is the question of how much care an orthopaedic surgeon is required to offer the uninsured. This has become more of an issue since the implementation of the 1986 Emergency Medical Treatment and Active Labor Act (EMTALA). This act mandates that emergency departments provide medical screening examinations to every person seeking treatment regardless of their ability to pay or whether it is the appropriate point of service. As a result of this law, many patients have also been seeking and receiving specialty care for nonemergent problems, although this was arguably not the original intent of this law. This consequence of EMTALA has left hospitals and physicians facing a crisis of overcrowded emergency departments and uncompensated care, which in turn threatens patient access to quality care.

Other current economic and political changes also have major impact on hospitals and health care providers, such as declines in Medicare payments for graduate medical education, lower disproportionate share payments, growth of Medicaid managed care, increased costs resulting from new government regulations such as the Healthcare Insurance Portability and Accountability Act (HIPAA) and Center for Medicare and Medicaid Services rules, increased costs of malpractice insurance, increased costs resulting from limited house staff duty hours and decreased payments for services provided from Medicare and other third party payers. These factors combined place a strain on orthopaedic surgeons, especially those in public and teaching hospitals that shoulder a disproportionate share of the care for the uninsured.

It appears appropriate to adopt a prudent stance toward providing services at no cost. Caring for the uninsured is an intrinsic part of orthopaedic surgery in a nation where a great number of people cannot afford even basic health care.

Table 2 | Why Physicians May Conceal a Medical Error

The medical profession values perfection

Feelings of shame or guilt

The admission may damage the physician's professional reputation

Possible drop in referrals or an impact on income

Desire to maintain the trust of the patient's family

Pressure felt from various sources:
  Managed care organizations
  Hospital administration
  Malpractice insurers

Fear of punishment or, in the case of trainees, dismissal

Fear of a malpractice lawsuit

(Adapted with permission from Selbst SM: The difficult duty of disclosing medical errors. *Contemp Pediatr* 2003;20:51-53.)

Table 3 | How To Approach Patients After a Medical Error

Notify professional insurer and seek assistance from those who might help with disclosure (for example, attending physician or risk manager)

Disclose promptly what is known about the event; concentrate on what happened and the possible consequences

Take the lead in disclosure; do not wait for the patient to ask

Outline a plan of care to rectify the harm and prevent recurrence

Offer to get prompt second opinions where appropriate

Offer the option of a family meeting and the option of having other representatives (for example, lawyers) present

Document important discussions

Offer the option of follow-up meetings and keep appointments

Be prepared for strong emotions

Accept responsibility for outcomes, but avoid attributions of blame

Apologies and expressions of sorrow are appropriate

(Adapted with permission from Selbst SM: The difficult duty of disclosing medical errors. *Contemp Pediatr* 2003;20:51-53.)

Disclosure in Medical Mistakes

Each year thousands of injuries and deaths in US hospitals result from medical errors. Errors involving medications have been reported in 4% to 17% of all hospital admissions. Although most of the information available about medical errors pertains to hospitalized patients, errors can occur anywhere in the health care system (operating room, office, clinic, emergency department, or elsewhere).

The AMA Code of Ethics provides important guidelines for professional practice including medical mistakes. The Joint Commission on the Accreditation of Healthcare Organizations requires health care workers to inform patients when they have been harmed by medical mistakes. However, this may not always occur as illustrated by one survey of house officers where they reported that they told an attending physician about serious mistakes only about half the time; errors were conveyed to patient or family in only 24% of the cases.

In one study, simulated case scenarios involving wrong medications were presented to 150 medical students, house officers, and attending physicians. The researchers found that as severity of injury increased, willingness to admit an error declined. About 95% of the students and physicians said they would admit an error to a patient when the outcome was minimal. However, only 79% said they would admit an error that resulted in the death of a patient. Another 17% said they would admit the error if they were asked directly about the event.

Although concealing a medical error violates ethical codes, fear of professional censure or medical malpractice lawsuits can pressure health care workers to be less than forthcoming when a mistake has occurred (Table 2).

In another study, three case scenarios were presented that varied in the degree of outcome severity to 400 patients. The respondents generally indicated that they would be more likely to file a lawsuit if the doctor withheld information about a mistake that subsequently surfaced. About 40% said they would stay with the physician after open disclosure of a mistake was made; however, only 8% said they would continue to see a doctor who did not disclose a mistake. Only 12% said they would sue if the physician informed them of a mistake that did not result in permanent aftereffects. However, 20% said they would sue if they found out about a mistake that the physician tried to cover up.

These results underscore the fact that patients generally appreciate an open, honest relationship with their physicians. In fact, a good doctor-patient relationship is one of the greatest factors that reduces the risk of a lawsuit if a poor outcome occurs. Prompt disclosure following a medical error will make the physician appear honest in the event of litigation and trial (Table 3). In contrast, nondisclosure can have significant negative legal implications as the legal statute of limitations may be extended if a physician is found to have knowingly and intentionally concealed information from a patient.

Evaluation of the Risk/Benefits Ratio in Patients With Difficult-to-Treat Problems

Acute, high-risk surgery involves operations on patients who often face a significant risk of morbidity and mortality without surgery, but for whom surgery itself involves a significant risk of morbidity and mortality as well. If nonsurgical management indeed involves a higher risk than surgery (for example, acute compartment syndrome, unstable 'open book' pelvis injury), the choice seems simple. However, most situations are not as straightforward. Informing the patient about surgical and nonsurgical statistics becomes important so that the pros and cons of surgery can be carefully weighed. In general, the "reasonable person standard" requires physicians to tell patients about a therapy's likely complications, especially if surgery is more likely to result in injury, disease, or a patient's death than an alternative treatment. The best interest for patients is then calculated by weighing the benefits against the burdens of treatment. If the treatment burdens outweigh the benefit, then the treatment is considered not to be in the patient's best interests. Benefits of treatment might include saving or prolonging life, alleviation of pain or restoration of function to an acceptable level or quality of life.

Relationships With Industry

Most orthopaedic surgeons foster active relationships with industry partners. Representatives of companies that produce prostheses, instrumentation, and other devices are frequent visitors to orthopaedic departments. Their companies regularly serve as sponsors of departmental functions and books for residents, and often fund clinical research when done to study their products. These types of financial relationships occur in every branch of medicine and are no less common in orthopaedic surgery. For orthopaedic surgeons, it is therefore important to be aware of the potential ethical problems these relationships can bring about, as such relationships may cause conflicting interests. These conflicts of interest may seriously compromise the integrity of clinical medicine, and may hamper the protection and safety of human research participants. The troublesome effects of conflicts of interest emerging from the research setting can be far-reaching, as published results often establish a standard that is followed by physicians treating patients worldwide.

A conflict of interest is defined here as any financial arrangement that compromises, has the capacity to compromise, or has the appearance of compromising trust in clinical care and/or clinical research. There are many different types of financial relationships that may surface between industry and orthopaedic surgeons and their institutions. For example, academic orthopaedic surgeons may be provided grants to study a sponsor's drug or product. Such grants may be a major source of salary support for investigators and their personnel. It is also often the case that device manufacturers offer investigators financial incentives for entering patients into a study. Although these "enrollment fees" are intended to cover the cost of the subject's participation, they typically exceed these costs. Academic orthopaedic surgeons may use the excess funds to support personnel, travel to meetings, or laboratory supplies and equipment, while in private practice these bonuses often remain with the researcher. Orthopaedic surgeons sometimes serve as consultants to companies whose products they are studying or join a company's advisory board and speakers' bureau, as well as enter into patent and royalty agreements, which may further complicate financial relationships. Arguably, such complex and considerable financial relationships may create some (perceived) dependency and/or loss of impartiality for the orthopaedic surgeon.

The appropriate ethical approach to take when faced with financial conflict of interest has been intensely debated, with editorialized pronouncements appearing in the nation's leading medical journals; societies and professional associations have addressed the issue of financial conflicts of interest in research.

For the moral orthopaedic surgeon, it is appropriate to be familiar with such professional statements, and to apply them to everyday practice and research as much as possible. Although financial conflicts of interest can probably never be fully eradicated, they can be diminished and brought to a morally more desirable level. One way this can be achieved is by meticulously disclosing all financial interests to patients and research subjects. Although disclosure is not a curative measure as advertising financial ties will not break them, it will lessen the potential for harm. In addition, orthopaedic surgeons should remain vigilant and cognizant of their ongoing relationships with industry, and regularly critically evaluate the extent of and the impact such ties have upon their practice and research.

Annotated Bibliography

General Reference

American Academy of Orthopaedic Surgeons (ed): *Guide to the Ethical Practice of Orthopaedic Surgery,* ed 4. Rosemont, IL, American Academy of Orthopaedic Surgeons, 2003.

The first edition of this booklet was published in 1991. The *Guide* provides standards of conduct and the essentials of ethical behavior for orthopaedic surgeons. This book can be considered required reading for the morally conscious orthopaedic surgeon and resident.

American Medical Association Council on Ethical and Judicial Affairs (ed): *Code of Medical Ethics: Current Opinions With Annotations.* Chicago, IL, American Medical Association, 2000-2001.

This text is presently the most comprehensive and current guide available to physicians in the United States. It is regularly revised and updated, and includes the seven basic principles of medical ethics and more than 180 opinions of the AMA's "EJA"-Council on a wide spectrum of topics.

Beauchamp TL, Childress JF: *Principles of Biomedical Ethics,* ed 5. New York, NY, Oxford University Press, 2001, pp 319-320.

This book is one of the most influential and important basic texts on bioethics, offering the theory of the four guiding principles: respect for autonomy, beneficence, nonmaleficence, and justice.

Surgical Ethics in the 21st Century

American Academy of Orthopaedic Surgeons Principles of Medical Ethics and Professionalism in Orthopaedic Surgery, 2002. Available at: http//www.aaos.org/wordhtml/papers/ethics/prin.htm. Accessed August 25, 2004.

These ten principles are standards of conduct that define the essential aspects of honorable behavior.

Moseley JB, O'Malley K, Petersen NJ, et al: A controlled trial of arthroscopic surgery for osteoarthritis of the knee. *N Engl J Med* 2002;347:81-88.

In this groundbreaking article the authors use sham surgery as a placebo in the randomized trial, concluding that arthroscopic knee surgery for this particular indication is no better than a placebo.

Satava RM: Disruptive visions. *Surg Endosc* 2003;17:104-107.

This visionary article paints a picture of the future of surgery, with technologies that seem like science fiction now but may very well be available within decades.

The Role of the Institutional Review Board in Modern Orthopaedics

United States Department of Health and Human Services Website. Protecting Personal Health Information in Research: Understanding the HIPAA Privacy Rule. Available at: http://privacyruleandresearch.nih.gov/pr_02.asp. Accessed February 2004.

The Department of Health and Human Services issued the Standards for Privacy of Individually Identifiable Health Information (the Privacy Rule) under the HIPAA of 1996 to provide the first comprehensive federal protection for the privacy of personal health information. Many of those who must comply with the Privacy Rule complied by April 14, 2003.

Department of Health and Human Services National Institutes of Health Office for Protection from Research Risks Website. Available at: http://ohrp.osophs.dhhs.gov/humansubjects/guidance/45cfr46.htm. Accessed February, 2004.

The Office of Human Research Protections (formerly the Office for Protection from Research Risks, OPRR), provides online decision charts, assisting prospective investigators in determining the need for IRB review and/or the subject's informed consent for research.

New Technology in Orthopaedic Surgery

American College of Surgeons Website. Statements on Principles. Revised March 2004. Available at: http://www.facs.org/fellows_info/statements/stonprin.html#top. Accessed August 25, 2004.

This website discusses codes of professional conduct and relationships between patients and surgeons.

Cronin DC II, Millis JM, Siegler M: Transplantation of liver grafts from living donors into adults: Too much, too soon. *N Engl J Med* 2001;344:1633-1637.

In this article, the rapid implementation of an experimental procedure into transplantation surgery is criticized.

Margo C: When is surgery research? Towards an operational definition of human research. *J Med Ethics* 2001;27:40-43.

This article analyzes the vague definition of clinical research in surgery and criticizes the wide implementation of so-called informal research.

Reitsma AM, Moreno JD: Ethical regulations for innovative surgery: The last frontier? *J Am Coll Surg* 2002;194:792-801.

This article discusses the regulatory gap between the protection of human subjects involved in research and those undergoing experimental surgery. Results of a survey among surgeons are presented.

Other Selected Ethical Issues in Orthopaedics

ABIM Foundation: American Board of Internal Medicine, ACP-ASIM Foundation, American College of Physicians, American Society of Internal Medicine, European Federation of Internal Medicine: Medical professionalism in the new millennium: A physician charter. *Ann Intern Med* 2002;136:243-246.

This article presents a discussion on professionalism, principles, and responsibilities for physicians.

American Academy of Orthopaedic Surgeons Website. American Academy of Orthopaedic Surgeons Advisory Statement: Preventing the Transmission of Bloodborne Pathogens. Available at: http://www.aaos.org/wordhtml/papers/advistmt/1018.htm. Accessed February, 2001.

Practical guidance for all clinically active orthopaedic surgeons infected with HIV, HBV, or HCV.

American Academy of Orthopaedic Surgeons Opinions on Ethics and Professionalism: Care and Treatment of the Medically Underserved. May 1998, revised May 2002. Available at: http://www.aaos.org/wordhtml/papers/ethics/1210eth.htm. Accessed August 25, 2004.

The AAOS applies its principles of medical ethics and professionalism in orthopaedic surgery to this pressing issue.

American Academy of Orthopaedic Surgeons Position Statement. Emergency Department On-Call Coverage. September 2002. Available at: http://www.aaos.org/wordhtml/papers/position/1157.htm. Accessed August 25, 2004.

A detailed statement explaining the various effects of EMTALA on orthopaedic surgeons and the Academy's stance towards it is presented.

Blendon RJ, DesRoches CM, Brodie M, et al: Patient safety: Views of practicing physicians and the public on medical errors. *N Engl J Med* 2002;347:1933-1940.

A scientific study of the subjective impact of medical errors as viewed by physicians and the public.

Meyer FN: Uninsured healthcare is a growing problem: Putting economic pressures on physicians. *AAOS Bulletin* 2003; August 51(4).

This article examines the growing concerns about issues related to uninsured health care in the United States.

Selbst SM: The difficult duty of disclosing medical errors. *Contemp Pediatr* 2003;20:51-53.

This article discusses how to manage medical mistakes and examines the reasons why disclosure is so difficult.

Tereskerz PM: Research accountability and financial conflicts of interest in industry sponsored clinical research: A review. *Account Res* 2003;10:137-158.

A discussion of financial conflicts of interest, research accountability, and other aspects of industry relationships are discussed.

United Kingdom Department of Health Website. HIV infected health care workers: A consultation paper on management and patient notification. Available at: www.doh.gov.uk/aids.htm. A list of exposure-prone procedures available at: www.doh.gov.uk/pub/docs/aids.pdf. Accessed February, 2004.

Although UK policy obviously does not apply to US surgeons, it is worthwhile to review the detailed list of exposure-prone procedures as a reference.

Wears RL, Wu AW: Dealing with failure: The aftermath of errors and adverse events. *Ann Emerg Med* 2002;39: 344-346.

This article discusses what happens after a medical mistake has occurred and how patients and health care workers can be guided through this situation.

Classic Bibliography

Aronheim JC, Moreno JD, Zuckerman C (eds): *Ethics in Clinical Practice,* ed 2. Gaithersburg, MD, Aspen Publishers, 2000, pp 17-50.

McCullough LB, Jones JW, Brody BA (eds): *Surgical Ethics*. New York, NY, Oxford University Press, 1998.

Recommendations for preventing transmission of human immunodeficiency virus and hepatitis B virus to patients during exposure-prone invasive procedures. *MMWR Recomm Rep* 1991;40(RR-8):1-9.

Recommendations for prevention and control of hepatitis C virus (HCV) infection and HCV-related chronic disease: Centers for Disease Control and Prevention. *MMWR Recomm Rep* 1998;47(RR19):1-39.

Statements on emerging surgical technologies and the evaluation of credentials: American College of Surgeons. *Bull Am Coll Surg* 1994;79:40-41.

Statement on Issues to be Considered Before New Surgical Technology is Applied to the Care of Patients: Committee on Emerging Surgical Technology and Education, American College of Surgeons. *Bull Am Coll Surg* 1995;80:46-47.

Sweet MP, Bernat JL: A study of the ethical duty of physicians to disclose errors. *J Clin Ethics* 1997;8:341-348.

US National Commission for the Protection of Human Subjects of Biomedical and Behavioral Research: The Belmont Report: Ethical Principles and Guidelines for the Protection of Human Subjects of Research. September 30, 1978. Superintendent of Documents, US Government Printing Office. Washington, DC, DHEW Publication No. 78-0013.

World Medical Association Recommendations Guiding Physicians in Biomedical Research Involving Human Subjects (document 17.1). Helsinki, Finland, June 1964.

Wu AW, Folkman S, McPhee SJ, Lo B: Do house officers learn from their mistakes? *JAMA* 1991;265:2089-2094.

Chapter 9

Outcomes Assessment and Evidence-Based Practice Guidelines in Orthopaedic Surgery

William A. Abdu, MD, MS

Outcomes Instruments in Orthopaedic Surgery

Traditional approaches to clinical research and reports of surgical interventions are commonly associated with the measurement of variables that are either easily available retrospectively from the medical record, or variables of primary interest to the researcher. These biologic, physiologic, and anatomic measures include mortality, strength measurement, range of motion, and radiographic findings. These examples of "hard" outcome measures or surrogate outcomes have a very weak association with the symptoms and functionality of the "end result" of therapeutic interventions and are only of modest relevance to patients and society. The perceived attractiveness of hard measures is that they are believed to be objective (unbiased judgment), have preservability (radiographs) and have dimension (measurement of radiographic findings). However, if the goal of treatment is to reduce pain and improve function, these constructs should be measured directly rather than assuming that surrogate hard measures will suffice.

More recently, the goals of clinical research have transitioned to the measurement of variables primarily critical to the patient, or "soft" outcome measures. These patient-reported outcomes of symptoms, physical function, and health may take several forms and include the assessment by disease-specific measures, general health measures, and satisfaction measures. These so-called soft outcomes measures are more reliable and more consistent than the traditional, hard measures. Outcomes research often refers to the study of a group or cohort of patients often with the same diagnosis, and relates their clinical and health outcomes to the care they received.

Outcomes research also includes methods of analysis for small (single site) and/or large (often multiple site) databases, small-area analysis, structured literature reviews (meta-analysis), prospective clinical trials, decision analysis, and guideline development. The focus of outcomes research is often on patient-centered outcomes of care (patient self-report) rather than on the process measures of care, which are not always under the patient's or the doctor's control.

An outcomes instrument is the survey tool or instrument used to measure these variables (Table 1). These measures are not designed or intended to substitute or replace the traditional measures or clinical end points, but are to be used in parallel with clinical measures.

An outcomes instrument, in order to be useful, should have clinical sensibility, meaning that the questionnaire includes relevant content and is appropriate for both the patient population and the setting in which it is to be used. The feasibility of the questionnaire is determined in part by its length, degree of respondent burden, ease of scoring and analyzing the results, and the costs of its use. In constructing a questionnaire, it must be reliable; the results must be reproducible from one time to another or between interviewers. The questionnaire must also have internal consistency. The instrument must be validated, meaning that there are correlations in the expected direction and magnitude with a variety of external measures that are somewhat different but are expected to have predictable associations. In addition, the instrument must be responsive, or have the ability to measure and detect small but clinically important differences between groups, or over time.

Outcomes instruments may be used for multiple purposes as outlined in Table 2. The increasing interest in the use of outcomes measures is relatively new and is a rapidly evolving methodology. Many issues remain controversial, raising several questions, such as: Which measurements are important? When and specifically how should they be measured? Are the outcomes instruments valid? Are there controls? What other factors (biologic, physiologic, environmental) may influence the measurement results? Are generic measures sufficient or are disease-specific measures also important? Over half a century ago, Lembcke noted that "the best measures of quality is not how well or how frequently a medical service is given, but how closely the result approaches the fundamental objectives of prolonging life, relieving stress, restoring function and preventing disability." The goal of outcomes research and the use of

Table 1 | Common Outcomes Survey Instruments

General health outcomes instruments
  Short Form-36 or Short Form-12 general health survey
  Health Related Quality of Life (HRQOL)
  Sickness impact Profile (SIP Nottingham Health Profile (NHP)
  Million Visual Analog Scale (VAS)
  Duke Health Profile
Patient satisfaction measures
  Patient Satisfaction Questionnaire (PSQ)
  Client Satisfaction Questionnaire (CSQ)
  Patient Satisfaction Survey (PSS)
Disease or condition specific instruments include
  Spine
    Oswestry Disability Index (ODI) for low back pain
    Roland-Morris Disability Questionnaire (RMDQ)
    Waddell Disability Index
    Low Back Pain Outcome Score (LBOS)
    Clinical Back Pain Questionnaire (CBPQ)
    Quebec Back Pain Disability Scale (QBPDS)
    Low Back Pain Rating Scale (LBPRS)
    North American Spine Society Lumbar Spine Questionnaire (NASS LSQ)
    Resumption of Activities of Daily Living Scale (RADL)
  Upper extremity
    Constant Shoulder Function Scoring System
    Carpal Tunnel Syndrome Evaluation
    Upper Extremity Disabilities of the Arm, Shoulder, and Head (DASH)
    Shoulder Pain Score
    Elbow questionnaire
  Lower extremity
    Western Ontario McMaster Universities Osteoarthritis Index (WOMAC)
    Harris Hip Score
  Trauma
    Short Musculoskeletal Function Assessment Questionnaire (SMAF)

Table 2 | Purposes for Outcomes Instruments

Study of populations in cross-sectional studies (at one point in time) to define the characteristics of a particular patient population with a specific condition, resource utilization, and baseline characteristics.

Determination of longitudinal impact on health change, function, and satisfaction in an individual patient's care for a specific disease process after intervention (such as elective surgery).

As measures for prospective clinical trials to determine the effectiveness of a particular intervention (for example, surgical versus nonsurgical treatment of a specific condition).

Development of disease-specific evidence-based medicine clinical pathways and guidelines for unifying the process of delivering effective medical care.

Table 3 | Key Factors in the Construct, Design, and Use of Outcomes Instruments

Content, Population, Setting, and Purpose

Which outcomes are to be measured (biologic, physiologic, function, general health, quality of life, satisfaction)?

Which population will be studied and in what setting (age, gender)?

What is the purpose of the study (to describe, predict, measure change, measure one point in time or change over time, or impact of an intervention)?

Content Validity

  What domains (health concepts) and items are included?

  Are there important omissions or inappropriate inclusions?

Face Validity

  Do these measures make good clinical sense?

  Is each question phrased in a suitable way?

  Are the response categories appropriate?

  Is there an overall score summarizing across questions, and how is this score calculated?

  Is there correlation with other outcomes measures?

  Are these measures predictive of future events?

Feasibility

  Is the instrument easy to use and understand?

  Is the instrument acceptable to the population and the clinician/investigator?

What is its format (self-administered, telephone, personal interview, computer, paper/pen)?

How long does it take to administer and report the results?

Responsiveness

  Is the instrument able to detect subtle but clinically relevant change over time or with intervention?

---

instruments can be divided into categories and are outlined in Table 3.

The major areas of interest in measuring patient-centered self-response measurements using outcomes instruments include measure of function (the ability to perform specific tasks, covering the domains of physical, social, role, and psychological function), general health perception (integrates the various aspects of health as reflected by the patient's subjective global rating), quality of life (general measure of a patient's overall well-being), and satisfaction (measure of treatment impact, process of care, results, and quality of life).

Although these factors are all distinct concepts, they may or may not tract together throughout the patient's course or treatment. For example, resolution of pain may not correlate with radiographic findings, ability to function, return to work, or satisfaction. Thus, outcomes should be measured in multiple dimensions. Compression of various dimensions of outcome into a single unidimensional scale obscures the detection of these possible variations in responses.

outcomes survey instruments is to help define the results of interventions and assess these desired end results.

The construct, design, and use of outcomes instruments are rapidly evolving. Key factors about outcomes

Outcomes measures are generally disease-specific or general health (generic) surveys. Disease-specific instruments such as the Oswestry Disability Questionnaire for low back pain are designed to measure disease-specific functional status, and have the advantage of capturing disease-specific dysfunction in greater detail. General health or generic surveys such as the Short Form-36 are important for detecting complications or ill effects of treatment that extend beyond a specific disease or condition. They also make it possible to compare the impact of treatments of specific disorders with the impact of treatment of other diseases. These surveys help determine the cost effectiveness of various treatments. A core set of survey instruments should include measures of symptoms, functional status, overall well-being, and work disability.

Several important factors must be considered for outcomes measures to be a valid indicator of health care quality. First, the process of medical care must actually affect the outcome. Second, the measure of outcome must be valid, reliable, and responsive to changes in a patient's health status. Third, sufficient information must be collected about comorbid conditions and patient demographics when studying the outcomes of a particular condition or treatment. Fourth, patient compliance and the timing of a survey are critical to obtaining representative measures. Finally, if the variable of interest is a rare event (such as death), then the population under study must be large enough to make valid comparisons between treatments or conditions.

Design of a Prospective Clinical Trial

The major source of information for clinicians is the published literature, and almost all knowledge in orthopaedics is based on information that has appeared in texts and journals. However, factors affecting the validity of many currently reported clinical studies include the lack of randomization of patients, inadequate study design, and missing sample size calculations, therefore rendering many studies unable to adequately answer the research question. Other factors include the lack of standardized study definitions and measures, poor descriptions of study patients and confounding variables, inadequate and unclear follow-up, and absence of patient-centered outcomes measures. Given the absence of a firm knowledge and research on which to base clinical decisions, it is no wonder that significant practice-pattern variation exists.

In order to be most efficient at designing and collecting the appropriate data elements, the clinician must give careful thought to the exact questions to be addressed and the study design to answer the research questions. The formulation of an appropriate research question informs the clinician and researcher about the most appropriate data elements to be collected, the pri-

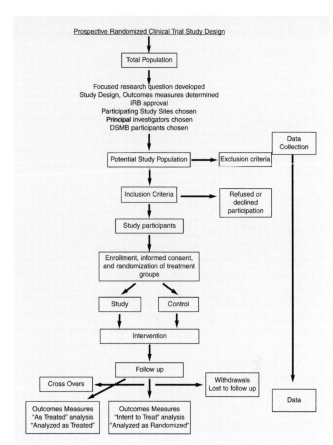

Figure 1 Basic design of a randomized clinical trial. IRB = Institutional Review Board; DSMB = Data and Safety Monitoring Board.

mary outcome of interest. In a prospective clinical trial, the researcher poses a question, intervenes, and follows the direction of inquiry forward. The events of interest occur after the onset of the study (Figure 1).

In clinical trials, the ability to determine the better of two treatments is the product of the trial hypothesis, the data elements chosen to evaluate the treatments in question, the magnitude of change in the scores over time needed to consider one treatment preference, and sample size for power of study. All research studies are subject to invalid conclusions because of bias, confounders, and chance. Bias is the nonrandom systematic error in study design. It is an unintentional outcome of factors such as patient selection, performance, and outcome determination. A confounder is a variable having independent associations with both the exposure and the outcome, and thus potentially distorts their relationship. Common confounders include age, gender, socioeconomic status, and comorbidities. Chance can lead to invalid conclusions based on the probability of type I error (concluding there is a difference when none exists equal to the p value) and type II error (concluding that there is no difference when one truly exists). Thus, the appropriate sample size and power calculation must be

Table 4 | Common Formulas for the Determination of Sample Size

Study Design and Type of Error	Sample Size Formula
Studies using paired *t* test (before and after studies) with alpha (type I) error only	$N = \dfrac{(z_a)^2 \cdot (s)^2}{(\bar{d})^2}$ = total number of subjects
Studies using *t* test (randomized controlled trials with one experimental and one control group, considering alpha error only)	$N = \dfrac{(z_a)^2 \cdot 2 \cdot (s)^2}{(\bar{d})^2}$ = number of subjects/ group
Studies using *t* test considering alpha and beta errors	$N = \dfrac{(z_a + z_b)^2 \cdot 2 \cdot (s)^2}{(\bar{d})^2}$ = number of subjects/ group
Tests of difference in proportions considering alpha and beta errors	$N = \dfrac{(z_a + z_b)^2 \cdot 2 \cdot \bar{p}(1-\bar{p})}{(\bar{d})^2}$ = number of subjects/ group

N = sample size, z_a = value for alpha error (equals 1.96 for $P = 0.05$ in two-tailed test), z_b = value for beta error (equals 0.84 for 20% beta error = 80% power in one-tailed test), $(s)^2$ = variance, p = mean proportion of success, d = smallest clinically important difference to be detected

determined before the initiation of the study to avoid chance, given the smallest clinically relevant differences in outcome and the variability in measures. It is necessary to have sufficient statistical power (the ability to detect a difference of the magnitude required if one truly exists) to determine whether the efficacy of one treatment is superior to another.

Sample Size Calculations

One of the more difficult issues determining the success of a study is sample size calculation, which must be done prior to the initiation of the clinical study. Sample size calculations are always an approximation, yet they are important in providing information about two study design questions. The first is how many subjects should participate in the intended study and second, is this study worth doing if only N number of subjects participate? In some cases the study may not be worth doing if the likelihood of demonstrating a significant clinical effect or difference between two treatments is very small or if the population needed to answer the question is extremely large. Variables critical to determining sample size include data type (paired data [observations before and after treatment in the same study group] and unpaired data [observations in an observation and control group], consideration of error type (beta errors [type II or false-negative errors] and alpha errors [type I or false-positive errors]), variance in data set (large and small), alpha level (usually set at $P = 0.05$ in the two-tailed test and confidence interval of 95%), beta level (usually set at 0.2), and determining the size of the detectable difference between groups.

Beta Error Importance

Statistical power refers to the sensitivity for detecting a mean difference in a clinical study, whereas sensitivity refers to the same difference in a clinical test (statistical power + beta error = 1.0). This means that the statistical power is equal to 1-beta error. Therefore, in calculating a sample size, if the investigators accept a 20% possibility of missing a true finding (beta error = 0.2), then the study should have a statistical power of 0.8 or 80%. That means that the investigators are 80% confident that they will be able to detect a true difference of the size that they specify with the sample size that they determine. By design, the investigator accepts a 20% chance of false-negative results. The best way to incorporate beta error into the study is to include it beforehand in the determination of sample size, which is simple to do, but it increases the sample size considerably. A large sample size can be viewed as a means of decreasing the false-negative results rate when a real treatment effect exists.

For the comparison of groups in which the data set variance is high, when the investigators want the answer to be close to the "true" value, and when the smallest clinically significant difference detected is to be extremely small, a large sample size will be required. In calculating the sample size, investigators must first determine the appropriate formula to be used, based on the type of study and the type of error to be considered. Four common formulas for the determination of sample size are listed in Table 4. As the complexity of the groups and error types increase, the N correspondingly increases.

The adverse affects of bias, confounding, and chance can be minimized by proper study design and statistical analysis. The purpose of prospective studies is to minimize bias from selection, information, recall, and nonresponder factors. Randomization minimizes selection bias and equally distributes the confounders. Random assignment implies that each individual has the same chance of receiving each of the possible treatments and that the probability that a given subject will receive a particular allocation is independent of the probability that any other subject will receive the same treatment assignment. The decision regarding study design and data collection may be the most critical part of planning a clinical trial. The study design is the map from which data collection follows, and which enables the physician to accurately produce data forms and collect data. The prospective randomized clinical trial with concurrent controls is the gold standard in clinical research. Traditional randomized trials tell about the efficacy (whether the treatment can work under ideal circumstances), whereas outcomes research more typically studies the effectiveness (how well a treatment works when applied in routine care). Effectiveness is a function of efficacy, but also of diagnostic accuracy, physician skill in applying treatment, and patient compliance with prescribed regimens. Any of these factors may create a gap between efficacy and effectiveness. The prospective randomized clinical trial provides not only qualitative conclusions about whether a treatment is better, but also quantitative estimates of the extent to which it is better.

Barriers to a Randomized Clinical Trial

There are many barriers that must be overcome to proceed with a prospective randomized clinical trial involving a surgical procedure (Table 5). History has not favored the validation of surgical procedures by randomized trials. Many commonly performed surgical procedures were introduced well before randomized trials became established in medicine. Once a procedure becomes accepted, it is difficult to test it against a control. For many common procedures performed, orthopaedic surgeons cannot fall back on history to explain the lack of rigor in surgical research.

Surgeons can be tempted to ignore evidence that threatens their personal interests because of competition and prestige. Objectivity about procedures central to a surgeon's reputation is difficult and randomized clinical trials may seem threatening. The literature must support and the investigators must feel comfortable with a state of equipoise, which is a point of maximum uncertainty, a state of balance or equilibrium between two alternative therapies such that there is no preference between treatments. Some also refer to this as the uncertainty principle in which clinicians, researchers, and patients acknowledge having hunches about a treatment's effectiveness, but that the boundaries (or confidence intervals) around their hunches may run from one extreme (extremely effective) to the other (harmful). If the answer to the clinical research question is clear, the randomized clinical trial cannot ethically proceed with the comparison of a known successful treatment with a known ineffective treatment.

The infrastructure within which to perform the study must be well planned and developed to function efficiently. This includes knowledge to obtain funding and to perform statistical analysis. A lack of education in

Table 5	Barriers to Overcome Before Proceeding With Prospective Randomized Clinical Trials Involving a Surgical Procedure
History
Competition
Equipoise/uncertainty
Infrastructure
Study design and statistics
Surgical trials
Events
Risk assessment
Commitment

clinical epidemiology can affect study design and statistics. The study design and implementation depends heavily on and will be most successful when a core multidisciplinary group of researchers (including clinicians, epidemiologists, and statisticians) all contribute their expertise to the project.

The inherent variability of surgery requires precise definitions of the diagnosis, interventions, and close monitoring of its quality. Surgical learning curves might cause difficulty in timing and performing randomized clinical trials. Blinding is often difficult in surgical trials, and it is not always possible or necessary. Events are conditions that may be emergent or life-threatening that may cause difficulties with recruitment, consent, and randomization of clinical trials. Multicenter studies are often required under these conditions. In addition, comparison of surgical and nonsurgical treatments with greatly different risks causes difficulties with patient equipoise, and thus recruitment. Finally, all involved must be absolutely committed to all aspects of the trial if it is to succeed.

These barriers to randomized clinical trials have stimulated some to question the need for randomized clinical trials in surgery, and the debate is substantial. For many medical questions, a large amount of evidence has been accumulated through nonrandomized studies. The risk of nonrandomized studies is that the studies may spuriously overestimate treatment benefits as they are more susceptible to unaccounted confounding, yielding misleading conclusions. Observational studies may provide sufficient evidence of a procedure's effectiveness, but the treatment effect of the procedure must be quite large, and the study well designed to be convincing. However, it is very difficult to use historical controls, obtained under less rigorous scientific standards of data collection, against which to test a new procedure. Many previously well established surgical procedures, once thought to provide significant clinical benefits in the hands of proponents, have been subsequently proven ineffective when tested rigorously in well-

Table 6 | Steps to be Taken Before Patients Are Enrolled in a Clinical Trial

Establish eligibility criteria that indicate the presence or required eligibility requirements and the absence of exclusion criteria.

Characterize the demographic and general health of the patients eligible for enrollment into the clinical trial.

Establish a research study database and include baseline data for assessment for changes in the outcome variable to be measured over the course of the clinical trial.

Recognize and account for stratification required in the randomization process (such as age, gender, race, diagnosis, smoking, education, body mass index, socioeconomic factors).

Develop a system for the determination of follow-up outcomes surveys and tracking patients throughout the trial duration.

Assess performance to the protocol and adherence to the clinical trial research protocol with quality checks of clinical sites and investigators.

Establish a Data and Safety Monitoring Board to independently monitor the progress and safety of the clinical trial.

designed studies. When comparisons of well-designed nonrandomized trials of selected medical topics with very narrow and specific selection criteria for the quality of the meta-analysis were compared with the results of randomized trials for the same diagnosis, very good correlation was observed between the summary odds ratios. However, the nonrandomized studies tended to show larger treatment effects, and the discrepancies beyond chance were less common when only prospective studies were considered.

The impact of the randomized clinical trial can be determined by four factors: the baseline control group's risk of an outcome event, the responsiveness of patients to experimental treatment, the potency of the experimental treatment, and the completeness with which the outcome events are ascertained and included. The goal of enrollment must be to enroll those most likely to have the events that are hoped to be prevented with the experimental treatment. Therefore, to measure the true success of the experimental treatment, these high-risk patients become the group most likely to benefit from participation in the trial and should be the target for enrollment. It is also critical that all attempts be made to preserve the sample size and prevent erosion of the participants by crossover or dropout in follow up. This allows the detection of events that otherwise might have been missed, and it increases the chances of being able to present a "worse-case scenario." This involves the process by which all experimental patients lost to follow up in a positive trial are assigned bad outcomes, and all lost controls are assigned a positive outcome. The loss of minimal patients to follow-up enhances the credibility of a trial's positive conclusions.

To ensure proper data collection to assess the impact of an intervention, study investigators must agree on the details of data collection, and the process by which the data are collected (paper, telephone, personal interview, computer). The schedule for data collection must be defined to determine when patients are to be surveyed throughout the study. To properly select appropriate outcome measures, the investigators must be thoroughly familiar with the disease process under investigation. This allows for the understanding of associated conditions, comorbidities, and other variables that are likely to influence the clinical results. These other associated conditions and variables (such as age, gender, body mass index, smoking, education level, medical comorbidities) must be measured to provide for statistical control for their influence (confounding effects) on the primary and secondary outcomes of interest.

Enrollment in a Clinical Trial

Before patients are enrolled in a clinical trial, several steps must be taken and these are outlined in Table 6. The enrollment process is best preceded by pilot testing of the procedures, survey instruments, and the overall process on test patients to resolve any potential problems before the initiation of the clinical trial with actual enrolled and randomized patients. When a patient is considered for the clinical trial, it is necessary to determine the patient's eligibility for participation. It is most efficient if all the initial required data are collected at a single visit, the recruitment/preenrollment/randomization visit, during which baseline data are obtained and treatment assignment occurs. The initial visit must also include a thorough explanation of the clinical trial, explaining the purpose and goals, and obtaining the informed consent for participation.

Once randomization occurs, the patient is a member of a treatment group to which they have been assigned. Postrandomization follow-up visits are then scheduled at predetermined times according to the data collection schedule. Completeness of the follow-up visits is critical to the success of the trial. Incomplete follow-up or withdrawals may bias the results. To ensure maximum follow-up participation, it is critical to minimize the burden on the patients by requiring only specific instruments to be completed at each visit. Subjects without telephones or those who plan to move are best excluded, and the addition of contact information including email addresses and names and contact information of family and friends is critical to maintaining contact. This information should be updated at each visit. Providing reminders for upcoming visits also ensures compliance with longitudinal follow up. Incentives are also helpful, whether they are financial or other tokens of appreciation for continued participation in the clinical trial.

Data collection and maintenance is critical to the success of a clinical trial. Data must be secure, safe, and protected. Computerized data must be backed up regularly. Specific identifying data for each patient is critical for providing and maintaining confidentiality and consistency. Dedicated personnel whose responsibilities are specific to data management infrastructure are critical to this process.

The role of maintaining the safety of the participants in the clinical trial is performed by the Data and Safety Monitoring Board (DSMB). This group is commonly composed of five non participating individuals who are knowledgeable about the disease process and statistical and study design. This committee reviews the summaries of safety, accrual and progress of the trial, the quality of the data, and blinded interim efficacy and effectiveness analyses and reports its findings to the principal investigator and executive working group. It is also responsible for interpreting data on adverse side effects. The DSMB meets every 6 months and makes recommendations to the principal investigator and executive working group regarding actions to ensure patient safety and that participants are not exposed to undue risks. The mandate of the DSMB should comply with the July 1, 1999 release of the National Institutes of Health policy for Data and Safety Monitoring, with the primary function being to "ensure the safety of participants and validity and integrity of the data." The DSMB has direct communications with the funding agency and can stop a clinical trial when public health or safety is at risk, or when study goals are not met.

Evidence-Based Medicine

Physicians seek to base their decisions on the best available evidence. Often this represents experience, teaching, and extrapolations of pathophysiologic principles and logic rather than established facts based on data derived from patients. The advent of randomized controlled clinical trials has led to an increase in the quality of evidence concerning clinical treatment interventions, making clinical reasoning more comprehensible. The ability to track down and critically appraise and incorporate evidence into clinical practice has been termed "evidence-based medicine." It is the conscientious, explicit, and judicious use of current best evidence in making decisions about the care of individual patients using patient-centered clinical and basic science research data along with the patient's values and expectations. Evidence-based medicine is not "cookbook" medicine. It is the integration of the best external evidence with individual clinical expertise and patients choice; neither alone is enough.

Many of these concepts were proposed by Codman in the early 1900s, who implemented the "end result" idea. Codman attempted to put into practice the notion that each hospital should follow every patient it treats, long enough to determine whether or not the treatment has been successful, and then to inquire "if not, why not"?

Evidence-based medicine is not restricted to randomized clinical trials and meta-analyses. It involves tracking down the best external evidence with which to answer the clinical questions. Best available external evidence includes clinically relevant research from both the basic sciences and patient-centered clinical research. It is when questions are asked about therapy that the nonexperimental approaches should be avoided, as these often lead to falsely positive conclusions about efficacy. The randomized clinical trial is the gold standard for judging whether a treatment does more harm than good. A systematic review of several randomized trials provides even greater degree of confidence in the level of evidence.

Without current best evidence, a clinical practice risks the possibility of rapidly becoming out of date, to the detriment of the patient. Three evidence-based medicine strategies have been developed to help the clinician maintain and expand clinically important knowledge: learning evidence-based medicine, seeking and applying evidence-based medicine summaries generated by others, and accepting evidence-based protocols and practice guidelines developed by others.

Classification of Study Strength

Evidence is a critical component in the decision-making process for delivering care to patients. For many questions, however, the amount of information is overwhelming and the conclusions often contradictory. Most surgeons would agree that to make the best decisions, evidence must be easily available in a comprehensive and timely fashion.

Levels of evidence, based on the rigor of the study design, are a way to sort through and evaluate the literature. Levels of evidence may also be used in the development of practice guidelines to weigh the strength of the recommendations, and should be used by practicing surgeons to wade through the multiple types of evidence to help determine which information is useful to them and their patients.

Levels of evidence provide only a rough guide to the study quality. Level I evidence may not be available for all clinical questions, and level II and III evidence can still have great value to the practicing surgeon. No single study will provide all the definitive answers.

The classification of levels of evidence was developed to minimize therapeutic harm to patients by using evidence that is least likely to be wrong. The Center for Evidence-Based Medicine (http://cebm.net/levels_of_evidence.asp) has created the categories for defining study strength (level of evidence) (Table 7) and grades (Table 8) for recommendations in common use today. Similar levels and grades have also been devel-

Table 7 | Oxford Centre for Evidence-Based Medicine Levels of Evidence and *Journal of Bone and Joint Surgery*: Instructions to Authors

	Therapeutic Studies: Investigating the Results of Treatment	Prognostic Studies: Investigating the Outcome of Disease	Diagnostic Studies: Investigating a Diagnostic Test	Economic and Decision Analysis: Developing an Economic or Decision Model
Level I	Randomized controlled trial Significant difference No significant difference but narrow CIs* Systematic review of Level I randomized controlled trials (studies were homogeneous)	Prospective study Systematic review of Level I studies	Testing of previously developed diagnostic criteria in series of consecutive patients (with universally applied reference "gold" standard") Systematic review of Level I studies	Clinically sensible costs and alternatives; values obtained from many studies; multiway sensitivity analyses System review of Level I studies
Level II	Prospective cohort study Poor-quality randomized controlled trial (eg, < 80% follow-up Systematic review Level II studies Nonhomogeneous Level I studies	Retrospective study Study of untreated controls from a previous randomized controlled trial Systematic review of Level II studies	Development of diagnostic criteria based on basis of consecutive patients (with universally applied reference "gold" standard") Systematic review of Level II studies	Clinically sensible costs and alternatives; values obtained from many studies; multiway sensitivity analyses System review of Level II studies
Level III	Case-control study Retrospective study Systematic review of Level III studies		Study of nonconsecutive patients (no consistently applied reference "gold" standard") Systematic review of Level III studies	Limited alternatives and costs; poor estimates Systematic review of Level III studies
Level IV	Case series (no, or historical, control group)	Case series	Case-control study Poor reference standard	No sensitivity analyses
Level V	Expert opinion	Expert opinion	Expert opinion	Expert opinion

*CI = Confidence interval

Table 8 | Oxford Centre for Evidence-Based Medicine Grades of Recommendation

A	Consistent Level 1 studies
B	Consistent Level 2 or 3 studies or extrapolations from Level 1 studies
C	Level 4 studies or extrapolations from Level 2 or 3 studies
D	Level 5 evidence or troublingly inconsistent or inconclusive studies of any level

oped by this group for evidence and actions in the domains: prognosis, etiology/harm, and economic analysis.

The Future of Evidence-Based Approaches in Orthopaedic Surgery

Efforts in improving the quality of care delivered to patients remains a continuous work in progress. The routine use of validated and standardized outcomes instruments, not primarily for research purposes but also for use in routine clinical practice, will provide data with which to assess interventions. It seems likely that there will be a growing and continued emphasis on evidence-based approaches in assessing functional status, symp-

toms, and health-related quality of life as relevant outcomes of clinical care. The growing efforts toward understanding the clinical study design and the implementation of multicenter prospective randomized clinical trials will provide the best evidence with which orthopaedic surgeons can develop practice guidelines, decrease practice variability, provide evidence-based quality care, and allow patients to make informed choices. The current mandate for quality, necessitating the measurements of results, provides an opportunity to develop a more focused approach to the delivery of care by orthopaedic surgeons and a means to document the quality of the end result.

Annotated Bibliography

Centre for Evidence-Based Medicine: Oxford-Centre for Evidence Based Medicine Web site. Levels of evidence and grades of recommendation. Available at: http://www.cebm.net/levels_of_evidence.asp. Accessed September 1, 2003.

This is a comprehensive Web-based resource on evidence-based medicine, including definitions and strategies for searching for literature on evidence-based medicine.

Ioannidis JP, Haidich A, Papa M, et al: Comparison of evidence of treatment effects in randomized and non-randomized studies. *JAMA* 2001;286:821-830.

In this review of 45 topics in selected medical topics, analysis of the results demonstrates larger treatment effects and discrepancy beyond chance nonrandomized studies compared with randomized trials.

Kocher MS, Zurakowski D: Clinical epidemiology and biostatistics: An orthopaedic primer. *J Bone Joint Surg Am* 2001; Orthopaedic Journal Club: 1-12.

This is a primer of clinical epidemiology and biostatistics for the orthopaedic surgeon.

McCulloch P, Taylor I, Sasako M, Lovett B, Griffin D: Randomised trials in surgery: Problems and possible solutions. *BMJ* 2002;324:1448-1451.

The quality and quantity of randomized trials in surgery is acknowledged to be limited. Some aspects of surgical trials present special difficulties for randomized trials and these difficulties and proposed solutions for improving the standards of clinical trials in surgery are discussed.

Sackett DL: Why randomized controlled trials fail but needn't: 2. Failure to employ physiological statistics, or the only formula a clinician-trialist is ever likely to need (or understand!). *CMAJ* 2001;165:1226-1237.

Causes of failure in randomized controlled trials is neither with the teacher nor the trialist, but lies in the mismatch between what is judged necessary to be learned about biostatistics and who learns it. Pitfalls in conducting clinical trials are discussed, along with appropriate sample size and eligibility and erosion of study participants.

Watters WC III: Evidence-based practice and the use of practice guidelines. *AAOS Bulletin*, August 2003, pp 15-16.

Scientific journals, textbooks, and presentations provide the cornerstone of good clinical decision making and patient care. The benefits and use of evidence-based medicine to produce and practice guidelines in the context of clinical quality improvement cycle is demonstrated.

Wright J: Summarizing the evidence. *AAOSBulletin*, June 2003, pp 51-52.

Evidence-based medicine, levels of evidence, and strategies for summarizing evidence are reviewed for the practicing orthopaedic surgeon faced with determining treatment recommendations.

Classic Bibliography

Bombardier C: Outcome assessments in the evaluation of treatment of spinal disorders. *Spine* 2000;25:3097-3099.

Daum WJ, Brinker MR, Nash DB: Quality and outcome determination in health care and orthopaedics: evolution and current structure. *J Am Acad Orthop Surg* 2000;8:133-139.

Deyo RA, Weinstein JN: Outcomes research for spinal disorders, in Herkowitz H, Garfin S, Balderston R, Eismont F, Bell G, Wiesel S (eds): *Rothman-Simeone: The Spine*, ed 4. Philadelphia, PA, WB Saunders, 1999.

Gartland JJ: Orthopaedic clinical research: Deficiencies in experimental design and determinations of outcome. *J Bone Joint Surg Am* 1988;70:1357-1364.

Hennekens C: Buring J: Interventional studies, in Mayrent S (ed): *Epidemiology in Medicine*. Boston, MA, Little, Brown and Company, 1987, pp178-212.

Jekel JJ, Elmore JG, Katz DL (eds): *Epidemiology, Biostatistics and Preventive Medicine*. Philadelphia, PA, WB Saunders, 1996, pp 160-171.

Kaska SC, Weinstein JN: Historical perspective: Ernest Amory Codman, 1869-1940: A pioneer of evidence-based medicine. The end result of an idea. *Spine* 1998;23:629-633.

Keller RB: Outcomes research in orthopaedics. *J Am Acad Orthop Surg* 1993;1:122-129.

Kopec JA: Measuring functional outcomes in persons with back pain: A review of back-specific questionnaires. *Spine* 2000;25:3110-3114.

Matthews DE, Farewell VT: *Using and Understanding Medical Statistics*. Basel, Germany, Karger, 1985, pp 184-195.

Rosenberg WM, Sackett DL: On the need for evidence-based medicine. *Therapie* 1996;51:212-217.

Sackett DL: Evidence-based medicine. *Spine* 1998;23:1085-1086.

Sackett DL: Why randomized controlled trials fail but needn't: 1. Failure to gain "coal-face' commitment and to use the uncertainty principle. *CMAJ* 2000;162:1311-1314.

Sackett DL, Rosenberg WM, Muir Gray JA, Hayes RB, Richardson WS: Evidence based medicine: What it is and what it isn't. *BMJ* 1996;312:71-72.

Ware JE, Snow KK, Kosinski M, Gandek B: *SF-36 Health Survey: Manual and Interpretation Guide*. Boston, MA, The Health Institute, New England Medical Center, 1997.

Weinstein JN, Deyo RA: Clinical research: issues in data collection. *Spine* 2000;25:3104-3109.

Chapter 10

Clinical Epidemiology: An Introduction

Karel G.M. Moons, PhD

Diederick E. Grobbee, MD, PhD

Introduction

The concept of evidence-based medicine implies that the medical care of individual patients should be based on results obtained from patient-oriented quantitative research, rather than on qualitative research or clinical experience. Patient-oriented quantitative research is also referred to as clinical epidemiologic research.

Traditionally, epidemiologic research focused on the occurrence of infectious diseases and tried to unravel determinants of infectious disease epidemics across populations. Over time, however, it has been shown that methods used for this type of epidemiologic research (population epidemiology) can be applied in a similar manner to investigate clinical questions. Clinical epidemiology is a term commonly used for epidemiology dealing with questions relevant to medical practice. Accordingly, evidence-based medicine is particularly served by results from clinical epidemiologic research. The distinction between clinical epidemiology and population epidemiology may be somewhat artificial because both types of studies use largely the same methods for design and analysis. To properly serve clinical practice and provide for evidence-based medicine, clinical epidemiologic studies should address relevant clinical questions, be validly executed, and should yield results with sufficient precision.

Clinical Epidemiologic Research Questions

Understanding the challenges related to clinical practice is essential for understanding the objectives of clinical epidemiologic research. Beginning with the patient-physician encounter, four principal challenges or questions in clinical practice can be defined. These questions relate back to Hippocrates and form the basis of the evidenced-based medicine movement. In hierarchical order these questions are: (1) What is the illness of the patient given the clinical and nonclinical profile? (2) Why did this illness occur in this patient at this time? (3) What will be the course of the patient with this illness and manifestations? (4) How can I, as a physician, improve the course of the patient with this illness and manifestations?

The first question asks for the most probable diagnosis or illness given the clinical (such as symptoms, signs, test results) and nonclinical (such as age, sex, and socioeconomic status) profile of the patient. The answer to the second question, which asks for the cause of the illness, is often impossible to give. Often, adequate care can be provided without knowing the cause of an illness. For example, a torn meniscus can effectively be treated by the orthopaedic surgeon without knowing how the injury occurred. The most challenging question concerns a prediction of the clinical course of the patient given the clinical and nonclinical profile, the underlying illness, and the possible etiology of that illness (question 3). This prediction of the patient's clinical course may be made without considering treatment (baseline prognosis) as well as with the consideration of the effects of possible treatments. Differences in the estimated course with and without treatment may guide the physician's decision on whether to initiate treatment and in the choice between various treatment options. For example, if in a patient with a torn meniscus the probability of an unfavorable outcome (such as pain with activity) is much higher without surgery (baseline prognosis) than with surgery, it is likely that surgery would be chosen as the proper course of action (question 4).

For a physician to meet the challenges of clinical decision making, quantitative or probabilistic knowledge is required. Diagnostic research yields quantitative knowledge about the probability of disease presence or absence given the patient's clinical and nonclinical profile (addressing question 1). Results from etiologic research help the physician to answer questions about the probability that a particular disease will occur when a particular risk factor is present (question 2). Prognostic research provides quantitative knowledge about the probability that a particular outcome (death, complication, recurrence, or improved quality of life) may occur over a particular period of time in relation to the patient's profile, illness, and etiology (question 3). Treatment decisions require knowledge about the probability

Table 1 | Main Design Characteristics of Diagnostic, Etiologic, Prognostic, and Therapeutic Studies

	Determinant(s)	Outcome	Occurrence Relation	Domain
General definition	Factor(s) under study that are related to the outcome occurrence	Health parameter (eg disease, survival, complication, quality of life) under study	Association between the outcome occurrence and the determinant(s)	Larger, theoretical population to whom the study results can be applied (generalized)
Type of research				
Diagnostic research	Test results under study	Presence/absence of target disease	Presence (prevalence) of disease in relation to combination of test results	Patients with particular symptom/sign suspected of particular disease
Etiologic research	Causal factor under study	Incidence of disease under study	Incidence of the outcome in relation to the causal factor, accounted for all possible confounders	Those potentially at risk to develop the outcome at interest
Prognostic research	Prognostic predictors under study	Incidence of disease (eg, disease, survival, complication, quality of life) under study	Incidence of the outcome in relation to combination of prognostic predictors	Patients potentially at risk to develop the outcome at interest
Therapeutic research	Treatment (relative to a control group) under study	Incidence of disease (eg, disease, survival, complication, quality of life) under study	Incidence of the outcome in relation to the treatment, accounted for all possible confounders	Patients with a particular disease for whom the treatment under study is indicated

or extent to which a treatment improves the prognosis (intended effect) and at what cost (such as treatment risks [unintended effects] and monetary costs).

In medical practice, few outcomes are certain or pathognomonic. Hence, the objective of clinical epidemiologic research is to provide probabilistic knowledge on diagnosis, etiology, prognosis, and treatment of illnesses as a means to enhance patient care. The design, conduction, and data analysis of clinical studies on diagnosis, etiology, prognosis, or treatment each have their own characteristics.

Basic Principles of Clinical Epidemiologic Studies

Research Question, Study Population, and Generalization

Any research question related to patient care is either diagnostic, etiologic, prognostic, or therapeutic in nature. Although each type of study has its own characteristics, every research question and thus each type of study addresses an association between the occurrence or probability of an outcome on one side and factors that are related to this outcome occurrence on the other side. These factors are commonly called determinants. Accordingly, central to clinical epidemiologic research is the occurrence relation or the association between the outcome occurrence and its determinant(s).

To quantify this relation requires empirical data, which in turn requires a study population. For each member or patient of the study population, both the presence of the determinant(s) and of the outcome

needs to be documented. From these empirical data, the true nature and strength of the association between determinant and outcome is quantified.

To apply the findings with confidence in patient care, the study results or estimated association need to be generalized to a larger population (domain) from which the patients of the study population were selected. The extent to which the results found in a particular study population can be applied to a larger (theoretical) patient population is called the generalizability of the study results.

Therefore, regardless of the question studied, each type of clinical epidemiologic study (diagnostic, etiologic, prognostic, or therapeutic) has certain basic elements: the occurrence relation, outcome, determinant(s), study population, and domain. These elements are described later in this chapter according to each type of study and also are outlined in Table 1.

Causal Versus Descriptive Research

A major distinction first should be made between causal and descriptive epidemiologic research, because of the major consequences for study design, conduction, and data analysis. The difference is directed by the determinant(s) under study. Although 'determinant' is a term that seems to refer to factors that cause the occurrence of an outcome, it should be stressed that a determinant, and therefore clinical epidemiologic research, may be causal or noncausal (descriptive).

Causal studies quantify whether a specific determinant is causally related to an outcome; for example, trauma as a causal factor for vertebral fractures or immobility as a causal factor for pulmonary embolism. The goal of causal studies is to explain the occurrence of an outcome in relation to a causal determinant. Treatment studies are also causal studies. A treatment cannot be effective if it does not interfere in some way in the causal pathway of the outcome, such as progress of the disease or complications. A treatment is also a causal determinant, although it does not induce outcome (such as trauma and immobility) but rather reduces the likelihood or prevents the occurrence of outcomes. The fact that therapeutic studies are causal studies is very important, as the design and data analysis of causal studies are quite different from the design and analysis of descriptive studies.

In descriptive studies, the occurrence of the outcome is only described by the determinant(s) at interest. The motive of descriptive studies is to quantify whether a determinant predicts rather than explains the occurrence of the outcome. Causality is not investigated. Consider, for example, a study to quantify whether the skin color of a neonate (one of the items of the Apgar score) is predictive for its survival (a prognostic study question). Skin color obviously is not causally related to mortality. Accordingly, prognostic research that does not involve questions about the effects of treatment is descriptive research. Diagnostic studies are descriptive as well. For example, in a patient who reports symptoms of a knee disorder, abnormalities on the MRI scan of the knee may predict the presence of knee arthrosis. Results of the MRI scan obviously are not the cause of the knee arthrosis, but may predict the likelihood of the presence or absence of the condition.

Therefore, etiologic and therapeutic research questions address causality between a determinant and outcome. To answer these questions requires a causal study design and causal data analysis. Diagnostic and prognostic research questions address the predictive value between determinants and outcome. Causality is not investigated. To answer diagnostic and prognostic research questions requires a descriptive study design and corresponding data analysis. The distinction between causal and descriptive research is further explained using clinical examples in the next section.

Characteristics of Diagnostic, Etiologic, Prognostic, and Therapeutic Studies
Diagnostic Research
Diagnosis in practice starts with a patient presenting with a particular set of symptoms or signs that lead the physician to suspect a particular disease, the so-called target disease. The goal of the physician is to estimate the probability of the presence of the underlying disease. This probability is (often implicitly) estimated using diagnostic test results. These test results are obtained from patient history (each question, including simple questions on age and sex, is a different diagnostic test), physical examination, and additional tests such as imaging, electrophysiology, and laboratory tests. Currently, many diagnostic tests are used, sometimes with considerable burden to patients and health care budgets. Therefore, it is important for physicians, patients, and health care providers to know which additional tests truly contribute to the distinction between disease presence and absence beyond the information obtained from patient history and physical examination. Quantitative diagnostic research is needed to acquire this knowledge. For example, a patient with low back pain who is suspected of having a herniated disk (target disease) is referred to an orthopaedic surgeon. A possible diagnostic question could concern which results from the patient's history (age, trauma, pain when seated) and from the physical examination (notably the Lasègue test) are relevant to predict or estimate the probability of the presence of a herniated disk. Also, does the conventional radiograph of the lower back provide added predictive value?

Occurrence Relation, Study Population, and Determinants
The occurrence relation of a diagnostic study to answer the above question would concern the frequency (or probability) of a herniated disk in relation to patient history, physical examination, and radiographic results. To study this relation, the study population should include a sufficient number of patients with low back pain who have suspected disk herniation. Each patient should undergo all diagnostic tests under study (all relevant tests indicated from patient history, physical examination, and lower back radiography). These tests are called the diagnostic determinants under study.

Outcome and Data Analysis
Subsequently, each study patient should undergo the reference or gold standard test to assess the patient's diagnostic outcome or "diagnostic truth." The procedure that is used in practice (at the time of study initiation) to ultimately determine the presence or absence of the target disease, should be used as a reference standard in a scientific diagnostic study. In the example of the herniated disk, MRI of the low back could be the reference standard. The results of the reference standard should always be interpreted without knowledge of the diagnostic tests or determinants under study, to prevent information bias. Some diseases may lack a single reference standard and sometimes it may be unethical or too costly to perform the reference standard in each patient. In such situations, a combination of tests or the so-called consensus diagnosis is commonly used to determine the diagnostic "truth" in each study patient.

Documented patient data from the study in the example can then be used to quantify the probability of a herniated disk in patients with particular symptoms and signs, and to quantify whether radiographs increase or decrease this probability, and to what extent. The latter reflect the added value of the radiographs beyond the information obtained from the history and physical findings. Causality between the determinants (test results) and outcome (final diagnosis) is not an issue. The only matter of importance is whether they predict the outcome presence. Diagnostic research is therefore descriptive or predictive research. To properly serve clinical practice, diagnostic studies should address multiple determinants or tests rather than one single test. In practice, any diagnosis is rarely set by a single test. Results from patient history and physical examination will always be considered before additional tests are applied.

Domain and Generalization

The domain or theoretical target population should be a defined group (such as all patients presenting in secondary care with symptoms or signs indicative of herniated disk) to which the results of the diagnostic study can be generalized. In general, the domain of a diagnostic study is first of all determined by the symptoms and signs exhibited by the study patients. The domain definition often includes the setting (primary, secondary, or tertiary care) as well.

The selection or recruitment of any study population is often restricted by logistic circumstances, such as necessity of patients to live nearby the research center or the availability of time to participate in the study. These characteristics, however, are unlikely to influence the applicability and generalization of clinical study results. It is important and challenging for the physician to appreciate which characteristics truly affect the generalizability of results obtained from a particular study population. This appreciation usually requires external knowledge of characteristics of the study population and of the research setting that may change the nature and strength of the estimated associations between determinant(s) and outcome. Therefore, generalizability or definition of the domain of a clinical study is not an objective process that can be framed in statistical terms. Generalizability is a matter of reasoning.

Etiologic Research

Clinicians and epidemiologists seem to be most familiar with etiologic research despite its limited direct relevance to patient care and its methodologic complexities. The goal of etiologic studies is to quantify whether a single, specific determinant is indeed causally related to the outcome under study. Consider, for example, a study to quantify whether frequent falling may cause hip fractures in the elderly.

Occurrence Relation, Study Population, and Determinants

The occurrence relation of this study would be the occurrence (probability) of hip fractures in relation to the frequency of falling. To study this relation, for example, a group (cohort) of study subjects (men and women older than 70 years who have not had a hip fracture) can be recruited and followed for a 5-year period. Each year, for example, the study subjects visit the research center so that the number of falls in the previous year can be assessed. In contrast to diagnostic and prognostic studies, etiologic studies focus on the quantification of the causal relation of a single determinant (falling) to the outcome (hip fractures).

Outcome and Data Analysis

During the study period, whether and when a hip fracture has occurred is documented for each subject. After the study period, the number of falls and whether a hip fracture has occurred is known for each subject. In the analysis, two determinant groups can be formed. One group includes subjects with a high frequency of falling (on average three or more times per year) and the other with a low frequency (less than three times per year). Accordingly, whether the occurrence of hip fractures is significantly higher in those with high versus low number of falls can be quantified. In addition, the data can be analyzed using a cutoff value other than three, or using more than two determinant groups (nonfallers, those with less than three falls, and those with more than three falls per year).

Domain

The domain to which the study result can be generalized will include all patients older than 70 years with no history of a hip fracture. In general, the domain of an etiologic study includes all persons who are potentially at risk to develop the outcome at interest. As stated earlier, other characteristics of the study population that may affect the generalizability of the estimated association also need to be considered in the domain definition. Such generalization remains a matter of subjective reasoning requiring external knowledge of the studied determinant-outcome or occurrence relation.

Confounders

In contrast to diagnostic and prognostic research, in etiologic research the role of confounders is an additional issue that must be considered. Suppose the example study would yield an incidence of hip fractures (within 5 years) of 6% among the frequent fallers and 3% among the nonfrequent fallers. The initial conclusion would be that frequent falling causes a twofold increased risk of hip fractures in subjects older than 70 years. This observation, however, might not be true. The observed difference in frequency of hip fractures could be caused by

Table 2	Hypothetical Example of the Distribution of Various Potential Confounders Across Subjects With a High (More Than Three Times Per Year) and Low (Less Than Three Times Per Year) Frequency of Falling		
Confounder	**Low Frequency of Falling** (n = 1,500)	**High Frequency of Falling** (n = 1,000)
Mean age (years)	74	83*
Current smoker	35%	36%
BMI (kg/m^2)	29	25*

*P value < 0.001

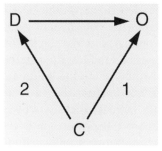

Figure 1 Diagram to determine whether a risk factor is a confounder of the studied association. D = determinant; O = outcome; C = potential confounder. 1 = the association between the potential confounder and the outcome; 2 = the association between the potential confounder and the determinant.

other risk factors that happened to be different across the two determinant groups. For example, it is known from the literature that increased age, smoking, and low body mass index (BMI) are also risk factors for hip fractures. If (by accident) in the study population these other risk factors are unequally distributed across the two groups of fallers, the observed difference of 3% in hip fractures could be caused by these other risk factors. In etiologic research these other risk factors of the outcome under study are called confounders.

Table 2 shows hypothetical results of the distribution of the other three risk factors of hip fractures across the two groups of fallers. Age was significantly higher and BMI significantly lower among the frequent fallers, whereas the smoking distribution was the same. The higher frequency of hip fractures among the frequent fallers could obviously not be caused by smoking (which was the same for both groups) but could be caused by their higher age and lower BMI compared with the infrequent fallers.

Note that a risk factor can only be a true confounder in an etiologic study, if it indeed has a causal association with the outcome, and is also (but not necessarily causally) associated with the determinant. The latter simply means that the confounder is unequally distributed across the two determinant groups. This situation is schematically shown in Figure 1. If association 1 and 2 exist in the data, C is a true confounder of the association between determinant and outcome. Because the goal of an etiologic study is to quantify whether there is a causal association between the determinant (falling) and outcome (hip fractures), the influence of any other risk factors that might confound this estimation must be ruled out or accounted for. If confounders are not accounted for in an etiologic study, then an observed association might not be the true association, and is therefore invalid. The association between the causal determinant and outcome without adjusting for confounders is called the crude association.

Accounting for Confounders

The most common and successful methods to account for confounding are randomization and adjustment in the analysis. Randomization means that the investigator randomly assigns the study subjects to the two (or more) determinant groups. Because of this process, the two determinant groups are by definition comparable for all other risk factors except for the determinant at issue, given that the groups are large enough. Randomization, however, is frequently not feasible or ethical. In the example study it is impossible to randomize subjects to frequent or nonfrequent falling groups. The same concept applies to causal studies investigating physiologic determinants such as blood pressure, cholesterol level, age, and bone mineral density. For ethical reasons, randomization is commonly not possible if the determinant increases the risk of the outcome at interest. For example, when studying the causal relationship between smoking and lung cancer, or alcohol consumption and hip fractures, subjects cannot be randomly assigned to years of smoking or alcohol consumption. Randomization is only possible for causal determinants that reduce the occurrence of the outcome at interest, and is mainly reserved for therapeutic determinants. Because therapeutic research is causal research, randomized studies particularly apply to therapeutic research.

In nonrandomized causal studies, accounting for confounding must be done in the data analysis. During the design phase, all potential risk factors of the outcome need to be defined beforehand such that association 1 in Figure 1 is fulfilled. This identification of the potential risk factors should be based on existing knowledge or "educated" reasoning. These other risk factors should then be measured in each study subject in addition to the determinant of interest. In the analysis it should be assessed whether association 2 in Figure 1 is indeed present in the data. If so, a so-called multivariable analysis is applied to adjust the crude association between the determinant and outcome (a difference of 3% hip fractures in the example) for all confounders. A determinant is called causally associated with an outcome, if the association remains after having accounted for all confounders in the data.

Note that adjustment for confounding might dilute but could also increase the crude association between the determinant and outcome, depending on the distribution of the confounders across the determinant categories and whether the confounder is a risk factor or preventive factor of the outcome. In the example study, adjustment for age and BMI would dilute the crude association of 3% difference in hip fractures because increased age and low BMI both increase the occurrence of hip fractures, and the frequent fallers were on average older and leaner than the nonfrequent fallers. Studies whose purpose is to quantify whether an unintended effect of a treatment is truly caused by that treatment are etiologic studies as well and should follow the above principles.

Prognostic Research

Prognostic research has received limited attention in applied medical research. In practice, to set a prognosis is to estimate the probability that a patient with a particular illness and clinical and nonclinical profile will develop a particular outcome (death, a complication, recurrence of disease, or a good quality of life) within a certain period of time. The prognostic probability could also be estimated given that the patient has undergone a particular treatment. Here, treatment is considered as one of the prognostic factors. Prognosis in practice does not simply imply the typical course of an illness or diagnosis; it refers to the course of a patient with particular clinical and nonclinical characteristics. Just as with diagnostic questions, it is relevant for physicians to know which information is truly needed to estimate a patient's prognosis. As with diagnosis, the probability should preferably be estimated with information or determinants that are easily obtainable from the patient using noninvasive, low-cost methods. The principles of design and analysis of prognostic research are similar to those of diagnostic research, because both can be grouped under the heading of descriptive or prediction research. Their study goal is to quantify the predictive association between the determinant(s) and the outcome; causal explanation of the outcome is not necessary.

An example of a prognostic question is whether preoperative patient characteristics are predictive for the occurrence of postoperative nausea and vomiting within 24 hours in patients undergoing orthopaedic surgery. If this occurrence can be estimated preoperatively, preferably using easily obtainable patient variables, the anesthesiologist or orthopaedic surgeon could perform a timely intervention in high-risk patients to reduce the risk of postoperative nausea and vomiting. For example, instead of using isoflurane, desflurane, or sevoflurane for general anesthesia, intravenous propofol, which has been proven to cause less postoperative nausea and vomiting could be used, or preemptive administration of antiemetics could be done.

Occurrence Relation, Study Population, and Determinants

The occurrence relation of a prognostic study to answer this example question would be the frequency (or probability) of postoperative nausea and vomiting within 24 hours in relation to multiple preoperative patient characteristics, such as planned duration of surgery, age, sex, history of postoperative nausea and vomiting, and smoking status. The study population could include patients at a particular hospital undergoing any orthopaedic surgery who are at risk of developing postoperative nausea and vomiting. All prognostic predictors of the outcome should be documented from each study patient. Similarly, as in diagnostic research, prognostic research should address multiple predictors rather than a single prognostic predictor because in practice, no prognosis is set by a single predictor.

Outcome and Data Analysis

Each patient should be followed up to measure whether the outcome has occurred. In the example, this measurement is done at 24 hours after surgery, using a simple questionnaire. As with diagnostic research, the person measuring the outcome must be blinded to the patient's predictor values to prevent information bias. Particularly in prognostic (and therapeutic) research, outcomes that are important to patients (such as degree of pain and quality of life issues) should be investigated. Researchers too often rely on so-called proxy outcomes such as duration of intensive care stay or intraoperatively measured physiologic parameters such as body temperature or blood pressure rather than on patient outcomes.

The preoperative predictors that truly have predictive value (that is, may predict the occurrence of postoperative nausea and vomiting within 24 hours) and which information actually is redundant to determine the patient's prognosis can be easily quantified from the data.

Domain

In general, the domain of a prognostic study is determined by the diagnosis or illness that places the patient at risk of developing the outcome at interest. As with diagnostic research, the setting (for example, primary or secondary) is often included if it is not inherent to the study population. Similarly, other characteristics of the study population that may affect the generalizability of the estimated association also need to be included. The domain of the example study would include all patients scheduled for orthopaedic surgery. However, there may be no reason to assume that the predictors estimated from the orthopaedic study population would not also apply to other surgical patients. Therefore, the results of the example study could perhaps be generalized to all types of surgery. However, as discussed previously, this generalization requires external knowledge and subjective judgment. The question to be asked is whether in these other types of surgery that were not included in the study population the same predictors would be found with the same predictive values.

The example study shows that as with diagnostic research, prognostic studies (apart from studies on treatment effects) aim to describe or predict the occurrence of a future outcome and possible given combinations of prognostic determinants. Causality between the determinants and outcome is not at issue. A similar approach as that described above has been applied to predict the need for intraoperative blood transfusion in orthopaedic and other types of surgery.

Therapeutic Research
Studies to quantify the intended effect of a treatment, including surgical treatment (further referred to as therapeutic or intervention studies) are the most popular form of clinical epidemiologic research. The methods for design and analysis of intervention studies, including the well-known Consolidate Standards of Reporting Trials (CONSORT), has been extensively documented in the literature. The principles of therapeutic research can be described by considering the following example of a study question: does arthroscopic débridement in patients with osteoarthritis of the knee reduce the occurrence of pain?

The question of how the clinical course of a patient with a particular illness and manifestations can be modified indicates that therapeutic research is a form of prognostic research. As stated earlier, the goal of a therapeutic study is to quantify whether an observed intended effect is truly caused by the treatment under study, excluding any other causes. Therapeutic studies are also a form of causal research and the characteristics described for etiologic research similarly apply to intervention research.

Occurrence Relation and Study Population
The occurrence relation of the example study question (regarding patients with osteoarthritis of the knee) would be the average level of pain at 24 months postoperatively in relation to arthroscopic débridement. Study subjects could include men and women of all ages, with osteoarthritis of the knee who have an indication for arthroscopy. The study subjects could be selected from four different hospitals, for example.

Determinant
Proper definition of the determinant in therapeutic studies requires some explanation. To quantify the effect of a treatment always requires a control group. A single group of patients that has been treated with the intervention under study, a so-called case series, is insufficient to properly quantify the treatment effect. Any ob-

served outcome could be caused by other factors such as natural course or, because the patient is aware of the treatment, change in patient perception and lifestyle changes that might influence the outcome occurrence. The latter is particularly the case when the study outcome is a subjective outcome requiring patient reporting, such as pain and quality of life. If the outcome, for example, is death, factors such as patient perception and lifestyle changes have much less influence on the outcome. In situations in which an extreme change in outcome is observed that is unlikely to be related to other factors, a controlled study may not be necessary. This situation, however, is rare in medicine. However, it may, for example, apply to the benefits of total hip replacement, which leads to such a dramatic change in mobility of a patient that the result can validly be assumed to be the consequence of the intervention. Generally, however, the determinant in a therapeutic study includes a group that receives the treatment (index group) and a control group that does not.

The control group may receive either placebo treatment or an existing treatment. A placebo treatment is exactly the same as the index treatment except that it does not include the effective part or substance of the treatment. Placebo treatment for a control group is common for drug therapies, but is also possible for non-pharmacologic or surgical interventions. The placebo drug has the same color, size, taste, or mode of use as the index drug, except that it does not include the pharmacologic substance. Administering one half of the study population the index and the other half the placebo treatment, and blinding the patient to the received treatment, excludes the influence of many factors that could influence the difference in outcome between the two groups. These factors include patient perception and lifestyle changes but also treatment-related factors such as taste, size, or mode of use of a drug. As both patient groups are unaware of the received treatment, the extent to which these factors operate will be the same across both groups and cannot cause any differences in outcome occurrence.

However, the use of a placebo treatment is not always feasible or ethical, especially for surgical therapies. For example, when quantifying the effect of coronary artery bypass grafting (CABG) it would be unethical to perform a placebo-CABG. Placebo-CABG would involve the same procedure as the index-CABG, including undergoing general anesthesia plus sternotomy, but without the bypassing which is in fact the effective ('pharmacologic') substance of the CABG treatment. Treatments or diseases that do not allow for a placebo comparison require comparison with an existing treatment. Existing treatment also could be no treatment (wait and see).

Besides ethical constraints, using an existing treatment as a control might also be favored to better reflect clinical practice. Using an existing treatment as control implies that all patients are aware of the received treatment; the patients are not 'blinded'. The influence of patient perception, lifestyle changes, and treatment factors other than the effective part, may thus be different across the new (index) and existing (control) treatment groups. However, all of these factors are considered as part of the total effect of each treatment strategy on the outcome. It merely reflects the real life situation of both treatments. Any difference in outcome between the two treatment groups will result from the overall difference between the two treatment strategies. It will be impossible to unravel which factors are responsible for the observed difference. Therapeutic studies using another (nonplacebo) treatment as control are called pragmatic studies. Placebo-controlled therapeutic studies are called explanatory studies, as any observed difference can be attributed to or explained by the difference in 'effective substance' between the two groups.

In the example, if a pragmatic trial would be desired, the determinant could include arthroscopic débridement versus no treatment (or wait and see). If a placebo-controlled study would be desired, the control group would include placebo arthroscopy, that is, without débridement. Such a study has recently been conducted.

Outcome

In the example study, the outcome is pain measured, for example, 1 and 2 years after surgery using a visual analog or verbal rating scale. As with prognostic research, patient-driven rather than intermediate outcomes should be chosen. Furthermore, as in all other types of research, the person who measures the outcome should be blinded to the treatment of the patient to prevent information bias, whether or not a pragmatic or placebo-controlled therapeutic study is performed.

Data Analysis and Confounding

As mentioned earlier, one of the most important aspects of causal research is to account for other risk factors of the outcome (such as confounders). Randomization is the best method to ensure that the compared groups are comparable on all risk factors except for the determinant under study. In therapeutic research, the benefits of the determinant (treatment) are supposed to outweigh its risks, making randomization feasible and ethical. Nevertheless, despite adequate randomization, an imbalance of confounders between the two treatment groups could still occur by chance, particularly when the number of patients is small. Therefore, in the analysis, investigators should first check other risk factors of the outcome to determine if they are indeed equally distributed. If not, adjustment in the analysis may sometimes be needed to account for confounding.

Domain

The domain to which the results of the example study can be generalized are patients who have osteoarthritis and an indication for arthroscopy.

Therapeutic research is causal research on the intended effects of treatments. The treatment under study may be compared with existing treatment including no treatment, or to a placebo treatment, depending on the research question. A pragmatic study approach will quantify the difference in effect between two treatment strategies. A placebo-controlled study quantifies the efficacy of the effective (pharmacologic) substance of the treatment under study. Blinding the patient is only at issue in placebo-controlled studies. In pragmatic and placebo-controlled studies, the treatments always should be allocated randomly to prevent confounding bias. If patient numbers are low, adjustment for confounding in the analysis may sometimes be necessary. Blinding the observer to the outcome is always desired except when the outcome under study is not sensitive to observer interpretation.

Summary

Clinical epidemiology attempts to provide quantitative answers to relevant questions to improve future medical care. Such questions arise from the patient-physician encounters and require either diagnostic, etiologic, prognostic, or therapeutic knowledge. Accordingly, the first step when designing a clinical epidemiologic study is to determine which of these four types of knowledge is addressed. Irrespective of the type of knowledge addressed, definition of the occurrence relation, outcome, and determinant applies to each type of study question. With etiologic or therapeutic research, the potential confounders of the determinant-outcome relationship should also be defined beforehand. It is also useful to initially define the domain of the studied occurrence relation because this process helps to select the suitable study population from that domain. Next, the determinant(s), confounders, and outcome should be measured from each study subject. Finally, the data should be analyzed, taking into account whether the goal is to predict the outcome (diagnostic or prognostic research) or to explain what actually causes the occurrence of the outcome (etiologic or therapeutic research).

Annotated Bibliography

General Reference

Greenhalgh T: *How to Read a Paper: The Basics of Evidence Based Medicine*, ed 2. London, England, BMJ Publishing Group, 2001.

This book provides a general introduction on the essentials of evidence-based medicine and guidelines for reading clinical epidemiologic studies.

Laupacis A: The future of evidence-based medicine. *Can J Clin Pharmacol* 2001;8(suppl A):6A-9A.

This article presents a state of the art review of evidence-based medicine and the challenges for the near future.

Clinical Epidemiologic Research Questions

Sackett DL: Clinical epidemiology: What, who, and whither. *J Clin Epidemiol* 2002;55:1161-1166.

A general introduction to the history of clinical epidemiology is presented.

Basic Principles of Clinical Epidemiologic Studies

Rothman KJ: *Epidemiology: An Introduction*. Oxford, England, Oxford University Press, 2002.

This book, which focuses on etiologic research, covers the field of epidemiology including history, study questions, and data analysis. A background in epidemiology is required.

Characteristics of Diagnostic Studies

Bossuyt PM, Reitsma JB, Bruns DE, et al: Towards complete and accurate reporting of studies of diagnostic accuracy: The STARD initiative: Standards for Reporting of Diagnostic Accuracy. *Clin Chem* 2003;49:1-6.

This article addresses a list of criteria that will enhance the reporting and conduction of diagnostic accuracy studies.

Knottnerus JA: *The Evidence Base of Clinical Diagnosis*. London, England, BMJ Publishing Group, 2002.

This book contains a series of *British Medical Journal* articles on the essentials of diagnostic studies, from study questions to analysis.

Moons KG, Grobbee DE: Diagnostic studies as multivariable, prediction research. *J Epidemiol Com Health* 2002;56:337-338.

A brief report discussing the need for studies that attempt to quantify the added value of new tests beyond existing tests (rather than estimating a test's sensitivity and specificity) is presented.

Moons KG, Harrell FE: Sensitivity and specificity should be deemphasized in diagnostic accuracy studies. *Acad Radiol* 2003;10:670-672.

This editorial on the Standards for Reporting of Diagnostic Accuracy initiative discusses why estimating a test's sensitivity has limited value for clinical practice.

Oostenbrink R, Moons KG, Bleeker SE, Moll HA, Grobbee DE: Diagnostic research on routine care data: Prospects and problems. *J Clin Epidemiol* 2003;56:501-506.

This article addresses the pros and cons of using routine care data for the evaluation of diagnostic tests.

Characteristics of Etiologic Studies

Hak E, Verheij TJ, Grobbee DE, Nichol KL, Hoes AW: Confounding by indication in non-experimental evaluation of vaccine effectiveness: The example of prevention of influenza complications. *J Epidemiol Community Health* 2002;56:951-955.

This article illustrates the problems of using data from a nonrandomized (observational) study to quantify the effectiveness of a therapy.

Kennedy KA, Frankowski RF: Evaluating the evidence about therapies: What the clinician needs to know about statistics. *Clin Perinatol* 2003;30:205-215.

The basics of data analysis of therapeutic studies is addressed in this article.

Lorenz JM, Paneth N: When are observational studies adequate to assess the efficacy of therapeutic interventions? *Clin Perinatol* 2003;30:269-283.

This article presents information on when and how nonrandomized (observational) study data can be useful to quantify the effectiveness of therapies.

Characteristics of Prognostic Studies

Concato J: Challenges in prognostic analysis. *Cancer* 2001;91(suppl 8):1607-1614.

This article enhances the understanding of studies that attempt to quantify the prognostic or predictive value of factors such as patient characteristics, etiologic factors, and diagnostic tests and results.

van Klei WA: Moons KG, Leyssius AT, Knape JT, Rutten CL, Grobbee DE: Reduction in type and screen: Preoperative prediction of RBC transfusions in surgery procedures with intermediate transfusion risks. *Br J Anaesth* 2001;87:250-257.

This article presents an example study that developed an easy applicable prognostic rule for surgeons or anesthesiologists to preoperatively predict which surgical patients would undergo perioperative blood transfusions.

van Klei WA, Moons KG, Rheineck-Leyssius AT, et al: Validation of a clinical prediction rule to reduce preoperative type and screen procedures. *Br J Anaesth* 2002; 89:221-225.

This article presents an example study that validated a developed prognostic rule to preoperatively predict which new surgical patients would undergo perioperative blood transfusions.

Vergouwe Y, Steyerberg EW, Eijkemans MJ, Habbema JD: Validity of prognostic models: When is a model clinically useful? *Semin Urol Oncol* 2002;20:96-107.

This article discusses an appealing method to determine whether a prognostic prediction rule is clinically useful.

Characteristics of Therapeutic Studies

Altman DG, Schulz KF, Moher D, et al: The revised CONSORT statement for reporting randomized trials: Explanation and elaboration. *Ann Intern Med* 2001;134: 663-694.

This article addresses a list of criteria that will enhance the reporting and conduction of randomized therapeutic studies.

Helms PJ: Real world pragmatic clinical trials: What are they and what do they tell us? *Pediatr Allergy Immunol* 2002;13:4-9.

This article presents a clear explanation of the differences between explanatory (such as placebo-controlled) randomized therapeutic studies and pragmatic randomized therapeutic studies.

Moher D, Schulz KF, Altman D: The CONSORT statement: Revised recommendations for improving the quality of reports of parallel-group randomized trials. *JAMA* 2001;285:1987-1991.

This article addresses a list of criteria to enhance the reporting and conduction of randomized therapeutic studies.

Moseley JB, O'Malley K, Petersen NJ, et al: A controlled trial of arthroscopic surgery for osteoarthritis of the knee. *N Engl J Med* 2002;347:81-88.

A good example of an explanatory (such as placebo-controlled) therapeutic study of a surgical intervention is presented.

Classic Bibliography

Apfel CC, Laara E, Koivuranta M, Greim CA, Roewer N: A simplified risk score for predicting postoperative nausea and vomiting: Conclusions from cross-validation between two centers. *Anesthesiology* 1999;91:693-700.

Charlton BG: Understanding randomized controlled trials: Explanatory or pragmatic? *Fam Pract* 1994;11:243-244.

Evidence-Based Medicine Working Group: Evidence-based medicine: A new approach to teaching the practice of medicine. *JAMA* 1992;268:2420-2425.

Grobbee DE, Miettinen OS: Clinical Epidemiology: Introduction to the discipline. *Neth J Med* 1995;47:2-5.

Guyatt GH, Sackett DL, Cook DJ: Users' guides to the medical literature: II. How to use an article about therapy or prevention: A. Are the results of the study valid?: Evidence-Based Medicine Working Group. *JAMA* 1993; 270:2598-2601.

Guyatt GH, Sackett DL, Cook DJ: Users' guides to the medical literature: II. How to use an article about therapy or prevention: B. What were the results and will they help me in caring for my patients?: Evidence-Based Medicine Working Group. *JAMA* 1994;271:59-63.

Hennekens CE, Buring JE: *Epidemiology in Medicine.* Boston, Massachusetts, Little, Brown & Co, 1987.

Jaeschke R, Guyatt GH, Sackett DL: Users' guides to the medical literature: III. How to use an article about a diagnostic test: A. Are the results of the study valid?: Evidence-Based MedicineWorking Group. *JAMA* 1994; 271:389-391.

Laupacis A, Sekar N, Stiell IG: Clinical prediction rules: A review and suggested modifications of methodological standards. *JAMA* 1997;277:488-494.

Laupacis A, Wells G, Richardson WS, Tugwell P: Users' guides to the medical literature: V. How to use an article about prognosis: Evidence-Based Medicine Working Group. *JAMA* 1994;272:234-237.

Levine M, Walter S, Lee H, Haines T, Holbrook A, Moyer V: Users' guides to the medical literature: IV. How to use an article about harm: Evidence-Based Medicine Working Group. *JAMA* 1994;271:1615-1619.

McAlister FA, Graham I, Karr GW, Laupacis A: Evidence-based medicine and the practicing clinician. *J Gen Intern Med* 1999;14:236-242.

Moons KG, van Es GA, Michel BC, Buller HR, Habbema JD, Grobbee DE: Redundancy of single diagnostic test evaluation. *Epidemiology* 1999;10:276-281.

Randolph AG, Guyatt GH, Calvin JE, Doig G, Richardson WS: Understanding articles describing clinical prediction tools. *Crit Care Med* 1998;26:1603-1612.

Reichenbach H: *The Rise of Scientific Philosophy.* New York, NY, Harper Row, 1965.

Roland M, Torgerson DJ: What are pragmatic trials? *BMJ* 1998;316:285.

Sackett DL, Haynes RB, Tugwell P: *Clinical Epidemiology: A Basic Science for Clinical Medicine.* Boston, Massachusetts, Little, Brown & Co, 1985.

Sackett DL, Rosenberg WM, Gray JA, Haynes RB, Richardson WS: Evidence based medicine: What it is and what it isn't. *BMJ* 1996;312:71-72.

Tinetti ME, Liu WL, Claus EB: Predictors and prognosis of inability to get up after falls among elderly persons. *JAMA* 1993;269:65-70.

Chapter 11

Musculoskeletal Imaging

John A. Carrino, MD, MPH

William B. Morrison, MD

Available Imaging Modalities

All medical imaging modalities that are available clinically have musculoskeletal applications. There have been significant technologic advancements in the areas of radiography, CT, ultrasound, nuclear medicine, and MRI.

Radiography

Digital radiography exists in the form of computed radiography or direct radiography. Image processing and distribution is achieved through a picture archiving and communication system. The images can be placed on a compact disk with an imbedded viewer. The widespread availability of computers with compact disk readers allows this method of image processing to be a more portable mechanism of transporting and managing images. Viewing the images in the soft copy environment allows for panning, zooming, windowing, and leveling so that the viewing experience and diagnostic yield are optimal. There are certain tradeoffs; the spatial resolution of digital radiography systems is not as great as that with film screen radiography. However, as additional experience and data are accumulated, it has been found that the improved contrast resolution is more important than spatial resolution for diagnostic efficacy, making less defined spatial resolution a reasonable trade-off (Figure 1).

Computed Tomography

The latest generation of CT scanners uses multiple detector row arrays. Multislice CT represents a major improvement in helical CT technology, wherein simultaneous activation of multiple detector rows positioned along the longitudinal or z-axis (direction of table or gantry) allows acquisition of interweaving helical sections. The principal difference between multislice CT and predecessor generations of CT is the improved resolution in the z-axis. More of the photons generated by the x-ray tube are ultimately used to produce imaging data. With this design, section thickness is determined by detector size and not by the collimator itself. Rapid data acquisition times are possible because of short gantry rotation intervals combined with multiple detectors providing increased coverage along the z-axis. Currently there are configurations with up to 64 channel detectors available. The data from a multislice CT scanner can be used to generate images of different thickness from the same acquisition. The minimum section thickness is reduced to approximately 0.5 mm and images can be reconstructed at this 0.5-mm interval. Isotropic (equal dimension) voxels measuring 0.5 mm in x, y, and z directions greatly improve the spatial resolution and the quality of reconstructing algorithms, allowing generation of exquisite multiplanar reformats (Figure 1) and three-dimensional images. These three-dimensional image processing and display techniques are particularly useful for regions of complex anatomy such as the pelvis, or for bones for which it is difficult to obtain isolated projections without overlap, such as the scapula or the cervical spine (Figure 2). Multiplanar reformats can be created in any plane or using a curved surface to reduce distortion. Other advantages include increased speed and increased total volume coverage. Therefore, a single pass whole body protocol may be feasible, particularly with 16-detector scanners that can image from the head vertex to below the hips in less than 1 minute. The ability to acquire high-quality images in the presence of hardware/joint implants has improved using multislice CT. Metal artifacts are caused by photopenic defects in the back projection and are displayed on CT images as streak artifact. With multislice CT, the holes in the filtered back projection are not as pronounced, resulting in a less severe streak artifact. This improvement is at the expense of excess tissue radiation along the penumbra of the beam, which is then picked up by adjacent detector channels filling in these photopenic defects in the projection. This technology has forced radiologists into redefining the image viewing process to a volumetric paradigm rather than a simple tile mode or section-by-section viewing. In addition, CT protocols have to be reformulated. There is also an expanded range of CT applications and indications. The challenges associated with multislice CT include selection of optimal imaging sequences, controlling radiation exposure to the patient,

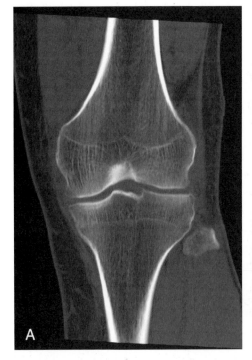

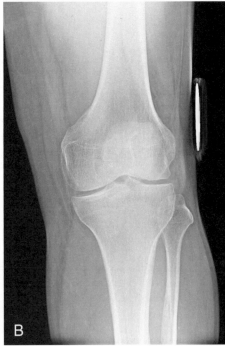

Figure 1 Digital radiography and multislice CT multiplanar reformat image quality. **A,** Anteroposterior projection of the knee performed with a direct radiography unit shows high-quality contrast. **B,** Multidetector CT coronal multiplanar reformat image shows exquisite trabecular detail similar to conventional radiography. Source images were acquired using isotropic 0.75-mm voxels.

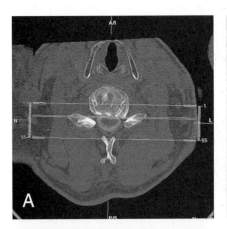

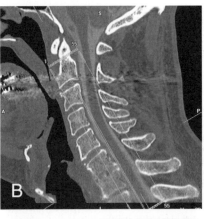

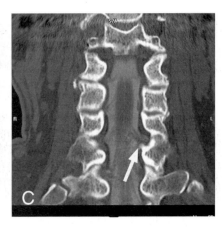

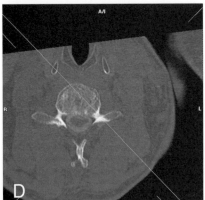

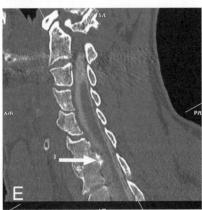

Figure 2 Position compensated multiplanar reformat. Cervical spine multislice CT myelography in a patient who underwent anterior cervical fusion: Sagittal and coronal multiplanar reformat images are created from an axial image **(A)** while adjusting the planes to correct for any rotation (double oblique prescriptions). Similar maneuvers are done for the sagittal **(B)** and coronal **(C)** planes to generate more useful sections based on true anatomic landmarks. Oblique axial images **(D)** are also used to generate sagittal oblique images **(E)** through the neural foramen at each level on each side to compensate for changes in orientation of the neural canal. Coronal and sagittal oblique multiplanar reformat images show an osseous ridge compressing the nerve roots (arrow in C and E).

and efficiently managing the large amount of data generated. Some disadvantages of multislice CT are high radiation dose to the tissue and potentially noisy images. Noise is inversely related to the number of photons per voxels; because smaller voxels tend to have fewer photons, increased image noise is the result. To keep the noise level reasonable, the exposure (and thus radiation dose) must be increased.

Ultrasound

Ultrasound is the medical imaging modality used to acquire and display the acoustic properties of tissues. A transducer array (transmitter and receiver of ultrasound pulses) sends sound waves into the patient and receives returning echoes that are converted into an image. Sound is mechanical energy that propagates through continuous, elastic medium by the compression and rarefaction of the "particles" that compose it (such as air). The resolution of the ultrasound image and attenuation of the ultrasound beam depend on the wavelength and frequency. A low frequency ultrasound beam has a longer wavelength and less resolution but greater depth of penetration. For musculoskeletal imaging of more superficial structures such as tendons and ligaments, a high frequency beam having a smaller wavelength provides superior spatial resolution and image detail. Thus, the creation of appropriate transducers is of critical importance in performing musculoskeletal imaging. Higher frequency transducers ranging from 7.5 MHz up to even 15 MHz are now available. Modern ultrasound scanners use phased array transducers with multiple piezoelectric elements to electronically sweep an ultrasound beam across the volume of interest, thus being able to create a three-dimensional image.

Applications of ultrasound include evaluation of tendon and muscle abnormalities such as rotator cuff tears. In addition, ultrasound has also been applied to evaluate the glenoid labrum and knee menisci. High-resolution ultrasound has the potential to be used for visualization of articular cartilage. Synovial effusions and proliferation can be evaluated using color Doppler imaging to determine the degree of hypertrophy and inflammation. Ultrasound has been used more often for diagnostic and therapeutic procedures because of improved transducer technology being better able to detect infrastructural detail. In addition, ultrasound is a more economical modality for assessing a specific clinical concern. Ultrasound is best used when the clinical question is specific and well formulated; the condition is dichotomous (is there a full thickness tear or not?); for characterizing a soft-tissue lesion (cystic or vascular); or for guiding particular interventions. Performing percutaneous interventions with ultrasound ensures accurate needle tip placement and helps direct the needle away from other regional soft-tissue structures and neurovascular bundles. The visualization of the needle tip in real time allows for reliable placement in the tendon sheath, bursa, or joint of interest. Intratendinous calcifications, the plantar fascia, and interdigital (Morton's) neuromas can also be visualized and injected directly under real-time guidance.

Nuclear Medicine and Positron Emission Tomography

The most significant recent advancement in nuclear medicine is positron emission tomography (PET) and the combination of PET CT scanners with important implications for oncology, especially for soft-tissue neoplasms or postoperative cancer patients. PET has only recently been widely used in clinical oncology. Short-lived positron emitting radioisotopes annihilate to form two photons with trajectories approximately 180° apart at a particular energy level (511 kev). The coincidental detection of these photons by a ring detector is reconstructed via a filtered backprojection (similar to CT) to form images of tracer distribution. [^{18}F] 2-deoxy-2-fluoro-D-glucose (FDG) is a metabolic tracer most widely used in clinical PET oncology. FDG accumulation reflects the rate of glucose utilization in a tissue because FDG is transported into a tissue by the same mechanisms of glucose transport and trapped in a tissue as FDG-6-phosphate, which is a poor substrate for the further enzyme systems of glycolysis or glycogen storage. The use of FDG in evaluation of the musculoskeletal system is based on increased glycolytic rate in pathologic tissues. Thus, PET has proved to be the gold standard in metabolic imaging. FDG provides a means of quantitating the glucose metabolism, with the amount of tracer accumulation reflecting the glucose metabolism. High-grade malignancies tend to have higher rates of glycolysis than do low-grade malignancies and benign lesions; therefore, high-grade malignancies have greater uptake of FDG than that of low-grade or benign lesions.

PET, as a metabolic imaging technique, has advantages over and complements structural imaging methods and also shows differences from conventional nuclear medicine. All of these factors have led to its growth in clinical applications in recent years. PET applications are evolving, but the technique has been approved for the diagnosis, staging, and restaging of many common malignancies and has shown efficacy for the detection of osseous metastasis from several malignancies, including lung and breast carcinomas and lymphoma. However, the significance of FDG PET in the evaluation of primary bone tumors and tumor-like lesions has not been extensively elucidated. Several investigators have reported the usefulness of FDG PET in oncologic applications for primary musculoskeletal tumors. Preliminary reports suggest a good correlation between glucose consumption measured by FDG PET and the aggressiveness of musculoskeletal tumors. However, a significant overlap exists between benign and malignant groups; therefore, PET is not a solo method for differential diagnosis of benign and malignant bone lesions. Both neoplastic and inflammatory processes can cause an increase in FDG activity; therefore, tissue sampling should be directed to the most metabolically active regions identified by PET (Figure 3). Therefore, PET has a role as a useful adjunct to anatomic imaging techniques because it can provide an in vivo method for quantifying functional metabolism in normal and diseased tissues.

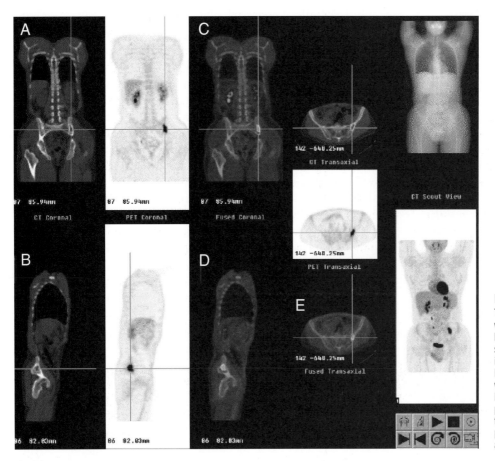

Figure 3 PET CT coregistration image fusion. The imaging studies are from a patient who was referred for evaluation for metastatic bone disease. Composite image: Coronal and sagittal maximum intensity projection FDG-PET images (**A** and **B**) show an area with abnormal FDG uptake in the pelvis that is not localized with certainty. Coronal, sagittal, and transaxial PET-CT fused images (**C**, **D**, and **E**) reveal a hypermetabolic focus corresponding to an osteolytic lesion, which was confirmed histopathologically by percutaneous biopsy to be adenocarcinoma.

Magnetic Resonance Imaging

Recent MRI technology developments include high field strength clinical systems for the entire body (3.0 Tesla) and dedicated extremity scanners operating at 1.0 Tesla, with improved gradients and radiofrequency (RF) coils. Parallel imaging and faster novel pulse sequences are addressing the time factor involved in obtaining an MRI scan. High spatial resolution imaging with improved signal-to-noise ratio has generated a new area of imaging known as magnetic resonance microscopy, used for the smaller and more complex articulations such as the hand, wrist, foot, ankle, and elbow. Expanding the types of three-dimensional pulse sequences available using fast spin-echo techniques afford the opportunity for isotropic voxel acquisition and better volumetric data rendering. Examination time can be reduced by using a single acquisition and reconstructing the plane of interest (similar to multislice CT). Currently the most useful sequences are two-dimensional. Because musculoskeletal imaging often relies on the depiction of particular anatomy, several planes are acquired using the same pulse sequence depending on the articulation, indication, and specific structure of interest.

Imaging of cartilage has been difficult; however, some new advances in MRI techniques, such as the use of biologically relevant elements such as hydrogen, oxygen-16, oxygen-17, fluorine-19, sodium-23, and phosphorus-31, will help in providing and interpreting these images. Most clinical MRI is hydrogen imaging; more recently, sodium and phosphorus images have been obtained in vivo. Sodium imaging can be used for estimating the glycosaminoglycan content of articular cartilage. Because of the low natural abundance of sodium in articular tissues, in vivo imaging is limited to high-field magnets (3.0 Tesla or greater). There are several pulse sequences that have been applied to cartilage imaging. Gradient-recall echo imaging has been used because of its three-dimensional capability and ability to provide high-resolution images. Fat-suppressed techniques are combined with gradient-recall echo imaging to increase the dynamic range and improve the detection of signal abnormalities in cartilage. However, scan acquisition time can be substantial (8 to 10 minutes), thus making the image prone to motion artifact. Magnetization transfer contrast creates tissue contrast by the exchange of magnetization between protons associated with macromolecules and bulk water protons by means of cross relaxation or chemical exchange. Magnetization transfer contrast acts as an off-resonant saturation pulse and may make cartilage lesions easier to see. Although this type of contrast is usually used in conjunction with the gradient echo techniques, some magnetization transfer occurs inherently with fast spin-echo or turbo spin-echo techniques. The driven equilibrium Fourier transform contrast method is another promising approach for imaging of cartilage disorders. This method produces image contrast that is a function of proton density, T1/T2 and echo time/repetition time (TE/TR). Many tissues have competing T1 and T2 contrast, so the T1 to T2 ratio for driven equilibrium Fourier transform contrast tends to be synergistic. Driven equilibrium Fourier transform contrast is well suited to imaging articular cartilage because synovial fluid is high and articular cartilage is intermediate in signal intensity; the osseous structures are dark and lipids can be suppressed using spectral fat saturation techniques. This creates an image in which cartilage is easily distinguishable from all adjacent tissues based on signal intensity alone, aiding segmentation and volume calculation.

Magnetic resonance arthrography has also been applied to the evaluation of cartilage and may be performed directly (a dilute gadolinium-containing solution is percutaneously placed into the joint via a needle) or indirectly (intravenous gadolinium is administered and allowed to diffuse into the joint). Gadolinium-enhanced imaging has the potential to monitor glycosaminoglycan (GAG) content within the cartilage. GAGs are fundamentally important for several reasons: they play a major mechanical support role, they are lost early in the course of cartilage degeneration, and may need to be replenished during the course of any effective cartilage treatment regimen. GAGs contribute strong negative charge to the cartilage matrix and mobile ions will distribute to reflect local GAG concentration. When GAGs are lost as part of the degenerative process, the negative charge conferred to the cartilage also is lost. Consequently, when a negatively charged contrast agent is administered (either intravenously or intra-articularly) it preferentially distributes into the degraded cartilage and the T1 effect of this contrast material can be qualitatively visualized and quantitatively measured. With direct magnetic resonance arthrography, it takes 3 hours for the contrast to sufficiently diffuse into the cartilage, whereas with indirect magnetic resonance arthrography it only takes approximately 1.5 hours.

Clinical higher field MRI systems, typically 3.0 Tesla (or 3T) are becoming widely available. The higher intrinsic signal-to-noise ratio of high-field strength MRI can be used to improve imaging speed or resolution but changes in relaxation time at 3T as well as increased artifacts must be considered. Nevertheless, 3T MRI offers the opportunity to explore physiologic imaging of joints as well as morphologic features. Tissues in a magnetic field are categorized by two types of relaxation: T1 (spin-lattice relaxation time) and T2 (spin-spin relaxation time). Manipulation of imaging parameters of the TE and the TR produce the various types of contrast

seen in MRI. T2 is fairly constant at different field strengths, but T1 increases with increasing field strength. Fat suppression is improved at 3T because the peaks between water and fat are further separated (greater chemical shift effect; the nature of the chemical shift phenomenon is that protons associated with long chain aliphatic fat molecules have precessional frequencies slightly lower than protons associated with mobile water molecules, which is field strength-dependent), providing more robust spectral fat suppression. The US Food and Drug Administration and manufacturers have mandated the use of power monitoring systems for 3T because of increased danger of RF burns. The more problematic sequences are fast spin-echo/turbo spin-echo (unless the refocusing pulse is reduced to less than 180°) and short TR spin-echo sequences (T1-weighted). Motion artifacts appear worse at 3T and may be because of the overall higher signal to noise ratio. Susceptibility artifacts will be increased, and postoperative imaging may be more problematic at higher field strengths. Increasing the receiver bandwidth may also help alleviate these artifacts. There are improvements in speed because the signal to noise ratio is proportional to the square of the imaging time, and therefore it is possible to go up to four times faster at 3T than 1.5T while maintaining an equal signal to noise ratio.

Another trend is the use of dedicated extremity scanners that typically operate at low field to midfield ranges. Low field open scanners or extremity scanners have been available for several years. However, recently a higher field extremity scanner at 1.0 T has become available (Orthone, ONI, Inc, Wilmington, MA). This unit can image the elbow, hand, wrist, knee, foot, and ankle but cannot acquire images of the shoulder, hip, or spine. Therefore, it is not considered a stand-alone unit but may be useful for a high volume site with a backlog of musculoskeletal patients to supplement a whole body unit. The site requirements are less than those for a conventional high field strength system, making it a more economical option. The image quality is much improved over the typical low field open MRI or very low field extremity scanners, and this type of device will likely have a niche role providing high-quality clinical images for the amenable body parts (Figure 4). It is also a useful option for claustrophobic patients. Larger and smaller diameter RF coils are available. Both coils are quadrature types of volume transmit-receive coils, which contribute to the improved image quality. There are certain advantages when this method is compared with traditional high field closed MRI systems. The images are of high quality despite the fact that the field strength is lower. Loss of signal to noise ratio and artifacts from off isocenter imaging are minimized. The majority of pulse sequences are available, including spectral fat suppression.

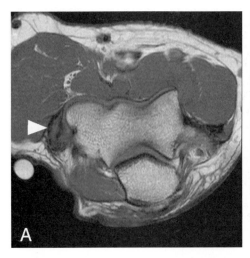
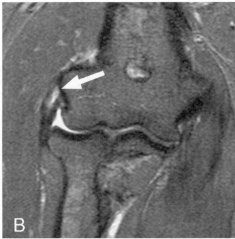
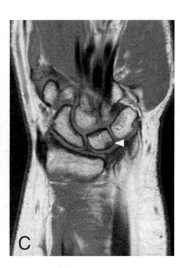

Figure 4 High-field open dedicated extremity MRI system. Elbow common extensor tendinopathy and partial tear: axial T1-weighted image **(A)** shows intermediate signal at the common extensor tendon ulnar attachment (arrowhead), coronal oblique T2-weighted image **(B)** with spectral fat suppression shows a small fluid gap (arrow) but not complete discontinuity of the common extensor tendon ulnar attachment reflecting a partial tear. Achilles tendinopathy (insertional tendinitis): axial T1-weighted image **(C)** through distal Achilles tendon (subjacent to marker) shows tendinosis manifested by enlargement (loss of the normal comma shape) and intermediate signal, sagittal T2-weighted image with spectral fat suppression. *(Images courtesy of Barbara N. Weissman, MD and Rosemary J. Klecker, MD, Harvard Medical School, Brigham and Women's Hospital.)*

Parallel imaging is a relatively new class of techniques capable of significantly increasing the speed of MRI acquisitions. Although a variety of different techniques have emerged, the common principle is to use the spatial information inherent in the elements of an RF coil array to allow a reduction in the number of time-consuming phase-encode steps required during the scan. Recent technical advances and increased availability to imaging centers place parallel imaging on the verge of widespread clinical use.

Imaging of Specific Orthopaedic Conditions
Spine

Disk Disease Nomenclature

Spine imaging can exquisitely provide information regarding pathoanatomy of degenerative disk disease but does not define a specific painful clinical syndrome because of the nonspecific appearance of painful versus painless degenerative conditions. However, abnormal imaging findings of the lumbar disks may be degenerative, adaptive, genetic, or a combination of environmental and determined factors. Many findings may simply represent senescent changes that are the natural consequences of stress applied during the course of a lifetime. The imaging appearance of lumbar spine degenerative disk disease has a similar incidence in symptomatic and asymptomatic patients. Therefore, the appropriate use of imaging modalities within a defined clinical context is paramount. For some patients with complicated or recalcitrant symptoms, the most useful aspect for advanced imaging techniques may be in the exclusion of more serious causes of axial low back pain such as infection, neoplasm, or fracture rather than the inclusion of any specific degenerative findings.

In terms of improving communications between providers there is a multispecialty, multisociety-endorsed nomenclature for the lumbar spine disk disease (some advocate that this system may be used for cervical and thoracic spine descriptors also). It is important to recognize that the definitions of diagnoses should not define or imply external etiologic events such as trauma, should not imply relationship to symptoms, and do imply need for specific treatment. Hence, the following are pathoanatomic descriptors that do not imply a specific pathoetiology or syndrome. Osteoarthritis or osteoarthrosis is a process of synovial joints. Therefore, in the spine it is appropriately applied to the zygoapophyseal (Z-joint, facet), atlantoaxial, costovertebral, and sacroiliac joints. Degenerative disk disease is a term applied specifically to intervertebral disk degeneration. The term spondylosis is often used in general as synonymous with degeneration, which would include both nucleus pulposus and anulus fibrosus processes, but such usage is confusing, so it is best that "degeneration" be the general term and spondylosis deformans a specifically defined subclassification of degeneration characterized by marginal osteophytosis without substantial disk height loss (reflecting predominantly anulus fibrosus disease). Intervertebral osteochondrosis is the term applied to the condition of mainly nucleus pulposus and the vertebral body end plate disease including annular fissuring (tearing).

Normally, the posterior disk margin tends to be concave in the upper lumbosacral spine (Figure 5, *A*), and is straight or slightly convex at L4-5 and L5-S1. The posterior margin typically projects no more than 1 mm beyond the end plate. An annular bulge is described as a generalized displacement (greater than 180°) of disk margin beyond the normal margin of the intervertebral

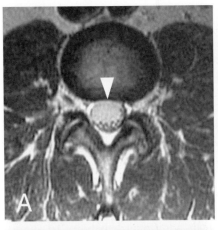

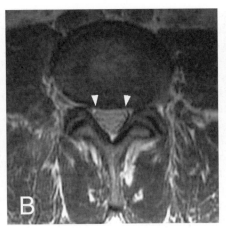

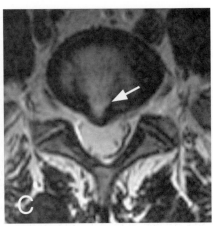

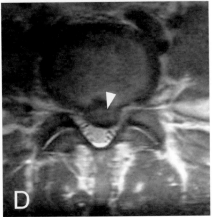

Figure 5 Lumbar disk contour abnormalities; all are axial T2-weighted images at the level of the intervertebral disk. **A,** Normal: the posterior disk margin (arrowhead) should have a slight concavity, with the exception of the lumbosacral junction, which may have a slight convexity. **B,** Annular bulge: There is generalized displacement (arrowheads) of greater than 180° of the disk margin beyond the normal margin of the intervertebral disk space and is the result of disk degeneration with an intact anulus fibrosus. **C,** Disk protrusion: The base against the parent disk margin is broader than any other diameter of the herniation. Extension of nucleus pulposus through a partial defect in the anulus fibrosus is identified (arrow) but the herniated disk is contained by some intact annular fibers. **D,** Disk extrusion: The base against the parent disk margin is narrower than any other diameter of the herniation (arrowhead). There may be extension of the nucleus pulposus through a complete focal defect in the anulus fibrosus. Substantial mass effect is present, causing moderate central canal and severe left lateral recess stenosis. (Reproduced with permission from Carrino JA, Morrison WB: Imaging of lumbar degenerative disk disease. *Semin Spine Surg* 2003;15:361-383.)

disk (Figure 5, *B*). The normal margin is defined by the vertebral body ring apophysis exclusive of osteophytes. The annular bulge can be the result of disk degeneration with a grossly intact anulus. Disk margins tend to be smooth, symmetric, or eccentric and nonfocal, and may have a level-specific appearance in the lumbar spine. Disk herniation is a localized displacement (less than 180° of the circumference) of disk material beyond the normal margin of the intervertebral disk space (Figure 5, *C*). This material may consist of nucleus pulposus, cartilage, fragmented apophyseal bone, or fragmented annular tissue. It is often the result of disk degeneration with some degree of focal annular disruption. The types of disk herniation are designated as protrusion, extrusion, and free fragment (sequestration). Protrusion refers to a herniated disk in which the greatest distance in any plane between the edges of the disk material beyond the disk space is less than the distance between the edges of the base in the same plane. It is characterized by the following: the base against the parent disk margin is broader than any other diameter of the herniation; extension of nucleus pulposus may occur through a partial defect in the anulus fibrosus but is contained by some intact outer annular fibers and the posterior longitudinal ligament. The types of protrusions may be broad based (90° to 180° circumference) or focal (less

than 90° circumference). Extrusion refers to a herniated disk in which, in at least one plane, any one distance between the edges of the disk material beyond the disk space is greater than the distance between the edges of the base in the same plane (Figure 5, *D*), or when no continuity exists between the disk material beyond the disk space and that within the disk space. An extrusion is characterized by the following: the base against the parent disk margin tends to be narrower than any other diameter of the herniation; extension of the nucleus pulposus through a complete focal defect in the anulus fibrosus. Extruded disks in which all continuity with the disk of origin is lost may be further characterized as sequestrated. Disk material displaced away from the site of extrusion may be characterized as migrated; it may stay subligamentous, contained by the posterior longitudinal ligament or may migrate widely. Schmorl's nodes are intervertebral disk herniations (transosseous disk extrusion). Herniation of the nucleus pulposus occurs through the cartilaginous end plate into the vertebral body. These herniations often have a characteristic round or lobulated appearance. They may enhance after contrast administration with ring-like enhancement being most common. They are often incidental and likely to be developmental or posttraumatic rather than purely degenerative or adaptive. There is now imaging evidence of a significant genetic association between the *COL9A3* tryptophan allele (*Trp3* allele), Scheuermann's disease, and intervertebral disk degeneration among symptomatic patients.

There are no formal staging systems for lumbar degenerative disk disease and most physicians will commonly report findings using the designations of mild, moderate, and severe disease. However, these designations will hold different meaning among physicians, especially with respect to degree of disk degeneration. The following scheme is used to define the degree of canal compromise produced by disk displacement based on the goals of being practical, objective, reasonably precise, and clinically relevant. Measurements are typically taken from an axial section at the site of the most severe compromise. Canal compromise of less than one third of the canal at that section is mild, between one and two thirds is moderate, and over two thirds represents severe disease. This scheme may also be applied to foraminal (neural canal) narrowing with the sagittal images also playing a useful role for defining the degree of narrowing. Observer interpretations are also made with various degrees of confidence. Statement of the degree of confidence is an important component of communication. The interpretation should be characterized as "definite" if there is no doubt, "probable" if there is some doubt but the likelihood is greater than 50%, and "possible" if there is reason to consider but the likelihood is less than 50%.

Positional, Load-Bearing, and Dynamic (Functional) Imaging

Because imaging in the supine position may not fully reveal the anatomic lesions, there has been an interest in performing functioning, positional, or load-bearing imaging of the spine. Spine imaging position options available are supine, supine with axial loading (simulated weight bearing), seated, or standing upright position. Noncompressive lesions on conventional MRI may show encroachment and neural element impingement on dynamic load-bearing (seated) scans. Fluctuating positional foraminal and central spinal canal stenosis has also been shown in the cervical spine between recumbent and upright neutral position. This situation has led to a concept of fluctuating kinetic central spinal canal stenosis (fluctuating fluid disk herniation) that can only be shown with these different positions. Cervical spine imaging in the recumbent position showing posterior osteophytes may only reveal cord compression with upright-extension positioning. Because of the prevalence of back pain that occurs in a nonsupine position and the inability of routine supine MRI to satisfactorily reveal clinical syndromes, it is likely that positional imaging will have a role in the future but how it exactly will be implemented is as yet undetermined; the role of imaging the hip, knee, and ankle under axial load also warrants further investigation. If the supine simulated weight-bearing paradigm becomes validated, then the currently installed base of magnets can be used without having to deploy new, costly space-occupying devices. Further studies comparing simulated weight-bearing versus upright imaging will be needed to show whether new magnets are required for this purpose.

Sports Medicine: Magnetic Resonance Arthrography

For any joint the placement of intra-articular contrast whether by direct or indirect means can be used to assist the evaluation of ligaments, cartilage, synovial proliferation, or intra-articular loose bodies. MRI provides cross-sectional and multiplanar imaging for precise spatial delineation and an additional capability to supply soft-tissue contrast outside of the joint cavity (tendons, muscles, and bone marrow) unavailable by any other modalities. Pertinent issues for optimizing diagnostic yield include technical considerations in performing magnetic resonance examinations, properly identifying structures of interest, and the clinical significance of the incidental findings. Magnetic resonance arthrography has been most extensively studied in the shoulder and to a lesser degree in the hip and the postoperative knee. Other joints in which it has been applied include the elbow and wrist and to a lesser degree the ankle.

Direct magnetic resonance arthrography, most often done with injection of diluted gadolinium or less often with saline solution, can be useful for evaluating certain pathologic conditions in the joints. Gadolinium-based contrast agents have not been approved by the US Food and Drug Administration for intra-articular injection but may be used clinically under the doctrine of the practice of medicine. These agents are most helpful for outlining labral-ligamentous abnormalities in the shoulder (Figure 6) and distinguishing partial-thickness from full-thickness tears in the rotator cuff, demonstrating labral tears in the hip, showing partial- and full-thickness tears of the collateral ligament of the elbow and delineating bands in the elbow, identifying residual or recurrent tears in the knee after meniscectomy (Figure 7), increasing the certainty of perforations of the ligaments and triangular fibrocartilage in the wrist, correctly identifying ligament tears in the ankle and increasing the sensitivity for ankle impingement syndromes, assessing the stability of osteochondral lesions in the articular surface of joints, and delineating loose bodies in joints. Direct magnetic resonance arthrography has become a well-established method of delineating various joint structures that otherwise show poor contrast on conventional MRI. However, direct magnetic resonance arthrography is minimally invasive and usually necessitates fluoroscopic guidance for joint injection (some authors have described doing blind injections or using other modalities such as ultrasound or MRI).

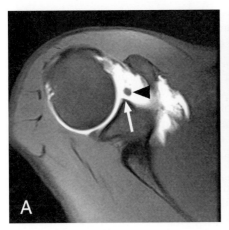
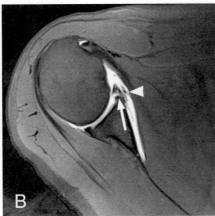
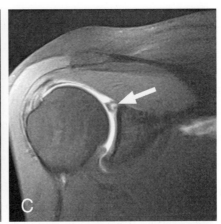

Figure 6 Direct magnetic resonance arthrography of the shoulder. T1-weighted fat-suppressed images obtained after the intra-articular injection of a dilute gadolinium solution. **A,** Buford complex: axial image at the level of the coracoid process shows a deficient anterosuperior labrum (white arrow) with a thick cord-like middle glenohumeral ligament (black arrowhead) reflecting a normal developmental variant. **B,** Bankart lesion: axial image caudal to the level of the coracoid process shows contrast intravasation into an irregular deformed anteroinferior glenoid labrum (arrow) distinct from the middle glenohumeral ligament (arrowhead). **C,** Superior labral anterior and posterior lesion: coronal oblique image posterior to the biceps attachment to the glenoid shows an irregular collection of contrast material (arrow) extending into the superior labrum with partial detachment.

Intravenous gadolinium-based contrast leaks from the capillary bed into the interstitial space of the synovium and then diffuses through the synovial lining into the joint cavity. Because the synovial membrane is highly vascular, intravenous gadolinium-based contrast material enhances the joint cavity, causing the arthrographic effect. This technique has developed as an alternative to direct magnetic resonance arthrography for imaging joints. The arthrographic effect is dependent on the degree of synovial enhancement and volume of synovial fluid. Synovial enhancement is poorer in noninflamed joints. Well-vascularized and inflamed tissues will show enhancement with this method. One limitation of indirect magnetic resonance arthrography is a lack of controlled joint distension compared with that of direct arthrography. Joint distension facilitates recognition of certain conditions such as capsular trauma or soft-tissue injury concealed by a collapsed capsule. Joints with a large capacity (knee, hip, shoulder) are less suited to indirect magnetic resonance arthrography because the larger volume necessitates a longer delay and leads to less predictable heterogeneous enhancement. Nonetheless, indirect magnetic resonance arthrography can provide diagnostic arthrogram-like images of the shoulder, elbow, wrist, hip, knee, and ankle joint if the technique is optimized. Fat saturation and joint exercise before imaging is critical to provide high signal intensity joint fluid. Diffusion is increased in joints, which are inflamed, or after gentle exercise, because of physiologic hyperemia. Factors affecting passage of contrast material between the blood vessels and synovial fluid include pressure differences between these spaces and the viscosity of the intra-articular fluid. The normal joint space is a low-pressure space, containing joint fluid of relatively low viscosity. Exercise not only increases vascular

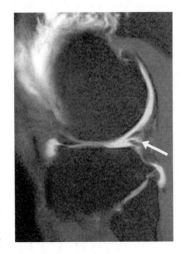

Figure 7 Direct magnetic resonance arthrography of the knee: Sagittal T1-weighted fat-suppressed spin echo images show a horizontal increased intrameniscal signal intensity similar to the contrast material extending to the free margin (arrow) of the posterior horn of the medial meniscus, reflecting a recurrent meniscal tear. The posterior horn of the medial meniscus is truncated from a prior partial meniscectomy. Extensive cartilage loss of the posterior aspect of the lateral femoral condyle is seen.

perfusion but also increases vascular pressure. Exercise also leads to motion within the joint fluid, thereby reducing the concentration of contrast adjacent to the synovial membrane and thus facilitating the diffusional effect. Increase in signal intensity of joint fluid has been reported to be four times greater in joints that were exercised 10° up to 15 minutes before imaging compared with joints that were not exercised. Without exercise the signal intensity increases slowly and reaches a maximum after approximately 60 minutes. In patients with osteoarthritis, maximum enhancement may occur as late as 90 minutes in the absence of joint motion. As contrast diffusion is based on the concentration difference between plasma and joint fluid, increasing the dose of contrast material administered intravenously may increase the diffusion gradient. However, double- and triple-dose intravenous injections have been shown to have a limited positive effect on indirect arthrography.

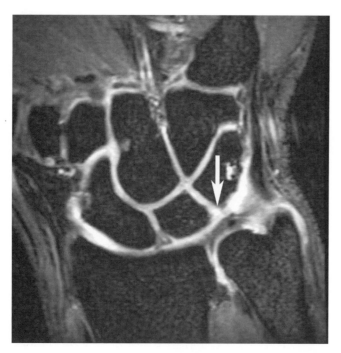

Figure 8 Indirect magnetic resonance arthrography of the wrist: lunotriquetral ligament tear. Coronal T1-weighted fat suppressed spoiled gradient recalled image obtained after the administration of a standard dose of intravenous gadolinium based contrast material and 10 minutes of exercise shows high signal equal to contrast material in the lunotriquetral interval (arrow) reflecting ligament disruption (normally there should be a low signal band at the base of the proximal carpal bones). Note the multicompartment enhancement.

Thus, a standard dose of gadolinium-based contrast injected intravenously is usually sufficient to attain a good signal to noise ratio and good contrast to noise ratio. It allows simultaneous assessment of both intra-articular and extra-articular soft tissues but the physician must be cognizant of the determinants of contrast enhancement not to be confounded by normally enhancing structures (Figure 8). Indirect magnetic resonance arthrography is a useful adjunct to conventional musculoskeletal MRI, may be preferable to the more invasive direct magnetic resonance arthrogram in certain applications, and often can be performed when direct arthrography is inconvenient or not logistically feasible (outpatient magnet). Although indirect magnetic resonance arthrography has some disadvantages, it does not require fluoroscopic guidance or joint injection and it is often superior to conventional MRI in delineating structures.

Hand/Upper Extremity: Internal Derangements of the Wrist

Challenges associated with MRI of the hand and upper extremity are related to the small compact complex anatomy and the high special resolution requirement. High signal-to-noise ratios are desired; however, thin section, small field of view, and high-resolution images all detract from signal-to-noise ratios. Off isocenter imaging, as is commonly done for the elbow and the wrist, can detract from quality because of artifacts related to reduced field homogeneity. Using a high-field dedicated extremity magnet can improve overall quality by having the structure of interest within the isocenter. High-quality surface RF coils should be used for wrist or elbow imaging and can improve the signal-to-noise ratios threefold to fivefold. Higher field strength with stronger gradients (increased slew rates) allows for thinner section acquisition, smaller field of views, and reduced scanner time. Conventional MRI systems have a 3-mm section limitation for two-dimensional pulse sequences because the amplifier can only deliver a fixed amount of power to the gradient coil. The addition of volumetric three-dimensional imaging can also be useful. The elbow and wrist are joints that contain compact anatomy and perform complex motions. Frequently, the structures of interest are not well shown in the standard planes of imaging and appropriate positioning at optimal planes needs to be acquired for each area. A three-dimensional pulse sequence that can be dynamically manipulated may be advantageous in this context. Contrast resolution issues are also extremely important and are related to determining the optimal pulse sequence. For certain structures in the wrist and elbow such as the fibrocartilage, ligaments, and capsule, there is a limited inherent contrast that normally exists. In this respect intra-articular contrast medium (magnetic resonance arthrography) greatly assists the conspicuity of findings. The contrast-to-noise ratio tends to improve by fat suppression because this alters the dynamic range by reducing the contribution of signal from fat with the smaller contrast differences rescaled across a broader range of signal intensity pixel values. The resulting effect is that the rescaling provides amplified contrast even with nonfat-containing structures (such as cartilage). Currently, gradient echo sequences can provide high-resolution imaging but there are significant contrast limitations. Spurious signals are often present in tendons and ligaments, particularly when they approach a 55° angle to the main magnetic field (causing magic angle artifact, a T2 shortening phenomenon manifested in short TE images). This is often the case in at least some portion(s) of some of the tendons given the complex anatomy in this region.

MRI of the hand, wrist, and elbow is useful for extra-articular pathology and in this sense is complementary to diagnostic arthroscopy. The reports for diagnostic performance of MRI for ligamentous wrist lesions in the literature are variable. Thus, MRI has not achieved a respected role in defining the biomechanically clinically significant lesions in the wrist. One mechanism to improve spatial resolution is to use dedicated high-resolution coils. Thin and contiguous slices are needed for adequate MRI of the wrist because many of the larger ligaments around the wrist are no greater than 1 to 2 mm thick. Recent magnetic resonance technology allows the use of a microscopy coil, which provides high-resolution MRI of the hand and wrist. High-resolution MRI with a microscopy coil is a promising method to diagnose triangular fibrocartilage complex and other ligament lesions. The limitation of microscopy coils is that the depiction of deep structures is inadequate. However, this may be resolved by combined positioning with a larger surface coil or a flexible coil. In addition, the limited sensitivity of microscopy coils may sometimes make accurate coil setting difficult over targeted structure or suspected lesions. The availability of superconducting coils has also been applied to small joint imaging. Overall, it is likely that advanced coil development will lead to improved diagnostic performance of MRI because high spatial resolution imaging is paramount to detect infrastructural features of the wrist and elbow when evaluating for internal arrangements.

Foot and Ankle: Bone Marrow Edema-Like Lesions

Bone marrow edema (BME)-like lesions are often observed on MRI. Although BME-like signal is not specific on MRI, additional morphologic findings are often useful to reveal the etiology of many BME patterns. Normal marrow constituents have three components: osseous, myeloid elements, and adipose cells. Hematopoietic (red) marrow has approximately 40% fat content and fatty (yellow) marrow has 80% fat content. The appendicular skeleton tends to have more fatty marrow than hematopoietic marrow and this serves as a natural contrast agent, showing bright T1 signal and suppression on fat saturation images. MRI to detect BME relies on fluid-sensitive sequences (short-tau inversion recovery [STIR] and fat suppressed T2-weighted images). T1-weighted images can supplement T2-weighted images and are very specific for the infiltrative process, but are not as sensitive if there is nonfat marrow or no substantial degree of edema. Gradient echo images are poor for assessing marrow because of increased susceptibility related to the interfaces between the trabecula and hematopoietic marrow. Gradient echo images can be useful to reveal other diagnoses such as lesions that contain iron, calcium, or hemosiderin (pigmented villonodular synovitis). Other novel MRI techniques that have been variably applied include chemical shift imaging, diffusion weighted imaging, and magnetic resonance spectroscopy.

BME lesions can reflect nonspecific response to injury or excess stress. The pathophysiology is related to the extracellular fluid, which can be affected by hypervascularity and hyperperfusion (hyperemia), an inflammatory infiltrate causing resorption, granulation (fibrovascular) tissue or an adaptive/reactive phenomena related to biomechanical alterations (MRI manifestation of Wolff's Law). The pathoetiologies are legion and

the signal intensity is directly proportional to the amount of extracellular water. Contrast enhancement occurs in areas of BME irrespective of etiology (benign or malignant, infectious or noninflammatory). The potential etiologies of BME include diseases in the category of trauma, biomechanical, developmental, vascular, neoplastic, inflammatory, neuropathic, metabolic, degenerative, iatrogenic, and potentially idiopathic conditions (transient BME syndromes).

Occult injuries result from an acute overt episode of trauma. The physician should suspect a fracture in these patients. The traditional modality applied to fracture detection has been radiography, which may be negative or indeterminate for nondisplaced fractures or a fracture plane that is not tangential to the x-ray beam. In this context MRI serves as a more sensitive technique for fracture detection and characterization. Contusions, also known as bone bruises, are considered microtrabecular fractures. On MRI there is no fracture line and the pattern may be a clue or secondary sign of ligament or tendon injury. These fractures often occur in a subarticular location from osteochondral impaction injuries.

In terms of developmental conditions the normal conversion of red marrow to yellow marrow sometimes has areas of slight T2 or STIR hyperintensity but these usually are not as bright as pathologic lesions. Areas of a developmental synchondrosis with failure of segmentation of the primitive mesenchyme may cause symptoms via abnormal biomechanics. Symptomatic fibrous or cartilaginous tarsal coalitions often show reciprocal areas of BME. Anatomic variants that can present as painful lesions may be considered a separate but related category. Those of chronic chondro-osseous disruption include bipartite patella, dorsal defect of the patella, and os subfibulare of the ankle. Those in the congenital synchondrosis category include accessory navicular bone and os trigonum. There are lesions that may predispose to premature degenerative joint disease; one example is the os intermetatarsarum, which can contribute to hallux valgus by causing excessive metatarsus varus. When these variants are symptomatic they often demonstrate BME-like signal about the abnormality, reflecting altered biomechanics, chronic stress, or sometimes areas of osteonecrosis. It is thought that MRI can form an objective basis for management of the lesions, particularly when surgery is considered.

The well-established vascular causes of BME-like signal may be related to either hyperemic or ischemic conditions. Of the hyperemic etiologies, inflammatory disorders that increase vascularity or disuse may cause subarticular BME patterns. The disuse pattern is also partly related to increased blood flow, can be characteristic and parallels the radiographic appearance of aggressive osteoporosis with diffuse or multiple rounded areas of fluid-like hyperintensity in a subarticular and metaphyseal distribution predominantly in the hindfoot

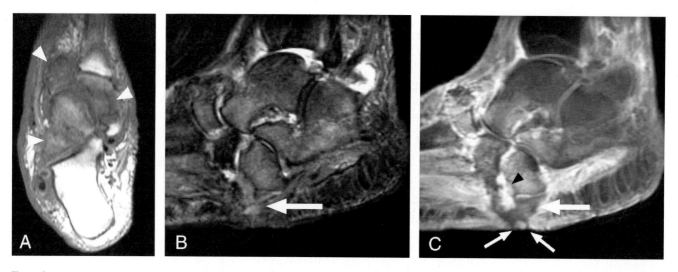

Figure 9 Osteomyelitis superimposed on neuropathic arthropathy. **A,** Axial T1-weighted spin-echo image of the midfoot reveals disorganization and dislocation of the Chopart joint, showing replacement of the normal marrow with diffuse infiltration of hypointense signal (arrowheads) in the tarsal bones. **B,** Sagittal T2-weighted fast spin-echo image reveals marrow edema in the midfoot and hindfoot bones, tarsus effusions, a rocker bottom deformity and fluid-like signal in the overlying subcutaneous tissues (arrow). **C,** Sagittal T1-weighted spin-echo contrast-enhanced image shows rim enhancement around plantar sinus tracts (small arrows) from the ulcer base and extending into midfoot reflecting a plantar space abscess (large arrow). The marrow edema is enhancing, which is nonspecific, but there is cortical irregularity of the anterior aspect of the cuboid adjacent to the soft-issue enhancement (arrowhead). The secondary signs of cutaneous ulcer, sinus tract, and cortical interruption have the highest positive predictive value for osteomyelitis.

and midfoot. In terms of ischemic lesions, the broad category of osteonecrosis (infarct, osteonecrosis) can have BME early in the course of the disorder associated with acute, painful symptomatology. Pain improvement usually parallels the resolution of the BME-like signal. The MRI pattern shows early BME with loss of subchondral fat signal intensity. The double line sign is specific and most often identified as a ring of T1 hypointensity and T2 hyperintensity. This likely reflects a reactive interface rather than chemical shift artifact. MRI signal of the necrotic segment may be reconstituted and appear fatty because of the lipid content (the signal is not significantly altered because of the reduced metabolic state). MRI findings may be seen as early as 10 to 15 days and for most patients within 30 days after the vascular insult. Transient osteoporosis or the MRI correlate, transient bone marrow edema syndrome, may occur in numerous other low extremity locations including the hip, knee, talus, cuboid, navicular, and metatarsals. In addition, it may be migratory and occur in a ray pattern. Some believe that these lesions may reflect salvaged osteonecrosis but it is likely that many of these lesions may simply be biomechanical in nature.

In the inflammatory category it is well established that infectious etiologies cause BME. One difficult differential diagnosis in the setting of diabetic neuropathy is distinguishing osteomyelitis from a Charcot joint. There are several MRI findings that may help in the differentiation. Osteomyelitis is more common in the phalanges, distal metatarsals, and calcaneus (secondary to overlying ulceration) whereas neuropathic disease is more common in the Lisfranc, Chopart, and ankle joints.

One notable exception is an ulceration that develops because of poorly fitting footwear, or foot deformity and altered weight bearing that can cause atypical location of osteomyelitis. However, there should be a soft-tissue defect identified over these areas to diagnose osteomyelitis. The epicenters of signal abnormalities can be useful. Neuropathic disease has an articular epicenter and usually multiple joints are involved with a regional instability pattern. Osteomyelitis has a marrow epicenter with focal centripetal spread throughout the bone. It is important to emphasize that transcutaneous spread is the route of inoculation in more than 90% of cases of osteomyelitis of the foot in patients with diabetes. Therefore, secondary soft-tissue signs are paramount; a subcutaneous ulcer with interruption of cutaneous signal, cellulitis, soft-tissue mass effect from a phlegmon, soft-tissue abscess (well-defined rim enhancing fluid collection) and particularly a sinus tract strongly support infection (Figure 9).

It has been recently recognized that degenerative conditions are associated with areas of BME. These degenerative conditions may occur with either primary or secondary osteoarthritis. Geodes (subchondral cysts) are one of the imaging hallmarks of osteoarthritis and can be identified on MRI. Early during the course of disease, ill-defined areas of BME appear and later form discrete cystic structures. Some of these areas with hyperintensity have been shown by pathologic studies not to reflect the fluid. It has been hypothesized that some of these findings are likely mechanical or adaptive responses related to the altered mechanics from the joint failure and may be considered the MRI manifestation

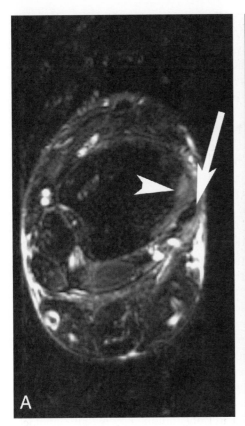
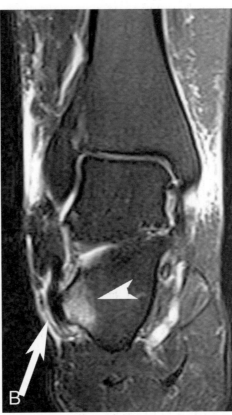

Figure 10 Tendinopathy-associated bone marrow edema. **A** and **B** are T2-weighted fat-suppressed fast spin-echo MRI. Posterior tibialis tendon dysfunction: axial image **(A)** shows medial malleolus marrow edema (arrowhead) immediately subjacent to the posterior tibialis tendon (arrow). Peroneal tendinopathy: coronal image **(B)** shows peroneus longus tendon tenosynovitis (arrow) with underlying subtendinous bone marrow edema in peroneal tubercle of the calcaneus (arrowhead).

of Wolff's Law. In the knee (and possibly in the ankle and foot) bone marrow findings are strongly associated with the presence of pain, and moderate or larger fusions in synovial thickening are more frequent among those with pain than those without pain adjusted for degree of radiographic osteoarthritis. In addition, focal subchondral BME may be a clue to focal cartilage defects (potential treatable cartilage defects), which presumably are posttraumatic events. The cartilage abnormality itself may be relatively inconspicuous on MRI pulse sequence selection or spatial resolution and therefore an area of subarticular flame-shaped BME in a nonarthritic joint can be a helpful secondary sign. Another recently described pattern of BME is a subtendinous location. This has been identified as a response to tendon abnormality and hypothesized to be from mechanical friction, hyperemia, or because of biomechanical reasons. A subtendinous location is most common in the lower extremity, particularly in the foot and ankle, and is most often seen with posterior tibialis tendon (PTT) dysfunction (Figure 10, *A*). The areas of edema related to PTT dysfunction are the medial tibia (malleolus), navicular tubercle, calcaneous, and talus. This finding is not seen in most people with PTT dysfunction but may be a sign for a more advanced stage and poorer tendon quality. Less frequently, BME may also be related to peroneal tendinopathy (Figure 10, *B*): typically in the lateral fibula (lateral malleolus) or lateral calca-

neus (along the peroneal tubercle). Noninfectious inflammatory enthesopathies such as psoriatic or reactive arthritis cause prominent flame-shaped BME patterns at the tendon-bone junction (enthesis) often with an associated erosion that may be better appreciated with radiography.

There are several miscellaneous but important causes of lower extremity BME patterns. Hematopoietic (red) marrow can sometimes be confused for an abnormal BME pattern. Hematopoietic marrow is most prominent in the pediatric population and there is a conversion pattern progression from distal to proximal. One important realization is that once an epiphysis is ossified, it should contain fatty signal with a couple of important exceptions (reconversion not infrequently occurs in proximal femoral epiphysis). In general, reconversion related to anemia or other conditions is in the opposite direction. In terms of marrow replacement disorders (leukemia and lymphoma) the pattern may be a diffuse or focal area of marrow signal abnormality. With infiltrative diseases, the marrow pattern tends to have some asymmetry and pathologic processes tend to have more T2 prolongation and higher signal intensity (brighter BME). Neoplasms often show lesional or perilesional BME. The signal intensities are unreliable for histology and there is substantial overlap between benign and malignant conditions. Metastatic deposits are hematogenous in origin and are predominantly located in red marrow areas (axial skeleton) but can also be present in the appendicular skeleton, especially for deposits from bronchogenic or breast carcinoma. For primary neoplasms, the degree of BME does not correspond to malignancy potential. There are several well-known benign lesions that are characterized by very prominent BME: chondroblastoma, osteoid osteoma, and Langerhans cell histiocytosis. Patients who have undergone radiotherapy or chemotherapy, those who are taking bone marrow recovery agents, and patients who have recently undergone débridement may show BME depending on the time course of the treatment.

Pediatrics: Physeal Lesions and Growth Arrest

The growing skeleton is susceptible to injury. Advances in pediatric musculoskeletal radiology have been made in imaging the cartilage, epiphysis, and physis. Closure disturbance of the long bones in children is frequently posttraumatic but also occurs because of physeal, epiphyseal, or metaphyseal ischemia. The growth mechanism represented by the cartilage structures at the ends of growing bones is not directly visible on radiography but is well visualized by MRI. Improved definition of cartilaginous abnormality by MRI may permit earlier detection and treatment of disorders and thus prevent bone deformity. The formation of physeal bars (bony bridges across the growth plate) is one active area of pediatric musculoskeletal radiology research. Premature bony fusion in children is most often posttraumatic and disproportionately involves the tibia and femur with bridges tending to develop as the site of earliest physiologic closures (anteromedially and centrally). The distal tibia, proximal femur, and proximal tibia physes are disproportionally at risk because of the complex geometry. The central undulations in the distal femur and Kump's bump in the distal tibia are sites of initial physiologic closure and the most frequently involved in the premature fusions. Animal studies with physeal and metaphyseal injuries have shown MRI can identify persistence of abnormality in the growth cartilage after physeal injuries and evolution of abnormalities after metaphyseal injury best seen on T2-weighted images. It has been shown on MRI in animal models that abnormalities in the physeal cartilage result in development of a transphyseal vascularity that precedes the formation of bony bridge after trauma. MRI can detect this transphyseal vascular lesion within the first 2 weeks of injury. In vivo studies in humans confirm that MRI defect abnormalities in the cartilage are associated with subsequent growth disturbances and provide accurate mapping of physeal bridging and associated growth abnormality in the posttraumatic population (Salter-Harris injuries). Contrast enhancement can be useful in showing reconstitution of metaphyseal vascularity after injury but does not reliably enable the detection of transphyseal vascularity after physeal injury until a distinct bony bridge is formed. Early MRI evaluation in children with lower extremity fractures can be prognostic. Physeal narrowing or tethering in the absence of growth arrest lines was found in those patients who subsequently required late surgical intervention. The MRI in acute phase provided accurate evaluation of physeal fracture anatomy and could often augment the staging of the Salter-Harris classification. The course and level of injury within the cartilage physeal fracture-separation can be defined with MRI. Extension into the juxtaepiphyseal region is another potential risk factor for growth arrest and is detectable by MRI. Early MRI can demonstrate transphyseal bridging or altered arrest lines in physeal fracture before they become manifest on radiographs. Physeal enhancement decreases with physeal closure as expected. In the marrow and the extremities, contrast enhancement is greater in the metaphyseal metathesis portion than the fatty epiphyseal portion. In both areas enhancement decreases as the marrow becomes more fatty. Local physeal widening in a growing bone may represent the imprint of the previous or ongoing interference with endochondral ossification. Widening can be seen on fluid-sensitive pulse sequences in physeal dysfunction without bridge formation. Physeal widening with focal palisading morphology, central distribution in the metaphysis and concomitant epiphyseal signal abnormalities are significant predictors of subsequent growth disturbance. Therefore, MRI should be considered as part of the evaluation for patients at high risk for growth disturbance, especially young children with extensive residual growth potential and those that involve particularly vulnerable growth plates (such as about the knee) and pediatric patients with severe complex fractures. MRI is now a standard of care and helps surgical management for these patient populations with cartilage-sensitive sequences, exquisitely showing the disturbance and associated abnormality that may follow physeal injuries.

Orthopaedic Oncology: Metabolic Imaging

Distinguishing benign from malignant soft-tissue lesions in the extremities is a difficult if not impossible task by imaging using either signal, morphologic, or enhancement criteria. Follow-up imaging for sarcoma patients is also complicated by complex prostheses, which can produce artifacts and limit visualization at the surgical site. PET scanning, discussed earlier in the chapter, holds promise in showing metabolically active areas and may be particularly suitable for monitoring patients after therapy (resection, chemotherapy, or radiotherapy).

Orthopaedic Traumatology: Multislice Computed Tomography

One of the most recently evident benefits of multislice CT is in the setting of appendicular and axial trauma. CT greatly improves the anatomic depiction of spinal injury when compared with projectional radiography. Compared with single detector helical CT scanners, multislice CT scanners have increased tube heating capacity and run at a higher table speed, allowing an increased volume of coverage with the same amount of scanning time. This makes screening examination of part of the spine or the entire spine feasible, which may eliminate screening radiographs in certain settings. Examinations of the thorax and the lumbar spine can be extracted from a CT examination of the chest abdomen and pelvis.

There are several pitfalls to be aware of but the most important image artifacts are not unique to multislice CT. These pitfalls include metal-induced streak artifact and patient motion. Because of the higher spatial resolution, vascular channels of the vertebral bodies are better appreciated and may be mistaken for normal structures. Multislice CT has some risk predominantly related to the radiation dose to the individual patient and to the population. The radiation dose of the patient increases as the volume of coverage increases. Multislice CT allows imaging of very thin sections quickly, much faster than previously possible, allowing for effective screening of spinal injuries and evaluating extremity injuries. Screening CT of the entire cervical spine is cost effective if high-risk criteria, such as focal neurologic deficit referable to the cervical spine, head injury (skull fracture, intracranial hemorrhage) or loss of conscious at the time of examination, and high-energy mechanism (motor vehicle accident at a speed of greater than 35 mm, pedestrian struck by a car, or a fall greater than 10 feet).

Diagnostic and Therapeutic Procedures
Spinal Injections
Epidural steroid injections, sacroiliac joint injections, zygapophyseal (facet) joint injections, diskography, and vertebral augmentation are image-guided procedures that are important components of a comprehensive management approach to spine pain syndromes for establishing a diagnosis, directing or administering therapy, and facilitating rehabilitation and functional restoration.

Demand for epidural injections is rapidly expanding. Patient satisfaction elicited from these procedures is often a direct result of imaging guidance, which can shorten and simplify procedures, minimize potential for complications, and verify accurate localization of the needle to selectively provide the lowest necessary dose of analgesic to the optimal area. These procedures can greatly contribute to patient management and surgical planning by determining sources of pain and treating pain generators. Participation of an experienced radiologist in performing these procedures optimizes patient care, because radiologists are trained in anatomy and image-guided needle localization procedures. However,

use of spinal injections should be considered a team effort in conjunction with an experienced clinical diagnostician who can accurately diagnose the patient's problem and recommend the appropriate procedure. Performance of these procedures requires an intimate knowledge of relevant anatomy, appropriate equipment and facilities, and apprenticeship with an experienced practitioner. Selective epidural injections can offer significant diagnostic and therapeutic benefit for patients with radicular pain. Attention to proper technique will minimize risk of complications from these procedures while maximizing their benefit.

Controversy and differences in opinion related to epidural steroid injections often revolve around choice of trajectory (transforaminal versus transflaval [translaminar, interlaminar]) and whether to use image guidance. Transflaval injections may be done with or without image guidance (using loss of resistance techniques), whereas transforaminal injections are done with image guidance. Studies reviewing the efficacy of epidural steroid injections favor it as a useful treatment overall. However, controlled clinical trials performed without fluoroscopic guidance are not unanimous in demonstrating the benefits of lumbar epidural steroid injections with a broad range of successful results, ranging from 18% to 90%. This broad range may be related to the actual location of medication deposition. The incidence of failure to reach the epidural space using a non–image-guided transflaval approach ranges from 13% to 30% and may target the wrong interlaminar space by one or more levels. The transforaminal approach demonstrates superior ventral opacification, whereas the transflaval method shows predominantly dorsal opacification (using CT as the reference standard to confirm contrast location after fluoroscopically-guided epidurography). Dorsal deposition may be less effective because the steroid is remote from the source of irritation (for example, disk herniation). There is an increased risk of a dural puncture (intrathecal administration), spinal headache (may require blood patch treatment), intrathecal administration of steroid or residual preservatives of local anesthesia leading to nerve root injury, hypotension, or dyspnea. For several reasons image-guided epidural steroid injection is favored; it adds only minimal risk (radiation) and may not add to the overall costs of spine injections but may even reduce costs by eliminating repeat injections (a nonimage-guided paradigm is to perform two to three successive transflaval epidural steroid injections because the miss rate of the epidural space is about 33%).

Intra-articular injections have an established role for identifying zygapophyseal (facet) and sacroiliac joint articulations as nociceptors. However, intra-articular injections with anesthetic or corticosteroid are often not sufficient for a long lasting therapeutic effect. Once a zygapophyseal joint has been implicated as a substantial

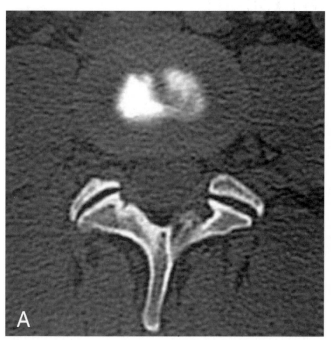
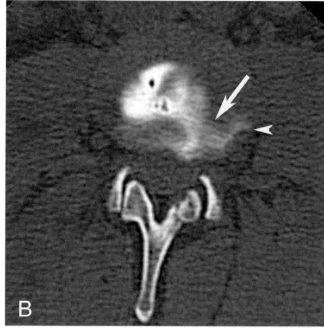

Figure 11 CT characterization after intradiskal contrast injection. Postdiskography transaxial CT images. **A,** Normal nucleogram characterized by central globule of contrast material that remains within the expected confines of the nucleus pulposus. **B,** Annular fissure. Contrast material is noted within the nucleus pulposus, but also extends in a radial fashion posterolaterally beyond the expected confines of the nucleus pulposus into the region of the anulus fibrosus (arrow). There is also a circumferential component noted in the anulus fibrosus (arrowhead).

or significant nociceptor then targeted therapy options exist that may include a neuroablative procedure (medial branch neurotomy) in conjunction with functional restoration via physical therapy. Sacroiliac joint treatment can be more problematic given the diffuse innervation of the articulation; however, sacroiliac joint fusion is a technique practiced by some orthopaedic surgeons. For true inflammatory sacroiliitis related to a spondyloarthropathy, there is good evidence from several clinical trials that intra-articular corticosteroid is proven to be an effective component of treatment. However, the data on the efficacy of steroid intra-articular injections for mechanical somatic dysfunction are conflicting. For an intracanalicular synovial cyst emanating from an adjacent zygapophyseal joint that is causing lateral recess stenosis with radicular symptoms, intra-articular injection with corticosteroid assists in decreasing the perineural inflammation, reducing the size of the cyst, and alleviating the radicular symptoms.

Diskography

The primary purpose for diskography is for documentation of the disk as a significant nociceptor. For patients who have chronic pain that is predominantly axial, nonmyelopathic, and nonradicular, imaging may be insufficient or equivocal for determining the nature, location, and extent of symptomatic pathology. A position statement regarding lumbar diskography from the North American Spine Society was published in 1995. Specific indications include patients with persistent pain in whom noninvasive imaging and other tests have not provided sufficient diagnostic information. In patients who are to undergo fusion, diskography can be used to determine if disks within the proposed fusion segment are symptomatic and if the adjacent disks are normal. Surgeons concerned with limiting the extent of fusion are interested in obtaining more evidence beyond MRI abnormalities to document what intervertebral disk levels are contributing to the painful syndrome. In postoperative patients who continue to experience significant pain, diskography can be used to assist in differentiating between postoperative scar and recurrent disk herniation (when MRI or CT is equivocal); or to evaluate segments adjacent to the arthrodesis. Postdiskography CT can also be used to confirm a contained disk herniation as a prelude to minimally invasive intradiskal therapy (Figure 11). Diskography is also being used as part of the selection criteria for many clinical trials assessing lumbar interbody fusion devices or percutaneous intradiskal treatments.

Annotated Bibliography

Available Imaging Modalities

Carrino JA: Digital imaging overview. *Semin Roentgenol* 2003;38:200-215.

This article provides an overview of the electronic imaging environment, including a review of the technologies behind picture archiving and communications systems and radiology information systems as well as practical information on implementation.

Horton KM, Sheth S, Corl F, Fishman EK: Multidetector row CT: Principles and clinical applications. *Crit Rev Comput Tomogr* 2002;43:143-181.

This article reviews the basic principles of multislice computed tomography. Scanner/detector design, beam collimation/slice thickness, radiation dose, data manipulation, and display are discussed.

Jadvar H, Gamie S, Ramanna L, Conti PS: Musculoskeletal system. *Semin Nucl Med* 2004;34:254-261.

In this article, the diagnostic utility of dedicated PET and PET combined with CT in the evaluation of patients with bone and soft-tissue malignancies is reviewed.

Recht M, Bobic V, Burstein D, et al: Magnetic resonance imaging of articular cartilage. *Clin Orthop* 2001; 391(suppl):S379-S396.

This article presents a review of procedures regarding MRI of articular cartilage and cartilage repair. Future directions in imaging strategies and ways to measure cartilage thickness and volume are discussed.

Sofka CM: Ultrasound in sports medicine. *Semin Musculoskelet Radiol* 2004;8:17-27.

Ultrasound plays an important role in the evaluation of injuries and painful conditions of the athlete. With portable ultrasound units, examinations can be performed on the playing field, immediately at the time of the acute injury, for rapid diagnosis. Ultrasound can be used to guide therapeutic procedures.

Yoshioka H, Stevens K, Hargreaves BA, et al: Magnetic resonance imaging of articular cartilage of the knee: Comparison between fat-suppressed three-dimensional SPGR imaging, fat-suppressed FSE imaging, and fat-suppressed three-dimensional DEFT imaging, and correlation with arthroscopy. *J Magn Reson Imaging* 2004;20:857-864.

In this study, signal to noise ratios and contrast to noise ratios were compared in various magnetic resonance sequences, including fat-suppressed three-dimensional spoiled gradient echo imaging, fat-suppressed fast spin echo imaging, and fat-suppressed three-dimentional driven equilibrium Fourier transform imaging. The diagnostic accuracy of these imaging sequences was compared with that of arthroscopy for detecting cartilage lesions in osteoarthritic knees. Fat-suppressed three-dimensional spoiled gradient echo imaging and fat-suppressed fast spin echo imaging showed high sensitivity and high negative predictive values, but relatively low specificity.

Imaging of Specific Orthopaedic Conditions
Aoki J, Endo K, Watanabe H, et al: FDG-PET for evaluating musculoskeletal tumors: A review. *J Orthop Sci* 2003;8:435-441.

Recent reports and experience suggest that FDG-PET cannot be a screening method for differential diagnosis between benign and malignant musculoskeletal lesions, including many neoplasms originating from different tissues. FDG-PET might not accurately reflect the malignant potential of musculoskeletal tumors, but rather might implicate cellular components included in the lesions. A high accumulation of FDG can be observed in histiocytic, fibroblastic, and some neurogenic lesions, regardless of whether they are benign or malignant. More specific uses of FDG-PET, such as grading, staging, and monitoring of musculoskeletal sarcomas, should be considered for each tumor of a different histologic subtype.

Ecklund K, Jaramillo D: Patterns of premature physeal arrest: MR imaging of 111 children. *AJR Am J Roentgenol* 2002;178:967-972.

The purpose of this study was to use MRI, especially fat-suppressed three-dimensional spoiled gradient-recalled echo sequences, to identify patterns of growth arrest after physeal insult in children. This method exquisitely shows the growth disturbance and associated abnormalities that may follow physeal injury, and guides surgical management.

Fardon DF, Milette PC: Nomenclature and classification of lumbar disc pathology: Recommendations of the combined task forces of the North American Spine Society, American Society of Spine Radiology, and American Society of Neuroradiology. *Spine* 2001;26:E93-E113.

This document provides a universally acceptable nomenclature that is workable for all forms of observation, that addresses contour, content, integrity, organization, and spatial relationships of the lumbar disk; and that serves as a system of classification and reporting built upon that nomenclature.

Karppinen J, Paakko E, Paassilta P, et al: Radiologic phenotypes in lumbar MR imaging for a gene defect in the COL9A3 gene of type IX collagen. *Radiology* 2003; 227:143-148.

The results of this study indicate that the presence of *Trp3* allele is associated with Scheuermann's disease and intervertebral disk degeneration. No associations were found for other radiologic phenotypes.

Ledermann HP, Morrison WB, Schweitzer ME: MR image analysis of pedal osteomyelitis: Distribution, patterns of spread, and frequency of associated ulceration and septic arthritis. *Radiology* 2002;223:747-755.

The purpose of this study was to evaluate the anatomic distribution of pedal osteomyelitis and septic arthritis in a large patient group with advanced pedal infection and to compare ulcer location with the distribution of osteomyelitis and septic arthritis. Pedal osteomyelitis results almost exclusively from contiguous infections and occurs most frequently around the fifth and first metatarsophalangeal joints. One third of patients with advanced pedal infection show evidence of septic arthritis on MRI.

Philipp MO, Kubin K, Mang T, Hormann M, Metz VM: Three-dimensional volume rendering of multidetector-row CT data: Applicable for emergency radiology. *Eur J Radiol* 2003;48:33-38.

This article presents a review of recent literature on volume-rendering technique and applications for the emergency department.

Steinbach LS, Palmer WE, Schweitzer ME: Special focus session: MR arthrography. *Radiographics* 2002;22:1223-1246.

Direct magnetic resonance arthrography with injection of saline solution or diluted gadolinium can be useful for evaluating certain pathologic conditions in the joints. Indirect magnetic resonance arthrography with intravenous administration of diluted gadolinium may be performed when direct magnetic resonance arthrography is inconvenient or not logistically feasible. Although indirect magnetic resonance arthrography has some disadvantages, it does not require fluoroscopic guidance or joint infection and is superior to conventional MRI in delineating structures when there is minimal joint fluid; vascularized or inflamed tissue will be enhanced with this method.

Zlatkin MB, Rosner J: MR imagingof ligaments an triangular fibrocartilage complex of the wrist. *Magn Reson Imaging Clin North Am* 2004;12:301-331.

This article summarizes the current diagnostic criteria that can be useful in interpreting abnormalities of the wrist ligaments and triangular fibrocartilage complex of the wrist.

Diagnostic and Therapeutic Procedures

Carrino JA, Chan R, Vaccaro AR: Vertebral augmentation: Vertebroplasty and kyphoplasty. *Semin Roentgenol* 2004;39:68-84.

Vertebroplasty and kyphoplasty (balloon-assisted vertebroplasty) have both led to good pain relief and improved function with minimal complication rates in appropriately selected patients when high-quality imaging and meticulous technique are used.

Classic Bibliography

Hoffman JR, Mower WR, Wolfson AB, Todd KH, Zucker MI: Validity of a set of clinical criteria to rule out injury to the cervical spine in patients with blunt trauma: National Emergency X-Radiography Utilization Study Group. *N Engl J Med* 2000;343:94-99.

Jensen MC, Brant-Zawadzki MN, Obuchowski N, et al: Magnetic resonance imaging of the lumbar spine in people without backpain. *N Engl J Med* 1994;331:69-73.

Karasick D, Wapner KL: Hallux valgus deformity: Preoperative radiologic assessment. *AJR Am J Roentgenol* 1990;155:119-123.

Lawson JP: International Skeletal Society Lecture in honor of Howard D. Dorfman: Clinically significant radiologic anatomic variants of the skeleton. *AJR Am J Roentgenol* 1994;163:249-255.

Martel W, Hayes JT, Duff IF: The pattern of bone erosion in the hand and wrist in rheumatoid arthritis. *Radiology* 1965;84:204-214.

Morrison WB, Schweitzer ME, Batte WG, Radack DP, Russel KM: Osteomyelitis of the foot: Relative importance of primary and secondary MR imaging signs. *Radiology* 1998;207:625-632.

Park YH, Lee JY, Moon SH, et al: MR arthrography of the labral capsular ligamentous complex in the shoulder: Imaging variations and pitfalls. *AJR Am J Roentgenol* 2000;175:667-672.

Stoller DW, Martin C, Crues JV III, Kaplan L, Mink JH: Meniscal tears: Pathologic correlation with MR imaging. *Radiology* 1987;163:731-735.

Weissman BN, Aliabadi P, Weinfeld MS, Thomas WH, Sosman JL: Prognostic features of atlantoaxial subluxation in rheumatoid arthritis patients. *Radiology* 1982;144:745-751.

Winalski CS, Aliabadi P, Wright RJ, Shortkroff S, Sledge CB, Weissman BN: Enhancement of joint fluid with intravenously administered gadopentetate dimeglumine: technique, rationale, and implications. *Radiology* 1993;187:179-185.

Chapter 12

Perioperative Medical Management

Gregory Argyros, MD

Introduction

Appropriate perioperative management of surgical patients is critical in ensuring the greatest likelihood of a successful patient outcome. It is important to understand the physiologic response to surgery and anesthesia, disease-related and procedure-related risk, prophylactic therapy to prevent perioperative problems, and postoperative medical complications. The medical consultant must determine exactly what is being requested—whether for surgical risk assessment, diagnostic or management advice, or documentation for legal reasons. The surgeon and the medical consultant must communicate directly to minimize the potential for misunderstanding.

Surgical risk is the probability of an adverse outcome or death associated with surgery and anesthesia. Surgical risk is categorized into four components: patient-related; procedure-related; provider-related; and anesthetic-related. Information from the medical history, physical examination, review of available data, and selectively ordered laboratory tests can be used to make an estimation of perioperative risk. The following factors must be considered: the patient's current health status; if there is evidence of medical illness, how severe it is and whether it will affect surgical risk; how urgent is the surgery; if surgery is delayed, will treatment of the medical illness lessen its severity; and, if there is no reason to delay the surgery, what changes need to be made perioperatively to maximize the patient's overall condition. Assessment of these factors will allow for a decision on whether the patient is in optimal medical condition to undergo the planned surgical procedure.

The Preoperative Evaluation

The practice of extensive testing of all patients before surgery can be expensive, both in terms of direct costs of the tests, but also for the follow-up of unanticipated minor abnormalities, many of which have no clinical relevance. Many studies have shown that preoperative routine testing of all patients is of limited value. Tests should be ordered based on history and physical examination findings that identify subgroups of patients who are more likely to have abnormal results. Tests should only be ordered if the result will influence management. If a test result is abnormal, documentation of the thought process regarding the planned response to the abnormality is critical. A summary of recommendations regarding testing before elective surgery is presented in Table 1.

Cardiac Risk Assessment and Optimization

The American College of Cardiology and the American Heart Association issued guidelines for perioperative cardiovascular evaluation of patients undergoing noncardiac surgery in 2002. They propose a stepwise strategy that relies on assessment of clinical markers, prior coronary evaluation and treatment, functional capacity, and surgery-specific risk. A framework for determining which patients are candidates for cardiac testing is presented in algorithmic form in Figure 1.

Clinical markers are divided into major, intermediate, and minor predictors of increased perioperative cardiovascular risk. Major clinical markers include an unstable coronary syndrome, such as a myocardial infarction, within 1 month of surgery, unstable or severe angina, evidence of a large ischemic burden by clinical symptoms or noninvasive testing, decompensated heart failure, significant arrhythmias, and severe valvular heart disease. Intermediate predictors are mild angina, a myocardial infarction occurring more than 1 month before surgery, compensated heart failure, a preoperative creatinine level greater than 2.0 mg/dL, and diabetes. Minor predictors are advanced age, abnormal electrocardiogram, heart rhythm other than sinus, low functional capacity, history of stroke, and uncontrolled hypertension.

Functional capacity can be expressed as metabolic equivalent (MET) levels. Increasing MET levels reflect a greater aerobic burden. Perioperative cardiac risk is increased in patients unable to meet a 4-MET demand during most normal daily activities. Activities such as light housework, climbing a flight of stairs, or walking

Table 1 | Recommendations for Preoperative Testing

Test	Indications
Hemoglobin	Anticipated major blood loss or symptoms of anemia
White blood cell count	Symptoms of infection, myeloproliferative disorder or myelotoxic medications
Platelet count	History of bleeding diathesis, myeloproliferative disorder, or myelotoxic medications
Prothrombin time	History of bleeding diathesis, chronic liver disease, malnutrition, recent or long-term antibiotic use
Partial thrombo-plastin time	History of bleeding diathesis
Electrolytes	Know renal insufficiency, congestive heart failure, medications that affect electrolytes
Renal function	Hypertension, age > 50 years, cardiac disease, major surgery, anticipated use of medications that may affect renal function
Glucose	Obesity or known diabetes
Liver function tests	No indication
Urinalysis	No indication
Electrocardiogram	Men > age 40 years, women > age 50 years, known coronary artery disease, diabetes, or hypertension
Chest radiograph	Age > 50 years, known cardiac or pulmonary disease, symptoms or examination suggestive of cardiac or pulmonary disease

on level ground at 4 miles per hour involve a 4-MET energy expenditure.

Surgery-specific risk is related to the type of surgery and the degree of hemodynamic compromise associated with the procedure. Most orthopaedic procedures are intermediate risk, with a cardiac risk generally less than 5%. Prolonged procedures associated with large fluid shifts and/or blood loss and emergency surgery are high risk, with a reported cardiac risk of greater than 5%.

Several trials have examined the impact of medical therapy begun before surgery on reducing cardiac events. Two randomized, placebo-controlled trials of β-blocker administration have been performed, with one showing reduced perioperative cardiac events and the other improved 6-month survival. When possible, β-blockers should be started far enough before elective surgery so that the dose can be titrated to achieve a resting heart rate between 50 and 60 beats per minute.

Pulmonary Risk Assessment/Optimization

The type of surgery performed and the anatomic location of the surgery are major determinants of risk in the development of postoperative pulmonary complications. Most orthopaedic procedures are associated with a very low incidence of pulmonary complications. Most of the complications that do occur involve either oversedation from pain medications that can result in atelectasis, or

postoperative deep venous thrombosis and pulmonary embolism.

Routine preoperative chest radiographs are not recommended for all patients. They should be obtained for all patients older than 50 years, those with known preexisting cardiopulmonary disease, and those with symptoms or findings on physical examination that suggest a likelihood of cardiopulmonary disease. Using these criteria, previously unrecognized abnormalities that may influence perioperative management will be detected in a small but clinically significant subset of patients.

The purpose of pulmonary function assessment in patients undergoing orthopaedic surgical procedures is not to preclude surgery but to help in anticipating and preventing complications. Preoperative pulmonary function studies are typically not indicated unless the patient is older than 60 years, has a history of pulmonary disease or smoking, or there is an anticipated anesthesia time of 2 hours or longer. Routine arterial blood gas assessments are not recommended.

If possible, elective surgery should be delayed if the patient exhibits evidence of active infection (such as a change in the character or amount of sputum). Also, surgery should be delayed if the patient has obstructive lung disease and is in the midst of an acute exacerbation. Although there is conflicting evidence regarding the benefits and ideal timing of smoking cessation before surgery, abstinence from smoking for at least 8 weeks before surgery is probably ideal for decreasing postoperative pulmonary complications, but an 8-week delay in surgery may not be feasible. Patients with obstructive lung disease who are receiving bronchodilator or inhaled anti-inflammatory therapy should continue this regimen throughout the perioperative period.

Although several abnormalities in pulmonary function have been noted in obese patients, studies have shown that obesity does not consistently contribute to significant pulmonary complications. In patients with known sleep apnea, perioperative airway management is paramount because perioperative continuous positive airway pressure may be required as these patients recover from anesthesia. It has not been determined whether screening patients with multiple risk factors for sleep apnea (obesity, increased neck circumference, craniofacial abnormalities, hypothyroidism) impacts postoperative pulmonary complications, but concerns about perioperative airway management difficulties should be raised.

Renal Risk Assessment/Optimization

In patients with chronic kidney disease, cardiac disease is the leading cause of death; therefore, a full cardiac risk assessment as previously described is needed. In addition, close attention must be paid to other manifestations of chronic kidney disease to include volume, elec-

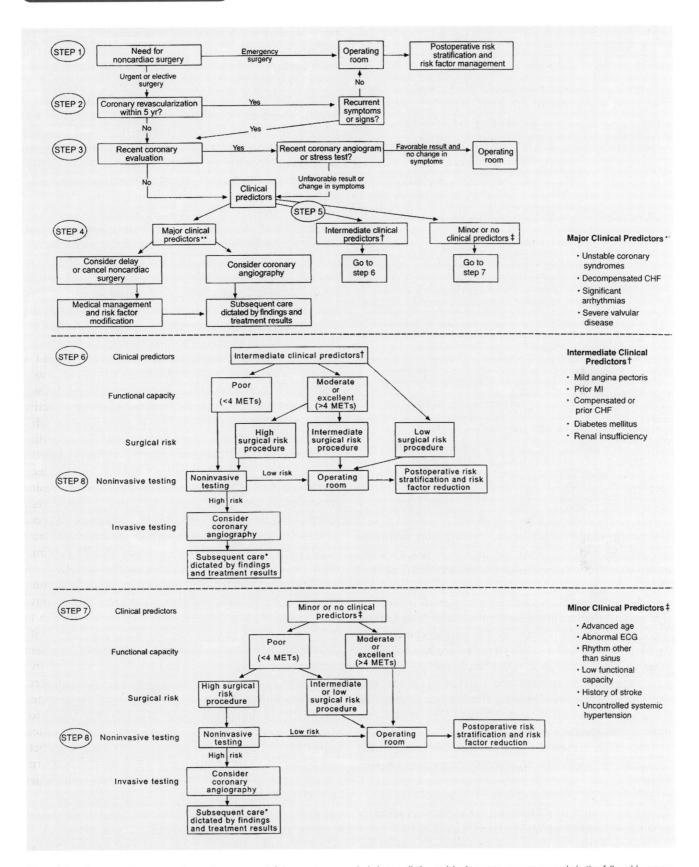

Figure 1 Stepwise approach to preoperative cardiac assessment. Subsequent care may include cancellation or delay in surgery, coronary revascularization followed by noncardiac surgery, or intensified care. *(Reproduced with permission from Eagle KA, Berger PB, Calkins H, et al: ACC/AHA guideline update for perioperative cardiovascular evaluation for noncardiac surgery: Executive summary. Circulation 2002;105:1257-1267.)*

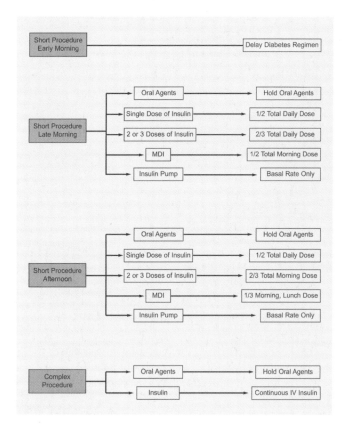

Figure 2 Summary of preoperative management recommendation based on therapeutic regimen and the complexity and scheduling of the surgical procedure. MDI indicates multiple doses of intravenous insulin; IV, intravenous. *(Reproduced with permission from Jacober SJ Sowers JR: An update on perioperative management of diabetes. Arch Intern Med 1999;159:2405-2411.)*

on microscopic evaluation of the urine. These patients require volume repletion with a bicarbonate-containing resuscitation fluid to maintain an alkalotic urine.

Diabetes Mellitus Risk Assessment and Optimization

Whenever possible, endocrine disorders should be identified and evaluated before surgery. The most common endocrine disorder by far is diabetes mellitus. Patients with diabetes have an increased risk of perioperative complications including infection, metabolic and electrolyte abnormalities, and renal and cardiac complications. The stresses of surgery and anesthesia cause several hormonal changes that contribute to hyperglycemia during and after surgery. The extent of the metabolic derangements is related to the type and length of surgery. Several of the most significant consequences of perioperative hyperglycemia include impaired wound healing and ability to fight infection. Patients with diabetes are also at risk for hypoglycemia in the perioperative period. This condition may go unrecognized in the patient under anesthesia if appropriate glucose monitoring is not performed. Factors that contribute to the risk of hypoglycemia perioperatively include prolonged fasting, use of oral hypoglycemic medications, inadequate nutritional state preoperatively, and postoperative gastrointestinal problems.

How a patient's diabetes is managed during surgery is dependent on several patient-specific and surgery-specific factors. Patient-related issues include whether treatment is with diet alone, with oral hypoglycemic agents, or with insulin, as well as the degree of glycemic control. Surgery-specific factors to consider are the type of anesthesia, whether major or minor surgery is scheduled, and how long the patient is expected to take nothing by mouth. Management algorithms for perioperative care of patients with diabetes are shown in Figures 2 and 3.

Rheumatologic Disease Risk Assessment and Optimization

Several unique perioperative issues must be addressed in the patient with rheumatologic disease. These issues are related to the disease itself, as well as the drug management of many of these disease processes. Patients with rheumatoid arthritis are unique in their high rate of cervical disk disease. When the ligaments, bones, and joints that maintain C1-C2 stability are eroded by synovitis, C2 can subluxate on C1 and cause spinal cord compression. Manipulating the neck for intubation during general anesthesia stresses this joint and can result in spinal cord injury. It is estimated that up to 25% of rheumatoid arthritis patients have cervical disk disease, and these patients should be evaluated preoperatively. Rheumatoid arthritis patients are also at risk for cricoarytenoid arthritis (seen in up to 50% to 80% in some

trolyte, and acid/base status, anemia, bleeding diatheses, the propensity for dramatic swings in blood pressure, and the need for dosage adjustments for many medications.

The high mortality rate of patients with postoperative acute renal failure makes prevention a key objective in overall management. Before surgery, particularly for those procedures capable of inducing renal ischemia, potential risk factors such as volume depletion, hypotension, nephrotoxin exposure, and preexisting chronic kidney disease must be identified. Elective surgery should be delayed until any abnormalities are improved. Common nephrotoxins include nonsteroidal anti-inflammatory drugs, including selective cyclooxygenase inhibitors, certain antibiotics, angiotensin-converting enzyme inhibitors, and radiocontrast. The use of these compounds must be monitored very closely and prophylactic regimens such as N-acetylcysteine before radiocontrast administration should be used.

Trauma patients with significant soft-tissue injury are at risk for developing acute renal failure from the myoglobin released from rhabdomyolysis. Acute renal failure should be suspected when dipstick urinalysis reveals the presence of heme when no red blood cells are seen series). This condition can also make intubation very difficult and, if suspected, indirect laryngoscopy should be performed preoperatively.

Anti-inflammatory drug and steroid use in patients with rheumatoid arthritis must be identified preoperatively. Salicylates or nonsteroidal anti-inflammatory drugs prolong bleeding time by inhibiting platelet aggregation. Relative risks of these medications vary with different surgical procedures, particularly if deep venous thrombosis prophylaxis is also going to be used. If possible, salicylates and long-acting nonsteroidal medications should be discontinued 7 to 10 days preoperatively. In this instance, low-dose prednisone can often control inflammatory symptoms.

Patients who have taken systemic steroid medications for more than 1 week in the 6 months before surgery should be considered for stress dosing of steroids during the perioperative period secondary to the risk of hypothalamic-pituitary-adrenal axis suppression. Based on the complexity/stress associated with the surgery, dosing recommendations can range from 100 mg of hydrocortisone given preoperatively, then every 8 hours for the first day, decreased by 50% per day, and then discontinued by the fourth day, to one dose of 50 to 100 mg of hydrocortisone immediately preoperatively as a single dose.

Perioperative Care in the Elderly

The perioperative management of the elderly has undergone major changes over the past 50 years because there has been a dramatic population shift. The age group 65 years and older is the fastest growing segment of the population in the United States, expected to comprise 20% of the population by 2025.

The contribution of individual patient conditions to surgical risk is related to a combination of physiologic changes associated with underlying diseases, combined to a lesser degree with age-related physiologic changes. Research has clarified that age alone is at most a minor risk factor for perioperative complications. Age-related cardiovascular, pulmonary, and renal changes have to be considered as well as recognition of altered pharmacokinetics in the elderly that can lead to an increase in complications and toxicity.

Several postoperative complications are more common in the elderly. Delirium is a clinical syndrome in which there is an acute disruption of attention and cognition. Orthopaedic patients, especially those with hip fracture, may have a 28% to 60% incidence of delirium. The development of postoperative delirium has been associated with increased morbidity and mortality, so it is critical to identify patients who may be at risk and focus interventions on this group. Risk factors that have been identified include a history of drug or alcohol abuse, preexisting cognitive dysfunction or physical impair-

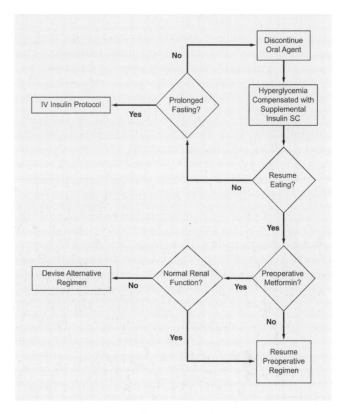

Figure 3 Management algorithm for oral hypoglycemic agents. SC indicates subcutaneously; IV, intravenous. *(Reproduced with permission from Jacober SJ Sowers JR: An update on perioperative management of diabetes. Arch Intern Med 1999;159:2405-2411.)*

ment, depression, polypharmacy, and the presence of metabolic abnormalities. Evaluation of the elderly patient who develops delirium requires consideration of preoperative, surgical, and postoperative factors. Preoperative risk factors identified above should be corrected as much as possible, medication lists should be reviewed, unnecessary medications stopped, and careful questioning about the use of over-the-counter medications and supplements should occur. Intraoperative factors associated with postoperative delirium include the type of surgery and anesthetic used. Hip fracture surgery (especially for femoral neck fractures) is a procedure with a high risk for delirium. Anticholinergic agents, barbiturates, and benzodiazepines may also play a role. Intraoperative hypotension or hypoxemia also are risk factors. Postoperative risk factors are similar to preoperative and intraoperative risk factors with reactions to pain medications, particularly meperidine, also playing a role. Sepsis, myocardial infarction, metabolic abnormalities, and withdrawal from drugs or alcohol must be considered. For a patient with preexisting impaired cognitive function, altered sensory input such as not having eyeglasses or hearing aids available, or environmental changes can contribute to the development of delirium.

Immobility, another postoperative complication that can be devastating in the elderly, can lead to pressure ulcers, increased risk for osteoporosis, pulmonary risks such as atelectasis, increased risk of aspiration and pneumonia, increased risk of venous thromboembolic disease, and gastrointestinal, genitourinary, and cardiovascular effects. Elderly patients require an aggressive, multidisciplinary mobilization strategy that starts early and continues as long as is necessary for maximal functional recovery.

In industrialized nations, the elderly are at perhaps the greatest risk of being malnourished, and it is important to identify these patients preoperatively. Elderly patients with preoperative malnutrition may develop protein-calorie malnutrition from the stress of surgery. Negative nitrogen balance depletes visceral protein stores, leading to a loss of muscle mass and less effective postoperative rehabilitation and ambulation. Nutritional status should be monitored and addressed from the first postoperative day and patients must not be allowed to fall behind nutritionally. Voluntary food intake should be monitored and nutritional supplements introduced promptly if necessary. Oral supplementation is usually adequate and parenteral feeding should be used only as a last resort for patients with altered gastrointestinal tract function.

Annotated Bibliography

The Preoperative Evaluation

Arozullah AM, Conde MV, Lawrence VA: Preoperative evaluation for postoperative pulmonary complications. *Med Clin North Am* 2003;87:153-174.

A review of the morbidity, mortality, and risk factors associated with postoperative complications is presented. Indications for preoperative tests and risk reduction strategies are discussed.

Eagle KA, Berger PB, Calkins H, et al: ACC/AHA guideline update for perioperative cardiovascular evaluation for noncardiac surgery: Executive summary. *Circulation* 2002;105:1257-1267.

This article presents an overview of cardiovascular risk stratification for patients undergoing noncardiac surgery.

Joseph AJ, Cohn SL: Perioperative care of the patient with renal failure. *Med Clin North Am* 2003;87:193-210.

A discussion of recognition and elimination of risk factors for development of acute renal failure is presented. Perioperative management of patient with end stage renal disease is reviewed.

Schiff RL, Welsh GA: Perioperative evaluation and management of the patient with endocrine dysfunction. *Med Clin North Am* 2003;87:175-192.

In this article, a discussion of current strategies for the perioperative evaluations and management of patients with diabetes mellitus is presented.

Perioperative Care in the Elderly

Beliveau MM, Multach M: Perioperative care for the elderly patient. *Med Clin North Am* 2003;87:273-290.

This article reviews perioperative strategies to decrease the risk of complications in this patient population.

Classic Bibliography

Cygan R, Waitzkin H: Stopping and restarting medications in the perioperative period. *J Gen Intern Med* 1987;2:270-283.

Goldman L: Cardiac risks and complications of noncardiac surgery. *Ann Intern Med* 1983;98:504-513.

Goldman L, Lee T, Rudd P: Ten commandments for effective consultations. *Arch Intern Med* 1983;143:1753-1755.

Kellerman PS: Perioperative care of the renal patient. *Arch Intern Med* 1994;154:1674-1688.

Kroenke K, Gooby-Toedt D, Jackson JL: Chronic medications in the perioperative period. *South Med J* 1998;91:358-364.

Mangano DT, Layug EL, Wallace A, et al: Effect of atenolol on mortality and cardiovascular morbidity after noncardiac surgery. *N Engl J Med* 1996;335:1713-1720.

Morrison RS, Chassin MR, Siu AL: The medical consultant's role in caring for patients with hip fracture. *Ann Intern Med* 1998;128:1010-1020.

Schiff RL, Emanuele MA: The surgical patient with diabetes mellitus: Guidelines for management. *J Gen Intern Med* 1995;10:154-161.

Smetana GW: Preoperative pulmonary evaluation. *N Engl J Med* 1999;340:937-944.

Sorokin R: Management of the patient with rheumatic diseases going to surgery. *Med Clin North Am* 1993;77:453-463.

Chapter 13

Work-Related Illnesses, Cumulative Trauma, and Compensation

Owen J. Moy, MD

Robert H. Ablove, MD

Introduction

It is difficult to estimate the overall cost of work-related illness. There is little doubt that the involved costs are extraordinary. Most economic studies of work-related illness focus on direct economic costs and disability duration. These studies place less emphasis on the significant social implications of these injuries, such as the impact on the surrounding family and community. These costs are also often high, on both a social and economic level.

The Workers' Compensation System

The origin of today's workers' compensation system in the United States dates back to the turn of the 20th century when laws were enacted at both state and federal levels to serve several purposes: paying workers' medical expenses, compensating workers for missed pay, and providing financial settlements for irrecoverable loss. Although there is considerable variation from state to state, the laws generally shield employers from charges of negligence, thus mitigating the possibility of civil litigation.

Workers' compensation tends to function as an advocacy system involving numerous parties, including the worker and possible legal representation, the treating physician, the employer, the employer's insurance carrier, case managers, and physicians performing independent medical examinations (IMEs). These examinations are usually performed at the request of either the insurance carrier or the patient's legal representation. Unfortunately, the parties involved often have conflicting goals.

Most patients wish to receive care and get better, although there are often some noninjury-related issues or barriers. On occasion patients may not want to return to work, because of issues as far ranging as a hostile work environment to possible secondary monetary gain. Most treating physicians desire to administer care as expeditiously as possible. Employers generally want employees to have as little sick or compensable time away as possible, while their insurance carriers endeavor to resolve

cases with as little expense as possible. The IME physician is usually paid by the insurance carrier, which can build further bias into the system. The fact that there are so many parties with different interests can ultimately delay treatment and in some cases affect the ultimate outcome. Several basic terms necessary for a discussion of this system are presented in Table 1.

Assessment of the Injured Worker

Several parties usually perform medical assessment of the injured worker. The treating physician evaluates the injured worker as he or she would any other patient, taking a thorough history of the injury, the patient's occupation, and any underlying conditions.

Social and psychological factors can play a large role in disability. Conflicts with supervisors or associates, workplace stress, emotional problems, and substance or alcohol abuse need to be explored and noted.

The physical examination is obviously an important part of the evaluation. Nonphysiologic findings need to be explored and noted as potential evidence of malingering. Waddell described a simple list of five physical signs to help establish a distinction between organic and nonorganic findings in patients with low back pain (Table 2). Findings of three or more positive signs are considered clinically significant.

Following a thorough physical examination, the physician formulates a treatment plan. In many cases, treatment cannot commence without permission of the insurance carrier. This is often the rate-limiting step in providing definitive care for an injured worker.

Depending on the cost of proposed treatment, the carrier may request an IME before initiation of nonurgent care. The physician administering that examination is theoretically rendering an independent opinion, but is being paid by the insurance carrier. At times, claimant attorneys may request additional "independent" examinations. It is important to remember that the insurance adjuster's main job is to limit the expense to the insurance company of the administered care and that the

Table 1	Basic Workers' Compensation Terms
Impairment	Deviation from normal function, which may be either permanent or temporary.
Disability	A nonmedical term pertaining to the loss or diminution of the ability to perform a function or functions. It is possible to be impaired without necessarily being disabled. A transcriptionist with a below-knee amputation has an impairment but is still able to perform all of his or her job functions. The terms are often incorrectly used interchangeably. Disability may be partial or total as well as temporary or permanent. Disability determinations help establish the amount of ongoing financial compensation received during periods of disability. The amount is usually a percentage of the regular salary.
Apportionment	A term referring to the relative contribution of different factors to overall disability. This applies in cases of either underlying illnesses or prior injuries that make the current disability materially and substantially greater than it would otherwise be. Both treating and independent medical physicians are often asked to assign fixed percentages to the relative contributing factors.
Loss of use	Usually refers to a permanent relatively static loss of function, usually of an extremity. This is a distinct category from disability. In certain states, loss of use determinations are used to help determine the appropriate lump sum settlement necessary to settle a case.
Maximal medical improvement	The point at which no further recovery from an injury or illness is expected.

Table 2	Waddell's Nonorganic Physical Signs in Low Back Pain
1. Tenderness	Tenderness related to physical disease should be specific and localized to specific anatomic structures. Superficial: tenderness to pinch or light touch over a wide area of lumbar skin. Nonanatomic: deep tenderness over a wide area, not localized to a specific structure.
2. Simulation Tests	These tests should not be uncomfortable. Axial loading – reproduction of low back pain with vertical pressure on the skull. Rotation – reproduction of back pain when shoulders and pelvis are passively rotated in the same plane.
3. Distraction Tests	Findings that are present during physical examination and disappear at other times, particularly while the patient is distracted.
4. Regional Disturbances	Findings inconsistent with neuroanatomy. Motor – nonanatomic "voluntary release" or unexplained "giving way" of muscle groups. Sensory – nondermatomal sensory abnormalities.
5. Overreaction	Disproportionate verbal or physical reactions.

IME physician may be under pressure to render a favorable decision for the carrier.

Functional capacity evaluations are an attempt to create an objective measurement of physical capabilities. They are a useful adjunct in determining work readiness and are at the very least more objective than arbitrary physician estimates. They also can provide evidence of submaximal or inconsistent patient effort, which may be of use in detecting malingering. Unfortunately, they also provide an additional layer of expenses to the care of injured workers.

Points of Documentation

Typically, the first step in the filing of a claim is to fill out an incident report. However, these reports are at times filed retrospectively after treatment has already been sought and possibly initiated, either via out-of-pocket expense or private insurance.

A detailed, specific occupational history including a list of current and previous occupations is paramount.

The occupational descriptions should include a list of the specific activities performed for each job, as well as their frequency and duration. It is also important to note any recreational activity involving significant physical exertion. Obviously, any history of other claims as well as nonwork-related injuries or illnesses should be documented.

Interacting With the Caseworker

Many insurance companies hire caseworkers to manage individual claims. Under ideal circumstances, they can expedite patient care, and manage the transition from rehabilitation to work hardening (discussed in more detail later in this chapter) to the ultimate return to work.

The caseworker's main role should be facilitating communication between the involved parties. To be effective, the caseworker needs to be conversant in orthopaedic and ergonomic issues (see next section). Specific ergonomic training increases caseworker effectiveness. The caseworker can accompany the patient to office visits and learn their specific work capabilities. A job site visit, including both an ergonomic assessment of the workstation and a discussion with the employer regarding availability of specific light duty positions, can help speed the return to work.

Patients need to be informed of the role of the caseworker as well as their own right to privacy. Given the organization of most current workers' compensation systems, caseworkers can be very effective. Because the employer's insurance carrier employs the caseworkers, it also is possible that bias can be introduced into the system.

Cumulative Trauma Disorders and Ergonomics
What is the Concept?
Cumulative trauma disorders (CTDs) is a term applying to health disorders arising from repetitive biomechanical stress. A discussion of ergonomics is central to this topic. Ergonomics is a relatively recent word, dating to approximately 1945, defined as a branch of ecology pertaining to human factors in machine design and operation as well as the physical environment. The Occupational Safety and Health Administration's (OSHA) current definitions of ergonomics listed on their website include both the science of fitting the job to the worker and the practice of designing equipment and tasks conforming to workers' capabilities.

The Occupational Safety and Health Act of 1970 states that it is the employer's responsibility to provide a workplace free from serious hazards. This includes the prevention of ergonomic hazards. To meet these goals, OSHA has developed a series of manuals and programs to help employers meet workers' ergonomic needs that include a generalized framework of health and safety programs as well as guidelines for specific industries. These guidelines have been developed with the assistance of the National Institute for Occupational Safety and Health, current scientific information, the medical literature, and OSHA's own enforcement experience.

Specifically, the guidelines include a process for protecting workers as well as a means of identifying specific problems and implementing solutions. There are also sections on task-specific training. Appropriately, most of the focus is on prevention.

CTDs refer to disorders from trauma occurring over time, rather than from one specific incident. In the early 1990s there was a significant increase in the reporting of CTDs. According to the Bureau of Labor, statistics from that time show that CTDs represented half of the occupational illnesses reported in their annual survey. The very term cumulative trauma disorder is fraught with controversy because it implies a level of a presumed knowledge regarding the etiology of certain conditions, which does not necessarily exist. OSHA literature now uses the less specific and therefore more benign term musculoskeletal disorders. OSHA manuals mention low back pain, sciatica, rotator cuff injuries, epicondylitis, and carpal tunnel syndrome as common musculoskeletal disorders, conceding that more needs to be learned about the connection between the workplace and these disorders.

Does This Exist and Is It an Epidemic?
There is little doubt that CTDs exist, but that does not mean that they are easy to describe or quantify. If a body is exposed to repetitive force over time, given enough repetitions the body will show signs of wear. Many CTDs have multifactorial causes and represent changes that may have occurred over a significant time period. Controversy exists because an immediate cause and ultimate responsibility for CTDs can therefore be hard to determine.

With carpal tunnel syndrome, for example, there is support in the literature for the role of extreme wrist position and vibration exposure in the development of the condition, both of which are potential occupational causes. Many nonoccupational causes exist, including gender, obesity, tobacco use, and diabetes. Therefore, it is difficult to ascribe causation to one particular factor. The situation is similar with other CTDs. This issue is paramount in workers' compensation because causation plays a key role in who ultimately pays for care.

Further epidemiologic study is necessary to estimate relative causation in diseases with more than one risk factor and ergonomic intervention needs to be preferentially directed toward high-risk groups. High-risk groups include patients with multiple claims, multiple medical problems, and prolonged absence from work.

Legal Issues in Occupational Medicine
Workers' compensation is generally set up as a no-fault system. As such, employers are legally shielded from being sued for negligence. Many of the legal issues focus therefore on causal relationship, degree of ongoing disability, and ultimate disability settlement.

Causal relationship is the key factor that determines who pays for care. The clinician must be careful to document any evidence of a presumed causally-related illness or injury. It is also important to document any history of prior illnesses and injuries, especially any that resulted in missed work. Patients' recreational and other nonoccupational activities need to be carefully noted. The duration and relative number of repetitions of both work and nonwork activities should be dutifully recorded. If there is any possible evidence that an injury is not causally related, an insurance carrier is likely to attempt to avoid payment for the condition. Direct communication with the insurance adjuster can sometimes help expedite care decisions.

Assignment of Disability
Disability Rating
Because disability is not a medical term, disability rating is not based solely on medical factors. Disability can be partial or total as well as temporary or permanent. Certain states publish guidelines giving criteria for types of partial disability. Ultimately, the physician makes a

somewhat arbitrary determination of whether or not the patient is capable of performing his or her job and to what degree. Administrative panels or workers' compensation judges often settle disputes and make final determinations.

Disputes can arise between worker and employer over the issue of partial disability. Insurance carriers often urge physicians to state that patients are available for light duty and thus not totally disabled. Unfortunately, they often make these urgings in the absence of firsthand knowledge regarding the workplace and the availability of specific types of light duty. Another problem with so-called light duty designations is that they are often not job-specific and only provide simple lifting and time restrictions. Caseworker jobsite visits and communication with the physician, patient, and employer can help resolve some of these issues.

Role and Certification of the Qualified Medical Examiner

The theoretical role of the qualified medical examiner is to provide an independent opinion regarding the patients' illness or injury as well as the care they have received. These are most commonly requested and paid for by the employer's insurance carrier. The typical assessment usually includes a history of present illness, past medical and surgical history, occupational and social history, record review, physical examination, and the formulation of an opinion. Examiners are usually asked to comment on specific issues requested by the carrier and not to offer unsolicited opinions. Commonly, opinions are requested regarding diagnosis, causal relationship, treatment to date, further treatment recommendations, and degree of disability. In certain instances where there have been prior injuries or underlying illnesses, examiners may comment on apportionment.

The IME is often a rate-limiting step of workers' compensation care. Insurance adjusters commonly refuse to authorize diagnostic testing as well as both surgical and nonsurgical care without a concurring independent opinion. If the treating and independent opinions differ, a compensation judge or administrative panel often has to settle the dispute. These steps can delay care for many months.

There continues to be a lack of consensus regarding how to manage workers' compensation claims. Typically and predictably, the more say patients have in their care the more satisfied they are with the outcome. However, this does not consistently result in measurable outcome differences. The prevailing fear against allowing more patient and physician autonomy is that costs will rise. However, experience has thus far not borne out this fear. In fact, there has been evidence that increased usage of musculoskeletal specialists tends to decrease overall costs. Additional prospective study is necessary.

One area of recent controversy has been documented reports of insurance companies altering reports as well as requesting specific opinions and wording from the examining physician. Presumably because of this, the state of New York recently changed regulations regarding reports, specifying that they can only be issued after being read and signed by the examining physician.

The certification process for qualified medical examiners is an evolving process and varies considerably from state to state. In the state of New York, laws have recently changed requiring that examining physicians be board certified. Ironically, there is no such requirement of treating physicians, allowing the possibility that a surgeon may legally operate on compensation patients, but not be able to render independent opinions.

In addition to orthopaedic board certification, there are other types of certification such as those by the board of disability examiners, which enable physician credentialing, and courses on occupational orthopaedics and workers' compensation.

Return to Work Strategies

The Maximal Medical Improvement Concept

As stated earlier, maximal medical improvement is the point at which no further improvement is generally expected. When this occurs, the patient is evaluated to determine if there is any permanent impairment. In cases of permanent impairment, a final settlement is made. Different criteria exist for establishing these settlements, which can be grouped into three main categories: functional, anatomic, and diagnostic.

The functional impairment system is based on what effect the impairment has had on the ability to work. The anatomic system is based on the loss of a body part. An amputation is a 100% loss; lesser injuries are quantified via mobility, sensibility, and strength measurements as compared with normal findings. The diagnostic system is based on the diagnosis code. All of these techniques are incorporated into the Fifth Edition of the *American Medical Association Guides to the Evaluation of Permanent Impairment.*

Generally, most states rely on some form of the anatomic system to determine final settlement sums. The state of New York divides final determinations into loss of use and disability. In static cases of extremity injuries in which patients are not completely disabled and further dramatic deterioration in function is not expected, a percentage loss of use is determined based on the involved body part. The award is then based on that percentage as well as the occupation and income level of the injured worker.

Patients with neck and back problems as well as extremity injuries involving ongoing significant disability, particularly where further deterioration is expected, may be classified as permanently disabled on either a partial or total basis.

Wisconsin uses a modification of the no-fault system. Awards can be increased or decreased in cases of unsafe work places and unsafe work practices, respectively.

Minnesota is one of the only states to rely on diagnosis codes to determine impairment, whereas California is one of the only states to rely on functional determination. Regardless of the system, one must remain cognizant of the distinction between disability and impairment and make a determination based on the guidelines of the particular system.

Work Hardening: How Does This Work?

Work hardening is an intermediate step between therapy and return to work. It has evolved over the past two decades as an outgrowth of traditional rehabilitation. A work-like environment is created for the recovering worker, who is then able to build both physical stamina and psychological confidence by replicating work activities in a controlled environment.

In this unique setting, the therapist provides occupation-specific ergonomic instruction, hopefully minimizing risk factors for re-injury upon return to work. Although additional prospective controlled efficacy studies of work hardening would be helpful, there already exists significant documented evidence of its benefits.

Summary

The intent of the workers' compensation system is admirable, namely treating and compensating workers for work-related injuries. Ultimately that intent is usually realized. Most of the patient and physician dissatisfaction with the system stems from the mode and timing of rendered care. Unfortunately, most state systems are cumbersome with multiple layers of administration, leading simultaneously to delayed care delivery and increased overall costs.

Several states have experimented with different models of administered care. Successful strategies include more integrated care, increased physician autonomy, increased specialist involvement, and use of well-trained case managers. Additional study is necessary. Hopefully, in the coming years, some of these strategies can be implemented on a larger scale.

Annotated Bibliography

Atcheson SG, Brunner RL, Greenwald EJ, Rivera VG, Cox JC, Bigos SJ: Paying doctors more: Use of musculoskeletal specialists and increased physicians pay to decrease worker's compensation cost. *J Occup Environ Med* 2001;43:672-679.

This article studies the effect of using visiting musculoskeletal specialists to assist primary care physicians. Claim costs were significantly lower in this system than in a typical workers' compensation managed care model.

Bernacki EJ, Tsai SP: Ten years experience using an integrated workers' compensation management system to control workers compensation costs. *J Occup Environ Med* 2003;45:508-516.

This article examines the positive effect of an integrative approach to managing workers' compensation claims. It presents 10 years of experience using a small group of health care providers who address both physical and psychological needs. It also illustrates the importance of maintaining open lines of communication between all involved parties.

Durand MJ, Loisel P, Hong QN, Charpentier N: Helping clinicians in work disability prevention: The work disability diagnosis interview. *J Occup Rehabil* 2002;12:191-204.

This article illuminates the multifactorial nature of musculoskeletal disorders. It describes the development of a work disability diagnosis interview as a means of helping detect prognostic factors in musculoskeletal pain patients.

Gross DP, Battie MC: Reliability of safe maximum lifting determinations of a functional capacity evaluation. *Phys Ther* 2002;82:264-271.

Functional capacity evaluations are evaluated for both interrater and test-retest reliability. Overall, functional capacity evaluations demonstrated excellent interrater and good test-retest reproducibility. The greatest source of variability was inconsistent patient performance.

Harper JD: Determining foot and ankle impairments by the AMA Fifth Edition guides. *Foot Ankle Clin* 2002;7:291-303.

This article describes how to determine impairments based on the American Medical Association Fifth Edition guide. It offers a good discussion of the different techniques of determining impairment and the difficulty of accounting for pain as part of this determination.

Lincoln AE, Feuerstein M, Shaw WS: MillerVI: Impact of case manager training on worksite accommodations in workers' compensation claimants with upper extremity disorders. *J Occup Environ Med* 2002;44:237-245.

This is a case control study that illustrates the effect of a two-day training course on the ability of nurse case managers to design and implement workplace changes. The trained nurses offered more specific accommodations and modifications whereas the untrained nurses more often recommended light duty and lifting restrictions.

Schonstein E, Kenny DT, Keating J, Koes BW: Work conditioning, work hardening and functional restoration for workers with back and neck pain, Cochrane Database System Review (on CD-ROM). 2003;(1) CD001822.

This article compares the effectiveness of management strategies for return to work in patients with back and neck pain. Patients with chronic back pain benefited from physical conditioning, even when non-job specific, having a reduced number of sick days compared with patients who did not undergo physical conditioning.

US Department of Labor: *Guidelines for Nursing Homes: Ergonomics for the Prevention of Musculoskeletal Disorders.* OSHA 2003;3182.

This manual is a one of a series for different industries commissioned by Elaine Chao, United States Secretary of Labor, as part of an overall strategy to reduce ergonomic injuries. It provides both a process for protecting workers and identifies solutions for specific work-related problems.

US Department of Labor: *All About OSHA Occupational Safety and Health Administration.* OSHA 2003; 2056-07R.

This manual describes the origin and function of OSHA. It also provides a concise summary of state programs, standards and guidance, as well as available programs and services.

Wickizer TM, Franklin G, Plaeger-Brockway R, Mootz RD: Improving the quality of workers' compensation health care delivery: The Washington State Occupational Health Services Project. *Milbank Q* 2001;79:5-33.

This is a summary of research and policy adopted in Washington State over recent years to identify and correct problems resulting in poor care and increased disability for injured workers. It points to a lack of integrative occupational health services as the most powerful predictor of adverse results.

Classic Bibliography

Cocchiarella L, Anderson GBJ (eds): *Guides to the Evaluation of Permanent Impairment*, ed 5. Chicago, IL, American Medical Association, 2000.

Creighton J: Workers' compensation and job disability, in Peimer CA (ed): *Surgery of the Hand and Upper Extremity*. McGraw Hill, 1996, pp 2345-2351.

Gordon SL, Blair SJ, Fine LJ (eds): *Repetitive Motion Disorders of the Upper Extremity*. Rosemont, IL, American Academy of Orthopedic Surgeons, 1995.

Lepping V: Work hardening: A valuable resource for the occupational health nurse. *AAOHN J* 1990;38:313-317.

Lieber SJ, Rudy TE, Boston JR: Effects of body mechanics training on performance of repetitive lifting. *Am J Occup Ther* 2000;54:166-175.

Luck JV Jr, Florence DW: A brief history and comparative analysis of disability systems and impairment rating systems. *Orthop Clin North Am* 1988;19:839-844.

Norris CR: Understanding Workers' Compensation Law. *Hand Clin* 1993;9:231-239.

US Department of Labor: *Ergonomics Program Management Guidelines for Meatpacking Plants*. (OSHA) 1993;3123.

Waddell G, McCulloch JA, Kummel E, Venner RM: Nonorganic physical sign in low back pain. *Spine* 1980;5:117-125.

Chapter 14

Medical Care of Athletes

Mark Anthony Duca, MD

Introduction

The physician's role in the medical care of athletes has become increasingly complex as the understanding of physiology and its application to athletic performance expands. With ever-developing technologies and ongoing research to improve the care of the athlete, the responsibilities of the team physician have grown rapidly.

The care of an individual athlete often requires a multidisciplinary approach. Expert opinions may be required from many medical specialties, and it is the role of the team physician to serve as the gatekeeper and liaison between the athlete and the health care system.

Medical care of athletes now not only requires an ability to assess and diagnose but a unique skill in coordinating an overall game plan for their management. The role of the team physician has evolved from one in which preparticipation qualification and game-time injury management were sole responsibilities to one in which coordination of medical expertise with other health-related professionals such as medical specialists, athletic trainers, nutritionists, pharmacists, physical therapists, and psychologists is essential. This dialog leads to the safe participation of the athlete and maximizing of their potential.

The medical management of the athlete not only requires the ability to coordinate the preparticipation assessment with management of on-the-field injuries, but also the skill to outline a plan for rehabilitation and return to participation after an injury or illness.

The team physician must also be adept with proper documentation when it comes to the care of athletes and equally skilled at communicating treatment plans with coaches, administrators, media, agents, and family members. The team physician must also communicate with others in a way that does not violate patient confidentiality and is in strict compliance with Health Insurance Portability and Accountability Act guidelines.

Athletic care from a medical standpoint, whether it be for an elite, recreational, or nonprofessional athlete, requires a detailed understanding of basic principles and standards of care.

The Preparticipation Evaluation

The goal of the preparticipation evaluation, defined as the assessment of an individual athlete's qualification to compete in a particular sport or activity, is multifaceted. The preparticipation evaluation must be comprehensive, yet at the same time sport-specific and focused, in an attempt to identify any illness or conditions that predispose the athlete to injury, assess appropriateness for participation, and identify athletes at risk for specific, sport-related injuries. For example, a detailed ocular and visual acuity examination would be much more important to the competitive archer than the Olympic swimmer; similar sports-specific factors should to be taken into consideration when preparing for the evaluation.

The timing and frequency of the preparticipation evaluation should be completed at least 4 to 6 weeks before competition. The optimal frequency of the examination has been debated in the literature. Annual examinations with health maintenance and training counseling have been advocated. Another approach has been a baseline examination at any new level of competition followed by interval history review at the beginning of each new season. The examination may need to be done much more frequently, particularly with athletes who participate in multiple sports throughout the year.

The examination is divided into the history and physical. Patient history is essential in identifying athletes at risk for a particular injury. A standardized, health-history questionnaire, completed by the athlete and reviewed by a health-related professional, can be very helpful (Figure 1). This tool can be modified for specific sports and improve the efficiency of the evaluation.

The physical examination is an assessment of overall general health, with specific focus on organ systems pertinent to the athlete's history or central to safe participation in their particular sport. Vital information including height, weight, blood pressure, heart and respiratory rates, and more recently, body mass index, should be recorded for every potential participant, and common

Preparticipation Physical Evaluation

History

Date _____

Name _____ Sex _____ Age _____ Date of birth _____

Grade _____ Sport _____ _____ _____

Personal physician _____ _____ _____
                                                        Address   Physician's phone

Explain "Yes" answers below:

		Yes	No
1.	Have you ever been hospitalized?	☐	☐
	Have you ever had surgery?	☐	☐
2.	Are you presently taking any medications or pills?	☐	☐
3.	Do you have any allergies (medicine, bees or other stinging insects)?	☐	☐
4.	Have you ever passed out during or after exercise?	☐	☐
	Have you ever been dizzy during or after exercise?	☐	☐
	Have you ever had chest pain during or after exercise?	☐	☐
	Do you tire more quickly than your friends during exercise?	☐	☐
	Have you ever had high blood pressure?	☐	☐
	Have you ever been told that you have a heart murmur?	☐	☐
	Have you ever had racing of your heart or skipped heartbeats?	☐	☐
	Has anyone in your family died of heart problems or a sudden death before age 50?	☐	☐
5.	Do you have any skin problems (itching, rashes, acne)?	☐	☐
6.	Have you ever had a head injury?	☐	☐
	Have you ever been knocked out or unconscious?	☐	☐
	Have you ever had a seizure?	☐	☐
	Have you ever had a stinger, burner or pinched nerve?	☐	☐
7.	Have you ever had heat or muscle cramps?	☐	☐
	Have you ever been dizzy or passed out in the heat?	☐	☐
8.	Do you have trouble breathing or do you cough during or after activity?	☐	☐
9.	Do you use any special equipment (pads, braces, neck rolls, mouth guard, eye guards, etc.)?	☐	☐
10.	Have you had any problems with your eyes or vision?	☐	☐
	Do you wear glasses or contacts or protective eye wear?	☐	☐
11.	Have you ever sprained/strained, dislocated, fractured, broken or had repeated swelling or other injuries of any bones or joints?	☐	☐

☐ Head ☐ Shoulder ☐ Thigh ☐ Neck ☐ Elbow ☐ Knee ☐ Chest
☐ Forearm ☐ Shin/calf ☐ Back ☐ Wrist ☐ Ankle ☐ Hip ☐ Hand ☐ Foot

		Yes	No
12.	Have you had any other medical problems (infectious mononucleosis, diabetes, etc.)?	☐	☐
13.	**Have you had a medical problem or injury since your last evaluation?**	☐	☐

14. When was your last tetanus shot? _____

When was your last measles immunization? _____

15. When was your first menstrual period? _____

When was your last menstrual period? _____

What was the longest time between your periods last year? _____

Explain "Yes" answers:

_____

_____

_____

_____

_____

_____

I hereby state that, to the best of my knowledge, my answers to the above questions are correct.

Date _____

Signature of athlete _____

Signature of parent/guardian _____

Figure 1 Sample preparticipation examination health questionnaire. *(Reproduced with permission from Fields KB: Preparticipation evaluation of the school athlete, in Richmond JC, Shahaday EJ, Fields KB (eds): Sports Medicine for Primary Care. Ann Arbor, MI, Blackwell Science, 1996, p 68.)*

Table 1 | Classification of Sports by Contact

Contact		Noncontact	
Collision/Contact	Limited Contact	Strenuous	Nonstrenuous
Basketball	Baseball	Dancing	Archery
Field hockey	Cycling	Discus	Bowling
Football	Diving	Javelin	Golf
Ice hockey	Fencing	Shot put	Rifle
Lacrosse	Field	Rowing	
Martial arts	High jump	Running/Cross	
Soccer	Pole vault	country	
Water polo	Gymnastics	Strength training	
Wrestling	Raquetball	Swimming	
	Skating	Tennis	
	Skiing	Track	
	Softball		
	Volleyball		

Table 2 | Medical Conditions Affecting Sports Participation

Conditions Requiring Clearance Before Sports Participation

Atlantoaxial instability
Hypertension
Dysrhythmia
Heart murmur/valvular heart disease
Diabetes mellitus
Heat illness history
Hepatomegaly, splenomegaly
History of repeated concussion
Asthma
Absent/undescended testicle
One-eyed athletes or athletes with vision < 20/40 in one eye
Bleeding diathesis
Congenital heart disease
Seizure disorder
Febrile illness
Eating disorders
One-kidney athletes
Malignancy
Organ transplant recipient
Obesity
Dermatologic disorder

general health problems such as obesity and hypertension should quickly be identified. Multiple studies have directly linked increased body mass indices with increased morbidity and mortality rates. Recent, stricter blood pressure screening guidelines established for the general public will no doubt affect preparticipation examinations as well.

The role of screening tests in the routine medical evaluation of athletes remains unproven. Many studies, looking at long-term benefits of screening modalities such as electrocardiograms, echocardiograms, or even urinalysis and chemistry screening profiles, have repeatedly failed to show any clear benefit. Thus, at this time these screening tests cannot be universally recommended unless specifically indicated by the history or physical examination.

Clearance for participation and fitness assessment is dependent on the preparticipation physical examination. The results of the examination then must be evaluated in conjunction with the specific demands of the sport before a final determination on clearance for participation can be made. Sport-specific requirements such as degree of exertion, degree of contact, agility, and environmental influences play a role in determining eligibility (Tables 1 and 2).

The team physician must be skilled and knowledgeable about acting on any clearance recommendations. A willingness to clearly communicate and document the results of the preparticipation evaluation with the athlete must be established. It is preferable that the examining physician coordinate any follow-up required to complete or change the clearance determination.

Conditioning and Preparation

Several basic principles of conditioning must be understood to provide medical consultation in the develop-

ment of a conditioning program. Whether it be sport-specific or for general overall fitness, concepts such as specificity, prioritization, periodization, and work overload need to be addressed. Also, it needs to be understood that conditioning and readiness is a combined product of overall general fitness, sport-specific fitness, and skills specific to the individual sport. Becoming familiar with calculation of workloads for the purpose of outlining a conditioning and fitness program using heart rates and metabolic measurements such as maximum oxygen consumption (MV_{O_2}) can be useful as well.

Conditioning specificity refers to the unique conditioning demands of an individual sport and the necessary adjustments an athlete has to make to accommodate those demands. Each sport has differences in muscle groups needed, aerobic capacity, flexibility, environmental and even psychological factors. Thus, the specifics of a conditioning program are adjusted to meet these particular demands.

Prioritization refers to different levels of emphasis placed on certain components of a conditioning program based on the athlete's preference with varying levels of input from coaches, trainers, and ultimately, physicians. Basketball players looking to improve their jumping ability may prioritize lower extremity strengthening and agility training much in the same way a baseball pitcher may emphasize upper extremity and arm flexibility workouts.

Periodization refers to a planned variation in intensity and duration of a specific workout over a predefined duration of time. A distance runner training for an upcoming marathon uses periodization as a conditioning method by changing the length in miles and intensity measured in speed at each training session before competition. The ultimate goal of periodization is obtaining maximal performance based on the concept of progressive overload, one at which conditioning is started at moderate tolerable levels of exertion and progressively pushed to maximum exertion. Multiple studies have demonstrated this method of conditioning is superior to training techniques in which intensity and duration of training are kept constant over a given period of time. Periodization cycles are defined by length of time and are referred to as macrocycles, mesocycles, or microcycles. Macrocycles generally refer to an entire training year (season to season), mesocycles 3 to 6 months, and microcycles 3 to 6 weeks. Multiple variables can be adjusted during a periodization cycle in addition to intensity and duration of a conditioning workout. They can include variations in types of exercises, number of repetitions of individual exercises, or length of rest periods between exercises.

Conditioning can be further defined as a product of aerobic capacity, strength, and flexibility. Aerobic capacity cannot only be subjectively measured by performance, but also objectively by measurement of the MVO_2 or VO_{2max}, referred to as maximum oxygen uptake. MVO_2 represents the maximum oxygen-carrying capacity of the oxygen transport system, which drives adenosine triphosphate (ATP) synthesis during aerobic metabolism. The oxygen transport system allows tissue to extract oxygen from oxygenated blood and synthesize ATP for energy for muscle activity. A very efficient system allows for maximum performance. The MVO_2 is defined as the product of heart rate (HR), stroke volume (SV), and the difference between arterial and mixed venous oxygen concentrations (a – VO_2), or: $MVO_2 = HR \times SV \times a - VO_2$.

HR times SV is referred to as the cardiac output, whereas SV is the difference in left ventricular volume between end diastole and end systole. Routine measurement of MVO_2 is not practical because it requires the use of a calorimeter, which may not be readily available.

Strength is an integral component to overall conditioning and fitness and is defined as the ability of a particular muscle or muscle group to perform work. Although specific strength training programs are beyond the scope of this chapter, the concepts mentioned earlier of specificity, periodization, and progressive work overload all apply here as well.

Flexibility training and development represents the final component of a total conditioning program. Flexibility is the ability of joints and particular muscle groups to maximize their natural range of motion without compromising strength and endurance. Certainly flexibility can vary from athlete to athlete. Thus, no set standard can be developed for outlining a flexibility program. A large body of evidence suggests that improved flexibility decreases risk for injury although few data exist to imply improved performance.

In contrast to flexibility, specific standards and guidelines can be developed for both aerobic capacity and strength training. For aerobic training, three methods are preferred to establish training guidelines. The first, which is relatively easy to calculate, uses the maximum heart rate as a predictor of intensity. The suggested intensity level is expressed as a percentage of the maximal predicted HR. The target HR for conditioning should be 60% to 90% of the maximum HR. A more highly competitive athlete would aim for a larger percentage of the maximum rate, whereas the daily jogger trying to stay in shape may use a lower percentage. For example, a 40-year-old recreational jogger may use 75% of his maximum HR to calculate his target HR. Calculation of the maximum predicted HR is done by subtracting his age from 220. In this instance it would be 180 beats per minute (bpm); 180 is then multiplied by 0.75 for a product of 135, which now becomes a projected target HR of 135 bpm. The second method requires a few simple calculations. First, the maximal predicted HR is established (example: age 40; 220 – 40 = 180 bpm HR maximum). Next, the HR reserve is calculated by subtracting the resting HR from the maximal predicted HR. The HR reserve is then multiplied by an intensity factor based on an individual athlete's goals and level of conditioning. A beginner should use an intensity factor in the range of 50% to 65% of HR reserve. A moderate conditioned or recreational athlete should use 65% to 75% of HR reserve. Finally, a highly conditioned athlete trying to maximize aerobic capacity for competition uses 75% to 85% of HR reserve. The product of the HR reserve and intensity factor (example: HR reserve 140 × 0.70 for a recreational athlete) is then added to the resting HR to calculate the target exercise HR.

A third method, which requires direct measurement of MVO_2 via calorimetry during maximal exercise stress testing, is less practical but ultimately more accurate than the second method. Similar to the HR method, the oximetry method establishes the target as a percentage of the MVO_2 obtained during maximum exercise testing. Similar intensity factors are used as guidelines for these percentages. For example, an elite athlete should target 75% to 85% of the MVO_2 as his conditioning intensity whereas an intermediate or novice athlete would target ranges from 65% to 75% and 55% to 65%, respectively. A relationship can then be established between heart rate and VO_2 during exercise testing to determine a target HR for training.

Much in the way HR or MV_{O_2} are central to developing guidelines for aerobic training, the repetition maximum (RM) can be used for developing strength-training guidelines. The repetition maximum, or 1-RM, is defined as the maximum amount of weight or resistance that can be lifted for one repetition. An RM also refers to a specific number of repetitions limited by a particular weight or resistance. For example, a weight that can be lifted 10 times until fatigue would be 10-RM. A preferable utilization of the RM allows the prescriber to establish an RM training zone based on the target goal of strength training. A training zone is usually a range of three RMs (eg, 8 to 10 RM), which reduces the need to exercise to fatigue with each set.

The concept of specificity mentioned earlier can be applied to strength training based on the goals and demands of an individual athlete's sport. Four common variables may be adjusted within the training program to achieve target goals. The RM, number of repetitions, number of sets, and rest period between sets can all be adjusted to optimize power, strength, and endurance. Exercises focusing on improvements in power use lower RMs (ie, higher weights or resistance), fewer numbers of repetitions, higher numbers of sets, and longer recovery times between sets. In contrast, training focusing on muscular endurance uses higher RMs (ie, lower weights or resistance), much higher number of repetitions, fewer number of sets and less recovery time in between sets. Strength training uses lower RMs than does power and endurance training with repetition numbers, set numbers, and recovery times being similar to that of power training.

Sideline Medicine

Sideline medicine is a phrase used to refer to the team physician's approach to handling game-time injuries and illnesses and developing a well-documented and organized plan for implementation at the site of competition and practices. From a consensus statement released in 2001 regarding sideline preparedness for the team physician, the definition of sideline medicine is the identification of and planning for medical services to promote the safety of the athlete. Goals are to limit injury and provide medical care at the site of competition. In addition, sideline medicine deals with three integrated aspects of athletic competition: preseason planning, game-day operations, and postseason evaluation.

Preseason planning involves the use of the preparticipation evaluation to identify potential problems during the season. The team physician must have access to any prior relevant health information before determining eligibility for participation. Timely completion of the preparticipation evaluation is advantageous because it allows treatment or follow-up to be initiated before competition, and involves review of the athlete's proposed competition schedule.

Medical care of the athlete involves coordination of administrative duties such as establishment and documentation of an emergency response plan for the seriously ill or injured competitor. Additionally, a policy to assess playing condition and environmental factors at the time of competition must be established, and a protocol involving administrators, competition officials, coaches, and staff to make an educated decision regarding safe competition conditions should be clearly delineated. Finally, medical record keeping is essential in the care of athletes and preseason planning should ensure that this takes place.

Game-day preparations and operations involve the assessment and management of game-day injuries and illnesses and final determinations on clearance for participation. A review of game-time playing conditions is conducted according to the established preseason policy and any concerns should be promptly brought to the attention of coaches, officials, and relevant staff. A well-prepared medical staff also needs to be familiar with medical equipment and examination and treatment facilities available. When traveling, game-time review of locations of examination areas, x-ray equipment, ambulances, and local hospitals with the hometown medical staff is essential to ensure a quick and efficient response to any athletic injuries. The team physician also needs to have a clear vantage point of the competition and easy access to the athletes competing. Return to competition decisions are a part of the game-day responsibilities. Evaluation of concussions, soft-tissue injuries, and eye trauma are a few examples where return to play decisions are made by the team physician during competition. Game-day assessment also requires a postcompetition review of all injuries and illnesses that have developed and an action plan to ensure necessary follow-up. The postcompetition assessment should involve the team physician, trainers, coaches, and relevant administrators.

The postseason evaluation involves a comprehensive summary of all athletic injuries and illnesses acquired during competition. It provides a good opportunity to collect data and identify trends during recent competition. It also is the time for the team physician to coordinate appropriate follow-up during the off-season.

Dehydration and Heat Syndromes

Dehydration is a loss of all body water caused by decreased intake or increased losses by evaporation and excretion. Prolonged dehydration can lead to tissue dysfunction and eventual hemodynamic collapse as the circulating intravascular volume drops to a critical level sufficient to lower cardiac output. As cardiac output decreases, so does blood supply to the skin, resulting in de-

Table 3 | Participants at Risk for Dehydration/Heatstroke

General
  Poorly acclimated or inexperienced competitors
  Obese or poorly conditioned
  Elderly
  Prior history of dehydration/heatstroke
Medication Usage
  Antihistamines
  Anticholinergics
  Diuretics
  Neuroleptics
Illness
  Acute febrile illness
  Recent vomiting or diarrhea
  Uncontrolled systemic condition (for example, diabetes mellitus or
    hypertension)

Table 4 | Total Body Water/Na⁺ Deficit Calculations

Calculation of Total Body Water Deficit

$$TBW = 0.6 \text{ (wt in kg)} \times \left(\frac{[Na^+]}{140} - 1\right)$$

Calculation of Na⁺ Deficit

$$\text{Meq Na}^+ \text{ deficit} = 0.6 \text{ (wt in kg)} (140 - [Na^+]) + (140) \times \text{(vol def in L)}$$

TBW = total body water; [Na⁺] = measured serum sodium concentration (mEq/L)

Table 5 | Clinical Estimates of Degree of Dehydration

% Dehydration (% wt)	Clinical Signs/Symptoms
3% to 5% (Mild to Moderate)	Orthostasis Thirst Decreased voiding Dry mucous membranes Reduced skin turgor Dry axillary folds

8% to 10% (Moderate to Severe)	All of the above plus:
	  Supine hypotension
	  Lethargy
	  Tachycardia
	  Tachypnea

12% to 15% (Severe)	Hemodynamic collapse

creased heat dissipation and a subsequent rise in core body temperature. At extremes of dehydration, sweating mechanisms cease in an attempt to preserve intravascular volume. This in turn can lead to further increases in core body temperature, which left unchecked can be fatal. As little as a 1% drop in total body water has been shown to affect performance.

Athletes are particularly at risk for dehydration and heat illnesses based on the increased demands of competition. It is not unusual for competitive athletes to lose as much as 1 to 2 L of sweat per hour with vigorous, intense exercise. Athletic participants at risk for dehydration and heatstroke are outlined in Table 3.

Aggressive volume replacement is essential during exercise. Rehydration also requires electrolyte replacement in addition to volume. Although electrolyte concentrations are highly variable, sodium is the cation excreted in the highest concentration, with lower concentrations of potassium usually found. Both electrolytes should be replaced, although the necessity is lessened in low-intensity or short-duration exercise and in those who consume a normal diet. At least 16 oz of fluid supplemented with sodium and potassium should be ingested for every pound of weight lost with exercise. Hypotonic salt, or isotonic, carbohydrate supplemented beverages referred to as "sports drinks" are effective rehydration solutions for palatability and rapid effective absorption. The presence of increased ingested sodium and glucose in the intestinal lumen promotes their cotransport for absorption in the small intestine. This active transport creates an osmotic gradient that enhances net water absorption by passive mechanisms. Plain water ingestion can be effective for maintaining hydration, but rehydration after exercise can be slowed by the drop in serum osmolality it may create. If allowed to progress, replacement of sweat losses with hypotonic fluid (water) leads to hyponatremia. Significant de-

creases in serum sodium levels can produce fatigue, lethargy, weakness, confusion, and even hemodynamic collapse and death. Salt loading is not recommended because of the plasma hypertonicity it may produce. Tables 4 through 7 serve as a brief guide for fluid and electrolyte replacement.

Thirst is a poor indicator of hydration status in humans and should not be used alone as a guide for volume replacement. Measurement of the weight of the athlete while unclothed, both before and after competition, is an excellent way to monitor fluid losses. Hydration before, during, and after exercise should be emphasized.

Overuse Injuries

Overuse injuries refer to musculoskeletal maladies that develop as a result of environmental, biomechanical, and equipment factors. They involve one of the following anatomic structures: bursae, tendons, bones, joints, and ligaments. Overuse injuries are often classified into four stages based on degree of pain. Stage 1 is mild pain that develops only after activity. Stage 2 is moderate pain that occurs during activity but does not restrict or interfere with performance. Stage 3 is moderate to severe pain that interferes with performance. Stage 4 is the most severe form of an overuse injury with signifi-

Table 6 | Approximate Deficits in Mild to Moderate Dehydration (5%)

Type of Dehydration	[Na$^+$] meq/kg	[K$^+$] meq/kg
Isotonic [Na$^+$] 134-145 meq/L	4-5	4-5
Hypertonic [Na$^+$] >145 meq/L	0-2	0-2
Hypotonic [Na$^+$] <134 meq/L	5-6	5-6

*Deficits are doubled for moderate-severe dehydration (10%)

Table 7 | Guide to Fluid/Electrolyte Replacement

Isotonic Dehydration: Serum [Na$^+$]134-145 meq/L
Net loss of solute and electrolytes equal to water loss
Ex: Common; healthy athlete with inadequate hydration
Tx: Replace sum of maintenance losses (30-35 mL/kg body weight), insensible losses (600-800 mL/day) and estimated water/electrolyte losses over first 24 h; replace 1/2 of volume within first 8 h, rest over next 16 h

Hypertonic Dehydration [Na$^+$] >145 meq/L
Net loss of water greater than solute
Ex: Inadequate hydration with strenuous exercise
Tx: Repair TBW deficit over 48 h; rate of reduction of serum Na$^+$ not to exceed 10 meq per/24 h

Hypotonic Dehydration [Na$^+$] < 134meq/L
Net loss of solute/electrolytes less than water
Ex: Unusual; seen in ultraendurance competitors who overhydrate
Tx: Do not replace more than one half total sodium deficit within first 24 h to avoid central pontine myelinolysis
3% NS used in rare situations with seizure
[Na$^+$] of NS 154 meq/L [Na$^+$] of ½ NS 77 meq/L [Na$^+$] of 3% NS 513 meq/L

Ex = example; Tx = treatment; TBW = total body water; NS = normal saline

cant pain even at rest. Table 8 outlines common overuse injuries.

Medical Care of the Female Athlete

Providing optimal medical care for the female athlete requires an understanding of unique gender-specific issues. A comprehensive review of these topics is beyond the scope of this chapter but topics such as exercise in pregnancy, postmenopausal fitness, the female triad (altered menstrual cycle, eating disorder, abnormal bone metabolism), and athletic injuries seen disproportionately in female competitors will be briefly reviewed.

Exercise during pregnancy is a vital part of the overall health of the mother and fetus. Recent studies have shown a decreased morbidity and mortality rate among expectant mothers who established a regular prepartum exercise regimen. Normal physiologic changes during pregnancy such as increased weight, increased intravascular volume, increased total body water content, and low back pain as a result of anatomic changes may make exercise more challenging during pregnancy. However, the intensity and frequency of exercise can be relatively maintained at prepregnancy levels until late in the pregnancy. Several modifications should be made. Pregnant women who exercise should be keenly aware of the propensity for thermal dysregulation and should make extra effort to ensure adequate hydration and provide an exercise environment that is optimal for adequate heat exchange. Pregnant women should be aware of increased caloric requirements, roughly 300 to 400 kcal/day, during pregnancy and adjust diet accordingly. Furthermore, because of diminished maternal aerobic capacity, the intensity of exercise may need to be modified. Exercise to exhaustion, even for elite athletes, is to be discouraged during pregnancy and maternal perceived exertion should be used as a guide for intensity levels. Certain specific types of exercises during pregnancy should be avoided. Any type of exercise with a chance of abdominal contact should be avoided. In general, complex exercises associated with a propensity for

falls should be avoided. Because of decreased venous return and a subsequent drop in cardiac output, exercise requiring prolonged, stationary standing after the first trimester should be avoided. It is also important to remember that physiologic changes may not occur for 6 to 10 weeks postpartum and that prepregnancy exercise practices should not be started immediately postpartum.

The benefits of regular exercise during pregnancy are numerous and include maintenance of a healthy weight and prevention of excess weight gain, more rapid postpartum recovery, improved posture and fewer musculoskeletal problems such as low back pain. Less peripheral edema, improved sleep quality, improved energy levels, and an improved overall sense of well-being contribute to a positive experience during the pregnancy. However, every physician supervising an exercise program during pregnancy should be aware of absolute and relative contraindications to exercise. Absolute contraindications include preexisting uncontrolled hypertension, diabetes mellitus, or valvular heart disease. Obstetrical specific contraindications include preeclampsia or pregnancy-induced hypertension, preterm labor with the current or previous pregnancy, premature rupture of membranes, second or third trimester bleeding, or incompetent cervix. Relative contraindications to exercise during pregnancy include history of multiple miscarriages, precipitous labor, breech fetal positioning, and multiple gestations.

The benefits of exercise in the postmenopausal female are just as clear. A regular aerobic exercise program

Table 8 | Common Overuse Syndromes

Structures Involved	Symptoms	Treatment
Bursae		
Prepatellar bursitis	Anterior/inferior knee pain and swelling	Protective padding, ice, NSAIDs, aspiration, corticosteriod injection
Greater trochanteric bursitis	Focal, lateral hip pain	Rest, ice, PT, local injection
Olecranon bursitis	Elbow pain, swelling	Protective padding, ice, NSAIDs, aspiration, corticosteroid injection
Pes anserine bursitis	Inferior knee pain	Ice, NSAIDs, aspiration, corticosteroid injection
Tendon		
Rotator cuff tendinitis	Nonlocalized shoulder pain	PT, rest, NSAIDs, corticosteroid injection
Biceps tendinitis	Localized anterior shoulder pain	Corticosteroid injection, rest, NSAIDs
Patellar tendinitis	Knee pain	PT, rest, NSAIDs
Achilles tendinitis	Heel pain	PT, rest, NSAIDs
Anterior tibialis tendinitis	Shin pain	PT, rest, NSAIDs
Medial/lateral epicondylitis	Focal medial/lateral elbow pain	Corticosteroid injection, PT, rest, NSAIDs
Bones		
Stress fractures Insufficiency fractures Apophysitis	Localized pain	Rest, correction of precipitating factors
Ligaments		
Plantar fasciitis	Heel, instep pain	PT, orthoses, splinting, ECSWT

NSAIDs = nonsteroidal anti-inflammatory drugs; PT = physical therapy; ECSWT = extracorporeal shock wave therapy

of intermediate intensity most days of the week combined with strength and flexibility exercises is essential to the health of the postmenopausal athlete. Improvements in bone density measurements, lipid profiles, body mass indices, and sleep quality, all problematic in postmenopausal females, are well established with regular conditioning.

The female athlete triad consists of abnormal bone metabolism, disordered eating, and abnormal menstrual function. The exact incidence of the disorder is unknown but several recent studies suggest that it may be as high as 12% of all competitive female athletes. Prevalence rates differ among individual components of the triad existing independently and also differ among individual sports. A prevalence rate of nearly 50% for menstrual dysfunction has been reported in some distance runners compared with a general prevalence rate of 2% to 5%.

Menstrual dysfunction comprises an entire spectrum of irregularity of menstruation. From delayed onset of menarche, defined as onset of menses after age 16 years, to complete amenorrhea, defined as the absence of 3 to 12 consecutive menstrual periods in the absence of pregnancy, to oligomenorrhea (irregular, infrequent menses), menstrual dysfunction is common in the female athlete. Females at risk tend to be younger, nulliparous, have lower body weights, and are involved with more strenuous, high-intensity sports. A poor dietary history is often central to the development of menstrual irregularities. Menstrual dysfunction is believed to be caused by a lack of a pulsatile release of gonadotropin-releasing hormone from the hypothalamus, which in turn leads to diminished release of luteinizing and follicle-stimulating hormone from the anterior pituitary gland. The exact cause of diminished gonadotropin-releasing hormone release is unclear but the role of circulating β-endorphins, cortisol, catecholamines, melatonin, and androgens are all currently under investigation. Treatment options include optimizing diet and nutritional status, exercise intensity modification, and hormone therapy.

Eating disorders encompass everything from restriction before competition to frank starvation or binging and purging, referred to as anorexia nervosa and bulimia nervosa, respectively. Signs and symptoms include a characteristically thin body habitus, thin hair and hirsute features, parotid gland hypertrophy, dental caries, subconjunctival hemorrhages, scarring on the dorsum of the hands, and rectal tears. Treatment depends on the severity of the condition and often involves a multispecialty approach including physicians, mental health specialists, and nutritionists. The exact prevalence of eating disorders among female athletes is unknown.

Regular exercise in females leads to increased bone density by increasing mechanical stress on bone. A low estrogen state seen with delayed or infrequent menarche, as is the case with the female triad, leads to poor primary bone mass accumulation and the early development of osteoporosis. If allowed to continue, the hypoestrogenic state promotes premature bone resorption, further compounding the problem. Combined with poor nutrition status, in particular a deficiency in calcium and vitamin D, the rate of bone loss can be startling. Several studies have recorded bone densities of female athletes in their 20s that were comparable to those of females in their 60s and 70s.

Although not exclusive to female athletes, several common musculoskeletal athletic injuries are often seen in females. Two ligamentous injuries more commonly seen in females include ankle sprains (particularly anterior talofibular) and anterior cruciate sprains and complete tears. Women are particularly vulnerable to anterior cruciate injuries but the exact cause is believed to be multifactorial. Hormonally-mediated ligamentous hyperlaxity, decreased ligament size, and a narrowed intercondylar notch have all been proposed as possible etiologic factors. Ankle sprains seem to be more easily explained because of the relatively reduced stability of the talus from an inflexible heel cord and the propensity of the female foot to favor a plantar-flexed position.

Lateral epicondylitis and rotator cuff tendinitis tend to be more prevalent in females, who are believed to be more susceptible to these injuries because of postural differences produced by strength deficiencies and soft-tissue laxity.

Overuse injuries of bone, particularly stress fractures, are more commonly encountered in females who comprise the classic triad. Healthy female athletes also are at increased risk because of hormonal factors and lower muscle to body mass ratios. Spondylolysis, a stress fracture to the pars interarticularis of the lumbar spine, is also seen more frequently in female athletes.

Mechanical low back pain is ubiquitous among females; the etiology is usually multifactorial. Two unique sources of back pain among women are the aforementioned spondylolysis and pelvic instability produced by sacroiliac joint dysfunction. Hormonal and mechanical (particularly the effects of childbirth) factors lead to increased laxity among the ligamentous, muscular, and joint structures that comprise the pelvic ring. This increased laxity leads to a propensity for subluxation, particularly anteriorly, that leads to pelvic ring asymmetry and subsequent back pain.

Patellofemoral syndrome is another athletic injury common in females. The athlete has anterior deep knee pain with varying degrees of swelling and pain that often is noted to be worsened by walking down steps. The increased propensity in females is believed to be the result of increased ligamentous laxity leading to abnormal lateral patellar tracking. A lack of flexibility and weakness of the hamstrings and vastus medialis obliquus also

contribute to abnormal patellar tracking. A wider pelvis and increased Q angles have also been proposed as possible etiologic factors. A propensity for plantar flexion leading to internal torsion of the tibia and femur accentuates lateral patellar tracking and is also believed to be a contributing factor. Treatment consists of biomechanical modification and physical therapy modalities.

Annotated Bibliography

Preparticipation Examination

Chobanian AV, Bakris GL, Black HR, et al: The Seventh Report of the Joint National Committee on Prevention, Detection, Evaluation, and Treatment of High Blood Pressure: The JNC 7 report. *JAMA* 2003;289:2560-2572.

This article presents new guidelines for hypertension management and prevention.

Carek PJ, Hunter L: The preparticipation physical examination for athletics: A critical review of current recommendations. *J Med Liban* 2001;49:292-297.

A critical review of current recommendations for the preparticipation examination is presented.

Seto CK: Preparticipation cardiovascular screening. *Clin Sports Med* 2003;22:23-35.

This review article advocates the standardization of the preparticipation examination.

Conditioning and Preparation

American Academy of Family Physicians, American Academy of Orthopaedic Surgeons, American College of Sports Medicine, American Orthopaedic Society for Sports Medicine, American Osteopathic Academy for Sports Medicine, American Medical Society for Sports Medicine: The team physician and conditioning of athletes for sports: A consensus statement. *Med Sci Sports Exerc* 2001;33:1789-1793.

This article presents a governing body consensus statement on conditioning principles for athletes.

Ebben WP, Blackard DO: Strength and conditioning practices of National Football League strength and conditioning coaches. *J Strength Cond Res* 2001;15:48-58.

A review of conditioning practices in the National Football League reveals 69% of conditioning coaches follow a periodization model.

Kraemer WJ, Knuttgen HG: Strength training basics: Designing workouts to meet patients goals. *Phys Sports Med* 2003;31:39-45.

Human power production capabilities and differences of physiologic response to varying intensities of exercise are outlined.

Sideline Medicine

Mellion M, Walsh WM, Shelton G: *The Team Physician's Handbook,* ed 3. Philadelphia, PA, Hanley & Belfus, 2001, pp 126-135.

This book chapter presents an outline for game day management for the team physician.

Stricker PR: The sports medicine kit: Basics of the bag. *Pediatr Ann* 2002;31:14-16.

A review of essential on-site materials for the team physician is presented.

Dehydration and Heat Syndromes

Burke LM: Nutritional needs for exercise in the heat. *Comp Biochem Physiol A Mol Integr Physiol* 2001;128: 735-748.

This article reviews the necessity for carbohydrate, volume, and electrolyte replacement for vigorous exercise.

Overuse Injuries

Maier M, Steinborn M, Schmitz C, et al: Extracorporeal shock-wave therapy for chronic lateral tennis elbow: Prediction of outcome by imaging. *Arch Orthop Trauma Surg* 2001;121:379-384.

Forty-two patients were assessed before and after extracorporeal shock wave therapy; 84% of men and 52% and of women showed a good outcome by MRI at 18 months. Tendons that were thickened and swollen were most likely to respond.

McFarlane D: Current views on the diagnosis and treatment of upper limb overuse syndromes. *Ergonomics* 2002;45:732-735.

Treatment remains focused on modification of biomechanical factors that precipitate these injuries.

Panni AS, Biedert RM, Maffulli N, Tartarone M, Romanini E: Overuse injuries of the extensor mechanism in athletes. *Clin Sports Med* 2002;21:483-498.

This article reviews the functional anatomy, pathophysiology, and overall management of overuse injuries of the extensor mechanism in athletes.

Medical Care of the Female Athlete

Brown W: The benefits of physical activity during pregnancy. *J Sci Med Sport* 2002;5:37-45.

Maintenance of a regular exercise program during pregnancy leads to improved maternal-fetal outcomes.

Burrows M, Nevill AM, Bird S, Simpson D: Physiological factors associated with low bone mineral density in female endurance runners. *Br J Sports Med* 2003;37: 67-71.

This article provides examples of very low bone mineral densities in a sample of 52 female endurance runners.

Classic Bibliography

American College of Sports Medicine Position Stand: The recommended quantity and quality of exercise for developing and maintaining cardiorespiratory and muscular fitness, and flexibility in healthy adults. *Med Sci Sports Exerc* 1998;30:975-991.

Anderson SD, Griesemer BA: Medical concerns in the female athlete. Pediatrics 2000;106:610-613.

Buettner CM: The team physician's bag. *Clin Sports Med* 1998;17:365-373.

Clapp JF III: Exercise during pregnancy. *Clin Sports Med* 2000;19:273-286.

Eichner ER: Treatment of suspected heat illness. *Int J Sports Med* 1998;19(suppl 2):S150-S153.

Grafe MW, Paul GR, Foster TE: The preparticipation sports examination for high school and college athletes. *Clin Sports Med* 1997;16:569-587.

Kurowski K, Chandran S: The preparticipation athletic evaluation. *Am Fam Physician* 2000;61:2683-2690.

Shirreffs SM, Maughan RJ: Rehydration and recovery of fluid balance after exercise. *Exerc Sport Sci Rev* 2000; 28:27-32.

Warren MP, Shantha S: The female athlete. *Baillieres Best Prac Res Clin Endocrinol Metab* 2000;14:37-53.

Chapter 15

The Polytrauma Patient

Hargovind DeWal, MD

Robert McLain, MD

Introduction

The management of the multiply injured or polytrauma patient requires a multidisciplinary approach integrating organ- and injury-specific treatment protocols. Multiple trauma—injury to multiple organ systems—can directly or indirectly trigger processes that may injure specific organs, disrupt metabolic processes, interrupt normal endocrine function, create hemodynamic and physiologic instability, and lead to highly lethal systemic diseases and multiple organ failure. By definition, multiple trauma is a life-threatening disorder.

Successful management of the polytrauma patient requires a team approach and a broad focus. Within a few days of injury, the polytrauma patient will be having or be at risk for a myriad of potentially serious disorders, in addition to their actual, initial injuries. A list of some of these disorders is found in Table 1.

The concept of a "damage control" approach to orthopaedic injuries is discussed in the recent literature and should be observed to minimize the risk of compounding systemic injury through added surgical injury. A dedicated intensivist, skilled anesthesia staff, trauma and orthopaedic trauma surgeons, nutritional support services, infectious disease specialists, and plastic and reconstructive surgeons may all play a role in the care of a single patient. It is imperative that all of these individuals buy into the principles of trauma management and communicate well with the other members of the team.

The environment for patient care must support the level of care required. Access to diagnostic studies, interventions, line care, and respiratory support must be immediate and available around the clock. Nursing staff must understand the fragility of the patient and recognize that changes in respiratory or circulatory parameters may require immediate attention and response. Staff must also be familiar with protocols for mobilization, deep venous thrombosis prophylaxis, and pulmonary and bowel care.

After the patient's condition is stabilized, attention to nutrition, infection control, pulmonary function, and skin care play an often underappreciated role in healing and rehabilitation. Psychological support, occupational and physical therapy programs, and multidisciplinary follow-up all contribute to full and timely recovery, and improve the likelihood of a satisfactory return to function and community life.

These patients often face some likelihood of permanent impairment and long-term disability. Advances have been made in all aspects of polytrauma care, ranging from improved prehospital care to more aggressive resuscitation and surgical management to aggressive physical therapy and spinal cord injury rehabilitation. The treating physician must be conversant in all of these areas, and keep an eye on all aspects of the patient's recovery if the best outcomes are to be obtained and the worst complications avoided.

Assessment of the Polytrauma Patient

An orderly, structured assessment of the polytrauma patient has been shown to improve care and reduce the likelihood of missed injuries. Patients with multiple injuries typically arrive in the emergency department under the care of another health care provider, most often a trained emergency medical technician, who will have assessed the patient in the field, established intravenous access, and may have intubated the patient to restore or maintain the airway. They will provide important information on the mechanism of injury, the patient's condition at the time of first contact, and evidence of neurologic function, respiratory status, and responsiveness at the time of initial resuscitation. Their initial observations may provide important perspective as to the patient's improvement or deterioration when compared with the initial assessment in the emergency department.

Once the patient arrives in the emergency department, resuscitation and a primary assessment begin simultaneously. These two processes are interdependent in that the purpose of the primary assessment is to find the causes of hemodynamic instability, respiratory impairment, and circulatory collapse at the same time others on the team are trying to restore those functions

Table 1 | Serious Disorders for Which the Polytrauma Patient is at Risk

Pulmonary contusions, aspiration, pneumonia	Cardiac ischemia, contusion, tamponade
Thromboembolic disease	Hypothermia
Urosepsis	Open, contaminated wounds, burns
Anemia	Spinal cord injury
Systemic hypotension and hemorrhagic shock	Acute pulmonary embolism
Renal insufficiency, acute tubular necrosis	Endocrine dysfunction
Immunosuppression	Hemothorax, pneumothorax, pyothorax
Malnutrition	Compartment syndrome
Pancreatitis	Multiple organ failure syndrome
Myonecrosis, myoglobinemia	Delirium
Coagulopathy	Ischemic brain injury
Electrolyte disturbances	Septic shock
Peptic ulcer disease	Iatrogenic injury
Gastrointestinal disease	Neurogenic shock
Decubitus ulcers	

through volume replacement, ventilation, and pharmacologic support. Once the primary survey is complete and the patient's condition begins to stabilize, a secondary, more complete survey is conducted, and the team can begin to formulate a plan for definitive care.

Primary Survey

Initial management of the polytrauma patient begins with an assessment of airway, breathing, and circulation, along with neurologic status (disability) and environmental exposure. Advanced Trauma Life Support guidelines set forth by the American College of Surgeons advocate use of both the primary and secondary survey to provide an orderly, consistent approach that will rapidly reveal life- and limb-threatening injuries. The secondary survey consists of a head-to-toe evaluation and history. Both the primary and secondary survey should be repeated as needed to ascertain any change in the patient's status. Initial radiographs should include those of the chest, pelvis, and cervical spine, all obtained immediately after the primary survey is complete.

Airway

Assessment of the airway and breathing begins immediately, in the field. The patient must be making an effort to breath, be successfully moving air, and be adequately transferring oxygen to the circulating blood. Evaluation of effort, chest wall excursion, and breath sounds should be done immediately on arrival. The physician should look for cyanosis and obtain an arterial blood gas sample. Mechanical obstruction should be addressed immediately, looking for loose teeth, dentures, blood, food, or

vomitus, and intubation performed as necessary. The arterial blood gas will assess degree of oxygenation. If oxygenation is inadequate, pulmonary function, including tension pneumothorax, hemothorax, and flail chest, should be reinvestigated.

Breathing: Thoracic Injuries

Signs of major thoracic injury during the primary survey, including tension pneumothorax, open pneumothorax, flail chest, massive hemothorax, and cardiac tamponade (discussed in the following section) should be noted.

Tension pneumothorax develops as air leaks into the chest cavity either through the chest wall or from the lung. The air enters via a "one-way valve" mechanism and does not exit the cavity. The affected lung collapses and as air continues to build up, the mediastinum is displaced to the contralateral side, impeding venous return and compressing the uninjured lung. The diagnosis is made on the clinical findings of absent breath sounds and a hyperresonant percussion note. A chest radiograph is not required before treatment is initiated. Treatment consists of immediate decompression by insertion of a large bore needle into the second intercostal space in the midclavicular line of the affected side, followed by chest tube placement.

Open pneumothorax results from large defects in the chest wall. Air will preferentially enter the chest cavity through the defect rather than the trachea when the diaphragm contracts. Initial management includes placement of an occlusive dressing covering the wound edges, taped on three sides, allowing the dressing to occlude the wound with each inhalation and allowing for air to escape during exhalation. A chest tube should be inserted at a site away from the wound as soon as possible.

Flail chest occurs in the presence of multiple rib fractures and is usually associated with an underlying pulmonary contusion. The flail chest segment demonstrates paradoxical chest wall motion with inspiration and expiration, impairing ventilation. The paradoxical motion is not solely responsible for the associated hypoxia. Pain results in restricted chest wall motion, and pulmonary contusion contributes significantly to development of hypoxia. Intubation and ventilation may be necessary if hypoxia is progressive and unresponsive to initial measures.

Massive hemothorax, the rapid accumulation of at least 1,500 mL of blood in the chest, may be the result of blunt or penetrating trauma. The blood loss may contribute to hypoxia, and initial management includes both restoration of blood volume and decompression of the chest cavity by chest tube placement. Massive hemothorax often requires thoracotomy to control the source of hemorrhage.

Circulation

Evaluation of circulation involves physical examination and an assessment of vital signs including blood pressure and heart rate. Intravenous fluid infusion is recommended in all patients, and is usually started before reaching the hospital. Resuscitation should be monitored by blood pressure, heart rate, perfusion, and urine output. If the extremities are cold, clammy, and/or cyanotic, the patient should be treated for hypovolemia irrespective of pulse or pressure. If brisk bleeding from an extremity or penetrating wound is encountered, direct pressure should be applied immediately.

Goals for urine output are 0.5 mL/kg/h in adults and 1.0 mL/kg/h in children. Central venous pressure will provide information regarding atrial-filling pressures. Elderly patients with severe thoracic trauma require a pulmonary artery catheter. The arterial-alveolar gradient should be calculated to detect ventilation-perfusion mismatches. Crystalloid infusion is used in the initial management of these patients, through large bore intravenous access. If intravenous access is not readily available, cutdown on the saphenous, femoral, or cubital veins may be necessary.

For patients who are experiencing exsanguination, immediate use of universal donor blood group (group O, Rh negative) is recommended. Thrombocytopenia is treated at levels below 50,000/mL.

Cardiac tamponade may result in circulatory failure in the face of normal blood volume. This condition usually results from penetrating injuries. The diagnosis is often difficult, and it must be distinguished from tension pneumothorax. The classic diagnostic finding of Beck's triad consists of (1) venous pressure elevation, (2) decline in arterial pressure, and (3) muffled heart tones. Kussmaul's sign, a rise in venous pressure with spontaneous inspiration, may be present in cardiac tamponade. An echocardiogram may aid in diagnosis, but a false-negative result may be seen in about 5% of patients. Examination of the pericardial sac may also be performed during a focused abdominal ultrasound. Prompt evacuation of the pericardial blood (usually by pericardiocentesis) is indicated for patients who do not respond to usual resuscitative measures. A pericardial window, thoracotomy and pericardiotomy, may be necessary.

Head Injury

All trauma patients should receive a minineurologic examination consisting of a Glasgow Coma Scale (GCS) score. This scoring system has prognostic value with regard to future neurologic function. A decline in the GCS score may indicate intracranial pathology. Reflexes of the triceps, biceps, knee, and ankle should be evaluated.

The minimum GCS score is 3 and is seen in flaccid patients who are unable to open their eyes spontaneously or speak. Patients who do open their eyes, obey commands, and are oriented score the maximum of 15 points. A GCS score of 8 or less corresponds to the generally accepted definition of coma.

Estimating Injury Severity

Grading the severity of multiple trauma is difficult. The Injury Severity Score (ISS) was the first scoring system to use anatomic criteria to assess the extent of injury. The ISS measures injury severity based on the abbreviated injury scale (AIS), developed in 1971 and revised in 1985. Injury severity in the AIS is graded on a scale of 1 to 5 for each organ system. As currently applied, the ISS is calculated by taking the AIS scores from the three most severely injured anatomic areas, squaring them, and adding the resultant figures. An ISS of 16 or more has been shown to be associated with a mortality of 10%, whereas a score greater than 40 predicts a 50% mortality. The ISS score has not been shown to accurately predict outcome for those individuals with a severe injury to a single body area.

Secondary Survey

During the secondary survey, thoracic trauma can be further defined. Injuries detected through the secondary survey include simple pneumothorax or hemothorax, pulmonary and cardiac contusion, tracheobronchial tree injuries, and diaphragmatic rupture. In all of these injuries hypoxia must be corrected before resuscitation is successful.

Abdomen

During the primary survey, assessment of circulation, especially in blunt trauma patients, includes a thorough abdominal examination to rule out hemorrhage. Peritoneal signs such as rigidity and rebound are useful to diagnose a surgical abdomen, but may not always be apparent in obtunded patients.

The Focused Assessment with Sonography for Trauma examination is now widely used to further evaluate the abdomen. This examination can be done quickly and does not require the transport of a critically injured patient. Ultrasound has a sensitivity, specificity, and accuracy comparable to diagnostic peritoneal lavage and CT scan, but the examination is operator dependent. Its utility is limited in obese patients, in the presence of subcutaneous air, and in patients who have had previous abdominal operations. One recent study found that the focused assessment with sonography for trauma examination underdiagnosed significant intra-abdominal trauma in one group of 372 patients.

CT scan is used only in patients who are hemodynamically stable and who have no immediate indication for a laparotomy. CT can evaluate the extent of a specific organ injury and can also help in the diagnosis of retroperitoneal and pelvic organ injuries not readily apparent on clinical examination. CT may also be performed serially to evaluate spleen, liver, and kidney injuries not requiring immediate surgical intervention.

Spine

Injuries to the spinal column should always be sought in polytrauma patients. Occult spinal injuries may be overlooked in patients with an altered level of consciousness. Inadequate immobilization and excessive manipulation may cause additional damage in a patient with spinal injury and may worsen the outcome. In hemodynamically unstable patients or patients with respiratory difficulty, exclusion of spine injury may be deferred as long as the patient's spine is safely immobilized and protected during the primary survey and initial care. Moreover, maintaining tissue perfusion and oxygenation will help stop progression of any existing cord injury.

The secondary spinal assessment should be performed once life-threatening issues have been dealt with. The goal of the secondary assessment is to identify and initially manage neurologically and mechanically unstable spinal injuries.

Log rolling the patient is essential for an adequate spinal examination. The soft tissues should be assessed for swelling, ecchymosis, wounds, deformity, or bogginess. Spinous processes should be palpated individually with particular emphasis placed on areas of tenderness.

A complete motor, sensory, and reflex examination should be performed, including tests for perianal sensation, rectal sphincter tone, and bulbocavernosus reflex. Serial examinations should be performed to document any progression of neurologic deficits. A neurologic deficit may be classified as complete, in which there is total absence of motor or sensory function below the level of injury, or incomplete. Identifying any distal motor or sensory sparing (incomplete injury) is essential, as these patients warrant treatment on a more urgent basis.

Spinal shock refers to the flaccidity and loss of reflexes, specifically sacral reflexes, after spinal cord injury. The return of these reflexes marks the end of spinal shock. The diagnosis of a complete neurologic injury cannot be made during spinal shock.

Neurogenic shock manifests itself through hypotension and bradycardia, and must be distinguished from cardiogenic shock, which is characterized by hypotension and tachycardia. Neurogenic shock should be treated with judicious use of fluid resuscitation and vasopressors. Atropine may be useful to treat the bradycardia.

It is unlikely that an awake, alert, neurologically normal patient without pain or tenderness along the spine has any spinal injury. However, patients with an altered level of consciousness (head injury, intoxication, hypoxia) need to have their normal radiographs corroborated via an adequate physical examination before neck injury can be formally ruled out (Figure 1).

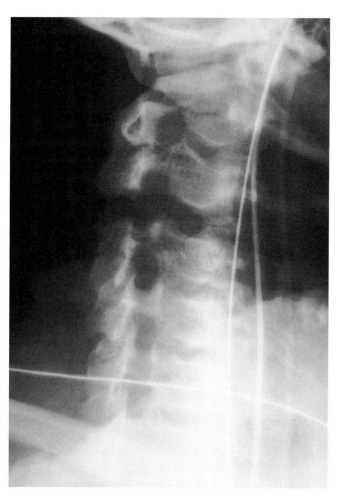

Figure 1 Radiograph of a patient who sustained multiple injuries during a head-on motor vehicle accident. Cognitively impaired because of head injury and intoxication, the patient was combative, denied neck or extremity pain, and demanded release from the cervical collar. Cervical precautions were maintained through resuscitation, emergent laparotomy, and multiple emergent studies. Definitive cervical radiographs demonstrated grossly unstable three-column cervical dissociation. The patient was treated definitively during the secondary stabilization period, with no neurologic injury or impairment.

A full radiographic spinal survey, including cervical, thoracic, and lumbosacral radiographs, is necessary in all patients with a suspected spinal cord injury. Patients with spinal cord injury at one level may have another injury at a noncontiguous level 5% to 20% of the time. Lateral cervical radiographs must show the cervicothoracic junction, or a lateral swimmer's view or CT should be obtained through this area. An AP odontoid view should also be obtained. Although patients with persistent pain despite normal radiographs may eventually benefit from flexion/extension views to identify ligamentous injury, there is rarely a role for flexion/extension radiographs in the initial evaluation of the trauma patient.

CT is useful in delineating the extent of bony injuries detected on plain radiographs. MRI is useful in patients with abnormal neurologic findings. In patients with specific lesions such as facet dislocations and who are undergoing closed reduction, MRI should be done to rule out extruded disks that may cause neurologic damage during closed reduction. MRI is indicated in any patient with a progressive neurologic deficit, or a deficit that does not match the level of the recognized spinal injury (C7 cord deficit in the face of a T10 burst fracture).

Pelvis

The primary survey of the pelvis involves mechanical assessment of stability and continuity: the physician quickly checks for fractures or disruption by medially compressing the iliac wings, applying an anterior-posterior stress through the ASIS, and by checking stability during hip range of motion. The secondary survey involves a more thorough history, physical examination, and analysis of an AP radiograph of the pelvis.

The history should determine the mechanism of injury. Higher energy injuries are more likely to be associated with an increased severity of fracture. Pelvic fractures occur more frequently with lateral impact than frontal impact. Patients on the side of impact are more likely to have a severe injury.

Physical findings of pelvic injury may include scrotal/labial swelling, open lacerations in the perineum and vagina or rectum, associated urologic or neurologic injuries, or excessive internal/external rotation of the lower extremity. Provocative maneuvers test the stability of the pelvis to internal and external rotation of the hip. The pelvis should move as a single unit. If a hemipelvis moves separately, the ring is disrupted and the pelvis is mechanically unstable. Once a pelvic injury is determined to be unstable, further manipulation that might dislodge clots that have formed within the fracture should be avoided.

Pelvic injuries can result in massive hemorrhage. In polytrauma patients, intrathoracic and intra-abdominal injuries are common, causing or contributing to hemorrhage and hypotension. Open wounds and long bone fractures such as femur fractures also contribute to blood loss. Hypotension caused specifically by a pelvic injury is invariably associated with a mechanically unstable pelvis, and may prove difficult to control until the pelvis is stabilized.

Early control of hemorrhage is crucial, in addition to staying ahead of volume requirements. Resuscitation of a hypotensive patient may result in hypothermia and acidosis. These factors may contribute to coagulopathy, complicating the existing problem and leading to further bleeding. Persistent hypotension can aggravate pulmonary and neurologic injury, and compromise renal, cerebral, and cardiac function. In addition, the risk of sepsis, adult respiratory distress syndrome (ARDS), and multiple organ failure is increased in these patients.

Particular attention should be paid to open pelvic injuries because they are associated with exceptional morbidity and mortality and will require emergent débridement. Rectal and vaginal examinations must be performed to rule out lacerations. Associated urologic injuries should be sought. Clinical findings that may indicate injury include blood at the urethral meatus, high-riding prostate, or inability to pass a Foley catheter. These patients will require retrograde urethrogram or cystogram, depending on the particular injury.

The AP radiograph of the pelvis is used in correlation with the physical examination to determine the stability of the pelvis. In a recent study, it was determined that physical examination was accurate in identifying injuries of the posterior pelvic ring. Signs of instability included more than 5 mm of displacement of the posterior sacroiliac joint, the presence of a posterior fracture gap, and the presence of an avulsion fracture of the transverse process of the fifth lumbar vertebrae. Pelvic ring injuries can be classified based on anatomic location, mechanism, or stability. The mechanistic classification can help predict blood loss and guide management. This classification as defined by Young and Burgess divides pelvic injuries into four mechanisms of injury: lateral compression, anteroposterior compression, vertical shear, and combined mechanism. Inlet and outlet radiographs as well as CT scan can help further clarify the degree of pelvic instability.

Classification of these injuries can help guide definitive management. (1) The estimated blood loss for a severe lateral compression injury is approximately 3.6 units whereas blood loss from an AP compression injury is 14.8 units. (2) AP compression injuries have a higher mortality and a higher incidence of shock and ARDS than lateral compression fractures. (3) Moderate lateral compression injuries have a higher incidence of brain injury, and vertical shear injuries also have a high incidence of associated injuries as well as mortality.

Lower Extremity Injuries

Femoral shaft fractures are high-energy injuries, usually occurring in the young patient population. Patients with bilateral fractures typically have a high ISS, higher mortality, and higher risk of ARDS. Early treatment of these injuries is important to survival and morbidity. An unsplinted closed femur fracture can lose up to four units of blood into the thigh. Tibial fractures are associated with severe soft-tissue and neurovascular trauma that can render the extremity dysfunctional or even nonviable.

Initial evaluation includes palpation of the entire extremity to the foot and a thorough neurovascular examination. Assessment of soft-tissue injury should be done to rule out an open fracture. AP and lateral radiographs should include the joints above and below the fracture. Special attention should be paid to the ipsilateral hip to

Table 2 | Factors in Severely Injured Patients That May Warrant a Damage Control Treatment Approach

Multiple injuries with an ISS > 20, and a thoracic trauma AIS >2

Multiple injuries with abdominal/pelvic trauma, and hemorrhagic shock (systolic BP < 90 mm Hg)

ISS > 40

Chest radiograph or CT evidence of bilateral pulmonary contusion

Initial mean pulmonary arterial pressure > 24 mm Hg

Pulmonary artery pressure increase during intramedullary nailing > 6 mm Hg

rule out an ipsilateral femoral neck fracture because this can be missed on initial examination.

Tibial shaft fractures can be caused by direct or indirect trauma. The limb should be inspected for evidence of open fractures. Soft-tissue injury can be classified according to the Tscherne classification: grade 0 has minimal soft-tissue injury whereas grade III represents a decompensated compartment syndrome requiring fasciotomy. Once the lower extremities have been surveyed, the evaluation should be repeated for the upper extremities. The physician should reduce dislocations as soon as possible, dress open fractures and wounds with saline-soaked gauze, and splint fractures at the first opportunity.

Open fractures are classified according to Gustilo, from type I (clean punctures) to type III (major disruption of the soft-tissue envelope). Type III injuries can be further classified according to the extent of neurovascular injury. Type IIIa injuries can be closed while type IIIb injuries require flap coverage, and type IIIc injuries require revascularization for limb salvage.

Vascular injury must be considered in any extremity injury, especially with knee dislocations. Pulses and perfusion must be checked, and if a pulse deficit is present, all correctable causes should be evaluated: fracture alignment should be corrected, traction released and restored, compartments checked, and hypotension corrected through resuscitation. Ankle-brachial index (ABI) may provide information about the perfusion of the limb. An ABI of 0.9 or higher will ordinarily rule out arterial injury. Angiography remains the gold standard, however. In the polytrauma patient, formal angiography may not be possible and a limited study may be performed in the operating room. Management of life-threatening injury takes priority over limb salvage.

Trauma Management

Management of the polytrauma patient requires a multidisciplinary approach because of multiple injuries requiring intervention from various disciplines including general surgery, neurosurgery, and orthopaedic surgery. The trauma surgery team is generally responsible for coordinating these efforts and obtaining the appropriate consultations. Most patients will benefit from rapid skeletal stabilization and mobilization, even when fixation procedures have to follow abdominal or thoracic surgery. Every patient must be assessed individually, however, to avoid serious complications.

The Concept of Damage Control

Although early stabilization of long bone fractures has been shown to reduce morbidity and length of hospital stay, there is a subset of patients who may deteriorate in the face of early, prolonged surgical intervention. The cause of this decompensation is always difficult to prove in patients with so many confounding issues, but several investigators have suggested that the trauma of surgery, with its systemic effects, superimposed on the initial trauma of injury, leads to an increased incidence of ARDS, multiple organ failure, and death. Patients at risk for these complications are more seriously injured and include patients with severe chest injuries and severe hemodynamic shock (Table 2). The development of these complications is thought to be linked to the proinflammatory cascades that develop as a result of injury, resuscitation efforts, and surgical interventions.

Although all polytrauma patients develop a systemic inflammatory response, the more seriously injured patients suffer from an increased inflammatory response and higher levels of cytokine release (interleukin [IL]-1, tumor necrosis factor) for longer periods of time. This prolonged inflammatory response is referred to as systemic inflammatory response syndrome. The inflammatory mediators such as IL-6 that are liberated during this cascade event may produce deleterious clinical effects, further impairing pulmonary function and precipitating organ failure in other systems. Surgical treatment of these severely injured patients may result in the release of additional inflammatory mediators, compounding the injury.

An increased awareness of the role of these proinflammatory cascades during surgery has led to the belief that the "second hit" or surgical intervention, taking place after the initial trauma ("first hit"), should be kept to a minimum in these severely compromised patients. This "damage control" concept was originally developed as an approach to managing severe abdominal trauma. As in the original concept, damage control orthopaedic care is delivered in three stages. The first stage involves immediate surgery to control bleeding, visceral injury, gross instability, and contamination. The second stage focuses on resuscitation and medical optimization. Definitive surgery to provide rigid fracture fixation, articular continuity, and soft-tissue coverage is reserved for the third stage.

The benefits of early skeletal stabilization are well recognized, and the impact of surgical trauma on polytrauma patients is far from proven. Several studies are available that suggest that other factors may be to blame for the increase in complications seen among these more seriously injured patients. Although many authors suggest that reamed intramedullary nailing is the culprit, particularly in the face of pulmonary trauma and contusion, comparative studies have shown no difference in the incidence of ARDS or mortality relative to that treatment. Similarly, the adequacy of early fluid resuscitation has long been believed to influence the recovery of these severely injured patients. Finally, studies of intramedullary fixation among severely injured patients have shown not only that the patients undergoing nailing had no increased risk compared with patients treated otherwise, but that, within these groups, the patients treated with immediate rodding had less pulmonary compromise and a lower incidence of ARDS than patients treated with intramedullary rodding on a delayed basis.

However, it may be inappropriate to attempt definitive procedures in some patients with severe chest trauma or hemodynamic instability. Damage control principles are well applied in these circumstances.

The first stage care of orthopaedic injuries consists of fracture and joint reduction, rapid skeletal stabilization, and control of hemorrhage. Wounds can generally be washed and superficially débrided as the patient is being resuscitated and ventilated, but procedures that generate more blood loss or tissue damage are avoided.

The second stage of damage control care focuses on resuscitation and optimization of the patient's medical status. This may require several days in an intensive care setting, but may also be accomplished over the course of a few hours without the patient ever leaving the resuscitation area or operating theater. The patient's condition may be considered stable for definitive care whenever specific parameters are met (Table 3). The trauma team may find circumstances under which it is believed worthwhile to push harder for stabilization of specific injuries to mobilize the patient and obtain a vertical chest for improved ventilation and pulmonary toilet. Spinal and pelvic stabilization are sometimes afforded priority to allow the patient to be safely moved and positioned. Similarly, rapid revascularization of a compromised extremity warrants additional consideration, and can be accomplished with a temporary shunt and external fixation.

It is in the third and final stage that delayed definitive care of individual fractures is performed. Two methods by which rapid, temporary fracture stabilization can be performed on the pelvis or long bones are external fixation and unreamed intramedullary fixation. External fixation can be accomplished rapidly, with minimal blood loss, and can be used to span simple, complex, and segmental fractures as well as traumatized joints. Conversion to an intramedullary nail or fixation plate is usu-

Table 3	Criteria for Adequate Resuscitation
Hemodynamically stable—warm and well perfused
Stable oxygen saturation
Lactate level < 2 mmol/L
No coagulopathy, INR < 1.25
Normal body temperature
Urine output > 1 mL/kg/h
Not requiring inotropic support

INR= International Normalized Ratio

ally straightforward and carries a low risk of infection within the first week of treatment. These methods of definitive fixation may be performed after the patient has achieved optimal medical status.

Prioritizing Orthopaedic Care
Early and stable fracture fixation is of utmost importance in the orthopaedic management of most polytrauma patients. If initial long bone stabilization is delayed the patient could be at risk for greater morbidity and mortality. It is useful to prioritize the orthopaedic problems of polytrauma patients with respect to four relative periods for intervention, as described by Tscherne: (1) acute care (first 3 hours after injury); (2) primary stabilization period (1 to 72 hours); (3) secondary stabilization period (3 to 8 days after injury); and (4) tertiary stabilization or rehabilitation period (after 6 to 8 days).

Acute Care
In the acute period, the primary survey and secondary assessment and hemodynamic resuscitation are accomplished. Head, chest, abdomen, and pelvic injury are all recognized and life-saving/limb-saving interventions are initiated. Significant epidural and subdural bleeding requires immediate evacuation. Once a hemothorax is diagnosed, a chest tube drainage should be placed. If more than 1,500 mL of blood is obtained through the chest tube or if drainage of more than 200 mL/h for 2 to 4 hours occurs, surgery should be considered. Continued hemorrhage into the peritoneal cavity of a hemodynamically unstable patient requires emergent laparotomy. Bleeding from the pelvic region must be ruled out before laparotomy is done.

External immobilization must be performed if the pelvic ring is determined to be unstable. Initial external immobilization consists of sandbags and straps, beanbags, or military antishock trousers. The use of military antishock trousers, however, has been associated with compartment syndrome and decreased respiratory ability. In the emergency department, external immobilization has been shown to decrease blood loss and to lower

ISS dependent mortality. Moreover, transfusion requirements are decreased in patients treated with external immobilization. External fixation can be applied in the emergency department or operating room in concert with other trauma surgery procedures.

Open fractures and joint injuries will require emergent débridement and stabilization. These wounds should not be closed primarily, and may require deep débridement and repeated irrigation when the patient is more stable. Open pelvic injuries require emergent débridement, and perineal wounds that communicate with the rectum or colon require diverting colostomy. Vaginal injuries associated with pelvic ring disruptions should be repaired to stop hemorrhage and to prevent the development of abscesses. Degloving injuries of the skin should be débrided.

Established or incipient compartment syndromes should be treated with adequate fasciotomy at the first opportunity. Although fully developed compartment syndrome is rarely seen at initial presentation, patients with severe crushing injuries or prolonged ischemia of the limb should undergo prophylactic fasciotomy under their first anesthetic, if at all possible.

Primary Stabilization Period

Maintaining adequate perfusion of the spinal cord helps to minimize secondary injury to the neural elements. Urgent care then focuses on methods of preventing further damage and rapid realignment of the spine to decompress neurologic structures. High-dose methylprednisolone is commonly used to treat patients presenting with a spinal cord injury with no contraindications to use. Despite widespread use and a perception that steroid therapy represents the standard of care for spinal cord injured patients, in reality steroid therapy simply represents a treatment option, and a controversial one at that. There is scant evidence that this intervention provides consistent or functionally significant improvement in neurologic outcomes. H2 blockers or proton pump inhibitors should be considered to prevent formation of gastric stress ulcers.

Compression of the neural elements from spinal malalignment such as a cervical spine facet dislocation should be addressed as soon as hemodynamic and respiratory stability has been achieved. Although a controversial issue, the use of MRI before reduction of dislocations to rule out disk extrusion that could compress the cord after reduction has been advocated. MRI also provides details of bone or disk fragments causing spinal cord compression or the presence of hematoma.

The issue of when to surgically stabilize patients with spinal injury and neurologic deficit remains controversial. Emergency surgery for spinal cord injury has not been clinically proven to be beneficial. However, some studies indicate that patients with incomplete lesions

probably benefit from early intervention to relieve persistent neurologic compression.

On the other hand, urgent surgical treatment (< 24 hours after injury) does not increase the risk to the spinal cord injured patient, compared with early care (1 to 3 days after injury), and can improve the overall outcome of the polytrauma patient. Urgent stabilization of the fractured spine allows immediate mobilization of the patient, reducing risks of prolonged recumbency (thrombophlebitis, pulmonary embolism, pneumonia, urosepsis, and ARDS). This appears to hold true for even the most severely injured patients. Urgent surgical stabilization among patients with a mean ISS of 40 or greater reduced overall mortality from expected, and reduced or eliminated pulmonary complications such as pneumonia, pulmonary embolus, and ARDS. Although this does not suggest that all spine fracture patients should be rushed to the operating room for urgent surgery, it does suggest that it is safe to proceed on an urgent basis when compelled to do so.

The benefits of early long bone stabilization have been well established. It has been shown that patients with femoral shaft fractures with an ISS greater than 18 who had early stabilization experienced a decrease in the incidence of ARDS, pulmonary complications, and length of intensive care unit stay.

Controversy exists regarding reaming during intramedullary nailing in patients with severe pulmonary injury. Marrow contents and bone fragments may embolize during reaming, and it has been proposed that embolization of such contents may lead to an inflammatory response as well as mechanical blockage, exacerbating the existing pulmonary injury. However, several recent studies have suggested that the extent of the primary pulmonary injury is the major determinant of pulmonary morbidity. As noted earlier, a study examining intramedullary fixation versus plating of femur fractures demonstrated no difference in pulmonary complications.

Vascular injury must be recognized immediately in injured extremities. Timely diagnosis and treatment can minimize ischemic injury. Although arterial reconstruction has high priority, bony stability may need to be achieved before vascular repair. If immediate repair is not possible, a temporary shunt may be placed. Compartment syndrome should be anticipated and treated immediately with fasciotomy. In obtunded polytrauma patients clinical examination may not prove to be reliable. Compartment pressures within 30 mm Hg of diastolic pressure are consistent with compartment syndrome and thus a fasciotomy should be performed.

Treatment of open fractures involves administration of antibiotics and extensive surgical débridement. Stable fixation of the fracture is advocated. Currently, extensive soft-tissue injuries and associated tibia and femur fractures (grade III) are safely treated with intramedullary nailing whereas in the past these injuries were treated with external fixation.

Soft-tissue injuries may require extensive débridement and reconstruction to ensure adequate coverage of bone, tendons, vessels, nerves, and implants. If a large soft-tissue defect is present, the decision on the type of reconstruction should be made at the second débridement or "second look," which is usually performed at 48 hours. Coverage with either a local or free vascularized flap should be performed within 72 hours of injury.

In the setting of multiple closed fractures, long bone fractures of the lower extremity should be stabilized first. Because of the extensive soft-tissue damage and blood loss associated with uncontrolled spasm and instability, femur and tibia fractures should be reduced and stabilized first, whereas fractures of the upper extremity can be splinted initially, with good results. Pelvic and spinal fractures may be definitively treated after treating the lower extremity fractures, in most cases, but unstable cervical injuries may warrant earlier treatment, maintaining the long bone fractures in traction until the spinal segment is adequately fixed. Upper extremity fractures may be definitively managed after addressing the above injuries.

Secondary Stabilization Period
During the secondary stabilization period, the patient is hemodynamically stable and surgical intervention is performed on a semielective basis. It is at this time that débridement of any areas of soft-tissue necrosis is performed. Secondary wound closure and some soft-tissue reconstructions may be achieved. Intra-articular reconstruction, hand, foot, and upper extremity fracture fixation, and complex spinal and pelvic and acetabular reconstruction may be performed at this time.

Tertiary Stabilization Period
Late reconstructive procedures may be performed in the tertiary stabilization period, including definitive closure of amputation sites or any procedure that may have been postponed during the secondary stabilization period. The prognosis of the patient is usually known.

If the patient is stable and is extubated, rehabilitation may begin. This process should be started on an inpatient basis and should be taken through the outpatient phase if necessary.

Long-Term Outcome
Advanced age and increased severity of injury is associated with increased mortality in the short term. Long-term outcomes of polytrauma patients vary with the severity of injury initially sustained. Severity of injury is associated with greater disability, higher rate of unemployment after injury, and lower quality of life. Studies examining both subjective and objective outcomes data

among patients with multiple extremity fractures have demonstrated that functional disabilities are greatest for injuries below the knee. Intra-articular injuries to the foot and ankle, in particular, tend to impair patients who have had an otherwise satisfactory recovery from trauma. Additionally, recent evidence indicates that polytrauma patients sustaining cord or cauda equina injury at the time of spinal fracture have poorer functional outcomes and poorer return to work, even among those with good neurologic recovery.

Annotated Bibliography

Bhandari M, Guyatt GH, Khera V, Kulkarni AV, Sprague S, Schemitsch EH: Operative management of lower extremity fractures in patients with head injuries. *Clin Orthop* 2003;407:187-198.

The authors compared femoral plating versus intramedullary nailing and tibial plating versus intramedullary nailing in head-injured patients. The study group included 119 patients with severe head injuries and lower extremity fractures. There was no significant difference in mortality rates between patients treated with intramedullary nailing or plating. The strongest predictor of mortality was the severity of the initial head injury.

Cook RE, Keating JF, Gillespie I: The role of angiography in the management of hemorrhage from major fractures of the pelvis. *J Bone Joint Surg Br* 2002;84:178-182.

This study examined 150 patients with unstable pelvic fractures and uncontrollable hypotension. In those patients undergoing angiography prior to external fixation or laparotomy, more than half of them died. The authors recommended that angiography be used in refractory cases after skeletal stabilization has been attempted in those patients with unstable pelvic injuries.

Giannoudis PV: Surgical priorities in damage control in polytrauma. *J Bone Joint Surg Br* 2003;85:478-483.

The author provides a review of the current trends and principles in orthopaedic management of polytrauma, including principles of damage control surgery.

Inaba K, Kirkpatrick AW, Finkelstein J, et al: Blunt abdominal aortic trauma in association with thoracolumbar spine fractures. *Injury* 2001;32:201-207.

The authors report their experience with blunt abdominal aortic disruption at regional trauma centers. Eight cases were identified, six of which were associated with thoracolumbar fractures, with a mean ISS of 42. All spinal fractures were associated with a distractive force pattern. The authors concluded that with all distractive thoracolumbar injuries, aortic disruption must be considered as this injury may occur as a result of similar distractive forces.

McCormick JP, Morgan SJ, Smith WR: Clinical effectiveness of the physical examination in diagnosis of posterior pelvic injuries. *J Orthop Trauma* 2003;17:257-261.

This article presents a prospective study evaluating the correlation of physical examination to radiographic studies in the diagnosis of posterior pelvic ring disruptions. Of those patients found to have posterior pelvic ring disruptions as shown on CT scan, 98% had posterior pelvic pain on examination. The authors concluded that physical examination was accurate in detecting injuries of the posterior pelvic ring.

Miller MT, Pasquale MD, Bromberg WJ, Wasser TE, Cox J: Not so FAST. *J Trauma* 2003;54:52-59.

The authors performed a study comparing a Focused Assessment with Sonography for Trauma with CT scan to compare accuracy in diagnosis of injury in patients sustaining blunt abdominal trauma. A total of 372 patients were studied and it was noted that the Focused Assessment with Sonography for Trauma examination underdiagnosed significant intra-abdominal trauma. The authors concluded that patients who are hemodynamically stable who sustain blunt abdominal trauma should undergo CT scan for further evaluation for more accurate diagnosis of intra-abdominal injuries.

Zalavras CG, Patzakis MJ: Open fractures: Evaluation and management. *J Am Acad Orthop Surg* 2003;11:212-219.

This article is a review of the literature regarding management of open fractures. The authors discuss the controversies regarding wound closure. Soft-tissue coverage of large and contaminated wounds is also discussed.

Classic Bibliography

Bohlman HH: Acute fractures and dislocations of the cervical spine: An analysis of three hundred hospitalized patients and review of the literature. *J Bone Joint Surg Am* 1979;61:1119-1142.

Bone L, Bucholz R: The management of fractures in the patient with multiple trauma. *J Bone Joint Surg Am* 1986;68:945-949.

Bone LB, Johnson KD, Weigelt J, Scheinbeng R: Early versus delayed stabilization of fractures: A prospective, randomized study. *J Bone Joint Surg Am* 1989;71:336-340.

Boulanger BR, Stephen D, Brennemann FD: Thoracic trauma and early intramedullary nailing of femur fractures: Are we doing harm? *J Trauma* 1997;43:24-28.

Chapman MW: The role of intramedullary fixation in open fractures. *Clin Orthop* 1986;212:26-34.

Civil ID, Schwab CW: The Abbreviated Injury Scale, 1985 revision: A condensed chart for clinical use. *J Trauma* 1988;28:87-90.

Gustilo RB, Anderson JT: Prevention of infection in the treatment of one thousand and twenty-five open fractures of long bones: Retrospective and prospective analyses. *J Bone Joint Surg Am* 1976;58:453-458.

Johnson KD, Cadambi A, Seibert GB: Incidence of adult respiratory distress syndrome in patients with multiple musculoskeletal injuries: Effect of early operative stabilization of fractures. *J Trauma* 1985;25:375-384.

McLain RF, Benson DR: Urgent surgical stabilization of spinal fractures in polytraumatized patients. *Spine* 1999;24:1646-1654.

Schwab CW, Shayne JP, Turner J: Immediate trauma resuscitation with type O uncrossmatched blood: A two-year prospective experience. *J Trauma* 1986;26:897-902.

Shackford SR, Hollingsworth-Fridlund P, Cooper GF, Eastman AB: The effect of regionalization on the quality of trauma care as assessed by concurrent audit before and after institution of a trauma system: A preliminary report. *J Trauma* 1986;26:812-820.

Tscherne H, Regel G, Pape HC, Pohlemann T, Kretteck C: Internal fixation of multiple fractures in patients with polytrauma. *Clin Orthop* 1998;347:62-78.

Winquist RA, Hansen ST Jr, Clawson DK: Closed intramedullary nailing of femoral fractures: A report of five hundred and twenty cases. *J Bone Joint Surg Am* 1984;66:529-539.

Chapter 16

Coagulation and Thromboembolism in Orthopaedic Surgery

Francis H. Shen, MD, FACS

Dino Samartzis, BS

Christopher J. DeWald, MD

Introduction

The coagulation pathway is a series of enzymatic processes whose final result is the formation of a thrombus (Figure 1). This cascade is the result of an equilibrium between prothrombotic and antithrombotic factors that occur in the bloodstream. The preferential occurrence of one process over the other can result in either a bleeding coagulopathy or thromboembolic disease.

Coagulopathies

Preoperative Assessment of Blood Clotting

Preoperative assessment begins with a thorough history, clinical examination, and appropriate laboratory studies. A history of easy, excessive, or spontaneous bleeding or bruising, previous need for blood transfusions, and/or a family history of bleeding disorders is suggestive of a clotting disorder. A review of the medical history preoperatively is imperative. Various conditions, such as chronic liver and renal disease, malnutrition, malabsorption, chronic antibiotic use, hematologic disorders, and drug or alcohol use may identify patients at risk for coagulopathies and these patients require additional evaluation. Although neither pathognomonic nor exclusionary, signs of potential bleeding or clotting problems should be investigated, such as bruising not associated with trauma, petechiae, and stigmata of liver disease and portal hypertension (for example, spider angiomata or caput medusa). Routine screening tests may include a complete blood cell count (CBC) and platelet count, and determination of prothrombin time (PT) and an activated partial thromboplastin time (PTT).

Work-Up of the Coagulopathic Patient

Most of the time, a CBC with platelet count, PT, and PTT are the only tests necessary during a routine preoperative screening. Other diagnostic testing, such as bleeding times, D-dimer, and assessment of specific factor deficiencies are not routinely recommended unless the patient history or clinical examination is suggestive. Differential diagnoses of common coagulopathies include quantitative or qualitative platelet disorders, disorders in the coagulation cascade, and coagulation factor deficiencies or dysfunction. Once a bleeding disorder is suspected then additional work-up is recommended.

Screening tests of the coagulation cascade include PT, which reflects deficiencies in factors II, V, VII, and X, whereas PTT reflects deficiencies of factor II, V, VIII, IX, X, XI, and XII. Isolated prolongation of the PTT is seen with factors VIII, IX, or XI deficiencies. Although also seen in patients with hereditary deficiencies of factor XII, these disorders are not usually associated with clinical bleeding. Isolated prolongation of PT usually reflects factor VII deficiency or low fibrinogen levels (< 1 g/L). Because isolated factor II, V, or X deficiencies are rare, prolongation of both PT and PTT are more commonly a reflection of multiple factor deficiencies as seen in disseminated intravascular coagulation or in hepatocellular dysfunction. Conversely, a normal PT and PTT does not automatically imply normal factor levels, because levels may have to drop below 30% of normal before elevated values are seen.

Quantitative and qualitative platelet dysfunctions may be more accurately identified with the use of bleeding times. Quantitative platelet disorders, such as idiopathic thrombocytopenic purpura, disseminated intravascular coagulation, and drug-induced thrombocytopenia are the result of peripheral platelet destruction and may be seen as multiple large, young platelets on a peripheral blood smear. Causes of qualitative platelet dysfunction with normal platelet numbers can occur in renal dialysis patients and are often drug-induced, as occurs with aspirin and other newer antiplatelet medications, such as clopidogrel and ticlopidine.

Treatment of Common Coagulopathies

Although uncommon in the general population (1 in 10,000), patients with hemophilia A (factor VIII deficiency) and B (factor IX deficiency) may be frequently seen by the orthopaedic surgeon. The gene for both factors is located on the X chromosome and affects males more than females. Hemarthrosis is one of the most common complications and first-line therapy is factor

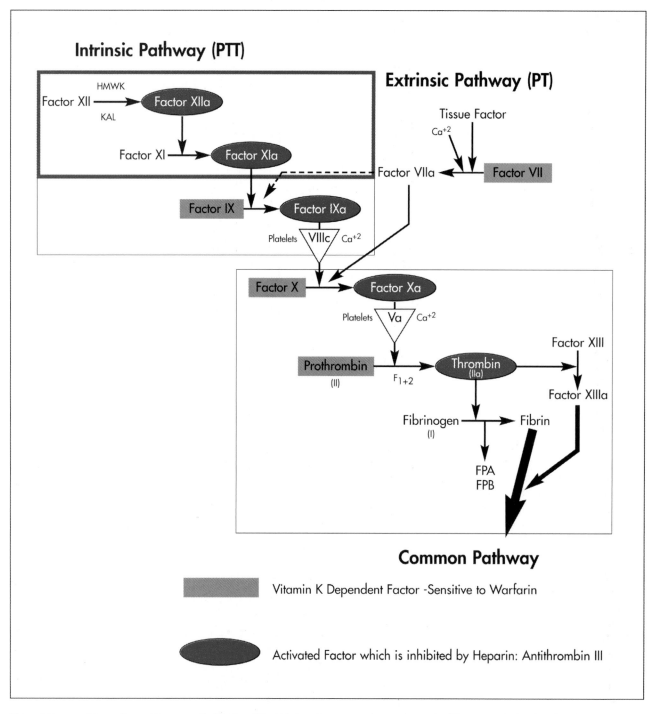

Figure 1 The coagulation pathways. PT measures the function of the extrinsic and common pathways, whereas the PTT measures the function of the intrinsic and common pathways. FPA = fibrinopeptide A; FPB = fibrinopeptide B. (Reproduced with permission from Stead RB: Regulation of hemostasis, in Goldhaber SZ (ed): *Pulmonary Embolism and Deep Venous Thromboembolism*. Philadelphia, PA, WB Saunders, 1985, p 32.)

replacement. In patients with spontaneous bleeds, the goal is to achieve circulating levels that are approximately 40% to 50% of normal. If surgical intervention is planned, the deficient factor should be replaced to levels near 100%. Continuous or intermittent boluses of high-purity plasma derivatives or recombinant factor concentrates can be given and have greatly reduced the risk of human immunodeficiency virus transmission. Although uncommon, hemophilia patients with factor inhibitors, antibodies that neutralize the coagulation factor, should be identified.

Various congenital bleeding disorders exist that may affect proper coagulation, the most common being von Willebrand's disease, an autosomal dominant disorder.

Table 1 | List of Common Antithrombotic Medications With Mechanism of Action and Laboratory Monitoring Method

Medication	Mechanism of Action	Laboratory Monitoring Method
Warfarin (Coumadin)	Prevents the vitamin K dependent γ-carboxylation of factors II, VII, IX, and X, proteins C and S, slowing thrombin production	Prothrombin time - International Normalized Ratio
Low molecular weight heparin (enoxaparin)	Upregulates the inhibitory effect of antithrombin on serine proteases thrombin, IXa, Xa, XIa, and XIIa with greatest effect upon Xa	None necessary in uncomplicated cases; Chromogenic anti-Xa assay available in complicated cases
Salicylates (aspirin)	Irreversibly inhibits cyclo-oxgenase activity in platelets and vascular endothelium	None necessary, although bleeding times may be prolonged
Traditional nonsteroidal anti-inflammatory drugs (ibuprofen)	Inhibition of COX-1 and 2, and leukotriene synthesis	None necessary, although bleeding times may be prolonged
Selective COX-2 inhibitors Celecoxib (Celebrex)	Selective inhibition of COX-2	None necessary, although bleeding times may be prolonged
Thienopyridines Ticlopidine (Ticlid) Clopidogrel (Plavix)	Binds to the GPIIb/IIIa receptor to irreversible blocking Adenosine diphosphate-induced platelet aggregation	None necessary, although bleeding times may be prolonged

It occurs secondary to a deficiency of von Willebrand's factor, which is important for promoting normal platelet function and stabilizing factor VIII. Although most patients will respond to desmopressin, a few may require the use of clotting factor concentrates.

Treatment of the acquired coagulopathies centers on identifying the cause. Prior to surgery, medications that inhibit platelet function and the coagulation pathway should be stopped if possible and blood work rechecked if necessary (Table 1). Nutrition should be optimized, especially in older patients. If necessary, platelets and fresh frozen plasma (FFP) should be available for infusion perioperatively. Because FFP contains only the normal amount of clotting factor per milliliter of plasma, achieving sufficient factor levels can require greater volumes.

Recombinant factor VII has been used in patients with a high titer inhibitor directed against factor V, VIII, or IX. More recent studies focus on the role of various recombinant factor concentrates to achieve hemostasis in patients demonstrating massive bleeding refractory to FFP and platelets. This may be the case in patients who develop consumptive coagulopathies secondary to massive bleeding from multitrauma or massive blood volume replacement postoperatively, and in patients who develop dilutional coagulopathies during prolonged surgeries. The lower volumes required with the use of these recombinant factors may result in less fluid overload, decreased fluid shifts, and anasarca in critically ill patients; however, additional studies are required to more clearly define the optimal dosing, safety, and efficacy of these recombinant factors before routine use is recommended.

Other areas of investigation include the local use of fibrin sealant and topical thrombin. Preliminary data suggest that in patients undergoing primary total knee arthroplasty, fibrin sealant may safely reduce postoperative wound drain output while maintaining higher postoperative hemoglobin levels.

Thromboembolic Disease

Thromboembolic disease refers to a group of disorders that includes thrombosis and embolic disorders, which can occur in either the arterial or venous system. In the orthopaedic patient, venous thromboembolic disease is more common, and includes deep venous thrombosis (DVT) and pulmonary embolism (PE).

Pathophysiology

In the 19th century, Virchow described the three major pathophysiologic factors (stasis, endothelial injury, and hypercoagulable states) contributing to thromboembolic disease. Thrombosis secondary to stasis occurs more commonly in the low-velocity, high capacitance venous system (venostasis) and is the result of a disruption of the normal laminar blood flow. These venous thrombi are typically composed of fibrin and trapped red cells and contain few platelets. Endothelial injury leads to thrombus formation secondary to traumatic exposure of extracellular matrix components (collagen) within the vessel walls to circulating platelets. Although this can occur in the venous system, it more typically is present in the high-velocity arterial system and is usually composed of platelets with little fibrin. The third cause, hypercoagulability, remains the least understood, and occurs in conditions such as malignancy, pregnancy, hormone replacement, in smokers, and during the postoperative state. Hereditary causes, such as resistance or deficiencies in antithrombin III, factor C, factor S, factor

V Leiden mutations, and antiphospholipid syndrome, have also been identified. Clinically, these patients are at increased risk for stroke and vascular and cardiac disease, and may have an increased risk of osteonecrosis, Legg-Calvé-Perthes disease, and other thrombotic disorders.

Epidemiology

Venous thromboembolic disease occurs for the first time in approximately 100 per 100,000 persons each year and increases exponentially with age from a negligible rate for those younger than 15 years up to 500 per 100,000 in individuals older than 80 years. Two thirds of symptomatic venous thromboembolic diseases present as a DVT, whereas one third present with PE. In large epidemiologic studies, the incidence is statistically higher among Caucasians and African Americans than in Hispanics and Asian-Pacific Islanders. Recurrence rates, even after successful anticoagulant therapy, are approximately 7% at 6 months after the initial event.

The risk of venous thromboembolic disease also varies depending on the procedure being performed. The reported rate of DVT in the total hip arthroplasty patient ranges from 15% to 25% and can be as high as 50% in the patient undergoing a total knee arthroplasty, whereas the risk of fatal PE without thromboprophylaxis is between 0.1% to 0.5%. The use of either chemical or mechanical prophylaxis has decreased these rates by half.

In patients with pelvic, acetabular, periacetabular, and hip fractures, reported DVT rates vary from 20% to 60% and increase when surgery is delayed by 2 days or longer. Although symptomatic PE rates range from 2% to 10%, fatal PE occurs in approximately 0.5% to 2%. In these patients, the occurrence of more proximal thrombi, particularly those in the pelvis, may result in a higher risk of embolization (up to 50%).

Identifying rates of thromboembolic disorders in the patient undergoing spinal surgery has been more difficult. Studies are limited, but reported rates of DVT range from 0.3% to 26%. In patients undergoing posterior spinal procedures alone there does not appear to be a difference in DVT rates when compared by sex, length of procedure, number of levels performed, and/or the addition of one- or two-level fusions. However, although still not clear, DVT rates may be higher in patients undergoing combined anterior and posterior spinal surgery than in those undergoing posterior-alone procedures.

In a prospective multicenter study of 2,733 patients who underwent foot and ankle surgery, the reported DVT rate was 0.22% with a 0.15% rate of nonfatal PE without occurrence of fatal PE. The authors did not find a statistical relationship with tourniquet use or history of thromboembolic disease. The only statistically significant relationship was the increased use of postoperative cast immobilization and no weight bearing, which increased the relative risk by 0.04%.

Treatment Strategies

Treatment consists of either thromboembolic disease prevention (thromboprophylaxis) or management of established thromboembolic disease. Because of high rates of venous thromboembolic disease in the orthopaedic patient, initial management should center on thromboprophylaxis. Treatment strategies include either mechanical or pharmacologic methods or a combination of both. Management techniques for the treatment of established thromboembolic disease is beyond the scope of this chapter.

Mechanical Approaches

Current mechanical options include pneumatic compression boots, plantar foot compression devices, and elastic compression stockings. Pneumatic compression boots reduce stasis by directly increasing the velocity of venous blood flow. Because these boots also increase the systemic release of endogenous fibrinolytic activity, their benefit can be realized even when used on a single limb or placed on the upper extremity. Plantar foot compression devices mimic the hemodynamic effects of ambulation, thus increasing venous return and decreasing venostasis. Although elastic compression stockings decrease lower extremity venous pooling and stasis, their use alone as an effective thromboprophylaxis is unclear. In patients undergoing combined anterior and posterior spinal procedures and in those who have had joint arthroplasty, if possible, elastic compressive stockings should be used in conjunction with other prophylactic agents.

The greatest advantages of these mechanical methods are that there is almost no risk of bleeding, minimal to no side effects, and they do not require laboratory monitoring. A less common, more invasive mechanical device is the inferior vena cava filter. This device can be associated with substantial morbidity; therefore, its routine use as a thromboprophylactic agent is not encouraged. However, it may have a role in management of patients with known DVT and recurrent PE despite adequate anticoagulant therapy, patients in whom anticoagulant therapy is contraindicated, and potentially in patients noncompliant with anticoagulant therapy. The use of temporary inferior vena cava filters (which are removed typically within 10 days from the time of insertion) is currently being investigated in various clinical scenarios, such as in the critically ill, multitrauma patient requiring multiple surgical interventions over a short time period.

Pharmacologic Approaches

At this time, common pharmacologic avenues for the treatment of thromboembolic disease include the use of warfarin, low molecular weight heparin (LMWH), and antiplatelet therapies (such as aspirin or thienopyridines). Warfarin exerts an anticoagulation effect by inhibiting the vitamin K-dependent clotting factors II, VII, IX, and X. Multiple studies have demonstrated warfarin's effectiveness in decreasing the rate of both DVT and PE in patients undergoing total joint arthroplasty. Because clinically significant bleeding occurs in 1% to 5% of patients, careful monitoring is necessary to maintain the international normalized ratio in a therapeutic range. The international normalized ratio was established by the World Health Organization as a way to standardize coagulation test results by using the international sensitivity index.

Some of the major disadvantages in the use of warfarin include the expense and inconvenience of monitoring, risk of bleeding, and multiple drug interactions. Although awareness has increased about the interaction of warfarin with many over-the-counter medications such as aspirin, ibuprofen, and other nonsteroidal anti-inflammatory drugs, many physicians and patients are still unaware of the potential interactions that can occur with various herbs and supplements such as ginger, ginkgo, ginseng, and St. John's Wort. Furthermore, patient education should include identification of foods high in vitamin K (such as broccoli and kale) that can reduce the effectiveness of warfarin.

The role of LMWH continues to evolve. LMWH is created by depolymerization of unfractionated heparin and contains compounds with molecular weights between 3,000 to 10,000 daltons. Because of the enhanced affinity for antithrombin III and activated factor X, LMWH is a more active agent than conventional heparin and intervenes at an earlier point in the clotting cascade. The dosages required for thromboprophylaxis do not increase PT or PTT values and therefore do not require monitoring. Disadvantages of LMWH include increased cost, parenteral administration, and the increased potential for bleeding. Therefore, LMWH should be considered with caution in patients undergoing spinal puncture or using epidural catheters as an anesthetic agent. LMWH appears to be effective in the management of venous thromboembolic disease in total joint arthroplasty patients and in the multitrauma patient. Ease of use and lack of need for monitoring may make LMWH an excellent medication for use in the outpatient setting, especially in patients who continued to be at risk for venous thromboembolic disease after being discharged from the hospital.

Currently, the use of aspirin as the sole thromboprophylactic agent is unclear. In doses greater than 100 mg per day, aspirin irreversibly binds and inactivates cyclooxygenase in both immature and circulating platelets, thereby inhibiting thrombus plug formation. Although some studies demonstrate that, compared with placebo, the use of aspirin in total joint arthroplasty patients decreases the rate of both proximal and distal DVTs, the question remains whether they are as effective as other methods in preventing fatal PE. In selected patients, the use of aspirin with or without other forms of prophylaxis may be acceptable; however, larger randomized controlled trials are necessary.

Newer agents continue to evolve and include medications such as direct thrombin inhibitors (lepirudin), direct and indirect factor Xa inhibitors, and heparinoids (danaparoid). At present, the role of such agents remains unclear and additional investigation is required before routine use is recommended.

Summary

Although consultation with an internist or hematologist may be necessary when complications arise, a basic knowledge of common bleeding disorders and thromboembolic disease is important for every orthopaedic surgeon to understand. Identification of possible coagulopathies begins with a careful history, examination, appropriate laboratory studies, and treatment directed toward management of the specific etiology. Newer recombinant factors that address various factors in the coagulation pathway are currently being developed.

Without thromboprophylaxis, the rate of thromboembolic disease in the orthopaedic population can be high. Early ambulation and mobilization should be encouraged and used in conjunction with other established prophylactic methods. The benefits of thromboprophylaxis should be carefully balanced with the risks of intervention and individualized to the patient being treated and be procedure-specific.

Annotated Bibliography

Coagulopathies

Eckman MH, Erban JK, Singh SK, Kao GS: Screening for the risk of bleeding or thrombosis. *Ann Intern Med* 2003;138:W15-W24.

For nonsurgical and surgical patients without synthetic liver dysfunction or a history of oral anticoagulant use, routine testing has no benefit in assessment of bleeding risk.

Hvid I, Rodriguiez-Merchan EC: Orthopaedic surgery in haemophilic patients with inhibitors: An overview. *Haemophilia* 2002;8:288-291.

Recombinant factor VIIa appears to be an efficient hemostasis product for patients with hemophilia A and B with inhibitors undergoing major elective orthopaedic procedures.

Shami VM, Caldwell SH, Hespenheide EE, Arseneau KO, Bickston SJ, Macik BG: Recombinant activated factor VII for coagulopathy in fulminant hepatic failure compared with conventional therapy. *Liver Transpl* 2003;9:138-143.

The authors found a statistically significant difference in correction of coagulopathy and decreased anasarca in patients with severe coagulopathy from fulminant hepatic failure after a single dose of recombinant activated factor VII compared with those receiving fresh frozen plasma alone.

Wang GJ, Hungerford DS, Savory CG, et al: Use of fibrin sealant to reduce bloody drainage and hemoglobin loss after total knee arthroplasty: A brief note on a randomized prospective trial. *J Bone Joint Surg Am* 2001; 83:1503-1505.

Preliminary data from a phase III trial of 53 patients undergoing unilateral primary total knee arthroplasty demonstrated a reduction in bloody drainage and higher postoperative hemoglobin in the fibrin sealant group than in the control group.

Thromboembolic Disease

Edelsberg J, Ollendorf D, Oster G: Venous thromboembolism following major orthopedic surgery: Review of epidemiology and economics. *Am J Health Syst Pharm* 2001;58(suppl 2):S4-S13.

A review of epidemiology of venous thromboembolic disease in joint replacement and hip fracture surgery is presented. Costs associated with the diagnosis, treatment, and recovery from venous thromboembolic disease is substantial, with the initial therapy consuming 90% of the total cost.

Fitzgerald RH Jr, Spiro TE, Trowbridge AA, et al: Prevention of venous thromboembolic disease following primary total knee arthroplasty: A randomized, multicenter, open-label, parallel-group comparison of enoxaparin and warfarin. *J Bone Joint Surg Am* 2001;83:900-906.

This article discusses a prospective, randomized, multicenter trial that compared the efficacy and safety of enoxaparin and warfarin in 349 patients undergoing total knee arthroplasties. The authors found enoxaparin administered twice daily to be more effective than warfarin in reducing the occurrence of asymptomatic venous thromboembolic disease.

Hyers TM: Management of venous thromboembolism: Past, present, and future. *Arch Intern Med* 2003;163:759-768.

A review of the state of current chemoprophylatic methods, including unfractionated heparin and low molecular weight heparin and their potential adverse effects and theoretical basis for failure is presented. Newer agents recently approved for venous thromboembolic disease, such as heparinoid, and selective Xa inhibitors are discussed.

Kim YH, Oh SH, Kim JS: Incidence and natural history of deep-vein thrombosis after total hip arthroplasty: A prospective and randomized clinical study. *J Bone Joint Surg Br* 2003;85:661-665.

The authors prospectively followed 200 patients who underwent primary total hip arthroplasties (THAs). DVT rates were 26% for bilateral THA and 20% for unilateral THA, but in the 72 patients with venogram confirmed thrombi, all thrombi had spontaneously and completely resolved at 6 months regardless of site and size.

Offner PJ, Hawkes A, Madayag R, Seale F, Maines C: The role of temporary inferior vena cava filters in critically ill surgical patients. *Arch Surg* 2003;138:591-595.

The authors concluded from a prospective cohort study of 44 patients at a level I trauma center that temporary inferior vena cava filters are a safe and effective approach to preventing venous thromboembolic disease in the multitrauma, critically ill surgical patient.

Samama CM: Venous thromboembolism deserves your attention. *Critical Care* 2001;5:277-279.

The author surveyed intensive care unit directors in Canada and reviewed the use of traditional and advanced compression techniques, as well as unfractionated versus low molecular weight heparin for the prevention and treatment of DVT and venous thromboembolic disease. The recommendations were that mechanical prophylaxis should be used alone or in combination with chemoprophylaxis in patients in the intensive care unit and that pharmacologic prophylaxis should always be combined with mechanical prophylaxis; however, large randomized controlled trials are needed.

Stannard JP, Riley RS, McClenney MD, Lopez-Ben RR, Volgas DA, Alonso JE: Mechanical prophylaxis against deep vein thrombosis after pelvic and acetabular fractures. *J Bone Joint Surg Am* 2001;83:1047-1051.

This article discusses a prospective, randomized, blinded study of the use of sequential and pulsatile mechanical compression devices for prophylaxis against DVT in 107 patients with pelvic or acetabular fractures that required surgical treatment. Pulsatile compression was associated with fewer instances of DVT than standard compression, but results did not reach significance.

White RH: The epidemiology of venous thromboembolism. *Circulation* 2003;107(suppl 23):I4-I8.

First-time venous thromboembolic disease occurs in approximately 100 per 100,000 persons each year and a recurrence rate of 7% has been reported. Risk factors identified from large epidemiologic studies include ethnicity, and advanced age. Gender does not appear to be a factor.

Classic Bibliography

Clagett GP, Anderson FA Jr, Geerts W, et al: Prevention of venous thromboembolism. *Chest* 1998;114(suppl 5): 531S-560S.

Coventry MB, Nolan DR, Beckenbaugh RD: Delayed prophylactic anticoagulation: A study of results and complications in 2,012 total hip arthroplasties. *J Bone Joint Surg Am* 1973;55:1487-1492.

Dearborn JT, Hu SS, Tribus CB, Bradford DS: Thromboembolic complications after major throacolumbar spine surgery. *Spine* 1999;24:1471-1476.

Freedman KB, Brookenthal KR, Fitzgerald RH Jr, Williams S, Lonner J: A meta-analysis of thromboembolic prophylaxis following elective total hip arthroplasty. *J Bone Joint Surg Am* 2000;82:929-938.

Geerts WH, Code KI, Jay RM, Chen E, Szalai JP: A prospective study of venous thromboembolism after major trauma. *N Engl J Med* 1994;331:1601-1606.

Geerts WH, Jay RM, Code KI, et al: A comparison of low-dose heparin with low-molecular-weight heparin as prophylaxis against venous thromboembolism after major trauma. *N Engl J Med* 1996;335:701-707.

Leclerc JR, Geerts WH, Desjardins L, et al: Prevention of venous thromboembolism after knee arthroplasty: A randomized, double-blinded trial comparing enoxaparin with warfarin. *Ann Intern Med* 1996;124:619-626.

Lieberman JR, Wollaeger J, Dorey F, et al: The efficacy of prophylaxis with low-dose warfarin for prevention of pulmonary embolism following total hip arthroplasty. *J Bone Joint Surg Am* 1997;79:319-325.

Lotke PA, Palevsky H, Keenan AM, et al: Aspirin and warfarin for thromboembolic disease after total joint arthroplasty. *Clin Orthop* 1996;324:251-258.

Mizel MS, Temple HT, Michelson JD, et al: Thromboembolism after foot and ankle surgery: A multicenter study. *Clin Orthop* 1998;348:180-185.

Montgomery KD, Geerts WH, Potter HG, Helfet DL: Thromboembolic complications in patients with pelvic trauma. *Clin Orthop* 1996;329:68-87.

NIH Consensus Development Conference Statement: *Prevention of Venous Thrombosis and Pulmonary Embolism.* Bethesda, MD, US Department of Health and Human Services, Office of Medical Application of Research, 1986, vol 6, no 2.

Pellegrini VD Jr, Clement D, Lush-Ehmann C, Keller GS, Evarts CM: Natural history of thromboembolic disease after total hip arthroplasty. *Clin Orthop* 1996;333:27-40.

RD Heparin Arthroplasty Group: RD heparin compared with warfarin for prevention of venous thromboembolic disease following total hip or knee arthroplasty. *J Bone Joint Surg Am* 1994;76:1174-1185.

Salvati EA, Pellegrini VD Jr, Sharrock NE, et al: Recent advances in venous thromboembolic prophylaxis during and after total hip replacement. *J Bone Joint Surg Am* 2000;82:252-270.

Sarmiento A, Goswami AD: Thromboembolic prophylaxis with use of aspirin, exercise, and graded elastic stockings or intermittent compression devices in patients managed with total hip arthroplasty. *J Bone Joint Surg Am* 1999;81:339-346.

Warwick D, Williams MH, Bannister GC: Death and thromboembolic disease after total hip replacement: A series of 1162 cases with no routine chemical prophylaxis. *J Bone Joint Surg Br* 1995;77:6-10.

Chapter 17

Blood Transfusion

John S. Xenos, MD

Andrew G. Yun, MD

Introduction

The perioperative management of blood products in the orthopaedic patient is becoming more sophisticated as new data and products become available. The drive for newer techniques of perioperative blood management is fueled by the desire to avoid transfusion of allogeneic blood products and thereby decrease risks associated with the use of these products, such as transmission of disease, immunosuppression, infection, and transfusion reactions.

Also, the supply of allogeneic blood products is expected to exceed demand in the future. According to a recent study, the domestic supply of blood in the United States in 1997 was found to be 5.5% less than in 1994, with the rate of whole blood collections being 12.6% lower in the population age 18 to 65 years. The red blood cell (RBC) transfusion rate remained the same, however, whereas the transfusion rates of platelets and plasma increased. Although the current margin of allogeneic blood supply is adequate, there is legitimate concern that the future demand for blood products will exceed supply.

Blood Products: Their Role and Indications

Blood products currently used in clinical practice include RBCs, platelets, fresh frozen plasma, and cryoprecipitated antihemophilic factor.

Red Blood Cells

RBCs are concentrated erythrocytes from whole blood either by an apheresis or by centrifuge. Packed red blood cells and red cells are terms synonymous with red blood cells. The typical preparation comprises RBCs with a hematocrit range of 60% to 70% and approximately 50 mL of acellular plasma, citrate for anticoagulation, and a preservative solution. ABO compatibility as well as compatibility with other antibodies must be established before transfusion.

The role of RBC transfusion is to replace deficient circulating RBC mass in the face of compromised oxygen-carrying capacity or tissue hypoxia. It is impor-tant to draw a distinction between the clinical manifestation of hypovolemia and anemia when considering transfusion of RBCs. Certainly, multiple patient-specific factors, such as cardiovascular status and other comorbidities that would affect the patient's ability to tolerate tissue hypoxia, come into play in this determination. The true limit of tolerance of anemia is not known. In healthy adults, hemoglobin levels as low as 6.0 g/dL may be tolerated and oxygen delivery is maintained.

One unit of RBCs transfused in a patient of normal size and not actively bleeding or in hemolysis should result in a 1.0-g/dL increase in hemoglobin. The current transfusion guidelines recommended by the American Society of Anesthesiologists are almost always to transfuse when the hemoglobin level is less than 6.0 g/dL and almost never when greater than 10.0 g/dL (Figure 1). A National Institutes of Health consensus document recommends that good clinical judgment should be the basis for appropriate perioperative transfusion rather than the use of a single criterion such as the hemoglobin level. In a 1999 study of patients undergoing total joint arthroplasty, a transfusion trigger of 7.0 g/dL was used unless symptoms were present in the face of higher hemoglobin levels. Most would agree that establishment of an absolute transfusion trigger based on hemoglobin is inappropriate and that avoidance of unnecessary transfusion is desirable.

The specific indications for transfusion in patients with hemoglobin levels between 6.0 g/dL and 10.0 g/dL should be based on the patient's risk associated with anemia after other measures, such as volume repletion, have been attempted. Patients should have adequate volume resuscitation before RBC transfusion is considered. Blood loss of less than 15% of total volume is well tolerated by most patients with minimal symptoms. In patients with 30% blood loss, tachycardia is present, and 30% to 40% loss of blood volume is associated with signs of severe shock. Invasive monitoring is the most effective method to assess tissue perfusion. Other measures to consider include heart rate, blood pressure, hemoglobin, and status of bleeding (active, controlled, or uncontrolled.)

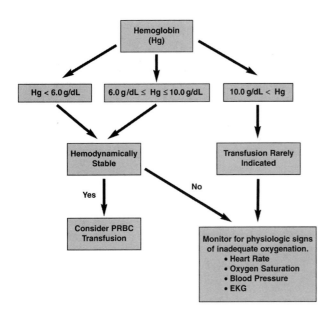

Figure 1 General transfusion guidelines. Use of an absolute "transfusion trigger" should be avoided. PRBC = packed red blood cell; EKG = electrocardiogram.

Platelets

Platelets, cells required for hemostasis, are prepared either as random donor platelets or as platelet pheresis also known as single donor platelets. Random donor platelets are derived from whole blood and usually contain approximately 7.5×10^{10} platelets per bag. Greater platelet quantities are obtained in single donor platelets preparations with approximately 4.5×10^{11} platelets per bag.

The primary indication for platelet infusion is when platelet counts are below 5,000/mm^3 regardless of bleeding. General guidelines call for platelet transfusion with counts less than 50,000/mm^3 before a major surgical intervention. Platelet infusions are not recommended for counts greater than 100,000/mm^3. The usual dosage of platelets is 6 units or 1 unit per 10 kg of body weight for random donor platelets or one apheresis unit. Reinfusion is generally required every 3 to 5 days in the absence of platelet consumption and more often when platelet consumption exists. Daily platelet counts should be monitored. Platelets should be administered to ABO-compatible patients as with RBC transfusions. Alloimmunized patients may require platelet apheresis units that have an HLA match.

Fresh Frozen Plasma

Fresh frozen plasma is the acellular component of blood and contains all of the peptide coagulation factors. It is separated from the RBCs and platelets and frozen at –18°C within 8 hours of collection. Use of fresh frozen plasma is indicated to address coagulopathy, docu-

mented clinically and/or with laboratory parameters. A prothrombin time greater than 18 seconds or 1.5 times normal, an activated partial prothrombin time above 55 to 60 seconds, or a coagulation factor assay demonstrating less than 25% activity are suggestive of coagulopathy. Other indications for fresh frozen plasma infusion include massive blood transfusion of greater than one blood volume with evidence of coagulopathy or documented coagulation factor deficiency before surgery, such as factor II, V, VII, X, XI, or XIII, von Willebrand's disease, or factor VIII deficiency when cryoprecipitate is not available. Conditions with multiple coagulation factor deficiencies as seen in liver disease or vitamin K deficiency may also require fresh frozen plasma infusion. The effects of warfarin may be reversed before an invasive procedure when the prothrombin time is greater than 18 seconds or the international normalized ratio is greater than 1.5. Fresh frozen plasma is not indicated for volume augmentation alone in the absence of coagulopathy. The usual dosage is 2 units, although correction of severe coagulopathy may require significantly greater doses of fresh frozen plasma. Monitoring should be performed with repeated laboratory parameters following fresh frozen plasma infusion.

Cryoprecipitated Antihemophilic Factor

Cryoprecipitated antihemophilic factor is the precipitable protein fraction derived from fresh frozen plasma. The typical preparation contains: factor VIII C, 80 to 120 units, von Willebrand's factor, 80 units, fibrinogen, 200 to 300 mg, and factor XIII, 40 to 60 units. Cryoprecipitated antihemophilic factor is considered to be acellular and does not require compatibility testing. Its use is indicated to address hypofibrinogenemia (rare), von Willebrand's disease, and hemophilia A. General indications are for use in patients with von Willebrand's disease not responsive to desmopressin, bleeding with von Willebrand's disease, or fibrinogen levels less than 80 to 100 mg/dL.

The dosage of cryoprecipitated antihemophilic factor required varies depending on the indications for usage. The recommended dosage for hypofibrinogenemia is one bag per 5 kg of body weight, whereas for von Willebrand's disease one bag per 10 kg body weight is usually required daily. Monitoring should be performed using measurement of ristocetin cofactor, factor VIII antigen, or von Willebrand's factor multimer levels. Cryoprecipitated antihemophilic factor is used in patients with hemophilia A to replace factor VIII C. Fifteen percent of hemophiliacs have inhibitors to factor VIII activity. The formula used to calculate dosage of the number of bags of antihemophilic factor for infusion is [(plasma volume in mL × % increase needed in factor VIII)/100]/80. Factor VIII activity is used to monitor therapeutic effect of the infused antihemophilic factor.

Assessment of the Patient During and After the Administration of a Blood Product

The transfusion of a specific blood product is indicated only when that blood product is deficient and the risk of transfusion is outweighed by the potential benefit. RBCs, fresh frozen plasma, cryoprecipitated antihemophilic factor, or platelets should never be used for volume expansion alone. Although a specific laboratory value as the sole basis for a transfusion decision is not appropriate, some general principles should be followed.

The patient's vital signs should be monitored closely during transfusion of a blood product, with close attention paid to temperature elevation, tachycardia, respiratory rate, blood pressure, and mental status. A significant temperature elevation of more than 2°C may indicate bacterial infection or an acute hemolytic reaction. Dyspnea, chest pain, or tachypnea may reflect fluid overload with subsequent pulmonary edema, which may occur especially in at-risk patients or patients given large transfusions over a short period of time. Pulmonary edema may not manifest clinically for up to 24 hours after transfusion. Hypothermia after rapid infusion of large blood volumes may result if the blood is chilled and an approved blood warmer is not used. Finally, metabolic complications may occur when the volume of transfused blood exceeds the patient's normal blood volume. These metabolic complications include hypokalemia or hyperkalemia, citrate toxicity, and ammonia toxicity with possible acidosis or alkalosis. In addition to measurement of circulating electrolytes and renal function, ionized calcium testing and electrocardiogram monitoring may be indicated.

Safety in Banking of Blood and Blood Products

The risks associated with blood transfusions include transmission of viral disease, hemolysis caused by ABO incompatibility, acute lung injury, transmission of bacteria or endotoxins, transmission of parasites, graft versus host disease, alloimmunization, allergic reaction, and immunosuppression.

Infectious Disease

Transmission of infectious disease via transfusion of human blood may be caused by known or unknown organisms. Current screening criteria exclude donors with human immunodeficiency virus (HIV), human T cell leukemia virus (HTLV), hepatitis, and other known agents. Blood is also screened for hepatitis B and C, HIV-1 and -2 including HIV antigen, and HTLV-I and HTLV-II. Although the risk of viral transmission has not been totally eliminated, the risk of transmission of hepatitis C and HIV has been decreased to less than 1:2 to 4

million using newer screening techniques such as nucleic acid testing.

Blood components containing white blood cells are unpredictably prone to contain cytomegalovirus, with up to 70% of donors positive for the disease. Transmission of cytomegalovirus is a concern primarily for immunocompromised patients. Some infectious agents, such as *Babesia* sp., *Bartonella* sp., *Borrelia* sp., *Brucella* sp., Colorado tick fever, *Leishmania* sp., *Parvovirus* sp., plasmodia, rickettsia, *Toxoplasma* sp., malaria, and some trypanosomes, are not screened for because pertinent tests are not available. Theoretically, Creutzfeldt-Jakob disease may also be transmitted through blood products.

Although rare, bacterial contamination may occur and may cause severe effects, including death. In the United States, septic reactions from bacterial contamination of blood components resulted in 77 of 694 transfusion-related deaths reported to the Food and Drug Administration (FDA) from 1985 to 1999. Platelets are the most likely among blood components to be contaminated. Skin flora are the most common pathogens. Endotoxemia may occur as a result of *Yersinia enterocolitica* contamination of RBC products.

Immunologic Complications

Immunologic complications can be acute or delayed and may vary significantly in clinical presentation. Although current cross-matching techniques minimize risk for immune reactions, the incidence has not been completely eliminated.

Hemolytic transfusion reactions usually occur as a result of antigen or ABO incompatibility of transfused RBCs, although nonimmunologic reactions may occur. Patient symptoms include elevated temperature and pulse, chest or back pain, and dyspnea. In unresponsive patients or patients under general anesthesia, disseminated intravascular coagulopathy may be the initial clinical presentation. Laboratory studies helpful to confirm the diagnosis include hemoglobin, serum bilirubin, and direct antiglobulin test. Delayed hemolytic reactions are possible in patients who are alloimmunized, with presentation of symptoms as late as 14 days after transfusion. In contrast to the potentially fatal course of acute hemolytic reactions, delayed hemolytic reactions do not require treatment and are usually benign.

Febrile nonhemolytic reactions and allergic reactions may also occur and are common. Febrile reactions occur in 1% of transfusions and require only antipyretics for palliative treatment. Most allergic reactions are minor with the primary report of urticaria and are adequately treated with antihistamines. Anaphylactic reactions, although rare, may also occur and require aggressive immediate treatment.

A potentially fatal immunologic complication is transfusion-related acute lung injury, which occurs through an unknown mechanism. This condition manifests within 6 hours (most often occurring within 2 hours) of transfusion and requires aggressive pulmonary treatment and maintenance of the hemodynamic status of the patient. Clinical manifestation of transfusion-related acute lung injury is the sudden onset of pulmonary edema, shortness of breath, hypotension unresponsive to intravenous fluids, and hypovolemia with or without fever. Rapid progression of severe hypoxia follows. Results from radiographic evaluation of the chest mimic adult respiratory distress syndrome. Although adult respiratory distress syndrome and transfusion-related acute lung injury are clinically identical, other causes of pulmonary edema should be excluded to confirm the diagnosis of transfusion-related acute lung injury. Risk factors for this condition are unknown and most patients have not been reported to have a previous history of transfusion reaction.

Other delayed immunologic complications are alloimmunization and graft versus host disease. Alloimmunization, which may occur after transfusion of any blood component and is asymptomatic, may result in shortened survival of subsequent blood products transfused, as in immune-mediated platelet destruction. Graft versus host disease may occur when T lymphocytes in the transfused component react to recipient tissue antigens.

Immunosuppression is associated with transfusion of allogeneic blood and is considered to be one of the greatest risks to the recipient. Although the mechanism is not well defined in humans, several studies have demonstrated transfusion of allogeneic blood to be an independent risk factor for development of postoperative infection in patients undergoing uncontaminated orthopaedic surgery. In a multicenter study of patients undergoing total joint arthroplasty, the infection rate in patients who had allogeneic blood transfusions was more than twice that of patients who did not undergo transfusion. Other studies suggest a range of risk of infection to be zero to 10 times greater in patients receiving allogeneic blood.

Trends in Transfusion Medicine

Preoperative assessment of the patient is important in determining the risk for postoperative transfusion. The most significant factor associated with risk of postoperative transfusion is preoperative hemoglobin. Most recent data indicate that a preoperative hemoglobin level of less than 13.0 g/dL carries a substantial increased risk of transfusion. Conversely, a preoperative hemoglobin level of more than 15.0 g/dL has a significantly diminished risk. Duration of surgery, smaller patient size, and female gender have also been associated with increased risk of transfusion in several studies. Preoperative patient assessment for transfusion risk is essential for im-

proved planning and minimizing the use of allogeneic blood. Effective perioperative blood management strategy may include use of agents that increase the preoperative hemoglobin level, agents or techniques that minimize intraoperative and postoperative blood loss, or protocols that allow for reinfusion of salvaged blood.

Recombinant human erythropoietin (EPO), a glycoprotein hormone secreted by the kidneys with a minor hepatic contribution in conditions of extreme stress, is responsible for regulation of erythropoiesis. Data suggest that there is a dose-related relationship between allogeneic transfusion and preoperative administration of EPO such that patients given higher doses of EPO are at lower risk of transfusion when undergoing major orthopaedic operations. Use of EPO is indicated for patients with a preoperative hemoglobin level between 10.0 g/dL and 13.0 g/dL and an expected blood loss of two units of blood. No significant adverse reactions have been associated with preoperative use of EPO in appropriate patients.

Reported use of EPO in athletes as a form of "blood doping" is of concern. The term "blood doping" refers to the use of blood transfusion as an ergogenic aid but has also been applied to use of EPO. Although banned by the International Olympic Committee, illicit use of EPO is difficult to detect. Urine tests that can differentiate recombinant human EPO and endogenous EPO have been described but have not yet been determined to be a reliable screening tool.

Perioperative use of pharmacologic therapies to reduce blood loss is an effective strategy to reduce risk of blood transfusion. Topical use of fibrin tissue sealants has been studied extensively. Fibrin tissue adhesive is composed of variable amounts of thrombin and fibrinogen. According to a 1999 study, use of fibrin tissue adhesive in total knee arthroplasty reduces postoperative blood loss and requirement for blood transfusions from 28% to 17%. Antifibrinolytic agents such as aprotinin, tranexamic acid, and aminocaproic acid have been shown to reduce surgical blood loss. Aprotinin is a naturally occurring broad-spectrum protease peptide that inhibits trypsin, plasmin, tissue kallikreins, and plasmin kallikreins. Although the exact mechanism of action is not known, aprotinin is thought to regulate fibrinolysis, stabilize platelet function, and modulate the intrinsic coagulation pathway. Aprotinin, used commonly in cardiothoracic surgery and liver transplantation, has been shown to have slightly better efficacy than the other antifibrinolytic agents. Aprotinin is also effective in orthopaedic surgery and has been determined to be a safe agent for maintaining hemostasis in total hip arthroplasty. There is a theoretical increased risk of deep venous thrombosis with this agent, however. Desmopressin is a valuable agent to minimize blood loss in patients with hemophilia A and von Willebrand's disease, but has not been shown beneficial in patients without coagulopathy undergoing elective surgery. Recombinant factor VIIa (eptacog alfa) is currently under investigation but preliminary data suggest that it may be effective in reduction of blood loss in surgical patients without coagulopathy.

Acute normovolemic hemodilution is a technique during which whole blood is drawn from the patient before or early in the surgical procedure, usually after initiation of anesthesia, while intravascular volume is maintained with a crystalloid and solutions. Thus, the blood loss during the procedure is diluted and the whole blood removed at the beginning of the procedure is re-infused. Acute normovolemic hemodilution has been shown to be as effective as preoperative autologous blood donation in patients undergoing total hip arthroplasty in the reduction of risk of allogeneic blood transfusion. Hypervolemic hemodilution has been found to be as beneficial as normovolemic hemodilution in one study and has the advantage of being simpler to perform without the need for blood withdrawal. Patients with cardiac disease may not be candidates for either technique.

Intraoperative salvage of shed blood that is spun and washed of contaminants and debris is well established as a means of avoiding blood transfusion. Comparison of different techniques of intraoperative cell salvage such as centrifuge, direct transfusion, and ultrafiltration has shown no difference in transfusion risk in each of these modalities. Cell salvage is generally considered in patients in whom intraoperative blood loss is expected to exceed 1,000 mL. Postoperative blood salvage requires transfusion of unwashed blood from a blood collection device. Several studies have indicated that postoperative blood salvage significantly reduces the risk for postoperative blood transfusion. The safety of this technique is somewhat controversial because there are increased risks of infection by contaminated blood, as well as reports of hyperthermia and hypotension.

Blood Substitutes

The ideal blood substitute would be readily available and without the associated risks of transfusion and transfusion-related infections. Blood alternatives are either plasma expanders or oxygen-based carrier substitutes. Blood volume expanders include crystalloid and colloid replacement. Crystalloid replacement with combinations of saline, lactated Ringer's solution, and glucose solutions are the first line of volume supplementation. Patients who are at risk of excessive intravascular volume overload may tolerate colloid replacement with albumin, dextran, or gelatins.

Oxygen-based carrier substitutes encompass a novel class of therapeutic agents. Hemoglobin-based preparations are either cell free or liposome enclosed as a substrate carrier. The molecules are genetically engineered

human hemoglobin from *Escherichia coli*, salvaged from expired human blood, or purified from bovine blood. The success of first-generation, cell-free preparations was marred by nephrotoxicity and excessive oxygen binding affinity. Some preparations have been discontinued after clinical trials demonstrated increased mortality in trauma patients with hemoglobin substitutes compared with placebo. The second-generation, liposome-based hemoglobin carriers currently demonstrate some promise in preclinical animal studies and phase 2 and 3 clinical trials.

Perfluorocarbon emulsions are another alternative to hemoglobin-based blood products and substitutes. These agents are hydrocarbon analogs substituting fluorine for hydrogen. Perfluorocarbons have 20 to 30 times the oxygen solubility of plasma. Fluosol-DA-20 is currently the only FDA-approved blood substitute. Its use, however, has been associated with hepatosplenomegaly, complement-induced hypertension, and anaphylactoid reaction.

Religious Practices and Transfusion Alternatives

The Jehovah's Witnesses is a growing religious group that originated during the Adventist movement of the 19th century. The Watchtower Bible and Tract Society is the controlling theological organization and has outlined rigid religious doctrine with specific relevance to medical care. Jehovah's Witnesses freely accept medical and surgical care, but most refuse the acceptance of blood and blood products based on their interpretation of the Old Testament. Deviation from this doctrine not only is believed to be a direct spiritual betrayal, but also carries profound social implications with "shunning" and excommunication from church and family.

Judicial precedent protects the sacrosanct position of Jehovah's Witnesses to refuse blood willingly against medical advice. Under the protection of informed consent, the Supreme Court and state courts have ruled repeatedly that the integrity of the medical profession cannot supersede the wishes or religious beliefs of the patient. The American Medical Association has likewise supported physicians and hospitals that provide care of Jehovah's Witnesses who provide informed consent.

Most Jehovah's Witnesses will not accept blood or most blood products, including whole blood, red blood cells, autologous blood donation, platelets, and plasma. Under specific circumstances outlined by the Watchtower Society, however, Jehovah's Witnesses may accept clotting factors, stem cells, bone marrow transplants, and separated plasma proteins of albumin, fibrin, and globulin. Jehovah's Witnesses may also accept dialysis, plasmapheresis, and intraoperative blood salvage where the extracorporeal circulation is uninterrupted. The medical team needs to consult with each patient to determine acceptable alternatives. The Watchtower Society readily provides patient resources through its Hospital Information Society and its regional Hospital Liaison Committees.

The surgical care of Jehovah's Witnesses can be successfully managed using anesthetic and pharmacologic alternatives. Many Jehovah's Witnesses will accept preoperatively the red cell production stimulating factor EPO and white cell stimulators granulocyte-colony stimulating factor and granulocyte-macrophage colony stimulating factor. Jehovah's Witnesses accept the use of fibrin glue as a hemostatic agent intraoperatively and the pharmacologic antifibrinolytics such as aprotinin and tranexamic acid. Proven anesthetic techniques in these patients involve hypotension, hypothermia, and acute normovolemic hemodilution. Intravascular volume can be acceptably maintained with colloid and crystalloid replacement.

With such protocols, major surgery on Jehovah's Witnesses has been successfully performed. The combined literature from cardiac, urologic, and obstetric surgery has demonstrated successful outcomes after major surgery without blood transfusion. Safe outcomes have also been reported after total joint surgery and major spine surgery. A study of 100 Jehovah's Witnesses undergoing total hip replacement reported no deaths, and smaller studies of spinal fusion for scoliosis have also reported success without mortality.

Controversy remains regarding the emergent care of the exsanguinating and obtunded patient and in the care of minors. A 1998 report determined that during a life-threatening emergency when the patient cannot provide informed consent and where there is no valid advance directive, emergency blood transfusions may be given until the patient's condition stabilizes. Interestingly, patients who are unconsciously transfused are not subject to religious sanction or the threat of excommunication. Regarding children, the American Academy of Pediatrics in 1997 stated that the "constitutional guarantees of freedom of religion do not permit children to be harmed through religious practice." Furthermore, an anonymous group of Jehovah's Witnesses called the Associated Jehovah's Witnesses for Reform on Blood Policy have voiced dissent over the religion's official blood policy. Consultation with the hospital ombudsman or ethics committee may be necessary to obtain consent in cases where life-saving transfusion is essential in a juvenile or incompetent patient whose guardian is a Jehovah's Witness.

Autologous Blood Donation: Current Trends

The impetus for the use of preoperative autologous blood donation in perioperative blood management in orthopaedic surgery is to avoid the major risks of allogeneic transfusions, especially the transmission of disease and immune-mediated transfusion reactions. The potential risk of transfusion error caused by clerical issues still exists with the use of preoperative autologous blood donation, but the major disadvantage is the cost related to this method. The high cost of preoperative autologous blood donation is magnified by the significant wastage of blood that occurs with preoperative autologous blood donation. Rates of discarded blood have been reported to be as high as 83% of units, with most studies demonstrating wastage in the 50% range. Better identification of patients likely to require transfusion before embarking on preoperative autologous blood donation is required to reduce the waste associated with this technique.

Most studies indicate that preoperative autologous blood donation is an effective way to minimize risk of allogeneic transfusion and lend support for its continued use. One concern related to preoperative autologous blood donation is donation-induced preoperative anemia. Blood donations within 2 weeks of surgery are more likely to result in preoperative anemia because of an insufficient erythropoietic response. A recent study of total joint arthroplasty patients presented convincing data that the use of EPO preoperatively in patients also undergoing preoperative autologous blood donation significantly decreased the allogeneic transfusion rate in patients either receiving EPO or using preoperative autologous blood donation alone. Patients with a hemoglobin level less than 10.0 g/dL are not considered candidates for preoperative autologous blood donation. Transfusion of autologous blood continues to be the most commonly used alternative to allogeneic transfusion.

Annotated Bibliography

Allain JP: Transfusion risks of yesterday and of today. *Transfus Clin Biol* 2003;10:1-5.

Improved screening techniques decrease risk of disease transmission with transfusion but may not be cost effective.

Bezwada HP, Nazarian DG, Henry DH, Booth RE: Preoperative use of recombinant human erythropoietin before total joint arthroplasty. *J Bone Joint Surg Am* 2003; 85:1795-1800.

In this prospective randomized study, the efficacy of erythropoietin and autologous blood in combination was demonstrated to have the lowest risk of allogeneic blood transfusion.

Cable R, Carlson B, Chambers L, et al (eds): *Practice Guidelines for Blood Transfusion: A Compilation From Recent Peer-Reviewed Literature.* Washington, DC, American National Red Cross, 2002, pp 1-48.

A thorough review of blood products, indications, and risks associated with transfusion is presented.

Dodd RY: Bacterial contamination and transfusion safety: Experience in the United States. *Transfus Clin Biol* 2003;10:6-9.

Septic transfusion reactions from 1985-1999 are reviewed.

Salido JA, Marin LA, Gomez LA, Zorrilla P, Martinez C: Preoperative hemoglobin levels and the need for transfusion after prosthetic hip and knee surgery: Analysis of predictive factors. *J Bone Joint Surg Am* 2002;84: 216-220.

The most important predictive factor related to risk of postoperative transfusion is preoperative hemoglobin. Duration of surgery, gender, and patient size were also predictive factors.

Sullivan MT, McCullough J, Schreiber GB, Wallace EL: Blood collection and transfusion in the United States in 1997. *Transfusion* 2002;42:1253-1260.

A review of supply and demand of blood products in 1994 and 1997 for comparison.

Classic Bibliography

Anders MJ, Lifeso RM, Landis M, Mikulsky J, Meinking C, McCracken KS: Effect of preoperative donation of autologous blood on deep-vein thrombosis following total joint arthroplasty of the hip or knee. *J Bone Joint Surg Am* 1996;78:574-580.

Bierbaum BE, Callaghan JJ, Galante JO, Rubash HE, Tooms RE, Welch RB: An analysis of blood management in patients having a total hip or knee arthroplasty. *J Bone Joint Surg Am* 1999;81:2-10.

Faris PM, Ritter MA, Abels RI: The effects of recombinant human erythropoietin on perioperative transfusion requirements in patients having a major orthopaedic operation: The American Erythropoietin Study Group. *J Bone Joint Surg Am* 1996;78:62-72.

Feagin BG, Wong CJ, Kirkley A, et al: Erythropoietin with iron supplementation to prevent allogeneic blood transfusion in total hip joint arthroplasty: A randomized, controlled trial. *Ann Intern Med* 2000;133:845-854.

Goodnough LT, Despotis GJ, Merkel K, Monk TG: A randomized trial comparing acute normovolemic hemodilution and preoperative autologous blood donation in total hip arthroplasty. *Transfusion* 2000;40:1054-1057.

Grosvenor D, Goyal V, Goodman S: Efficacy of postoperative blood salvage following total hip arthroplasty in

patients with and without deposited autologous units. *J Bone Joint Surg Am* 2000;82:951-954.

Hatzidakis AM, Mendlick R, McKillip T, Reddy RL, Garvin KL: Preoperative autologous donation for total joint arthroplasty: An analysis of risk factors for allogeneic transfusion. *J Bone Joint Surg Am* 2000;82:89-100.

Levy O, Martinowitz U, Oran A, Tauber C, Horoszowski H: The use of fibrin tissue adhesive to reduce blood loss and the need for blood transfusion after total knee arthroplasty. *J Bone Joint Surg Am* 1999;81:1580-1588.

Lundberg GD: Practice parameter for the use of fresh-frozen plasma, cryoprecipitate, and platelets. *JAMA* 1994;271:777-781.

Migden DR. Braen GR: The Jehovah's Witness blood refusal card: Ethical and medicolegal considerations for emergency physicians. *Acad Emerg Med* 1998;5:815-824.

Murkin JM, Haig GM, Beer KJ, et al: Aprotinin decreases exposure to allogeneic blood during primary unilateral total hip arthroplasty. *J Bone Joint Surg Am* 2000;82:675-684.

NIH Consensus Statement available on perioperative red cell transfusion. *Am J Public Health* 1988;78:1588.

Practice guidelines for blood component therapy: A report by the American Society of Anesthesiologists Task Force on Blood Component Therary. *Anesthesiology* 1996;84:732-747.

Religious objections to medical care: American Academy of Pediatrics Committee on Bioethics. *Pediatrics* 1997;99:279-281.

Simon TL, Alverson DC: AuBuchon J, et al: Practice parameter for the use of red blood cell transfusions: Developed by the Red Blood Cell Administration Practice Guideline Development Task Force of the College of American Pathologists. *Arch Pathol Lab Med* 1998;122: 130-138.

Sparling EA, Nelson CL, Lavender R, Smith J: The use of erythropoietin in the management of Jehovah's Witnesses who have revision total hip arthroplasty. *J Bone Joint Surg Am* 1996;78:1548-1552.

Spence RK: Surgical red blood cell transfusion practice policies. *Am J Surg* 1995;170(suppl 6A):3S-15S.

Section 3

Systemic Disorders

Section Editors:
Kristin L. Carroll, MD
Brian K. Kwon, MD

Chapter **18**

Bone Metabolism and Metabolic Bone Disease

Mary A. Murray, MD

Introduction

Osteoporosis is a major public health care issue. In the United States, the cost of fracture treatment is estimated at $10 to $15 billion annually. Although bone mineral density (BMD) is the current measure of fracture risk, it is becoming evident that there is much that remains to be learned about predicting fracture occurrence. BMD is not the sole determinant of fracture risk—anatomic considerations, ethnicity, and lifestyle all are contributing factors.

Age-related bone loss is universal; therefore, factors that compromise the ability to attain peak bone mass in young adult life increase the likelihood of osteoporosis with aging. Osteoporosis may represent one of several adult diseases in which intervention during the pediatric and adolescent years may alter the course of the disease. Strategies to increase peak bone mass may include maximizing calcium and vitamin D intake, minimizing the use of drugs that inhibit normal bone growth and formation, encouraging weight-bearing activities, and ensuring normal sex steroid exposure. Various professional societies have recently established working groups whose goals are to better characterize and understand pediatric and adolescent bone health and formation and their effects on adult bone health.

Basic Science Aspects of Bone Metabolism

The three basic functions of bone are (1) mechanical support and locomotion, (2) protection of the internal organs, and (3) metabolic activities to maintain calcium homeostasis. Bone is responsive to hormonal signals at all stages of life. The cellular constituents that mediate hormonal signals within the bone are osteoblasts and osteoclasts.

Osteoblasts are derived from a mesenchymal cell lineage and are mainly responsible for synthesizing the organic, nonmineralized bone matrix. They are cuboidal cells aligned in layers along the osteoid and possess features consistent with protein-producing and -secreting cells. Osteoblasts differentiate under the influence of growth factors including fibroblast growth factor (FGF)

and bone morphogenetic proteins. They synthesize and secrete type I collagen and other matrix proteins. Osteoblasts contain receptors for most of the systemic mediators of bone remodeling (parathyroid hormone [PTH], sex steroids, glucocorticoids, 1, 25-dihydroxyvitamin D_3 [$1,25(OH)_2D_3$], insulin, and thyroid hormone) as well as local factors such as cytokines and interleukins. Osteoblasts can stimulate osteoclastogenesis by secretion of factors that act in a paracrine manner, such as colony-stimulating factor-1, osteoprotegerin, and receptor activator of nuclear factor-kappaB ligand (RANKL). A membrane rich in alkaline phosphatase is the hallmark of the osteoblast cell. Alkaline phosphatase is released into the serum and is elevated at times of increased bone formation (such as pubertal growth acceleration). At the end of its life cycle, an osteoblast becomes either a flat lining cell or an osteocyte.

Osteocytes are differentiated osteoblasts that are incorporated into the bone matrix during bone formation. They possess long cytoplasmic arms that provide a mechanism for intercellular communication. Osteocytes possess cell surface receptors for PTH and respond to receptor binding with a release of calcium from the bone into the circulation. Osteocytes also respond to mechanical signals and transfer stress and strain indices to surrounding cells to effect bone remodeling. Mechanical stimulation has been shown to increase the production of prostaglandin E_2 by cells of the osteoblastic lineage; this substance stimulates both bone formation and bone resorption.

Osteoclasts are large, multinucleated giant cells formed by fusion of mononuclear cells; they are responsible for bone resorption. They are derived from hematopoietic cells related to monocyte/macrophage lineages and are found within Howship's lacunae in contact with calcified bone. Osteoclasts have a ruffled border surrounded by a clear zone (ring of actin) that attaches the cell to the bone surface and seals off the resorption compartment. Attachment is accomplished through integrin receptors that bind to specific matrix proteins in response to specific signaling molecules. Osteoclasts express high levels of tartrate-resistant acid phosphate and

Table 1 | Factors That Influence Renal Resorption of Calcium

Factors That Increase Renal Calcium Resorption	Factors That Decrease Renal Calcium Resorption
PTH	Increased sodium intake
PTH-related peptide	Increased calcium intake
1,25-dihydroxyvitamin D	Metabolic acidosis
Calcitonin	Phosphate depletion
Increased phosphate intake	Glucocorticoids
Chronic thiazide diuretic use	Furosemide (loop diuretics)
	Cyclosporin A

cathepsin K through the ruffled border. The bone resorption compartment contains lysosomal enzymes and the bony substrate in acidic pH. The acidic pH causes dissolution of hydroxyapatite crystals; the lysosomal enzymes digest matrix proteins resulting in resorption of bone within the attachment site of the osteoclast.

Hormonal Regulation of Cell Differentiation
Calcium and Phosphorus Metabolism

Calcium is important in regulating muscle contraction, coagulation, intracellular signal transduction, and control of cell membrane potentials. Calcium balance is regulated by intestinal absorption of dietary intake, excretion by the kidney, and storage in the skeleton. Normal serum calcium levels are tightly regulated with a normal range of 8.5 to 10 mg/dL (2.2 to 2.5 mmol/L). In the pediatric population calcium levels reach a nadir at 1 week of age (range, 7.5 to 10 mg/dL, 1.9 to 2.5 mmol/L) and then increase to a slightly higher level than the normal adult range (range, 9.0 to 11.0 mg/dL, 2.3 to 2.8 mmol/L). In the circulation, calcium exists approximately equally in the free (ionized) form and the protein-bound form (the major binding protein is albumin). A small portion is bound to anions, such as phosphate. The skeleton acts as a reservoir for calcium that can be metabolized to maintain circulating concentrations.

Dietary calcium absorption in the intestines occurs in the duodenum and the jejunum and is a function of active, saturable transport regulated by vitamin D and passive, gradient dependent transport. Calcium absorption is regulated by $1,25(OH)_2D$ concentration and by calcium intake. Both increased calcium intake and increased $1,25(OH)_2D$ serum concentrations act to increase intestinal calcium absorption. In an average adult, calcium loss in the stool exceeds calcium absorption if calcium intake is less than 200 mg/day (5 mmol/day). To maintain calcium balance, an average adult must consume more than 400 mg/day (10 mmol/day). As calcium intake increases, the efficiency of absorption de-

creases such that net intestinal absorption tends to plateau at about 300 mg/day when intake exceeds about 1,000 mg/day (25 mmol/day); however, there is wide variability in net absorption at higher calcium intake that probably reflects differences in active transport rather than passive diffusion. The activated form of vitamin D, $1,25(OH)_2D$, regulates active transport of calcium in the intestine. Elevated concentrations act to increase the intestinal absorption at all calcium intake levels.

The kidney also regulates calcium balance. To maintain net calcium balance, the renal tubules must resorb 98% of the filtered calcium. Approximately 70% of the filtered calcium is resorbed in the proximal tubule primarily via passive diffusion. About 20% of calcium resorption takes place in the thick ascending loop of Henle driven by positive voltage in the lumen generated by the Na-K-2Cl transporter. The absorption in this portion of the kidney is impaired by loop diuretics such as furosemide. A calcium-sensing receptor (CaSR) along the basolateral surface of the cells responds to alterations in the peritubular concentration of calcium. Some paracellular transport takes place in the tight junctions via the protein paracellin-1. Remaining resorption occurs in the distal convoluted tubule, which is the major site for regulation of calcium excretion; here calcium enters the cytosol via the renal epithelial calcium channel down an electrical and chemical gradient. It is then shuttled through the cytoplasm bound to calbindin-D_{28K}, a vitamin D-dependent protein, without altering the intracellular free calcium concentration. At the basolateral membrane, calcium is actively transported across the large chemical gradient to the interstitium by a magnesium-dependent adenosine triphosphatase.

Various factors influence the renal resorption of calcium (Table 1). Genetic mutations that alter renal tubular handling of calcium have been described and some have been localized to the proteins involved in the transport of calcium through the renal cells.

Phosphorus also is necessary for adequate mineralization of bone; approximately 85% is present in crystalized form in the skeleton. The remaining 15% is present largely in extracellular fluid and intracellular phosphorylated intermediates. Phosphorylated intermediates are important in multiple processes of intermediary metabolism including the production of intracellular energy and intracellular signaling. Absorption is dependent on passive diffusion and active transport; the serum concentration is less tightly regulated than is calcium concentration. Serum concentrations range between 2.7 to 4.5 mg/dL (0.81 to 1.45 mmol/L) in adults; concentrations are higher in infants and young children and decrease by late adolescence to normal adult levels. Passive transport is directly related to the intraluminal concentration of phosphate after eating.

Phosphate absorption is decreased in the vitamin D-deficient individual. Phosphorus resorption takes place primarily in the proximal tubule (85%) against an electrochemical gradient. Three sodium gradient-dependent phosphate transporters have been described (Npt1, Npt2, and Npt3). Npt2 is highly regulated and responsible for most phosphorus transport. FGF-23 has been identified as a regulator of Npt2. The *PHEX* gene product metabolizes FGF-23 and mutations in the *PHEX* gene can cause hypophosphatemia because of the inability to metabolize FGF-23 (X-linked hypophosphatemic rickets).

Hormonal Regulation of Calcium and Phosphorus Metabolism

Parathyroid Hormone

The principal regulators of calcium metabolism are PTH and vitamin D. PTH acts in the bone to stimulate the release of calcium and phosphorus into the circulation and in the renal tubules to increase the resorption of calcium and the excretion of phosphorus. It also increases the 1-α hydroxylase activity, thereby raising the concentration of $1,25(OH)_2D$, which acts to enhance the intestinal absorption of calcium and phosphorus.

The major physiologic regulator of PTH secretion is the extracellular calcium concentration. Low calcium concentrations increase, and high calcium concentrations decrease the PTH secretory rate, PTH gene expression, and parathyroid cell proliferation. The CaSR appears to be the principal mediator of calcium concentration and PTH response. The CaSR is a G-protein coupled receptor; binding activates several intracellular signaling pathways including protein kinase C and inositol triphosphate, which increase cytosolic calcium concentrations and several mitogen-activated protein kinases. These changes modulate the expression of genes controlling cell proliferation, differentiation, and apoptosis. CaSR also stimulates the influx of extracellular calcium ions through a mechanism that is not yet fully understood. In the parathyroid gland, CaSR has three key regulatory actions: PTH secretion, PTH gene expression, and cell proliferation. Mouse gene knockout studies and human gene mutations both have shown the key role of CaSR in the regulation of PTH. A drop in serum calcium concentration, perceived by the CaSR, is translated into a rapid release (in seconds) of PTH, a decreased intracellular PTH degradation rate that increases the amount of bioavailable PTH for release (in minutes), increased transcription of the PTH gene (in hours to days) and eventually increased proliferation of parathyroid cells (in days to weeks).

PTH has complex actions in bone with a net result that may be either anabolic or catabolic. Chronic PTH exposure leads to a catabolic state; increased numbers of osteoclasts and osteoclast activity increase degradation of bone and the release of calcium, phosphate, and matrix proteins into the circulation. PTH stimulates expression of RANKL on the cell surfaces of osteoblasts, and stimulates synthesis of macrophage colony-stimulating factor, which act together to stimulate maturation of osteoclasts. PTH also inhibits the expression of osteoprotegerin, a decoy protein that blocks the effect of RANKL; this action further increases osteoclastogenesis and the activity of mature osteoclasts. Intermittent PTH exposure, however, appears to result in increased bone remodeling and a net increase in trabecular bone. The mechanisms by which PTH increases bone formation are not fully understood. PTH increases the number of osteoblasts and may act by increasing local concentrations of growth factors, such as insulin-like growth factor-I (IGF-I) and FGFs, which then exert paracrine actions on the bone to stimulate growth and new bone formation. This observation of the anabolic actions of PTH may lead to new therapies for the treatment of osteoporosis.

Vitamin D

Vitamin D is a classic steroid hormone that is derived from cholesterol and undergoes hydroxylation in the liver and kidney to its biologically active form, $1,25(OH)_2D$. The primary role of vitamin D is to maintain calcium levels within the normal range by increasing intestinal absorption of calcium and by increasing maturation of osteoclasts to mobilize calcium from the bone when needed. In addition, vitamin D has effects on cell differentiation and proliferation and on the immune system. It enhances insulin secretion and downregulates the renin-angiotensin system. Vitamin D is produced in the skin during exposure to sunlight (ultraviolet B, 290 to 315 nm) and absorbed from dietary intake. The production of vitamin D by sunlight exposure is severely impaired by the use of sunscreens. Natural dietary sources of vitamin D are limited to oily fish such as mackerel and salmon. Dietary vitamin D is also available from fortified foods such as milk and orange juice, and from multivitamins. A recent increase in the incidence of rickets in children has led the American Academy of Pediatrics to release new recommendations for the intake of vitamin D in infants.

Sex Steroids/Estrogen

Adolescence is a time of rapid increase in skeletal mass resulting from the concurrent release of sex steroids and an increase in the growth hormone secretory rate. Up to 25% of peak bone mass is accumulated during the peak of pubertal growth. At peak height velocity, adolescents have reached 90% of adult height but only 57% of peak bone mass. Over the next several years, the bone density increases.

Adult women, at the end of the reproductive life cycle, experience rapid loss of bone mass associated with menopause and declining estrogen production. Bone loss also occurs in men, although at a slower rate, as testosterone production declines. Evidence suggests that it is the circulating estradiol concentration in men that is most correlated with bone loss. Both osteoblasts and osteoclasts possess estrogen receptors. Estrogen promotes the differentiation of osteoblasts and suppresses osteoclast activity in part by increasing osteoclast apoptosis. Estrogen may also act through the stromal cells in the bone marrow to decrease cytokine production, which decreases osteoclast recruitment.

In the elderly population, growth hormone secretion also declines and may contribute to decreased bone mineralization. In response to decreased growth hormone levels, IGF-I concentration is reduced. The magnitude of the decrease of human growth hormone and IGF-I on bone loss is unclear. Glucocorticoids inhibit bone formation by shortening osteoblast lifespan via a combination of decreased replication and increased apoptosis and decreased transcription of type I collagen, osteocalcin, and other matrix proteins. Glucocorticoids suppress IGF-I and insulin-like growth factor binding protein expression in osteoblasts. IGF-I and insulin-like growth factor binding protein act in a paracrine manner to increase bone formation. Glucocorticoids increase bone resorption, decrease sex steroid concentrations, and inhibit calcium absorption in the intestine. All of these factors result in increased bone resorption and subsequent osteoporosis.

Metabolic Bone Disease

Bone formation and bone resorption pathways are tightly coupled. When there is a disruption in either component of bone formation or bone resorption, the result is metabolic bone disease. Depending on the nature of the disturbance, either bone formation or bone resorption will predominate, resulting in increased or decreased bone formation.

Osteoporosis

Osteoporosis is a global problem that is becoming more prevalent with the increasing age of the population. The major clinical outcome of osteoporosis is fracture, but multiple factors contribute to fracture risk. The most readily available and best standarized clinical measure of osteoporosis is the BMD measurement; BMD is strongly correlated with bone strength and is a predictor of fracture risk. The World Health Organization has defined osteopenia and osteoporosis based on BMD values, which are defined in adult women by a T score. A T score of 0 is equal to the mean for age. A T score of –1.0 to –2.5 defines osteopenia, and a T score of less than –2.5 defines osteoporosis. Osteoporosis and os-

teopenia can be defined for both the lumbar spine and for the femoral neck. There are inherent limitations in BMD measurements that limit their applicability in defining standards of osteopenia and osteoporosis in adults, and even more so in pediatric patients. Dual-energy x-ray absorptiometry (DEXA) scans interpret the bone density unicompartmentally with no ability to evaluate the cortical density separately from the trabecular density, although each may respond differently to disease state or therapy. Response of one compartment rather than another could potentially alter outcomes. A DEXA scan provides limited information on bone integrity and is unlikely to impart the complete status of bone health.

In postmenopausal women, the mainstay of treatment of osteoporosis has been hormone replacement therapy (HRT) using an estrogen preparation. Because bone loss resumes when estrogen therapy is stopped, it was believed by some physicians that therapy should be lifelong. Recently that recommendation has been questioned by the results of the Women's Health Initiative. This long-term study was designed to compare treatment of postmenopausal women with an estrogen and progestin combination arm, an unopposed estrogen arm, and a placebo arm; outcome measures were incidence of colorectal cancer, breast cancer, heart disease, and fractures. After 5 years, the study arm using the estrogen and progestin combination was terminated early when an interim analysis indicated evidence of an increased risk for breast cancer. This finding, along with evidence of some increased risk for cardiovascular disease, stroke, and pulmonary embolism, outweighed the benefits of a reduced risk for fractures and the possible benefits in preventing colorectal cancer. The study arm using estrogen alone is continuing. The study has significant limitations, but it is likely to discourage some women from using postmenopausal HRT.

Authors of a recent meta-analysis of pooled results from randomized studies concluded that multiple therapies, including vitamin D, calcitonin, raloxifene, and alendronate decrease the incidence of vertebral fractures. Based on the quality of the available studies, the magnitude of the treatment effects, the narrow confidence intervals, and the consistent positive results throughout each study, the authors of this meta-analysis concluded that the evidence most strongly supports the effect of alendronate and risedronate for reducing vertebral fractures; the effects of other agents remain unclear. The data on HRT indicate a confidence interval that includes a possible increase in risk for vertebral fractures. It has been shown that HRT increases BMD; studies of longer duration may ultimately prove that it also decreases the incidence of vertebral fractures. Large randomized controlled studies, such as the Women's Health Initiative, are needed to definitively determine the benefit and risk/benefit ratio. Most studies that have shown an impact for HRT have been case controlled or cohort studies.

Pediatric Bone Health

Osteoporosis has been considered to be a disease of adulthood; however, there is increasing evidence that the roots of osteoporosis begin much earlier in life. Osteoporosis is often assumed to be the result of bone loss in the older patient, however, a patient who does not attain optimal bone mass is at increased risk for accelerated bone loss and premature osteoporosis. Peak bone mass is attained as a result of bone mass acquisition during childhood and adolescence. Therefore, any factors that inhibit the maximal acquisition of bone mass can contribute to lower peak bone mass and the subsequent development of osteoporosis and its inherent health consequences. Attainment of peak bone mass is a function of intrinsic, unalterable factors such race, gender, and genetics, and extrinsic or alterable factors such as diet, participation in weight-bearing exercise, the effects of illness, and the use of certain medications.

It is more difficult to assess bone health in children than in adults because there is limited information about normal or average bone mass acquisition and virtually no data correlating fracture incidence with BMD. Fracture incidence during childhood may not be the correct end point to assess bone health. The DEXA scan is more difficult to interpret in children and adolescents because diagnostic standards developed by the World Health Organization are based on adult bone mass and are not applicable to pediatric and adolescent patients, who are still acquiring bone. For the pediatric and adolescent patient, it is crucial to have the DEXA scan done on a machine that has a pediatric software database and to have the scan interpreted by a health professional experienced with pediatric scans. Pediatric BMD measurements are subject to many variables not encountered in the adult population. During puberty, there is a substantial increase in skeletal mass and mineralization exerted by the growth stimulating effects of the sex steroids (estrogen and testosterone) and by growth hormone. The timing of peak growth velocity and peak bone mass is different in males and females with peak growth of the skeleton preceding the attainment of peak bone mass. Pubertal status has a major effect on bone mineralization; it may be more appropriate to compare patients by pubertal stage (Tanner stage) rather than by chronologic age. Some centers with large databases can provide that information.

All pediatric DEXA scans must be interpreted with a Z score rather than a T score. The T score relates the patient's BMD measurement with an adult reference standard. The Z score relates the patient's BMD to age- and gender-matched controls. The use of adult reference data to interpret pediatric scans will result in an underestimate of BMD, leading to misdiagnosis of osteoporosis and osteopenia. Incorrect diagnoses of these conditions in children and teens may lead to excessive parental concern, increased health care expenditures, and unnecessary therapy. Unnecessary restrictions on patient activity could prove detrimental rather than helpful.

The lack of diagnostic criteria for osteoporosis is a major limitation to the usefulness of DEXA data in the pediatric population. Currently, BMD data will allow comparison of a pediatric patient with an age-matched, gender-matched, and possibly a pubertal stage-matched average; however, this comparison does not allow for the prediction of fracture risk. Studies that correlate BMD with fracture incidence in the pediatric population are ongoing, but data are not yet available.

Serum and urine markers of bone formation and resorption have been used in adult patients to determine the etiology of bone loss and to follow up on treatment effectiveness (Table 2); however, the data are of limited use in the pediatric and adolescent populations. Reference ranges must be determined for age and pubertal status and any values must be interpreted with knowledge of the patient's pubertal status. The fact that peak growth and bone mineral acquisition correlates with increased bone turnover and net bone formation, should be reflected in the markers of bone metabolism and will alter the reference range for a child of any age. As better standards are developed, bone markers in conjunction with an imaging modality may help to identify children with bone mass acquisition deficiencies and assist in determining therapeutic plans.

Rickets

Rickets is a disease of growing bone resulting in decreased mineralization of new bone, which can ultimately limit peak bone mass if not recognized and treated. The deficiencies that cause rickets are present long before physical signs are evident. Rickets easily can be diagnosed with a radiograph of the wrist or knee and laboratory evaluation, which is essential to determine the etiology of the disease (Tables 3 and 4).

In the past several years, a resurgence of nutritional rickets has become evident. In response to this resurgence, the American Academy of Pediatrics published new guidelines in 2003 for the intake of vitamin D in infants and children (Table 5). The increase in the incidence of rickets is probably a consequence of several factors. (1) There has been an increased emphasis on breastfeeding infants. Human breast milk typically has a low concentration of vitamin D (< 136 IU/L), which is limited even with maternal supplementation. Also, many women do not maintain an adequate intake of calcium and vitamin D during lactation. (2) Over the years, it

Table 2 | Markers of Bone Metabolism Measurable in Serum and Urine

Bone Formation Markers

Alkaline phosphatase	Serum	Most extensively used; 80% of activity is derived from bone
Osteocalcin	Serum	Available from specialized reference laboratories; must use age-appropriate reference ranges for the pediatric population
Bone-specific alkaline phosphatase	Serum	Available from specialized reference laboratories
Procollagen type I carboxyterminal propeptide	Serum	Cleavage product from formation of type I collagen; other sources of type I collagen besides bone hamper test specificity
Procollagen type I amino-terminal propeptide	Serum	Cleavage product from formation of type I collagen; other sources of type I collagen besides bone hamper test specificity

Bone Resorption Markers

Tartrate-resistant acid phosphatase	Serum	Produced by osteoclasts; assay available in reference laboratories; data on normal values are scarce
Collagen type I cross-linked C-telopeptide	Serum	Fragment from cross-linking peptides within collagen; assay available in reference laboratories, data on normal values are scarce
Hydroxyproline	Urine	Amino acid component of collagen; specificity is hindered by wide variation in day-to-day values and effects from dietary sources
Pyridinoline/deoxypyridinoline	Urine	Cross-linking peptides within collagen; good specificity; standard is to assay on first morning void
Collagen type I cross-linked N-telopeptide	Urine	Fragment from cross-linking peptides within collagen; good specificity; values strongly affected by puberty, standard is to assay on second morning void

Table 3 | Laboratory Diagnosis of Rickets

	Ca++	Phosphorus	Alkaline Phosphorus	PTH	25-D	1,25-D
Nutritional	normal/low	normal/low	high	high	low	normal/low
Hypophosphatemic (x-linked)	normal	low	high	normal	normal	normal
VDDR I (1-α hydroxylase deficiency)	low	normal	high	high	normal	low
VDDR II (1,25 D receptor defect)	low	normal	high	high	normal	high

VDDR = vitamin D-dependent rickets

was assumed that normal casual sunlight exposure in older children and adolescents ensured adequate vitamin D production (especially in areas of the country that enjoy many days of bright sunlight throughout the year). However, it is difficult to quantify the amount of sunlight exposure of any individual and to determine the amount of sunlight necessary to ensure adequate vitamin D production. This situation is further complicated by the American Academy of Pediatrics' recommendation for sunscreen use on children and for the limitation of sunlight exposure in very young children to decrease the risk of skin cancer. The use of sunscreens markedly decreases skin production of vitamin D; application of a 5% *p*-aminobenzoic acid solution (sun protection factor 8) blocks over 95% of the conversion of 7-dehydrocholesterol to previtamin D in the skin. Even in regions with high amounts of sunlight, it is likely that the proper use of sunscreens will markedly reduce the endogenous production of vitamin D in children. (3) Dietary calcium deficiency may contribute to the increase in the number of observed cases of rickets. Many children who are breast fed for most of the first year of life are being weaned from breast milk to nondairy drinks; many children drink little or no milk and some consume virtually no dairy products. Older toddlers are at risk for developing rickets because of inadequate calcium intake compounded by marginal vitamin D status. Surveys of children and teens have repeatedly documented calcium intake of less than 50% of the American Dietetic Association guidelines (Table 6).

Table 4 | Laboratory Tests to Evaluate Suspected Rickets

Assay/Test	Purpose
Calcium, phosphorus	Assess for deficiency
Alkaline phosphatase	High level indicates increased bone turnover
Blood urea nitrogen, creatinine, bicarbonate	Evaluate renal function
$25(OH)D$, $1,25(OH)_2D$	Assess for deficiency and vitamin D metabolism
PTH	Evaluate PTH response
Urine calcium: creatinine ratio	Rule out hypercalciuria; young child has higher levels than does older child or adult (normal values < 0.25 in older child or adult)
Tubular resorption of phosphorus	Assess for renal phosphorus wasting

Table 5 | The 2003 American Academy of Pediatrics Guidelines for Vitamin D Intake for Infants and Children

The ingestion of 200 IU of vitamin D per day is recommended for healthy infants and children

A supplement of 200 IU of vitamin D per day is recommended for:

All breastfed infants unless they are weaned to at least 500 mL per day of vitamin-D fortified formula or milk

All nonbreastfed infants who are ingesting less than 500 mL per day of vitamin-D fortified formula or milk

Children and adolescents who do not get regular exposure to sunlight and who do not ingest at least 500 mL per day of vitaminD- fortified milk

Table 6 | Recommendations for Daily Calcium Intake

Age Range (years)	Adequate Intake* (mg/d)	Age Range (years)	Recommended Intake[†] (mg/d)
0.0 to 0.5	210	0.0 to 0.5	400
0.5 to 1.0	270	0.5 to 1.0	600
1.0 to 3.0	500	1.0 to 5.0	800
4.0 to 8.0	800	6.0 to 10.0	800 to 1,200
9.0 to 13.0	1,300	11.0 to 18.0	1,200 to 1,500
14.0 to 18.0	1,300		

*Institute of Medicine

[†] National Institutes of Health Guidelines

The American Academy of Pediatrics' guidelines on vitamin D intake in infants and children (Table 5) are designed for these patients to achieve a serum concentration of vitamin D greater than 11 ng/mL. This is a conservative target and was determined from studies that evaluated the dosage required to prevent rickets. Traditionally, serum levels or 10 to 12 ng/mL have been considered adequate for sufficient vitamin D stores; however, most endocrinologists now recommend serum levels of at least 15 to 20 ng/mL. Based on serum vitamin D levels and studies on the use of supplemental vitamin D, an intake of 300 to 400 IU/day is probably necessary to maximize bone health in the absence of sunlight. In the presence of sunlight, the requirement for dietary vitamin D may be lower. Nutritional rickets is a preventable disease. The cost of prevention is low and the safety profile of vitamin D is good.

Renal Osteodystrophy

Impaired renal function results in disordered mineral metabolism that is manifested in multiple tissues. Renal osteodystrophy includes multiple disorders of bone metabolism associated with chronic renal disease. Chronic renal disease leads to altered PTH synthesis and secretion, parathyroid gland hyperplasia, abnormal calcium and vitamin D metabolism, chronic acidosis, and inhibition of growth hormone action. All of these effects alter bone metabolism and manifest in renal bone diseases. The spectrum of renal bone disease includes both increased and decreased turnover states. In general, high turnover states are associated with increased PTH levels and low turnover states with normal or low PTH levels. The definitive method for determining the type of renal disease is bone histology.

High turnover renal bone disease is a consequence of sustained high PTH levels. Secondary hyperparathy-roidism is a result of several factors including hypocalcemia and hyperphosphatemia, decreased $1,25(OH)_2D$ production by the kidney, skeletal resistance to PTH action, altered PTH gene transcription, and reduced expression of CaSR and vitamin D receptors on the parathyroid cells. With sustained elevation of serum PTH levels, osteoblastic and osteoclastic activity in bone increases and results in increased bone turnover.

Low turnover bone disease occurs when the PTH level is normal or minimally elevated. This disease had previously been associated with aluminum toxicity. Currently, low turnover bone disease is more likely to be associated with diabetes, corticosteroid use, or advanced age. The recent use of large doses of oral calcium and active vitamin D analogs can lead to lowered PTH levels and decreased stimulus for bone turnover; this situation probably accounts for the increase in adynamic disease, which is histologically evidenced by increased osteoid and undermineralized bone collagen. The long-term consequences of low turnover renal osteodystrophy are unknown.

Hyperparathyroidism

Hyperparathyroidism is characterized by hypercalcemia resulting from excessive PTH secretion. The normal feedback control of PTH secretion is disrupted, leading to increased secretion that is not normally responsive to an increased calcium concentration. Most patients (80%) with primary hyperparathyroidism have solitary adenoma in one parathyroid gland. In about 15% of patients, hyperparathyroidism is a consequence of four-gland hyperplasia, which can occur in conjunction with multiple endocrine neoplasia type 1 or type 2. Very rarely (in < 1% of patients), it is a result of parathyroid carcinoma. The exact molecular basis for primary hyperparathyroidism is unknown. Familial causes of hyperparathyroidism include multiple endocrine neoplasias (1 and 2A). Germline mutations in a nuclear protein tumor suppressor gene encoded on chromosome 11 have been described in patients with both familial and sporadic multiple endocrine neoplasm 1. Multiple endocrine neoplasm 2 is caused by mutations in the *RET* proto-oncogene.

Primary hyperparathyroidism is treated by removal of the abnormal parathyroid tissue. Medical management is more difficult but bisphosphonates can be used to acutely lower serum calcium levels. Over the long course, bisphosphonates may help protect bone density in patients with hyperparathyroidism who cannot have or choose not to have surgery.

Osteopetrosis

Osteopetrosis (marble bone disease) is a disorder characterized by increased bone mass. It can result from a defect in a variety of genes or gene products, but the final common pathway is a failure of osteoclast mediated bone resorption.

Infantile osteopetrosis is evident in infancy and is rapidly fatal. Cranial nerve deficits, delayed dental eruption, hypersplenism, and hemolysis may occur. Treatment may include bone marrow transplant, high-dose glucocorticoids, limitation of dietary calcium, and high-dose calcitriol.

Intermediate osteopetrosis causes short stature, recurrent fractures, and possible cranial nerve deficits. One variant of intermediate osteopetrosis is caused by carbonic anhydrase II deficiency; it is characterized by osteopetrosis, renal tubular acidosis, and cerebral calcifications and is inherited in an autosomal recessive pattern.

Some individuals with adult osteopetrosis are asymptomatic, whereas others have facial cranial nerve involvement, carpal tunnel syndrome, slipped capital femoral epiphysis, and osteoarthritis.

Iatrogenic suppression of osteoclast activity is another potential etiology of osteopetrosis. Because of promising results seen with the use of bisphosphonates in the treatment of children with osteogenesis imperfecta, the use of bisphosphonates in treating children with a variety of conditions has increased. However, few data are available from randomized clinical trials for the use of bisphosphonate treatment in children and teenagers. Although bisphosphonates may prove beneficial, they should be used with extreme caution. Growing bone requires coordination of bone resorption and bone formation. Bone formation predominates in children and teens, and thus the pharmacologic suppression of resorption may have different consequences than seen in adult patients. Also, the half-life of the bisphosphonates is nearly a decade. Treating a young woman before or during childbearing years may have unforeseen consequences for the fetus and mother. It is important to select patients for treatment in whom the risk to benefit ratio is apparent; this information should be clearly communicated with the parents and the child or teen.

Paget's Disease

Paget's disease is a localized disorder of bone remodeling; it has a familial pattern of aggregation, but no single gene abnormality has been implicated in the etiology. Infectious agents have also been implicated as a possible cause. The initial defect in Paget's disease is increased bone resorption associated with abnormalities of osteoclasts found in the lesion. Osteoclasts in a Paget's lesion are more numerous and contain more nuclei than normal. Early lesions usually contain abundant osteoblasts and increased new bone formation. The increased bone turnover is manifested by increased urinary excretion of biomarkers indicative of increased bone resorption. Paget's disease is slightly more predominant in men than in women and occurs most often in patients older than 40 years of age. The most common presenting symptom is bone pain. The diagnosis is usually evident from the radiographic appearance of a localized lesion consisting of cortical thickening, cortical expansion, mixed areas of lucency and sclerosis, and laboratory evaluation showing increased markers of bone resorption in the urine and increased alkaline phosphatase in the serum.

The treatment of Paget's disease is directed at decreasing the activity of the pagetic osteoclasts. Approved pharmacologic therapies include the bisphosphonates and calcitonin. Medical treatment is indicated for patients with painful lesions in the long bones, skull, and vertebrae, which may cause neurologic damage or secondary arthritis. Although intended to alleviate pain and to prevent complications, few data exist to show that pharmacologic intervention actually prevents complications from this metabolic bone disease.

Future Directions
Bone Mineral Density

BMD has been a useful tool in the understanding of bone health and in identifying patients with osteoporosis. It is also increasingly clear that there are limitations to the use of DEXA as a device to measure bone health. Better studies correlating DEXA data with fracture risk in adults and especially in children and teens are necessary. Alternate imaging modalities may become more useful in understanding the determinants of fracture risk and in improving the understanding of how different therapies alter bone characteristics and strength. One of the major weaknesses of DEXA is its inability to separate and assess cortical bone and trabecular bone compartments. Imaging modalities such as peripheral quantitative CT can be used to evaluate both compartments individually and may prove useful in the next few years to determine the effects of medications, growth, and aging on bone and to help evaluate various treatment modalities.

New Medications

The current predominant therapy for altering bone metabolism is directed at bone resorption (for example, bisphosphonate therapy). Developing medications that increase bone formation also may prove to be a means to improve systemic therapy for those with osteoporosis or genetic syndromes. Recently, recombinant human parathyroid hormone (1-34) [rhPTH(1-34)] has been approved by the Food and Drug Administration for the treatment of osteoporosis. When present continuously, PTH causes demineralization of bone; when present intermittently or episodically, it increases bone mineralization. In animal studies, intermittent rhPTH exposure increases osteoblast numbers without a concomitant increase in osteoclasts and has been shown to increase bone mass, vertebral strength, and trabecular number in monkey studies. In a fracture prevention study of women with postmenopausal osteoporosis, rhPTH increased the BMD of patients in the spine and hip and decreased vertebral fractures; there are no data available regarding use in children. During the next several years, more information, including data on optimal dosage and timing will become available and may offer new alternatives for the treatment of osteoporosis.

The effect of bisphosphonates on postoperative healing needs to be studied. The healing of bone after fractures or surgical intervention (such as cervical spine fusion) is a tightly coupled balance of bone resorption and formation. Treatment with bisphosphonates has the potential to alter that balance. Fracture healing does not seem to be impaired in children with osteogenesis imperfecta who are being treated with bisphosphonates; however, this finding may not be applicable for bisphosphonate treatment in elderly patients. It is imperative that fracture and postoperative healing in patients treated with bisphosphonates be monitored over the next several years because these findings may significantly impact the decision on how to treat some patients.

Pediatric Bone Health

Pediatric bone metabolism is very different than adult bone metabolism, most notably because bone formation is predominant. Impaired bone formation during childhood has long-term effects that may set the stage for premature osteoporosis in adulthood. Better definitions of normal pediatric bone health and the effects of chronic illness on bone health are needed to ensure that all children achieve peak bone mass and minimize the risks for the bone diseases of adulthood.

Annotated Bibliography

General Reference

Proceedings of the Surgeon General's Workshop on Osteoporosis and Bone Health, December 12-13, 2002. Washington, DC, Department of Health and Human Services.

A summary of a meeting held to provide an opportunity for key stakeholders to provide input as to the most important priorities for the Surgeon General's report on osteoporosis and bone health is presented.

Basic Science Aspects of Bone Metabolism

Favus MJ (ed): *Primer on the Metabolic Bone Diseases and Disorders of Mineral Metabolism,* ed 5. Washington, DC, American Society for Bone and Mineral Research, 2003.

A comprehensive review of bone metabolism and bone disease is presented.

Ma YL, Bryant HU, Zeng Q, et al: New bone formation with teriparatide (human parathyroid hormone-(1-34) is not retarded by long-term pretreatment with alendronate, estrogen, or raloxifene in ovariectomized rats. *Endocrinology* 2003;144:2008-2015.

This article discusses the ability of teriparatide to induce bone formation.

Vahle JL, Sato M, Long GG, et al: Skeletal changes in rats given daily subcutaneous injections of recombinant human parathyroid hormone (1-34) for 2 years and relevance to human safety. *Toxicol Pathol* 2002;30:312-321.

This article discusses effects of daily subcutaneous injections of rhPTH(1-34). Results indicated increased bone mass and BMD.

Hormonal Regulation of Cell Differentiation

Leonard MB, Zemel BS: Current concepts in pediatric bone disease. *Pediatr Clin North Am* 2002;49:143-173.

A description of expected gains in bone size and mass during childhood and adolescence is presented. The article discusses modifiable determinants of bone mineralization during growth and the impact of osteopenia on childhood and lifetime fracture risk.

Metabolic Bone Disease

Anderson JB: Calcium requirements during adolescence to maximize bone health. *J Am Coll Nutr* 2001;20(suppl 2):186S-191S.

A review of information on the calcium needs of children and young adults from approximately 9 to 20 years of age is presented. It was concluded that children and teens are not getting the recommended daily amounts of calcium and vitamin D in their diets and that it is increasingly important to provide counseling to families about the appropriate calcium and vitamin D intake required to maximize bone mineralization.

Bilezikian BP (ed): *Endocrinology and Metabolism Clinics of North America.* Philadelphia, PA, WB Saunders, 2003.

This book summarizes important developments in the detection and treatment of osteoporosis. The areas with the most significant advances are identified.

Cranney A, Guyatt G, Griffith L, et al: Meta-analyses of therapies for postmenopausal osteoporosis: IX. Summary of meta-analyses of therapies for postmenopausal osteoporosis. *Endocr Rev* 2002;23:570-578.

Cranney A, Tugwell P, Adachi J, et al: Meta-analyses of therapies for postmenopausal osteoporosis: III. Meta-analysis of risedronate for the treatment of postmenopausal osteoporosis. *Endocr Rev* 2002;23:517-523.

Cranney A, Tugwell P, Wells G, Guyatt G: Osteoporosis Methodology Group and The Osteoporosis Research Advisory Group: Meta-analyses of therapies for postmenopausal osteoporosis: I. Systematic reviews of randomized trials in osteoporosis: Introduction and methodology. *Endocr Rev* 2002;23:496-507.

Cranney A, Tugwell P, Zytaruk N, et al: Meta-analyses of therapies for postmenopausal osteoporosis: IV: Meta-analysis of raloxifene for the prevention and treatment of postmenopausal osteoporosis. *Endocr Rev* 2002;23: 524-528.

Cranney A, Tugwell P, Zytaruk N, et al: Meta-analyses of therapies for postmenopausal osteoporosis: VI. Meta-analysis of calcitonin for the treatment of postmenopausal osteoporosis. *Endocr Rev* 2002;23:540-551.

Cranney A, Wells G, Willan A, et al: Meta-analyses of therapies for postmenopausal osteoporosis: II. Meta-analysis of alendronate for the treatment of postmenopausal women. *Endocr Rev* 2002;23:508-516.

Papadimitropoulos E, Wells G, Shea B, et al: Meta-analyses of therapies for postmenopausal osteoporosis: VIII. Meta-analysis of the efficacy of vitamin D treatment in preventing osteoporosis in postmenopausal women. *Endocr Rev* 2002;23:560-569.

Shea B, Wells G, Cranney A, et al: Meta-analyses of therapies for postmenopausal osteoporosis: VII. Meta-analysis of calcium supplementation for the prevention of postmenopausal oseoporosis. *Endocr Rev* 2002;23: 552-559.

Wells G, Tugwell P, Shea B, et al: Meta-analyses of therapies for postmenopausal osteoporosis: V. Meta-analysis of the efficacy of hormone replacement therapy in treating and preventing osteoporosis in postmenopausal women. *Endocr Rev* 2002;23:529-539.

The previous nine bibliographic entries comprise a series of articles describing the principles of a meta-analysis (Section I) and the results of a meta-analysis of many large published studies and some unpublished observations that were designed to evaluate therapies for osteoporosis. This series compared placebo controlled studies and showed that the results of large, randomized studies may be different from case controlled studies.

Rossouw JE, Anderson GL, Prentice RL, et al: Risks and benefits of estrogen plus progestin in healthy postmenopausal women: Principal results from the Women's Health Initiative randomized controlled trial. *JAMA* 2002;288:321-333.

An interim analysis of the Women's Health Initiative led to early termination of one arm of the study and has had a significant impact on the treatment of osteoporosis. The results are summarized in this article.

Whyte MP, Wenkert D, Clements K, McAlister WH, Mumm S: Bisphosphonate-induced osteopetrosis. *N Engl J Med* 2003;349:457-463.

A case report of bisphosphonate-induced osteopetrosis in a 12-year-old boy is presented. This article shows the consequences of overtreatment with bisphosphonates in the pediatric population.

Future Directions

Deal C, Gideon J: Recombinant human PTH 1-34 (Forteo): An anabolic drug for osteoporosis. *Cleve Clin J Med* 2003;70:584.

This article presents a discussion of the use of forteo, a genetically engineered fragment of parathyroid hormone, in the treatment of osteoporosis.

Steelman J, Zeitler P: Osteoporosis in pediatrics. *Pediatr Rev* 2001;22:56-65.

A description of determinants of bone mass, pediatric populations at risk for osteoporosis, test procedures for assessing bone quality and quantity, and available treatments are presented.

Chapter 19

Musculoskeletal Oncology

Richard D. Lackman, MD

Introduction

The evaluation of a patient with a bone tumor involves the collection of data from several sources that can impact the differential diagnosis; these sources include patient history, physical examination, and imaging studies. Ultimately, if it is determined that histologic confirmation is required, careful evaluation of lesional tissue will confirm a specific diagnosis.

The history associated with the presence of a musculoskeletal tumor defines the clinical context of the lesion. Patient age, sex, duration of symptoms, presence and quality of pain, and history of trauma, weight loss, smoking, and prior malignancy all are important factors. The knowledge that the early symptoms associated with skeletal neoplasms mimic all types of ordinary musculoskeletal disorders is critical to the early diagnosis of a skeletal tumor. Any pain that extends beyond the expected duration associated with a provisional, nonmalignant diagnosis may indicate an underlying tumor. Night pain is a red flag that may lead to the supposition of an occult lesion; however, it should be recognized that many nonneoplastic conditions may also result in pain at night.

A history of trauma in a patient with an occult tumor may delay an accurate diagnosis. Patients will often experience some mild trauma to the affected area and then notice pain, which would probably not have occurred in the absence of an underlying lesion. The patient may directly attribute the local symptoms and findings to the traumatic event, which then influences the treating physician to initially concentrate on the local symptoms. Eventually it will become obvious that the true nature of the lesion is more involved than a minor trauma. An example of this scenario is that of a waiter who kicked a kitchen door to open it while carrying a heavy tray. The door was stuck and did not move, resulting in an apparent calf injury. When the pain did not resolve, a compartment syndrome was suspected; it was not until several months later that tissue was obtained revealing an underlying lymphoma. Similar is the example of an elderly woman taking full-dose warfarin after implantation of a mechanical heart valve who bumps her thigh on a kitchen table and discovers months later that the resulting large anterior thigh mass is a soft-tissue sarcoma and not a simple hematoma. It is only through intellectual discipline and diligence that early diagnoses of occult tumors can be accomplished in patients with a history of trauma involving the affected area.

To assemble a complete differential diagnosis it is helpful to memorize or to have readily available a reasonable list of common lesions to review when a set of radiographs is examined. Without such mental organization, it is difficult or impossible to assemble a comprehensive differential diagnosis of a particular lesion. Table 1 lists three categories of lesions that should be individually considered each time a radiograph is reviewed to ensure the inclusion of the most relevant lesions in a specific differential diagnosis.

Table 1 | Tumors and Common Lesions to Consider When Reviewing Radiographs for a Differential Diagnosis

Bone-Forming Tumors	Cartilage-Forming Tumors	Other Tumors and Lesions
Osteoid osteoma	Osteochondroma	Lesions caused by infection
Osteoblastoma	Chondroblastoma	Metastatic lesions
Osteochondroma	Chondromyxoid fibroma	Round cell tumors
Osteosarcoma	Enchondroma	Unicameral (simple) bone cyst
Blastic metastasis	Chondrosarcoma	Aneurysmal bone cyst
Paget's disease		Nonossifying fibroma
		Fibrous dysplasia
		Giant cell tumor
		Langerhans cell histiocytosis
		Stress fracture
		Lesions caused by metabolic condition

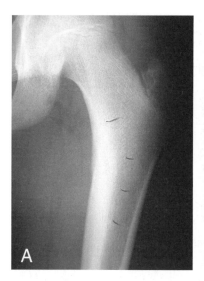
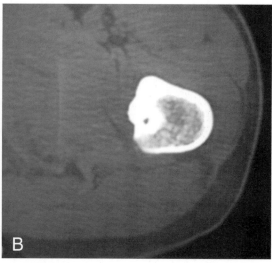

Figure 1 A, Radiograph of osteoid osteoma showing lytic nidus and surrounding sclerosis. **B,** CT scan of osteoid osteoma showing lytic nidus.

Bone-Forming Tumors

Osteoid Osteoma

Osteoid osteoma most commonly occurs during the first two decades of life and appears as a small lytic nidus, often with a target appearance surrounded by significant sclerosis (Figure 1). The nidus may be very tiny and difficult to find on a radiograph. MRI scans will show extensive edema, which may be mistaken for a marrow replacing neoplasm. A CT scan with fine cuts (for example, 1 mm) is the study of choice for locating the lesion. Bone scintigraphy shows focal intense uptake. Osteoid osteomas are associated with a classic pattern of constant pain secondary to prostaglandin secretion. For this reason, pain resulting from these lesions is relieved significantly for short periods by drugs such as aspirin or ibuprofen that inhibit prostaglandin synthesis.

Osteoblastoma

Osteoblastoma is a rare neoplasm most often occurring in the posterior elements of the spine or in the metadiaphyseal region of long bones. This tumor has a variable appearance, may be blastic or lytic, and is rarely diagnosed correctly before histologic material is reviewed. The classic appearance is that of a calcified lesion in the posterior elements of the spine (Figure 2).

Osteochondroma

Osteochondromas are formed by radial growth of bone during childhood and are characterized by a lesion that grows away from the bone at an angle from the adjacent growth plate. The hallmark of an osteochondroma is that, because it grows away from the underlying bone, the cortex of the lesion is confluent with the cortex of the bone of origin and it pulls medullary bone up into itself (Figure 3). A tumor that is located on an intact cortex is never an osteochondroma. Osteochondromas can be sessile or pedunculated and many that grow out

of the flat bones or the proximal femur can be very large and take on a cauliflower appearance. Secondary chondrosarcomatous degeneration occurs in less than 1% of patients and should be suspected in any osteochondroma that grows after puberty or has a cartilage cap of greater than 3 cm during adulthood.

Osteosarcoma

Osteosarcoma usually occurs during the first through third decades of life with a second peak in occurrence after the sixth decade. These tumors present as permeative metaphyseal lesions with soft-tissue extension and new bone formation (Figure 4). Periosteal reaction is common and frequently takes on a sunburst or "hair on end" appearance. Osteosarcoma needs to be considered in the differential diagnosis of every aggressive lesion seen in bone in patients of all ages. It may appear as a purely lytic lesion with no radiographically apparent bone formation.

Blastic Metastasis and Paget's Disease

Blastic metastasis is most frequently seen with prostate and breast carcinoma and typically presents as a permeative lesion with infrequent soft-tissue extension. Paget's disease may mimic other conditions and can exhibit a variety of radiographic appearances. Early stage Paget's disease is characterized by lytic bone, whereas in late stage Paget's disease, bone is blastic with coarse trabeculae and thickened cortices (Figure 5).

Cartilage-Forming Tumors

Chondroblastoma

Chondroblastoma usually appears as a painful lytic lesion in the epiphysis of a child; significant edema is seen on an MRI scan. In older adolescents, it can occasionally grow across an old epiphyseal line to involve the adjacent metaphysis. This classic picture of a painful epiphy-

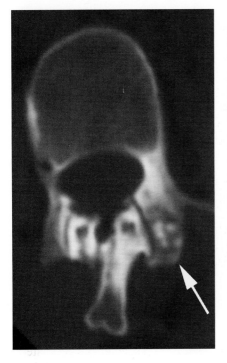

Figure 2 CT scan of the spine showing osteoblastoma (arrow) in the posterior elements.

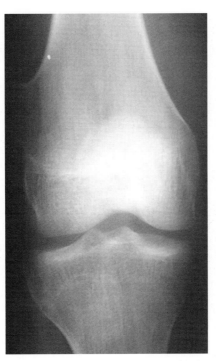

Figure 3 Radiograph showing a typical osteochondroma.

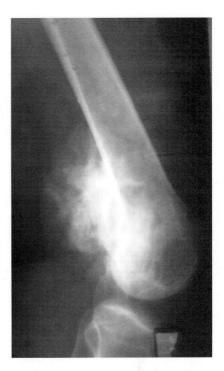

Figure 4 Radiograph showing a typical osteoblastic osteosarcoma.

seal lytic lesion with abundant edema may cause this lesion to be confused with infection or osteochondritis dissecans.

Chondromyxoid Fibroma

Chondromyxoid fibroma is a rare tumor usually presenting as a lytic metaphyseal lesion with cortical thinning but no periosteal reaction (Figure 6). This tumor usually occurs during the first through third decades of life and is most often located in the proximal tibia. It frequently has the appearance of a very large nonossifying fibroma.

Enchondroma

An enchondroma is a nest of cartilage tissue typically found in a metaphyseal region and is usually discovered as an incidental finding in adult patients. These lesions are commonly found when a radiograph of the adjacent joint is obtained for reasons unrelated to the enchondroma itself. Enchondromas tend to be noncalcified or minimally calcified in young adults and usually show an increase in calcification but not an increase in size with long-term follow-up. The calcification has a typical stippled or popcorn pattern. These lesions usually do not cause pain but typically appear hot on a technetium bone scan. Unlike chondrosarcomas, enchondromas do not damage the host bone because they do not cause cortical thinning or expansion. They may cause some slight scalloping; however, the scallops seen on radiographs are usually short and less than 1 cm each. When enchondromas occur in thin or small bones such as the fibular head or scapula, some expansion may be seen in the radiographic appearance. Because "enchondromas do not know what bone they are in," some cortical expansion in small or thin bones may be present when the lesion grows to a typical size.

Chondrosarcoma

Unlike enchondromas, chondrosarcomas are active lesions that grow and alter the host bone over time (Figure 7). Working from the inside of the bone to the outside, the changes associated with chondrosarcomas include intralesional lysis, endosteal scalloping, cortical thinning, and expansion. Most chondrosarcomas show chondroid calcification but some may appear purely lytic; they also cause pain.

Other Tumors

Lesions Caused by Infection

Infection can also mimic the appearance and symptoms of other lesions and can exhibit a variety of radiographic appearances from geographic to permeative and from lytic to blastic. Periosteal reaction is commonly seen on radiographs; localized heat and erythema are often found on physical examination.

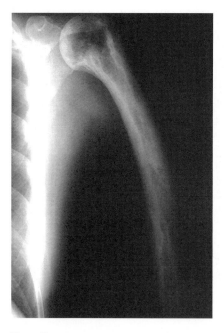

Figure 5 Radiograph showing typical findings of late Paget's disease including cortical thickening and coarse trabeculae.

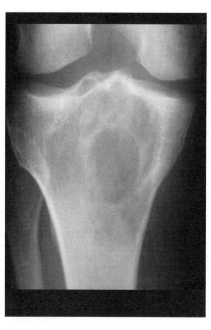

Figure 6 Radiograph showing chondromyxoid fibroma of the proximal tibia.

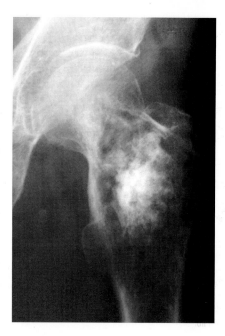

Figure 7 Radiograph of chondrosarcoma of the proximal femur.

Metastatic Lesions

Metastatic lesions are the most common, aggressive, destructive lesions in adults and can exhibit a variety of radiographic appearances from lytic to blastic. Metastasis frequently results in multiple lesions and may be the first presentation of the underlying neoplasm. Although some metastatic bone lesions, especially those from kidney and lung tumors, may grow beyond the confines of the bone involved, the presence of an associated soft-tissue mass should increase the suspicion of a sarcoma.

Round Cell Tumors

Pediatric round cell tumors include Ewing's sarcoma and metastatic neuroblastoma. Ewing's sarcoma classically presents as a diaphyseal permeative lesion with "onion skin" periosteal reaction and a large associated soft-tissue mass. Alternatively, Ewing's sarcoma may be more metaphyseal and destructive, and it should be considered in the differential diagnosis of such a lesion (Figure 8). Twenty percent of patients with Ewing's sarcoma will have associated systemic symptoms such as fever, chills, and a high white blood cell count, which may cause the lesion to mimic osteomyelitis. Neuroblastoma (Figure 9) appears as a permeative lesion with medullary bone replacement and varying degrees of osteolysis. Adult round cell lesions include myeloma and lymphoma. Myeloma occurs as solitary or multiple medullary lytic lesions with sharp margins but little reaction (Figure 10). Whereas most myeloma patients present with multiple lesions, a small percentage will have a sol-

itary bone lesion. If no other bone lesions are found and a random bone marrow aspirate from another bone shows fewer than 5% plasma cells, then a solitary plasmacytoma exists and the prognosis is much better than for a patient with multiple myeloma. Only 25% of patients with solitary plasmacytoma will have a positive serum or urine myeloma protein (m-protein) whereas most patients with multiple myeloma will have measurable m-proteins detected by serum and urine protein electrophoresis. The levels of these m-proteins are useful for tumor staging and also for assessing response to treatment. MRI scans, especially of the spine, are useful screening studies; technetium bone scans are usually normal in patients with multiple myeloma. Lymphoma is typically a very permeative but minimally destructive lesion, which usually progresses by filling the medullary canal and then growing into the surrounding soft tissues while causing little destruction of the bone itself (Figure 11). Radiographs may be remarkably normal, whereas MRI scans show marrow replacement and often an associated soft-tissue mass.

Unicameral (Simple) Bone Cyst

Unicameral bone cysts are usually found in the proximal humerus; are always central, full width lesions; may cause cortical thinning and minimal expansion; and usually have no associated periosteal reaction. The widest portion of these lesions is usually no wider than the widest portion of the adjacent metaphysis (Figure 12).

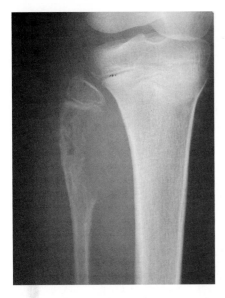

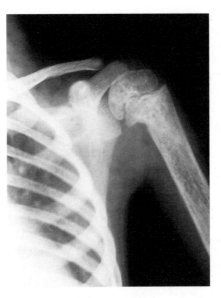

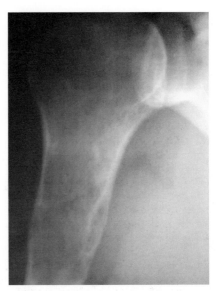

Figure 8 Radiograph of Ewing's sarcoma of the proximal fibula.

Figure 9 Radiograph of metastatic neuroblastoma in the proximal humerus of a child.

Figure 10 Radiograph of myeloma of the proximal humerus.

Aneurysmal Bone Cyst

Aneurysmal bone cysts (ABCs) are usually very expansile and occur as eccentric metaphyseal lesions in patients during the first 3 decades of life (Figure 13). These lesions frequently have a delicate rim of expanded cortical bone, which may be seen best on a CT scan. Fluid-fluid levels are frequently present but are not diagnostic of primary ABC because areas of secondary ABC formation may exist in other lesions such as osteosarcomas and giant cell tumors.

Nonossifying Fibroma

Nonossifying fibromas that occur in children are usually eccentric metaphyseal lesions that grow to varying sizes (Figure 14). As skeletal growth continues and external remodeling occurs, lesions that were previously intramedullary in the metaphysis become intracortical in the metadiaphysis. This cortical disruption creates a mechanical insufficiency and causes the bone to replace the lesion with new bone formation as the lesion heals.

Fibrous Dysplasia

The classic fibrous dysplastic lesion presents as a long lesion in a long bone with ground-glass textured medullary calcification and cortical thinning but no periosteal reaction (Figure 15). Fibrous dysplasia can have a variable appearance and should be included in the differential diagnosis of every benign-appearing lesion in bone.

Giant Cell Tumor

A giant cell tumor presents as a juxta-articular lytic lesion and frequently has a moth-eaten or irregular margin, cortical thinning, and expansion; and may have soft-tissue extension, but usually without a periosteal reaction (Figure 16). It very rarely occurs before the growth plates are closed or after the age of 50 years.

Langerhans Cell Histiocytosis

Langerhans cell histiocytosis is an inflammatory condition that usually presents as intramedullary lysis in patients during the first three decades of life. This condition includes three separate clinical entities: eosinophilic granuloma, Hand-Schüller-Christian disease, and Letterer-Siwe disease. These diseases have different clinical courses and prognoses but share identical histologic findings. Eosinophilic granuloma is the most common and mildest form of this disease and usually occurs as a solitary lesion in bone. The larger the lesion grows and the closer to a cortex it becomes, the more likely it is to show some associated sclerosis. These lesions also may occur on the surface of a bone where they occasionally elicit an aggressive-appearing periosteal reaction, which can be mistaken for a malignant tumor on radiographic evaluation. Histiocytosis must be considered in the differential diagnosis of any intramedullary lesion in a patient younger than 30 years of age.

Factors to Consider in the Differential Diagnosis

Metabolic Conditions and Trauma

Metabolic conditions include a wide variety of underlying diseases such as osteoporosis, osteomalacia, and renal osteodystrophy that affect bone formation and healing. Such conditions should be considered when forming a differential diagnosis.

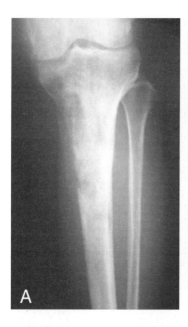

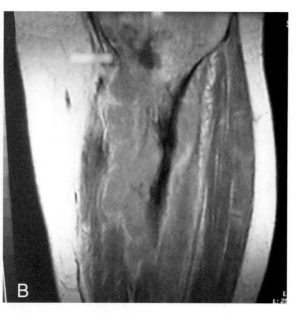

Figure 11 A, Radiograph of lymphoma of the proximal tibia. **B,** MRI scan of lymphoma of the proximal tibia.

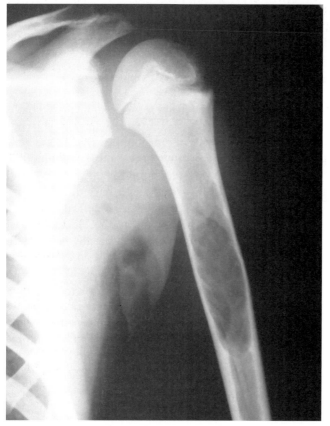

Figure 12 Radiograph of a unicameral bone cyst of the proximal humerus.

Obvious blunt, acute trauma does not usually mimic tumors, whereas patients with chronic stress factures may present with bony reaction that can mimic and be confused with lesions such as lymphoma, osteoid osteoma, metastasis, or infection.

Radiographic Findings

Certain radiographic findings are important to consider when making a specific differential diagnosis. By using the information described in Table 2, a very complete differential diagnosis of most lesions should be possible. For example, the radiograph in Figure 17 shows a juxta-articular lytic lesion in the proximal tibia with a moth-eaten margin, cortical thinning, and no periosteal reaction in a 19-year-old man with a 6-week history of progressive knee pain that is worse at night and with weight bearing. A reasonable differential diagnosis using the lists in Table 1, and taking into consideration the patient's age, includes osteosarcoma, infection, Ewing's sarcoma, giant cell tumor, and ABC. Biopsy proved the lesion to be a giant cell tumor. If the same radiograph had been taken of a 50-year-old man, the differential diagnosis would include osteosarcoma, chondrosarcoma, metastasis, myeloma, lymphoma, and giant cell tumor. In either case, having a list of lesions to mentally review greatly increases the completeness of a radiographic differential diagnosis and is helpful in ensuring that relevant lesions are considered in the diagnosis.

Imaging Studies
Computed Tomography

The major role of a CT scan is to show bony detail including bone formation as well as bone destruction. CT scans are the best study for determining the amount of bone destruction and the presence of soft-tissue calcification. The ability of CT scans to detect the extent of a permeative lesion in bone, soft-tissue extension from a bone lesion, or the extent of a lesion in soft tissue is less than optimal.

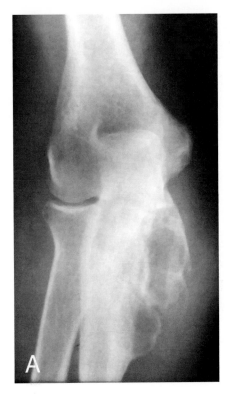 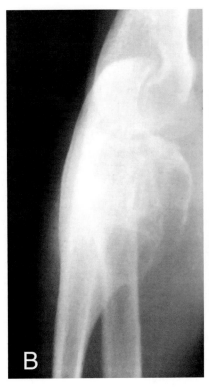 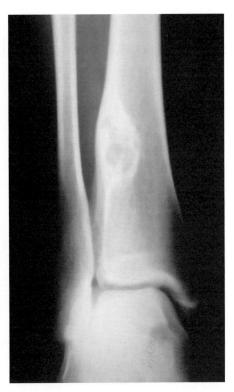

Figure 13 A and **B,** Radiographs of an aneurysmal bone cyst of the proximal ulna.

Figure 14 Radiograph of a nonossifying fibroma of the distal tibia that is spontaneously resolving.

Magnetic Resonance Imaging

MRI scans are excellent for showing the extent (starting and stopping points) of a lesion in bone. They are also excellent for showing the presence and extent of edema within bone and the presence or absence of an associated soft-tissue extension. MRI is the study of choice for any soft-tissue lesion. The addition of contrast to an MRI scan can help distinguish areas of cyst formation (which do not enhance with contrast but may show rim enhancement) from areas of solid tumor (which do enhance). One exception to this generalization are chondroid lesions, such as low grade chondrosarcomas, which may also show rim enhancement with little internal enhancement and, in this regard, may mimic a cyst. Care must be taken to differentiate edema in bone and tumor in bone. Lymphoma frequently presents as high signal in marrow and must be included in the differential diagnosis of traumatic marrow lesions such as stress fractures or bone bruises.

Technetium Bone Scan

Technetium bone scans are most useful as a skeletal survey tool to determine the total number of lesions present or to locate a single lesion that is suspected but not seen on the initial radiograph. All active bone-forming lesions appear hot, whereas some lytic lesions, which engender no bone reaction, may be normal or cold (for example, myeloma). Sclerotic lesions, which

are normal on bone scan, are usually old and inactive. Most metastatic carcinomas and sarcomas in bone are hot on bone scans, although this finding is not a constant.

Biopsy

If after careful clinical evaluation and imaging studies a diagnosis has not been confirmed, a biopsy is the next step. The ideal biopsy provides all of the tissue needed to establish a histologic diagnosis without affecting subsequent treatment options. Biopsy has caused much concern among clinicians and several studies have reported the problems caused by poorly planned and executed biopsies. There is disagreement on whether a community orthopaedic surgeon or a specialized orthopaedic oncologist should perform a biopsy. If the diagnosing physician deems that referral to a tumor specialist for treatment would be appropriate, the physician should defer performing the biopsy. The physician who will ultimately treat the lesion should determine if and how a biopsy is performed. For example, in a 17-year old boy with a large painful mass about the distal femur and radiographic findings indicative of osteosarcoma, most orthopaedic surgeons would not perform the resection and reconstruction of such a lesion. Therefore, the patient should be referred to a subspecialist who will perform the biopsy in a manner that will not compromise the definitive treatment. It is understood that the treating surgeon should be familiar with the

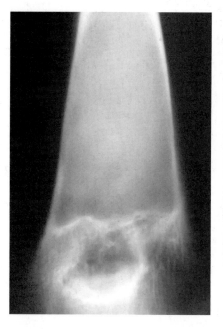

Figure 15 Radiograph of fibrous dysplasia of the distal humerus showing the "ground glass" appearance.

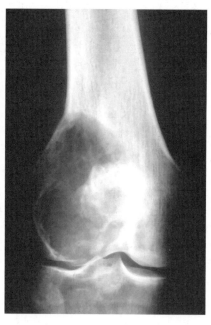

Figure 16 Radiograph of a giant cell tumor of the distal femur.

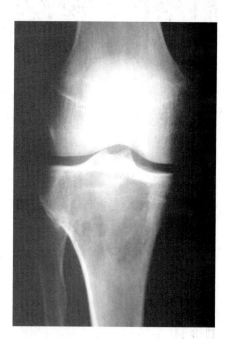

Figure 17 Radiograph of a giant cell tumor of the proximal tibia.

guidelines concerning the type of biopsy to be performed and the appropriate biopsy techniques.

Current biopsy options include both open and needle techniques. The advantage of percutaneous needle biopsies is that they cause little soft-tissue contamination and require little or no anesthesia. They are frequently performed under CT scan or ultrasound guidance, which can direct a biopsy needle into an underlying lesion. The disadvantage of percutaneous needle biopsy is that only a small amount of tissue is obtained for the pathologist to review. Such biopsies can frequently be nondiagnostic. More importantly, primary bone tumors are notoriously heterogeneous, thereby creating a great potential for sampling error with closed techniques. Needle biopsies are optimal for initial sampling of lesions in anatomically inaccessible areas such as the spine or pelvis. In most locations, however, the carefully performed open biopsy is still the gold standard. Important rules that should be considered when performing an open biopsy are outlined in Table 3.

Histologic Evaluation

The histologic diagnosis of musculoskeletal tumors is difficult and complicated; one of the difficulties encountered in musculoskeletal pathology is the large number of potential diagnoses. If all lesions are considered separately, it may be very difficult for the orthopaedist to place a specific lesion into a reasonable differential diagnosis. By considering trends and patterns of groups of histologic lesions and as the relationship of histologic findings to a differential diagnosis based on available imaging studies, the whole spectrum of histologic diagnoses, at least at an elementary level, is more understandable.

Bone-Forming Tumors

Bone forming tumors, including fracture callus, myositis ossificans, osteoid osteoma, osteoblastoma, fibrous dysplasia, parosteal osteosarcoma, and osteosarcoma, typically contain woven bone and a spindle cell stroma, each of which needs to be scrutinized to understand the nature of the lesion. Histologic evaluation of bone-forming lesions requires an understanding that the bone differentiates reactive from neoplastic lesions and the stromal cells differentiate benign from malignant neoplasms. First, the bone produced by a specific lesion should be examined. Figure 18, *A* shows lamellar bone with a surrounding round cell infiltrate (Ewing's sarcoma) in which the lines of individual bone lamellae can be seen. Lamellar bone is rarely produced by tumors and is usually just native host bone entrapped in a lesion or part of a mature bone reaction. However, woven bone can be either neoplastic or reactive, which is determined by the presence or absence of osteoblastic rimming. Typically, woven bone with significant osteoblastic rimming is reactive and indicative of fracture callus, periosteal reaction, or myositis ossificans (Figure 18, *B*). In such lesions, spindled stromal cells also may be present and have some mild atypia (especially in early myositis or early fracture callus). In contrast, woven bone that shows no osteoblastic rimming is usually neoplastic in origin and is seen with both benign and malignant bone-forming neoplasms (Figure 19, *A*). Neoplastic woven bone (bone with no osteoblastic rimming) found in association with a benign spindle cell stroma is indicative of a benign bone-forming neoplasm. Such lesions include osteoid osteoma, osteoblastoma, and fibrous dysplasia. Also included in this histologic differential diagnosis is parosteal osteosarcoma, a grade 1 malignant tumor, which presents with a stroma with little overt atypia. The final pattern seen in bone-forming lesions is the presence of neoplastic woven bone in association with a malignant spindle cell stroma that constitutes osteosarcoma (Figure 19, *B*). The findings that make a spindle cell stroma appear malignant include increased cellularity, spontaneous necrosis, the presence of significant atypia or pleomorphism, and a high mitotic rate with many abnormal mitoses.

These bone-forming lesions tend to look very different radiographically; therefore, a radiographic differential diagnosis integrated into the histologic differential diagnosis helps to determine the final diagnosis.

Cartilage-Forming Tumors

There are three histologic patterns of cartilage tumors: (1) benign cartilage (enchondroma) merging into low-grade cartilage which merges into intermediate and high grade chondrosarcoma; (2) chondroblastoma that is characterized by cobblestone chondroblasts and intervening chicken-wire calcification with immature cartilage; (3) chondromyxoid fibroma that is a benign spindle cell lesion with some areas of immature cartilage.

In the first histologic pattern, it is essential to understand the spectrum of cartilage appearances that match the spectrum of histologic grading. Normal cartilage has two components: cells and matrix. Both are important when evaluating cartilage histologically. Normal cartilage is sparsely cellular (Figure 20, *A*). The cells have small oval (pyknotic) nuclei and only one nucleus per cell. There is only one cell per lacuna and there are rarely cells outside of the lacunae. The matrix is well-formed and regular with no areas that are loose or falling apart (myxoid change).

As cartilage changes from benign to low grade the following changes occur—increased cellularity, the presence of plump nuclei, occasional binucleate cells, more than one cell in some lacunae, some cells outside the lacunae, and myxoid change in the matrix.

The finding of low-grade cartilage includes the spectrum of lesions ranging from cellular or active enchondromas to what are sometimes called grade one-half chondrosarcoma, to grade 1 chondrosarcoma. It is critical to appreciate that tumors in this range have a variable biologic potential in terms of their propensity for

**Table 2	Important Radiographic Findings for Making a Specific Differential Diagnosis**	
Finding	**Differential Diagnosis**
Sclerotic soap bubble lesion in the anterior cortex of the tibial shaft	Adamantinoma Cortical fibrous dysplasia
Small sclerotic lesion with a central lytic nidus	Osteoid Osteoma Stress fracture Infection
Changes that indicate edema in bone*	Intramedullary changes caused by lymphoma Intramedullary edema caused by a bone bruise or stress reaction
Cauliflower exophytic lesion†	Cauliflower osteochondroma Secondary chondrosarcoma arising in an osteochondroma
Multiple bone lesions	Metastases Myeloma Enchondromas Histiocytosis Fibrous dysplasia Nonossifying fibromas
Lytic lesion in the humeral shaft of a child with no periosteal reaction	Simple bone cyst
Lytic lesion in the sacrum	Chordoma Chondrosarcoma Giant cell tumor Metastasis Myeloma
Calcified lesion on the bone surface	Osteochondroma Periosteal osteosarcoma Parosteal osteosarcoma Myositis ossificans Periosteal chondroma Periosteal chondrosarcoma
Aggressive metaepiphyseal lesion in patients younger than age 30 years	Osteosarcoma Ewing's sarcoma Infection Aneurysmal bone cyst Giant cell tumor
Aggressive metaepiphyseal lesion in patients 30 years of age or older	Osteosarcoma Chondrosarcoma Metastasis Adult round cell tumor Giant cell tumor
Lytic lesion in the epiphysis of a child with edema seen on MRI	Chondroblastoma Infection

*Sequential MRI scans of lymphomas show stable or progressive marrow replacement, whereas sequential MRI scans of stress reaction or a bone bruise show a decrease in bone edema over time

†It is important to measure the thickness of the cartilage cap

continued growth. Throughout this range of histologic appearance, pathologists have no effective means of predicting growth; therefore, an attempt to artificially

Table 3 | Important Rules to Consider When Performing an Open Biopsy

Rules Regarding the Incision

The smallest possible incision should be made over the lesion

The incision on the extremities should be longitudinal; the incision on the trunk should be planned to be part of a resection incision

The use of an Esmarch tourniquet wrapped over a tumor may rupture the tumor into the surrounding tissues and should be avoided; it is reasonable to use an extremity tourniquet proximal to a tumor of the extremity (particularly to minimize blood loss)

A small incision should be made into the capsule of a tumor so that it can be easily closed; a small incision is especially important when no tourniquet is used because a large incision can cause appreciable bleeding that is difficult to control

The size of the incision into the tumor should be no larger than the surgeon can fill with a fingertip—this will allow a rapid, temporary hemostasis; if excessive bleeding does not occur, a larger incision can then be made

Rules Regarding Avoidance of Contamination

Care should be taken to prevent direct contamination of the neurovascular bundle

Care should be taken to prevent the violation of major flap structures (eg, gluteus maximus) or functionally important structures (eg, rectus femoris)

Minimal retraction should be used to limit soft-tissue contamination

It is preferable to go through a single muscle belly (if it is large enough) than to go between two structures, which could contaminate both

Good hemostasis must be obtained by meticulous, multilayered watertight closure; large tumors may put the point of closure under pressure and the vascularity that is present may predispose the area to subsequent drainage and breakdown

Rules Regarding Conditions During and After Open Biopsy

Wound complications should be avoided because they increase the risk of secondary infection and may delay subsequent chemotherapy or radiation

Drains should not be used routinely; if needed, they should be thin and should exit 1 to 2 cm beyond one end of the incision so that the drain track can be resected easily with the biopsy track

A frozen section should be obtained when feasible to ensure that diagnostic material is present; the necrotic nature of tumors may require a large volume of tissue to ensure that diagnostic material is obtained

Sending biopsy material for culture and sensitivity should be considered if there is suspicion that the lesion is neoplastic or infectious

When performing a diagnostic open biopsy, the operating surgeon should accompany the specimen to the pathology department if feasible; the pathologist and surgeon should then review imaging studies, the specimen, frozen section slides, and the patient's clinical history

determine where cellular enchondroma ends and low-grade chondrosarcoma begins would be arbitrary. The term low-grade cartilage tumor has become popular, denoting the fact that the pathologist is acknowledging the position of the tumor somewhere within this spectrum of behavior. The key for the treating physician is to evaluate the clinical history and imaging studies and to determine a reasonable course of treatment. Options may range from careful observation, to curettage, to resection depending on a host of factors including the presence or absence of pain, the age of the patient, the bone involved, and the presence or absence of radiographic changes typical of chondrosarcomas.

Chondrocytes look less normal and behave in a less normal fashion with increasing grades of malignancy; the chondrocytes develop dark, plump nuclei, cellularity increases appreciably, and mitoses become more common. The cells make less or no matrix, or may produce an abnormal matrix, which may look nothing like recognizable chondroid. Associated with this histologic progression is a progressive increase in biologic potential in terms of local aggressiveness and metastatic behavior.

The second histologic pattern in chondroid lesions is seen in chondroblastoma. This lesion is often suspected even before histologic material is examined because of its characteristic radiographic and clinical features (for example, a painful lytic lesion in the epiphysis of a child). Histologically, a pattern of cobblestone chondroblasts (polygonal cells with well-defined cell borders) are seen (Figure 20, *B*). In association with these cells, a branching pattern of calcification referred to as chicken wire is also common, as is the presence of immature chondroid matrix. These histologic findings in association with an epiphyseal lytic lesion in a child yield a fairly straightforward diagnosis of chondroblastoma.

The third histologic pattern seen in cartilage tumors is found in chondromyxoid fibroma. This is a rare lesion that is composed of benign spindle cells in a collagenous matrix with varying amounts of immature chondroid (Figure 20, *C*). This histologic pattern in association with the typical radiographic findings helps in determining the diagnosis.

Many bone- and cartilage-forming lesions can be accurately diagnosed by first assembling a radiographic differential diagnosis via the radiology lists and then assessing the histologic spectrum of bone and cartilage forming lesions using a knowledge of simple trends and pattern recognition. For example, in a 40-year-old woman with a recent history of knee pain who has otherwise been in good health, radiographs show an aggressive lytic lesion in the distal femur with cortical bone destruction and soft-tissue extension. The radiographic

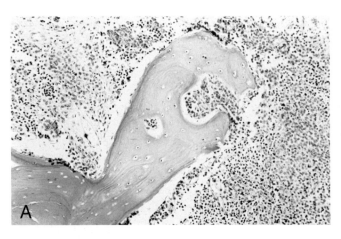
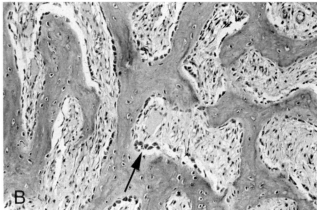

Figure 18 A, Lamellar bone with a surrounding round cell tumor. **B,** Reactive woven bone showing abundant osteoblastic rimming (*arrow*) of trabecular surfaces.

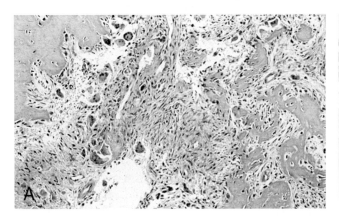
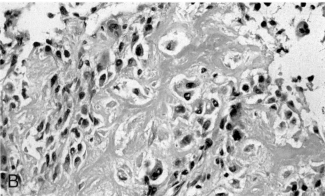

Figure 19 A, Neoplastic woven bone showing the absence of osteoblastic rimming and the presence of an associated benign spindle cell stroma typical of a benign bone forming neoplasm. **B,** Osteosarcoma showing neoplastic woven bone in association with a malignant spindle cell stroma.

differential of this lesion includes osteosarcoma, chondrosarcoma, metastasis, myeloma, lymphoma, and giant cell tumor. The histology shows woven bone with no osteoblastic rimming compatible with neoplastic woven bone (Figure 19, *B*). A malignant spindle cell stroma is also seen histologically. The final diagnosis, osteosarcoma, is compatible with the radiograph. Although this system cannot encompass and diagnose every musculoskeletal lesion, it can provide a framework for developing an approach to these diagnoses.

Other Tumors
Round Cell Tumors
Round cell tumors are another group of bone lesions and include Ewing's sarcoma and neuroblastoma in children and myeloma, lymphoma, and small round cell metastatic carcinomas in adults. Also included in the differential diagnosis of this group of tumors are nonmalignant lesions such as Langerhans cell histiocytosis and infection. The common thread between all of these lesions is that they are composed in part or in whole of small round cells. When round cell infiltrate is present in a histologic slide from a bone lesion, the following classes of

disorders should be considered: infection (ie, osteomyelitis), Langerhans cell histiocytosis, primary round cell tumors, and small round cell metastatic carcinomas.

The histology of bone infection includes the presence of acute and chronic inflammatory cells. Whereas lymphocytes, which tend to be associated with chronic inflammatory conditions, may resemble lymphoid cells seen in lymphoma, polymorphonuclear leukocytes are usually easy to see and, when present in large numbers, indicate a diagnosis of infection. When a round cell infiltrate is seen and most of the cells can be shown to be polymorphonuclear leukocytes, then infection is the likely diagnosis. Confirmation requires culture of an appropriate pathogenic microorganism.

Langerhans cell histiocytosis is also a type of inflammatory condition in bone and can present as a round cell infiltrate. As the name implies it is composed of foci of proliferating histiocytes; varying numbers of small round cells including lymphocytes, neutrophils and, most notably, eosinophils are also present. Histiocytes are large cells with ill-defined cytoplasmic borders and an oval or indented nucleus and are often difficult for a nonpathologist to recognize. Eosinophils are distinctive

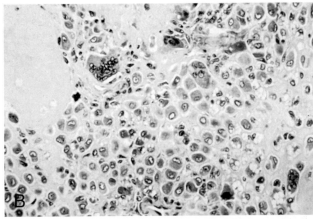

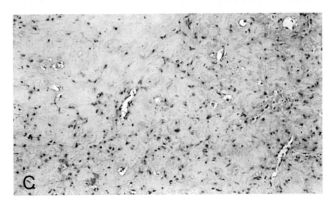

Figure 20 A, Normal cartilage showing sparse cellularity and good matrix production. **B,** Chondroblastoma showing cobblestone chondroblasts and a chondroid matrix. **C,** Chondromyxoid fibroma showing bland spindle cells in a chondroid matrix.

small round cells with bilobed nuclei and red cytoplasm on hematoxylin-eosin staining. When diagnosing histiocytosis, pathologists tend to look for histiocytes whereas orthopaedists look for eosinophils.

Pediatric round cell tumors occurring in bone include Ewing's sarcoma and metastatic neuroblastoma. Ewing's sarcoma is a malignant tumor of unknown histogenesis composed of uniform sheets of small round blue cells. These cells show round or oval nuclei of uniform size with poor delineation of cytoplasm. Stains for intracellular gly-

cogen are typically positive. A neuroblastoma occurring in bone is usually a metastasis from a primary tumor in the midline. The cells of a neuroblastoma look similar to those of Ewing's sarcoma but show the presence of pseudorosettes, which appear as circles of round cells surrounding a pink ground substance. Thus, in pediatric round cell tumors, small round blue cells with no pseudorosette formation is typical of Ewing's sarcoma whereas similar appearing cells that also show pseudorosette formation are typical of neuroblastoma.

Adult round cell tumors include myeloma, lymphoma, and small round cell metastatic carcinomas. Usually, myeloma is easily recognizable (when well differentiated) because it is composed of sheets of plasma cells. Plasma cells have a single round or oval nucleus with eccentric cytoplasm. The cell outlines are distinct and the nuclei often show prominent clumping of chromatin, which produces a clock face or wheel spoke appearance.

Lymphoma and small round cell carcinoma metastases are much more difficult to differentiate by routine light microscopy and may require immunohistochemical stains for final verification. As such, metastases usually stain positive for cytokeratin, whereas lymphomas will stain positive for lymphoid markers such as leukocyte common antigen or B or T cell markers. Thus, with adult round cell tumors, sheets of plasma cells indicate myeloma whereas round cells, which are not plasma cells and look more lymphocytic, are either lymphoma or a small round cell carcinoma.

Unicameral and Aneurysmal Bone Cysts
Bone cysts include unicameral or simple bone cysts and aneurysmal bone cysts. As previously noted, these lesions appear different radiographically. Histologically, unicameral bone cysts appear as a thin layer of fibrous tissue lining large empty spaces. Benign giant cells, hemosiderin pigment, and a few chronic inflammatory cells also may be present. Aneurysmal bone cysts have a different histologic appearance and are characterized by the presence of blood-filled cavernous spaces with walls that lack the normal features of blood vessels. There is some overlap between these two lesions however, and some cysts will have characteristics of both. This situation is most evident in cysts directly abutting the growth plate in skeletally immature patients, especially in young children. In these instances, the cyst is often central as opposed to eccentric and often minimally expansile. These lesions can have a very aggressive course, particularly the aneurysmal bone cysts, which may be unresponsive to percutaneous treatments and often require open treatments such as curettage, bone grafting, and embolization. Great care needs to be directed toward preservation of the adjacent growth plate.

Giant Cell Tumor

Giant cell tumor of bone is a lesion with a variable biologic potential. Although this is typically an aggressive benign lesion, 2% of patients with histologically benign giant cell tumor of bone will have pulmonary metastases; several of these patients will die from progressive metastatic disease. In other patients, however, the metastases will not have an aggressive course. The diagnosis of benign giant cell tumor is usually fairly simple when the histologic findings are coupled with typical radiographic changes. The radiographs usually show a juxta-articular lytic lesion with a moth-eaten margin, cortical thinning or erosion, and no periosteal reaction. Histologically, the lesion is composed of multinucleate giant cells and mononuclear stromal cells. The characteristic finding is that the nuclei of the giant cells look identical to the nuclei of the stromal cells. Mitotic figures may be found in all of these lesions and may be prominent in some. Small areas of woven bone also may be seen along with areas of spindle cells with spindled nuclei. Whereas the diagnosis of most of these lesions is straightforward, there are some giant cell rich osteosarcomas that are indistinguishable from benign giant cell tumor. In these lesions, it is often only a malignant pattern of subsequent growth and metastasis that elucidates the true nature of the neoplasm. When evaluating a probable benign giant cell tumor of bone, it is recommended that the possibility of giant cell rich osteosarcoma be considered, realizing that the ultimate differentiation may be difficult or impossible.

Nonossifying Fibroma (Metaphyseal Fibrous Defect)

A nonossifying fibroma is a common lesion that only rarely requires surgical intervention. Most of these lesions are incidental findings and require no specific treatment other than occasional radiographs to document stability and healing; however, they occasionally may be large enough to cause mechanical pain and limit the ability of the child or adolescent to participate in desired activities. When this occurs or when the specific diagnosis remains elusive, open biopsy with curettage and some form of bone grafting is reasonable. Histologically, these lesions have a characteristic appearance showing benign spindle cells with frequent benign giant cells. After surgical excision and grafting, these lesions will usually heal completely in about 8 weeks, whereas such healing would commonly take 2 years or more without surgical intervention.

Adamantinoma

Adamantinoma is a characteristic lesion usually found in the anterior cortex of the midshaft of the tibia. It usually appears as a "soap bubble" sclerotic lesion and can mimic cortical fibrous dysplasia. Cortical fibrous dysplasia occurs predominately in males in the first and second decades of life, whereas adamantinoma occurs in both genders and all age groups usually occurring during the first through fourth decades of life. Histologically, adamantinoma is a low-grade spindle cell sarcoma with islands of epithelial cells that may resemble cutaneous basal cells. A second histologic pattern for this lesion consists of islands of neoplastic cells surrounded by columnar cells in a palisading fashion. These findings are usually fairly diagnostic when seen with the usual radiographic presentation.

Immunohistochemistry

One of the major advances in diagnostic pathology that has occurred over the past two decades has been the development of sophisticated immunohistochemical techniques. These stains have greatly improved the diagnostic acumen of tissues seen via light microscopy and have added a new area of classification based on specific cell proteins. Although a detailed knowledge of this field is not essential, these stains are commonly referred to in pathology reports of musculoskeletal lesions and should be familiar at a basic level to all orthopaedic surgeons.

Immunohistochemical stains are available to identify specific intermediate filament proteins, which are basic structural components of all human cells. These proteins include distinct moieties that are separated biochemically and include vimentin, desmin, keratins, and neurofilament, glial fibrillary, and lamin filament proteins (nuclear envelope proteins). In terms of cell function, the intermediate filament proteins serve a nucleic acid binding function and may also act as modulators of nuclear function at a translational or transcriptional level. It should be emphasized that whereas certain tumors have typical immunohistochemical profiles, the profiles vary from tumor to tumor as individual tumors exhibit specific genotypes and phenotypes.

Keratins

Keratins are usually seen in epithelial tissues and cells. As a diagnostic marker in bone tumors, keratins are the classic markers of metastatic carcinomas. In rare instances, however, they may be seen in almost any form of sarcoma. Keratins are also commonly seen in the epithelial component of those sarcomas that show some epithelial differentiation, including synovial sarcoma, adamantinoma, and epithelioid sarcoma.

Vimentin

Vimentin is a protein typically found in tumors with a mesothelial origin. Immunohistochemical staining of vimentin is positive in almost all sarcomas but usually negative in carcinomas. Because its presence is widespread among sarcomas, it is not a useful marker to distinguish between specific sarcoma types.

Desmin and Actin

Desmin is typically found in muscle cells and in tumors with myodifferentiation. Such tumors most commonly

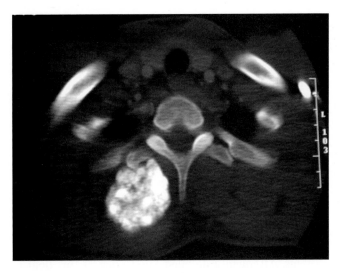

Figure 21 Radiograph of a densely calcified synovial sarcoma mimicking myositis ossificans.

present in soft tissue and include rhabdomyomas, rhabdomyosarcomas, leiomyomas, and leiomyosarcomas. Desmin is also occasionally present in desmoid tumors and in primitive neuroectodermal tumors. Like desmin, actin is indicative of myogenous differentiation and its tissue-specificity parallels that of desmin.

S-100

S-100 is a protein that derives its name from the fact that it is soluble in 100% solution of ammonium sulfate. It has a wide distribution in human tissues and the stains indicating the presence of this protein are most commonly associated with neural, chondroid, or melanocytic differentiation.

Factor VIII Related Antigen

Factor VIII related antigens (also called von Willebrand's factor) are found in lesions with vascular differentiation. These antigens are typically seen in benign and low-grade vascular lesions such as hemangiomas and hemangioendotheliomas; they usually are not present in high-grade angiosarcomas.

Soft-Tissue Tumors

Soft-tissue tumors, like bone lesions, require a systematic approach for diagnosis. These lesions have a limited number of clinical presentations. Histologically, however, they form a large and diverse group with fewer trends in their histologic appearance than those found in bone tumors.

Clinical Presentation

Most soft-tissue tumors present with pain and/or a mass. As noted previously, there is often a history of trauma as patients tend to relate the emergence of a mass lesion with even trivial local trauma. It is also remarkable that soft-tissue masses including sarcomas can grow to a very large size and yet cause minimal or no symptoms. Many patients falsely assume that because the lesion is painless it must also be harmless. Although this assumption is incorrect, it is often responsible for long delays in diagnosis. Ironically, the lesions in soft tissue that are usually painful are the benign soft-tissue tumors including desmoid tumors, hemangiomas, benign nerve sheath tumors, and soft-tissue infections.

Radiographic Evaluation

Most soft-tissue masses are seen poorly or not at all on plain radiographs; however, those with calcification will be more apparent. Although myositis ossificans is the most common lesion characterized by soft-tissue calcification, synovial sarcoma may present in this manner also. The calcification seen in synovial sarcomas can vary considerably from minute, almost imperceptible calcifications to very dense calcification, which may mimic a benign lesion (Figure 21).

MRI Findings

MRI is the gold standard for the evaluation of lesions in soft tissue. MRI is quite useful in locating a lesion but less useful in delineating the nature of the lesion. There are, however, some notable exceptions to this generalization. The classic MRI finding in most soft-tissue tumors is that of a lesion that is well circumscribed and showing dark signal on T1, and high signal on T2, fat-suppressed T2, or short-tau inversion recovery (STIR) views (Figure 22). The possible etiology of such a lesion includes benign tumor, malignant tumor, abscess, cyst, and hematoma. It is often incorrectly believed that soft-tissue sarcomas are grossly invasive whereas benign lesions are radiographically distinct and encapsulated. Most soft-tissue sarcomas are very distinct and often show some edema in the compartment in which they occur, whereas many benign lesions including desmoid tumors, hemangiomas, inflammation, injury, and infection are poorly marginated on MRI scans. Lesions with a characteristic MRI appearance include lipomas, atypical lipomas, myositis ossificans, and hemangiomas.

Lipoma

Lipoma is one of the few histologic diagnoses that can be made confidently on the basis of MRI and clinical findings alone. Benign lipomas appear as masses of uniform fat density and parallel the appearance of normal subcutaneous fat on all sequences. They are bright on T1 and T2 views (Figure 23) but suppress, as does normal fat, on fat-suppressed T2 and STIR views. A mass seen on MRI as a uniform fat density with no interstitial markings is diagnostic of benign lipoma.

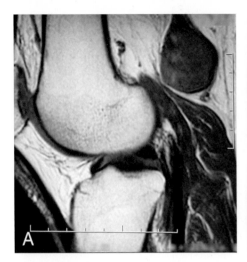 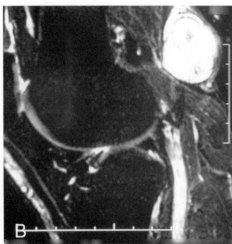

Figure 22 A soft-tissue tumor showing the typical findings of low signal on T1 **(A)** and high signal on T2 **(B)**. This lesion is a benign schwannoma.

Atypical Lipoma

Atypical lipoma is also called well-differentiated liposarcoma and lipoma-like well-differentiated liposarcoma. It is a fat-containing lesion characterized by lobules of fat signal on MRI with surrounding layers of fibrous tissue, which appear as thin layers of high signal (Figure 24). The critical difference between this lesion and higher-grade liposarcoma is that the lobules in this lesion appear fatty on MRI. Ordinary liposarcoma looks like the typical nonlipomatous lesion, which appear dark on T1 and bright on T2 and fat-suppressed T2 views, and on STIR views. Although atypical lipomas do not metastasize, they present a 10% risk of malignant transformation, usually to high-grade liposarcoma.

Myositis Ossificans

Late inactive myositis ossificans lesions present radiographically as uniform, well marginated, and benign appearing calcification in soft tissue. The calcification often is more prominent peripherally and is termed eggshell calcification (Figure 25). Early lesions show little or no calcification but do show tremendous inflammation and edema in the adjacent soft tissues. In such cases, the area of edema is much larger in volume than the area of the lesion itself.

Hemangioma

Hemangiomas are typically diffuse heterogeneous lesions with serpiginous borders (Figure 26). The classic findings of a hemangioma include the presence of a painful lesion in soft tissue which presents with a soft-tissue mass seen on MRI scan but with no mass effect. Atrophy, underlying pain, and smooth soft-tissue calcifications (phleboliths) are common.

Histology of Soft-Tissue Tumors

The histology of soft-tissue tumors has fewer common trends compared with the histology of bone lesions.

Table 4 │ Surgical Steps for Effective Intralesional Surgery
Extensive soft-tissue exposure
Create a large bone window to completely expose all surfaces of the underlying cavity
Wide resection of any area of soft-tissue extension
Complete curettage of all gross tumor in the cavity
Burring of the perimeter of the bony cavity to extend the curettage beyond all visible areas of tumor extension
Pulsatile lavage to expose clean surfaces of adjacent bone
Cauterization of the bony surface of the cavity using 90% phenol or liquid nitrogen
Reconstruction with bone cement or bone graft with or without internal fixation as needed for bony stability and joint surface support

There are many specific tumors to consider and the range of lesions goes beyond the scope of this chapter.

Treatment of Musculoskeletal Tumors

Several treatment options are available for musculoskeletal tumors. Lesions in bone may be treated with options ranging from simple curettage, to aggressive intralesional excision, to wide and radical resection. Simple curettage is sufficient for lesions that tend to be self-limited such as nonossifying fibroma and eosinophilic granuloma. Aggressive benign lesions such as giant cell tumor, aneurysmal bone cyst, chondromyxoid fibroma, and osteoblastoma require a more aggressive surgical technique entailing several steps, which together allow the surgeon to control the tumor bed and result in a high likelihood of local control. These steps for aggressive intralesional excision are shown in Table 4. It is only through the meticulous and methodic application of these steps that eradication of the underlying lesion can be reliably achieved.

Soft-tissue tumors may be treated with a full range of surgical options including debulking, marginal excision,

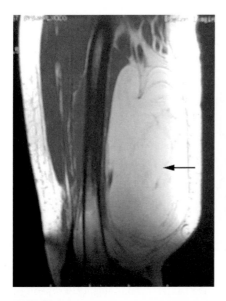

Figure 23 A benign lipoma (*arrow*) of the thigh showing a uniform fat density with no interstitial markings.

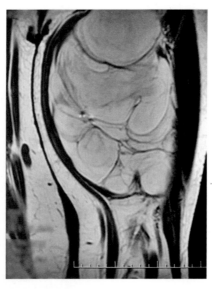

Figure 24 An atypical lipoma (well-differentiated liposarcoma) showing lobules of fat with surrounding fibrous strands.

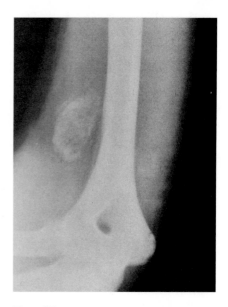

Figure 25 Myositis ossificans of the elbow with typical "eggshell" calcification.

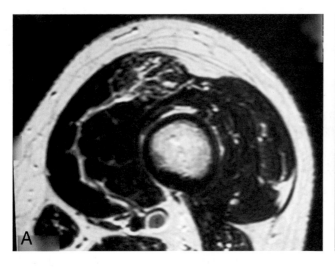

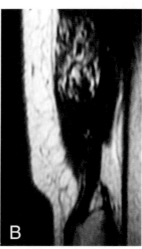

Figure 26 A benign hemangioma showing extensive infiltration within the forearm. **A,** Axial view. **B,** Sagittal view.

wide resection, and radical resection. Most benign soft-tissue masses such as lipomas, schwannomas, and myxomas can be easily excised. Soft-tissue tumors with a greater tendency for local invasion and infiltration can be very challenging to treat and may require a variety of treatment modalities beyond simple surgical techniques. Benign vascular lesions, for example, have a high rate of recurrence following surgical excision and often involve such large areas of tissue that excision is not reasonable. These lesions may be treated with a variety of nonsurgical techniques such as embolization or direct alcohol injection. Many patients with benign vascular lesions such as hemangiomas and arteriovenous malformations are difficult to cure; many will have prolonged symptoms and disability despite therapeutic intervention. Desmoid tumors are another example of benign yet problematic

lesions in soft tissue. Like hemangiomas, these lesions have a very high rate of recurrence following even aggressive attempts at local resection and are often large and may involve significant portions of major functional structures. The idea of a major and morbid resection for a benign lesion is often unacceptable. Nonsurgical options exist and have replaced surgery in many centers. Treatment using low-dose chemotherapy with methotrexate, vinblastine, or vinorelbine has been reported by several authors and achieves a high rate of local control with minimal morbidity. Radiation is also a reasonable option but is a cause for concern for subsequent malignant transformation because of the young age of most patients with desmoid tumors.

The treatment options for sarcomas of bone and soft tissue are summarized in Table 5. The therapeutic strategy is to apply treatments to specific lesions that respond to that type of treatment and to avoid options that are not effective. The differentiation of local versus systemic treatments is also important. Local treatment options include surgery and radiation. In the context of sarcoma treatment, surgery usually refers to procedures that achieve wide margins around the tumor. Current musculoskeletal oncology surgery infrequently requires amputation or radical margin surgery for extremity sarcomas. The primary indication for such procedures would involve long-neglected lesions or lesions with the direct involvement of neurovascular structures, whose resection would preclude the maintenance of a functional limb. Adjuvant treatments such as chemotherapy and radiation have permitted wide margins to become increasingly thin, especially along neurovascular structures. These surgical procedures allow functional preservation and still achieve good rates of local control that are not statistically different from those obtained with amputation. Both surgery and radiation are aimed at local control and do not affect the systemic tumor burden. Chemotherapy is a systemic treatment that has the potential to act effectively against tumor cells throughout the body even if they cannot be detected by current imaging techniques. Chemotherapy may affect the local tumor as well as any distant disease. Low-grade malignant tumors tend to metastasize at a lower rate than do high-grade lesions; therefore, it is reasonable to approach the former with local treatments only. High-grade lesions, which carry a high likelihood of metastasis, are best treated with a systemic treatment designed to cure systemic spread and increase the resectability of the primary lesion, followed by local treatment designed to remove the primary tumor.

Low-grade bone sarcomas such as chondrosarcoma, chordoma, and adamantinoma respond poorly to radiation and chemotherapy, making surgery the best treatment option. High-grade bone sarcomas such as osteosarcoma and Ewing's sarcoma respond well to chemotherapy and it is therefore a consistent part of treatment protocols. Other high-grade bone sarcomas such as malignant fibrous histiocytoma in bone, high-grade chondrosarcoma, and dedifferentiated chondrosarcoma present a challenge because of their predilection to metastasize. Although less data are available than for osteosarcoma, chemotherapy is often used in an attempt to both increase resectability and decrease the appearance or progression of systemic spread. Radiation is still a possible local treatment choice for Ewing's sarcoma, but usually has been replaced by surgery because of the potential for postradiation morbidity and malignant transformation. Despite these concerns, radiation is still used and reasonable in patients where resection carries the risk for unacceptable morbidity or when surgical margins are closer than desired. These principles also apply to other high-grade bone sarcomas; a treatment

Table 5 | Sarcoma Treatment Modalities

	Radioresistant Tumors	Radiosensitive Tumors
Low Grade	Surgery Chondrosarcoma Chordoma Adamantinoma	Surgery + Radiation Low-grade soft-tissue sarcomas
High Grade	Surgery + Chemotherapy Osteosarcoma Ewing's sarcoma Other high grade bone sarcomas	Surgery + Radiation + Chemotherapy High-grade soft-tissue sarcomas

plan should be individualized for each patient with consideration for the potential benefits of each treatment option.

Low-grade soft-tissue sarcomas respond well to a combination of wide resection surgery and local radiation. The radiation can be given either preoperatively or postoperatively because there is no difference in local control if the treatments are well planned. The major advantage to preoperative radiation is that the presence of the lesion in situ allows the radiation oncologist to concentrate the field of radiation on the lesion, which usually allows treatment of a smaller field size than in patients where the lesion has been removed. Radiation also has beneficial effects on the local tumor, which usually will decrease in size and vascularity and increase in firmness, thereby greatly facilitating resection. The disadvantage of preoperative radiation treatment is that it necessitates working with tissues that have been damaged by radiation (usually 50 cGy [5,000 rads] of radiation); this carries a 20% risk of major wound complications in most series.

High-grade soft-tissue sarcomas still present a major challenge to the oncology team. Local control can be achieved with radiation and wide resection as with the low-grade malignant lesions. Ideally, the high-grade lesions should also receive systemic treatment in the form of chemotherapy because of the higher rate of metastasis associated with high-grade histology. Although these patients are usually treated with protocols that include multidrug chemotherapy, the results of this treatment in terms of improved survival are not as dramatic as would be hoped. Chemotherapy for high-grade soft-tissue sarcomas continues to be a controversial topic and the subject of much research. It is hoped that new findings regarding the molecular and genetic bases of these diseases will spawn new drug treatments for all types of sarcomas and further improve the survival of these patients.

Emerging Concepts and Future Directions

There are several areas in orthopaedic oncology where promising new discoveries may advance current treatment and diagnosis. From a surgical perspective, one of the practical problems that has impeded the use of prostheses for segmental replacement has been the inability of current designs to optimize soft-tissue attachment, thus presenting a major challenge for treatment of the greater trochanter, the patellar tendon, and the shoulder capsule. On the horizon are promising new fiber metals that promote scar invasion and perhaps even bone ingrowth, especially when combined with biologic stimulants of bone formation. These new materials may allow for much firmer and more consistent attachment of important tendons and ligaments, which in turn will promote joint stability and function.

Advances in several fields will facilitate a deeper understanding of our present classification of tumors and will aid in tumor diagnosis. Newer immunohistochemical stains simplify the job of classifying tumors, which may be difficult to label based on light microscopy alone. In addition, ongoing research into the genetic makeup of musculoskeletal tumors is proceeding. This work, aided by microarray and comparative genetic hybridization techniques, is beginning to identify genetic defects as well as individual genes that are upregulated and downregulated in different tumor types. This increased knowledge will aid in subclassifying tumors based on their genetic makeup and should suggest new treatment options directed against specific genetic targets.

Annotated Bibliography

Factors to Consider in the Differential Diagnosis

Muscolo DL, Ayerza MA, Makino A, Costa-Paz M, Aponte-Tinao LA: Tumors about the knee misdiagnosed as athletic injuries. *J Bone Joint Surg Am* 2003;85: 1209-1214.

Of 667 tumors evaluated, 25 (3.7%) were initially misdiagnosed as athletic injuries. Oncologic surgical treatment was affected in 15 of the 25 patients.

Imaging Studies

Aboulafia AJ, Levin AM, Blum J: Preferential evaluation of patients with suspected bone and soft tissue tumors. *Clin Orthop* 2002;397:83-88.

This article concludes that many unnecessary imaging studies are often obtained in the initial work up of suspected musculoskeletal tumors especially in those that are found to be benign.

Treatment of Musculoskeletal Tumors

Aboud JA, Patel RV, Donthineni-Rao R, Lackman RD: Proximal tibial segmental prosthetic replacement without the use of muscle flaps. *Clin Orthop* 2003;414:189-196.

Twenty-two patients with tibial bone tumors were treated with proximal tibial segmental replacement prostheses by direct reattachment of the patellar tendon to the prosthesis without the use of muscle flaps. Functional results were comparable to patients treated with the use of flaps.

Bickels J, Wittig JC, Kollender Y, et al: Distal femoral resection with endoprosthetic reconstruction. *Clin Orthop* 2002;400:225-235.

A review done at one center of distal femoral replacement prostheses that included 110 reconstructions with 7.8-year follow-up is presented. Important statistics include a 5.4% infection rate, 5.4% local recurrence rate, and 10.8% revision rate for aseptic loosening or polyethylene failure.

Jung ST, Ghert MA, Harrelson JM, Scully SP: Treatment of osseous metastases in patients with renal cell carcinoma. *Clin Orthop* 2003;409:223-231.

A good review, including survival statistics, of 99 patients with metastatic renal cell tumors is presented. A reasonable argument is presented for wide resection of solitary bone lesions in patients with no other metastatic locations.

Les KA, Nicholas RW, Rougraff B, et al: Local progression after operative treatment of metastatic kidney cancer. *Clin Orthop* 2001;390:206-211.

Twenty-two of 41 patients (53%) treated with intralesional procedures required reoperation whereas only 1 of 37 patients (3%) treated with wide or marginal resection required repeat surgery.

Malo M, Davis AM, Wunder J, et al: Functional evaluation in distal femoral endoprosthetic replacement for bone sarcoma. *Clin Orthop* 2001;389:173-180.

A multicenter review of 56 patients compared outcomes for 31 patients treated with an uncemented Kotz prostheses with outcomes for 25 patients treated with cemented modular replacement prostheses. Functional scores were significantly better with the cemented modular replacement system prostheses.

Rougraff BT, Kling TJ: Treatment of active unicameral bone cysts with percutaneous injection of demineralized bone matrix and autogenous bone marrow. *J Bone Joint Surg Am* 2002;84:921-929.

Twenty-three patients with active unicameral bone cysts were treated with percutaneous injections of demineralized bone matrix and autogenous bone marrow. Only 5 of 23 required a second injection and patients returned to full activity at an average follow-up of 6 months.

Turcotte RE, Wunder JS, Isler MH, et al: Giant cell tumor of long bone: A Canadian Sarcoma Group study. *Clin Orthop* 2002;397:248-258.

A multicenter study of 186 patients with giant cell tumor of long bone showed a local recurrence rate of 18% after curettage and 16% after resection. The nature of the filling material or adjuvant uses did not alter recurrence risk.

Zeegen EN, Aponte-Tinao LA, Hornicek FJ, Gebhardt MC, Mankin HJ: Survivorship analysis of 141 modular metallic endoprostheses at early followup. *Clin Orthop* 2004;420:239-250.

A review done at one center of endoprostheses about the hip, knee, and shoulder, which included a short mean follow-up of less than 2 years, is presented. Statistical data and Kaplan-Meier analyses are presented and provide a good indication of short-term complications and short-term prosthetic survival.

Emerging Concepts and Future Directions

Bacci G, Ferrarri S, Bertoni F, et al: Histologic response of high-grade nonmetastatic osteosarcoma of the extremity to chemotherapy. *Clin Orthop* 2001;386:186-196.

In 510 consecutive patients with high-grade osteosarcoma of the extremity, the histologic response to chemotherapy depended on the number of drugs given and the histologic subtype of the tumor. Four drug regimens and telangiectatic tumors each correlated with an improved prognosis.

Classic Bibliography

Consensus Conference: Limb-sparing treatment of adult soft-tissue sarcomas and osteosarcomas. *JAMA* 1985;254:1791-1794.

Enneking WF, Dunham W, Gebhardt MC, Malawar M, Pritchard DJ: A system for the functional evaluation of reconstructive procedures after surgical treatment of tumors of the musculoskeletal system. *Clin Orthop* 1993;286:241-246.

Enneking WF, Spanier SS, Goodman MA: A system for the surgical staging of musculoskeletal sarcoma. *Clin Orthop* 1980;153:106-120.

Glasser DB, Lane JM: Stage IIB osteogenic sarcoma. *Clin Orthop* 1991;270:29-39.

Mankin HJ, Gebhardt MC, Tomford WW: The use of frozen cadaveric allografts in the management of patients with bone tumors of the extremities. *Orthop Clin North Am* 1987;18:275-289.

Mankin HJ, Lange TA, Spanier SS: The hazards of biopsy in patients with malignant primary bone and soft-tissue tumors. *J Bone Joint Surg Am* 1982;64:1121-1127.

Mankin HJ, Mankin CJ, Simon MA: The hazards of the biopsy, revisited: Members of the Musculoskeletal Tumor Society. *J Bone Joint Surg Am* 1996;78:656-663.

Nelson TE, Enneking WF: Staging of bone and soft-tissue sarcomas revisited, in Stauffer RN (ed): *Advances in Operative Orthopedics.* St. Louis, MO, Mosby Year-Book, 1994, vol 2, pp 379-391.

Pisters PW, Leung DHY, Woodruff J, Shi W, Brennan MF: Analysis of prognostic factors in 1041 patients with localized soft tissue sarcomas of the extremities. *J Clin Oncol* 1996;14:1679-1689.

Simon MA, Aschliman M, Thomas N, Mankin HJ: Limb-salvage treatment versus amputation for osteosarcoma of the distal end of the femur. *J Bone Joint Surg Am* 1986;68:1331-1337.

Winkler K, Beron G, Delling G, et al: Neoadjuvant chemotherapy of osteosarcomas: Results of a randomized cooperative trial (COSS-82) with salvage chemotherapy based on histological tumor response. *J Clin Oncol* 1988;6:329-337.

Chapter 20

Infection

Michael J. Patzakis, MD

Charalampos Zalavras, MD, PhD

Introduction

Infections of the musculoskeletal system are associated with considerable morbidity and can be challenging to treat. Prompt diagnosis, aggressive eradication of infection using appropriate antibiotic administration and surgical débridement, and the restoration of function constitute the principles and goals of treatment. The resistance of pathogens and the tissue loss resulting from infection or from surgical débridement are common clinical problems that complicate the achievement of these goals.

New diagnostic techniques and new classes of antibiotics have been introduced and serve as a useful adjunct to surgical management; however, the importance of prevention cannot be overemphasized. Minimization of nosocomial contamination, judicious use of antibiotic prophylaxis, and proper surgical technique are key factors in preventing the development of orthopaedic infections.

Pathogenesis of Musculoskeletal Infections

The pathogenesis of musculoskeletal infections involves inoculation of the microorganism in musculoskeletal tissues and interaction of the microorganism with the host environment, resulting in the clinical picture of infection.

Staphylococcus aureus is the most common organism responsible for musculoskeletal infections; however, any organism is capable of causing infection depending on the source of inoculation and the host environment. The microorganism may gain access to musculoskeletal tissues through three principal mechanisms: hematogenous spread, spread from a contiguous source of infection, or direct inoculation during trauma or surgical procedures.

The complex interaction of the inoculated microorganisms with the local and systemic host environment will determine the occurrence and severity of infection. Microorganisms adhere to host tissues, begin proliferating and colonizing the involved area, and result in an inflammatory response and host tissue damage. The ability of the organism to overcome the host defenses and

cause infection is termed virulence. Virulence is a key mechanism leading to infection, and varies among and within organism species. *S aureus* has a multitude of mechanisms that enable the organism to survive and cause infection. *S aureus* initially expresses receptors for host extracellular matrix proteins such as fibronectin, thereby facilitating adhesion of the pathogens on host tissues and colonization of bone, joints, and implants. Subsequently, the organism releases toxins that damage host cells and stimulate a systemic inflammatory reaction. *S aureus* is protected from host immune defenses by several mechanisms including the excretion of protein A, which inactivates immunoglobulin G; production of a capsular polysaccharide, which reduces opsonization and phagocytosis of the organism; and the formation of a biofilm, which secludes the organism from host defense mechanisms. The biofilm is an aggregation of microbe colonies embedded within a glycocalyx matrix that usually develop on implants or devitalized bone surfaces.

Local and systemic host factors play a major role in the outcome of the microorganism and host interaction. Local host factors that facilitate infection include reduced vascularity (resulting from arterial disease, venous stasis, irradiation, scarring, and smoking), neuropathy, trauma, and the presence of implants. Trauma predisposes a patient to infection by compromising the soft tissues, by creating a dead space with hematoma accumulation, and in patients with open fractures, by direct inoculation of tissues. The presence of implants promotes adherence of microbes, biofilm formation, and adversely affects phagocytosis, thereby facilitating development of infection. Early postoperative infections in the presence of implants usually result from contamination of the surgical wound. Late infection usually results from hematogenous seeding of the implant; *S aureus* and *Staphylococcus epidermidis* are the most common pathogens.

Systemic host factors that may reduce the ability of the immune system to respond to the pathogen include renal and liver disease, malignancy, diabetes mellitus, alcoholism, malnutrition, rheumatologic diseases, and an immunocompromised status (such as in patients with acquired immunodeficiency syndrome or those receiving immunosuppressive therapy). Intravenous drug users experience multiple episodes of bacteremia and are at increased risk for hematogenous infections.

Antibiotic Therapy and Antibiotic Resistance

The selection of appropriate antibiotic therapy from the many available agents is dependent on knowledge of the microbiology of musculoskeletal system infections (Table 1). Antibiotic therapy should initially cover the most probable pathogens until culture and sensitivity results are available; the antibiotic regimen then should be reevaluated and modified if necessary. Table 2 summarizes the microbiology of common pathogens and the suggested empiric antibiotic therapy.

Although a pathogen may initially be susceptible to an antibiotic, resistance may gradually develop by either spontaneous mutation or by acquisition of new DNA in the form of plasmids. A plasmid is a construct of autonomously replicating DNA that is distinct from the normal genome of bacteria, spreads from organism to organism, and can be incorporated in the organism's genome. The emergence of resistance is facilitated by the suboptimal use of antibiotics for both the prophylaxis and treatment of infection; this would include unnecessary use of antibiotics, empiric administration of wide-spectrum agents when a narrow spectrum agent is appropriate, and inadequate dosage or duration of treatment. Resistance is also promoted by prolonged antibiotic therapy in patients with immunosuppression or multiple comorbidities, and in patients who had inadequate débridement leading to recurrence of infection. Noncompliance with measures to prevent infection (such as hand washing and isolation of patients with resistant pathogens) spreads these organisms from one patient to another. The use of antibiotics in livestock to promote growth is another factor contributing to antibiotic resistance.

In 1999 in the United States, 52% of infections that occurred in intensive care units were caused by strains of methicillin-resistant *S aureus* (MRSA), and 25% of enterococci infections resulted from vancomycin-resistant enterococci (VRE). These resistance rates represent a 37% and 43% increase, respectively, compared with the period from 1994 to 1998. Infection with a resistant organism requires modification of antimicrobial therapy, patient isolation, and implementation of contact precautions to prevent nosocomial spread. MRSA infections can be treated with vancomycin; however, *S aureus* with intermediate resistance to vancomycin has been reported. Two newer antimicrobial agents, linezolid and quinupristin-dalfopristin, appear promising in the treatment of MRSA and VRE infections.

Diagnostic Modalities

Diagnosis of musculoskeletal infection is facilitated by laboratory tests, imaging modalities, histology, Gram stain and culture of specimens, and molecular techniques. The erythrocyte sedimentation rate (ESR) and the C-reactive protein (CRP) are markers of the acute phase response secondary to infection or the noninfectious inflammatory processes. The ESR is elevated in approximately 92% of pediatric patients with osteomyelitis. It rises within 2 days from the onset of infection, continues to rise for 3 to 5 days after appropriate antibiotic treatment is instituted, and returns to normal after approximately 3 weeks. In contrast, the CRP is elevated in approximately 98% of pediatric patients with osteomyelitis, begins rising within 6 hours, reaches a peak within 36 to 50 hours, and returns to normal approximately 1 week after successful therapy. Surgical treatment prolongs the peak and normalization times of both the ESR and CRP. The CRP shows a closer temporal relationship to the course of infection; therefore, it is the preferred marker for early diagnosis and for monitoring the response to treatment. In periprosthetic infections, studies have shown that the sensitivity and specificity of the ESR was 82% and 85%, respectively, whereas that of the CRP was 96% and 92%, respectively. An elevated peripheral blood white blood cell (WBC) count with increased polymorphonuclear cells is indicative of infection, but is only elevated in up to 50% of patients; therefore, its absence does not rule out infection.

Radiographs may show soft-tissue swelling, bone changes (resorption, periosteal new bone formation), and may disclose the presence of a fracture or tumor mimicking infection. In arthroplastic infections, radiographs may show lucency around the implants; however, this may also result from aseptic loosening. Bone scintigraphy using technetium Tc 99m evaluates the perfusion and osteoblastic activity of the skeleton, and is especially useful in localizing the pathologic process to an anatomic area. Indium-111-labeled leukocyte scans help distinguish between an infectious and noninfectious etiology and have 83% to 85% sensitivity and 75% to 94% specificity. Bone scintigraphy with indium-111-labeled immunoglobulin has 90% to 93% sensitivity and 85% to 89% specificity. In patients who have had a hip arthroplasty, bone scans may be positive in the presence of aseptic loosening and may also be positive for up to 2 years postoperatively in a well-fixed prosthesis. However, the combination of results from technetium Tc 99m and indium-111-labeled leukocyte scans show 88% sensitivity and 95% specificity in the diagnosis of infection around hip and knee arthroplasties. Positron emission tomography with F-18 fluorodeoxyglucose is a new modality that has shown 100% sensitivity and 88% specificity for chronic musculoskeletal infection. MRI can detect marrow changes secondary to infection at a

Table 1 | Antibiotics Commonly Used in Musculoskeletal Infections

Antibiotics	Adult Dosage	Spectrum of Activity
Beta-Lactam Antibiotics (active against cell wall)		
Penicillin G	2,000,000 IU every 4 hours, IV	*S pyogenes, S pneumoniae,* Anaerobes
Penicillinase-resistant penicillins Oxacillin, nafcillin	1 to 2 g every 4 hours, IV	*S aureus* (β-lactamase producing) Other gram-positive cocci
Aminopenicillins Ampicillin	1 to 2 g every 4 to 6 hours, IV	Non β-lactamase producing gram-positive cocci Gram-negative organisms (not *Pseudomonas*), Anaerobes

Aminopenicillins and β-lactamase inhibitors
  Ampicillin-sulbactam
  Amoxicillin-clavulanate
	1.5 to 3 g every 6 hours, IV
	250 to 500 mg every 8 hours, PO
		Coverage expanded to β-lactamase producing organisms

Antipseudomonal penicillins
  Piperacillin
  Ticarcillin
	3 g every 6 hours, IV
	3 g every 6 hours, IV
		Non β-lactamase producing gram-positive cocci
		Gram-negative organisms (including *Pseudomonas*)
		Anaerobes

Antipseudomonal penicillins and β-lactamase inhibitors
  Piperacillin-tazobactam
  Ticarcillin-clavulanate
	3.75 g every 6 hours, IV
	3 g every 6 hours, IV
		Coverage expanded to β-lactamase producing organisms

Cephalosporins: first generation Cefazolin	1 to 2 g every 6 to 8 hours, IV	Gram-positive cocci (β-lactamase producing)
Cephalosporins: second generation Cefuroxime	1.5 g every 8 hours, IV	Gram-positive cocci (β-lactamase producing) Gram-negative organisms (not *Pseudomonas*)
Cephalosporins: third generation Ceftriaxone	2 g every 24 hours, IV	Gram-negative organisms Gram-positive cocci (β-lactamase producing)
Cephalosporins: fourth generation Cefepime	2 g every 8 to 12 hours, IV	Gram-positive cocci (β-lactamase producing) Gram-negative organism (including *Pseudomonas*)
Carbapenems Imipenem-Cilastatin	500 mg every 6 hours, IV	Gram-positive and gram-negative organisms Anaerobes
Monobactam Aztreonam	1 to 2 g every 8 to 12 hours, IV	Gram-negative organisms (including *Pseudomonas*)
Aminoglycosides (active against ribosomes)		
Gentamicin	3 to 5 mg/kg/day (in a single dose or divided into three doses), IV	Gram-negative organisms (including *Pseudomonas*), Gram-positive cocci
Tobramycin	3 to 5 mg/kg/day in a single dose or divided into three doses), IV	
Fluoroquinolones (active against DNA)		
Ciprofloxacin	500 to 750 mg every 12 hours, PO	Gram-positive cocci
Levofloxacin	500 to 750 mg every 24 hours, PO/IV	Gram-negative organisms (including *Pseudomonas*)
Glycopeptides (active against cell wall)		
Vancomycin	1 g every 12 hours, IV	Gram-positive cocci (including MRSA and *Enterococci*), *Clostridium difficile*
Lincosamides (active against ribosomes)		
Clindamycin	900 mg every 8 hours, IV	Gram-positive cocci, anaerobes
Streptogramins (active against ribosomes)		
Quinupristin-dalfopristin	7.5 mg/kg every 8 to 12 hours, IV	Gram-positive cocci (including MRSA, VRE)
Oxazolidinones (active against ribosomes)		
Linezolid	600 mg every 12 hours, PO/IV	Gram-positive cocci (including MRSA, VRE)

IV = intravenously; PO = by mouth; MRSA = methicillin-resistant enterococci *S aureus*; VRE = vancomycin-resistant enterococci

Table 2 | Most Common Pathogens and Suggested Empiric Antibiotic Therapy in Musculoskeletal Infections

Infection and Clinical Setting	Most Common Pathogens	Empiric Antibiotic Therapy
Osteomyelitis and septic arthritis		
Infant	S aureus S pyogenes S pneumoniae Gram-negative organisms	Penicillinase-resistant penicillin and aminoglycoside or ceftriaxone
Child younger than age 3 years	S aureus S pneumoniae H influenzae (if nonimmunized)	Ceftriaxone
Older child	S aureus	Cefazolin or Penicillinase-resistant penicillin
Child with sickle cell disease	Salmonella species S aureus	Ceftriaxone
Adult	S aureus Suspected MRSA	Penicillinase-resistant penicillin Vancomycin or clindamycin
Immunocompromised adult or child	Gram-positive cocci Gram-negative organisms	Penicillinase-resistant penicillin and aminoglycoside
Septic arthritis in sexually active patients	S aureus N gonorrhoeae	Ceftriaxone
Diskitis	S aureus	Penicillinase-resistant penicillin
Lyme disease	B burgdorferi	Amoxicillin-doxycycline
Clenched-fist bite wounds	E corrodens P multocida Anaerobes	Ampicillin-sulbactam or piperacillin-tazobactam
Nail puncture wounds	S aureus P aeruginosa	Penicillinase-resistant penicillin and aminoglycoside or piperacillin-tazobactam
Necrotizing fasciitis	Streptococcus group A beta-hemolytic Gram-positive cocci, anaerobes ± Gram-negative organisms	Penicillin and Clindamycin ± Aminoglycoside

very early stage and is a highly sensitive modality for detecting osteomyelitis with a sensitivity approaching 100%. The increased water content secondary to edema and hyperemia results in a decreased marrow signal in T1-weighted images, and an increased signal in T2-weighted images, respectively. In the diagnosis of septic arthritis, studies have shown that MRI has 97% sensitivity and 92% specificity. It allows for the detection of increased intra-articular fluid, and for the evaluation of potential spread of infection into adjacent bone or soft tissue.

Identification of organisms following Gram stain of specimens from the involved area occurs in approximately one third of cases. Despite its low yield, the Gram stain examination can be useful because it is highly specific and may help the physician to determine the most appropriate antibiotic for initial therapy. For infections occurring after hip arthroplasty, evaluation of inflamed tissue specimens with Gram staining has a 19% sensitivity and a 98% specificity; frozen section histologic examination for the presence of more than five polymorphonuclear cells per high-power field has an 80% sensitivity and a 94% specificity.

Cultures remain the gold standard for establishing the diagnosis of infection. However, the prior administration of antibiotics, inadequate specimen sampling, or improper handling of specimens may preclude the growth of pathogens.

Molecular diagnostic techniques are available and may improve diagnostic efficacy in the future. A recent study indicates that polymerase chain reaction (PCR) can amplify and detect bacterial DNA, potentially leading to an earlier diagnosis compared with cultures. Another advantage of this technique is that the results are not affected by the concurrent use of antibiotics because PCR does not depend on in vitro growth of the organism. However, concerns about false-positive results secondary to contamination still exist.

Osteomyelitis in Adults

Osteomyelitis (bone inflammation secondary to the presence of microbial pathogens) can be classified based on the pathogenesis (hematogenous, traumatic, contiguous spread), the duration of the process (acute, subacute, chronic), and the age of the patient (adult versus pediatric).

Osteomyelitis in adults usually results from trauma (open fractures), surgical procedures (postoperative infections after open reduction and internal fixation of fractures), or contiguous spread from adjacent infections. The tibia is the most common site of adult osteomyelitis. Hematogenous osteomyelitis is uncommon in adults but may occur in intravenous drug users. The most common pathogen is *S aureus;* however, a variety of organisms may be involved depending on the clinical setting. *Pseudomonas aeruginosa* or other gram-negative organisms may be responsible for the infection in intravenous drug users, and less virulent microbes or fungi in immunocompromised patients. Adult osteomyelitis can be staged with the Cierny-Mader classification system, which evaluates the anatomic type of bone involvement (medullary, superficial, localized, diffuse) and the physiologic class of the host (A: normal; B: systemic, local, or combined compromise of the host; C: morbidity of treatment worse than that of disease).

A diagnosis is based on clinical findings (pain, erythema, draining sinuses, systemic symptoms), laboratory tests (elevated CRP, ESR), imaging modalities (radiographs, MRI, scintigraphy), Gram stain, and cultures. It should be noted that osteomyelitis may be clinically silent, so a high index of suspicion is warranted in situations such as atrophic nonunions after an open fracture or internal fixation of a closed fracture. Chronic draining sinuses may be complicated by malignant transformation and development of squamous cell carcinoma (Marjolin's ulcer) in approximately 1% of patients.

Osteomyelitis can be a limb-threatening condition. Treatment may be prolonged and financially and socially demanding for the patient; therefore, amputation may be a reasonable option in some complex cases. Treatment of osteomyelitis with a limb-salvage protocol consists of débridement, systemic and local antibiotic treatment, skeletal stabilization, soft-tissue coverage, and treatment of bone defects and nonunited fractures. These principles can be incorporated in a staged protocol.

The first stage of a limb salvage protocol includes radical débridement of all nonviable tissues and skeletal stabilization. Débridement should proceed until bleeding, definitively viable tissue is present at the resection margins. Inadequate débridement leads to recurrence of infection despite antibiotic therapy, because pathogens form biofilms on nonviable tissue and escape antibiotic therapy and host defense mechanisms. Specimens of pu-

rulent fluid, soft tissue, and bone from the affected area require aerobic, anaerobic, mycobacterial, and fungal cultures. The latter two cultures are especially important in immunocompromised patients or those with chronic osteomyelitis. The wound is copiously irrigated with saline; antibiotics may be added to the irrigation fluid.

The dead space that results from débridement is filled with physician-made polymethylmethacrylate beads impregnated with antibiotics such as tobramycin, vancomycin, cefepime, or other microbial-specific antibiotics available in powder form. Elution of antibiotics depends on the surface area and characteristics of the antibiotic delivery vehicle, the type and concentration of the antibiotic(s) used, the presence of fluid, and the rate of fluid turnover. Local antibiotic delivery is a useful option resulting in high local concentration and low systemic side effects and can supplement systemic therapy, provided the pathogen is susceptible to the eluted antibiotic. Nonabsorbable antibiotic delivery vehicles may require revision for removal. Intravenous administration of antibiotics for 4 to 6 weeks is the recommended therapy and can be accomplished on an outpatient basis. Oral administration of linezolid or quinolones can achieve adequate blood and tissue concentration levels and may be a useful alternative to intravenous therapy. Antibiotic administration is a key part of the treatment but will not be effective without adequate débridement. Development of resistant organisms may occur.

Skeletal stabilization in the presence of fractures that have not yet united is necessary for infection control. The optimal method of stabilization depends on the involved bone and the condition of its soft-tissue envelope. The need for careful consideration of the soft tissue when planning fixation constructs cannot be overemphasized.

The second stage of the protocol consists of wound management. If the soft-tissue envelope is adequate, delayed closure can be performed. In the presence of compromised soft tissues, coverage should be achieved by local or free muscle flaps, depending on the location and extent of the soft-tissue defect. Muscle flaps eliminate dead space, provide soft-tissue coverage, prevent contamination with new pathogens, improve the local vascularity and biologic environment, assist the host defense mechanisms, enhance antibiotic delivery, and promote the healing process. Flap coverage is usually done 3 to 7 days after the initial débridement. Local muscle flaps used for coverage of the tibia include the gastrocnemius for proximal third defects and the soleus for middle third defects. It is important to consider the biologic status of the local muscle to be transferred to avoid using muscle that has itself been compromised by the injury or by ischemic changes. In patients with distal third tibial defects, a free muscle flap is necessary.

The third stage of the treatment regimen consists of management of existing bone defects, usually by autogenous bone grafting, which is performed when the soft-tissue envelope has healed (usually 6 to 8 weeks after the muscle transfer). At this stage, viability of the flap and control of infection have been determined. For anterior defects and most nonunions of the tibia, the muscle flap is elevated and the graft is placed at the site of the nonunion or defect. Posterolateral tibia bone grafting is an alternative if there is no anterior sequestrum or need for a soft-tissue procedure anteriorly. The usefulness of bone graft substitutes as void fillers in a defect of infectious etiology is still being evaluated. Bone defects greater than 6 cm require specialized reconstructive procedures such as vascularized bone grafts or distraction osteogenesis. Limb salvage can result in a satisfactory functional outcome. An outcomes study of patients with chronic osteomyelitis of the tibia done in 2000 showed that at a mean follow-up of 5 years, 39 of 46 patients (85%) were able to ambulate independently without pain. Patient age (advanced age) and a history of smoking adversely affected the outcome.

Septic Arthritis in Adults

The portals of pathogen entry in patients with septic arthritis include hematogenous inoculation, spread from an adjacent area of infection, or inoculation by a penetrating or surgical wound. Susceptibility to septic arthritis is increased in immunocompromised hosts, patients with preexisting joint pathology, and patients with frequent bacteremic episodes. Microorganisms trigger an inflammatory response that recruits polymorphonuclear cells. Enzymes released by bacteria and polymorphonuclear and synovial cells promote the degradation of glycosaminoglycans and the subsequent loss of collagen, which results in gross damage to the articular cartilage.

Neisseria gonorrhoeae is the most common pathogen causing septic arthritis in otherwise healthy adults; women are more frequently affected than men. Clinical symptoms of disseminated disease include migratory polyarthritis, rash, and tenosynovitis of the dorsal aspect of the wrist and hand. Septic involvement of a single joint also may occur with the knee joint most commonly affected. *S aureus* is the second most common pathogen causing adult septic arthritis. Immunocompromised hosts may have infections with gram-negative organisms, or unusual pathogens, such as mycobacteria or fungi. Intravenous drug users, in addition to being susceptible to *S aureus*, are prone to infections with *Pseudomonas aeruginosa* or *Serratia marcescens*.

Septic arthritis is more common in joints of the lower extremity, with the knee most frequently involved. The affected joint is painful, swollen, has limited range of motion, and is often erythematous. The CRP and ESR are generally elevated, and the WBC count is elevated in approximately 50% of patients. Radiographs help assess bone involvement and ultrasound is useful in detecting a joint effusion. MRI, in addition to detecting a joint effusion, delineates any bone and soft-tissue involvement.

Aspiration of the involved joint always should be done to establish the diagnosis and to identify the pathogen. The joint aspirate should be sent for Gram stain, cultures, sensitivity testing, WBC count with differential, and crystal analysis. A WBC count greater than 50,000 cells/mm^3 and a differential with polymorphonuclear leukocytes exceeding 75% indicate septic arthritis; however, lower values do not preclude the diagnosis. Synovial fluid cultures are positive in approximately 90% of patients with nongonococcal arthritis, compared with 25% of those with gonococcal arthritis. Blood cultures are positive in approximately 50% of patients with nongonococcal arthritis, whereas the yield is only 10% in those with gonococcal arthritis.

Surgical decompression by arthrotomy of a septic joint relieves pressure and evacuates enzymes, inflammatory mediators, and bacteria from the joint to minimize cartilage damage. Arthroscopic irrigation may be an alternative. Repeated joint aspirations may be satisfactory in some knee infections but should not be used for infections of the hip or small joints. Synovial biopsy for culture and histology is recommended for joints undergoing arthrotomy. In chronic or recurrent infections, a complete synovectomy is warranted. Septic arthritis after anterior cruciate ligament reconstruction occurs in approximately 0.2% to 0.5% of patients. According to one recent study, the rate of infection after anterior cruciate ligament reconstruction was 0.14% in 3,500 consecutive procedures. In early (occurring from up to 4 to 6 weeks) postoperative infections, graft retention may be possible with prompt irrigation, débridement, and antibiotic therapy.

Empiric systemic antibiotic therapy should be started immediately after cultures have been collected and should cover the most likely pathogens based on the clinical setting. In otherwise healthy adults, both *N gonorrhoeae* and *S aureus* should be covered, usually with a third generation cephalosporin. Immunocompromised hosts and intravenous drug users should receive coverage for both *S aureus* and *P aeruginosa*. The duration of antibiotic therapy is usually 4 weeks for nongonococcal arthritis and 1 week in gonococcal arthritis that responds well to therapy.

Lyme disease is a multisystem spirochetal disorder caused by *Borrelia burgdorferi*, which is transmitted by the bite of an infected tick. It usually occurs in the Northeast, Midwest, and Northwest regions of the United States. The disease occurs in three clinical stages. In the first stage (early localized disease) a pathognomonic skin lesion (erythema migrans) emerges and progressively increases in size. The second stage (early disseminated disease) is characterized by neurologic and cardiac manifestations. In the third stage (late disease) musculoskeletal symptoms develop in 80% of untreated patients and include arthralgia, intermittent episodes of arthritis, and subsequently chronic monoarthritis, usually of the knee. Acute monoarthritis may clinically resemble septic arthritis. The synovial fluid in acute noninfectious monoarthritis usually has a WBC count of 10,000 to 25,000 cells/mm^3 with an increased number of polymorphonuclear cells; a higher count may be present, creating a resemblance to a more typical bacterial infection. Chronic Lyme arthritis is rarely destructive and has been associated with HLA-DRB1*040, thereby suggesting an autoimmune mechanism. Enzyme-linked immunosorbent assay establishes the diagnosis. Oral antibiotic therapy with amoxicillin or doxycycline for approximately 4 weeks is recommended. Intravenous therapy with ceftriaxone may be used for patients with recurrent episodes of arthritis and for those with neurologic involvement. A single 200-mg dose of doxycycline given within 72 hours after a tick bite that occurs in an endemic area can prevent the development of Lyme disease.

Tuberculosis should be considered in the differential diagnosis of arthritis and chronic osteomyelitis, especially in immunocompromised patients and in patients from areas endemic for tuberculosis outside of the United States. Tubercular arthritis usually affects the hip and the knee, and is characterized by an insidious onset, subtle inflammatory signs, and disproportionately extensive bone involvement relative to the symptoms present. Radiographic changes include subchondral bone erosions and joint space narrowing. Synovial biopsy, acid-fast stains, and cultures help to establish the diagnosis. Growth of the organism in solid medium culture requires up to 8 weeks and sensitivity testing should always be performed. Therapy for tuberculosis should include a multidrug regimen with isoniazid, rifampin, pyrazinamide, and ethambutol. When sensitivity results are available, ethambutol can be discontinued if the organism is fully susceptible. The duration of therapy ranges from 6 to 9 months.

Pediatric Musculoskeletal Infections
Osteomyelitis in Children

Osteomyelitis in children is usually hematogenous in origin. Osteomyelitis is more common in males, the lower extremity, and increases in incidence during the warmer months. The most common organism causing pediatric osteomyelitis is *S aureus*. Neonates may also have infections with group B *Streptococci* or gram-negative pathogens. *Haemophilus influenzae* type B was previously a common musculoskeletal pathogen in children between 1 and 4 years of age, but vaccination against this organism has almost eliminated its role in pediatric osteomyelitis. In children younger than 3 years of age, the most common pathogens include *S aureus*, *Streptococcus*

pneumoniae, and *Streptococcus pyogenes*. Children with sickle cell disease are more prone to infections from the *Salmonella* species compared with the normal pediatric population. Similarly, immunocompromised children are more susceptible to osteomyelitis from less virulent microbes or fungi than patients with uncompromised immune systems.

Pediatric acute hematogenous osteomyelitis has a predilection for the metaphysis of long bones. The metaphysis is perfused by end-arteries that enter large venous sinusoids. The sluggish circulation and defective phagocytosis in the capillary loops allow bacteria to inoculate in the metaphyseal area by the physeal plate. The infection subsequently may spread through Volkmann's canals of the metaphyseal bone to the subperiosteal region where a resultant abscess may elevate the periosteum and devitalize cortical bone. Osteomyelitis may spread to the epiphysis, especially in infants because of their distinct vascular pattern with metaphyseal vessels traversing into the epiphyseal area. Septic involvement of the adjacent joint occurs in 33% of patients with metaphyseal osteomyelitis. The most commonly affected joint is the knee. Joint involvement is facilitated if the metaphysis is intra-articular (proximal femur, proximal humerus, proximal radius, distal lateral tibia). Therefore, careful evaluation of the adjacent joint should be an important part of the evaluation for any child with osteomyelitis. The infectious process may also spread to the surrounding soft tissues and to the medullary canal. Acute hematogenous osteomyelitis in older children usually involves a single site. However, in neonates, polyostotic involvement occurs in 30% of patients, and may be identified with a bone scan.

Clinical findings of acute hematogenous pediatric osteomyelitis include pain, refusal to bear weight, inability to use the affected extremity, and fever. Previous trauma to the affected site is present in 30% to 50% of patients. The patient history should include the presence of medical conditions (useful for assessing the likely pathogen) and any recent antibiotic administration (likely to alter the clinical presentation). Diagnosis can be challenging in neonates because the clinical picture is often subtle. The proximal femur and hip joint are most commonly involved and a high index of suspicion is needed for early diagnosis; pseudoparalysis in a neonate should be carefully evaluated.

Laboratory tests include a WBC count and differential, ESR, and CRP. Bone aspiration and blood cultures are essential. Bone aspiration or intraoperative cultures identify the pathogen in 48% to 85% of patients, whereas blood cultures are positive in 30% to 60%. The combination of data from bone aspiration and blood cultures is important to achieve accurate diagnosis. Radiographs show soft-tissue swelling but are of limited value in identifying osseous changes, which typically do not occur until 7 to 14 days later. Bone scanning is useful when the location of the pathology is uncertain or multiple locations are suspected, such as in the neonate. In children with sickle cell anemia, osteomyelitis can be differentiated from bone infarction with acute bone pain by a combination of sequential bone marrow and bone scintigraphy.

Treatment of pediatric acute hematogenous osteomyelitis consists of prompt systemic antibiotic administration and close monitoring of the patient. Surgical treatment is based on the presence of an abscess. In approximately 50% of patients, surgery is not necessary because early antibiotic therapy contains the infectious process before an abscess can form. Surgical intervention is warranted if an abscess is present (diagnosed by aspiration, or MRI), if the adjacent joint is septically involved, or if changes are present on plain radiographs, indicating late presentation.

Antibiotics should be given immediately after bone aspiration and blood cultures have been obtained. Empirical antibiotic administration while the culture results are pending should target the most likely pathogens based on the age of the child and should always cover *S aureus*, which is the most frequent pathogen in all age groups. Systemic antibiotics can be substituted with oral therapy provided the patient is afebrile, shows considerable clinical improvement, and in whom CRP levels have normalized or considerably decreased. Antibiotics are usually given for 4 to 6 weeks.

In some patients subacute osteomyelitis may insidiously develop over a period of months until the patient develops symptoms, such a pain and limp. The radiographic appearance of subacute osteomyelitis may resemble a tumor, and biopsy is frequently necessary to establish the diagnosis.

Chronic Recurrent Multifocal Osteomyelitis

Chronic recurrent multifocal osteomyelitis is characterized by bilateral, usually symmetric bone involvement. The onset is insidious and inflammatory symptoms may wax and wane over time. The clavicle and the metaphyses of long bones usually are affected; lytic and sclerotic changes are seen on radiographs. A pustular rash on the palms and soles may be present. Cultures are negative and the diagnosis is one of exclusion after microbial osteomyelitis or bone tumors are ruled out. No effective treatment exists; however, anti-inflammatory medication may relieve symptoms. Antibiotics are not needed if cultures are negative. Although symptoms tend to recur over a 2-year period, the long-term prognosis appears to be good.

Septic Arthritis

Septic arthritis is usually hematogenous in origin, is caused by pathogens similar to those involved in hematogenous osteomyelitis, and commonly occurs in the knee and hip joints. Septic arthritis may originate from contiguous spread of adjacent infection or osteomyelitis. In neonates, osteomyelitis in the metaphysis can spread to the epiphysis via blood vessels traversing the physis, and then to the joint space via the thin bone cortex. Pathogens also may be directly inoculated into the joint by a penetrating injury.

Clinical symptoms include fever, pain, inability to use the upper extremity (pseudoparalysis), or refusal to walk when the lower extremity is affected. The range of motion of the involved joint is markedly decreased and painful. In septic arthritis of the hip, the joint is positioned in external rotation, abduction, and mild flexion to increase joint volume and release tension on the capsule.

An elevated CRP and ESR are present in at least 90% of patients with septic arthritis, whereas the WBC count is elevated in approximately 50%. MRI shows fluid collection in the joint and also is useful in elevating any adjacent bone or soft-tissue involvement. Ultrasonography can detect a joint effusion. Scintigraphy is useful for the evaluation of multiple joints when the pathologic process cannot be localized to a single joint, or when the joint involved is not clinically apparent. Joint aspiration should always be performed. Fluoroscopic or ultrasonographic guidance is useful for hip aspiration. The joint aspirate should be sent for a Gram stain, cultures, sensitivity testing, and WBC count and differential. A WBC count greater than 50,000/mm^3 is found in approximately 50% of patients.

Transient synovitis of the hip in a young child (age 3 to 8 years) may present as an acutely irritable hip with an effusion; the clinical presentation may be indistinguishable from septic arthritis. The presence of a fever, the inability to bear weight, an ESR greater than 40 mm/h, and a peripheral WBC count greater than 12,000 cells/mm^3 are independent variables that can help distinguish the two conditions. According to a 1999 study, the probability of a correct diagnosis of septic arthritis was found to be 99.6% for children with all four factors, 93.1% for those with three factors, 40% for those with two factors, and 3% for those with only one factor.

Inflammatory arthritides, such as juvenile rheumatoid arthritis, poststreptococcal arthritis, and rheumatic fever should be included in the differential diagnosis of pediatric arthritis with joint effusion. Juvenile rheumatoid arthritis may present as a single acutely swollen and painful joint. However, in juvenile rheumatoid arthritis the onset is usually gradual, the patient may be able to walk, systemic symptoms are milder, the joint fluid WBC count is usually less than 50,000 cells/mm^3, and the Gram stain and cultures are negative.

Surgical decompression of a septic joint may be accomplished by open arthrotomy or arthroscopy. Repeated joint aspiration may be an alternative in some patients in whom the affected joints are easily accessible; however, failure to respond to nonsurgical treatment within 24 to 48 hours warrants surgical intervention. In patients with a septic hip, prompt surgical arthrotomy, irrigation, and débridement are mandatory because delayed or incomplete decompression impairs perfusion of the femoral head and may cause further morbidity, such as osteonecrosis, hip dislocation, and osteomyelitis. The anterior approach is preferred to avoid any damage to the vascularity of the femoral head.

Antibiotic therapy should be started immediately after cultures have been collected and should target the most probable pathogens based on the child's age and the clinical setting. In sexually active adolescents *N gonorrhoeae* is a potential pathogen. Systemic antibiotics can be converted to oral therapy as the patient clinically improves. The total duration of therapy is usually 3 weeks. Contiguous osteomyelitis should be suspected if the clinical course is not dramatically improved after drainage of the septic joint and the CRP remains elevated.

Diskitis

Diskitis is a hematogenous infection involving the disk and vertebral body. *S aureus* is the most common pathogen. Clinical symptoms may be insidious and may include back pain, abdominal pain, or inability to walk. Tenderness is present over the involved vertebrae. Systemic symptoms and signs of infection may be absent; ESR and CRP are usually elevated but the WBC count may be normal. Radiographs are initially noncontributory but subsequently show disk space narrowing. MRI reveals early changes in the disk and the adjacent vertebral bodies. Bone scintigraphy may be helpful when the location of the pathologic process is uncertain. Blood cultures should be obtained. Needle or open biopsy and cultures may be helpful if the diagnosis is uncertain; however, the yield (as low as 27%), the potential complications of biopsy, and the preponderance of *S aureus* infections do not justify routine biopsy. Although the infectious nature of diskitis has been questioned based on the low yield of biopsy cultures and the resolution of symptoms with rest alone, treatment should include rest and antibiotic therapy with an antistaphylococcal agent.

Sacroiliac Joint Infection

Sacroiliac joint infection may present with a variety of symptoms including back pain, abdominal pain, pain in the gluteal area, limp, fever, malaise, and tenderness over the involved area. The FABER test (flexion, abduction, external rotation) and compression of the pelvis elicit pain. MRI is useful in determining the location of the infectious process and the extent of bone and soft-tissue involvement. *S aureus* is the most common pathogen and should be covered by initial antibiotic therapy.

Surgical débridement is seldom necessary, except in the presence of an abscess.

Wound Infections

Wound infections involve a wide spectrum of anatomic locations and etiologic mechanisms. An awareness of the potential for infection in particular wounds, such as clenched-fist injuries and nail puncture wounds, is needed for proper treatment. Identification and prompt treatment of severe life-threatening infections, such as necrotizing fasciitis, are essential to reduce mortality and morbidity.

Clenched-fist injuries represent human bite wounds with a high potential for damage of underlying tissues and infection. Violation of the joint capsule of the metacarpophalangeal joints occurs in 68% of patients. *Eikenella corrodens* and *Pasteurella multocida* are gram-negative, facultative anaerobes, often found in human mouth flora. All patients with clenched-fist lacerations or puncture wounds over joints should be treated with surgical débridement and exploration of the deep structures, including the joint and the extensor tendon, at the time of initial medical care. The wound should not be closed primarily. Antibiotic therapy consisting of wide-spectrum antibiotics active against anaerobes should be administered.

Nail puncture wounds to the foot may lead to bone or joint penetration and predispose the patient to osteomyelitis and/or septic arthritis. The area overlying the metatarsal neck region and extending distally to the toes carries the highest risk for infection, because the metatarsal heads are a major weight-bearing area with a limited amount of overlying tissue. Approximately 97% of patients requiring hospitalization for septic complications had sustained a puncture wound through this region. *P aeruginosa* is the most common pathogen involved, especially if the nail enters through an athletic shoe; the exact reason for this is unknown. If increasing tenderness is present over a puncture wound area, admission to the hospital is needed for antibiotic therapy and surgical débridement.

Necrotizing fasciitis involves the fascia and overlying tissues but spares the muscles. Although group A streptococcus is often involved, the disease may be polymicrobial. Immunocompromised hosts and children with varicella infections are at increased risk for developing the disease. Necrotizing fasciitis initially may resemble cellulitis, but the edema and induration extend beyond the area of erythema. The infection rapidly spreads along fascial planes, results in septic shock, and does not respond to antibiotic therapy alone. Emergent surgical débridement is warranted. The disease carries a high mortality rate ranging from 6% to 76%, especially if surgical treatment is delayed.

Infection in the Setting of Internal Fixation

In the presence of internal fixation, microorganisms grow in a biofilm that adheres to the implant surface and protects them from host defense mechanisms and antibiotics. The choice of retaining or removing infected implants depends on several factors including time since fracture fixation, stability provided by the hardware, and bone healing status. In the early postoperative period, before the fracture is united, internal fixation is necessary to maintain reduction of the fracture. Treatment should include irrigation, débridement, intraoperative cultures, brushing of exposed implants, and antibiotic therapy for 6 weeks. If the fracture is healed, internal fixation is removed. Loose hardware that does not provide stability should be removed regardless of the time frame. If the fracture is not healed, it should be stabilized with another device, preferably an external fixator for the tibia and an intramedullary rod for the femur. In intra-articular united fractures, internal fixation should not be removed or replaced unless it is loose and not providing stability.

Infection in the Setting of Arthroplasty

Infection occurs in approximately 1% of patients who have undergone total joint arthroplasty, with *S epidermidis* and *S aureus* the most common infecting organisms. The pathogenesis of infection involves either direct inoculation of the organisms (during the procedure and in the early postoperative period) or hematogenous spread (at any point during the life of the implant).

The clinical indicators of periprosthetic infection may be straightforward and consist of pain, decreased range of motion, drainage, and systemic symptoms. However, the clinical picture is often subtle with pain as the only symptom. Laboratory tests (ESR and CRP), bone scintigraphy, and joint aspiration are useful. The combination of normal ESR and CRP levels reliably predicts the absence of infection. Aspiration has 86% sensitivity and 94% specificity in the absence of existing antibiotic therapy and should be used when the ESR or the CRP level is elevated or when a clinical suspicion of infection remains. In addition, intraoperative tests, such as cultures (94% sensitivity and 97% specificity), and frozen sections evaluating the number of polymorphonuclear leukocytes per high-power field (80% sensitivity and 94% specificity) can be helpful in equivocal cases. The Gram stain is unreliable (19% sensitivity and 98% specificity) for determining the presence of periprosthetic infection.

Treatment options, in addition to administration of systemic antibiotics for 4 to 6 weeks, include irrigation and débridement with retention of components, or exchange arthroplasty (one-stage versus two-stage). Salvage procedures include permanent resection or arthrodesis. Chronic antibiotic suppression or amputation may

be considered in selected patients. Treatment choice depends on duration of infection, virulence of the organism, implant stability, the patient's immune and medical status, and the condition of the local soft-tissue envelope. Staging systems may be useful to evaluate these factors, compare results among treatment centers, and to establish guidelines for care.

Irrigation, débridement, exchange of the polyethylene liner, and retention of the components are options for patients who develop infections in the early postoperative period (less than 1 month), and in patients with acute hematogenous infections (symptoms of duration less than 2 to 4 weeks in a previously well-functioning patient) with well-fixed components. Component retention is associated with lower rates of infection control (50% to 71%), possibly because of concurrent hematogenous seeding and osteomyelitis of adjacent bone, biofilm formation, and limited débridement.

Exchange arthroplasty is the preferred option for patients with chronic late-developing infections (developing more than 1 month after the procedure with indolent course and duration greater than 2 to 4 weeks), and for those with acute hematogenous infections with implant loosening (provided that the patient is in good condition and the bone stock is adequate or reconstructible). Flap coverage may be warranted for treatment of an infected arthroplasty with a poor soft-tissue envelope. Following irrigation and débridement, the exchange arthroplasty can be performed at the same time (one stage), or preferably as a subsequent procedure with an interval of 6 weeks or longer (two stage). Local antibiotic delivery during the reimplantation interval can be accomplished by using antibiotic-impregnated spacers. Two-stage exchange arthroplasty has a higher rate of eradication of infection (88% to 95%) compared with the one-stage technique (70% to 85%).

Reimplantation of a prosthesis may not be possible because of a severely compromised host, deficient bone stock, poor condition of the soft tissues, the presence of infection with resistant organisms, or repeated failed exchanged arthroplasties. In this situation, resection arthroplasty is an option. Arthrodesis may be a preferable choice for use in the lower extremity of active patients, because it offers improved function compared with resection arthroplasty. Chronic antibiotic suppression is an option for severely compromised patients, or for patients with limited life expectancy, provided the infecting organism is sensitive to oral antibiotics. Amputation of the extremity may be needed for persistent uncontrolled infection in a severely compromised patient.

Episodes of bacteremia may cause hematogenous seeding of implants; therefore, patients should be in good dental health before a total joint arthroplasty is done and should maintain good oral hygiene after the procedure. Single-dose antibiotic prophylaxis with cephalosporin or amoxicillin (clindamycin in patients allergic to penicillin) is recommended when a dental procedure with high risk for bacteremia, such as dental extraction, is performed on a patient with increased risk for hematogenous infection (such as immunocompromised patients, or those with comorbidities) within 2 years from the date of arthroplasty.

Future Directions

The goal of future research is improved prevention, diagnosis, and treatment of musculoskeletal infections. Immunization against pathogens and development of implant materials resistant to infection may aid prevention. Refinement of diagnostic methods, such as PCR, will lead to early and accurate diagnoses. Development of new antibiotics, biodegradable materials for local antibiotic delivery, and pharmacologic improvement of host defenses (such as by granulocyte stimulating hormone), may make treatment more effective. Genetic interventions may help fight infection by the alteration of resistant organisms and, in combination with tissue engineering, may find application in the restoration of damaged host tissue.

Annotated Bibliography

Pathogenesis of Musculoskeletal Infections

Elasri MO, Thomas JR, Skinner RA, et al: Staphylococcus aureus collagen adhesin contributes to the pathogenesis of osteomyelitis. *Bone* 2002;30:275-280.

The authors created an *S aureus* strain that was mutant for collagen-binding adhesin. The mutant strain, which was able to bind fibronectin but not collagen, resulted in hematogenous osteomyelitis in 5% of injected mice, compared with 70% when the nonmutant strain was used.

Antibiotic Therapy and Antibiotic Resistance

Birmingham MC, Rayner CR, Meagher AK, Flavin SM, Batts DH, Schentag JJ: Linezolid for the treatment of multidrug-resistant, gram-positive infections: Experience from a compassionate-use program. *Clin Infect Dis* 2003;36:159-168.

The authors evaluated the role of linezolid in 796 patients with multidrug-resistant, gram-positive infections, mostly from vancomycin-resistant enterococci and methicillin-resistant staphylococci. Linezolid use resulted in high rates of clinical and microbiological cure with good overall tolerance.

Diagnostic Modalities

Tarkin IS, Henry TJ, Fey PI, Iwen PC, Hinrichs SH, Garvin KL: PCR rapidly detects methicillin-resistant staphylococci periprosthetic infection. *Clin Orthop* 2003; 414:89-94.

PCR successfully predicted the presence of methicillin-resistant staphylococci infections in a septic arthritis model and gave results concordant with culture results in 34 of 35 samples obtained during revision arthroplasty.

Septic Arthritis in Adults

Indelli PF, Dillingham M, Fanton G, Schurman DJ: Septic arthritis in postoperative anterior cruciate ligament reconstruction. *Clin Orthop* 2002;398:182-188.

The rate of infection after anterior cruciate ligament reconstructions in 3,500 consecutive procedures was found to be 0.14%. All patients had arthroscopic débridement followed by 6 weeks of intravenous antibiotics. In four patients the grafts were retained and full range of motion was achieved.

Pediatric Musculoskeletal Infections

Khachatourians AG, Patzakis MJ, Roidis N, Holtom PD: Laboratory monitoring in pediatric acute osteomyelitis and septic arthritis. *Clin Orthop* 2003;409:186-194.

A review of 50 children with osteomyelitis, septic arthritis, or both showed that surgical intervention resulted in postoperatively increased levels of ESR and CRP and an increase in the amount of time to peak and normalization of ESR and CRP values.

Skaggs DL, Kim SK, Greene NW, Harris D, Miller JH: Differentiation between bone infarction and acute osteomyelitis in children with sickle-cell disease with use of sequential radionuclide bone-marrow and bone scans. *J Bone Joint Surg Am* 2001;83:1810-1813.

The combination of sequential bone marrow scans and bone scintigraphy was used in 79 episodes of acute bone pain in children with sickle cell anemia and reliably differentiated osteomyelitis from a bone infarction.

Wound Infections

Wong CH, Chang HC, Pasupathy S, Khin LW, Tan JL, Low CO: Necrotizing fasciitis: Clinical presentation, microbiology, and determinants of mortality. *J Bone Joint Surg Am* 2003;85:1454-1460.

The authors reviewed 89 patients with necrotizing fasciitis. Only 13 patients had an admitting diagnosis of necrotizing fasciitis. A delay in surgery of more than 24 hours resulted in increased mortality. A high index of suspicion and prompt treatment are essential for this condition.

Infection in the Setting of Arthroplasty

American Academy of Orthopaedic Surgeons Website. Advisory Statement: Antibiotic Prophylaxis for Dental Patients with Total Joint Replacements: American Dental Association and American Academy of Orthopaedic Surgeons. Available at: http://www.aaos.org/wordhtml/papers/advistmt/1014.htm. Accessed February, 2004.

This advisory statement updates recommendations for antibiotic prophylaxis in patients with total joint replacements who are undergoing dental procedures.

Kilgus DJ, Howe DJ, Strang A: Results of periprosthetic hip and knee infections caused by resistant bacteria. *Clin Orthop* 2002;404:116-124.

The authors reviewed 70 periprosthetic infections and reported successful retention of the prosthesis or reimplantation in 48% of hips and 18% of knees infected with methicillin-resistant *S aureus* or *S epidermidis*, compared with 81% of hips and 89% of knees infected with antibiotic-sensitive organisms.

Lehman CR, Ries MD, Paiement GD, Davidson AB: Infection after total joint arthroplasty in patients with human immunodeficiency virus or intravenous drug use. *J Arthroplasty* 2001;16:330-335.

Patients infected with the human immunodeficiency virus and/or intravenous drug users are susceptible to deep periprosthetic infection. The infection rate was 14% (4 of 28) in human immunodeficiency virus-positive patients undergoing total joint arthroplasty and 25% (2 of 8) in intravenous drug users.

Classic Bibliography

Cierny G III, Mader JT, Penninck JJ: A clinical staging system for adult osteomyelitis. *Contemp Orthop* 1985;10: 17.

Costerton JW, Stewart PS, Greenberg EP: Bacterial biofilms: A common cause of persistent infections. *Science* 1999;284:1318-1322.

Kocher MS, Zurakowski D, Kasser JR: Differentiating between septic arthritis and transient synovitis of the hip in children: An evidence-based clinical prediction algorithm. *J Bone Joint Surg Am* 1999;81:1662-1670.

Mazur JM, Ross G, Cummings J, Hahn GA Jr, McCluskey WP: Usefulness of magnetic resonance imaging for te diagnosis of acute musculoskeletal infections in children. *J Pediatr Orthop* 1995;15:144-147.

McPherson EJ, Tontz W Jr, Patzakis M, et al: Outcome of infected total knee utilizing a staging system for prosthetic joint infection. *Am J Orthop* 1999;28:161-165.

Perlman MH, Patzakis MJ, Kumar PJ, Holtom P: The incidence of joint involvement with adjacent osteomyelitis in pediatric patients. *J Pediatr Orthop* 2000;20:40-43.

Scott RJ, Christofersen MR, Robertson WW Jr, Davidson RS, Rankin L, Drummond DS: Acute osteomyelitis in children: A review of 116 cases. *J Pediatr Orthop* 1990;10:649-652.

Siegel HJ, Patzakis MJ, Holtom PD, Sherman R, Shepherd L: Limb salvage for chronic tibial osteomyelitis: An outcomes study. *J Trauma* 2000;48:484-489.

Spangehl MJ, Masri BA, O'Connell JX, Duncan CP: Prospective analysis of preoperative and intraoperative investigations for the diagnosis of infection at the sites of two hundred and two revision total hip arthroplasties. *J Bone Joint Surg Am* 1999;81:672-683.

Tsukayama DT, Estrada R, Gustilo RB: Infection after total hip arthroplasty: A study of the treatment of one hundred and six infections. *J Bone Joint Surg Am* 1996; 78:512-523.

Unkila-Kallio L, Kallio MJ, Eskola J, Peltola H: Serum C-reactive protein, erythrocyte sedimentation rate, and white blood cell count in acute hematogenous osteomyelitis of children. *Pediatrics* 1994 ;93:59-62 .

US Department of Health and Human Services, Public Health Service, Centers for Disease Control and Prevention (CDC): Semiannual Report: Aggregated data from the National Nosocomial Infections Surveillance (NNIS) System, March 2000.

Chapter 21

Arthritis

Kam Shojania, MD, FRCPC

John M. Esdaile, MD, MPH

Nelson Greidanus, MD, MPH, FRCSC

Introduction

Arthritis encompasses a heterogeneous group of more than 100 diseases that involve the synovial joints and the periarticular structures. The exact pathoetiologic mechanisms underlying most of these disorders are uncertain; however, pathology of the synovium, articular cartilage, and their subcomponents are believed to be the primary cause of the most common types of arthritis. Correct diagnosis relies primarily on clinical features that may be both musculoskeletal and nonmusculoskeletal in nature. Patients with arthritic involvement of their joints have significant pain, loss of motion, deformity, and instability. The mainstay of contemporary treatment is nonsurgical and includes patient education, lifestyle and activity modifications, and pharmacologic agents. Surgical intervention, particularly in the hip and knee, may be necessary for the treatment of severe symptoms, and occasionally may be indicated as a preventive measure. Pain relief remains the most predictable result of reconstructive surgery and represents the primary indication for most surgical interventions. Restoration of motion and function is less predictable; therefore, preoperative assessments need to be individualized and patients should be counseled concerning functional expectations. The development of novel pharmacologic strategies is underway to treat and possibly alter the natural history of these disorders. Innovations in prosthetic design and surgical technique are improving the outcomes for patients requiring surgical intervention.

Cartilage Structure and Physiology

The two major types of articular cartilage are fibrocartilage and hyaline cartilage. Menisci are typical examples of fibrocartilage. Hyaline cartilage, which is the predominant form of articular cartilage, covers the cortical bone ends and protects them by absorbing force, providing an extremely low coefficient of friction, and improving joint stability (Figure 1). Articular hyaline cartilage is securely fastened to cortical bone by a layer of calcified cartilage. The low friction joint surface helps to withstand the high shear forces created by the muscles that typically insert near the joint with short lever arms.

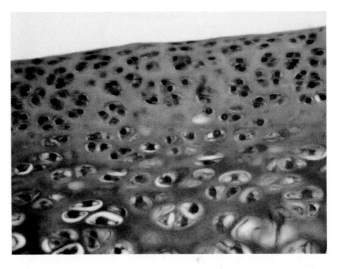

Figure 1 High power photomicrograph of normal cartilage from a rat knee. *(Courtesy of Dr. Michael Nimmo.)*

Chondrocytes

Chondrocytes are isolated cells within cartilage that function to produce, maintain, and remodel the extracellular matrix constituents. Chondrocyte activity is regulated by mechanical factors, cytokines, and growth factors. For example, interleukin (IL)-1 can stimulate chondrocytes to produce proinflammatory mediators such as matrix metalloproteinases (MMPs), while transforming growth factor beta stimulates chondrocytes to differentiate and produce type II collagen and proteoglycans. IL-4 is a chondroprotective cytokine that is activated with mechanical loading of the chondrocyte. Mechanical forces across the cartilage stimulate chondrocyte synthesis of proteoglycan and collagen; conversely, prolonged inactivity contributes to degenerative changes in the cartilage through reduction in extracellular matrix synthesis by chondrocytes.

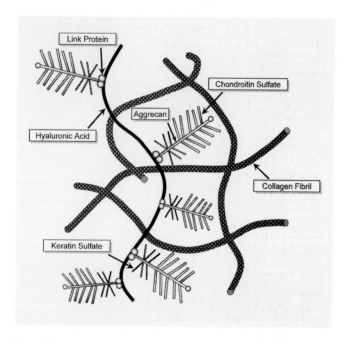

Figure 2 Diagram of aggrecan, collagen. *(Courtesy of Dr. Andrew Thompson.)*

Collagen

Collagen provides tensile strength to the cartilage and provides the extracellular matrix architecture for the proteoglycans and chondrocytes to fill (Figure 2). Type II collagen comprises 90% of the articular cartilage with additional small amounts of collagen type IX and XI. Type II collagen is oriented tangentially to the articular surface in the superficial zone of the articular cartilage. This orientation allows the cartilage to withstand the high-intensity shearing forces in this area. Collagen fibers curve downward to form vertical sheets through the middle and deep zones of articular cartilage to provide further vertical tensile strength. Type IX collagen helps to maintain the orientation of the ubiquitous type II collagen network.

Proteoglycans

Aggrecan, biglycan, and decorin are the three main proteoglycans in the extracellular matrix. Aggrecan, the predominant proteoglycan and thereby the best studied, is a large aggregation of long-chain, negatively charged glycosaminoglycan molecules attached covalently to a protein core that itself attaches via a link protein to hyaluronic acid (Figure 2). The glycosaminoglycan molecules are composed of chondroitin sulfate and keratan sulfate. A single hyaluronic acid chain will have many aggrecan molecules linked to it. Biglycan and decorin are nonaggregating proteoglycans that have roles in the cartilage matrix structure.

Aggrecan provides elastic strength to articular cartilage, and as a polyanionic molecule attracts water, which allows the cartilage to swell. The swelling, however, is

limited to about 20% of its potential volume because the network of collagen fibers in the articular cartilage restricts absorption of water. Pressure on the articular cartilage causes aggrecan to release water from the cartilage into a thin film on the articular surface. This film of water provides a surface of minimal friction for smooth articular motion. The release of the pressure on the articular surface allows fluid to be drawn back into the cartilage, bringing nutrients to the chondrocytes. Because cartilage is avascular, this fluid is its only source of nutrition.

Synovial Fluid

Synovial fluid is an acellular plasma ultrafiltrate that protects the subchondral structures and lubricates the joint. Its high viscosity gives it important mechanical properties and is related to large amounts of polymerized hyaluronic acid.

Cartilage Homeostasis

In the normal joint, there is a homeostasis between the breakdown of cartilage matrix and the formation of newly synthesized matrix. Growth factors stimulate chondrocytes to produce matrix constituents whereas cytokines such as IL-1 and tumor necrosis factor-alpha (TNF-α) stimulate matrix degradation. When this balance is disturbed, there is a shift toward excessive degradation, which causes disruption of the structural and functional integrity of the cartilage.

Collagenase, stromelysin, and gelatinase are MMPs that act as degradative enzymes. They contain zinc at the active site and are produced by the chondrocyte as part of the cartilage development process. The cytokine IL-1 stimulates production of MMPs by infiltrating leukocytes and connective tissue cells. MMP activity is inhibited by tissue inhibitor of metalloproteinase located in the cartilage. The complex interplay between MMPs, tissue inhibitor of metalloproteinase, and the various cytokines that mediate chondrocyte activity will influence the overall structural integrity of the articular cartilage.

Osteoarthritis

Epidemiology

Osteoarthritis (OA) is the most common form of arthritis and a leading cause of disability in the developed world. Hip and knee OA rarely occur before the age of 50 years. The prevalence of clinically apparent knee OA is 30% in the population older than 75 years; OA of at least one joint occurs in 80% of this population. Autopsy and radiographic studies show a much higher rate of OA than do epidemiologic studies. The fact that the incidence of OA increases significantly with age has led to the erroneous conclusion that OA is simply an age-related degenerative condition. The prevalence of OA increases with age because of ligamentous laxity, a failure of the periarticular structures such as muscles and proprioceptors to function appropriately, a reduction in matrix production by chondrocytes, or decreased responsiveness of chondrocytes to growth factors. Other risk factors for OA include gender, genetic predisposition, obesity, higher than normal bone mineral density, and joint trauma. The incidence of OA is higher in women than in men, especially after the age of 50 years.

Etiology

OA is likely a genetically heterogeneous disease where local factors (such as excessive load) act within the context of a systemic susceptibility (such as a genetic predisposition). OA can be classified as primary (idiopathic) or secondary (Table 1). Secondary causes of OA can result from highly intense or abnormal chronic forces across the joint (for example, from trauma or occupational overuse) or from a disorder in a joint constituent (for example, hemochromatosis, chronic inflammatory arthritis, chronic crystal joint disease, septic arthritis). The incidence of OA is increased with certain occupations. Farmers and miners have an increased incidence of hip OA. Occupations that require regular kneeling and squatting are correlated with an increased incidence of knee OA. Elite athletes, but not recreational athletes, have an increased incidence of knee OA.

Pathogenesis

In the common forms of OA such as polyarticular small joint nodal arthritis in women, there is a familial component. However, in rare subtypes of OA (such as osteochondrodysplastic syndromes), genetic susceptibility may follow mendelian inheritance modes, and often involve the genes that code type II collagen. Mutations in the *COL2A1* gene (type II procollagen) were found in rare types of OA in certain families. Mutations in this same gene have been found to cause skeletal dysplasias that clinically resemble OA. However, in families with common forms of OA there were no mutations in the *COL2A1* gene.

Obesity is an important, modifiable risk factor for bilateral knee OA in both the patellofemoral joint and tibiofemoral joint. Fortunately, weight loss reduces the risk of knee OA. The association of obesity and knee OA is stronger in women than in men. Obesity may increase the incidence of knee OA by increasing force across the knee, by increasing bone density (which may be independently associated with OA), or by the adipose tissue increasing production of OA-causing growth factors or hormones. Obesity is also associated with OA in the hand, which suggests that weight is not the sole explanation linking obesity and knee OA. Obesity has not been consistently associated with hip OA.

Higher bone density has been linked to OA of the hip and knee, but not the hand. The relationship of higher

TABLE 1 | Classification of Osteoarthritis

Primary (idiopathic)
Peripheral joints
  Nodal (at PIP and DIP joints)
  First CMC and first MTP
  Large joints (hip and knee)
Spine
Variant OA
  Inflammatory OA
  Generalized OA
  Diffuse idiopathic skeletal hyperostosis
Secondary
Traumatic (occupational, sports)
Local joint disorders
  Osteonecrosis
  Postinfectious
Diffuse joint disorders
  Rheumatoid arthritis
  Hypermobility syndrome
Endocrine disorders
  Diabetes
  Acromegaly
Systemic metabolic diseases
  Hemochromatosis
  Ochronosis
  Wilson's disease
Crystal joint disease
  Gout
  Calcium crystal diseases
    Calcium pyrophosphate dihydrate
    Calcium apatite
Neuropathic diseases (Charcot joint)
  Tabes dorsalis
  Diabetes mellitus

PIP = proximal interphalangeal; DIP = distal interphalangeal; CMC = carpometacarpal; MTP = metatarsophalangeal

bone density with OA of weight-bearing joints may be the result of the presence of stronger, stiffer subchondral bone, which deforms less under loading, therefore increasing stress to the cartilage.

Several local factors may play a role in the incidence or progression of OA including knee injury, which has been associated with a subsequent increase in the incidence of both hip and knee OA. Abnormal knee alignment also increases the incidence of OA. A varus or valgus deformity of 4° to 5° results in a fourfold increase in the risk of medial and lateral knee OA. Weakness of the quadriceps plays a small role in OA in women, but not in men. Conversely, increased hand muscle strength is associated with hand OA in men. Development abnormalities, such as acetabular dysplasia and slipped capital femoral epiphysis, frequently lead to premature OA of the hip.

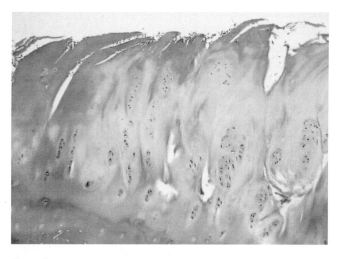

Figure 3 Low power photomicrograph of OA cartilage shows fibrillation of the cartilage surface. *(Courtesy of Dr. Michael Nimmo.)*

The chondrocyte is key in the development of OA. In response to mechanical stress and to cytokines such as IL-1 and TNF-α, chondrocytes release MMPs that degrade the extracellular matrix. The cytokines stimulate prostaglandin release, which may cause the pain and stiffness of OA. Microscopic examination of the cartilage shows fibrillation (Figure 3). Subcortical bony sclerosis and osteophytosis reduce bone elasticity and transfer more force across the articular cartilage. Chondrocytes attempt to repair the damaged type II cartilage; however, the repair is inadequate and the new cartilage contains type I collagen and increased fibronectin. This new cartilage lacks the low friction and elastic properties of healthy cartilage. Further breakdown ushers the beginning of clinical OA.

Biomarkers

Biomarkers, including markers for type II collagen and aggrecan turnover, cartilage oligomeric matrix protein, MMPs, and tissue cytokines, monitor the progression of OA on cartilage, adjacent bone, and synovium. Changes in certain biomarkers occur within weeks of surgical or nonsurgical trauma to articular cartilage; such injuries are associated with subsequent OA. It has not yet been established which markers are best suited to provide an early diagnosis of OA and which will correlate with treatment response or disease progression. The study of such biomarkers is currently an area of intense research.

Treatment

Nonsurgical and Nonpharmacologic Treatment

In most patients, OA has usually been present for several years with resultant muscle deconditioning, increased weight, and radiographic changes before a physician is consulted. The goals of treatment are to reduce pain, improve function, and delay progression of the disease. Non-pharmacologic interventions have been shown to be beneficial for patients with OA; the most important is patient education. Several studies that have evaluated the effectiveness of arthritis self-management programs have shown improvements in pain scores, function, therapy compliance, and quality of life. Weight loss reduces the symptoms of OA in weight-bearing joints. Physical therapy and regular exercise improve function and pain scores and prevent disability caused by muscular deconditioning. Exercise may also reduce the progression of OA in joints that are presymptomatic. Reduced-load and low-impact exercises (such as cycling, swimming, or tai chi preceded by an aerobic warm-up if thought to be safe from a cardiovascular standpoint) are most beneficial. To improve symptoms of medial joint compartment knee OA, lateral wedge orthotics or knee bracing for more muscular, younger patients may provide symptomatic improvement; knee braces often are not tolerated in the elderly. The use of a cane is beneficial.

Therapies that have little or conflicting supportive data include dietary supplements and passive modalities such as ultrasound and transcutaneous electrical nerve stimulation. There is conflicting data on the use of oral glucosamine to treat OA pain or reduce OA joint damage. Commercial preparations of glucosamine are not standardized and may not contain the amount of glucosamine indicated on the package. Few data exist to support the use of chondroitin sulfate in patients with OA. Additional studies are necessary before glucosamine or other dietary supplements can be routinely recommended.

Pharmacologic Treatment

The goal of pharmacologic therapy is to reduce pain and improve function; the ability to significantly alter the progression of OA has not been clearly shown for any agent. Initial treatment is with acetaminophen (up to 4 g/day). If this treatment is unsuccessful, or if there are features of local inflammation such as joint warmth or effusion, a nonsteroidal anti-inflammatory drug (NSAID) would be appropriate. Whereas OA is typically considered to be a noninflammatory arthropathy, the induction of prostaglandin E_2 in OA provides some rationale for the use of NSAIDs in this context. NSAIDs exert a peripheral role in the reduction of OA pain; they also may contribute to pain reduction by their action on the central nervous system.

NSAIDs are superior to acetaminophen in the symptomatic treatment of knee OA, but can cause increased gastrointestinal (GI) side effects such as pain and dyspepsia. More serious GI side effects include peptic ulcer, perforation, obstruction, or hemorrhage which occur in 2% to 4% of chronic NSAID users each year and in a higher percentage for those patients with several risk factors (Table 2). Unfortunately, half of GI ulcers are silent. In high-risk patients, it is prudent to avoid

TABLE 2 | Relative Risk of Traditional NSAID-Induced GI Complications

Risk Factor	Relative Risk	95% CI
Age (> 60 years)	5.5	4.6 to 6.6
Prior GI event	4.8	4.1 to 5.6
Severe RA	2.3	1.1 to 4.7
Concurrent corticosteroids	4.4	2.0 to 9.7
Concurrent anticoagulants	12.7	6.3 to 25.7

CI = confidence interval

TABLE 3 | Recommended Dosage for Coxibs Available in the United States

Coxib	OA dose	RA dose
Celecoxib	100 to 200 mg/day	200 mg/bid
Valdecoxib	10 mg/day	20 mg/day

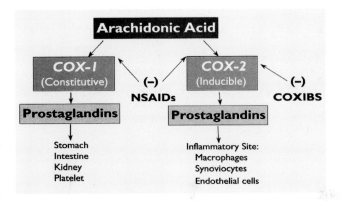

Figure 4 Diagram of COX-1 and -2.

NSAIDs; however, if an NSAID is required, the newer selective cyclooxygenase-2 (COX-2) inhibitors will reduce the incidence of ulcers and upper GI bleeding by approximately 50%. Alternatively, an NSAID can be given with a proton pump inhibitor.

Coxibs In the early 1990s, it was recognized that two separate proteins, cyclooxygenase enzymes (COX-1 and COX-2) were responsible for both the benefits and the toxicity of traditional NSAIDs (Figure 4). It was found that the COX-1 enzyme protected the upper GI tract and promoted platelet aggregation. The inducible COX-2 enzyme was found to be primarily responsible for promoting pain and inflammation. Traditional NSAIDs inhibit both COX-1 and COX-2. NSAIDs that inhibit COX-2 with little or no effect on COX-1 are called coxibs or COX-2 specific inhibitors. The selective inhibition of COX-2 still provides an anti-inflammatory benefit in joints while reducing the upper GI complications (caused by the inhibition of COX-1) seen with traditional NSAIDs. Coxibs that are currently available in the United States include celecoxib and valdecoxib (Table 3). Etoricoxib, lumiracoxib, and parecoxib are other coxibs that may be available soon.

Coxibs have no appreciable effect on platelet function, which allows the use of these medications preoperatively and perioperatively with improved postoperative pain control. All NSAID and COX-2 inhibitors may cause cardiovascular and renal side effects in higher risk patients such as the elderly, those on diuretics, or those with preexisting cardiovascular or renal dysfunction. In October 2004, Merck withdrew the coxib rofecoxib from the worldwide market. This decision was based on data from a randomized controlled trial looking at the use of 25 mg of rofecoxib in patients with gastrointestinal polyps. Results of the study showed a significant increase in myocardial infarction in patients after 18 months (1.48% in the rofecoxib group compared with 0.75% in the placebo group). Other rofecoxib studies have shown an increase in serious cardiovascular events. The issue of cadiovascular safety for the currently available coxibs (celecoxib and valdecoxib) especially in comparison to

naproxen, is unclear. Therefore, for patients who require anti-inflammatory medications, it would be reasonable to use coxibs in patients with higher GI risk but lower cardiovascular risks. Animal and in vitro studies have shown an impairment of bone healing with the use of NSAIDs and COX-2 inhibitors, probably caused by the inhibition of prostaglandins. Prostaglandins are an integral component in the stages of bone healing from the initial inflammatory phase, followed by bone resorption (osteoclasts), and new bone formation (osteoblasts). Although there are data from animal studies suggesting that the effects of COX-2 inhibitors are both dose-dependent and reversible, it is recommended that short-term administration or other analgesics be used in the treatment of these patients until sound clinical evidence becomes available.

Intra-Articular Injections If acetaminophen or NSAIDs are not beneficial or are contraindicated, an intra-articular corticosteroid injection may help up to half of affected patients. The risk of sepsis is about 1 in 10,000. Intra-articular injections of a hyaluronic acid preparation have been used in knee OA. Although side effects are uncommon, the data on efficacy are conflicting and the magnitude of clinical improvement is small.

Other Analgesics Tramadol is an analgesic medication that works through several mechanisms. It has activity at the Mu opioid receptors but also inhibits serotonin and norepinephrine uptake. Opioid analgesics are useful for OA flare-ups if other therapies have not been adequate.

TABLE 4 | 1987 Revised Criteria for the Classification of RA*

Criteria	Definition
(1) Morning stiffness	Morning stiffness in and around the joints, lasting at least 1 hour before maximal improvement
(2) Arthritis of three or more joint areas	At least three joint areas simultaneously have had soft-tissue swelling or fluid (not bony overgrowth alone) observed by a physician; The 14 possible areas are right or left PIP, MCP, wrist, elbow, knee, ankle, and MTP joints
(3) Arthritis of the hand joints	At least one area swollen (as defined above) in a wrist, MCP, or PIP joint
(4) Symmetric arthritis	Simultaneous involvement of the same joint areas (as defined in [2]) on both sides of the body (bilateral involvement of PIPs, MCPs, or MTPs is acceptable without absolute symmetry)
(5) Rheumatoid nodules	Subcutaneous nodules, over bony prominences, or extensor surfaces, or in juxta-articular regions, observed by a physician
(6) Serum rheumatoid factor	Demonstration of abnormal amounts of serum rheumatoid factor by any method for which the result has been positive in < 5% of normal subjects
(7) Radiographic changes	Radiographic changes typical of rheumatoid arthritis on PA hand and wrist radiographs, which must include erosions or unequivocal bony decalcification localized in or most marked adjacent to the involved joints (OA changes alone do not qualify)

*Requirements: A patient shall be said to have RA if he/she has satisfied at least four of the seven criteria. Criteria 1 through 4 must have been present for at least 6 weeks. Patients with two clinical diagnoses are not excluded. Designation as classic, definite, or probable RA is not to be made.

PIP = proximal interphalangeal; MCP = metacarpophalangeal; MTP = metatarsophalangeal

(Reproduced with permission from Arnett FG, Edworthy SM, Bloch DA, McShane OJ, et al: The American Rhematism Association 1987 Revised Criteria for the Classification of Rheumatoid Arthritis. Arthritis Rheum 1988;31:315-324.)

Short- or long-acting codeine, oxycodone, or propoxyphene can be used, preferably on a fixed interval basis for less than 2 weeks at a time. Patients with severe OA who are not surgical candidates and have severe pain that is unresponsive to other agents should be treated with appropriate long-term opioid analgesics. Although there are limited data to suggest that combination medications containing caffeine may have additional analgesic properties, caffeine has significant side effects including sleep disturbances and withdrawal headache.

Surgical Management

The goals of surgical intervention in OA are to decrease or eliminate pain and to improve function. The success of joint arthroplasty in achieving these goals has resulted in substantial investment in and development of prosthetic joints and techniques for their implantation. However, it is important to consider that other procedures that decrease pain and improve function by restoring, resecting, or replacing the joint also have a role and are attractive alternatives for young patients who do not desire a prosthetic joint or for patients with less advanced joint degeneration who want to maintain a high level of activity.

Procedures to treat OA by preserving or restoring articular cartilage surfaces include osteotomies and muscle releases, joint débridement, partial resection or perforation of subchondral bone to stimulate fibrocartilage healing, resection arthroplasty, and the use of various autografts and allografts. Joints compromised by adjacent bony deformity may be appropriate for osteotomy. Arthrodesis may be most appropriate for joints that are severely compromised or in patients too young for successful prosthetic arthroplasty. Prosthetic joint arthroplasty is often recommended for patients with advanced OA and/or advanced symptoms of OA that are no longer responding to maximal nonsurgical modalities. Although complication rates are low in prosthetic hip and knee joints, prosthetic elbow and ankle joints have higher complication rates.

The ability of the prosthetic arthroplasty intervention to alleviate pain and improve function has been described as one of the great advances in 20th century health care. Whereas traditional indications for prosthetic arthroplasty included incapacitating symptoms, old age, and sedentary lifestyle, contemporary advances in arthroplasty technique and prosthetic design have expanded the indications to younger patients with intractable symptoms.

Rheumatoid Arthritis
Epidemiology

Rheumatoid arthritis (RA) is an autoimmune disease that affects 1% of the white population. All racial groups are affected but aboriginal North Americans have a higher prevalence. RA is a chronic, fluctuating polyarthritis that is symmetric, erosive, and eventually deforming (Table 4).

Clinical Features

In most patients, RA manifests over weeks to months with an insidious onset of fatigue and joint pain, which

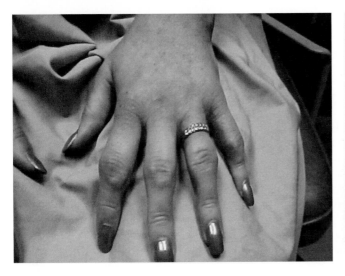

Figure 5 Photograph showing early RA of the hand.

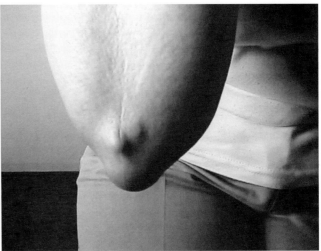

Figure 6 Rheumatoid nodules are shown.

TABLE 5 | Extra-Articular Manifestations of RA

Organ System	Manifestations
Pulmonary	Cricoarytenoid cartilage, interstitial lung disease, bronchiolitis obliterans, pleural effusion, rheumatoid nodules
Skin	Rheumatoid nodules, cutaneous vasculitis, pyoderma gangrenosum
Cardiac	Pericardial effusions
Neurologic	Myelopathy resulting from atlantoaxial instability, entrapment neuropathies, mononeuritis multiplex, peripheral sensory neuropathy
Hematologic	Felty's syndrome (neutropenia, splenomegaly), anemia, thrombocytosis
Ocular	Episcleritis, scleritis, corneal melt, keratoconjunctivitis sicca

TABLE 6 | Infectious Agents That May Be An Environmental Trigger for RA

Viral
  Epstein-Barr virus
  Parvovirus
  Rubella
Cytomegalovirus
Bacteria
  Escherichia coli
  Proteus mirabilis
Mycoplasma
Mycobacteria

Extra-articular manifestations of RA are summarized in Table 5.

may be transient early in the course of the disease. However, 10% of patients will experience an acute onset of symptoms that occurs within days. Eventually, joint inflammation becomes more persistent with warmth, effusion, tenderness, and loss of function. Early morning joint stiffness occurs in most patients and improves with physical activity. Morning stiffness usually exceeds 60 minutes and its duration correlates with the extent of synovial inflammation. Classic areas of symmetric polyarthritis are the wrists, metacarpophalangeal (MCP), metatarsophalangeal (MTP), and proximal interphalangeal (PIP) joints of the hands and feet (Figures 5 through 7). Structural damage to the joints, once believed to occur only after 1 or more years, has been shown by MRI to occur within months of RA onset.

Rheumatoid Factor

Rheumatoid factors are immunoglobulin M antibodies directed against the constant fragment region of the immunoglobulin G molecule. Rheumatoid factor is present in as few as half the patients with early RA, is found in 5% of healthy individuals, and is found in a host of chronic inflammatory and infectious conditions. Therefore, as a diagnostic test, rheumatoid factor has been overvalued; however, its presence has some prognostic value because a positive test portends a more aggressive course of RA with a higher morbidity and mortality.

Etiology

Although the exact etiology of RA is unknown, genetic susceptibility and environmental factors have some demonstrable importance. Compared with a prevalence of

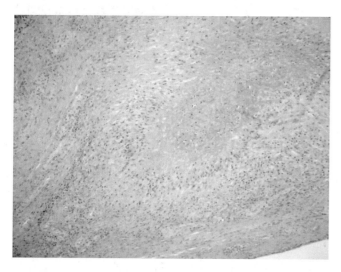

Figure 7 Medium power photomicrograph of rheumatoid nodule depicting palisading histiocytes and central fibrinoid necrosis. *(Courtesy of Dr. Michael Nimmo.)*

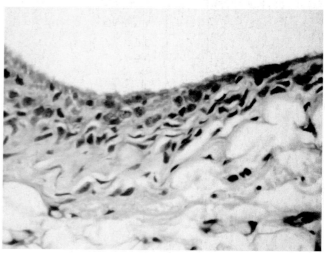

Figure 8 High power photomicrograph of normal synovium showing a thin layer of cells. *(Courtesy of Dr. Michael Nimmo.)*

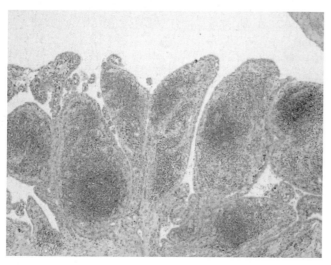

Figure 9 Medium power photomicrograph of pannus. Thick villi of synovium with neovascularization and lymphoid aggregates are seen. *(Courtesy of Dr. Michael Nimmo.)*

1% in the general population, the concordance rate in monozygotic twins is 12% to 15%, and is 2% to 5% for dizygotic twins and siblings. About half of the genetic susceptibility resides within the major histocompatibility complex class II loci, in which the DR4β chains with the greatest association with RA are *DRB*0401* and *DRB*0404*. The remaining genetic predisposition is believed to lie within other loci that are currently being investigated. Such loci include the major histocompatibility complex class III genes for TNF-α, heat shock protein 70 (*HSP70*), and complement C4, as well as genes not included in the major histocompatibility complex such as T cell and immunoglobulin genes.

Geographic clusters of erosive arthritis have been found in ancient archaeological sites in North America; however, no convincing findings of RA in Western Europe have been found that predate the settlement of the New World. This finding suggests an infectious etiology for RA. Several potential agents have been proposed, but none has yet been proven (Table 6). There is no consistent evidence of a specific microorganism in RA synovium, which may indicate that the infectious trigger is subclinical, outside the synovium, or precedes the RA by a long latent period before clinically evident joint inflammation.

Pathogenesis

RA probably begins with an antigen-mediated activation of T cells in an immunogenetically susceptible host, which then initiates a cascade of events including endothelial cell activation, proliferation of type A and B synoviocytes, and recruitment of additional inflammatory cells from the bone marrow. TNF-α and IL-1 are the apex of a cytokine cascade leading to the production of proteases and autoantibodies. When the immune response is triggered by the antigen, additional antigens may be created and recognized by the T cell to create an ongoing immune response. The synovium is transformed from a thin layer only several cells deep (Figure 8), to a proliferative and invasive synovium (pannus) composed of synoviocytes, T cells, and macrophages (Figure 9). The synovitis and vascular proliferation invade adjacent cartilage and bone. TNF-α and IL-1 stimulate chondrocytes to degrade cartilage and osteoclasts to promote periarticular bony erosion and osteopenia.

A significant humoral component may be involved in the pathogenesis of RA. Whereas T cells outnumber B cells in the synovium, there are active plasma cells in the synovium and the expanded B lymphocyte pool, which exhibits an origin from a limited number of B cell clones. It is intriguing that the B cell-depleting therapy, rituximab, has shown remarkable preliminary benefits in the treatment of RA and has provided further evidence that B cells are important in the pathogenesis of RA. The improved understanding of RA pathogenesis has resulted in important therapeutic breakthroughs.

Pharmacologic Therapy

The traditional approach to the treatment of early RA has been the use of analgesics and NSAIDs to reduce symptoms. Such pharmacotherapies, however, do not prevent joint erosion and articular damage. MRI has shown that joint erosions can occur within months of symptom onset, and the rate of progression of erosions is highest in the first 3 years after RA onset. The recognition of these early changes has resulted in a dramatic shift in treatment philosophy for patients with RA. RA must be treated early and aggressively. The evidence is overwhelming that a delay in instituting disease-modifying antirheumatic drug (DMARD) therapy or a failure to maintain disease suppression with DMARDs can result in irreversible joint destruction and disability.

DMARDs, previously considered second-line drugs, are currently the mainstay of the pharmacologic treatment of RA. This heterogeneous group of medications reduces inflamed joint counts, acute phase reactants, and erosion scores and stabilizes or even improves functional status and reduces long-term disability (Table 7). Methotrexate is the most commonly used DMARD in North America. It is relatively potent compared with the other DMARDs and more patients will continue to use methotrexate over the long term than other traditional DMARDs. About 50% of patients who begin treatment with methotrexate will remain on the medication after 5 years compared with 20% of patients who are initially treated with intramuscular gold or sulfasalazine. Newer DMARDs include leflunomide and anticytokine agents.

In addition to beginning early treatment with DMARDs, a new but well-established development is the early use of combination drug therapy. Established examples of drugs used in combination with methotrexate are hydroxychloroquine, sulfasalazine, gold, cyclosporine, and anti-TNF-α agents.

Understanding the cytokine cascade in RA has helped in the development of novel new therapies that target these factors. TNF-α and IL-1 are key proinflammatory cytokines in RA. In clinical studies, inhibition of TNF-α has resulted in a dramatic reduction in the symptoms of RA, an improvement in function, and a retardation of radiographic progression. Etanercept, infliximab, and adalimumab are the available anti-TNF-α agents. The mode of action and route of administration of these anticytokine DMARDs are shown in Table 8.

Compared with traditional DMARDs, these agents have remarkable efficacy with minimal adverse events in the treatment of RA. Immunosuppression and the risk of infection (including reactivation of mycobacterium tuberculosis) are potential complications with all anti-TNF-α drugs. There have been rare reports of demyelinating diseases with the use of etanercept. Infliximab must be given concomitantly with methotrexate or azathioprine (in the methotrexate intolerant patient), whereas etanercept and adalimumab can be given as monotherapy or in combination with methotrexate. Infliximab has been shown to exacerbate congestive heart failure.

Anakinra is the only IL-1 inhibitor currently available. There is less reduction of inflammation with anakinra than with the anti-TNF-α agents; however, anakinra has a good safety profile. Injection site reactions with anakinra are frequent, but are generally mild and self-limiting. Anakinra use is also associated with a small increase in the incidence of pneumonia and urinary tract infections.

There is no perioperative standard of practice to guide the use of anticytokine DMARDs. It is recommended that surgery be performed when presumed levels of the therapies are at their lowest—2 weeks prior to the infliximab infusion; 3 days after the etanercept injection; 10 days after the adalimumab injection. Some physicians will postpone resumption of the medications for 1 to 2 weeks postoperatively, in the hope that the reduced immunosuppression therapy will reduce the risk of subsequent postoperative infection. However, this approach may necessitate the use of perioperative corticosteroids or cause a flare of synovitis, which could contribute to a poor postoperative recovery and an increased risk of infection. The other approach is to continue the use of DMARDs unless there are contraindications (such as an active infection). There is no consensus on which of these two methods is safer; few data are currently available.

Glucocorticoids

The DMARDs generally have a slow onset of action, and although they are effective in reducing pain and inflammation, patients usually require ongoing analgesic and anti-inflammatory medication. While waiting for DMARDs to take effect, some rheumatologists prescribe a course of "bridging" glucocorticoid (GC) medication such as prednisone (10 mg daily) on a tapering dose over several weeks to months. GCs are powerful suppressors of inflammation, but long-term side effects and an absence of disease modifying benefits preclude their long-term use. GCs can be given orally, parenterally, and intra-articularly. High-dose parenteral GC can be used to treat severe extra-articular manifestations such as interstitial lung disease, ocular inflammation, or vasculitis. Intra-articular therapy causes few systemic

TABLE 7 | Common Disease-Modifying Antirheumatic Drugs

Drug	Onset of Action	Relative Effectiveness	Half Life	Monitoring	Usual Dose
Hydroxychloroquine	2 to 6 months	weak	Up to 50 days	Visual changes, funduscopic examination and visual fields every 6 to 12 months	< 6.5 mg/kg/day of ideal body weight
Minocycline	2 to 6 months	weak	15 hours		200 mg/day
Sulfasalazine	2 to 3 months	moderate	10 hours	CBC, liver enzymes every 2 weeks for first 2 months then every 3 months	Gradual increase to 1 to 1.5 g/bid
Azathioprine	2 to 3 months	moderate	3 hours	Monthly CBC, liver enzymes, but more frequent when dose increased	Start at 1 mg/kg/day and slowly increase as needed to 2.5 mg/kg/day
Methotrexate	2 to 3 months	strong	3 to 10 hours	Monthly CBC, liver enzymes, albumin, creatinine	7.5 mg to 15 mg by mouth or subcutaneously weekly Increase to response or to 25 mg/wk
Parenteral gold salts	2 to 6 months	strong	Up to 27 days	CBC, urinalysis and serum creatinine every second injection	50 mg/wk intramuscularly for first 6 months, then slow taper if response occurs
Leflunomide	2 to 3 months	strong	15 days, but enteropathic circulation may increase half life	Monthly CBC, liver enzymes, creatinine If toxicity or pregnancy occurs, must wash out with cholestyramine	Loading dose of 100 mg/day for 3 days then 10 to 20 mg/day
Cyclosporine	2 to 3 months	strong	Up to 18 hours	CBC, creatinine, blood pressure, liver enzymes every 2 weeks until steady dose then monthly	Start at 1.5 mg/kg/day and increase to 4 mg/kg/day

CBC = complete blood count

side effects and can be particularly useful for patients with a few resistant, inflamed joints.

Nonsteroidal Anti-Inflammatory Drugs

NSAIDs are useful for reduction of pain and inflammation in RA; however, their use in RA as in OA is complicated by GI and other toxicities. Patients with RA are more prone to developing symptomatic GI ulcers than patients with OA. GCs also increase the incidence of GI ulcers independently. Therefore, if anti-inflammatory medications are indicated in a patient with RA, a coxib is the preferential therapy. Although anti-inflammatory medications reduce the symptoms of RA, they do not prevent the progression of damage and therefore should not be the only therapeutic agent used.

Surgical Management of Rheumatoid Arthritis

Because patients with RA often have special needs because of multiple joint involvement, it is important that a multidisciplinary team (surgeon, rheumatologist, nurse, physiotherapist, occupational therapist, and social worker) be consulted before surgical intervention. The team should ensure that planning, staging, and rehabilitation after surgery is appropriate and that the patient is provided with optimal information on goals, expectations, and opportunities to improve outcome and minimize complications.

TABLE 8 | Anticytokine DMRDs

Anticytokine DMARDs	Mechanism of Action	Route and Dosage
Etanercept	Human soluble p75 TNF-α receptor fusion protein	25 mg subcutaneously twice weekly
Infliximab	Chimeric (human/murine) IgG1 monoclonal antibody to TNF-α	3mg/kg intravenously at 0, 2, 6, then every 8 weeks Can be increased up to 10 mg/kg every 4 weeks
Adalimumab	Human IgG1 monoclonal antibody to TNF-α	40 mg subcutaneously every 2 weeks Can be increased to weekly
Anakinra	Human IL-1 receptor antagonist	100 mg/daily subcutaneously

Before any surgical intervention, it is imperative that the patient receive a comprehensive preoperative evaluation. If acute joint inflammation is apparent, it is prudent to first optimize medical treatment and resolve the acute synovitis. Surgical, chemical, or radioactive synovectomy can be considered if the synovitis does not adequately respond to medication and there is no structural damage to the joint. It is unlikely that synovectomy will alleviate all symptoms if significant structural damage to the joint has already occurred. If structural joint damage exists and patient symptoms of synovitis do not respond to conventional medical treatment, surgical intervention with arthrodesis or arthroplasty may be indicated. Patients with multiple joint involvement should receive staged surgical reconstruction to avoid prolonged periods of hospitalization and immobility.

Extensive RA involvement of the shoulder, elbow, or wrist may compromise any anticipated postoperative use of crutches or a walker for patients needing lower extremity surgery. Therefore, it may be necessary to treat the involved joints of the upper extremity before proceeding with lower extremity surgery (for example, wrist arthrodesis may facilitate the use of crutches for lower extremity reconstruction). However, the completion of lower extremity reconstruction before treatment of upper extremity joints may be most appropriate if it is anticipated that the patient's need for a walking device in the postoperative period could overload delicate arthroplasties in the elbow and/or hand. Patients unable to attain at least 100° of flexion of the knee require maximal assistance from the upper extremities in rising from a seated position. If the upper extremities cannot withstand these forces, then maximal hip and knee flexion must be a goal of surgery.

Prior to surgery, the patient should be in optimal medical condition. The patient should be taking the lowest possible dose or should discontinue taking corticosteroids and certain DMARDs before surgery to minimize any increased risk of postoperative infection from use of these medications. Any other sites, or potential sites, of infection in the patient should be resolved before surgical intervention. For example, coexisting dental infections, skin ulcers, and urinary tract infections can all increase the risk of infection in the joint targeted for surgery. The rehabilitation team should perform a comprehensive preoperative assessment to ensure that the patient is motivated and able to participate in the expected postoperative program. Instructing the patient in the use of a walker, crutches, or a cane before surgery may help to facilitate an uneventful transition to these devices in the immediate postoperative period.

Significant cervical spine involvement exists in up to 40% of patients with RA. Because this involvement is frequently asymptomatic, preoperative evaluation with lateral cervical spine flexion and extension radiographs are necessary to document the existence of C1-C2 or subaxial instability that might compromise the spinal cord during routine intubation.

The perioperative use of antirheumatic drugs should be managed to minimize the risk of bleeding or infection while optimizing patient comfort and pain relief. The rheumatologist, surgeon, and patient should work together to determine the ideal individualized drug treatment plan. The use of anti-inflammatory medication in the perioperative period is also important. Most NSAIDs should be discontinued a minimum of at least five half-lives before surgery, and aspirin should be discontinued at least 7 to 10 days before surgery to decrease bleeding associated with the surgical procedure. Coxibs such as celecoxib and valdecoxib have no significant effect on platelet activity and can be continued. Antimalarial agents, gold salt injections, auranofin, sulfasalazine, and penicillamine may be continued during the preoperative and immediate postoperative periods. It is sometimes recommended that methotrexate be temporarily discontinued for 1 to 2 weeks during the immediate preoperative period and during hospitalization because of fluid balance alterations and immunesuppressant effects. Azathioprine may be continued in the preoperative period if the patient's leukocyte count remains greater than 3,500 mm³; however, it should be discontinued while the patient is in the hospital after surgery. GCs can be reduced in the preoperative period, but there is a potential for adrenal suppression in longstanding use. It is currently recommended that most patients taking oral corticosteroids receive stress coverage the day of surgery and for the following 24 hours.

TABLE 9 | Juvenile Idiopathic Arthritis: 1997 Durban Classification Compared With the ARA/ACR Classification

ILAR Classification of JIA		ARA/ACR 1972 Classification of JRA
Type	Subtype	
Systemic		Systemic onset Still's disease
Polyarthritis	RF positive RF negative	Polyarticular JRA (RF positive)
Oligoarthritis	Persistent Extended	Pauciarticular JRA
Psoriatic arthritis		
Enthesitis-related arthritis		
Other (does not meet criteria for any of the above categories)		

ARA = American Rheumatism Association; ACR = American College of Rheumatology

Juvenile Idiopathic Arthritis

Juvenile idiopathic arthritis (JIA) is a new term that was first proposed at the 1997 International League of Associations for Rheumatology (ILAR) meeting. The classification was revised at the ILAR meeting in 2001. JIA has replaced the older term juvenile rheumatoid arthritis (JRA) that was used primarily in North America and the term juvenile chronic arthritis that had been used in Europe. The new classification also incorporates other idiopathic arthritides. These heterogeneous diseases have diverse prognoses, treatments, and long-term outcomes. Table 9 compares the ILAR classification with the American College of Rheumatology classification. The onset of JIA must be before the age of 16 years and must persist for at least 6 weeks. The new classification system specifically excludes arthritis of a known cause, such as reactive arthritis.

Systemic JIA (formerly, systemic onset JRA or Still's disease) includes children with rash, daily high fever, and any number of inflamed joints. These children appear quite ill with anemia and a high white cell count and may have serositis, hepatosplenomegaly, and lymphadenopathy. An infection or a hematologic malignancy usually must be ruled out when making this diagnosis. Children with this subtype of arthritis have the highest likelihood of systemic complications and internal organ involvement.

Childhood polyarthritis includes children with the previous diagnosis of polyarticular JRA with some modifications. This disease has been divided into rheumatoid factor (RF) positive and RF negative polyarthritis. A family history of psoriasis is a specific exclusion. Childhood polyarthritis is characterized by the involvement of more than four joints in the first 6 months of the disease. Both large and small joints are involved. Patients who are older than 10 years of age at onset and who have a positive RF, have disease characteristics much like adult patients with RA.

Childhood oligoarthritis includes children with the previous diagnosis of oligoarticular (pauciarticular) JRA. It is the most common type of JIA and affects approximately 50% of JIA patients. This type of arthritis is characterized by the involvement of four or fewer joints in the first 6 months of the disease; the extended subtype encompasses children who develop more inflamed joints after 6 months of the disease. The peak incidence occurs in the second or third years of life and affects more girls than boys. Childhood oligoarthritis usually involves large joints other than the hip. The child typically presents with a limp that improves during the day. Other than uveitis, which occurs in about 20% of patients with childhood oligoarthritis, there are few systemic manifestations. The uveitis is more frequently associated with a positive antinuclear antibody (ANA) and is clinically silent in the early, reversible stages. Thus, children with childhood oligoarthritis who are ANA positive should have ocular screening every 4 months and those who are ANA negative should be screened every 6 months to prevent long-term ocular damage. A leg-length discrepancy is another common complication of childhood oligoarthritis, which is caused by the increased blood flow to the inflamed joint that results in increased length and width of the bone. A single inflamed knee can result in a significant leg-length discrepancy.

Childhood psoriatic arthritis includes children with arthritis and psoriasis and also includes children without psoriasis who have arthritis with dactylitis or characteristic fingernail abnormalities (onycholysis or nail pitting), or a first degree relative with psoriasis.

Childhood enthesitis-related arthritis was previously called childhood spondyloarthropathy. Children with this disease have arthritis and enthesitis, or enthesitis with at least two of the following other symptoms or characteristics: sacroiliac or inflammatory lumbosacral pain; acute, symptomatic anterior uveitis; a positive HLA-B27; a family history of spondyloarthropathy.

The monitoring and treatment of children with JIA depends on the severity and type of disease and extra-articular involvement. Some types of JIA may go into remission and some may recur in adulthood. Medical therapy, such as DMARD use, does not always mirror the same use as in adult therapy. For example, DMARDs are used more often in patients with the polyarticular type of JIA than in those with the oligoarticular type. Also, some drugs commonly used to treat adult arthritis, such as the coxibs, have not been adequately studied for use in children (yet are frequently prescribed). Corticosteroids may cause significant side effects in both adults and children, but children may also be affected by marked growth retardation. A pediatric rheumatologist is the best resource in treating children with JIA.

Patients with JIA often have unique perioperative challenges. The temporomandibular joint is frequently involved and, when combined with micrognathia, intubation and postextubation ventilation can be difficult. Fiberoptic intubation may be necessary.

Seronegative Spondyloarthropathies

Clinical Features

The seronegative spondyloarthropathies are a group of four conditions: ankylosing spondylitis (AS), psoriatic arthritis (PsA), reactive arthritis (ReA), and arthritis associated with inflammatory bowel disease. AS is a chronic inflammatory disease of the axial skeleton. The major symptoms of AS are back pain with prolonged (longer than 1 hour) morning stiffness and progressive loss of motion of the axial spine. Other clinical features that help to distinguish AS from the much more common mechanical back pain are back pain that awakens the patient at night and pain that is relieved by light exercise. The hallmark radiologic findings are sacroiliitis and progressive fusion of the spine (called a bamboo spine), which occurs in a later stage of the disease. AS typically affects young adults between 15 and 35 years of age. The onset of axial symptoms is insidious. Other symptoms include frequent peripheral joint inflammation (usually oligoarticular and asymmetric), acute, unilateral anterior uveitis, and rarely, cardiac and pulmonary disease.

There are five types of PsA. The most common is an oligoarticular, asymmetric pattern. Other types include a polyarticular symmetric arthritis similar to RA, a pattern of axial involvement similar to AS, a distal interphalangeal joint involvement pattern, and arthritis mutilans with telescoping digits. PsA usually is preceded by cutaneous psoriasis, but in about 20% of patients, the arthritis precedes the psoriasis. PsA usually is associated with nail pitting (Figure 10) and patients may have dactylitis (sausage digit) with a fusiform swelling of the entire digit.

ReA was previously called Reiter's syndrome and is triggered by a sexually transmitted disease (infecting bacteria—*Chlamydia*) or a bowel infection (infecting bacteria—*Yersinia, Salmonella, Campylobacter, Shigella*). Typical features of ReA include asymmetric lower limb oligoarthritis, conjunctivitis, and dysuria. The dysuria can be either caused by a *Chlamydia* pyuria or by a sterile pyuria that can be triggered by a bowel infection.

Approximately 20% of patients with inflammatory bowel disease will develop an inflammatory arthritis with axial and/or peripheral joint involvement. The peripheral joint inflammation often can flare with bowel disease activity, whereas the axial inflammation does not flare in conjunction with the inflammatory bowel disease.

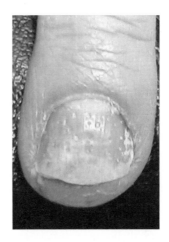

Figure 10 Photograph of nail pits in a patient with psoriatic arthritis.

These four spondyloarthropathies often have overlapping symptoms of axial inflammation including sacroiliitis and enthesitis. The enthesis is the structure that includes the ligament and tendon attachment to the bone as well as the extension into the bone cortex. Enthesitis is a characteristic finding.

Human Leukocyte Antigen-B27

The major factor in the pathogenesis of the spondyloarthropathies is the class I major histocompatibility antigen, HLA-B27. HLA-B27 is present in 5% to 8% of the general population, but is present in 95% of white patients and 50% of black patients with AS. This antigen also is found in 50% to 80% of patients with other seronegative spondyloarthropathies. The presence of HLA-B27 is not needed to confirm a diagnosis of AS; however, it can be used as a diagnostic test in children and young women who may have normal radiographs and in patients who have an atypical presentation.

Treatment

Treatment protocols of the spondyloarthropathies include maintenance of posture, back range-of-motion exercises, and the use of NSAIDs. If there is chronic peripheral joint involvement, methotrexate and sulfasalazine are frequently used to reduce joint erosions and damage, similar to the therapy used for RA (Table 7). Local GC injections may be useful for large joint involvement, but systemic steroids are not often used. For patients with ReA, the triggering infection should be treated. If the joint inflammation persists after the infection has been eradicated, long-term antibiotic use has not been shown to be effective. Studies of the use of anti-TNF-α therapies for patients with PsA have found remarkable improvement in joint pain, damage control, and function, as well as in the psoriasis lesions. In resistant patients with AS, anti-TNF-α can cause dramatic clinical improvement. No treatment has been shown to prevent the ankylosis of the axial spine; however, current studies show that the anti-TNF-α agents used in the treatment of AS are promising.

Surgical Management

The protocols for the perioperative use of DMARDs and NSAIDs in RA also apply to their use in treatment of the spondyloarthropathies. Additional surgical issues need to be considered for AS patients. These patients have diminished chest excursion, which creates a greater risk for postoperative pulmonary complications. Intubation also may be extremely difficult because of cervical spine rigidity; fiberoptic intubation may be necessary. Ossification of the anulus fibrosus and spinal ligaments may make administration of spinal anesthetic difficult. When such patients are positioned on the operating table, great care must be exercised to ensure that the spine is adequately padded and supported, particularly if a significant kyphotic deformity exists. Patients with AS often fail to fully regain the same range of motion after joint reconstruction in comparison with other groups of patients. Although postoperative range of motion may be less, it is still often adequate to significantly improve the patient's ability to perform activities of daily living. Patients with AS may have an increased risk of heterotopic ossification. Indomethacin or perioperative radiation may be used to decrease this risk.

Patients with PsA may have skin involvement in the area of the proposed surgical incision. Because local bacterial contamination may increase the risk of infection, it is recommended that the skin be treated aggressively with topical agents or ultraviolet light before any surgical procedure. In addition, patients should use antimicrobial soaps before surgery.

Emerging Concepts and Future Directions

There is increasing knowledge about the systemic risk factors of OA and the modification of these risk factors to prevent OA. The search for the first disease-modifying OA drug (similar to a DMARD in RA) continues; this process will be facilitated by the increased understanding of the molecular basis of articular cartilage degradation. Possible candidates for such a disease-modifying agent include the combination cyclooxygenase/lipoxygenase inhibitors, MMP inhibitors, IL-1, and nitric oxide blockade.

Although the anti-TNF-α therapies have dramatically improved function and quality of life for patients with RA, the use of these agents has not led to a permanent remission of inflammation in RA patients. There are probably other factors contributing to the persistent systemic inflammation in RA. Other cytokine inhibitors are currently in clinical trials and are showing good preliminary results. B cell inhibition is a promising treatment of RA that is currently under investigation. Although the treatment of RA has advanced greatly in recent years, the possible causes of RA are still unknown. Understanding the causes of RA offers the best chance for finding a cure or a preventive therapy.

Treatment of the spondyloarthropathies also will benefit from the anti-TNF-α research in RA. These agents may be the first to actually reduce long-term progression of axial disease. Investigating the trigger for the spondyloarthropathies may lead to the identification of other infectious organisms, similar to those found in ReA.

Stem cell transplant has been tested in patients with RA, JIA, and other autoimmune diseases with the goal of replacing most of the activated cells with uncommitted stem cells (based on the assumption that the original triggers for the disease are no longer present). A recent study noted that positive responses were found with 59% remission for up to 4 years in patients with JIA. Transplant mortality was 1.4% for RA patients and 12.5% for those with JIA. Most RA patients who did not experience remission regained sensitivity to antirheumatic medications, allowing for better disease control. There is one report of the development of RA after autologous peripheral blood stem cell transplantation.

Annotated Bibliography

Osteoarthritis

Brown KN, Saunders MM, Kirsch T, Donahue HJ, Reid JS: Effect of COX-2-specific inhibition on fracture-healing in the rat femur. *J Bone Joint Surg Am* 2004;86:116-123.

The results of this study on rats with nondisplaced fractures of the femur showed that a traditional NSAID (indomethacin) delayed fracture healing more than a coxib (celecoxib) or placebo.

DeGroot J, Bank RA, Tchetverikov I, Verzijl N, TeKoppele JM: Molecular markers for osteoarthritis: The road ahead. *Curr Opin Rheumatol* 2002;14:585-589.

This is an excellent recent summary of the developments made in the study of molecular markers for osteoarthritis.

DeMaria AN, Weir MR: Coxibs: Beyond the GI tract: Renal and cardiovascular issues. *J Pain Symptom Manage* 2003;25(suppl 2):S41-S49.

This article presents an important review of the clinical implications of the use of coxibs on the renal and cardiovascular systems. The article also reviews the lack of platelet effect of the coxibs and the role of supplemental acetylsalicylic acid in those patients who require an antiplatelet agent for cardiovascular prophylaxis.

Fries JF, Lorig K, Holman HR: Patient self-management in arthritis: Yes! *J Rheumatol* 2003;30:1130-1132.

This article reviews the importance of patient self-management in arthritis. Patients who learn about their arthritis and who take an active role in the management of this chronic condition have better long-term outcomes.

Jordan JM, Kraus VB, Hochberg MC: Genetics of osteoarthritis. *Curr Rheumatol Rep* 2004;6:7-13.

This article provides a perspective on the various genetic studies of OA and the limitations of these studies given the variation in study populations and diagnostic criteria.

Rheumatoid Arthritis

Alderman AK, Ubel PA, Kim HM, Fox DA, Chung KC: Surgical management of the rheumatoid hand: Consensus and controversy among rheumatologists and hand surgeons. *J Rheumatol* 2003;30:1464-1472.

This article describes the large discrepancy in communication between rheumatologists and hand surgeons and knowledge of timing and options in hand surgery.

Cannella AC, O'Dell JR: Is there still a role for traditional disease-modifying antirheumatic drugs (DMARDs) in rheumatoid arthritis? *Curr Opin Rheumatol* 2003;15:185-192.

This article reviews recent and relevant trials in the treatment of RA, suggests a treatment algorithm, and argues that traditional disease-modifying antirheumatic drugs continue to play a pivotal role in treatment. A more aggressive approach using combination DMARDs and biologics in the treatment of early RA is discussed.

Laine L, Bombardier C, Hawkey CJ, et al: Stratifying the risk of NSAID-related upper gastrointestinal clinical events: Results of a double-blind outcomes study in patients with rheumatoid arthritis. *Gastroenterology* 2002; 123:1006-1012.

The risks of traditional NSAIDs in the treatment of RA is investigated with a review of the recent literature.

Mohan AK, Cote TR, Siegel JN, Braun MM: Infectious complications of biologic treatments of rheumatoid arthritis. *Curr Opin Rheumatol* 2003;15:179-184.

Authors from the United States Food and Drug Administration present a review of the infectious complications from the use of the biologic therapies as reported in the medical literature from November 2001 through October 2002.

Juvenile Idiopathic Arthritis

Petty RE, Southwood TR, Manners P, et al: International League of Associations for Rheumatology classification of juvenile idiopathic arthritis: Second revision, Edmonton, 2001. *J Rheumatol* 2004;31:390-392.

An excellent review of the classification of JIA that includes the rationale for the choice of subtypes is presented.

Ravelli A: Toward an understanding of the long-term outcome of juvenile idiopathic arthritis. *Clin Exp Rheumatol* 2004;22:271-275.

This article presents an analysis of the outcome of JIA in terms of clinical remission, physical disability, and radiographic damage. The extensive prognostic indicators and the subtypes that persist into adulthood are reviewed.

Seronegative Spondyloarthropathies

Davis JC Jr, Van Der Heijde D, Braun J, et al: Recombinant human tumor necrosis factor receptor (etanercept) for treating ankylosing spondylitis: A randomized, controlled trial. *Arthritis Rheum* 2003;48:3230-3231.

This study of patients with moderate to severe ankylosing spondylitis showed that etanercept was highly effective and well tolerated. Patients showed a dramatic improvement in symptoms and measures of spinal mobility. It also had a good safety profile.

Emerging Concepts and Future Directions

Edwards JC, Leandro MJ, Cambridge G: B lymphocyte depletion therapy with rituximab in rheumatoid arthritis. *Rheum Dis Clin North Am* 2004;30:393-403.

Most of the current DMARD therapy for RA focuses on T cell inhibition. This article discusses the concept of B-cell inhibition with rituximab as a promising new therapy for RA.

Furst DE: The status of stem cell transplantation for rheumatoid arthritis: A rheumatologist's view. *J Rheumatol Suppl* 2001;64:60-61.

Stem cell transplantation may become an important therapy for the treatment of certain subtypes of RA. This review discusses specific selection criteria and outcome measurements.

Wulffraat NM, Brinkman D, Ferster A, et al: Long-term follow-up of autologous stem cell transplantation for refractory juvenile idiopathic arthritis. *Bone Marrow Transplant* 2003;32(suppl 1):S61-S64.

This review discusses the outcome of autologous stem cell transplantation in 31 children with JIA from eight pediatric European transplant centers.

Classic Bibliography

Bathon JM, Martin RW, Fleischmann RM, et al: A comparison of etanercept and methotrexate in patients with early rheumatoid arthritis. *N Engl J Med* 2000;343:1586-1593.

Bresnihan B, Alvaro-Gracia JM, Cobby M, et al: Treatment of rheumatoid arthritis with recombinant human interleukin-1 receptor antagonist. *Arthritis Rheum* 1998; 41:2196-2204.

Maini R, St Clair EW, Breedveld F, et al: Infliximab (chimeric anti-tumour necrosis factor alpha monoclonal antibody) versus placebo in rheumatoid arthritis patients receiving concomitant methotrexate: A randomised phase III trial. *Lancet* 1999;354:1932-1939.

Oliveria SA, Felson DT, Reed JI, Cirillo PA, Walker AM: Incidence of symptomatic hand, hip, and knee osteoarthritis among patients in a health maintenance organization. *Arthritis Rheum* 1995;38:1134-1141.

Recommendations for the medical management of osteoarthritis of the hip and knee: 2000 update: American College of Rheumatology Subcommittee on Osteoarthritis Guidelines. *Arthritis Rheum* 2000;43:1905-1915.

Shojania K: Rheumatology: 2. What laboratory tests are needed? *CMAJ* 2000;162:1157-1163.

Watterson JR, Esdaile JM: Viscosupplementation: Therapeutic mechanisms and clinical potential in osteoarthritis of the knee. *J Am Acad Orthop Surg* 2000;8:277-284.

Chapter 22

Connective Tissue Diseases

Jacques L. D'Astous, MD, FRCSC

Kristen L. Carroll, MD

Introduction

Connective tissue disorders such as Ehlers-Danlos syndrome (EDS), osteogenesis imperfecta (OI), and Marfan syndrome are phenotypic expressions of inherited collagen and/or fibrillin anomalies. The errors of the extracellular matrix of the involved tissues in these diseases lead to pathology within the bone, vascular system, and viscera. Although the genetics and pathophysiology are different, the underlying similarity of abnormal genetic expression leading to systemic disease is unmistakable.

Ehlers-Danlos Syndrome

EDS includes a group of the most common heritable disorders of the connective tissue. Although all have features of skin and joint hypermobility, they are a heterogenous group presently classified based on genetic transmission, biochemical anomaly, and major and minor clinical findings. The previous classification system of 11 different types has been reduced to 6 in the present Villefranche classification system (Table 1).

Classic

Classic EDS includes the former type I (gravis) and type II (mitis) subsets. The classic type combined with hypermobility and vascular types are by far the most common, comprising more than 90% of all types of EDS. The classic form is an autosomal dominant condition with 40% to 50% of patients manifesting a *COL5A1* or *COL5A2* gene mutation of type V collagen. The major clinical diagnostic criteria include skin hypermobility, widened atrophic scars, and joint hypermobility. Up to 33% of patients will have aortic root dilatations and therefore, echocardiography is suggested. Other minor criteria include velvety skin, spheroids, hypotonia, and tissue fragility. Nearly 30% of patients will have scoliosis, with most having the thoracic or thoracolumbar type. Tower vertebra may be seen (Figure 1). More than 50% of these patients may have chronic musculoskeletal pain.

Hypermobility

The hypermobility subtype (formerly type III) is the most orthopaedically debilitating of all forms of EDS, and the most likely to require orthopaedic surgical intervention. It is an autosomal dominant variant of unknown molecular basis; therefore, no diagnostic test presently exists. Clinically, these patients present with soft skin and both small and large joint hypermobility; recurrent and/or chronic dislocations may also be present. Up to 20% of patients may have aortic root anomalies. Multidirectional instability of the shoulder, patella subluxation, and chronic ankle instability are common. A snapping of the iliotibial band is often misinterpreted as a dislocated hip, although true dislocations can occur (albeit rarely) even in the presence of radiographically normal bony architecture (Figure 2). Surgical interventions such as capsular shift or plication should be undertaken only if physical therapy is ineffective. Excellent results are elusive. Bracing is frequently used, especially of the hands because of finger instability. Nearly 90% of patients have debilitating pain, often with abnormal gait or the need for assistive devices.

Vascular

The vascular subtype (formerly type IV) is most often autosomal dominant and occasionally autosomal recessive. Biochemically, a defect in the *COL3A1* gene for type III collagen is present in more than 90% of the patients. As in the other EDS subtypes, hypermobility of the small joints and clubfoot may be present. However, the hallmark of the vascular subtype is malignant involvement of the viscera and arteries. These patients have thin, translucent skin, and may experience spontaneous rupture of the bowel, uterus, or large arteries. Aortic root dilatation is present in more than 75% of patients. Twenty-five percent of women die during pregnancy because of complications, most often uterine rupture. Life expectancy is 45 to 50 years.

Kyphoscoliosis

This rare subtype (previously type VI) is an autosomal recessive disorder with a biochemical deficiency in lysyl

TABLE 1 | Ehlers-Danlos Classification

Villefranche Classification (1998)	Berlin Classification (1988)	Genetics	Major Symptomatic Criteria	Biochemical Defects (Minor Criteria)
Classic	Type I (gravis) Type II (mitis)	AD	Hyperextensible skin, atrophic scars, joint hypermobility	*COL5A1, COL5A2* mutations (40% to 50% of families) Mutations in type V collagen
Hypermobility	Type III (hypermobile)	AD	Velvety soft skin, small and large joint hypermobility and tendency for dislocation, chronic pain, scoliosis	Unknown
Vascular	Type IV (vascular)	AD (rarely) AR	Arterial, intestinal and uterine fragility, rupture, thin translucent skin, extensive bruising	*COL3A1* mutation, abnormal type III collagen structure of synthesis
Kyphoscoliosis	Type VI (ocular-scoliotic)	AR	Severe hypotonia at birth, progressive infantile scoliosis, generalized joint laxity, scleral fragility, globe rupture	Lysyl hydroxylase deficiency, mutations in the *PLOD* gene
Arthrochalasis	Type VIIA, VIIB	AD	Congenital bilateral hip dislocation, hypermobility, soft skin	Deletion of type I collagen exons that encode for N-terminal propeptide (*COL1A1, COL1A2*)
Dermatosparaxis	Type VIIIC	AR	Severe sagging or redundant skin	Mutations in type I collagen N-terminal peptidase

AD = autosomal dominant; AR = autosomal recessive

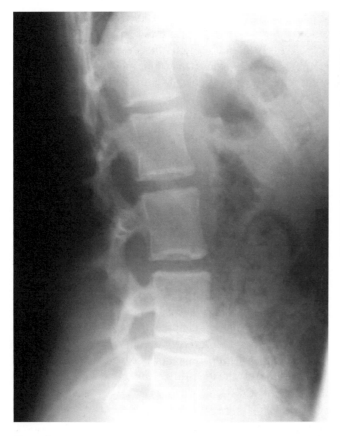

Figure 1 Radiograph of the lateral lumbar spine of a 16-year-old girl with classic (previously type II) EDS. Note the high vertebral height known as tower vertebra.

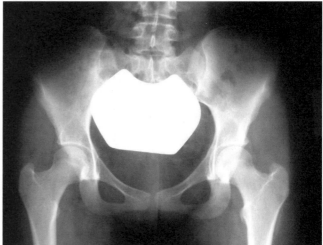

Figure 2 Radiograph of an 18-year-old woman who required three closed reductions of the hip following ground level falls. As seen here and confirmed by MRI, the bony (and labral) architecture of the hip appear normal.

hydroxylase, an enzyme that modifies collagen. Major diagnostic criteria include muscle hypotonia at birth and a progressive scoliosis; most of the curves are double thoracic in pattern. There is generalized joint laxity. Ocular findings such as scleral fragility and globe rupture are found in 50% of patients. Minor criteria include bruising, tissue fragility, osteopenia, and arterial rupture. Kyphoscoliosis EDS may be confused with Marfan syn-

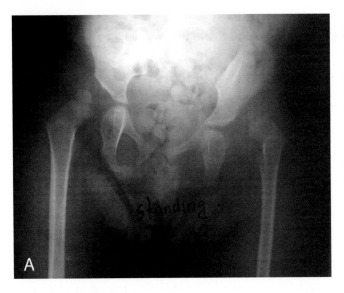

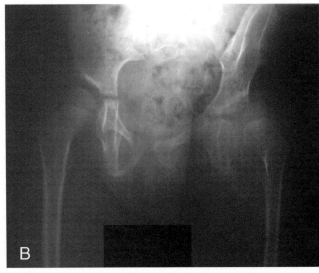

Figure 3 A and **B**, Radiographs of a 3-year-old girl with bilateral developmental dysplasia of the hip, a family history of EDS, and arthrochalasis. After bilateral reduction of the hip through an anterior approach and capsulorrhaphy, the left hip has resubluxated.

drome as patients have scoliotic, cardiac, and ocular involvement and often a tall, thin body habitus.

Arthrochalasis

This extremely rare form of EDS was previously classified as types VIIA and VIIB. This autosomal dominant form is characterized by a deficiency in the pro-α I or pro-α 2 collagen type I chains at their N-terminal end. Children with arthrochalasis type EDS are born with bilateral developmental dysplasia of the hip that is often recalcitrant to surgical intervention (Figure 3). They may also, as minor criteria, display skin hyperextensibility, muscle hypotonia, osteopenia, and kyphoscoliosis. Easy bruising and tissue fragility also exist.

Dermatosparaxis

Dermatosparaxis is a rare, autosomal recessive form of EDS (formally known as type VIIC) notable for a deficiency of procollagen I N-terminal peptidase. Patients have redundant, severely fragile, and often sagging skin. Premature rupture of fetal membranes, large hernias, and easy bruising also may be seen.

Other Forms

In addition to the six major forms of the Villefranche classification, other forms of EDS exist encompassing previous types V, VIII, and X and include those with periodontal friability (VIII), and the poor clotting/ fibronectin deficient type (X). In addition, a form of EDS with symptoms similar to the classic form exists, but with an X-linked inheritance pattern. This was formerly type V EDS and has been described in only a single family.

Osteogenesis Imperfecta

OI is a hereditary condition resulting from an abnormality in type I collagen that is manifested by an increased fragility of bones and low bone mass (osteopenia). It is estimated that in the United States alone, 20,000 to 50,000 people are affected with OI.

Eighty percent to 90% of patients with OI can be grouped into the Sillence type I to IV categories and have mutations of one of the two type I collagen genes. (Recently, types V, VI, and VII have also been added). The *COL1A* gene encodes the pro-α1(I) protein chain and the *COL2A* gene encodes pro-α2(I) protein chain of type I procollagen. The etiologies of the remaining 10% to 20% remain unclear.

Iliac crest biopsies of patients with OI show a decrease in cortical widths and cancellous bone volume, with increased bone remodeling. There is a direct relationship between the increase in bone turnover and the severity of the disease.

The clinical features of OI are osteopenia, bone fragility, and fractures and may include some or all of the following: joint laxity, gray-blue sclerae, dentogenesis imperfecta, premature deafness, kyphoscoliosis, and basilar invagination (prolapse of the upper cervical spine into the base of the skull). In OI, the bones can be biologically "soft," producing deformities such as protrusio acetabuli in the pelvis and basilar invagination at the craniovertebral junction. It is believed that repeated microfractures in OI bone combined with healing and remodeling is responsible for the "soft" bones.

Symptoms of basilar invagination in OI typically occur in the third and fourth decades but may be present during the teenage years. These symptoms include brainstem dysfunction such as apnea, altered consciousness,

TABLE 2 | Types of OI Modified From Sillence

Type	Transmission	Biochemistry	Orthopaedic Manifestation	Miscellaneous
I A I B	AD	50% amount of type I collagen	Mild to moderate bone fragility, osteoporosis, late fractures	Blue sclerae, hearing loss, easy bruising, normal life expectancy More severe than IA with dentinogenesis imperfecta, slightly decreased life expectancy
II II A II B II C II D	AD, AR and mosaic	Unstable triple helix	Multiple intrauterine fractures, extreme bone fragility, beaded ribs, broad bones, platyspondyly Severely osteopenic with generally well formed skeleton, normally shaped vertebrae and pelvis	Usually lethal in perinatal period, delayed ossification of skull, blue sclerae
III	AD and AR	Abnormal type I collagen	Progressive deforming phenotype, severe bone fragility with fractures at birth, "popcorn" epiphyses/metaphyses, scoliosis and platyspondyly, severe osteoporosis, extreme short stature	Hearing loss, blue sclerae becoming less blue with age, shortened life expectancy, dentinogenesis imperfecta, relative macrocephaly with triangular faces
IV A IV B	AD AD	Shortened pro-α1 chain	Mild-moderate bone fragility, osteoporosis, bowing of long bones, scoliosis	Light sclerae, normal hearing, normal dentition Same as IVA plus dentogenesis imperfecta present, slight decreased life expectancy
V	AD	Irregular mesh-like lamellar bone, lack of parallel organization of collagen fibers	Hypertrophic callus after fractures, calcification of interosseous membrane	
VI		Mineralization defect, abundance of osteoid, fish-scale organization of lamellae	Low bone mineral density, frequent fractures, vertebral compressions, long bone deformities	Normal vitamin D levels, absence of hypocalcemia and hypophosphatemia
VII	AR		Rhizomelic limb shortening	

AD = autosomal dominant; AR = autosomal recessive

lower cranial nerve deficits, myelopathy, and ataxia. Neurologic abnormalities are consequences of direct neural compression, altered cerebrospinal fluid flow, or vascular compromise. The recommended treatment of basilar invagination in OI consists of extensive removal of bony compression by a transoral approach followed by a posterior fusion and posterior rigid fixation that transfers the weight of the head to the thoracic spine.

Although it may be difficult, determining the clinical distinction between children with OI and those with nonaccidental trauma has obviously important implications. Skin biopsies and fibroblast cultures may be helpful, but are only positive in 80% of patients with type IV OI (the most commonly confused with nonaccidental trauma) (Table 2).

Nonsurgical Treatment

The medical treatment of OI involves strategies to improve bone mass. Recombinant human growth hormone has been used in the past because of its anabolic effects on bone; however, clinical studies showed no increase in bone mass or change in natural history. For the past 10 years, bisphosphonates have been used to treat patients with types III and IV OI. Bisphosphonates decrease the resorption of bone by suppressing the activity of osteoclasts. Pamidronate, an injectable bisphosphonate, increases cortical bone thickness and, in severe forms of OI, improves overall bone mass. Pamidronate therapy decreases the incidence of fractures, relieves chronic bone pain, increases activity levels, decreases the reliance on mobility aids, and increases the height of the collapsed vertebral bodies. Unfortunately, there has been no decrease in the incidence of scoliosis. Radiographically, pamidronate therapy creates growth lines in the bone (Figure 4). These radiodense areas of bone probably represent the inhibition of osteoclastic resorption, whereas the clear areas between the lines represent the interval growth between treatment cycles.

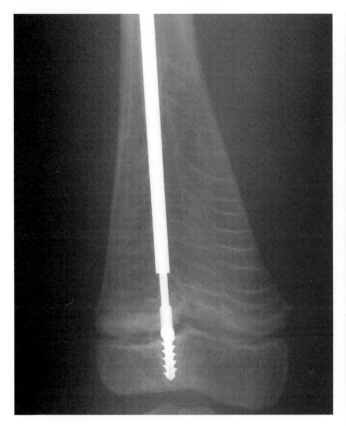

Figure 4 Growth lines secondary to pamidronate therapy.

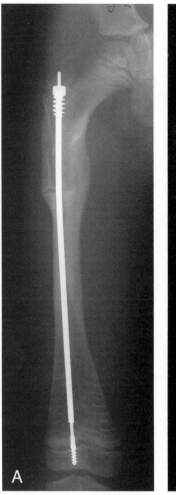
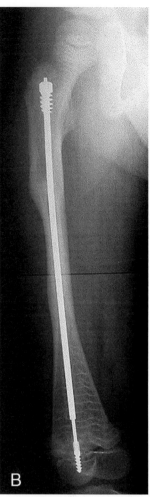

Figure 5 **A** and **B,** The Fassier-Duval telescopic nail obtains purchase in the greater trochanter and femoral epiphysis without requiring an arthrotomy. **A,** The limb is shown shortly after corrective osteotomy and instrumentation. **B,** Note interval extension of rod with growth.

Newer, more potent forms of bisphosphonates (for example, zoledronate) that require fewer injections are being evaluated. There is concern, however, that bisphosphonates may make bone more brittle. Bone marrow transplantation, which introduces normal marrow stem cells that could potentially differentiate into normal osteoblasts, has been used with some success for severely affected patients with OI. Problems of graft rejection and graft versus host reactions limit this approach.

Orthotic devices are indicated to stabilize lax joints, prevent progression of deformity and fractures, and allow early weight bearing following surgical intervention.

Surgical Treatment

The mainstay of surgical treatment of patients with OI is realignment osteotomy, which is performed to improve the mechanical axis of appendicular bones. In addition to decreasing the risk of fracture, the goals and principles of realignment surgery are to allow for early weight bearing and to achieve union. The realignment osteotomies should be performed through small incisions in an attempt to preserve the blood supply, and then stabilization should be achieved with intramedullary devices, of which there are both telescopic and nontelescopic forms. The most commonly used nontelescopic devices include Rush rods and Williams rods. The use of telescopic rods appears to decrease the incidence

of re-rodding to accommodate for growth, (51% for simple rods versus 27% for telescopic rods) and therefore are preferred for use when possible. The Sheffield rod and the newly developed Fassier-Duval rod represent an improvement over the older Bailey-Dubow rod (Figure 5).

The treatment of spinal deformities in OI can be challenging. It is impossible to effectively push on the spine through the ribs because of the fragility of the rib cage and the possibility of further aggravating the thoracic deformity. When the curves approach 45° in the mild forms of OI and 30° to 35° in the severe forms, a posterior spinal fusion with segmental instrumentation to prevent progression of the curve should be considered (Figure 6). Because of bone fragility, it may be necessary to reinforce the upper and lower hook claws with bone cement or use Mersilene tape instead of sublaminar wires. Because of the paucity of bone in the iliac crest, allograft bone should be used. Anterior spinal fu-

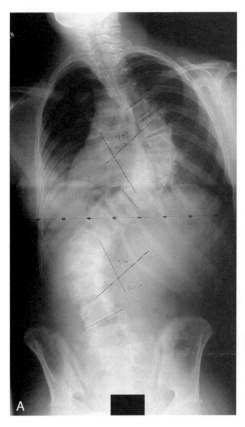
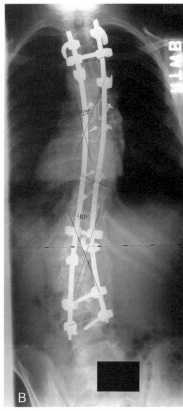

Figure 6 Preoperative **(A)** and postoperative **(B)** radiographs showing scoliosis in a patient with type IV OI treated by posterior spinal fusion.

sion may be considered in the very young patient to prevent crankshafting of the spine. Surgery for basilar invagination is indicated for patients with radiographic progression or with neurologic deficits resulting from brainstem and high cervical cord compression.

Marfan Syndrome

Marfan syndrome is an inherited connective tissue disorder that is usually transmitted as an autosomal dominant trait. Approximately 25% of cases arise from new mutations. The incidence is roughly 1:10,000 with approximately 200,000 people in the United States having Marfan syndrome. There is no ethnic or gender predilection.

The genetic mutation of Marfan syndrome is on the fibrillin-1 (*FBN1*) gene located on chromosome 15q21. More than 135 mutations in the *FBN1* gene have been identified. The genetic heterogenicity explains the pleiotropic manifestations of Marfan syndrome with variable phenotypic expression. *FBN1* is the main component of the 10 to 20 nm extracellular microfibrils that are important for elastogenesis, elasticity, and homeostasis of elastic fibers.

The clinical features include increased height, disproportionately long, gracile limbs (dolichostenomelia), arachnodactyly with a positive wrist (Walker) and thumb (Steinberg) sign, an arm span greater than height (span to height ratio > 1.05), anterior chest wall defor-

mity (pectus excavatum > pectus carinatum), generalized ligamentous laxity, severe planovalgus, and/or long thin feet with a disproportionately long great toe. Scoliosis is seen in 60% to 70% of patients (right thoracic lordotic curves are the most common); males and females are equally affected. The head and neck reveal a high arched palate, myopia, corneal flatness, dislocation of lenses (ectopia lentis) and iridodonesis (tremor of the iris secondary to lens dislocation). Cardiac manifestations include mitral valve prolapse, mitral regurgitation, dilatation of aortic root, aortic regurgitation, aortic dissection, and aortic aneurysm. Marfan syndrome may lead to spontaneous pneumothorax secondary to lung bullae and striae distensae.

A severe neonatal form of Marfan syndrome exists. These children are identified within the first few months of life by serious cardiac abnormalities and congenital contractures. This form of the syndrome is believed to result from a spontaneous mutation in the *FBN1* gene.

The diagnosis of Marfan syndrome is based on family history, evaluation of six organ systems, and molecular data. The Ghent system outlines diagnostic criteria for both the index patient (the first case in a family) and for subsequent relatives (Table 3). To establish the diagnosis of Marfan syndrome in the index case, the patient must fulfill one major criteria in at least two different organ systems and have involvement of a third system. To establish the diagnosis in a relative of an index case,

TABLE 3 | Marfan Syndrome

System	Major Criteria	Minor Criteria
Musculoskeletal*	Pectus carinatum; pectus excavatum requiring surgery; dolichostenomelia; wrist and thumb signs; scoliosis > 20° or spondylolisthesis; reduced elbow extension; pes planus; protrusio acetabuli	Moderately severe pectus excavatum; joint hypermobility; highly arched palate with crowding of teeth; facies (dolichocephaly, malar hypoplasia, enophthalmos, retrognathia, down-slanting palpebral fissures)
Ocular†	Ectopia lentis	Abnormally flat cornea; increased axial length of globe; hypoplastic iris or hypoplastic ciliary muscle causing decreased miosis
Cardiovascular‡	Dilatation of ascending aorta ± aortic regurgitation, involving sinuses of Valsalva; or dissection of ascending aorta	Mitral valve prolapse ± regurgitation
Family/Genetic history§	Parent, child, or sibling meets diagnostic criteria; mutation in *FBN1* known to cause Marfan syndrome; or inherited haplotype around *FBN1* associated with Marfan syndrome in family	None
Skin and integument‖	None	Stretch marks not associated with pregnancy, weight gain, or repetitive stress; or recurrent incisional hernias
Dura§	Lumbosacral dural ectasia	None
Pulmonary‖	None	Spontaneous pneumothorax or apical blebs

*Two or more major or one major plus two minor criteria required for involvement
†At least two minor criteria required for involvement
‡One major or minor criterion required for involvement
§One major criterion required for involvement
‖One minor criterion required for involvement

(Adapted from Miller NH: Connective tissue disorders, in Koval KJ (ed): Orthopaedic Knowledge Update: 7. Rosemont, IL, American Academy of Orthopaedic Surgeons, 2002, pp 201-207.)

a major criterion in the family history needs to be present, the individual must have one major criterion in any organ system and involvement of a second organ system.

Marfan syndrome must be differentiated from the MASS phenotype, an acronym assigned to the following clinical features: mitral valve prolapse, aortic root diameter at the upper limits of normal, stretch marks, and skeletal features of Marfan syndrome (including scoliosis, pectus excavatum or carinatum, and joint hypermobility). The aortic root diameter may be at the upper limits of normal for body size, but there is no progression to aneurysm or predisposition to dissection. Ectopia lentis does not occur. MASS patients therefore have a better prognosis than those with classic Marfan syndrome. This condition can be inherited within families and has been shown to result from mutations in the *FBN1* gene.

In addition to the MASS phenotype, the differential diagnosis of Marfan syndrome includes congenital contractural arachnodactyly (Beals' syndrome), Stickler's syndrome, arthrochalasis type EDS, hypermobility syndrome, and homocystinuria.

There are no specific laboratory investigations for Marfan syndrome, although genetic testing is now available in some centers. Prenatal molecular diagnosis is possible only if the family's mutation is known or several affected family members are available for genetic linkage analysis.

Radiographic analysis of Marfan syndrome may reveal the presence of scoliosis, protrusio acetabuli, chondrolysis, and high-grade spondylolisthesis (Figure 7). MRI reveals dural ectasia in more than 60% of patients. Other important investigations include transesophageal echocardiogram, electrocardiogram, slit lamp examination, and keratometry.

The medical treatment of Marfan syndrome includes the use of β-blockers to slow the progression of aortic dissection. Aortic replacement is indicated if aortic diameter is greater than 5 cm. Pregnant women with aortic dilatation should have a cesarean section at 38 weeks. The success rate for bracing of spinal deformities is much lower than in adolescent idiopathic scoliosis. Curves greater than 25° in children with Risser grade II skeletal maturity will likely require surgery despite bracing. Preoperative imaging of the spine with MRI to identify dural ectasia and CT to assess fixation points

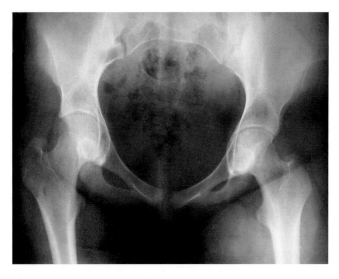

Figure 7 Radiograph of the hip of a 13-year-old girl with Marfan syndrome showing classic protrusio acetabuli.

are essential. Preoperative cardiopulmonary evaluation is mandatory. There is an increased incidence of pseudarthrosis in posterior spinal fusion. Closure of the triradiate cartilage to treat protrusio acetabuli also has been proposed.

If untreated, the life expectancy of a patient with Marfan syndrome is 30 to 40 years, with death resulting from aortic dissection, aortic rupture, or valvular induced cardiac failure. With modern cardiovascular treatment regimens, the average lifespan is now 70 years. It is important to remember that the tall, agile, athletic patient with Marfan syndrome is at risk for aortic dissection and sudden death. It is imperative to educate patients about the signs and symptoms of aortic and cardiac disease, and to counsel them on activity restriction and the possibility of genetic transmission.

Future Directions

As recent studies indicate, an advanced understanding of the genetic basis behind inherited connective tissue disorders will potentially allow for intervention at a molecular level with gene therapy. Although a safe mode of introducing genetically modified collagen for patients with EDS, osteoblasts for those with OI, or fibrillin for those with Marfan syndrome is presently elusive, it should become a reality. Several new strains of Marfan mice have recently been developed with mutant fibrillin-1 proteins to further clarify the mechanism of disease and eventually its treatment.

While awaiting interventions that address the molecular causes of connective tissue disease in these patients, the treatment of their symptoms has become more comprehensive. For patients with OI, advances in the pharmacologic treatment has and will continue to lead to de-

creased pain, increased ease of drug administration, and a reduction in fractures and deformity. For patients with Marfan syndrome, advances in cardiothoracic surgery have doubled the lifespan, and new drugs such as deoxycycline and losartan may decrease the incidence of aortic aneurysms. Ophthalmologic interventions and rigorous slit lamp screening have decreased the incidence of blindness. As the knowledge of the genetics and biochemical anomalies of connective tissue disorders expands, patient care improves.

Annotated Bibliography

Ehlers-Danlos Syndrome

Wenstrup RJ, Meyer RA, Lyle JS, et al: Prevalence of aortic root dilatation in the Ehlers-Danlos syndrome. *Genet Med* 2002;4:112-117.

Twenty-eight percent of all EDS patients have aortic root dilatation (25% in classic form, 17% in the hypermobile form). Patients without the vascular form of EDS also should be carefully monitored for this complication.

Osteogenesis Imperfecta

Cole WG: Advances in osteogenesis imperfecta. *Clin Orthop* 2002;401:6-16.

This article presents a review of the current state of knowledge regarding collagen mutations in OI.

Glorieux FH: The use of bisphosphonates in children with osteogenesis imperfecta. *J Pediatr Endocrinol Metab* 2001;14(suppl 6):1491-1495.

One of the more recent reviews on the use of bisphosphonates for patients with OI is presented by the group who first studied the use of bisphosphonates for this condition.

Osteogenesis imperfecta. NIH Medline Plus Website. Available at: http://www.nlm.nih.gov/medlineplus/osteogenesisimperfecta.html. Accessed June, 2004.

A complete, up-to-date review of all aspects of OI is presented, with numerous links to related websites.

Osteogenesis Imperfecta Foundation Website. Available at: http:/www.oif.org/. Accessed June, 2004.

The OI foundation's official site presents a wealth of information for health professionals and families dealing with all aspects of OI.

Pattekar M, Caccrarelli A: Osteogenesis imperfecta. eMedicine Website. Available at: http:/www.emedicine.com/ped/topic1674.htm. Accessed June, 2004.

This thorough review of OI is available online and includes excellent photographs.

Zeitlin L, Fassier F, Glorieux FH: Modern approach to children with osteogenesis imperfecta. *J Pediatr Orthop B* 2003;12:77-87.

This article reviews the molecular pathogenesis of OI. It also summarizes the most recent medical and surgical management of patients with OI and describes three new types of OI.

Marfan Syndrome

Channell K, Washington E: Marfan syndrome. eMedicine website. Available at: http://www.emedicine.com/orthoped/topic414.htm. Accessed June, 2004.

A complete review of all aspects of Marfan syndrome is presented.

Chen H: Marfan syndrome. eMedicine Website. Availabe at: http://www.emedicine.com/PED/topic1372.htm. Accessed June, 2004.

All aspects of Marfan syndrome are reviewed.

Giampietro PF, Raggio C, Davis JG: Marfan syndrome: Orthopedic and genetic review. *Curr Opin Pediatr* 2002; 14:35-41.

This review summarizes recent developments in the genetic and orthopaedic aspects of Marfan syndrome.

Jones KB, Erkula G, Sponseller PD, Dormans JP: Spine deformity correction in Marfan syndrome. *Spine* 2002; 27:2003-2012.

A recent review of 39 patients with Marfan syndrome treated for spinal deformities with a discussion on preoperative planning, complications, and outcomes is presented.

Loeys BL, Matthys DM, de Paepe AM: Genetic fibrillinopathies: New insights in molecular diagnosis and clinical management. *Acta Clin Belg* 2003;58:3-11.

This article provides an overview of the current diagnostic criteria and medical management of fibrillinopathies, estimates the role of fibrillin-1 mutation analysis, sheds new light on genotype-phenotype correlations, and summarizes new insights on the pathogenesis of this disorder based on mouse models.

The National Marfan Foundation Website. Available at: http://www.marfan.org/. Accessed June 2004.

The latest information concerning the genetic aspects of Marfan syndrome is presented.

Nollen GJ, Groenink M, van der Wall EE, Mulder BJ: Current insights in diagnosis and management of the cardiovascular complications of Marfan syndrome. *Cardiol Young* 2002;12:320-327.

This article presents a review of new advances in surgical and medical treatment for cardiovascular complications of Marfan syndrome that have dramatically improved the prognosis.

Robinson PN, Booms P: The molecular pathogenesis of the Marfan syndrome. *Cell Mol Life Sci* 2001;58:1698-1707.

This article provides an overview of the clinical aspects of Marfan syndrome and current knowledge concerning the pathogenesis of this disorder.

Future Directions

Turgeman G, Aslan H, Gazit Z, Gazit D: Cell-mediated gene therapy for bone formation and regeneration. *Curr Opin Mol Ther* 2002;4:390-394.

This article reviews the most recent studies related to cell-mediated gene therapy for bone formation and regeneration.

Classic Bibliography

Beighton P, De Paepe A, Steinman B, Tsipouras P, Wenstrup RJ: Ehlers-Danlos syndromes: Revised Nosology: Ehlers-Danlos National Foundation (USA) and Ehlers-Danlos Support Group (UK), Villefranche, 1997. *Am J Med Genet* 1998;77:31-37.

Byers PH: Osteogenesis imperfecta: Perspectives and opportunities. *Curr Opin Pediatr* 2000;12:603-609.

Collod-Beroud G, Le Bourdelles S, Ades L, et al: Update of the UMD-FBN1 mutation database and creation of an FBN1 polymorphism database. *Hum Mutat* 2003; 22:199-208.

De Paepe A, Devereux RB, Dietz HC, Hennekam RC, Pyeritz RE: Revised diagnostic criteria for the Marfan syndrome. *Am J Med Genet* 1996;62:417-426.

Dietz HC, Mecham RP: Mouse models of genetic diseases resulting from mutations in elastic fiber proteins. *Matrix Biol* 2000;19:481-488.

Harkey HL, Capel WT: Bone softening diseases and disorders of bone metabolism, in Dickman CA, Spetzler RF, Sonntag VKH (eds): *Surgery of the Craniovertebral Junction*. New York, NY, Thieme, 1998, pp 197-202.

Harkey HL, Crockard HA, Stevens JM, Smith R, Ransford AO: The operative management of basilar impression in osteogenesis imperfecta. *Neurosurgery* 1990;27: 782-786.

Joseph KN, Kane HA, Milner RS, Steg NL, Williamson MB, Bowen JR: Orthopaedic aspects of the Marfan phenotype. *Clin Orthop* 1992;277:251-261.

Kocher MS, Kasser JR: Orthopaedic aspects of child abuse. *J Am Acad Orthop Surg* 2000;8:10-20.

Lubicky JP: The spine in osteogenesis imperfecta, in Weinstein SL (ed): *The Pediatric Spine: Principles and Practice*, ed 2. New York, NY, Raven Press, 2001.

Niyibizi C, Smith P, Mi Z, Robbins P, Evans C: Potential of gene therapy for treating osteogenesis imperfecta. *Clin Orthop* 2000;379(suppl):S126-S138.

Pyeritz RE: The Marfan syndrome. *Annu Rev Med* 2000; 51:481-510.

Sillence DO, Senn A, Danks DM: Genetic heterogeneity in osteogenesis imperfecta. *J Med Genet* 1979;16:101-116.

Sponseller PD, Bhimani M, Solacoff D, Dormans JP: Results of brace treatment of scoliosis in Marfan syndrome. *Spine* 2000;25:2350-2354.

Stanitski DF, Nadjarian R, Stanitski CL, Bawle E, Tsipouras P: Orthopaedic manifestations of Ehlers-Danlos syndrome. *Clin Orthop* 2000;376:213-221.

Section 4

Upper Extremity

Section Editors:
Mark D. Lazarus, MD
Joseph F. Slade III, MD

Chapter 23

Shoulder and Elbow Injuries in the Throwing Athlete

Patrick J. McMahon, MD
Michael Gilbart, MD
Brian S. Cohen, MD
Anthony A. Romeo, MD

Introduction

Athletic injuries to the upper extremity are much less common and receive significantly less attention in the literature than lower extremity injuries. Unfortunately, compared with lower extremity injuries, upper extremity injuries can be just as devastating to the overhead athlete. The shoulder and elbow of the overhead athlete are subject to a tremendous amount of force during overhead "throwing" that an average patient's shoulder and elbow never experience. Although completely different in their anatomic structure (shoulder: ball and socket joint; elbow: hinged joint), both areas are most susceptible to injury during the late cocking and early acceleration phases of throwing. It is during these phases of throwing that the tensile and compressive forces peak, placing potentially pathologic stresses on both areas. As a result of the repetitive nature of overhead sports, "overuse disease" can exacerbate an essentially benign problem into a full-blown disabling condition.

Shoulder

History and Physical Examination

In overhead throwing athletes, grouping symptoms according to a specific phase of throwing, as well as localizing the pain to the front or back of the shoulder, may help in determining the etiology of the injury (Table 1). Physical examination of the shoulder, as with all areas, should begin with visual inspection and should include a comparison of the contralateral or normal side. Examination of the 'joint' above (cervical spine) and the 'joint' below (elbow) should also be included in a comprehensive evaluation of the patient with a shoulder disorder. The general posture of the shoulder should be assessed. It is not uncommon for the overhead athlete to have overdevelopment of the shoulder musculature and humeral head in the throwing extremity. Evaluation of both active and passive motion is critical in assessing shoulder function; specifically, observing the patient from behind to assess scapular motion particularly looking for scapular winging, which can be the result of weakness of the scapular stabilizers. Increased external rotation and decreased internal rotation can be a normal finding in an athlete's throwing shoulder. This increase in external rotation may be related to greater laxity of the anterior ligaments from the deforming forces of overhead throwing, or an increase in the amount of humeral retroversion (little leaguer's shoulder) that represents an adaptive change that probably occurs through the physis. This change has two benefits: first, it allows for increased external rotation during throwing; and second, it acts as a protective mechanism against impingement of the greater tuberosity on the posterior superior glenoid rim during throwing. A greater loss of active motion compared with passive motion within the same shoulder may be the result of pain, rotator cuff pathology, or neurologic compromise. Palpation of specific areas, such as the acromioclavicular (AC) joint and biceps, may help to further localize contributing pathology, whereas specific provocative testing such as the apprehension and relocation tests, the Neer and Hawkins impingement signs, and the O'Brien's and Speed's tests can also contribute to the establishment of the correct diagnosis.

Internal Impingement

Internal impingement is defined as abnormal contact between the rotator cuff undersurface and the posterosuperior glenoid rim, resulting in tearing of the rotator cuff and labrum. Presently, there is no consensus on the treatment of this condition. The etiology of posterosuperior glenoid impingement has also been the source of much debate. Internal impingement has been attributed to anterior microinstability and tightness of the capsule posteriorly. Others argue that posteroinferior capsular contracture results in posterosuperior instability and a peel-back to the superior labrum (a posterior subtype [B] of a type II superior labrum anterior and posterior [SLAP] lesion) and a partial-thickness tearing of the rotator cuff.

On physical examination, the patient's pain is usually posterior and will be reproduced with the arm in the abducted, externally rotated, extended position. Patients may experience pain during an apprehension maneuver, which may be relieved by the relocation test.

Radiographic evaluation will show cystic and sclerotic changes in the greater tuberosity of nearly half of the patients with internal impingement and there may be evidence of rounding of the posterior glenoid rim in one third of patients; both are nonspecific findings. MRI evaluation may show partial undersurface rotator cuff tears and often reveal a pathologic insertion of the supraspinatus tendon. A magnetic resonance arthrogram with an abduction-external rotation view is a useful diagnostic test, revealing posterior-superior labrum abnormalities with an associated "kissing lesion" of articular-sided rotator cuff fraying.

Initial treatment focuses on rehabilitation protocols that improve the function of the dynamic stabilizers and, at the same time, stretch the posterior capsule. Another approach, based on study of baseball pitchers, focused on adjusting throwing mechanics to avoid shoulder extension beyond the plane of the scapula during the cocking phase and through most of the acceleration phase. This phenomenon was termed hyperangulation. The correction of this abnormality in the throwing mechanics of these patients resulted in elimination of their symptoms.

Surgical treatment is reserved for those patients who fail to improve following a well-executed rehabilitation program. Arthroscopic treatment of this disorder focuses on débridement of the partial-thickness rotator cuff tear and associated posterior glenoid labral lesion. Tightening of the anterior capsuloligamentous structures is also performed either by thermal capsulorrhaphy or with a suture plication technique. If internal rotation of the abducted shoulder is diminished, a con-

comitant posterior capsular release may be necessary. Following this procedure, a well-planned rehabilitation program is needed that allows for tissue healing (6 to 8 weeks), followed by restoration of motion and strength (8 to 12 weeks), and concluding with proprioception training and a gradual return to sport-specific activities, with a return to competitive throwing at about 4 to 6 months.

Another procedure that is available, but is used as a last resort, is a humeral derotational osteotomy. This procedure is reserved for patients in whom conservative management and/or arthroscopic treatment have failed and who are faced with either additional surgery or permanent cessation of throwing. This procedure has a high complication and reoperation rate, and, therefore, requires that the patient be thoroughly educated on expected outcomes before surgery. The goal of the surgery is to obtain a postoperative humeral retroversion of 30°. The amount of correction needed is determined from a preoperative CT arthrogram. Overcorrection can cause impingement of the lesser tuberosity on the anterior glenoid with consequent loss of internal rotation. Postoperatively, external rotation is limited for the first 4 weeks to allow for subscapularis healing. Active range of motion is permitted at 4 weeks, and resistive exercises are permitted at 8 weeks. Return to overhead throwing activity is accomplished at about 6 months. Results following this procedure have been mixed. The procedure was performed in 20 throwing athletes; 11 patients returned to their sport at their preinjury level. However, the complication rate was high, with 16 patients requiring removal of hardware for pain in the biceps area or problems associated with anterior forward elevation.

Instability
Anterior Glenohumeral Joint Instability
When the shoulder is repetitively forced beyond the limit of its normal range of motion, displacement of the articular surface of the humeral head from the glenoid may occur. Anterior instability occurs in athletes when the abducted shoulder is repetitively placed in the anterior apprehension position of external rotation and horizontal abduction. Two lesions may occur to the anteroinferior capsulolabrum with anterior instability. The first is the Bankart lesion, which is an avulsion of the anteroinferior capsulolabrum from the anteroinferior glenoid rim. The other lesion associated with recurrent anterior instability in athletes results from stretching of the anteroinferior capsulolabrum.

The history given by the athlete as to when they experience their symptoms may help to determine the direction of their instability. Throwers with anterior instability will report a sensation that the shoulder wants to slide out the front during the late cocking phase of throwing, whereas athletes with posterior laxity will report shoulder discomfort and instability symptoms on the follow-through phase of throwing. The "dead arm syndrome" may occur after anterior joint instability. An overhead throwing athlete with transient anterior instability may experience sudden, sharp pain associated with loss of control of the extremity, numbness, and an inability to throw the ball. These symptoms are transient, and usually resolve within a few seconds to minutes.

The apprehension test is useful in assessing for anterior instability. The examiner applies an anteriorly directed force to the humeral head with the shoulder in abduction and external rotation. A positive test results with the patient having apprehension that the joint will dislocate. This maneuver mimics the position of instability and causes reflex guarding. The relocation test is positive if relief occurs when a posteriorly directed force is applied to the humeral head.

Treatment, especially in patients who have symptomatic laxity as the result of repetitive microtrauma, should focus on a rehabilitation program that avoids the provocative position during the first 6 to 8 weeks and incorporates a strengthening program to enhance the function of the dynamic stabilizers. Following a period of tissue healing, proprioception training followed by a slow return to sport-specific activities should occur.

Surgical intervention should be reserved for patients in whom conservative treatment is unsuccessful, or who represent a population with a high risk of failure, such as young patients with a history of a traumatic anterior dislocation. Identification of the pathoanatomy is essential for relieving the athlete's instability; a patient-specific selective capsular repair can be done, along with refraining from addressing all instability problems with a single type of surgical procedure. Arthroscopically, patients with a history of a traumatic anterior event can have their Bankart lesion repaired anatomically with suture anchors. Treatment of specific capsuloligamentous structures for predetermined directional instabilities can be accomplished with arthroscopic techniques of suture plication, thermal capsulorrhaphy, and, when necessary, closure of the rotator interval.

Posterior Glenohumeral Joint Instability

Posterior instability results either from avulsion of the posterior glenoid labrum from the posterior glenoid, or stretching of the posterior capsuloligamentous structures. Posterior instability is often difficult to diagnose. No single test has high sensitivity and specificity. During the circumduction test, the patient actively rotates the shoulder from the side to an internally rotated and cross-body position, to a fully elevated position, to an abducted and externally rotated position, and then returns the arm to the side. The examiner stands behind the patient and palpates the posterior shoulder. If posi-

tive, the joint subluxates in the internally rotated, cross-body position, and reduction occurs with further rotation. The posterior apprehension test is performed by applying a posterior force to the shoulder with the arm in a forward flexed and internally rotated position. In the Jahnke test, a posterior directed force is applied to the forward flexed shoulder. The shoulder is then moved into the coronal plane as an anterior-directed force is applied to the humeral head. A clunk occurs as the humural head reduces from the subluxated position.

The sulcus sign is used to evaluate inferior laxity and associated inferior instability. The test is performed with the athlete in a sitting position with the arm at the side. A distraction force is applied longitudinally along the humerus. The magnitude of displacement and the presence of discomfort or apprehension is compared with that of the contralateral limb.

Initial treatment should be nonsurgical, consisting of rehabilitation of the glenohumeral and scapular muscles, and surgical treatment should be considered if nonsurgical treatment fails. Posterior stabilization may be performed with arthroscopic or open techniques, and includes repair of the posterior labral avulsion and plication of the stretched posterior capsuloligamentous structures. Special attention should be sought for associated inferior instability and rotator internal lesions should be repaired if present. Patient selection is important, because those with a traumatic etiology and no evidence of generalized ligamentous laxity have the best prognosis.

Superior Labral Anterior and Posterior Lesions

The SLAP lesion was first described in 1985. A more extensive injury pattern was subsequently identified that involved the superior labrum; four basic types were described (Figure 1). Type II lesions were further subdivided into a type II lesion with an anterior component (A), a posterior component (B), or a combined anteroposterior lesion (C). A peel-back phenomenon was described that is part of the pathoanatomy associated with type II SLAP lesions that have a posterior component (B or C), which is observed arthroscopically in the abducted and externally rotated position and may contribute to posterosuperior glenohumeral instability. Anatomic repair of the SLAP lesion has been shown to eliminate the dynamic peel-back of the posterior superior labrum.

The diagnosis of a SLAP lesion is difficult because the injury may be caused by either the repetitive nature of overhead throwing, or as the result of a traumatic event. SLAP lesions are commonly associated with other injuries and usually have overlapping, nonspecific symptoms. The patient may have difficulty describing their pain. The discomfort is typically associated with

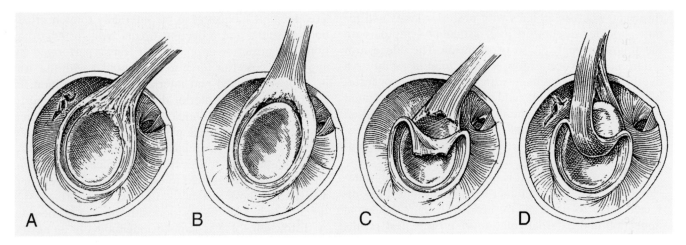

Figure 1 SLAP classification. **A**, Type I: fraying and degeneration of the superior labrum with a normal biceps tendon anchor. **B**, Type II: pathologic detachment of the labrum and biceps anchor from the superior glenoid. **C**, Type III: vertical tear of the superior labrum analogous to a bucket-handle tear. **D**, Type IV: tear extending into biceps tendon. *(Reproduced with permission from Snyder SJ, Karzel RP, Del Pizzo W, et al: SLAP lesions of the shoulder. Arthroscopy 1990;6:274.)*

the late cocking phase of throwing as the arm begins to accelerate forward. The patient may feel a sudden, sharp pain in the extreme abducted and externally rotated position followed by a "dead arm" sensation. These symptoms usually result in an inability to throw with preinjury velocity.

No finding on physical examination has been found to be specific for identifying patients with a SLAP lesion. Provocative tests that have been suggestive of the existence of superior labral pathology include Speed's test, the O'Brien test, and the Jobe relocation test. The O'Brien test (active compression test) may be the most useful. The internally rotated shoulder is forward flexed to 90° and brought across the body in horizontal abduction about 10°. The test is positive if the patient has pain with resisted forward flexion that is relieved by external rotation of the shoulder. It should be noted that a positive relocation test for patients with superior labral pathology is highlighted by posterosuperior glenohumeral joint pain with the arm in the abducted and externally rotated position that is relieved by the relocation maneuver. Imaging studies including plain radiographs and MRI evaluation should be done to rule out coexisting pathologies. A magnetic resonance arthrogram may help in the diagnosis of a SLAP lesion. Diagnostic arthroscopy remains the best means to definitively diagnose SLAP lesions.

Because patient complaints can be nonspecific with no preceding traumatic event, treatment generally begins with a physical therapy program focusing on strengthening of the dynamic stabilizers with the goal of improving joint stability during overhead throwing. Surgical intervention is usually reserved for patients in whom conservative management has failed and is accomplished through an arthroscopic approach. Meaningful detachment of the capsulolabral structures requires

repair to the bony glenoid rim. Lesions producing significant defects extending into the biceps tendon may require biceps tenotomy, with or without tenodesis.

Rehabilitation following a SLAP repair allows for a 6-week interval for tissue healing. During this time, patients are in a gentle range-of-motion program with set limitations, followed by a progressive strengthening program. Sport-specific activities are begun at about 3 to 4 months with a return to sports activity at approximately 6 months. Success following this procedure has been reported to be as high as an 87% return to preinjury level of competition.

Rotator Cuff Tears

Rotator cuff pathology in the overhead throwing athlete is seen primarily as a partial-thickness articular-sided tear of the supraspinatus and, to a lesser extent, the infraspinatus tendons. Factors that predispose the rotator cuff to this injury include not only the abnormal contact between the greater tuberosity and posterosuperior glenoid rim, but also a less vascular articular cuff surface, a higher modulus of elasticity, higher eccentric forces, and a less favorable stress-strain curve than on the bursal side. Full-thickness tears are less common in the overhead throwing athlete and can be the result of a partial-thickness tear progressing to a full-thickness tear or the result of a traumatic event.

Acromioclavicular Joint

Repetitive overhead throwing can result in microtraumatic wear and tear of the AC joint resulting in osteolysis of the distal end of the clavicle. Patients report pain localized to the AC joint that becomes worse with both overhead motion and cross-body adduction. Physical examination reveals tenderness at the AC joint, and pain with a cross-body adduction compression test. Radiographic evaluation of the AC joint with a Zanca view may show osteolysis or arthritic changes. Diagnosis and treatment can be accomplished by performing a local injection into the AC joint with a combination of a local anesthetic and a corticosteroid.

Patients who fail to improve with conservative treatment will benefit from a distal clavicle resection, which can be done either through an open or arthroscopic approach. If there is concern about additional shoulder pathology, arthroscopic evaluation of the glenohumeral joint and the subacromial space is recommended before the distal clavicle is resected. Although the best amount of resection is unknown, between 5 and 10 mm is acceptable. Postoperatively, patients are placed in a physical therapy program with the goal of regaining motion and strength; cross-body adduction should be avoided for 6 weeks. A slow progression to sport specific activities is followed by a return to sports activity in about 2 to 3 months.

Suprascapular Neuropathy

Suprascapular neuropathy is a rare condition in overhead throwing athletes. In elite volleyball players, it may result from a stretch injury or direct compression of the nerve. A paralabral ganglion cyst compression at the transverse scapular ligament or the spinoglenoid notch is possible. Proximal compression at the suprascapular notch will result in denervation of the supraspinatus and infraspinatus muscles. Distal compression at the spinoglenoid notch results in denervation of the infraspinatus only. In the late cocking phase of throwing, the medial tendinous margin between the supraspinatus and infraspinatus may compress the infraspinatus branch of the suprascapular nerve against the scapular spine.

Patients with suprascapular neuropathy present with a history of weakness and dull shoulder pain. On physical examination, weakness of the supraspinatus and infraspinatus muscles correlates with the location of nerve compression. Chronic injuries are associated with muscular atrophy. MRI will help to identify a ganglion cyst, which will appear as high signal intensity on a T2 image, and aids in ruling out a rotator cuff tear as the etiology of weakness. Electrodiagnostic studies confirm the diagnosis. Increased latency on the affected side is consistent with nerve impairment and can be used to localize the suprascapular nerve compression.

When an anatomic reason cannot be identified, conservative treatment with a well-organized physical therapy program is helpful for most patients. When compression is localized to an anatomic reason, surgical decompression is recommended. Ganglion cysts in the spinoglenoid notch can be treated with an arthroscopic technique. Because the cyst usually originates from the glenohumeral joint, a repair of the labrum may be required to prevent recurrence. For patients with compression at the suprascapular notch, possibly from a hypertrophied transverse scapular ligament, decompression is best with an open technique.

Vascular Injuries

Vascular injuries in the overhead throwing athlete are rare, and include digital vessel thrombosis, proximal thrombosis with distal embolization, aneurysms, and vessel compression such as thoracic outlet syndrome and quadrilateral space syndrome.

Aneurysms in overhead throwing athletes have been reported in the subclavian artery, axillary artery, and the posterior humeral circumflex artery. It is believed that these injuries occur as a result of repetitive trauma or impingement during the throwing motion. The pectoralis muscle and humeral head have both been implicated as a source of the traumatic impingement when the arm is in the abducted and externally rotated position.

Quadrilateral space syndrome is another neurovascular compression syndrome that appears to be unique to overhead throwing athletes. The quadilateral space is the area bordered by the teres minor superiorly, the humeral shaft laterally, the teres major inferiorly, and the long head of the triceps medially. Arteriograms have documented compression of the posterior humeral circumflex artery with abduction and external rotation, but it is believed that the symptoms are caused by compression of the axillary nerve, which runs with the artery.

Conservative management is the standard of care focusing on stretching of both the posterior capsule and the teres minor. Patients in whom conservative management has failed can undergo open decompression of the quadrilateral space, which has proved to be a successful procedure for resistant cases.

Elbow

In the overhead throwing athlete, most injuries seen in the elbow are related to the repetitive nature of throwing, and are best characterized as medial tension and lateral compression injuries. During the late cocking and early acceleration phases of throwing, the medial elbow is subject to significant tensile forces, whereas the lateral elbow experiences considerable compressive forces. Unlike the shoulder, the elbow derives most of its stability from its bony configuration. The ligaments surrounding the elbow help to further stabilize the joint. It is the ulnar or medial collateral ligament (MCL) on the medial side that functions as the primary stabilizer to valgus stress, whereas the lateral collateral ligament resists both varus and external rotation stresses. Dynamic muscle contraction also contributes to elbow stability by increasing the joint compression forces during muscle contraction. Repetitive trauma to the MCL allows for increased secondary compression at the radiocapitellar joint on the lateral side, which can ultimately lead to

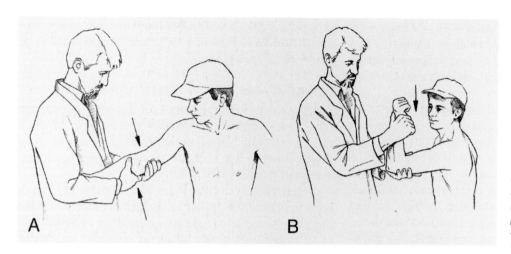

Figure 2 Tests for medial UCL injury. **A,** Valgus stress test. **B,** Milking maneuver. The patient's elbow is flexed beyond 90° while a valgus stress is applied. *(Reproduced from Chen FS, et al: Medial elbow problems in the overhead throwing athlete.* J Am Acad Orthop Surg 2001;9: 102.)

chondromalacia about the elbow and possibly loose body formation.

Medial Elbow Pain

The MCL is divided into three segments: the anterior bundle, the posterior bundle, and the transverse segment. It is the primary stabilizing structure to valgus stresses about the elbow and is most often injured during the late cocking and acceleration phases of throwing. About one third of patients will not report a preceding acute event, and in those who do, a subset of them will describe a period of nondescript elbow discomfort before the traumatic event. Pain is usually localized to the medial side of the elbow. Athletes with chronic MCL incompetence may develop concomitant ulnar nerve neuritis, and this neuritis may be accompanied by posterior elbow pain caused by posteromedial olecranon impingement.

On physical examination, patients with an acute injury may develop medial-sided ecchymosis. Tenderness to palpation on the medial side will lend support to the diagnosis, but positive results on provocative testing are also required. The valgus stress test is positive if the applied valgus stress reproduces the symptoms of medial elbow pain, and the valgus laxity is greater on the affected side than the uninjured side. This test must be done with the elbow flexed 20° to unlock the olecranon from within the olecranon fossa. A gravity stress test is performed with the athlete supine, the shoulder externally rotated to 90°, and the elbow flexed 20° so that gravity is used to elicit the valgus stress. If the ulnar collateral ligament (UCL) has been injured but remains intact, stress testing may elicit pain but no instability. The milking maneuver will also elicit pain along the medial side of the elbow (Figure 2). An additional test recently described, called the moving valgus stress test, reproduces the patient's medial elbow pain and symptoms by rapidly extending the elbow from a starting position of full flexion while maintaining a constant valgus torque.

Radiographs may be normal. In patients with chronic MCL injuries, radiographs may show calcification of the MCL, medial spurs on the humerus and ulna, posterior spurs on the olecranon tip, and loose bodies within the joint. AP stress radiographs of the elbow are useful when a wider medial opening in the unstable elbow is found compared with the contralateral normal side. When the history and physical examination support the diagnosis of an MCL injury, a magnetic resonance arthrogram is especially useful if a T sign of ulnar avulsion or if humeral avulsion or a midsubstance tear is found.

MCL injuries initially can be treated with a conservative approach focusing on a rehabilitation program that incorporates modality treatments such as phonophoresis, electrical stimulation, and iontophoresis, a stretching program, and a strengthening protocol focusing on the medial side flexor-pronator muscle mass. Sport-specific throwing, beginning with soft tossing of the ball, usually starts 3 months after initiation of treatment. Adjustments in the athlete's mechanics during throwing may further support a return to previous levels of competition.

Overhead throwing athletes with MCL injuries who continue to throw run the risk of developing posteromedial olecranon impingement and subsequent ulnohumeral arthritis. Surgical treatment is recommended for athletes who wish to continue sports participation and in whom conservative management has failed, and for elite athletes who are unable to throw at their normal level. Surgical treatment consists of reconstruction of the MCL with a tendon graft. Direct repair should be considered only in those patients who sustain an acute traumatic avulsion injury. Graft options include the ipsilateral or contralateral palmaris longus tendon, the fourth toe extensor tendon, the plantaris tendon, and the gracilis tendon.

Approximately 40% of athletes requiring an MCL reconstruction reportedly have ulnar nerve symptoms, yet surgical treatment is rarely needed. Only patients who demonstrate muscle involvement on physical examination or electrodiagnostic testing, or experience pain from ulnar nerve subluxation require treatment. More than 70% of throwers who have undergone an MCL reconstruction are able to return to their previous level of competition.

Posterior Elbow Impingement

Impingement may result from mechanical abutment of bone and soft tissues in the posterior elbow. This condition may or may not be associated with injury of the MCL. Pure hyperextension injuries associated with an intact MCL occur in gymnasts, football linemen, and weightlifters. The lesion is usually located in the center of the posterior elbow and is reproduced by forcible extension of the elbow. In athletes with MCL insufficiency, as often occurs with overhead throwing athletes, the posterior elbow impingement occurs posteromedially. Then, the impingement is located between the medial aspect of the olecranon and the lateral side of the medial wall of the olecranon fossa. Pain may be reproduced with the valgus stress test as previously described for valgus instability, but the pain is posteromedial as well as medial. Clinically, a flexion contracture is commonly present. Radiographs, including AP, lateral, and oblique views, may show osteophytes of the olecranon fossa.

Elbow Injuries in the Skeletally Immature Throwing Athlete

Little Leaguer's Elbow

Overhead throwing exposes the elbow of skeletally immature athletes to specific pathology. As in the mature thrower, the elbow is exposed to tension injuries on the medial side and compression injuries on the lateral side. On the medial side, the medial epicondyle growth plate (apophysis) is weaker and therefore more susceptible to trauma than the MCL. Patients may experience medial-sided elbow pain from apophysitis, or little leaguer's elbow that occurs during the cocking and acceleration phases of throwing, partly from tension in the MCL, and partly from the pronator flexor muscle pull that occurs during throwing. The medial epicondyle growth plate is vulnerable to injury in athletes between the ages of 11 and 13 years when the growth plate is beginning to close. Avulsion of the medial epicondyle may also be the result of a sudden muscle contraction or a traumatic event. Physical examination reveals point tenderness at the medial epicondyle, which is often associated with a 10° to 15° flexion contracture of the elbow. Radiographic evaluation may show widening of the medial epicondyle apophysis compared with the contralateral side. Patients are treated with a period of rest. Throwing is avoided for 2 to 3 months and normal growth plate closure is usually completed within 1 year. Avulsion of the medial epicondyle is confirmed on radiographic examination. Patients are usually treated with surgery if the epicondyle is displaced greater than 1 cm, ulnar neuropathy exists, valgus instability is documented, or the medial epicondyle displaces into the elbow joint. The surgical technique is open reduction with internal fixation with Kirschner wires or a single screw.

Osteochondritis Dissecans

On the lateral side, the repetitive compression loads experienced during throwing result in microtrauma of the articular cartilage that may lead to focal osteonecrosis of the capitellum or the radial head. Osteochondritis dissecans of the capitellum is seen in throwing athletes 13 to 15 years of age. The exact cause is still unknown, but the pathology is attributed to trauma, vascular insult resulting from the trauma, and family predisposition. Osteochondritis dissecans may be associated with the development of loose bodies, which can cause mechanical symptoms. Patients usually present with activity-related pain that resolves with rest. If loose bodies are present, patients may report clicking, catching, or locking. Radiographs will show irregularities of the capitellum, typically with a defect seen on the AP view, and possibly loose body formation. The initial treatment of osteochondritis dissecans is rest until symptoms resolve. Surgical treatment is reserved for those patients with loose bodies, which can be successfully removed using an arthroscopic technique. Microfracture of the defect to obtain a fibrocartilage scar may also be helpful. Fixation of osteochondral fragments can be attempted if they are large enough.

Annotated Bibliography

Shoulder

Altchek DW, Hatch JD: Rotator cuff injuries in overhead athletes. *Oper Tech Orthop* 2001;11:2-16.

A review of the diagnosis and treatment of rotator cuff injuries in the overhead throwing athlete, with a focus on the surgical technique for treating partial-thickness and full-thickness rotator cuff tears.

Andrews JR, Cain EL: Open treatment of anterior shoulder instability in the overhead athlete. *Oper Tech Orthop* 2001;11:9-16.

This article presents a review of the diagnosis and treatment of anterior shoulder instability in the overhead throwing athlete, focusing on the technique of open surgical stabilization procedures.

Cohen B, Cole BJ, Romeo AA: Thermal capsulorrhaphy of the shoulder. *Oper Tech Orthop* 2001;11:38-45.

The diagnosis of shoulder instability, including anterior, posterior, and multidirectional instability, and the treatment of these different instabilities with thermal capsulorrhaphy, is discussed.

Fealy S, Altchek DW: Athletic injuries and the throwing athlete: Shoulder, in Norris TR (ed): *Orthopaedic Knowledge Update: Shoulder and Elbow 2.* Rosemont, IL, American Academy of Orthopaedic Surgeons, 2002, pp 117-127.

This chapter provides an extensive review of shoulder injuries in the overhead throwing athlete. Diagnosis, treatment, and outcomes are presented.

Parten PM, Burkhart SS: The relationship of superior labral anteroposterior (SLAP) lesions and pseudolaxity to shoulder injuries in the overhead athlete. *Oper Tech Sports Med* 2002;10:10-17.

This article reviews the three subtypes of a type II SLAP lesion and how this condition contributes to the pathomechanic changes experienced by patients with internal impingement. Diagnosis and surgical treatment of patients with type II SLAP lesions are also reviewed.

Pinto MC, Snyder SJ: SLAP lesions: Current operative techniques and management. *Oper Tech Orthop* 2001;11: 30-37.

A review of SLAP lesions with a focus on diagnosis and treatment of the four types of SLAP lesions, and a technique review of the surgical repair of type II and IV lesions is presented.

Elbow

Bennett JB, Mehlhoff TL: Immature skeletal lesions of the elbow. *Oper Tech Sports Med* 2001;9:234-240.

Pathologic entities in the young throwing athlete, including how to make the diagnosis and how to treat the problem, are discussed.

Conway JE, Lowe WR: Elbow medial ulnar collateral ligament reconstruction. *Oper Tech Sports Med* 2001;9: 196-204.

This article discusses the anatomy of the MCL of the elbow, and the diagnosis of its injury, treatment, and outcomes.

Fealy S, Rohrbough JT, Allen AA, Altchek DW, Drakos MC: Athletic injuries and the throwing athlete: Elbow, in Norris TR (ed): *Orthopaedic Knowledge Update: Shoulder and Elbow 2.* Rosemont, IL, American Academy of Orthopaedic Surgeons, 2002, pp 297-311.

Elbow injuries in the throwing athlete including diagnosis, treatment, and outcomes are discussed.

Gabel GT: Operative management of ulnar neuropathy at the elbow in the throwing athlete. *Oper Tech Sports Med* 2001;9:225-233.

The anatomy of the ulnar nerve and the diagnosis and treatment of ulnar neuropathy in the throwing athlete are reviewed.

Thompson WH, Jobe FW, Yocum LA, Pink MM: Ulnar collateral ligament reconstruction in athletes: Muscle-splitting approach without transposition of the ulnar nerve. *J Shoulder Elbow Surg* 2001;10:152-157.

In this study, reconstruction of the UCL using a muscle-splitting approach resulted in a decreased rate of postoperative complications and improved outcomes compared with results of previous procedures.

Williams RJ III, Urquhart ER, Altchek DW: Medial collateral ligament tears in the throwing athlete. *Instr Course Lect* 2004;53:579-585.

Surgical treatment of MCL injuries, specifically using reconstruction of the MCL using a single ulnar tunnel and single humeral tunnel performed through a muscle-splitting approach, is discussed.

Yadao MA, Field LD, Savoie FH III: Osteochondritis dissecans of the elbow. *Instr Course Lect* 2004;53:599-606.

A discussion of the natural history, clinical presentation, classification, and treatment of osteochondritis dissecans of the elbow is presented.

Classic Bibliography

Antoniadis G, Richter HP, Rath S, Braun V, Moese G: Surprascapular nerve entrapment: Experience with 28 cases. *J Neurosurg* 1996;85:1020-1025.

Azar FM, Andrew JR, Wilk KE, Groh D: Operative treatment of ulnar collateral ligament injuries of the elbow in athletes. *Am J Sports Med* 2000;28:16-23.

Conway JE, Jobe FW, Glousman RE, Pink MM: Medial instability of the elbow in throwing athletes: Treatment by repair or reconstruction of the ulnar collateral ligament. *J Bone Joint Surg Am* 1992;74:67-83.

DaSilva MF, Williams JS, Fadale PD, Hulstyn MJ, Ehrlich MG: Pediatric throwing injuries about the elbow. *Am J Orthop* 1998;27:90-96.

Edelson G, Teitz C: Internal impingement in the shoulder. *J Shoulder Elbow Surg* 2000;9:308-315.

Jobe CM: Posterior superior glenoid impingement: Expanded spectrum. *Arthroscopy* 1995;11:530-536.

Jobe CM, Pink MM, Jobe FW, Shaffer B: Anterior shoulder instability, impingement and rotator cuff tears, in Jobe FW, Pink MM, Glousman RE, Kvitne RS, Zemel NP (eds): *Operative Techniques in Upper Extremity Sports Injuries.* St Louis, MO, Mosby-Year Book, 1996, pp 164-177.

Kuhn JE, Bey MJ, Huston LJ, Blasier RB, Soslowsky LJ: Ligamentous restraints to external rotation of the humerus in the late-cocking phase of throwing: A cadaveric biomechanical investigation. *Am J Sports Med* 2000;28:200-205.

Lester B, Jeong GK, Weiland AJ, Wickiewicz TL: Quadrilateral space syndrome: Diagnosis, pathology, and treatment. *Am J Orthop* 1999;28:718-725.

Martin SD, Warren RF, Martin TL, Kennedy K, O'Brien SJ, Wickewicz TL: Suprascapular neuropathy: Results of non-operative treatment. *J Bone Joint Surg Am* 1997;79:1159-1165.

McFarland EG, Hsu CY, Neira C, O'Neil O: Internal impingement of the shoulder: A clinical and arthroscopic analysis. *J Shoulder Elbow Surg* 1999;8:458-460.

Schneider K, Kasparyan NG, Altcheck DW, Fantini GA, Weiland AJ: An aneurysm involving the axillary artery and its branch vessels in a major league baseball pitcher: A case report and review of the literature. *Am J Sports Med* 1999;27:370-375.

Chapter 24

Shoulder and Arm Trauma: Bone

Robert P. Lyons, MD

Mark D. Lazarus, MD

Clavicle Fractures

The clavicle constitutes the only bony connection between the axial skeleton and the upper extremity. Displaced clavicle fractures risk injury to the cords of the brachial plexus and subclavian artery and vein, which pass between the medial curvature of the clavicle and the first rib. Allman's classification system for clavicle fractures is the most common and divides the clavicle into thirds. Although somewhat arbitrary, this system provides an efficient framework to stratify treatment options and prognosis.

Midshaft Fractures

Acute Fractures

Fractures to the middle third segment are most common and account for 81% of all clavicle fractures. Most middle third fractures heal with a sling or figure-of-8 dressing that is provided for symptomatic relief. An epidemiologic study of 535 isolated clavicle fractures found that 48% of middle third clavicle fractures were displaced (using 3 mm as the displacement criterion), 19% were comminuted, 68% of patients were men, and 61% of fractures involved the left side.

A study of 1,430 clavicles from adult skeletons identified 73 clavicular fractures, of which 54 were malunions. In middle third fractures, the lateral shaft fragment was consistently displaced posteriorly to the medial shaft fragment. In contrast, most medial third fractures showed anterior displacement of the lateral fragment, often forming a prominent anterior spike. Twenty-four of 36 clavicles with significant shortening had overriding of the bone fragments and angulation, which tended to increase in severity the more lateral the fracture. The maximal amount of angulation occurred at the coracoclavicular junction, presumably because of the deforming force of the upper extremity's weight transmitted through the coracoclavicular ligamentous complex. Although standing AP radiographs of clavicle fractures display the inferior displacement of the lateral fragment, this study suggests that the principal deformity in malunions is anterior angulation. Mild fixed scapular winging was a common finding accompanying clavicular malunions.

Indications for open reduction and internal fixation (ORIF) of acute fractures include open fractures, neurovascular injury, or widely displaced fractures that tent, and may compromise, the overlying skin. Some consider wide displacement and comminution a relative indication for ORIF, citing impaired long-term function and an increased chance of nonunion. However, the absolute amount of shortening that can be accepted without functional deficit has not been definitively established. Techniques for fixation include plating or intramedullary pinning.

Recent studies documenting the patient-based outcomes following nonsurgical treatment of clavicular fractures have shown that results are not as good as once believed, with 31% of patients reporting shoulder weakness and fatigability, paresthesias of the hand and forearm, and an asymmetric or ptotic shoulder. Fractures with greater than 2 cm of shortening have been associated with a poor outcome. In addition, significant comminution associated with displacement also may be an indication for ORIF.

Another study compared 40 patients who received nonsurgical treatment with a figure-of-8 bandage with 40 patients who underwent open reduction and intramedullary fixation with a 2.5-mm threaded pin. Each group consisted of a similar profile of uncomplicated midclavicular fractures. The group that underwent surgery experienced a high rate of complications including eight superficial infections, three refractures, two delayed unions with pin breakage, and two nonunions. These results suggest that nonsurgical treatment appears more advantageous than open intramedullary fixation for the treatment of most midclavicular fractures.

Malunions and Nonunions

The incidence of clavicular nonunions has been reported between 0.1% and 15%. Factors that predispose patients to the development of a clavicular nonunion include open fractures, comminuted fractures, or initial shortening greater than 2 cm. Anteroinferior plating of

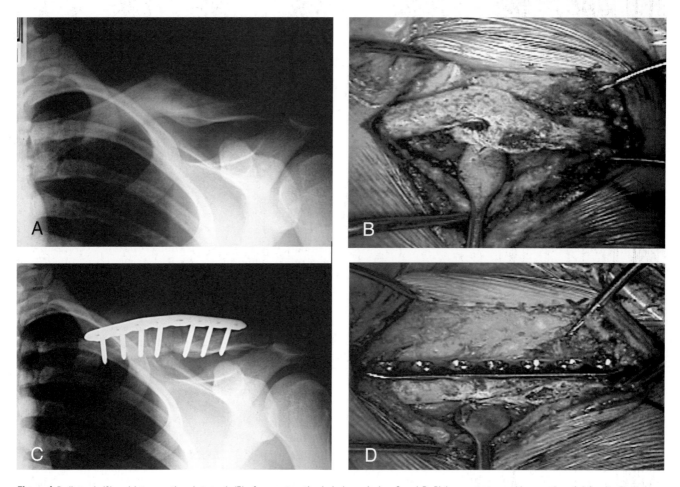

Figure 1 Radiograph (**A**) and intraoperative photograph (**B**) of a symptomatic clavicular malunion. **C** and **D**, Biplanar osteotomy with correction of deformity. Fixation was achieved with a 3.5 mm dynamic compression locking plate. No intercalary graft was required.

midshaft clavicular nonunions with a 3.5-mm pelvic reconstruction plate, lag screw, and bone graft has been described and resulted in a 100% union rate in 12 patients. The advantages of this technique include a longer bicortical screw purchase because the anteroposterior diameter of the clavicle is much greater than its supero-inferior dimension. The plate in this position acts as a buttress with theoretically less risk of screw pullout from the lateral fragment and less chance of neurovascular injury during screw placement. Alternatively, a superiorly placed dynamic compression plate in compression mode can be used for more transverse fracture patterns. The newer AO locking plates may be particularly advantageous for this indication. Care must be taken to restore clavicular length and alignment during nonunion correction. Prior reports have described the use of a locked intramedullary device; however, the restoration of length with this device is more difficult. Finally, the use of a vascularized fibula graft to salvage a recalcitrant clavicular nonunion with segmental bone loss was described in three patients. Both pain and shoulder function were improved and all patients achieved union.

A recent patient-based outcome study of 15 patients with clavicular midshaft malunion revealed a mean 2.9 cm of clavicular shortening. All patients had major functional deficits including chronic pain, shoulder weakness, and thoracic outlet symptoms for 1 year after injury. After corrective osteotomy, it was possible to appose two fresh osseous surfaces in all patients without the need for intercalary bone graft. The distal fragment was typically rotated such that the flat superior surface faced anteriorly, and this malrotation was corrected before fixation with a 3.5-mm limited contact dynamic compression plate, using a minimum of six holes. This plate was believed to be stronger than the reconstruction plate and easier to contour than the standard compression plate. Postoperatively the mean degree of shortening was 0.4 cm and most patients were satisfied with the result (Figure 1).

Distal Third Fractures

Neer classified distal third clavicle fractures into three types. Type I fractures are the most common and remain stable as the conoid and trapezoid ligaments remain intact. Type II fractures occur medial to the coracoclavicu-

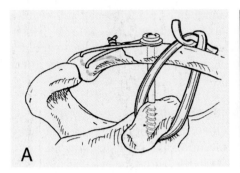 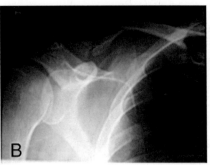 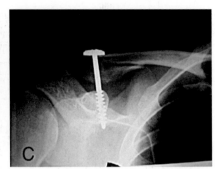

Figure 2 **A** through **C**, fixation methods for type II distal clavicle fractures include coracoclavicular stabilization, using screws or tapes, with or without tension band fixation of the distal clavicular segment. *(Reproduced with permission from Lazarus MD: Fractures of the clavicle, in Bucholz RW, Heckman JD (eds): Rockwood and Green's Fractures in Adults, ed 5. Philadelphia, PA, Lippincott Williams & Wilkins, 2001.)*

lar ligaments, thus the lateral fragment is usually unstable and displaced inferiorly with a high incidence of nonunion. Type III fractures extend into the acromioclavicular joint and usually do not involve ligamentous injury.

Distal third fractures account for 15% of clavicular fractures, and type II distal third fractures have a rate of delayed union and nonunion between 30% and 45%. Fixation techniques described in the literature include transacromial Kirschner wires, coracoclavicular screws, plates, Dacron tapes, and tension wires (Figure 2). Fixation between the clavicle and coracoid or clavicle and acromion will often fail because it interferes with the normal rotation of the clavicle that occurs with arm elevation. Thus, a second operation is required to remove the fixation before full mobilization is commenced. A modification of Neviaser's technique has been described, in which two No. 1 polydioxanone sutures are used as a superior figure-of-8 tension band between the fracture fragments. If the distal fragment is too small, the lateral drill hole can be passed through the acromion because the fixation is absorbable and the acromioclavicular joint is not violated. All fractures healed at 6 weeks with no complication.

A retrospective comparison of type II distal clavicle fractures treated nonsurgically versus those that underwent open reduction and coracoclavicular stabilization was reported. Nonsurgical treatment resulted in a 43% nonunion rate; however, the nonunion had no significant effect on functional outcome or strength. This study suggests that most type II distal clavicle fractures can be treated nonsurgically.

Scapula Fractures
Epidemiology
Scapula fractures account for 3% to 5% of all fractures involving the shoulder girdle. Injury to the scapula is rare because it is enveloped by a well-developed muscular layer and lies flush with the thorax. However, other injuries occur concomitantly in patients with scapula

fractures and these may delay the diagnosis. The associated mortality rate is 10% to 15% and this outcome usually is secondary to pulmonary sepsis or head injury. Half of all patients with scapula fractures have other insults to the ipsilateral extremity, including vascular and brachial plexus injuries in 13%. Other associated injuries include hemopneumothorax, pulmonary contusion with rib fractures, and spinal cord injury. Ninety percent of scapula fractures are minimally displaced or nondisplaced, and thus can be treated nonsurgically.

Classification
The classification of glenoid fossa fractures was recently modified to better estimate scapular body involvement and provide more consistent guidance for choosing a surgical approach. Type I injuries represent isolated involvement of the anteroinferior articular surface and may be associated with a glenohumeral dislocation. Treatment is based on instability criteria with fracture fixation, either arthroscopically or through a deltopectoral approach, indicated for fractures that involve more than 25% of the articular surface. Type II fractures involve the superior one third to one half of the articular surface in continuity with the coracoid. Types I and II can be treated surgically via a standard deltopectoral approach. A Schanz screw used as a joystick or a dental pic may aid reduction before fixation with 2.7-mm or 3.5-mm cortical screws.

Types III, IV, and V fracture patterns involve a variable portion of the lateral border of the scapula and usually require the posterior approach described by Judet. Type V patterns, which involve a large separate coracoid or superior articular surface fragment, may require a combined Judet and deltopectoral approach. Surgical indications for glenoid fractures have been described as displacement greater than 5 mm or any displacement associated with subluxation of the humeral head. For scapula neck fractures, surgery has been recommended if the glenoid is medially displaced greater than 2 cm or if there is more than 40° of angular displacement. Surgical indications for type V fractures include articular step-off of 5 mm or greater, severe diastasis of the articular surfaces, inferior displacement of the glenoid fragment with inferior subluxation of the humeral head, or severe disruption of the superior shoulder suspensory complex.

Glenoid Fractures

Glenoid fractures are rare injuries that account for only 9% to 20% of all scapula fractures, and only 10% of glenoid fractures are substantially displaced. Common surgical indications for extra-articular glenoid fractures include angulation greater than 40°, displacement of the glenoid segment greater than 1 cm, or a fracture associated with ipsilateral clavicle fracture (such as floating shoulder). Surgical indications for intra-articular glenoid rim fractures include displacement greater than 10 mm, recurrent glenohumeral instability, or for fractures involving more than 25% of the anterior rim or 33% of the posterior rim. Complex intra-articular fractures are treated with surgery when there is greater than 5 mm displacement or persistent glenohumeral subluxation. Nonsurgical treatment of minimally displaced fractures has been successful. Thus, the decision for surgery must be based not only on fracture character but also on patient age, hand dominance, and activity level.

Arthroscopic fixation of a displaced posterior glenoid rim fracture involving more that one third of the glenoid cavity has been described. Ligamentotaxis on the surgical extremity held in lateral decubitus traction was believed to have assisted reduction.

Glenoid neck fractures are best visualized through a posterior approach, which includes the more limited muscle-sparing, or the extensile Judet approaches. A muscle-sparing approach can be used for isolated posterior glenoid rim or isolated glenoid neck fractures.

The incision for the Judet approach begins at the posterolateral corner of the acromion, extends along the scapular spine, and then curves inferiorly along the medial scapular border. The deltoid is detached from the scapular spine and reflected laterally. The infraspinatus is then elevated from the scapular body on its neurovascular pedicle and reflected laterally, giving wide exposure to the posterior scapula. The fracture is identified and directly reduced. Provisional fixation can be obtained with Kirschner wires by passing them through the acromion into the glenoid fragment from a superior direction. A 3.5-mm reconstruction plate is contoured and applied to the lateral scapular body and posterior glenoid. Intraoperative radiographs or fluoroscopy is used to confirm anatomic reduction and prevent intra-articular screw penetration.

Postoperative stiffness is a concern. Prophylaxis against heterotopic ossification should be considered in all patients with closed head injury. Despite early mo-

tion, a significant number of patients may still require surgical intervention for postoperative stiffness. Unfortunately, associated injuries, especially those to the peripheral or central nervous system, will negatively affect rehabilitation.

Superior Shoulder Suspensory Complex Injuries

The superior shoulder suspensory complex is a bony soft-tissue ring made up of the glenoid, coracoid, acromion process, distal clavicle, acromioclavicular joint, and coracoclavicular ligaments. The superior strut is the middle clavicle and the inferior strut is the lateral scapula. Injury to any two of these elements is believed to result in the potential for a large amount of scapula fracture displacement with resultant disability to the patient. It is generally believed that displacement of the scapular neck will alter the relationship of the glenohumeral joint with the acromion and create a functional imbalance. However, the exact amount of displacement or angulation required to create this functional imbalance has not been quantified. Abduction weakness, decreased range of motion, and nonunion are the frequently implicated complications of nonsurgical treatment.

Floating Shoulder Injuries

The floating shoulder constitutes a double disruption of the superior shoulder suspensory complex and occurs in only 0.1% of all fractures. In the past, this injury has been considered unstable and thought to require surgical stabilization of one or both elements. Most glenoid neck fractures exit the superior scapular border medial to the base of the coracoid process, near the suprascapular notch. This results in a distal fragment consisting of the glenoid and coracoid process, and a proximal fragment consisting of the acromion, scapular spine, and scapular body. The distal fragment is still attached to the proximal fragment by the coracoacromial ligament, and through the coracoclavicular ligament and distal clavicular fragment by the acromioclavicular capsular ligaments.

In one study, 20 patients with a floating shoulder were treated nonsurgically and functional scores were equivalent to those from studies involving surgery. Although most of the scapula fractures in this study were minimally displaced, the five patients who did have severe displacement of both scapula and clavicle fractures had outcomes comparable to those with minimal displacement. Nonsurgical treatment of floating shoulder injuries, especially those with less than 5 mm displacement, is recommended. The criteria for surgical intervention needs better delineation.

A recent study was the first to directly compare the functional and clinical outcomes of surgical versus nonsurgical treatment of displaced ipsilateral fractures of the clavicle and glenoid neck. The surgically treated patients, in whom clavicle and glenoid fractures were fixed, had significantly better forward elevation but had weaker external rotation (possibly related to the surgical approach). It was concluded that patient satisfaction can be achieved with either surgical or nonsurgical care; thus, the decision must be individualized for each patient. However, type of treatment was based on surgeon preference, and the severity of fractures in each group was not specified.

A masked retrospective radiographic review of 20 patients found that scapular neck fracture displacement, angulation, and anatomic classification showed moderate interobserver reliability by plain films, which was not enhanced by CT. CT may be helpful to assess possible intra-articular extension of a glenoid neck fracture or occult injury to the superior shoulder suspensory complex. However, whether such an injury would render the shoulder unstable and require surgical fixation has yet to be clarified.

A recent biomechanical cadaver study testing medial stability of ipsilateral fractures of the clavicular shaft and scapular neck did not demonstrate instability (floating shoulder) without additional disruption of the coracoacromial and acromioclavicular capsular ligaments. Although not included in the original description of the superior shoulder suspensory complex, the coracoacromial ligament is believed to be an important stabilizer of scapular neck fractures because it is the only direct ligamentous connection between proximal and distal fragments.

Proximal Humeral Fractures

Epidemiology

Fractures of the proximal humerus account for 4% of all fractures. The current incidence is 70 fractures per 100,000 people and is likely to increase because these fractures are related to both patient age and osteoporosis. Eighty-five percent of these fractures are nondisplaced or minimally displaced and respond to treatment with immobilization followed by early motion.

Risk factors for fracture of the proximal humerus were evaluated with data collected from the European Patient Information and Document Service study, which prospectively followed 6,901 white women who lived independently at home. Overall, the incidence of proximal humeral fracture was 6.6 per 1,000 person-years, which occurred at a mean age of 82.2 years. The incidence of proximal humeral fracture in women with osteoporosis and a low fall risk score (5.1 per 1,000 woman-years) was only slightly higher than in women who did not have osteoporosis (4.6 per 1,000 woman-years), and similar to the incidence in women without osteoporosis but a high fall risk score (5.5 per 1,000 woman-years).

Classification

Under Neer's criteria a segment is nondisplaced when radiographs reveal less than 1 cm of displacement or less than 45° angulation of any one fragment with respect to the others. The number of fracture lines is important only if the displacement criteria are fulfilled. A one-part fracture is nondisplaced and is the most common type. There are four types of two-part fractures: anatomic neck, surgical neck, greater tuberosity, and lesser tuberosity. Three-part fractures involve either a greater or lesser tuberosity fracture in conjunction with a fracture of the surgical neck. Four-part fractures have displacement of all four segments. Articular surface and head-splitting fractures are also included in this category. Neer also characterized fracture-dislocations as either anterior or posterior dislocation of the articular segment. Two-, three-, and four-part fractures can occur as fracture-dislocations.

The AO/Orthopaedic Trauma Association classification system emphasizes the vascular supply to the articular segment. Type A fractures are the least severe and involve only one tuberosity with no isolation of the articular segment. Type B fractures are extra-articular, involve both tuberosities, and constitute a low risk of osteonecrosis. Type C are intra-articular fractures involving the anatomic neck and carry a high risk of osteonecrosis. Each type is further classified into three subtypes. The complexity of this classification system has limited its widespread appeal.

Much attention has been given to the poor interobserver reliability of Neer's classification documented by some studies. However, a recent study showed that kappa values for interobserver variation improved substantially among physicians who underwent two 45-minute training sessions compared with a control physician group who did not receive training in the Neer system. Another study showed that 8 of 22 patients who underwent surgery for three- and four-part fractures of the proximal humerus did not correspond to any category of the Neer or AO classification system. Articular surface orientation on plain radiographs (medially oriented or not) appeared to be more indicative of remaining soft-tissue attachments to the head. Whether this factor has validity in predicting osteonecrosis or functional outcome has yet to be determined.

Two-Part Surgical Neck Fractures

In the two-part surgical neck fracture, the pectoralis major acts as a deforming force and displaces the shaft medially and anteriorly. Closed reduction is often possible. If the fragments are impacted, axial traction is applied. Then a gentle posteriorly and laterally directed force is applied to the upper arm as the shaft is flexed and brought underneath the head. The fragments are then impacted and stability is evaluated. The surgeon should

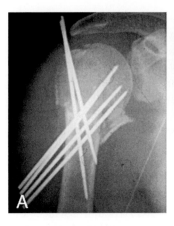

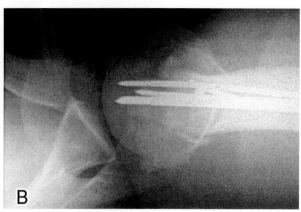

Figure 3 AP (**A**) and axillary (**B**) radiographs of a three-part proximal humeral fracture treated with percutaneous pinning.

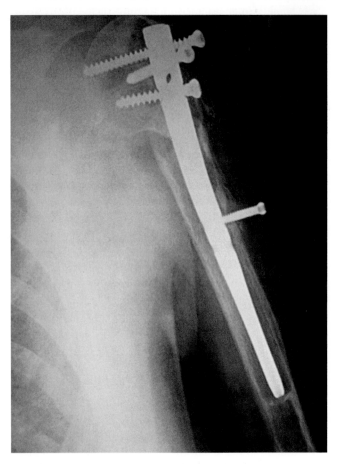

Figure 4 Pullout of an antegrade intramedullary humeral nail in an elderly patient.

be aware of an oblique surgical neck fracture pattern (low anteromedial to high posterolateral), which is usually irreducible by closed means. If the reduction cannot be maintained, then either closed reduction with percutaneous pinning or ORIF is performed.

Percutaneous pinning also carries a risk to neurovascular structures. At risk are the main trunk of the axillary nerve and posterior humeral circumflex artery from the greater tuberosity pin, the anterior branch of the axillary nerve from the proximal lateral pin, and the cephalic vein, biceps tendon, and musculocutaeous nerve from the anterior pin. The shoulder should be externally rotated during placement of greater tuberosity pins and these pins should engage the cortex of the humeral neck 20 mm from the inferior most aspect of the humeral head. Finally, great care should be used to place threaded pins into but not through the subchondral region of the humeral head (Figure 3).

Intramedullary rodding has been advocated by some and has shown an 85% success rate in younger patients. However, concerns over poor proximal locking-screw purchase and subsequent proximal rod migration in older patients with osteoporotic bone limit its appeal in this patient population (Figure 4). In addition, antegrade intramedullary rods violate the rotator cuff and articular cartilage. Locked intramedullary nailing of proximal humeral fractures is best indicated for use in patients with multiple trauma or pathologic fracture.

Heavy nonabsorbable sutures have been shown to be an attractive choice for fixation of two- and three-part fractures, especially in those patients with osteoporotic bone. The use of sutures allows the incorporation of the rotator cuff as a fixation point and precludes any chance of hardware failure.

Two-Part Greater Tuberosity Fractures

Isolated fractures of the greater tuberosity are frequently missed. In one study, 58 of 99 fractures (58%) were initially overlooked. There was a 64% rate of missed diagnoses in one-part (nondisplaced greater tuberosity fracture) compared with a 27% rate of missed diagnoses in Neer two-part fractures. The presence of tenderness on the lateral wall of the greater tuberosity (distal to the insertion of the rotator cuff) is an effective clinical sign to confirm the correct diagnosis. Greater tuberosity fractures occur in 5% to 15% of anterior glenohumeral dislocations. After age 50 years, the incidence of nerve injury with proximal humeral fracture-dislocations as determined by somatosensory-evoked potentials is 50%, and this includes axillary nerve as well as infraclavicular brachial plexus injuries. Displaced greater tuberosity fractures can be associated with rotator cuff tears, but in many surgical cases, the cuff remains intact and only a capsular rent is observed. If radiographs do not adequately show the fracture displacement, a CT scan may be necessary. In addition, ultrasound can detect occult nondisplaced greater tuberosity fractures.

Most authors advocate conservative treatment of fractures with less than 5 mm displacement and surgery for displacement greater than 5 mm. Given the literature to date, any greater tuberosity fracture displaced 5 mm or more should be treated with reduction and fixation.

Isolated screw fixation of greater tuberosity fractures should be used only in younger patients because, with aging, the bone of the tuberosity becomes fragile and prone to comminution. The fracture can be fixed percutaneously with arthroscopic assistance. The superior approach typically permits easier fragment reduction, whereas the deltopectoral approach allows easier suture placement. The edge of the fragment can be aligned with the edge of the fracture bed of the proximal humerus. The sutures are passed around the greater tuberosity and through the attachment of the rotator cuff tendons and then cross in a figure-of-8 fashion across the fracture site to avoid overreduction of the fragment. Because no hardware is used, there is no concern about hardware failure. Subacromial scarring, even without displacement and capsular contracture, may limit motion postoperatively. This complication is best avoided by initiating passive range-of-motion exercises early in the postoperative period.

Three- and Four-Part Fractures

In three-part fractures, one tuberosity is displaced and there is a displaced unimpacted surgical neck fracture that allows the head to be rotated by the attached tuberosity. Four-part fractures involve displacement of all four segments (the greater and lesser tuberosities, the articular segment, and the shaft), and the articular fragment is usually devoid of soft-tissue attachments. Three- and four-part fractures represent 13% to 16% of proximal humeral fractures. Surgical modalities have included plates, pins, screws, staples, intramedullary nails, wires, sutures, or any combination of these, and arthroplasty. Neer preferred ORIF for two- and three-part fractures and arthroplasty for four-part fractures. Others have approached all three- and four-part fractures that are amenable to stable internal fixation with minimal osteosynthesis.

Osteonecrosis of the humeral head after four-part fracture of the proximal humerus has an incidence of 21% to 75%, which is believed to be the result of the injury pattern itself. It is important to preserve the ascending branch of the anterior humeral circumflex artery, which is the primary vessel supplying the humeral head. The posteromedial vessels may preserve some

blood flow to the humeral head when the anterior humeral circumflex artery has been interrupted. Plates were applied lateral to the bicipital groove to avoid injury to the anterior humeral circumflex artery. No significant relationship was found between the method of fixation (cerclage wire versus plate) and the development of osteonecrosis. Although most patients in this study who had four-part fractures developed osteonecrosis, the results were generally good.

Newer fixation devices have led to improved techniques for ORIF of two-, three-, and four-part fractures of the proximal humerus. The use of a blade plate and interfragmentary sutures has been shown to provide firm fixation and a good functional result in the treatment of 34 three-part and 8 four-part fractures of the proximal humerus in elderly patients. The blade plate has primarily been used for two-part surgical neck fractures. The use of a blade plate and autogenous cancellous bone graft resulted in good or excellent results in 80% of patients with two-part nonunions (and in 90% of low two-part nonunions). Low two-part nonunions were easier to treat because the proximal fragment is larger and thus easier to secure.

The advent of the locking compression plate, with a plate specifically designed for the proximal humerus, is an excellent new option for ORIF of proximal humeral fractures. With this technique, it is crucial that the surgical approach preserve soft-tissue attachments as much as possible. It is mandatory to use the drill guide that threads directly into the screw hole in the plate because this ensures that the screw threads will engage precisely with the plate threads. Locking screws will not bring the plate to the bone, which is not a critical feature of the technique (as opposed to the standard dynamic compression plate) and may actually increase the blood supply to the bone and enhance the biology of healing.

Some plate-bone contact may be required to improve fracture alignment and diminish the prominence of the implant. This goal can be accomplished by using a few standard (nonlocking) screws. A mechanical study in cadavers showed that the locking compression plate for the proximal humerus was a more elastic implant than the spiral blade, T-plate, and humeral nail, a property making this plate less likely to fail in osteoporotic bone, compared with the other implants.

Valgus-Impacted Three- and Four-Part Fractures

The valgus-impacted pattern of a proximal humeral fracture is characterized by preservation of the posteromedial capsular attachments to the humeral articular surface. Radiographically, this pattern is defined by the alignment between the medial shaft and head segments. The results of treatment of the three-part valgus-impacted fracture variant are better than for the standard Neer three-part fracture. The intact posteromedial soft tissue supplying residual perfusion to the humeral head is presumably responsible for a better prognosis with the valgus-impacted fracture. In a recent study, 80% of patients had a good or excellent result by Neer's outcome criteria with nonsurgical care. Patients will regain only 80% of abduction and flexion strength but do not require full motion or strength to return to daily activities.

A new technique of minimal fixation for valgus-impacted fractures of the humeral head has been introduced. An open technique without any sharp deep soft-tissue dissection was used, and the split between the tuberosities was opened to allow elevation of the impacted humeral head fragment. The tuberosities were reduced to hold the humeral head fragment in place and repaired with heavy absorbable suture (No. 2 Vicryl) between the rotator cuff insertions. No bone grafting, Kirschner wire, or additional fixation was used. No attempt was made to secure the head to the shaft because the fracture configuration was considered stable. For 11 patients with an average age of 55 years, the mean follow-up was 69 months. The mean Constant-Morley score as a percentage compared with the opposite side was 86%. One patient (9%) developed osteonecrosis. This rate of osteonecrosis was similar to other reported rates using closed techniques. Most of the soft-tissue dissection occurred at the time of fracture, so if the principle of minimal further disruption of the soft tissues is adhered to, an open technique such as this should not increase the rate of osteonecrosis.

Role of Arthroscopy

Arthroscopy was used to preoperatively assess 80 shoulder fractures, including 52 proximal humerus fractures, 20 fracture-dislocations, and 8 glenoid and/or scapula fractures. Overall, 20% of fractures were found to have a full-thickness supraspinatus and/or infraspinatus cuff tear and 30% had partial tears. Eighteen percent had subscapularis tendon tears. Two-part fractures had a 31% incidence of complete labral tear, whereas only 10% of three- and four-part fractures had a complete labral tear, presumably because more energy is dissipated at the fracture site in the more complex patterns. Proximal humeral fracture-dislocations showed a 56% incidence of complete labral tear.

Role of Arthroplasty

Incongruity of the humeral head or complete detachment of the articular blood supply are the main indications for humeral arthroplasty, which typically includes some three-part fractures, most four-part fractures, humeral head-splitting injuries, and humeral head impression defects involving greater than 40% of the articular surface. Other factors that may favor arthroplasty include excessive comminution, inadequate bone quality

to allow for stable fixation, tuberosity fragments that include a substantial portion of the articular surface, and inability to obtain an acceptable reduction. These patients are best treated with hemiarthroplasty or total shoulder arthroplasty depending on the condition of the glenoid surface and rotator cuff.

Hemiarthroplasty is primarily indicated for displaced four-part fractures. Tuberosity osteolysis, malunion, and nonunion are implicated as the main causes of failure. Late arthroplasty after failed primary treatment of proximal humeral fractures improves pain, range of motion, and function, but most authors have found that the results of late arthroplasty are inferior compared with proximal humerus fractures treated acutely with humeral head replacement.

Prognostic factors in prosthetic replacement for acute proximal humeral fractures were studied in 32 patients retrospectively. Fracture type, gender, and type of prosthesis were found to be irrelevant with respect to outcome. Increased age and an increased preoperative delay correlated with a poorer clinical outcome. Patients who had surgery within 14 days had a better general outcome. This study showed a strong correlation between the radiologic position of the tuberosities and the quantitative as well as qualitative clinical outcome. Tuberosity complications were the most common complication and were seen in 50% of patients. Humeral offset is defined as the distance between the geometric center of the humeral head and the lateral edge of the greater tuberosity. The average humeral offset of patients with a good or excellent outcome (25.39 mm) was significantly higher than the average offset in patients with unsatisfactory outcomes (20.20 mm). Patients with a humeral offset of 23 mm or more had a significantly better outcome. Also, patients with a head height of 14 mm or less had a better outcome. Lateralizing the tuberosities results in a better outcome and their distal transfer causes a poorer outcome. Stable fixation and anatomic repositioning of the tuberosities must be achieved during surgery.

In a similar study reviewing outcome of hemiarthroplasty for fractures of the proximal humerus, it was determined that early surgical intervention within 2 weeks of injury and accurate tuberosity reconstruction were two factors that were found to have the greatest impact on functional outcome. The height of the superior humeral articular surface with respect to the greater tuberosity is termed the head-to-tuberosity distance (HTD) and is 8 ± 3 mm as measured in cadaver specimens. The tuberosity was considered malreduced if the fragment was superior to the humeral head or if the HTD was greater than 20 mm.

Proper height was established by placing the articular surface of the prosthetic head at the midpoint of the glenoid, and with gentle traction, the prosthetic head remained within the glenoid fossa. The humeral component was cemented in all patients and the tuberosities were then reconstructed so that the greater tuberosity was overlying the lateral fin or was repaired to the anterior fin in a three-fin design. Other studies indicate that when a prosthesis is inserted for fracture, the lateral fin should be a mean distance of 5.2 ± 2.6 mm from the posterior edge of the bicipital groove. In a recent biomechanical study, it was shown that a horizontal circumferential cerclage suture passed through the medial hole of the prosthesis and around the tuberosity fragments substantially improves fracture stability, and, in theory, minimizes the potential for nonunion of the tuberosities.

Another study considered an HTD of 3 to 20 mm as an anatomic reconstruction. Acceptable alignment and position of the tuberosities was achieved in 79% of patients. The most common complication was malreduction of the greater tuberosity in the vertical plane. In patients with a nearly anatomic reduction of the greater tuberosity, American Shoulder and Elbow Surgeons and the Simple Shoulder Test scores, patient satisfaction, and motion were all significantly better than in those patients in whom an anatomic reduction was not achieved. Superior migration was associated with pain, impingement, and motion loss. These patients either had a malunion or nonunion of the tuberosities. It is now recommended that the greater tuberosity be placed 10 mm below the superior articular surface of the humeral head, but not overreduced, as this places the supraspinatus under increased tension and jeopardizes tuberosity fixation. Technical errors that can result in an increased HTD include humeral lengthening by cementing the prosthesis proud, using a head segment that is too thick, and overreduction of the greater tuberosity distal to its normal anatomic location.

Reasons for poor outcomes after hemiarthroplasty for displaced fractures of the proximal humerus have been analyzed. Initial tuberosity malposition was found to be present postoperatively in 27% of patients and tuberosity detachment and migration were noted in 23%. Final tuberosity malposition was present in 50% and correlated with an unsatisfactory result, superior migration of the prosthesis, stiffness, weakness, and pain. The worst association was a prosthesis that was too high and too retroverted with a low greater tuberosity. This "unhappy triad" was associated with migration of the greater tuberosity and proximal migration of the prosthesis under the acromion in all cases. The functional results after hemiarthroplasty for three- and four-part proximal humerus fractures are directly associated with tuberosity osteosynthesis. Lengthening of the prosthesis greater than 10 mm because of a proud prosthesis significantly correlated with tuberosity detachment and proximal migration of the prosthesis. The most common mistake was excessive retroversion of the prosthesis. All patients with retroversion exceeding 40° relative to the

transepicondylar axis had posterior migration of the greater tuberosity and a poor functional result.

In a related study, shoulder arthroplasty for the treatment of sequelae of fractures of the proximal humerus was evaluated. The most significant factor affecting functional outcome was greater tuberosity osteotomy. All patients who underwent greater tuberosity osteotomy had either fair or poor results and did not regain active elevation above 90°. Whenever possible, osteotomy of the greater tuberosity should not be done, and the prosthesis should be implanted by attempting to adapt the implant to the modified anatomy. This goal is accomplished by changing the inclination or offset of a modular prosthesis. All complications concerning the greater tuberosity (nonunion, bone resorption, and tuberosity migration) occurred after osteotomy. Another study showed that 10 of 24 patients who underwent osteotomy had a complication related to tuberosity nonunion, malunion, or resorption.

A promising surgical option for severe tuberosity nonunions or long-standing surgical neck nonunions may be a reverse prosthesis. In theory, by placing a "glenosphere," the proximal humerus can gain a motion fulcrum without the necessity of a rotator cuff centering force. There are long-term risks associated with this implant, including glenoid notching and fracture and loosening of the glenoid component. Also, implantation is technically demanding. Long-term efficacy studies are needed to determine if a reverse prosthesis is the answer for these difficult reconstructive cases.

Nerve Injury
A prospective study of 143 consecutive proximal humerus fractures found evidence of nerve injury by electromyography in 67% of patients. The axillary nerve was involved in 58% and the suprascapular nerve in 48%. A combination of nerve lesions was frequently seen. As might be expected, nerve lesions were more common in displaced fractures. Although the nerve lesions recovered in all patients, restoration of shoulder function was less favorable. This finding has implications for patients treated both surgically and nonsurgically.

Humeral Shaft Fractures
Acute Fractures
Since Sarmiento's original description in 1977, functional bracing has been considered the gold standard treatment for acute humeral shaft fractures. One recent study revealed a 95% union rate in patients. The rate of nonunion has been reported as low as 1.5% for closed fractures and 5.8% for open fractures with the brace removed between 10 and 13 weeks. Varus angulation after treatment with functional bracing is common. However, the angulation in most patients is usually functionally and cosmetically acceptable. The high rate of union and

no chance of postsurgical infection imply an earlier return to daily function and a lower cost of care.

Transverse fracture patterns are the most likely to develop angular deformity. Axial distraction between the fragments implies a high level of soft-tissue injury, and these fractures are more likely to develop delayed union or nonunion. In general, fractures at various levels heal at the same speed and with similar degrees of angulation. It is not necessary for the brace to fully cover every proximal or distal fragment. The brace should begin approximately 1 inch (2.5 cm) distal to the axilla and should terminate 1 inch proximal to the humeral condyles. Supra-acromial and supracondylar extensions are unnecessary. Active exercises may begin as soon as symptoms allow. However, active abduction and elevation of the shoulder must be avoided until after the fracture is clinically stable because these movements may produce angular deformities.

Indications for surgical intervention include open fractures, segmental and pathologic fractures, bilateral humeral fractures, fractures associated with vascular injuries, fractures where radial nerve palsy develops after reduction, multiple trauma with substantial chest/head injuries, floating elbow injuries (ipsilateral fractures of both forearm and arm), obesity that prevents adequate reduction, severe neurologic disorder, and inability to maintain satisfactory alignment. For a patient in the recumbent position for an extended period, it is difficult to control the fracture with closed treatment. Also, patients with concomitant chest injury are poor candidates for sling and swathe treatment. Alignment is considered acceptable with up to 20° anterior angulation, 30° of varus angulation, and 3 cm of shortening.

A radial nerve palsy sustained during humeral fracture is not an indication for exploration of the nerve or for internal fracture fixation. However, whenever the nerve is explored and the fracture is not healed, internal fixation is recommended. Patients with associated brachial plexus injury should undergo internal fixation because stabilization of the humeral fracture allows earlier rehabilitation of the injured extremity. Fractures that occur in the proximal and distal quarters of the humerus without an intervening diaphyseal fracture component should be treated separately. These fractures are exposed through separate incisions and fixed with separate plates.

Plate osteosynthesis has been the most accepted method for surgical treatment of both acute humeral shaft fractures and nonunions. The rate of union after compression plate fixation has been reported to be greater than 95%. The disadvantages include considerable soft-tissue stripping, poor screw purchase in osteoporotic bone, difficulties in complex fractures, and the risks associated with hardware removal.

Closed intramedullary nailing is considered for pathologic fractures, segmental fractures, fractures of osteopenic bone, and in patients with overlying burns and in those with multiple traumas. The advantages of intramedullary nailing over plate fixation include preservation of fracture hematoma and local blood supply, smaller surgical incision, a load-sharing as opposed to a stress-shielding device, and the theoretical advantage of earlier weight bearing. However, immediate weight bearing in acutely plated fractures has also been shown to have no detrimental effect.

Recent biomechanical studies show increased initial fracture stability when nails are inserted antegrade for proximal humeral shaft fractures and retrograde for distal humeral shaft fractures. Intramedullary nails can be inserted for shaft fractures in the region 2 cm distal to the surgical neck and 3 cm proximal to the olecranon fossa. The nonunion rate for intramedullary nailing was shown to be 5.6%, a rate comparable to that for plating. However, a complication rate of 19% for humeral locked nailing indicates that the procedure is not simply benign and noninvasive. Antegrade nailing carries the risk of shoulder pain and disability in 16% to 37% of patients. Retrograde nailing has a significantly higher risk of surgical comminution, and this comminution significantly increases the risk of nonunion. Great care must be taken to avoid anterior cortical notching during retrograde reaming. In addition, radial nerve exploration has been recommended before intramedullary rodding of distal third spiral fractures regardless of the presence or absence of nerve palsy because the radial nerve is in imminent danger when intramedullary rodding is attempted with this fracture pattern.

Several studies in recent years have compared plate fixation of humeral shaft fractures with intramedullary devices and have reached different conclusions. In reports in which plate and intramedullary rod fixation are directly compared, the rate of complications associated with intramedullary rodding appears higher than that associated with plate fixation. The complications associated with intramedullary rodding are related to rates of union (which appear to be somewhat lower than after plate fixation) and increased functional symptoms such as shoulder pain and weakness. Complications such as infection, radial nerve palsy, delayed union, and failure of fixation seem to occur at an equivalent rate with both types of intervention.

A prospective multicenter study reported the first clinical results of the Locking Compression Plate (Synthes, Paoli, PA) in 169 fractures in 144 patients, including 45 humeral fractures. In 86% of all fractures treated, healing occurred within the expected time period and without complication. The 1.5% infection rate was low considering the heterogenous sample with numerous open fractures and many revision surgeries. This report provided several guidelines regarding when to use compression technique or a bridging technique with the locking compression plate. Compression technique can be used for joint fractures and simple metadiaphyseal fracture patterns. The bridging technique is recommended for multifragmentary metadiaphyseal and diaphyseal fractures. A combined approach is warranted in only two situations: (1) in joint fractures with multifragmentary metadiaphyseal components, the compression technique should be used for the joint and bridging technique used for the metadiaphyseal segment; (2) in two-level fractures with different fracture patterns, the compression technique is used for the simple fracture part and the bridging technique for the multifragmentary segment.

Nonunion

Nonunion is defined as lack of union after 24 weeks. Nonunion of the humeral shaft occurs in 2% to 10% of nonsurgically treated fractures and up to 15% of fractures treated by primary ORIF. An increased incidence of nonunion can be seen with open fractures, high-energy injuries, bone loss, soft-tissue interposition, unstable or segmental fracture patterns, impaired blood supply, infection, and initial treatment with a hanging arm cast. Preexisting elbow or shoulder stiffness can cause increased motion at the fracture site and predispose to nonunion. Obesity, osteoporosis, alcoholism, malnutrition, smoking, and noncompliance are all patient factors that may increase the risk of nonunion.

A 98% consolidation rate was reported after ORIF of humeral nonunion using an anterolateral approach and autogenous bone grafting. A wave plate was applied in two instances when an intramedullary nail was in place and its removal was believed to be too hazardous. Only 2 of 51 patients had a transient sensory radial neuropathy. An anterolateral approach with routine identification and ample release of the radial nerve well beyond the nonunion ensures a very low rate of radial nerve injury. This broad exposure allows a plate of sufficient length to be applied, which increases the probability of union.

A recent study reported on results of the use of wave-plate fixation and autologous bone grafting in the management of humeral nonunion with a retained intramedullary nail. None of the patients had a prominent nail, which might represent a source of shoulder pain. Healing occurred in all six patients at a mean of 16 weeks postoperatively. The 4.5-mm wave plates were bent at two different locations so that the middle portion of the plate was standing 5 to 10 mm off the bone at the level of the nonunion. At least three bicortical screws were applied proximally and distally. Autologous cancellous graft was packed under the elevated portion of the plate at the site of nonunion. A high rate of nonunion has been shown after exchange nailing of humeral fractures, which is in contrast to the good results achieved for exchange nailing of femoral and tibial nonunions.

Humeral nonunion defects of 6 cm or greater present a reconstructive challenge. A vascularized bone graft remains alive, does not resorb, maintains its structural characteristics, and can hypertrophy, thus increasing its structural integrity. The healing of a vascularized bone graft is a process similar to acute fracture healing, in contrast to the long-standing process of creeping substitution, which must be endured with a nonvascularized allograft. The technique involves the creation of an intramedullary dowel of the vascularized fibula graft that is placed in the medullary canal of the humerus. The graft is impacted 1 to 2 cm at each end and the construct is stabilized with a 4.5-mm dynamic compression plate (Synthes, Paoli, PA). The fibula is applied as an onlay graft if the construct is already stable, as with a retained intramedullary rod. The peroneal artery is usually anastomosed end-to-side with the brachial artery. The peroneal vein is anastomosed end-to-side with either the venae comitantes of the brachial artery, or the basilic or cephalic vein. According to one recent study, 11 of 15 humeral nonunions united with this technique. Three of these 11, however, sustained a fracture of the fibula transplant at a mean of 8 months postoperatively and required additional bone grafting and plating but progressed to healing. Three other patients with early fixation failure underwent plating and bone grafting and eventually healed. One patient developed an infection and required a second vascularized fibula graft. Three patients had early revision of the venous anastomosis because laser Doppler readings were below 40% of the initial reading for 30 minutes and clinical observation of the skin island showed questionable perfusion. Only 5 of 15 patients regained nearly normal function, illustrating the complexity of the humeral reconstruction.

Annotated Bibliography

Clavicle Fractures

Edelson JG: The bony anatomy of clavicular malunions. *J Shoulder Elbow Surg* 2003;12:173-180.

Seventy-three fractures and 54 malunions were found in a study of 1,430 clavicles from adult skeletons. A consistent pattern of clavicular shortening involving anterior-posterior angulation is described.

Grassi FA, Tajana MS, D'Angelo F: Management of midclavicular fractures: Comparison between nonoperative an open intramedullary fixation in 80 patients. *J Trauma* 2001;50:1096-1100.

This study compared figure-of-8 bandaging to intramedullary fixation for midclavicular fractures and found that nonsurgical treatment appeared more advantageous for most patients with midclavicular fractures.

Levy O: Simple minimally invasive surgical technique for treatment of type 2 fractures of the distal clavicle. *J Shoulder Elbow Surg* 2003;12:24-28.

A minimally invasive technique is described in 12 patients, which uses absorbable suture fixation to treat Neer type II distal clavicle fractures. Union was achieved in all fractures with no complications.

McKee MD, Wild LM, Schemitsch EH: Midshaft malunions of the clavicle. *J Bone Joint Surg Am* 2003;85-A:790-797.

Fifteen patients who had a malunion following nonsurgical treatment of a clavicle fracture underwent corrective osteotomy through the original fracture line and internal fixation without bone graft. The mean amount of clavicular shortening was 2.9 cm preoperatively and 0.4 cm after surgery.

Postacchini F, Gumina S, DeSantis P, Albo F: Epidemiology of clavicle fractures. *J Shoulder Elbow Surg* 2002;11:452-456.

An epidemiologic study of 535 isolated clavicle fractures during an 11-year period was performed. Most patients (68%) were men. The left side was involved in 61% and fractures of the middle third were the most common (81%).

Rokito AS, Zuckerman JD, Shaari JM, Eisenberg DP, Cuomo F, Gallagher MA: A comparison of nonoperative and operative treatment of type II distal clavicle fractures. *Bull Hosp Joint Dis* 2002;61:32-39.

This retrospective study compared nonsurgical and surgical treatment of type II distal clavicular fractures. At an average follow-up of 53.5 months, 7 of 16 patients that were treated nonsurgically had a nonunion. However, nonunion had no significant impact on functional outcome or strength.

Scapula Fractures

Egol KA, Connor PM, Karunakar MA, Sims SH, Bosse MJ, Kellam JF: The floating shoulder: Clinical and functional results. *J Bone Joint Surg Am* 2001;83-A:1188-1194.

Nineteen patients with a floating shoulder injury were compared with respect to fracture healing, functional outcome, patient satisfaction, and muscular strength. Treatment was nonsurgical in 12 patients and surgical in 7 patients. There was no significant difference between groups with regard to the three functional outcome measures.

McAdams TR, Blevins FT, Martin P, DeCoster TA: The role of plain films and computed tomography in the evaluation of scapular neck fractures. *J Orthop Trauma* 2002;16:7-10.

Scapular neck fracture displacement, angulation, and anatomic classification showed moderate interobserver reliability by plain films and was not enhanced when supplemented with CT. CT may be useful to assess associated injuries to the superior shoulder suspensory complex, which could be missed when using plain films alone.

Schandelmaier P, Blauth M, Schneider C, Krettek C: Fractures of the glenoid treated by operation: A 5 to 23 year follow-up of 22 cases. *J Bone Joint Surg Br* 2002;84:173-177.

The results after ORIF of 22 displaced glenoid fractures with a mean follow-up of 10 years is described. At follow-up, the median Constant score was 94%. The score was less than 50% in four patients, including two patients who developed an infection.

Williams GR Jr, Naranja J, Klimkiewicz J, Karduna A, Iannotti JP, Ramsey M: The floating shoulder: A biomechanical basis for classification and management. *J Bone Joint Surg Am* 2001;83-A:1182-1187.

After a standardized neck fracture was made in 12 cadaver shoulders, the resistance to medial displacement was determined following sequential creation of an ipsilateral clavicle fracture, coracoacromial ligament disruption, and acromioclavicular capsular disruption. In another group, resistance to medial displacement was determined following sequential release of the coracoacromial and coracoclavicular ligaments. Ipsilateral scapular neck and clavicle fractures do not produce a floating shoulder until the coracoacromial and acromioclavicular capsular ligaments are disrupted.

Proximal Humeral Fractures

Boileau P, Krishnan SG, Tinsi L, Walch G, Coste JS, Mole D: Tuberosity malposition and migration: Reasons for poor outcomes after hemiarthroplasty for displaced fractures of the proximal humerus. *J Shoulder Elbow Surg* 2002;11:401-412.

The results of hemiarthroplasty for displaced proximal humeral fractures is evaluated. Final tuberosity malposition occurred in 33 patients (50%) and correlated with superior migration of the prosthesis, stiffness, weakness, and persistent pain.

Boileau P, Trojani C, Walch G, Krishnan SG, Romeo A, Sinnerton R: Shoulder arthroplasty for the treatment of sequelae of fractures of the proximal humerus. *J Shoulder Elbow Surg* 2001;10:299-308.

Seventy-one sequelae of proximal humeral fractures were treated with shoulder arthroplasty with the same modular prosthesis (Aequalis) in this multicenter study. The most significant factor affecting functional outcome was greater tuberosity osteotomy. Surgeons should accept the distorted anatomy of the proximal humerus and adapt the prosthesis to the modified anatomy if possible, to avoid tuberosity osteotomy.

Brorson S, Bagger J, Sylvest A, Hobjartsson A: Improved interobserver variation after training of doctors in the Neer system: A randomized trial. *J Bone Joint Surg Br* 2002;84:950-954.

Fourteen doctors were randomly assigned to two training sessions or to no training and asked to categorize 42 pairs of plain radiographs of proximal humerus fractures according to the Neer system. The kappa value for interobserver variation improved (especially for specialists) from 0.30 to 0.79 with formal training in the Neer system.

Court-Brown CM, Cattermole H, McQueen MM: Impacted valgus fractures of the proximal humerus. The results of non-operative treatment. *J Bone Joint Surg Br* 2002;84:504-508.

In this retrospective study of 125 patients with valgus-impacted fractures of the proximal humeral, all were treated nonsurgically. At 1-year follow-up, 80.6% of patients had a good or excellent result.

Demirhan M, Kilicoglu O, Altinel L, Eralp L, Akalin Y: Prognostic factors in prosthetic replacement for acute proximal humerus fractures. *J Orthop Trauma* 2003;17:181-189.

This retrospective study investigated the effect of radiologic and other factors on the outcome of prosthetic replacement in 32 patients with acute proximal humeral fractures. The humeral offset was directly correlated to the amount of forward elevation and Constant score. The head height was inversely correlated to the same parameters.

Frankle MA, Ondrovic LE, Markee BA, Harris ML, Lee WE III: Stability of tuberosity reattachment in proximal humeral hemiarthroplasty. *J Shoulder Elbow Surg* 2002;11:413-420.

This biomechanical study compared the stability of different reconstructive techniques of tuberosity reattachment for proximal humeral head replacement in four-part fractures using eight fresh-frozen cadaver shoulders. Mercury strain gauges were used to measure bony fragment displacement during cyclic loading. Repairs that used a medial circumferential cerclage had significantly lower displacements and strains.

Hockings M, Haines JF: Least possible fixation of fractures of the proximal humerus. *Injury* 2003;34:443-447.

An open technique with no deep dissection is described for the fixation of valgus-impacted proximal humeral fractures. No bone grafting, Kirschner wires, or other fixation was used. The mean Constant-Murley score as compared with the opposite side was 86%.

Lee SH, Dargent-Molina P, Breart G: Risk factors for fractures of the proximal humerus: Results for the EPIDOS prospective study. *J Bone Miner Res* 2002;17:817-825.

The EPIDOS study evaluated 6,901 white women age 75 years and older. The examination included measurements of femoral neck bone mineral density, calcaneal ultrasound parameters, a functional clinical examination, and lifestyle questionnaire. The incidence of proximal humerus fractures was greatly increased in women who had osteoporosis and a high risk score for falling.

Mighell MA, Kolm GP, Collinge CA, Frankle MA: Outcomes of hemiarthroplasty for fractures of the proximal humerus. *J Shoulder Elbow Surg* 2003;12:569-577.

Eighty shoulders that had been treated with hemiarthroplasty for proximal humeral fractures were reviewed. Tuberosity complications occurred in 16 shoulders. Healing of the greater tuberosity more than 2 cm below the humeral head correlated with a worse functional result.

Ogawa K, Yoshida A, Ikegami H: Isolated fractures of the greater tuberosity of the humerus: Solutions in recognizing a frequently overlooked fracture. *J Trauma* 2003;54:713-717.

Isolated greater tuberosity fractures were overlooked in 58 of 99 shoulders (59%) that had been initially examined at other clinics. A smaller fragment correlated with a higher rate of missed diagnosis. The presence of tenderness on the lateral wall of the greater tuberosity is a clinically effective method to avoid a missed diagnosis.

Park MC, Murthi AM, Roth NS, Blaine TA, Levine WN, Bigliani LU: Two-part and three-part fractures of the proximal humerus treated with suture fixation. *J Orthop Trauma* 2003;17:319-325.

The radiographic and clinical outcomes of patients with displaced two- and three-part proximal humeral fractures that were treated with nonabsorbable cuff-incorporating sutures were reviewed. Both groups had similar outcomes; some residual deformity did not preclude an excellent outcome.

Ring D, McKee MD, Perey BH, Jupiter JB: The use of a blade plate and autogenous cancellous bone graft in the treatment of ununited fractures of the proximal humerus. *J Shoulder Elbow Surg* 2001;10:501-507.

A blade-plate with autogenous cancellous graft was used to treat proximal humeral nonunions in 25 patients with a mean age of 61 years. Union was achieved in 23 of 25 patients (92%). The results were classified as good or excellent in 20 of 25 patients.

Robinson CM, Page RS: Severely impacted valgus proximal humerus fractures. *J Bone Joint Surg Am* 2003;85-A:1047-1055.

Twenty-five patients with severely impacted valgus proximal humeral fractures were treated with open reduction, fixation with screws or a buttress plate, and the fracture defect was filled with Norian Skeletal Repair system bone substitute. All fractures united within the first year and no patient had signs of osteonecrosis at latest follow-up. The functional result continued to be satisfactory for the 12 patients who were followed for 2 years.

Rowles DJ, McGrory JE: Percutaneous pinning of the proximal part of the humerus: An anatomic study. *J Bone Joint Surg Am* 2001;83-A:1695-1699.

In 10 fresh-frozen cadaver shoulders the intact proximal humerus was pinned using fluoroscopic guidance and a standard published technique. The specimens were dissected to determine the distance of each pin from vital neurovascular structures. Some modifications of technique and a knowledge of local anatomy are needed to avoid injury to the axillary nerve, musculocutaneous nerve, and biceps tendon.

Stoffel K, Dieter U, Stachowiak G, Gachter A, Kuster MS: Biomechanical testing of the LCP: How can stability in locked internal fixators be controlled? *Injury* 2003;34(suppl 2):B11-B19.

A biomechanical analysis including axial stiffness and torsional rigidity, fatigue testing, and finite element analysis were undertaken to evaluate the locking compression plate. Optimal use of the locking compression plate as it relates to biomechanical principles is discussed. For comminuted fractures of the humerus, it is recommended that innermost screws be placed as close to the fracture as practicable. The distance between the plate and the bone should be kept small. Long plates should be used to provide sufficient axial stiffness.

Visser CP, Coene LN, Brand R, Tavy DL: Nerve lesions in proximal humeral fractures. *J Shoulder Elbow Surg* 2001;10:421-427.

Fourteen consecutive proximal humeral fractures were evaluated with electromyograms in this prospective study. The electromyogram showed denervation in 96 patients (67%), with the axillary (58%) and the suprascapular nerves (48%) most frequently involved.

Wijgman AJ, Roolker W, Patt TW, Raaymakers EL, Marti RK: Open reduction and internal fixation of three and four-part fractures of the proximal part of the humerus. *J Bone Joint Surg Am* 2002;84-A:1919-1925.

The long-term results were assessed for 60 patients with a three- or four-part fracture of the proximal humerus who had undergone ORIF with cerclage or a T-plate. Thirty-seven percent of patients had development of osteonecrosis and 77% of these had a good or excellent Constant score.

Humeral Shaft Fractures

Gerber A, Marti R, Jupiter J: Surgical management of diaphyseal humeral nonunion after intramedullary nailing: Wave-plate fixation and autologous bone grafting without nail removal. *J Shoulder Elbow Surg* 2003;12: 309-313.

Sic patients with a nonunion of the humeral diaphysis after intramedullary nailing were treated with a wave-plate and autologous bone grafting. Union can be achieved without removal of the intramedullary device.

Heitmann C, Erdmann D, Levin LS: Treatments of segmental defects of the humerus with an osteoseptocutaneous fibular transplant. *J Bone Joint Surg Am* 2002;84-A:2216-2223.

Fifteen patients with an average 9.3-cm segmental humeral defect were treated with osteoseptocutaneous fibular transplant. This treatment can be successful but has a high rate of complications.

Koch PP, Gross DF, Gerber C: The results of functional (Sarmiento) bracing of humeral shaft fractures. *J Shoulder Elbow Surg* 2002;11:143-150.

Sixty-seven humeral shaft fractures were treated by Sarmiento bracing over a 15-year period. At a mean of 10 weeks, 87% had healed clinically. Among nine cases of delayed or nonunion leading to surgery, there were six cases with transverse fractures. Reasons for failed nonsurgical treatment included incorrect indication, significant axial deformity, and a hyperextended position of the fracture fragments.

Lin J, Shen PW, Hou SM: Complications of locked nailing in humeral shaft fractures. *J Trauma* 2003;54:943-949.

Delayed unions, nonunions, and acute humeral shaft fractures in 159 patients were treated with humeral locked nails and followed for an average 25.4 months. Surgical comminution was significantly higher in retrograde nailing and surgical comminution and significantly increased the risk of nonunion. Other complications included functional shoulder impairment, angular malunion, and postnailing radial nerve palsy.

Marti RK, Verheyen CC, Besselaar PP: Humeral shaft nonunion: Evaluation of uniform surgical repair in fifty-one patients. *J Orthop Trauma* 2002;16:108-115.

This article presents a review of the standard treatment of aseptic humeral shaft nonunions involving an anterolateral approach, radial nerve identification, compression plating, and autogenous bone grafting. This approach is reliable and achieves union without a significant risk of complications.

Ring D, Jupiter JB: Internal Fixation of the humerus with locking compression plates. *Tech Shoulder Elbow Surg* 2003;4:169-174.

The drawbacks of previous methods of internal fixation for humeral fractures and nonunions is discussed. The advantages of and technique for the application of Locking Compression Plates to humeral fractures and nonunions is presented. Preliminary results are also discussed.

Sommer C, Gautier E, Muller M, Helfet DL, Wagner M: First clinical results of the Locking Compression Plate (LCP). *Injury* 2003;34(suppl 2):B43-B54.

A prospective multicenter study of the combined European and American experience with the new locking compression plate system used to treat various fractures in 144 patients is presented. In this study, tibial fractures (n = 46) and humeral fractures (n = 45) predominated. General principles for the application of the locking compression plate to different fracture configurations as well as to humeral fractures, are discussed. The low infection rate (1.5%) in this heterogenous sample with numerous open fractures and revision procedures attests to the good "biology" of the implant.

Stannard JP, Harris HW, McGwin G Jr, Volgas DA, Alonso JE: Intramedullary nailing of humeral shaft fractures with a locking flexible nail. *J Bone Joint Surg Am* 2003;85-A:2103-2110.

A flexible humeral nail is described that allows both antegrade and retrograde insertion and static locking without violating the rotator cuff or humeral articular surface. Although the nail functioned well in most patients, the use of the smaller (7.5 mm) nail was associated with a higher complication rate. This implant should be used with caution in any patient with a medullary canal diameter of 8 mm or less.

Classic Bibliography

Chapman JR, Henley MB, Agel J, Benca PJ: Randomized prospective study of humeral shaft fracture fixation: Iintramedullary nails versus plates. *J Orthop Trauma* 2000;14:162-166.

Edwards SG, Whittle AP, Wood GW II: Nonoperative treatment of ipsilateral fractures of the scapula and clavicle. *J Bone Joint Surg Am* 2000;82:774-780.

Galatz LM, Iannotti JP: Management of surgical neck nonunions. *Orthop Clin North Am* 2000;31:51-61.

Herscovici D Jr, Saunders DT, Johnson MP, Sanders R, DiPasquale T: Percutaneous fixation of proximal humerus fractures. *Clin Orthop* 2000;375:97-104.

Hintermann B, Trouillier HH, Schafer D: Rigid internal fixation of fractures of the proximal humerus in older patients. *J Bone Joint Surg Br* 2000;82:1107-1112.

Mayo KA, Benirschke SK, Mast JW: Displaced fractures of the glenoid fossa: Results of open reduction and internal fixation. *Clin Orthop* 1998;347:122-130.

McCormack RG, Brien D, Buckley RE, McKee MD, Powell J, Schemitsch EH: Fixation of fractures of the shaft of the humerus by dynamic compression plate or intramedullary nail: A prospective, randomized trial. *J Bone Joint Surg Br* 2000;82:336-339.

Momberger NG, Smith J, Coleman DA: Vascularized fibular grafts for salvage reconstruction of clavicle nonunion. *J Shoulder Elbow Surg* 2000;9:389-394.

Schai PA, Hintermann B, Koris MJ: Preoperative arthroscopic assessment of fractures about the shoulder. *Arthroscopy* 1999;15:827-835.

Tingstad EM, Wolinsky PR, Shyr Y, Johnson KD: Effect of immediate weightbearing on plated fractures of the humeral shaft. *J Trauma* 2000;49:278-280.

Webber MC, Haines JF: The treatment of lateral clavicle fractures. *Injury* 2000;31:175-179.

Chapter 25

Shoulder Instability

Andrew D. Pearle, MD

Frank A. Cordasco, MD

Natural History

The glenohumeral joint is the most mobile articulation in the body and the most commonly dislocated diarthroidal joint, with peaks in the incidence of dislocation occurring during the second and sixth decades of life. Instability of the glenohumeral joint ranges from subtle increased laxity to recurrent frank dislocation. No single disease or lesion is responsible for all types of shoulder instability, and treatment has evolved to anatomically address specific lesions.

Traumatic injury is the major cause of shoulder instability, accounting for approximately 95% of shoulder dislocations. The sequela of traumatic anterior dislocation is associated with the age of the patient at the time of initial dislocation and the degree of injury. Age at the time of the initial dislocation is inversely related to the recurrence rate. In patients younger than 20 years of age, recurrent dislocation rates may be as high as 90% in the athletic population. The rate of recurrences drops to 50% to 75% in patients 20 to 25 years of age. In patients older than 40 years, anterior dislocation is associated with lower rates of redislocation, but high rates of rotator cuff tears. Although the incidence of rotator cuff tears in patients older than 40 years at the time of initial dislocation is 15%, this incidence reaches 40% in patients older than 60 years. The degree of injury (presence and size of Bankart tear, presence and size of osseous lesions including Hill-Sachs defects and osseous Bankart lesions, capsular tears such as a humeral avulsion of the glenohumeral ligament, and the presence of associated rotator cuff pathology) is directly related to the recurrence rate.

Pathophysiology

The normal humeral head translates only 1 mm from the center of the glenoid during active motion. The glenohumeral joint is stabilized by both static and dynamic stabilizers. The static restraints consist of the glenoid labrum, the articular anatomy, negative intra-articular pressure, joint fluid adhesion, and the capsuloligamentous structures. Dynamic stabilizers of the joint include

the rotator cuff muscles, biceps, and periscapular muscles. In general, the capsular ligaments provide stability at end range of motion; however, during midrange of motion, the capsuloligamentous structures are lax and the joint is stabilized by dynamic joint compression. Glenohumeral instability occurs when there is a deficiency in the bony, soft-tissue, or dynamic muscular restraints to translation of the humeral head on the glenoid. Rehabilitation following instability episodes is directed toward optimizing the dynamic stabilizers, whereas surgical intervention restores the static stabilizers.

The oval glenoid is longest in its inferior-superior diameter and has a nearly flat articular surface. Although the osseous shape of the glenoid does not contribute greatly to stability, the peripheral chondral surface of the glenoid is thickened, creating a concave articular surface that augments glenohumeral stability. The labrum is a fibrous structure firmly bound to the glenoid at its inferior margin and bound more loosely superiorly, where it is confluent with the origin of the tendon of the long head of the biceps. The labral tissue contributes to glenohumeral stability by deepening the glenoid by approximately 50%. The labrum is thought to act as a "chock block" and has been shown to decrease resistance to humeral translation by 10% to 20%. In addition, the labrum serves as an attachment site connecting the glenoid to the capsule, ligaments, and biceps tendon.

The capsule of the glenohumeral joint is lax under normal circumstances, which allows for great range of motion of the joint. The capsule attaches medially to the glenoid and labrum and extends lateral to the surgical neck of the humerus. In addition to providing structural stability, the capsule maintains the negative joint pressure, which creates a negative vacuum that augments joint stability.

The ligaments of the glenohumeral joint are discrete bands that insert onto the glenoid labrum. The most important ligaments in the glenohumeral joint are the superior glenohumeral ligament (SGHL), the middle glenohumeral ligament (MGHL), and the inferior glenohumeral ligament complex (IGHLC) (Figure 1).

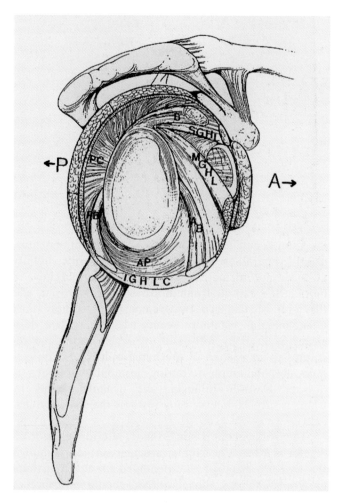

Figure 1 Schematic drawing of the shoulder capsule showing the glenohumeral ligaments highlighting the IGHLC. A, anterior; P, posterior; B, biceps tendon; AB, anterior band; AP, axillary pouch; PB, posterior band; and PC, posterior capsule. *(Reproduced with permission from O'Brien SJ, Neves MC, Arnoczky SP, et al: The anatomy and histology of the inferior glenohumeral ligament complex of the shoulder. Am J Sports Med 1990;18:449-456.)*

The SGHL originates on the superoanterior rim of the glenoid, just anterior to the biceps origin, and courses across the rotator interval to the lesser tuberosity adjacent to the bicipital groove. The SGHL is the primary static restraint to inferior translation of the adducted shoulder. The coracohumeral ligament (CHL) is an extra-articular structure that arises from the base of the coracoid and passes between the supraspinatus and subscapularis, forming the roof of the rotator interval. It is composed of an anterior and posterior band that inserts onto the lesser and greater tuberosity, respectively. The CHL is a static restraint to anteroinferior translation in the adducted shoulder.

The MGHL has the most variable morphology of the ligaments; however, no distinct variation in its structure has been correlated with increased rates of instability. The MGHL normally originates in the upper third of the anterior glenoid rim and labrum and courses obliquely across the subscapularis tendon to its humeral

attachment on the lesser tuberosity. A Buford complex is a normal anatomic variant defined by the absence of the superoanterior aspect of the labrum and a broad, cord-like MGHL. The MGHL prevents anterior translation when the shoulder is externally rotated and in the middle range of abduction.

The IGHLC is the major static anterior stabilizer of the glenohumeral joint, especially during abduction and external rotation (Figure 2). The complex consists of an anterior and posterior band as well as the axillary pouch. It originates from the inferior labrum and inserts on to the humeral neck. Detachment of the anterior labrum and anterior IGHLC is referred to as a Bankart lesion and has classically been understood as the "essential" lesion in traumatic anterior instability (Figure 3). However, in cadaveric models, minimal translation has been noted with recreation of this lesion, suggesting that capsular and ligamentous plastic deformation is an important pathologic component of instability. In a recent study using MRI to quantitate the amount of capsular elongation in patients with recurrent anterior dislocations, the authors showed that the anterior and inferior portions of the shoulder capsule are elongated an average of 19% compared with the unaffected contralateral shoulder.

A recent cadaveric study has demonstrated that the posterior band of the IGHLC shows greatest strain in flexion and internal rotation, the provocative positions for posterior instability. This finding suggests that the posterior band of the IGHLC is a static posterior stabilizer and should be firmly repaired in patients with posterior instability.

Dynamic stabilization of the glenohumeral joint occurs through joint compression by the rotator cuff, primarily the subscapularis and infraspinatus. Dynamic joint compression from the rotator cuff musculature limits superior-inferior translation and imparts stability during abduction. The dynamic joint compression force from the rotator cuff muscles is more important for stability than the static glenohumeral ligaments. The scapular stabilizers, including the trapezius, rhomboids, latissimus dorsi, serratus anterior, and levator scapulae position the glenoid in an anteverted and superior position and provide dynamic coverage for the retroverted humeral head; this increases the posterior and inferior stability of the glenohumeral joint during motion.

The biceps tendon is thought to be a dynamic stabilizer of the joint, particularly at middle and lower elevation angles. The tendon provides stability in the anterior and superior direction, imparting more posterior stability in external rotation of the humerus and anterior stability with internal rotation. In addition, because of the intimate association of the bicipital anchor and the SGHL and MGHL, lesions that involve the bicipital anchor, such as superior labral anterior and posterior

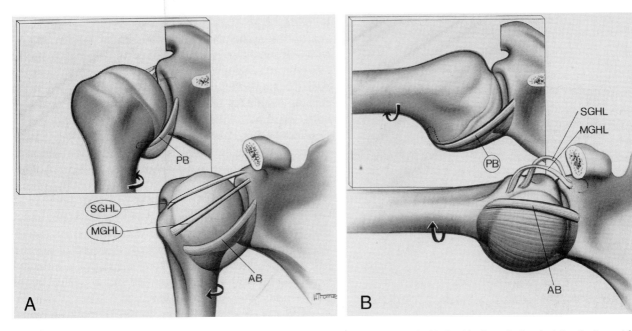

Figure 2 The glenohumeral ligaments provide static restraint in different functional positions. **A,** With the shoulder in adduction and external rotation, the ligament SGHL and MGHL are taut while the anterior band (AB) and posterior band (PB) of the IGHLC are lax. **B,** With the shoulder in abduction and external rotation, the AB of the IGHLC tightens and the SGHL and MGHL become lax. *(Reproduced with permission from Warner JP, Boardman ND III: Anatomy, biomechanics, and pathophysiology of glenohumeral instability, in Warren RF, Craig EV, Altcheck DW (eds): The Unstable Shoulder. Philadelphia, PA, Lippincott-Raven, 1999, pp 51-76.)*

(SLAP) tears, may increase anteroposterior as well as superoinferior glenohumeral translation.

Patient Evaluation

Multiple static and dynamic structures contribute to shoulder stability; therefore, proper classification of shoulder instability is essential to identify injured structures and plan treatment. Shoulder instability is classified by the degree, frequency, etiology, and direction of instability (Table 1). Patient history and physical examination should focus on accurately classifying the instability pattern.

History

A careful history is essential to begin to classify the patient's instability. The etiology of the instability may be readily apparent as the patient may describe a frank traumatic dislocation event, history of repetitive microtrauma with overhead activity, or generalized laxity that is familial. Patients are usually able to clearly describe the frequency and chronicity of instability episodes. Pain or instability with particular movements or positions may reveal the direction of instability. Patients with anterior instability report symptoms with the arm in an abducted and externally rotated position. Posterior instability often occurs with the arm flexed, internally rotated, and adducted. Patients may experience symptoms while pushing open a door or heavy object. Patients with inferior instability often have pain while carrying heavy objects; they may also experience traction paresthesias.

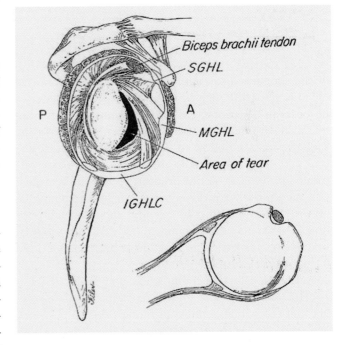

Figure 3 Schematic drawing of the anatomy of the Bankart lesion demonstrating avulsion of the capsulolabral structures off the inferior rim of the glenoid. A = anterior; P = posterior l*(Reproduced with permission from Warner JP, Caborn DNM: Overview of shoulder instability. Crit Rev Phys Rehabil Med 1992;4:145-198.)*

Physical Examination

Examination of shoulder instability begins with a thorough evaluation of the cervical spine. Careful inspection

Table 1 | Classification of Shoulder Instability

Degree
  Dislocation
  Subluxation
    Microinstability
Frequency
  Acute (primary)
  Chronic
    Recurrent
    Fixed
Etiology
  Traumatic (macrotraumatic)
  Atraumatic
    Voluntary (muscular)
    Involuntary
  Aquired (microtrauma)
Direction
  Unidirectional
    Anterior
    Posterior
    Inferior
  Bidirectional
    Anterior-inferior
    Posterior-inferior
  Multidirectional

(Reproduced with permission from Backer M, Warren RF: Glenohumeral instabilities in adults, in DeLee JC, Drez D Jr, Miller MD (eds): DeLee and Drez's Orthopaedic Sports Medicine: Principle's and Practice. Philadelphia, PA, Saunders, 2003, pp 1020-1034.)

of the shoulder girdle and upper extremity may reveal obvious deformity such as an acute dislocation. Anterior dislocations are characterized by prominence of the humeral head anterior, medial, and often inferior to the shoulder joint, a hollow region beneath the lateral deltoid, and the arm held in an abducted, slightly externally rotated position. Posterior dislocations may be less obvious but a posterior prominence is usually noted and the arm is held in an internally rotated and adducted position. The coracoid is prominent as well. More subtle findings on inspection of a reduced but unstable joint include muscle atrophy caused by general neurologic conditions, local nerve compression, and tendon tears.

The strength of the muscles surrounding the shoulder and the patient's range of motion should be tested and compared with the contralateral side. The function of the axillary nerve should be evaluated by testing the function of the deltoid and the sensation on the lateral aspect of the shoulder.

Provocative tests for shoulder instability allow the examiner to further classify the instability. Evaluation of the contralateral side should be conducted for comparison. Tests that reproduce the symptoms of instability include the apprehension test and the posterior load and shift test.

Imaging

Acute traumatic shoulder dislocations are evaluated with a trauma series that includes an AP, transscapular (Y) lateral, and an axillary view. The axillary view is especially important to confirm reduction. In more chronic instability, additional views are useful to assess bony anatomy and identify characteristic pathologic lesions. The West Point axillary view, which is taken with the patient prone, the arm in 90° of abduction and neutral rotation, and the x-ray beam directed 25° posterior to the horizontal plane and 25° medial to the vertical plane, shows the anterior glenoid rim and may reveal bony Bankart lesions. The Stryker notch view, taken with the patient supine and the hand placed on top of the head, shows the posterosuperior humeral head and Hill-Sachs lesions. CT scans can be helpful in selected patients with complex bony injuries and in evaluation of glenoid and humeral head version.

MRI has become a helpful tool to evaluate patients with acute and chronic shoulder instability. With MRI, capsular and ligament detachments, labral lesions, rotator cuff tears, and bony trauma can be identified with more accuracy than with radiographs or CT scan.

Examination Under Anesthesia and Arthroscopy

Although classification of the frequency, etiology, and direction of instability may be evaluated with a thorough history and physical examination, the degree of instability is often best appreciated with examination under anesthesia or during arthroscopy. The axial load test is used and the degree of instability in each direction is graded.

Arthroscopic examination allows for complete assessment of injured structures in the glenohumeral joint. The articular surfaces, labrum, glenohumeral ligaments, integrity of the capsular tissue, biceps tendon, and rotator cuff should be carefully inspected and probed.

Treatment of Acute Dislocation

Acute dislocations should be reduced as quickly and atraumatically as possible. After a trauma series is obtained, closed reduction is performed with the patient relaxed with sedation or local anesthetics.

A recent MRI study has shown that the conventional position of immobilization in adduction and internal rotation results in significantly more separation and displacement of a Bankart lesion than immobilization in adduction and external rotation.

In the young, highly active athletic population with a traumatic anterior dislocation, primary surgical intervention may be warranted. Several studies from the US Military Academy at West Point have reported recurrent dislocation rates of 80% to 92% for cadets treated with physical therapy after initial traumatic shoulder dislocation. In this population, surgical intervention has been advocated. In a recent prospective randomized clinical trial comparing arthroscopic stabilization with nonsurgical treatment of first-time shoulder dislocations in active duty soldiers, 75% of the nonsurgically treated patients developed recurrent instability, versus 11% of the arthroscopy treated patients. Average follow-up was 3 years. In another study from the US Military Academy at West Point, the recurrence rate of instability after primary arthroscopic repair of initial anterior shoulder dislocations at 2- to 5-year follow-up was 12%.

Treatment of Recurrent Traumatic Instability

Whereas the goal of rehabilitation is the enhancement of the dynamic stabilizers of the shoulder, the aim of surgical intervention is the restoration of disrupted static restraints. Primary stabilization should be considered for first-time traumatic shoulder dislocation with a Bankart lesion confirmed by MRI in the athletic population younger than 25 years old. These patients have a low rate of return to previous activity level if managed with rehabilitation alone. In the older or less athletic population, the primary indication for surgical stabilization is recurrent instability despite an appropriate rehabilitation program.

The goals for treatment of shoulder instability are identical whether the procedure is arthroscopic or open. Anatomic repair of the static stabilizers involves identification and reattachment of disrupted structures with minimal disturbance of the length and attachments of uninvolved tissues (Figure 4).

An open Bankart repair involves an anterior approach to the glenohumeral joint and repair of the detached capsulolabral structures to the glenoid through drill holes or with suture anchors. With this time-honored procedure, the expected success rate is approximately 90% to 95%. Because the capsule is opened during the approach and may be retensioned, imbricated, or shifted, open repair is traditionally favored in situations of multiple recurrences with increased capsular laxity. In addition, open repair is generally considered a more durable procedure for patients who wish to return to contact sports.

Arthroscopic stabilization techniques involve anatomic repairs without the takedown and reattachment of the subscapularis tendon as required in the open procedure. The arthroscopic techniques have improved greatly. Fixation devices for reapproximation of the capsulolabral lesions have evolved from staples to transglenoid sutures to cannulated bioabsorbable screws and suture anchors. In addition to shorter hospitalization times and less postoperative pain, results of arthroscopic procedures show increased external rotation compared with open techniques. The major disadvantage of arthroscopic techniques has been a higher recurrence rate in comparison with open procedures. In most studies using

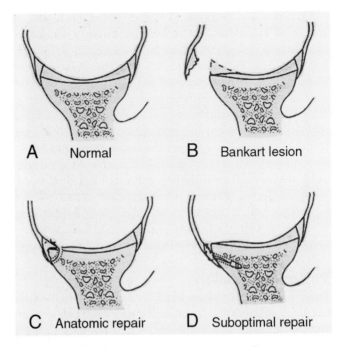

Figure 4 A, In the normal shoulder, the capsule and labrum serve to deep glenoid. **B,** This effect is lost in the presence of a Bankart lesion. **C,** Anatomic repair restores effective depth of glenoid concavity. **D,** Nonanatomic repair does not restore normal "chock-block" effect of the capsulolabral structure. *(Reproduced with permission from Matsen FA III, Lippitt SB, Sidles JB. Harryman DT II: Stability, in Matsen FA III (ed): Practical Evaluation and Management of the Shoulder. Philadelphia, PA, WB Saunders, 1994, p 59.)*

older techniques for arthroscopic fixation, the recurrence rate has been between 10% to 20%, approximately twice as high as with open procedures. However, in a recent review of the outcomes of 167 arthroscopic Bankart repairs using suture anchor techniques, recurrence of instability was 4% at a mean postoperative follow-up of 44 months with a mean loss of external rotation of 2°.

Recently there have been two prospective studies comparing open procedures with arthroscopic stabilization with biodegradable tacks for shoulder instability in patients with Bankart lesions. In a prospective, randomized multicenter study, 30 patients were treated with arthroscopic stabilization and 26 patients were treated with an open procedure. At 2-year follow-up, the recurrence rate in the arthroscopic group was 23% versus 12% in the open group. In another study, which was not randomized, patients were evaluated at 3-year follow-up. The patients in open and arthroscopic groups had similar demographics, although patients who underwent open procedures had a greater number of dislocations before surgery. In this study, the recurrence rate, including subluxations or dislocations, was 15% in the arthroscopic group compared with 10% in the open group. The external rotation in abduction averaged 90° in the arthroscopic group compared with 80° in the open group.

Traumatic glenohumeral defects have been associated with failed Bankart repairs, particularly when performed arthroscopically. Two bony lesions in particular, the engaging Hill-Sachs lesion and the inverted-pear glenoid, have been associated with high rates of recurrent instability after arthroscopic repair, particularly in athletes who participate in contact sports. In the engaging Hill-Sachs lesion, the orientation of the Hill-Sachs lesion is such that it engages the anterior glenoid in abduction and external rotation. In the inverted-pear glenoid, the normal pear-shaped configuration of the glenoid is altered because of significant anteroinferior bone loss, which creates an inverted pear appearance. With these osseous findings, open procedures with reconstruction of the osseous defects may be warranted.

Posterior Instability

Posterior instability occurs in 2% to 4% of patients with shoulder instability. Causative factors for posterior instability include major trauma, repetitive microtrauma as in overhead athletes, and generalized ligamentous laxity. Acute posterior dislocations occur with load to a flexed, adducted, and internally rotated upper arm and are commonly missed at initial presentation. Patients present with an adducted, internally rotated arm and are unable to externally rotate the shoulder. The classic radiographic findings on the AP view include a loss of the humeral neck profile, a vacant glenoid sign, and an anterior humeral head compression fracture (reverse Hill-Sachs lesion). After recognition, gentle reduction should be performed with lateral traction, external rotation, and abduction. Initial treatment after radiographic confirmation of reduction is immobilization in slight extension and external rotation followed by physical therapy.

Most authors recommend a prolonged period of rehabilitation for symptoms of posterior instability. In patients who do not respond to nonsurgical treatment, a variety of surgical and arthroscopic interventions have been described. Open procedures include posterior capsulorrhaphy, bone block procedures, and glenoid or humeral osteotomy. One study reported results of open posterior capsulorrhaphy for traumatic recurrent posterior subluxations in athletic patients; good or excellent results were achieved in 13 of 14 patients. Arthroscopic procedures include posterior capsular plication, thermal shrinkage, and capsulolabral repair. In a recent retrospective review of 27 shoulders treated with arthroscopic repair using bioabsorbable tack fixation for a posterior capsulolabral detachment (posterior Bankart lesion), symptoms of pain and posterior instability were eliminated in 92% of patients at a mean follow-up of 5.1 years. In another review of patients with traumatic unilateral posterior instability, 27 patients with posterior Bankart lesions underwent arthroscopic repair using su-

ture anchor fixation. At a mean follow-up of 39 months, 96% of these patients had a stable shoulder and were able to return to their prior sports activity with few or no limitations.

Multidirectional Instability

There is a common misconception that multidirectional instability is limited to young sedentary patients with generalized ligamentous laxity, an atraumatic history, and bilateral symptoms. Although a subgroup of such patients exists, shoulders with multidirectional instability are often seen in athletic patients, many of whom have had an injury. Activities such as gymnastics or butterfly swimming may have resulted in repetitive microtrauma that selectively stretched out the shoulders, and other joints may not be lax on examination. Additionally, Bankart lesions and humeral head impression defects may be present in patients with multidirectional instability, although less commonly than in patients with unidirectional traumatic instability.

Symptoms typically include episodes of pain and instability that are positional or occur after minimal force. The lesion in multidirectional instability was classically thought to be a loose redundant inferior pouch with a large rotator interval. However, the etiology of multidirectional instability appears to be multifactorial and may include aberrant muscle firing patterns and abnormal connective tissue. In a recent MRI study, isometric muscle activity leads to an off-centered humeral head position in patients with multidirectional instability compared with a recentered humeral head position during muscle firing in patients with traumatic instability. Initial treatment focuses on rehabilitation, which has a greater than 80% success rate if sustained for 6 to 12 months.

The goal of arthroscopic and open procedures is to reduce the capsular volume of the joint while maintaining motion. Capsular shift, performed anteriorly or posteriorly, has an 85% to 90% success rate. Humeral-based as well as glenoid-based shift procedures have been described and have yielded similar success rates.

Arthroscopic techniques include capsular plication, rotator interval closure, and thermal capsular shrinkage. Various arthroscopic devices have been developed to deliver heat to capsular tissue. Investigators have noted a 15% to 40% reduction in the length of collagenous tissue when it is heated to 65° to 72°C. This reduction in length has been shown to be caused by thermal denaturation of the collagen triple helix structure with subsequent reorganization into a random coil formation at a shorter length. A recent retrospective review of the results of arthroscopic laser-assisted capsular shrinkage in 27 shoulders with multidirectional instability has shown an overall success rate of 81.5% (with recurrent instability as a measure of failure) at an average follow-up of

28 months. In another study using arthroscopic thermal capsulorrhaphy to treat multidirectional instability in 30 shoulders, 76% of patients had a good or excellent result at an average follow-up of 3 years. The long-term sequela of thermal shrinkage techniques is not known. Recent studies of the behavior of lax ligaments treated with electrothermal shrinkage in animal models have found that although thermal shrinkage reduced laxity, there was increased potential for creep and failure at low physiologic stresses. A recent histologic analysis of the capsule from seven patients after failed thermal capsulorrhaphy showed denudation of the synovial layer and morphologic changes in the collagen layer that included, in some cases, a hyalinization appearance. Although no pathognomonic histologic changes were identified, the study demonstrated that histologic abnormalities may be present for years after failed thermal capsulorrhaphy.

Failed Instability Surgery

Recurrent instability after surgical treatment of instability may occur because of new trauma, incomplete treatment of pathologic lesions, poor rehabilitation, abnormal host healing response, or diagnostic error. Treatment of recurrent stability after surgical stabilization is difficult. Prior to surgical intervention, careful evaluation by history, physical examination, and diagnostic imaging should be performed to identify the cause of the recurrence. Recurrent instability after failed stabilization should be classified according to direction, degree, and frequency of instability.

Initial treatment almost always consists of extensive rehabilitation. New traumatic lesions may heal, and strengthening and improved control of the dynamic muscular stabilizers may make the instability more tolerable.

Surgical intervention should be directed by the etiology of the recurrent instability. Common findings at revision surgery include excessive capsular redundancy, uncorrected Bankart lesions, and bone loss from the glenoid or from the humeral head. Incomplete correction of pathologic lesions, particularly Bankart lesions, should be repaired anatomically. An inferior capsular shift should be performed in patients with capsular laxity, particularly in those with a patulous axillary pouch.

One retrospective review investigated the outcome of 50 patients who underwent revision anterior stabilization. Forty-nine of the procedures involved an open capsular shift, and 23 shoulders underwent concomitant repair of a Bankart lesion. At an average 4.7-year follow-up, good or excellent results were obtained in 78% of patients. The authors identified factors associated with poor results of the revision procedure that included atraumatic causes of failure, voluntary dislocations, and multiple prior stabilization attempts.

Irreparable capsular deficiency after failed stabilization procedures presents a particularly challenging situation. Capsular deficiency has been described after open procedures because of subscapularis tendon incompetence and after arthroscopic thermal capsulorrhaphy caused by excessive thermal injury and tissue necrosis. Deficiencies of the subscapularis tendon can be reconstructed using a transfer of the sternal head of the pectoralis major tendon. Capsular deficiencies can be reconstructed with a portion of the subscapularis tendon, autograft tissue, or allograft tendon. A recent report in which the iliotibial band was used to reconstruct the deficient capsular tissues in seven patients showed the elimination of instability and the maintenance of a physiologic range of motion.

Osseous deficiency of the humerus or of the glenoid is a rare etiology of recurrent instability after failed stabilization. Bone procedures to reconstruct osseous deficiencies include the Latarjet and the Bristow procedures in which a portion of the coracoid is used to reconstruct an inferior glenoid deficiency. Hill-Sachs lesions, an impaction fracture of the posterolateral margin of the humeral head, are found in more than 80% of patients with traumatic anterior instability. These lesions are thought to play a significant role in recurrent instability if they comprise more than 30% of the proximal humerus articular surface or if they engage the glenoid. Large Hill-Sachs lesions that engage the glenoid and contribute to recurrent instability may be treated with osteochondral allografts.

In patients with multiple failed stabilization procedures and recurrent, debilitating instability, arthrodesis may be considered as a salvage procedure. A recent study evaluated the efficacy of shoulder arthrodesis performed after an average of seven failed stabilization attempts. The results of eight patients were reviewed at a mean follow-up of 35 months. All patients had achieved bony union and all patients reported that they would repeat the surgery.

Chronic Dislocations

The diagnosis of chronic locked anterior or posterior shoulder dislocations may be made after physical examination and proper radiographic analysis. Nonsurgical treatment may be considered in elderly patients with poor general mental status, especially when the condition is associated with limited pain. Surgical treatment is necessary for reduction of the joint. Humeral head impaction fractures (Hill-Sachs lesions with chronic anterior dislocations and reverse Hill-Sachs lesions with chronic posterior dislocations) may preclude stable reduction.

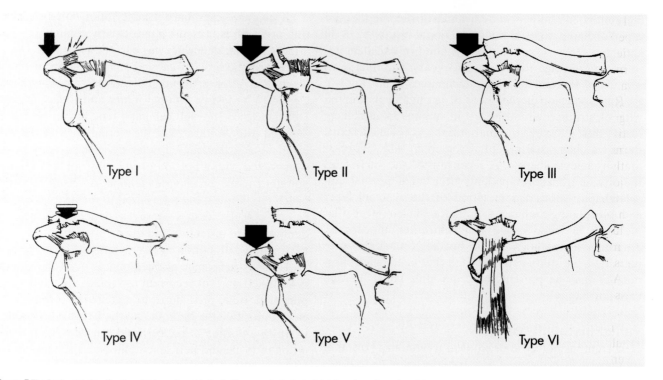

Figure 5 The Rockwood classification of ligamentous injuries to the acromioclavicular joint. Type I, no disruption of the acromioclavicular or coracoclavicular ligaments. Type II, disruption of the acromioclavicular ligament (coracoclavicular ligaments remain intact.) Type III, disruption of the acromioclavicular and coracoclavicular ligaments. Type IV, disruption of the acromioclavicular and coracoclavicular ligaments, and the distal end of the clavicle is displaced posteriorly into or through the trapezius muscle. Type V, disruption of the acromioclavicular and coracoclavicular ligaments, along with disruption of the muscle attachments and creation of a major separation between the clavicle and the acromion. Type VI, disruption of the acromioclavicular and coracoclavicular ligaments. Inferior dislocation of the distal clavicle in which the clavicle is inferior to the coracoid process and posterior to the biceps and coracobrachialis tendons. *(Reproduced with permission from Rockwood CA, Williams GR, Young DC: Shoulder instability, in Rockwood CA, Green DP, Bucholz RN, Heckman JD (eds): Rockwood and Green's Fractures in Adults. Philadelphia, PA, Lippincott-Raven, 1996, p 1354.)*

Acromioclavicular Separations

The acromioclavicular (AC) joint is a sturdy structure that affixes the clavicle to the scapula. Injury to the AC joint is common (comprising approximately 9% of shoulder girdle injuries) and occurs most often in males in their 20s. The AC joint is surrounded by and stabilized by a capsule and AC ligaments (superior, inferior, anterior, and posterior). Additional joint stability is provided by the coracoclavicular ligaments (trapezoid and conoid) as well as the coracoacromial ligament.

Injury to the AC joint is understood as a sequential loss of AC stabilizers. The classification of AC joint instability reflects this anatomic progression of injury (Figure 5) and is useful in directing treatment.

Radiographic evaluation of the AC joint may be performed with standard AP and lateral views of the shoulder. However, improved visualization of the AC joint is achieved with a Zanca view, performed by tilting the beam 10° to 15° cephalad. Additionally, only one third to one half of the penetration strength for a standard AP of the glenohumeral joint is used to more precisely visualize the AC joint; standard shoulder radiographic penetration will overpenetrate the less dense AC joint. Stress views, using 5-lb weights placed on the wrist and comparing both AC joints, have been advocated in the

past to help distinguish between type II and type III AC joint separation; however, this technique is no longer favored because it usually does not influence the choice of treatment.

Type I and II AC separations are considered incomplete lesions and may be treated conservatively with ice, rest, and a brief period of immobilization followed by therapy. Types IV, V, and VI are complete injuries that usually require surgical reconstruction. Treatment of type III injuries remains controversial.

Sternoclavicular Dislocations

The sternoclavicular joint is the only true articulation between the clavicle and the axial skeleton. Sternoclavicular dislocations are usually the result of high-energy force sustained during a motor vehicle accident or during contact sports activity.

Classification of sternoclavicular dislocations is based on anatomic findings. Anterior dislocations are most common and are present when the medial end of the clavicle is displaced anterior or anterosuperior to the sternum. Patients with anterior dislocations have a palpable medial clavicular head mass that may be more pronounced with abduction and elevation. Posterior dislocations are uncommon but more concerning. The medial end of the clavicle is displaced posteriorly or postero-superiorly and may impinge on vital structures. The patient presents with a hollow region just lateral to the sternum, and may also present with dyspnea or dysphagia.

Radiographic evaluation involves standard chest radiographs as well as the serendipity view obtained by directing the x-ray beam 40° cephalad to visualize both sternoclavicular joints. CT scan and/or MRI are currently the best techniques to evaluate the sternoclavicular joint and clearly distinguish the direction of the dislocation as well as any associated fractures. In patients with posterior dislocation, CT and/or MRI allow for the evaluation of mediastinal structures and visualization of the medial clavicular head in relationship to these structures.

Acute reduction of anterior sternoclavicular dislocations may be attempted with traction of the extended arm. Residual anterior instability is well tolerated but may result in persistent deformity. Posterior dislocations should be reduced in the operating room with care taken to avoid damage to the mediastinal structures.

Annotated Bibliography

Pathophysiology

Urayama M, Itoi E, Hatakeyama Y, Pradhan RL, Sato K: Function of the 3 portions of the inferior glenohumeral ligament: A cadaveric study. *J Shoulder Elbow Surg* 2001;10:589-594.

The strain of the three portions or sections of the inferior glenohumeral ligament in 17 fresh-frozen cadaveric shoulders was studied during elevation and rotational maneuvers. The anterior band and axillary pouch showed the greatest strain in abduction and external rotation, confirming their role as anterior stabilizers. The posterior band showed the greatest strain with flexion and internal rotation, suggesting a key role as a posterior stabilizer.

Urayama M, Itoi E, Sashi R, Minagawa H, Sato K: Capsular elongation in shoulders with recurrent anterior dislocation: Quantitative assessment with magnetic resonance arthrography. *Am J Sports Med* 2003;31:64-67.

Magnetic resonance arthrography was used to evaluate the length of the anteroinferior, inferior, and posteroinferior capsule in 12 patients with unilateral recurrent anterior instability. Unaffected shoulders were used as controls. The anteroinferior and inferior portions of the shoulder capsule were elongated an average of 19% in shoulders with recurrent anterior dislocation compared with the unaffected shoulders.

Treatment of Acute Dislocation

Bottoni CR, Wilckens JH, DeBerardino TM, et al: A prospective, randomized evaluation of arthroscopic stabilization versus nonoperative treatment in patients with acute, traumatic, first-time shoulder dislocations. *Am J Sports Med* 2002;30:576-580.

Twenty-one active duty military personnel between the ages of 18 and 26 years with primary, traumatic shoulder dislocation were randomized to nonsurgical treatment or arthroscopic Bankart repair using a bioabsorbable tack. At an average of 3 years follow-up, 75% of patients treated nonsurgically versus 11% of the patients treated with arthroscopic repair developed recurrent instability. Six of nine patients treated nonsurgically who developed recurrent instability required subsequent open Bankart repair.

Buss DD, Lynch GP, Meyer CP, Huber SM, Freehill MQ: Nonoperative management for in-season athletes with anterior shoulder instability. *Am J Sports Med* 2004;32:1430-1433.

Thirty in-season athletes with either acute or recurrent anterior instability were treated with physical therapy and, if appropriate, bracing. Eighty-seven percent of athletes were able to return to their sport in season and an average of 1.4 recurrent instability episodes per season per athlete occurred. No further injuries were attributable to the shoulder instability. Fifty-three percent of patients had subsequent surgical stabilization in the off-season.

DeBerardino TM, Arciero RA, Taylor DC, et al: Prospective evaluation of arthroscopic stabilization of acute, initial anterior shoulder dislocations in young athletes: Two- to five-year follow-up. *Am J Sports Med* 2001;29:586-592.

Forty-eight cadets at the US Military Academy with 49 anterior dislocations were treated with primary arthroscopic repair using bioabsorbable tacks. At an average follow-up of 37 months, the average Rowe score was 92%, and 88% of shoulders remained stable. Factors associated with failure included a history of bilateral shoulder instability, a 2+ sulcus sign, and poor capsulolabral tissue at the time of repair. All patients with stable shoulders returned to their preinjury levels of athletic activity. These results are favorable compared with nonsurgical treatment in young, active adults at the US Military Academy.

Itoi E, Hatakeyama Y, Kido T, et al: A new method of immobilization after traumatic anterior dislocation of the shoulder: A preliminary study. *J Shoulder Elbow Surg* 2003;12:413-415.

Forty patients were randomly assigned to immobilization in external rotation versus immobilization in internal rotation for 3 weeks after initial anterior dislocation. The average ages in the internal and external groups were 38 years and 40 years, respectively, with similar numbers of patients under the age of 29 years. At approximately 1-year follow-up, the recurrence rate was 30% in the internal rotation group and 0% in the external rotation group. Anterior apprehension was positive in 14% of the internal rotation group without recurrence and 5% of the external rotation group.

Miller SL, Cleeman E, Auerbach J, Flatow EL: Comparison of intra-articular lidocaine and intravenous sedation for reduction of shoulder dislocations: A randomized, prospective study. *J Bone Joint Surg Am* 2002;84: 2135-2139.

In a prospective study, 30 patients with anterior glenohumeral dislocation were randomized to receive either intra-articular lidocaine or intravenous sedation before relocation using the Stimson method. There was no significant difference between the two groups with regard to pain, success of the Stimson technique, or time required for reduction of the shoulder. The lidocaine group spent significantly less time in the emergency department and required less nursing resources.

Treatment of Recurrent Traumatic Instability

Karlsson J, Magnusson L, Ejerhed L, Huttenheim I, Lundin O, Kartus J: Comparison of open and arthroscopic stabilization for recurrent shoulder dislocation in patients with a Bankart lesion. *Am J Sports Med* 2001; 29:538-542.

One hundred eight shoulders with symptomatic, recurrent anterior instability and a Bankart lesion underwent either open stabilization or arthroscopic stabilization with bioabsorbable tack fixation. At a mean follow-up of 28 months, the recurrence rate, including both dislocations and subluxations, was 9 of 60 (15%) in the arthroscopic group, compared with 5 of 48 (10%) in the open group. No significant differences were found between the study groups for the Rowe or Constant scores at follow up. The only significant difference in range of motion assessment was in external rotation in abduction, which was 90° (range, 50° to 135°) in the arthroscopic group and 80° (range, 25° to 115°) in the open group. The treatment groups in this study were not randomized.

Kim SH, Ha KI, Cho YB, Ryu BD, Oh I: Arthroscopic anterior stabilization of the shoulder: Two to six-year follow up. *J Bone Joint Surg Am* 2003;85:1511-1517.

One hundred sixty-seven patients with traumatic recurrent anterior instability were treated with arthroscopic Bankart repair using suture anchors. At a mean follow-up of 44 months, the rate of postoperative recurrence of instability was 4% with a mean loss of external rotation of 2°. Postoperative recurrence was related to an osseous defect of more than 30% of the glenoid circumference. These results compare favorably with historical results of open stabilization.

Sperber A, Hamberg P, Karlsson J, Sward L, Wredmark T: Comparison of an arthroscopic and an open procedure for posttraumatic instability of the shoulder: A prospective, randomized multicenter study. *J Shoulder Elbow Surg* 2001;10:105-108.

Fifty-six patients with anterior instability and a Bankart lesion were randomized to either open stabilization or arthroscopic stabilization with the use of bioabsorbable tacks. Patients were evaluated at 2, 12, and 24 months postoperatively. Thirty patients were surgically treated with the arthroscopic technique and 26 patients with the open technique. In the arthroscopic group, there were recurrences in 7 of 30 patients

(23%) at a mean of 13 months (range, 5 to 21 months) after surgery. In the open group, there were recurrences in 3 of 26 patients (12%) at a mean of 10 months (range, 2 to 23 months) after surgery (*P* = not significant). A tendency toward more redislocations in the arthroscopic group was noted.

Posterior Instability

Kim SH, Ha KI, Park JH, et al: Arthroscopic posterior labral and capsular shift for traumatic unidirectional recurrent posterior subluxation of the shoulder. *J Bone Joint Surg Am* 2003;85:1479-1487.

Twenty-seven patients with unidirectional posterior instability were treated with arthroscopic labral repair and posterior capsular shift using suture anchors. At a mean postoperative follow-up of 39 months, all patients had a stable shoulder by subjective and objective measurements except for one patient who had recurrent subluxation. Twenty-six patients returned to prior sports activity with few or no limitations. The authors also describe arthroscopic findings in traumatic unidirectional recurrent posterior instability.

Williams RJ III, Strickland S, Cohen M, Altchek DW, Warren RF: Arthroscopic repair for traumatic posterior shoulder instability. *Am J Sports Med* 2003;31:203-209.

Twenty-seven shoulders in 26 patients with traumatic posterior shoulder instability were treated with arthroscopic repair using bioabsorbable tack fixation. At a mean follow-up of 5.1 years, no patients showed a range-of-motion deficit. There was no instability greater than 1+ in the anterior, posterior, or inferior directions. Symptoms of pain and instability were eliminated in 24 patients (92%). Two patients (8%) required additional surgery after arthroscopic repair of the posterior Bankart lesion.

Multidirectional Instability

Favorito PJ, Langenderfer MA, Colosimo AJ, Heidt RS Jr, Carolonas RL: Arthroscopic laser-assisted capsular shift in the treatment of patients with multidirectional shoulder instability. *Am J Sports Med* 2002;30:322-328.

Twenty-seven shoulders in 25 patients with multidirectional shoulder instability were treated with an arthroscopic laser-assisted capsular shift procedure. At an average follow-up of 28 months, 22 shoulders had no recurrent symptoms and required no further surgical intervention. In five shoulders, treatment was considered a failure because of recurrent pain or instability and the need for an open capsular shift procedure. With recurrent instability as a measure of failure, the overall success rate was 81.5%.

Fitzgerald BT, Watson BT, Lapoint JM: The use of thermal capsulorrhaphy in the treatment of multidirectional instability. *J Shoulder Elbow Surg* 2002;11:108-113.

Thirty shoulders with multidirectional instability were treated with arthroscopic thermal capsulorrhaphy. At a mean follow-up of 36 months (range, 24 to 40 months), 3 excellent, 20 good, and 7 poor results were reported using the University of California at Los Angeles score. Twenty-three patients (76%) returned to full activity.

McFarland EG, Kim TK, Banchasuek P, McCarthy EF: Histologic evaluation of the shoulder capsule in normal shoulders, unstable shoulders, and after failed thermal capsulorrhaphy. *Am J Sports Med* 2002;30:636-642.

Shoulder capsules were evaluated histologically in 12 patients with traumatic anterior instability and in 7 patients who experienced recurrent instability after a thermal capsulorrhaphy. The capsules of six fresh-frozen cadavers with no shoulder lesions were used as controls. In patients who had a history of traumatic instability, a denuded synovial layer was present in 58%, subsynovial edema in 58%, increased cellularity in 25%, and increased vascularity in 83%. At the time of surgery, five of seven shoulders in the failed thermal capsulorrhaphy group (71%) were subjectively felt to be thin and attenuated. Denuded synovium was found in 100% of these patients, subsynovial edema in 43%, and changes in the collagen layer in 100%. Changes in the collagen layer in these patients included the appearance of hyalinization in five patients (71%), increased collagen fibrosis in two patients (29%), and increased cellularity in two patients (29%).

von Eisenhart-Rothe RM, Jager A, Englmeier KH, Vogl TJ, Graichen H: Relevance of arm position and muscle activity on three-dimensional glenohumeral translation in patients with traumatic and atraumatic shoulder instability. *Am J Sports Med* 2002;30:514-522.

Open MRI and three-dimensional post processing technique was used to evaluate glenohumeral translation with different arm positions with and without muscle activation in 12 patients with traumatic and 10 patients with atraumatic instability. In patients with traumatic instability, increased translation was observed only in functionally important arm positions, whereas intact active stabilizers showed sufficient recentering. In patients with atraumatic instability, a decentralized head position was recorded also during muscle activity, suggesting alterations of the active stabilizers.

Wallace AL, Hollinshead RM: FrankCB: Electrothermal shrinkage reduces laxity but alters creep behavior in a lapine ligament model. *J Shoulder Elbow Surg* 2001;10:1-6.

Using a lapine medial collateral ligament laxity model, the acute effects of radiofrequency shrinkage were assessed. Thermal treatment resulted in restoration of laxity but a significant increase in the cyclic and static creep strains compared with control sides. The authors concluded that radiofrequency electrothermal shrinkage is effective at reducing laxity but significantly alters viscoelastic properties, posing a risk of recurrent stretching-out at physiologic loads.

Failed Instability Surgery

Diaz JA, Cohen SB, Warren RF, Craig EV, Allen AA: Arthrodesis as a salvage procedure for recurrent instability of the shoulder. *J Shoulder Elbow Surg* 2003;12:237-241.

Eight patients with recurrent shoulder instability with an average of seven prior stabilization attempts were treated with glenohumeral arthrodesis. The average time to bony union after arthrodesis was 3.5 months (range, 2.5 to 5 months). At mean follow-up of 35 months, the patients reported significant overall subjective improvement as a group after fusion. None of the patients reported instability postoperatively. All eight patients stated that they would repeat the surgery again under similar preoperative circumstances.

Iannotti JP, Antoniou J, William GR, Ramsey ML: Iliotibial band reconstruction for treatment of glenohumeral instability associated with irreparable capsular deficiency. *J Shoulder Elbow Surg* 2002;11:618-623.

Seven patients with recurrent anterior instability after failed surgery complicated by the loss of capsular tissue underwent reconstruction of the capsular ligaments using the iliotibial band. After iliotibial band reconstruction, the patients showed significant improvement in their American Shoulder and Elbow Surgeons score ($P = 0.0004$), and no patient had any persistent symptoms of instability. Physiologic range of motion and function were maintained. The authors describe their surgical technique for iliotibial band reconstruction for capsular deficiency.

Acromioclavicular Separations

Schlegel TF, Burks RT, Marcus RL, Dunn HK: A prospective evaluation of untreated acute grade III acromioclavicular separations. *Am J Sports Med* 2001;29:699-703.

Twenty patients with acute grade III AC separations were treated nonsurgically with a sling for comfort through progressive early range of motion as tolerated and completed a 1-year evaluation and strength-testing protocol. Subjectively, 4 of the 20 patients (20%) thought that their long-term outcome was suboptimal, although 3 of them did not believe that the outcome should warrant surgery. Objective examination and strength testing of the 20 patients revealed no limitation of shoulder motion in the injured extremity and no difference between sides in rotational shoulder muscle strength. The bench press was the only strength test that showed a significant short-term difference, with the injured extremity being an average of 17% weaker.

Classic Bibliography

Bankart ASB: The pathology and treatment of recurrent dislocation of the shoulder-joint. *Br J Surg* 1938;26:23-29.

Burkhart SS, DeBeer JF: Traumatic glenohumeral bone defects and their relationship to failure of arthroscopic Bankart repairs: Significance of the inverted-pear glenoid and humeral engaging Hill-Sachs lesion. *Arthroscopy* 2000;16:677-694.

Curl LA, Warren RF: Glenohumeral joint stability: Selective cutting studies on the static capsular restraints. *Clin Orthop* 1996;330:54-65.

Hovelius L, Augustini BG, Fredin H, Johansson O, Norlin R, Thorling J: Primary anterior dislocation of the shoulder in young patients: A ten-year prospective study. *J Bone Joint Surg Am* 1996;78:1677-1684.

Neer CS II, Foster CR: Inferior capsular shift for involuntary inferior and multidirectional instability of the shoulder: A preliminary report. *J Bone Joint Surg Am* 1980;62:897-908.

O'Brien SJ, Neves MC, Arnoczky SP, et al: The anatomy and histology of the inferior glenohumeral ligament complex of the shoulder. *Am J Sports Med* 1990;18:449-456.

Rowe CR, Patel D, Southmayd WW: The Bankart procedure: A long-term end-result study. *J Bone Joint Surg Am* 1978;60:1-16.

Speer KP, Deng X, Borrero S, Torzilli PA, Altchek DA, Warren RF: Biomechanical evaluation of a simulated Bankart lesion. *J Bone Joint Surg Am* 1994;76:1819-1826.

Thomas SC, Matsen FA III: An approach to the repair of avulsion of the glenohumeral ligaments in the management of traumatic anterior glenohumeral instability. *J Bone Joint Surg Am* 1989;71:506-513.

Tossy JD, Mead NC, Sigmon HM: Acromioclavicular separations: Useful and practical classification for treatment. *Clin Orthop* 1963;28:111-119.

Weaver JK, Dunn HK: treatment of acromioclavicular injuries, especially complete acromioclavicular separation. *J Bone Joint Surg Am* 1972;54:1187-1194.

Wheeler JH, Ryan JB, Arciero RA, et al: Arthroscopic versus nonsurgical treatment of acute shoulder dislocations in young athletes. *Arthroscopy* 1989;5:213-217.

Zabinski SJ, Calloway HG, Cohen S, Warren RF: Revision shoulder stabilization 2 to 10 year results. *J Shoulder Elbow Surg* 1999;8:58-65.

Chapter 26

Shoulder Reconstruction

Leesa M. Galatz, MD

Rotator Cuff Tear

Pathophysiology

The etiology of rotator cuff tears has not been clearly elucidated. Focus has centered primarily on intrinsic and extrinsic mechanisms of generating rotator cuff tears, with reports in the early literature primarily focused on an extrinsic mechanism. Three types of acromial morphology were defined (types I, II, and III), with increasing curvature of each type. Type III acromions, with maximal curvature or hooking of the undersurface, were associated with an increased incidence of rotator cuff tears resulting from increased mechanical contact of the cuff with the bone. Recent studies have provided data that do not substantiate this early information and suggest a much more complex etiology for rotator cuff tears.

Attention has focused on the role and contribution of plain radiographic imaging for the diagnosis and detection of full-thickness rotator cuff tears. Acromial osteophytes or spurring, acromioclavicular degeneration, and lateral clavicular and acromial sclerosis seen on plain radiographs have been correlated with age rather than rotator cuff disease. Rotator cuff disease, especially involving full-thickness tears, has also been correlated with age, complicating the issue. Although some cadaveric studies have demonstrated an association between spurring of the anterior acromion and the acromioclavicular joint and rotator cuff tears, a direct causal relationship between degenerative radiographic changes and full-thickness tears has not been definitively proven. One recent study of radiographic changes in 40 patients with full-thickness cuff tears and a large group of age-matched controls found no association between acromial morphology and rotator cuff tears. Findings that were indicative of cuff tears included sclerosis, osteophytes, subchondral cysts, and osteolysis of the greater tuberosity. There was no relationship between any of these findings in the greater tuberosity and tear size.

Intrinsic mechanisms of rotator cuff degeneration have been implicated in the etiology of rotator cuff tears. Histologic changes in chronic rotator cuff tissue tears have shown degenerative changes, but there is little evidence of acute inflammation. This finding reinforces the notion that changes in proteoglycan and other extracellular matrix protein content in the aging tendon may have a role in attritional changes leading to tears. More research is necessary to make definitive conclusions regarding the true etiology, and it is likely that both intrinsic and extrinsic mechanisms as well as patient-related factors contribute to the development of rotator cuff disease.

After a rotator cuff is torn, several changes can occur in the shoulder joint. Clinically these changes manifest as pain and decreased strength and range of motion. Radiographic changes can include proximal migration of the humeral head, narrowing of the acromial-humeral interval, sclerosis of the undersurface of the acromion and superior humeral head, acetabularization or rounding of the undersurface of the acromion such that it is congruent with the humeral head, and degenerative changes of the glenohumeral joint. Most of these changes occur only with massive, long-standing rotator cuff tears. These structural changes to the joint with rotator cuff tears result from kinematic changes secondary to loss of the normal muscle forces about the shoulder. The purposes of the rotator cuff are to keep the humeral head centered on the glenoid (termed concavity compression) by counteracting the superior vector of the deltoid, and to add strength and dynamic stability to glenohumeral motion.

Several recent basic science studies have been performed to investigate the changes in forces and motion patterns associated with rotator cuff tears. One cadaveric study examined the effect of rotator cuff tears on joint reaction forces at the glenohumeral joint. There were no significant differences in joint reaction force magnitude or direction with abduction motion between the intact state, partial supraspinatus tear, or complete supraspinatus tear. Extension of tears beyond the supraspinatus tendon resulted in a significant decrease in the magnitude of the joint reaction force. Additionally, the vector of the force changed direction toward the deficient area. Clinically, this finding may explain why some patients with fairly large tears may still maintain function. The critical tear size at which the force couple of the remaining musculature is overcome and pseudoparalysis of the shoulder results is yet to be determined, and clinically seems to differ between individuals.

Another cadaveric study was performed to compare the effects of supraspinatus detachments, tendon defects, and muscle retraction. Simply detaching a portion of the supraspinatus tendon had no effect on the force transmitted by the rotator cuff. Detaching or creating a defect of the entire supraspinatus tendon led to a moderate decrease in force transmission (11% and 17%, respectively). However, when the investigators simulated muscle retraction of the tendon by incising medially to detach the tendon from adjacent tendon tissue, there were substantial reductions in force transmission (58% with involvement of the entire supraspinatus). Side-to-side repair of smaller defects restored force capability, but a deficit remained even after side-to-side repair of the entire supraspinatus tendon retraction simulation. This study supports the cable concept of force transmission of the rotator cuff, and suggests that the amount of retraction and not just transverse diameter may be an important factor in functional deficit after a rotator cuff tear.

Natural History

The severity of rotator cuff disease ranges from painful cuffs without tears to partial-thickness tears to full-thickness tear. It is not known whether this is a continuous spectrum in which a patient will go from one stage to the next as part of the natural history of their condition or whether some patients present at one stage, never progressing to another. One longitudinal ultrasonographic study showed that over a time period of 5 years, approximately 28% of patients had an increase in size of known full-thickness rotator cuff tears. Additionally, more recent data show a high prevalence of full-thickness tears in the opposite shoulders of patients with full-thickness tears, and this was also seen more often as patients get older. Research on the natural history of tears is ongoing and more information will likely be available in the near future.

Evaluation

History and Examination

Patients with rotator cuff tears report a history of shoulder pain and/or weakness. Pain associated with rotator cuff tears is usually located on the anterolateral aspect of the shoulder and often radiates distally toward the deltoid insertion. Pain that radiates below the elbow to the hand should raise suspicion of cervical radiculopathy or peripheral nerve compression.

Examination should begin with an inspection of both shoulders to detect asymmetry or muscle atrophy. The examiner should stand behind the patient and observe the scapulae during overhead elevation for winging and motion pattern. Range of motion should be recorded for elevation in the scapular plane, external rotation at the side, and external rotation in abduction to fully examine the anterior capsule. Internal rotation can be tested by internal rotation of the shoulder with the arm in 90° of abduction and by asking the patient to reach behind the back. Side-to-side comparison is critical to determine normal motion, as range of motion differs between individuals.

Supraspinatus strength is tested by external rotation with the arm at the side with the shoulder in neutral or slight internal rotation. Testing external rotation with the shoulder in external rotation allows substitution by the posterior deltoid. Placing the arm in 90° of abduction in the scapular plane with the thumbs down and asking the patient to resist downward pressure is another way to isolate the supraspinatus. This test (Jobe's) is useful for both strength and pain. A lag sign (for testing the posterosuperior rotator cuff) is performed by placing the arm in maximal external rotation. A patient with a large or massive tear will not be able to maintain the arm in this position and the hand will swing toward neutral rotation. In a patient with a massive tear, including the teres minor, the hornblower's sign will be positive (the patient is unable to externally rotate the arm to 90° with the arm in abduction). Positive results from these two tests are usually associated with massive tears and there is correlation with fatty degeneration of the cuff musculature.

Subscapularis integrity is tested using the lift-off test and the abdominal compression test. The lift-off test involves placing the arm behind the back, at the midline, at waist level. The patient is asked to raise the hand off the back, a motion requiring an intact subscapularis. An abdominal compression test is performed by placing the hand flat on the abdomen with a straight line between the hand, wrist, and elbow. A patient with a torn subscapularis will either bend the wrist to keep the hand on the abdomen or lose contact. Internal strength can be tested in this position as well.

The Neer and Hawkins impingement signs are used to detect pain related to rotator cuff disease by provoking impingement in the subacromial space by internally rotating the shoulder, bringing the greater tuberosity underneath the acromion, and minimizing space available for the cuff. A thorough examination should also include evaluation of the acromioclavicular joint for pain on direct palpation and pain with cross-body adduction. Biceps tendon pathology is often associated with rotator cuff tears. The Speed and Yergason tests are sensitive for biceps tendon pain.

Diagnostic Studies

Plain radiographs should be the initial radiographic study of choice. A standard series should include an AP radiograph of the shoulder with the arm in internal rotation, an AP radiograph of the scapula with the arm in neutral or slight external rotation, an outlet view, and an axillary view. The acromioclavicular joint is best visualized on the AP view of the shoulder. The glenohumeral joint space is assessed on the scapular AP and the axillary views, in which degenerative changes are best detected. The outlet view enables evaluation of acromial morphology. MRI is valuable for evaluating the soft tissues about the shoulder and is a sensitive and specific test for rotator cuff pathology. The role of ultrasonography in the evaluation of the rotator cuff has gained popularity in recent years because it is highly accurate in making the diagnosis of full-thickness and partial-thickness tears. Because the reliability of ultrasonography is operator-dependent, significant experience should be gained before this study is used independently. MRI has largely replaced arthrography, which is rarely used; however, arthrography remains a good alternative if an MRI evaluation cannot be obtained and an ultrasound is not available.

Treatment of Partial-Thickness Rotator Cuff Tears

Partial-thickness tears are often managed successfully with nonsurgical treatment. An exercise program focuses on range of motion, stretching, and strengthening of the rotator cuff, deltoid, and scapular stabilizers. Partial-thickness tears that do not become asymptomatic with nonsurgical treatment can be effectively treated surgically. Arthroscopic treatment entails débridement of the tear after careful inspection of both the articular and bursal sides. In general, if the tear involves less than 50% of the thickness of the cuff, débridement should be adequate. If the tear involves more than 50% of the thickness of the cuff or the remaining tissue is degenerative and easily débrided, then the tear is expanded to a full-thickness tear and healthy tissue is repaired primarily. Recently, several arthroscopic methods of imbricating partial-thickness tears and repairing laminated flaps have been described, and offer promising options in the management of partial-thickness tears.

Treatment of Full-Thickness Rotator Cuff Tears

Nonsurgical treatment for full-thickness tears is the same as for partial-thickness tears in terms of exercise and pain control measures. Surgical treatment of symptomatic full-thickness rotator cuff tears is indicated in patients in whom nonsurgical treatment has failed and who are candidates for surgery, those with acute tears, and patients with tears associated with a sudden loss of strength and function. Relative indications include younger people of working age with a painful tear. Factors to consider include the following: (1) tears are easier to repair when they are smaller, and there is documented evidence that tear size can increase with time; (2) there is a higher recurrence rate after repair of large and massive tears; (3) long-standing chronic tears are associated with muscle atrophy and fatty degeneration, which are irreversible changes that can compromise functional outcome after repair; and (4) there may be attritional changes in the tendon edge of chronic tears that may compromise healing potential.

Surgical Approaches

An open surgical approach involves an incision and removal of the anterior deltoid origin from the acromion to maximize exposure. The major advantage of an open repair is the extensive exposure and ability to mobilize the cuff under direct observation. It also requires no arthroscopic skills. A mini-open repair is alternatively performed through a deltoid split rather than removing the deltoid origin. To achieve a repair using a mini-open approach, arthroscopic assistance is used. Because exposure is more limited, inspection, cuff mobilization, and the acromioplasty are performed with the use of the arthroscope, obviating the need for a more extensile approach. The major advantage of a mini-open repair is that the deltoid is not removed from the acromion. Removal of the deltoid is one of the more painful aspects of the open procedure, and failure of the deltoid repair is a serious and painful complication for which there is no reliable option for correction.

Arthroscopic repair of full-thickness tears has gained recent popularity. As equipment and techniques continue to advance, this approach will likely continue to become easier and more achievable with advanced arthroscopic skills. Potential advantages of an arthroscopic approach include decreased scarring, easier rehabilitation, decreased pain, and improved cosmesis. Damage to the deltoid is minimized with an arthroscopic approach. One disadvantage to an arthroscopic repair may be a higher recurrence rate after repair of large and massive tears. The procedure requires advanced arthroscopic skills, which may be considered by some to be a disadvantage of using the procedure; however, the use of minimally invasive approaches is becoming mainstream.

Role of Acromioplasty

An acromioplasty has historically been a standard aspect of a rotator cuff repair based on Neer's classic description of impingement syndrome and the theory that contact with the rigid coracoacromial arch is the mechanical impetus for rotator cuff tears. An acromioplasty entails takedown of the coracoacromial ligament from the anterior acromion and removal of bone from the undersurface of the acromion to increase the space available for the rotator cuff. Historically, removal of large amounts of bone, including full-thickness removal

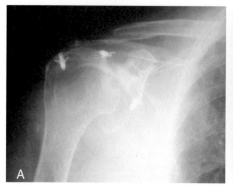 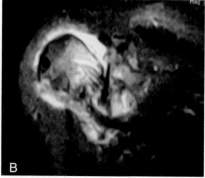 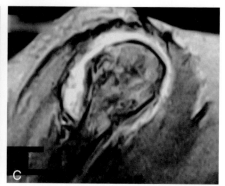

Figure 1 A, Radiograph of a shoulder after failed rotator cuff repair and distal clavicle resection. The anchors have failed, the humeral head has migrated anteriorly and superiorly, and degenerative changes have begun to involve the glenohumeral joint. **B,** MRI of the shoulder demonstrates the massive rotator cuff tear and proximal migration. **C,** A sagittal oblique cut of the MRI demonstrates the cuff insufficiency as well as the deltoid attenuation.

of bone from the anterior acromion in some instances, was recommended. The more recent trend for acromioplasty is to remove enough bone to make the undersurface of the acromion flat to protect the origin of the deltoid. One anatomic study found that the average thickness of the acromion was 7 mm. Therefore, removal of large amounts of bone, as had been previously recommended, could potentially compromise the acromion and deltoid origin.

Results of Treatment

Rotator cuff repair has historically been a reliable option for pain relief over time. This finding has been substantiated by two long-term follow-up studies. In a recent study, results of a large number of patients treated with open cuff repair, V-Y plasty, tendon transposition, and reinforcement with fascia lata were reported. Tear size was the most important determinant of outcome with regard to active motion, strength, rating of the result, patient satisfaction, and need for another operation. Another recent study reported over 90% good to excellent results in a prospective series of patients after open cuff repair on the shoulder. These patients were studied longitudinally over a 10-year period. Outcome at 10 years had not deteriorated from the 2-year results, demonstrating the longevity of results after rotator cuff repair.

One recent study showed 46 of 48 good to excellent results after arthroscopic repair of medium to large full-thickness rotator cuff repairs. Forty-four of 45 patients were satisfied with the results. Another study reported on the results of arthroscopic rotator cuff repair of large and massive chronic tears. Despite a high rate of satisfaction and significantly improved functional outcome, ultrasonographic analysis revealed 17 of 18 patients had recurrent tears. These results suggest that success in terms of functional outcome and pain relief may not correlate with anatomic healing of the rotator cuff. In a

series of tears involving the subscapularis, a lower Constant score correlated with duration of symptoms longer than 6 months and the appearance of fatty degeneration and atrophy of the subscapularis muscle as detected by MRI. The authors recommended repair of the subscapularis before 6 months of symptoms to maximize functional outcome.

Complications

The rate of complications after rotator cuff repair is low in most series. Potential complications include stiffness, infection, deltoid dehiscence after open repair, failure of repair, and less commonly, neurovascular injury. Although the incidence of infection is low after rotator cuff repair, recently one organism, *Propionibacterium acnes*, has gained attention as a frequent cause of infection in the shoulder. This is a low virulence organism that was found in the few infections in a large series of mini-open rotator cuff repairs.

Another complication that has become increasingly recognized is anterior-superior instability in the shoulder associated with massive, irreparable cuff tears. This complication results from a combination of rotator cuff insufficiency, disruption of the coracoacromial arch, and anterior deltoid dehiscence. Anterior-superior instability usually is an iatrogenic complication after open cuff repair and subacromial decompression where the deltoid and rotator cuff repair have failed (Figure 1). Clinically, it is recognized by proximal and anterior migration of the humeral head to the subcutaneous position and obligates extension of the shoulder with attempted overhead elevation. This condition occurs because the intact posterior and lateral deltoid exert a superior vector on the humerus, with no rotator cuff or coracoacromial arch to keep the head contained. Surgical attempts at coracoacromial arch reconstruction and muscle transfers for treatment of this problem have met with unpredictable results and limited success.

Treatment of the Massive Rotator Cuff Tear

Treatment of the massive rotator cuff tear is a controversial issue. It is important to consider that the massive tear does not equal the irreparable tear. Many massive tears are easily repairable, and some smaller tears and many massive tears can be irreparable. Preoperative evaluation of the massive tear should give some indication as to the likelihood of successful repair. MRI demonstrating significant atrophy and fatty degeneration of the musculature (Figure 2) along with a history consistent with a chronic tear can indicate a difficult if not impossible repair. Most studies that have examined the anatomic results after rotator cuff repair have demonstrated a higher rate of recurrence with larger tears. Therefore, preoperative discussions with patients should include a discussion of these results as well as patient goals and expectations after surgery. Overall, repair of a massive tear can be potentially predictable for pain relief, but it is much less reliable for restoring lost strength.

Nonsurgical treatment should be attempted initially, especially in the older patient with lower physical demands. Younger patients of working age in whom strength is more important are exceptions; early intervention should be considered in these patients to avoid future irreversible, degenerative changes that compromise results. Physical therapy helps to strengthen the remaining musculature about the shoulder and improve kinematics to facilitate or regain range of motion. Nonsteroidal anti-inflammatory drugs and cortisone injections are options for providing pain relief.

Surgical treatment options include open or mini-open repair, débridement, and arthroscopic repair. Most studies of open and mini-open repair have found that an increasing tear size correlates with inferior results. Simple débridement and acromioplasty have been advocated, especially for irreparable tears, with a reported 83% satisfaction rate for this procedure at an average 6.5-year follow-up. In other studies, it was shown that the results of treatment with débridement were inferior to results in a series in which the cuffs were repaired. Results of débridement deteriorated with time, and a comparison of results of débridement with those of open repair found that patients who had open repair had better strength, function, and outcome scores, although patient satisfaction was comparable.

Arthroscopic treatment is particularly advantageous in the management of massive rotator cuff tears because it allows assessment of whether the tear is repairable before an open incision and splitting or detaching of the deltoid is performed. An intact deltoid is critical for a good result in a patient with a massive tear, whether or not it is repaired. Limited, early results of arthroscopic repair are promising. In a previously mentioned study of arthroscopic repair of large and massive tears, there was

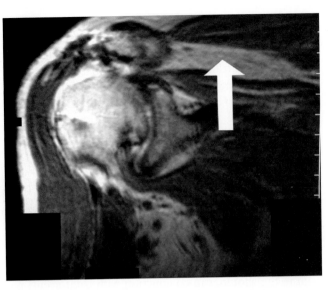

Figure 2 An MRI of a massive cuff tear. The cuff has retracted to the level of the superior glenoid rim. The muscle belly has undergone severe atrophic changes and a widened subtrapezial fat space (arrow) is evident. There is also proximal migration of the humeral head relative to the glenoid.

a significant improvement in functional outcome and pain relief, and a high degree of patient satisfaction despite a high recurrence rate. The margin convergence technique has been used in patients undergoing arthroscopic repair of massive tears, with an improvement in range of motion and high degree of patient satisfaction. One recent study reported on the results of tuberoplasty, a procedure in which the bony excrescences of the greater tuberosity are débrided such that the humeral head conforms to the rounded undersurface of the acromion. No subacromial decompression was performed in this series. Although the long-term results of arthroscopic treatment in patients with massive tears are not yet available, early results suggest that it can play a role in the management of this challenging problem. A repair should be performed if possible. The role of an acromioplasty alone in the treatment of a massive rotator cuff tear remains debatable, but it is clear that excessive bone removal along with compromise of the anterior deltoid leads to significantly inferior results and is therefore contraindicated. If an acromioplasty is performed, an arthroscopic approach and conservative bone removal, if any, are recommended.

The final option for treatment of a massive rotator cuff tear is a muscle transfer. A transfer of the pectoralis major is performed for a chronic irreparable subscapularis tear, and a latissimus transfer is used for posterior and superior cuff insufficiency. Other transfers have been described, but results are not as favorable and they are rarely used today. Indications for a latissimus transfer for an irreparable tear involving supraspinatus, infraspinatus, and teres minor tears are primarily pain and loss of function. Relative indications are a young, active patient and an intact subscapularis. Inferior results are reported for patients with concurrent subscapularis tears. The deltoid must also be intact and functioning well. A muscle transfer is a major reconstructive procedure with a long period of rehabilitation, and should only be considered as a salvage operation for patients willing and able to undergo the operation and comply with the rehabilitative program.

Role of the Biceps Tendon

The role of the long head of the biceps tendon continues to generate interest and controversy. Its exact function, if any, in the shoulder is a subject of debate with both cadaveric and clinical studies that support several differing viewpoints. Nevertheless, the long head of the biceps tendon is an increasingly recognized source of pain in the shoulder in conjunction with rotator cuff pathology. The synovial lining of the glenohumeral joint is continuous with the tenosynovium of the proximal biceps so any inflammatory process involving the joint can affect the biceps tendon as well.

The biceps tendon should be carefully inspected during any rotator cuff repair to rule out any concurrent pathology. This evaluation is generally performed as part of the arthroscopic assessment. The portion of the biceps tendon from the intertubercular groove should be pulled into the joint for inspection as well. Lesions of the tendon can include inflammation of the tendon, tearing, or instability relative to the intertubercular groove. Instability is always associated with subscapularis tears or tears of the rotator interval. In some circumstances, the tendon may have already ruptured. This condition is more common in conjunction with larger tears.

Minor fraying involving only a minimal amount of the tendon proper can be débrided; however, a tear involving 50% or more of the tendon should be treated with tenotomy or tenodesis. Any instability of the tendon should also be treated in this fashion. The issue of whether to use tenotomy or tenodesis of the long head of the biceps tendon is also a subject of debate. In general, tenodesis is indicated in younger patients (younger than 55 years) because of concerns about muscle cramping and cosmesis. Potential disadvantages are increased length of the procedure, possible pain at the tenodesis site, and the possibility of an additional incision. Older patients have done well with simple tenotomy, with little to no noticeable deformity, but it is important to discuss the possibility of either procedure with patients preoperatively.

Recently, biceps tenotomy has been performed as part of the surgical procedure for massive rotator cuff tears. In one series containing the largest number of patients treated with tenotomy for rotator cuff tears, tenotomy was found to be particularly effective for massive tears.

Glenohumeral Joint Arthritis
Etiology

Glenohumeral joint arthritis results from multiple different etiologies, including primary osteoarthritis, the synovial-based arthroses such as rheumatoid arthritis, osteonecrosis, posttraumatic arthritis, malunion or nonunion of the proximal humerus, rotator cuff arthropathy, and arthritis associated with instability or surgery for instability. The etiology of shoulder arthritis is important because each of these entities is associated with certain characteristics that impact the technique and/or outcome of the surgery.

Primary osteoarthritis is associated with osteophyte formation and posterior glenoid wear. Posterior wear can make glenoid implantation very challenging and at times can even preclude glenoid insertion. One solution to this problem is bone grafting the glenoid with internally fixed corticocancellous bone. A recent report on this procedure in 21 shoulders with an average correction of 33° demonstrated that this is a technically demanding procedure with failure in eight patients. Rheumatoid arthritis, on the other hand, can be associated with osteophyte formation but more typically presents with central wear of the glenoid, osteopenia, bone erosions, and subchondral cyst formation.

Arthritis secondary to previous instability surgery is thought to arise because of an imbalance in the soft tissues surrounding the shoulder. This condition most often occurs after older instability procedures that involved transfer or imbrication of the subscapularis have been done, leaving the shoulder extremely deficient in external rotation. These shoulders also have large osteophyte formation and preferential posterior glenoid wear. The soft-tissue contractures and scarring about the shoulder make the approach and exposure for shoulder arthroplasty extremely difficult. Static posterior subluxation of the humeral head has recently been recognized as a possible etiology of early glenohumeral arthritis in young adults. One recent article discussing a small group of men (average age, 40 years) with early arthritis found an increase in mean glenoid retroversion and marked static posterior subluxation. The condition was unresponsive to surgical treatment, and could indicate a risk for the development of glenohumeral arthritis in some patients.

Arthroplasty after nonunion or malunion of the proximal humerus is another very difficult problem to manage. The outcome is better if the reconstruction does not involve osteotomy of the tuberosities. Therefore, every effort should be made to accommodate the abnormal bony anatomy with a modular prosthesis (Figure 3). Osteonecrosis is characterized by sclerosis early, bone collapse at the later stages, and degenerative changes on both the glenoid and humeral sides at the last stage. Stiffness is often a prominent characteristic of arthritis associated with osteonecrosis.

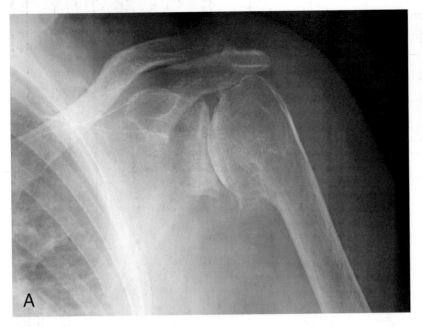
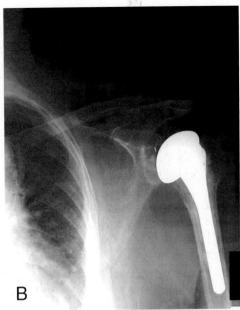

Figure 3 A, A healed proximal humerus fracture has left the surgical neck with a varus malunion. The glenohumeral joint shows evidence of posttraumatic arthritis. **B,** A prosthesis has been placed without osteotomy of the surgical neck or greater tuberosity. Modularity of the prosthesis facilitates an attempt to recreate normal anatomy.

Surgical Treatment

Indications and Contraindications

The main indication for shoulder arthroplasty is end-stage arthritis associated with pain unresponsive to non-surgical measures. Contraindications include active infection, absence of both deltoid and rotator cuff musculature, neuropathic arthropathy such as a Charcot joint, and intractable instability. Relative contraindications to glenoid implantation include young patients, excessive bone loss from the glenoid, and rotator cuff arthropathy.

Prosthetic Arthroplasty: Hemiarthroplasty Versus Total Shoulder Arthroplasty

Prosthetic replacement for primary osteoarthritis has historically been associated with extremely favorable results. Whether to use hemiarthroplasty or total shoulder arthroplasty remains a topic of debate. Advantages cited for performing a hemiarthroplasty include less lateralization of the joint line, less time spent in the operating room, less blood loss, easier procedure, and the fact that conversion to total shoulder arthroplasty can be performed at a later date. Advantages of glenoid implantation include better pain relief and longer survival of the arthroplasty. Various authors have reported good results using both techniques. Most of the recent literature however, supports the use of glenoid components because the results are better for pain relief in long-term follow-up. One prospective, randomized study showed superior results in the total shoulder group, with a 12% revision rate in the hemiarthroplasty group at an average follow-up of 35 months. In this study, the only fac-tors that made hemiarthroplasty advantageous over to-tal shoulder replacement were shorter operating room time and less blood loss. Another study of the long-term follow-up of both procedures cited the 15-year survival rate as 93% for the patients who had total shoulder arthroplasty and 75% for the patients who underwent hemiarthroplasty.

Results of conversion of a hemiarthroplasty to a to-tal shoulder arthroplasty at a later date has not proved to be as satisfactory as originally thought. There is often severe bone loss on the glenoid side after a hemiarthro-plasty, which makes glenoid implantation more chal-lenging (Figure 4). Pain relief in this group of patients is not as predictable; additional surgery is often required. In one series of 18 conversions, there was marked pain relief and increased range of motion; however, results were unsatisfactory in 7 because of limited motion and additional surgery. Overall, although some controversy still exists, total shoulder replacement including implan-tation of a glenoid component is emerging as the stan-dard for the treatment of primary osteoarthritis.

It is well established in the literature that pain relief is much better with total shoulder arthroplasty for rheu-matoid arthritis. A recent study of 105 shoulder arthro-plasties in patients with rheumatoid arthritis showed no statistical difference in Constant score between humeral head replacement and total shoulder arthroplasty. The group that underwent total shoulder arthroplasty had a high rate of glenoid lucencies (58%), but none required revision, demonstrating excellent longevity of the gle-noid in this population. Of significance, in the group that had humeral head replacement, there was superior

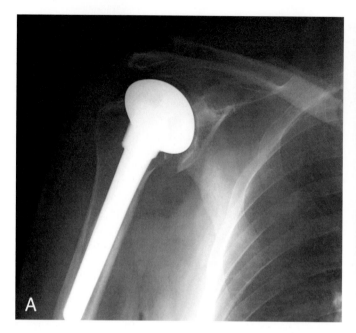

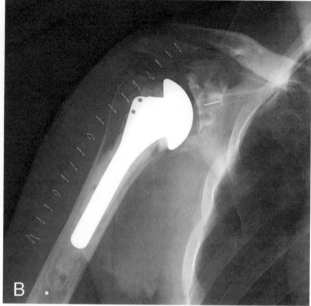

Figure 4 A, A hemiarthroplasty was placed for osteoarthritis in this patient, without relief of pain. The head is slightly proud and asymmetric glenoid wear has occurred such that the center of the glenoid is worn to the base of the coracoid. **B,** The hemiarthroplasty was converted to a total shoulder arthroplasty. A pegged glenoid component was inserted to restore joint space and help lateralize the joint line to a more anatomic location.

migration of the humeral component by more than 5 mm in 28% and medial migration by more than 2 mm in 16%. This migration did adversely affect the outcome in these patients. Overall, the 8-year survival rate was 92% in this population. The issue of bone wear in rheumatoid arthritis remains a critical complication in terms of potential reconstruction. Rheumatoid shoulders tend to have central wear of the glenoid, which can eventually preclude implantation of a prosthetic component. Therefore, at this point, the standard of care is to perform a total shoulder arthroplasty in a rheumatoid shoulder unless severe bone wear already makes this impossible.

When osteonecrosis is diagnosed at an early stage before the development of degenerative changes on the glenoid, the results of hemiarthroplasty have been consistently favorable. In patients with long-standing disease with radiographic involvement of the glenoid or in patients in whom cartilage wear is discovered at the time of surgery, total shoulder arthroplasty is recommended.

Glenoid implantation is generally not recommended in patients with rotator cuff arthropathy. These shoulders are characterized by severe degenerative changes to the glenohumeral joint, with complete loss of the joint space in combination with a massive rotator cuff tear with subsequent loss of rotator cuff function, resulting in proximal migration of the humeral head such that it articulates with the undersurface of the acromion. There also is often a slight anterior superior subluxation. Glenoid implantation during arthroplasty for ro-

tator cuff arthropathy has historically been discouraged because of concerns over early loosening. Earlier recommendations were to oversize the humeral head in these shoulders. The technique of humeral head replacement has evolved, however, and anatomic head sizing is now advised. Overstuffing the joint has been associated with painful arthroplasty because of soft-tissue stretch. This overstuffing also lateralizes the deltoid insertion, compromising its function. Preservation of the coracoacromial arch is critical during humeral head replacement for rotator cuff arthropathy to prevent anterior-superior instability. Bipolar components have not demonstrated improved results in these cases and are rarely used. Reverse ball and socket prostheses are still under investigation and may hold promise for future use in treating rotator cuff arthropathy.

Total Shoulder Arthroplasty
Total shoulder arthroplasty is a reliable operation for pain relief and good function can be anticipated. Recently, a large study reported the results of arthroplasty for osteoarthritis using a third generation, anatomically designed shoulder prosthesis. Patients were evaluated using the age-adjusted Constant score an average of 30 months postoperatively. The score improved from an average of 37 to 97 postoperatively. Good or excellent results were obtained in 77% of patients, and 94% were satisfied or very satisfied. Forward elevation was 145°.

Another recent study investigated the effect of rotator cuff disease on the outcome of total shoulder arthroplasty. Rotator cuff tears are uncommon in patients with osteoarthritis, occurring in less than 5%. In this series of 514 patients, 41 had a partial-thickness tear and 42 had a full-thickness tear. Supraspinatus tears did not adversely affect outcome, satisfaction, or mobility. Treatment of the tears did not change outcome parameters. However, shoulders with moderate or severe fatty degeneration of the infraspinatus were associated with poorer results. This study suggests that small tears limited to the supraspinatus do not negatively affect the outcome; however, more global degenerative changes in the rotator cuff musculature will.

Another prospective study further substantiates the fact that small tears of the supraspinatus do not adversely affect the outcome after total shoulder arthroplasty. This study was performed to determine the effect of tears, preoperative glenoid bone erosion, and radiographic evidence of subluxation of the humeral head on the outcome of shoulder arthroplasty. Tears of the supraspinatus tendon did not adversely affect the outcome. Radiographic posterior subluxation of the humeral head was associated with a lower outcome score, and patients with moderate to severe glenoid erosion did much better after total shoulder arthroplasty than humeral head replacement. Based on these data, the use of a glenoid component is recommended in shoulders with preoperative glenoid erosion.

Glenohumeral arthritis can occur after surgery for shoulder instability, and in general occurs more often after nonanatomic repairs where there is excessive shortening of the anterior capsule and subscapularis resulting in severe limitation of external rotation. The reported results for arthroplasty for arthritis of this etiology are not as good as those for primary arthritis. One reason may be that the patients are in general younger, and have higher physical demands and expectations. Two recent studies showed definite improvements in range of motion and pain relief. However, both studies had relatively high revision rates and some unsatisfactory results. The survivorship of the components at 10 years was 61% and is significant because the average age of patients undergoing arthroplasty was 46 to 47 years in both studies.

Glenoid component loosening has been recognized as one of the most common reasons for revision shoulder arthroplasty surgery. Although radiolucency around the glenoid component occurs in a much higher number of patients than the number that ultimately require revision for glenoid loosening, the glenoid component remains the most likely to fail of the shoulder arthroplasty components. It has been shown in a series of 48 shoulders undergoing glenoid component revision surgery that satisfactory pain relief was achieved in a much higher percentage of patients that had a new glenoid component inserted than in those who had glenoid component removal without reimplantation. Patients who did not have reinsertion of a component underwent

bone grafting of the defects; these patients may be candidates for glenoid component placement after graft consolidation.

Nonprosthetic Treatment Options for Glenohumeral Arthritis The role of arthroscopy in the treatment of glenohumeral joint arthritis remains unknown and recent studies of results in the knee joint have made this a controversial topic. Nevertheless, there are several recent reports of small studies of arthroscopic treatment of arthritis in the shoulder suggesting favorable short-term results. Indications for arthroscopic surgery for arthritis are ill defined, but generally include younger patients in whom it is desirable to prolong the need for prosthetic arthroplasty, and those with concentric wear of the glenoid, absence of severe joint contracture, loose bodies, and minimal if any bone loss. Arthroscopic treatment is most useful in alleviating mechanical symptoms from loose cartilage fragments or interposed soft tissue. Contraindications to arthroscopy for the treatment of arthritis include older patients with global arthritis who are candidates for shoulder arthroplasty, marked posterior or otherwise nonconcentric wear of the glenoid, severe joint contracture, and bone loss on the humeral side. Other arthroscopic procedures such as microfracture arthroplasty and glenoidplasty (burring nonconcentric wear) have been suggested, but their usefulness has not yet been substantiated in the peer-reviewed literature.

Soft-Tissue Resurfacing With or Without Hemiarthroplasty Soft-tissue interposition arthroplasty has received significant attention in recent years, given the complications associated with early glenoid wear and the frequency of radiolucencies associated with glenoid implantation. The two most common materials used are fascia lata, both allograft and autograft, and allograft knee meniscus. One early report of fascia lata interposition is promising, with failure in only one patient in whom the graft was found to have lost fixation at the time of revision surgery. However, the numbers are small and follow-up has been short term.

More recently, several centers have successfully used the lateral knee meniscus as an interposition tissue. The rationale for the use of the lateral meniscus is that it is tissue designed to withstand significant load with weight bearing under normal physiologic conditions. The lateral meniscus is used because it is more discoid in shape and gives better glenoid coverage. It is secured to the glenoid surface in place of a prosthetic component using bone anchors in the glenoid in a circumferential fashion. Early results show maintenance of the joint space radiographically and excellent functional results. Long-term survival analysis of this construct is still not available. The effect of severe posterior glenoid wear is also not clearly delineated at this point, but it may be a relative contraindication to the use of soft-tissue interposition because of the risk of continued bone loss that may make future reconstructive options difficult or impossible.

The primary indication for soft-tissue interposition arthroplasty is young patients with severe arthritis who are candidates for arthroplasty, but have a high likelihood of needing revision surgery in the future because of their young age. In general, this includes patients in their 40s and active, higher-demand patients in their early 50s. There is always a small risk of disease transmission with use of allograft material, and recipients should be made aware of this risk. Although the long-term results of this procedure are still not available and the indications are still developing, soft-tissue interposition in the shoulder holds significant promise for the treatment of arthritis in the young patient.

Acromioclavicular Joint Arthritis

Symptomatic acromioclavicular joint arthritis is a clinical rather than a radiographic diagnosis. Examination findings include tenderness with palpation at the acromioclavicular joint and pain with cross-body adduction. Radiographic changes are extremely common and do not correlate with symptomatic pathology that requires treatment. Nonsurgical treatment of isolated acromioclavicular joint pain includes nonsteroidal anti-inflammatory drugs, rest from inciting activity, and corticosteroid injections. If the condition is associated with rotator cuff pathology, physical therapy may be of benefit. Nonsurgical treatment of at least 3 to 6 months is generally recommended before surgical treatment should be considered.

A persistently painful acromioclavicular joint that is not responsive to nonsurgical treatment is surgically treated with a distal clavicle resection that can be performed through an open or an arthroscopic approach. If the procedure is performed through an open incision, care should be taken to repair the acromioclavicular ligaments. The superior and posterior acromioclavicular ligaments are the most important for maintaining stability. Disadvantages of the open approach are that the ligaments must be violated and subperiosteally removed from the distal clavicle. A portion of the deltoid is also removed from the anterior acromion and clavicle. This removal is of little consequence if appropriately repaired, but failure to do so results in significantly compromised outcome.

An arthroscopic distal clavicle resection is performed with the arthroscope in the posterior or posterolateral portal into the subacromial space. The working instruments are inserted through the rotator interval portal redirected into the subacromial space or through a separate portal to access the acromioclavicular joint. This approach allows excision of the clavicle without disturbing the ligaments and deltoid. Care must still be taken not to violate the ligaments with the arthroscopic instruments. The surgeon must adequately assess for complete bone removal. The most commonly missed bone is located superiorly and posteriorly, and symptoms may continue if resection is not thorough.

Annotated Bibliography

Rotator Cuff Tear

Cofield RH, Parvizi J, Hoffmeyer PJ, Lanzer WL, Ilstrup DM, Rowland CM: Surgical repair of chronic rotator cuff tears. *J Bone Joint Surg Am* 2001;83:71-77.

This is a prospective long-term study examining the results of open surgical repair and acromioplasty of chronic rotator cuff tears. Satisfactory pain relief was obtained in 96 of 105 shoulders. Tear size was the most important determinant of outcome with regard to active motion, strength, rating of results, patient satisfaction, and need for revision.

Fenlin JM Jr, Chase JM, Rushton SA, Frieman BG: Tuberoplasty, creation of an acromiohumeral articulation: A treatment option for massive, irreparable rotator cuff repairs. *J Shoulder Elbow Surg* 2002;11:136-142.

The authors discuss results of tuberoplasty in 20 patients. Overall results (improved pain relief and return to daily activities) were good.

Galatz LM, Griggs S, Cameron BD, Iannotti JP: Prospective longitudinal analysis of postoperative shoulder function: A ten-year follow-up study of full-thickness rotator cuff tears. *J Bone Joint Surg Am* 2001;83:1052-1056.

The authors reported that early results of rotator cuff repairs do not deteriorate with time in this prospective longitudinal study.

Halder AM, O'Driscoll SW, Heers G, et al: Biomechanical comparison of effects of supraspinatus tendon detachments, tendon defects, and muscle retractions. *J Bone Joint Surg Am* 2002;84:780-785.

The effects of supraspinatus tendon detachments, tendon defects, and muscle retraction on in vitro force transmission by the rotator cuff to the humerus were compared.

Murray TF, Lajtai G, Mileski RM, Snyder SJ: Arthroscopic repair of medium to large full-thickness rotator cuff tears: Outcome at 2- to 6-year follow-up. *J Shoulder Elbow Surg* 2002;11:19-24.

Forty-eight arthroscopic repairs of medium to large rotator cuff tears were evaluated 2 to 6 years after surgery. There were 35 excellent, 11 good, 2 fair, and no poor results. Only one patient had clinical evidence of failed repair.

Parsons IM, Apreleva M, Fu FH, Woo SL: The effect of rotator cuff tears on reaction forces at the glenohumeral joint. *J Orthop Res* 2002;20:439-446.

Results from this study of nine cadaveric upper extremities indicate that the integrity of the rotator cuff has a significant effect on joint reaction forces.

Pearsall AW IV, Bonsell S, Heitman RJ, Helms CA, Osbahr D, Speer K: Radiographic findings associated with symptomatic rotator cuff tears. *J Shoulder Elbow Surg* 2003;12:122-127.

Radiographs of 40 patients with a documented rotator cuff tear were compared with those of asymptomatic age-matched control patients. Results indicate that radiographs of patients with rotator cuff tear have greater tuberosity radiographic abnormalities that are not seen in the asymptomatic patients.

Postacchini F, Gumina S: Results of surgery after failed attempt at repair of irreparable rotator cuff tear. *Clin Orthop* 2002;397:332-341.

This is a study of a small number of patients who had an open attempt at rotator cuff repair including deltoid detachment and acromioplasty. At the time of surgery, the tears were found to be irreparable. Shoulder function deteriorated in 11 patients. The authors recommended against attempted open repair of irreparable cuff tears because the functional results are generally poor.

Warner JJ, Higgins L, Parsons IM IV, Dowdy P: Diagnosis and treatment of anterosuperior rotator cuff tears. *J Shoulder Elbow Surg* 2001;10:37-46.

According to results of this study, repair within 6 months of subscapularis tear may produce a better functional outcome.

Yamaguchi K, Tetro AM, Blam O, Evanoff BA, Teefey SA, Middleton WD: Natural history of asymptomatic rotator cuff tears: A longitudinal analysis of asymptomatic tears detected sonographically. *J Shoulder Elbow Surg* 2001;10:199-203.

The natural history of asymptomatic rotator cuff tears was studied over a 5-year period to determine risk of tear progression and development of symptoms.

Glenohumeral Joint Arthritis

Antuna SA, Sperling JW, Cofield RH, Rowland CM: Glenoid revision surgery after total shoulder arthroplasty. *J Shoulder Elbow Surg* 2001;10:217-224.

Glenoid component revision surgery was performed on 48 shoulders. The indications for surgery were glenoid component loosening in 29 shoulders, implant failure in 14, and component malposition or wear leading to instability in 5 shoulders. Satisfactory pain relief was acute in 86% of patients who had another glenoid component inserted and in 66% of patients who underwent glenoid component removal. Patients who have bone grafting may be candidates for glenoid component placement after graft consolidation.

Edwards TB, Boulahia A, Kempf J-F, Boileau P, Nemoz C, Walch G: The influence of rotator cuff disease on the results of shoulder arthroplasty for primary osteoarthritis: Results of a multicenter study. *J Bone Joint Surg Am* 2002;84:2240-2248.

Rotator cuff tears are uncommon in primary glenohumeral arthritis. This study examined the effect of full-thickness tears, partial-thickness tears, and fatty degeneration of the rotator cuff on the outcome. Supraspinatus tears were not found to influence the postoperative outcome. Additionally, treatment of these tears did not influence outcome parameters. However, shoulders with severe and moderate fatty degeneration of the infraspinatus had poorer results.

Godeneche A, Boileau P, Favard L, et al: Prosthetic replacement in the treatment of osteoarthritis of the shoulder: Early results of 268 cases. *J Shoulder Elbow Surg* 2002;11:11-18.

This is a study reporting the results of 268 shoulder arthroplasties for primary osteoarthritis. Good to excellent results were observed in 77% of patients and there was a 94% satisfaction rate. Mean active forward elevation was 145° postoperatively. In this study, glenoid radiolucent lines were present in 58% of cases and were associated with a less satisfactory result. Patients who underwent biceps tenodesis had better pain relief. Complications occurred in 8.6% of cases.

Hill JM, Norris TR: Long-term results of total shoulder arthroplasty following bone grafting of the glenoid. *J Bone Joint Surg Am* 2001;83:877-883.

Bone grafting of the glenoid can restore bone stock in patients with structural defects.

Iannotti JP, Norris TR: Influence of preoperative factors on outcome of shoulder arthroplasty for glenohumeral osteoarthritis. *J Bone Joint Surg Am* 2003;85:251-258.

The purpose of this study was to evaluate the influence of full-thickness rotator cuff tears, preoperative erosion of glenoid bone, radiographic evidence of subluxation of the humeral head, and preoperative range of motion on the outcome of shoulder arthroplasty. Repairable full-thickness tears of the supraspinatus tendon did not affect outcome. Shoulders with severe or moderate glenoid erosion had better results with total shoulder arthroplasty than hemiarthroplasty. Based on these results, it is recommended that a glenoid component be inserted in shoulders with glenoid erosion. A repairable tear of the supraspinatus tendon is not a contraindication to the use of a glenoid component.

Sperling JW, Antuna SA, Sanchez-Sotelo J, Schleck C, Cofield RH: Shoulder arthroplasty for arthritis after instability surgery. *J Bone Joint Surg Am* 2002;84:1775-1781.

Arthroplasty was associated with significant pain relief. There was not a significant difference between the hemiarthroplasty and total shoulder arthroplasty groups with regard to external rotation, abduction, or pain. The survival of the components at 10 years was 61%. The data from these studies suggest that arthroplasty in this particular group of patients is associated with good pain relief; however, there were high rates of revision surgery and unsatisfactory results because of component failure instability and glenoid arthritis in the hemiarthroplasty group.

Trail IA, Nuttall D: The results of shoulder arthroplasty in patients with rheumatoid arthritis. *J Bone Joint Surg Br* 2002;84:1121-1125.

A clinical and radiologic analysis of 105 shoulder arthroplasties in patients with rheumatoid arthritis was performed. Constant scores and American Shoulder and Elbow Surgeons scores were improved, and both scores were statistically significant.

Classic Bibliography

Bigliani LU, Cordasco FA, McIlveen SJ, Musso ES: Operative repair of massive rotator cuff tears: Long term results. *J Shoulder Elbow Surg* 1992;1:120-130.

Brenner BC, Ferlic DC, Clayton ML, Dennis DA: Survivorship of unconstrained total shoulder arthroplasty. *J Bone Joint Surg Am* 1989;71:1289-1296.

Burkhead WZ Jr, Hutton KS: Biologic resurfacing of the glenoid with hemiarthroplasty of the shoulder. *J Shoulder Elbow Surg* 1995;4:263-270.

Gartsman G, Khan M, Hammerman S: Arthroscopic repair of full-thickness tears of the rotator cuff. *J Bone Joint Surg Am* 1998;80:832-840.

Gartsman GM, Roddey TS, Hammerman SM: Shoulder arthroplasty with or without resurfacing of the glenoid in patients who have osteoarthritis. *J Bone Joint Surg* 2000;82:26-34.

Gerber C, Fuchs B, Hodler J: The results of repair of massive tears of the rotator cuff. *J Bone Joint Surg Am* 2000;82:505-515.

Goutallier D, Postel JM, Bernageau J, Lavau L, Voisin MC: Fatty muscle degeneration in cuff ruptures: Pre- and postoperative evaluation by CT scan. *Clin Orthop* 1994;304:78-83.

Hawkins RJ, Angelo RL: Glenohumeral osteoarthrosis: A late complication of the Putti-Platt repair. *J Bone Joint Surg Am* 1990;72:1193-1197.

Iannotti JP, Bernot MP, Kuhlman JR, Kelley MJ, Williams GR: Postoperative assessment of shoulder function: A prospective study of full-thickness rotator cuff tears. *J Shoulder Elbow Surg* 1996;5:449-457.

Neer CS II: Replacement arthroplasty for glenohumeral osteoarthritis. *J Bone Joint Surg Am* 1974;56:1-13.

Neer CS II, Watson KC, Stanton FJ: Recent experience in total shoulder replacement. *J Bone Joint Surg Am* 1982;64:319-337.

Rodosky M, Bigliani L: Indications for glenoid resurfacing in shoulder arthroplasty. *J Shoulder Elbow Surg* 1996;5:231-248.

Rokito AS, Cuomo F, Gallagher MA, Zuckerman JD: Long-term functional outcome of repair of large and massive chronic tears of the rotator cuff. *J Bone Joint Surg Am* 1991;81:991-997.

Walch G, Boileau P: Prosthetic adaptability: A new concept for shoulder arthroplasty. *J Shoulder Elbow Surg* 1999;8:443-451.

Chapter 27

Elbow and Forearm: Adult Trauma

David Ring, MD

Jesse B. Jupiter, MD

Distal Humeral Fractures

Fractures Involving the Metaphyseal Columns of the Distal Humerus

Fractures of the distal humerus are usually bicolumnar, and most will involve the articular surface. Although often depicted as Y- or T-shaped fractures with a simple articular split, it is becoming evident that these relatively simple fracture patterns are not as common as the more complex metaphyseal and articular fractures. Most fractures involve one of the following factors that increase the challenge of surgical treatment: (1) low (distal) fracture of one or both columns (at the level of the base of the olecranon fossa); (2) metaphyseal fragmentation of one or both columns; (3) complex fragmentation of the articular surface, including entirely or nearly entirely articular fragments (especially those with a coronal plane fracture line).

The surgical treatment of fractures of the distal humerus remains unsatisfactory in approximately 25% of patients in most reported series. Some series have reported a greater complication rate in older patients, probably because of poor bone quality, but perhaps also resulting from more difficult injury patterns. On the other hand, two recent series evaluated the results of treatment using the Disabilities of the Arm, Shoulder, and Hand outcomes instrument and found reasonably good restoration of function from the patient's perspective.

Olecranon osteotomy for exposure of fractures of the distal humerus has waned in popularity primarily because of problems related to the wires or screws used to repair the osteotomy. Alternative exposures commonly in use include the recently introduced triceps-reflecting anconeus pedicle modification of the triceps elevating exposure of Bryan and Morrey; the traditional Campbell exposure (midline triceps split), with additional elevation of the triceps off of the proximal ulna; and the reintroduced Allonso-Llamas exposure (in which the triceps is elevated off of the back of the humerus, but its insertion onto the olecranon is preserved). However, a recent cadaver study showed that olecranon osteotomy provides the best exposure of the distal humerus. The authors of this study also report that with attention to detail in the creation and repair of the olecranon osteotomy the rate of complications and revisions specifically to address prominent wires is acceptable.

The use of two plates in orthogonal planes has become well established in the treatment of fractures of the distal humerus. However, there is biomechanical support for the use of parallel plates placed on the direct medial and lateral aspects of the columns, and this configuration is often better suited to the treatment of complex fracture patterns. Newer plate designs include precontoured shapes and smaller 2.7-mm screws placed distally to facilitate internal fixation.

Total elbow arthroplasty is now an accepted treatment option for older, less active patients with fractures of the distal humerus. Several studies, including a recent comparative study of arthroplasty and plate and screw fixation, document very good early results; however, long-term follow-up is needed because elbow arthroplasties have a limited life span and eventually wear out. In addition, patients who undergo total elbow arthroplasty require a 5-kg lifting restriction, and patients who undergo this procedure are more prone to infection and other complications than those who undergo total hip or knee arthroplasty. The best candidate for total elbow arthroplasty is an older, infirm, and inactive patient with a fracture of the distal humerus, or a patient with a fracture of the distal humerus with an elbow joint that is already compromised by rheumatoid arthritis.

Fractures Involving Primarily the Articular Surface

The discussion of fractures involving primarily the articular surface of the distal humerus is often limited to fractures of the capitellum. It is now known that isolated fractures of the capitellum are uncommon. An apparent fracture of the capitellum nearly always extends into the lateral trochlear lip (the so-called coronal shear fracture) and may also involve a fracture of the lateral epicondyle, impaction of the posterior aspect of the lateral column, fracture of the posterior aspect of the tro-

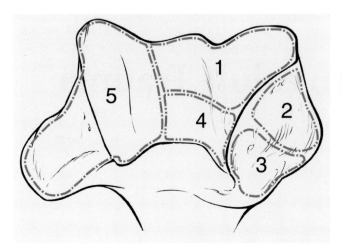

Figure 1 Illustration of the lateral lip of the trochlea (1), lateral epicondyle (2), posterior aspect of the lateral column (3), posterior trochlea (4), and medial epicondyle (5). Apparent fractures of the capitellum usually involve region 1, and injuries with greater complexity can involve fractures in regions 2 through 5. (© Copyright D. Ring, MD & J.B. Jupiter, MD.)

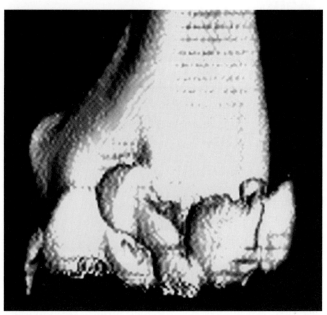

Figure 2 Three-dimensional reconstruction of a CT image; this is useful for understanding complex articular fractures of the distal humerus and planning surgical treatment. (© Copyright D. Ring, MD & J.B. Jupiter, MD.)

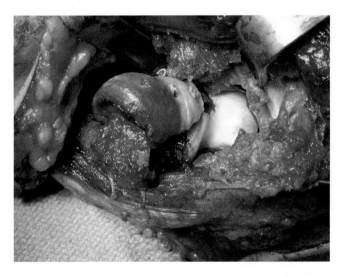

Figure 3 When the articular fragments do not fit, as shown in this photograph, there is impaction of the posterior aspect of the distal humerus, which must be elevated to allow accurate reduction of the articular fragments. (© Copyright D. Ring, MD & J.B. Jupiter, MD.)

chlea, and fracture of the medial epicondyle (Figure 1). Other variations such as fractures involving primarily the trochlear side of the joint are occasionally encountered.

When a semicircular fracture fragment is identified anterior to the distal humerus on the lateral radiograph of a patient with an injured elbow, surgeons should look for a second arc or semicircle on the fragment, which indicates that the fracture involves the trochlea. A trochlear defect is often apparent on the AP view. Because these features and the more complex fractures of the distal humeral articular surface can be difficult to detect on standard radiographs, CT is especially helpful in diagnosing these injuries. In particular, three-dimensional

CT reconstructions with the ulna and the radius subtracted from the image are invaluable for understanding the injury and planning surgical treatment (Figure 2). Traction radiographs and fluoroscopy can help define the fracture pattern, but they are not as useful for preoperative planning as three-dimensional CT reconstructions because they are usually obtained at the time of surgery after the administration of anesthesia.

Surgical fixation can usually be achieved through a lateral muscle interval with elevation of the extensor carpi radialis brevis and part of the extensor carpi radialis longus off of the supracondylar ridge and anterior humerus. If the lateral collateral ligament and epicondyle are intact, it is often possible to work through an interval anterior to the lateral collateral ligament (through the common extensor muscles) and rely on reduction of the metaphyseal fracture lines. For patients with more complex fractures, there is nearly always a fracture of the lateral epicondyle, which can be mobilized along with the origins of the lateral collateral ligament and common extensor muscles. The elbow joint can then be subluxated, allowing a good view of the anterior articular surface of the distal humerus. If the posterior aspect of the trochlea or the medial epicondyle is fractured, exposure through an olecranon osteotomy may be preferable.

If the fracture fragments do not seem to fit back onto the intact portions of the distal humerus, additional impaction of the intact distal humerus should be suspected (Figure 3). In this situation, it will be necessary to hinge open the posterior aspect of the lateral column and the posterior aspect of the trochlea to properly realign the anterior fracture fragments. The articular fragments are secured with countersunk screws (screws with threads on the head, such as Herbert screws, can be used), small threaded Kirschner wires, or screws entering from the nonarticular parts of the distal humerus, such as the posterior aspect of the lateral column. The lateral epicondyle is secured with a tension band wire to incorporate the common extensor fascia; a screw or a plate is also used if the fragment is large enough.

Ideally, active-assisted exercises and use of the arm for light daily activities are started the day after surgical fixation of a fracture of the distal humerus. However, if the fracture is complex or the bone quality is poor and the fixation is therefore not optimal, it may be preferable to immobilize the elbow for 4 weeks before initiating exercises. A healed stiff elbow will be easier to salvage than a nonhealed elbow, particularly in patients with complex fractures.

Radial Head Fractures

Isolated radial head fractures usually involve part of the radial head and heal well with nonsurgical treatment. Sometimes they are displaced enough to block forearm rotation and benefit from surgical treatment. The most important complication of isolated partial radial head fractures is elbow stiffness, and the most important aspect of treatment is mobilization of the elbow.

As documented in two recent case series, nonsurgically treated minimally displaced fractures of the radial neck will occasionally fail to heal. The prevalence of nonunion is obscured for several reasons: (1) nonunion of the radial head is usually asymptomatic; (2) radiographs are rarely obtained until union in the treatment of patients with this type of fracture; and (3) a fracture of the radial head that is unhealed 1 year after the injury may still eventually heal 2 years or longer after the injury.

Fractures of the radial head—particularly complex fractures involving the entire head and neck—are often associated with one of the following five injury types: (1) an Essex-Lopresti fracture-dislocation of the forearm or a variant thereof; (2) rupture of the medial collateral ligament complex; (3) dislocation of the elbow; (4) dislocation of the elbow with fractures of the radial head and coronoid process—the so-called terrible triad of the elbow; and (5) an olecranon fracture-dislocation—usually with an apex posterior fracture of the proximal ulna or olecranon (the so-called posterior Monteggia lesion). In each type, the associated fractures and ligament injuries may compromise forearm or elbow instability, thereby increasing the importance of the radial head.

Although the classification system of Mason is still used, it is often modified. The Mason classification distinguished nondisplaced fractures (type 1), partial head

fractures (type 2), and complete head fractures (type 3). There are few data in the literature to support any subclassification based on the size or displacement of partial head fractures. Several important factors are not accounted for in this classification system, and they are only partially accounted for in the more recent comprehensive classification of fractures, including: (1) the number of fracture fragments; (2) lost or unrecoverable articular fragments; (3) central impaction and deformation of the radial head; (4) the quality of the fracture fragments (amount of subchondral bone, osteoporosis); and (5) metaphyseal comminution. These factors all will have a substantial impact on attempts at surgical repair of a radial head fracture. In particular, a recent study suggested that patients with fractures of the entire radial head that create more than three articular fragments have high rates of early failure, nonunion, and poor forearm rotation after surgical fixation.

Excision of a complex fracture of the radial head without prosthetic replacement is still a viable treatment option. To do this safely, surgeons must make sure that there is no forearm ligament injury by using the recently described radius pull test and ensure that there is no fracture of the coronoid (terrible triad). Although it is usually preferable to treat an elbow fracture-dislocation with either repair or replacement of the radial head, reasonable results have been reported after radial head resection as long as the coronoid is not also fractured. Excision of the radial head without prosthetic replacement is considered primarily in older patients with limited demands and simple injury patterns.

Partial excision of the radial head has traditionally been associated with less optimal results. Even a small portion of the radial head can be important to stability of the forearm or elbow. In the setting of an unstable fracture-dislocation of the forearm or elbow, if a partial radial head fracture has inadequate fragments for repair, it may be preferable to proceed with prosthetic replacement.

Surgical repair should be used only for patients with simple fractures with three or fewer fragments with good quality bone and little or no impaction. The implants must be placed directly laterally, with the arm in neutral rotation to avoid impingement on the ulna with forearm rotation. Another rough guide for placement is provided by the arc defined by the radial styloid and Lister's tubercle. Implants placed on the articular surface of the radial head must be countersunk beneath the articular surface.

Several metal radial head prostheses are in common use. Two studies support the use of a loose-stemmed metal prosthesis that acts as a stiff spacer, and another study supports the use of a bipolar prosthesis that is cemented into the neck of the radius. Surgeons should be careful not to place a prosthesis that is too long or wide and always err toward using a slightly smaller prosthesis

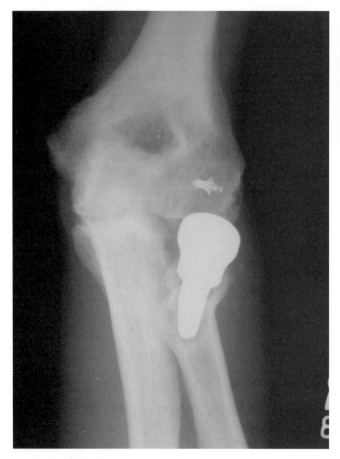

Figure 4 Radiograph showing wear of the capitellum that can result when a metal radial head prosthesis is too long; the medial side of the ulnohumeral joint will be hinged open in such instances. Therefore, it is important not to place too large an implant. (© Copyright D. Ring, MD & J.B. Jupiter, MD.)

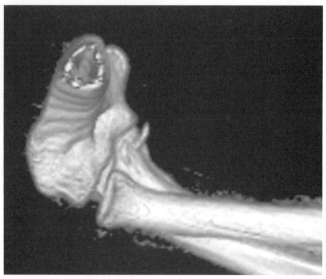

Figure 5 Three-dimensional reconstruction of a CT image showing that even very small coronoid fractures can be associated with recurrent elbow instability, particularly when they involve the anteromedial facet of the coronoid. (© Copyright D. Ring, MD & J.B. Jupiter, MD.)

because the major problem is overstuffing of the joint, which can lead to problems with wear of the capitellar cartilage and potential instability or malalignment of the elbow (Figure 4). Some of the older prosthetic designs had stems that were too big for the average radial neck, which could result in inadequate placement with the radial head not well seated into the shaft. Biomechanical studies have confirmed the ability of metal radial head prostheses to restore near-normal stability to the elbow after radial head excision.

Elbow Dislocations

It is now well recognized that elbow dislocations are associated with complete or near-complete disruption of the capsuloligamentous stabilizers of the elbow and that the progression of injury is typically from lateral to medial. It is possible to dislocate the elbow with the anterior band of the medial collateral ligament still intact. The focus of treatment has shifted from the medial to the lateral collateral ligament complex. The medial collateral ligament is repaired only if treatment of associated fractures and the lateral collateral ligament fails to restore stability.

The lateral collateral ligament characteristically fails by avulsion of its lateral epicondylar origin, with midsubstance tears and avulsion from the ulna occurring less commonly. This facilitates repair with either suture anchors or drill holes through the bone of the lateral epicondyle. Instability after dislocation of the elbow is usually associated with fracture of the radial head and coronoid process. Elbow dislocations without major associated fractures are also occasionally unstable. Whether they occur in older or younger patients after a high-energy injury, there are usually extensive avulsions of the common extensor and flexor muscles from the distal humerus. Older patients may have primarily lateral-sided injuries, with a tendency for the elbow to rotate on the relatively preserved medial soft tissues. Some patients with unstable elbow dislocations have a small fracture of the anteromedial facet of the coronoid process—a variant of posteromedial varus rotational instability pattern injuries (Figure 5). Unstable elbow dislocations are treated with either extensive soft-tissue reattachment to the distal humerus, cross pinning of the elbow joint, or hinged external fixation.

Coronoid Fractures

Although a recently published biomechanical cadaver study suggested a limited effect of small coronoid fractures on elbow instability, clinical data document that even very small fractures can lead to troublesome elbow instability. For instance, although the coronoid fractures associated with terrible triad pattern fracture-dislocations of the elbow are nearly always transverse fractures that are less than 30% of the coronoid height, terrible triad elbows can dislocate in spite of cast immobilization, are prone to dislocation after surgical treatment (particularly if radiocapitellar contact is not restored), and can have a high prevalence of unsatisfactory treatment results. Because of the poor results associated with the treatment of this type of fracture, many surgeons are routinely repairing the coronoid fracture, usually with suture placed through drill holes in the ulna.

Fractures of the anteromedial facet of the coronoid process are usually associated with injury to the lateral collateral ligament complex and can be difficult to manage. These have been labeled posteromedial varus rotational instability pattern injuries. This type of fracture is repaired with a plate and screws through a medial exposure between the two heads of the flexor carpi ulnaris (where the ulnar nerve usually sits), more anteriorly through a split in the flexor pronator mass, or both.

Large coronoid fractures are nearly always associated with an olecranon fracture-dislocation. These fractures typically involve multiple fragments, particularly when part of a posterior olecranon fracture-dislocation. They can be accessed and manipulated through the olecranon fracture itself and fixed with a dorsal plate and screws with or without an additional medial plate. The results of treatment of anterior transolecranon fracture-dislocations have been quite good, whereas the treatment of posterior olecranon fracture-dislocations has been associated with a greater number of complications and revisions and diminished results. Patients with large fractures with complex comminution or poor bone quality may occasionally benefit from protection with hinged external fixation.

Olecranon Fractures

The Mayo classification of olecranon fractures characterizes fractures based on the three most important factors in treatment considerations: comminution, displacement, and fracture-dislocation.

There is wide variation regarding the treatment of olecranon fractures. A biomechanical study found that a large screw was best for internal fixation of olecranon fractures, but reported that the stability was insufficient to allow active elbow exercises. Conversely, internal fixation of olecranon osteotomies and fractures with small caliber wires with immediate active mobilization has been shown to be very successful in practice, at least when specific techniques are used.

The major disadvantage of tension band wiring continues to be a high rate of subsequent surgical procedures for removal of symptomatic prominent hardware, which has been reported in one long-term study as ranging between 43% and 81% (depending on technique); however, in another study, it was reported to be only 13% when specific techniques intended to limit the prominence of the wires were used. Plates are becoming a more popular treatment option for fixation of even

simple olecranon fractures, and good results have been reported; however, 20% of patients had a second surgery for plate removal. Furthermore, it may not be wise to rely on screws to secure a small osteopenic proximal fragment. The long-term results of successful surgical repair of olecranon fractures are good.

Diaphyseal Forearm Fractures
Mechanics

Several recent studies have examined the impact of rotational malalignment of the radius and ulna on forearm rotation. These studies consistently show that rotational malalignment of the ulna has less impact on forearm rotation than radius malrotation. In both the radius and the ulna, forearm motion was not impacted unless there was substantial malalignment (at least 30° malrotation)—an amount of malalignment that is unlikely to occur in the management of patients. Prior studies have shown a more substantial impact with even minor angular malalignments of the radius and ulna, particularly loss of the normal radial bow.

A biomechanical study of dynamic compression plates applied to transverse diaphyseal osteotomies of the radius showed that even relatively small plates could achieve a bending stiffness comparable to that of the intact bone and that longer plates with bicortical screws at the ends of the plates had better torsional stiffness. This is consistent with the findings of previous studies and emphasizes the advantages of longer plates and bicortical screws in a setting with substantial torsional stresses such as the forearm. These advantages may be even more pronounced in patients with comminuted fractures.

Ulnar Fractures

Two recently published meta-analyses of the treatment of isolated fractures of the ulnar diaphysis (the so-called nightstick fracture) identified only retrospective case series and therefore could not make definitive recommendations regarding treatment. Fractures with greater than 50% of displacement or 10° of angulation can impact forearm rotation. Because surgical treatment of these fractures is straightforward, it is recommended that surgeons have a low threshold for surgical treatment for displaced fractures. For less displaced fractures, nonsurgical treatment—even simple symptomatic treatment—will usually result in union with good function, but the time to complete healing can be quite prolonged. Therefore, surgical treatment is also a reasonable option for motivated patients with less displaced fractures.

Diaphyseal ulnar fractures with anterior or lateral dislocation of the proximal radioulnar joint (anterior or lateral Monteggia lesions) are uncommon in adults. Plate and screw fixation of the ulna in anatomic alignment usually restores good function. Open reduction of the proximal radioulnar and radiocapitellar joints is rarely necessary. Residual malalignment of these joints usually reflects residual malalignment of the ulna.

Posterior Monteggia fractures occur more commonly in adult patients, particularly when posterior olecranon fracture-dislocations are included. Few of these injuries occur at the diaphyseal level. Most occur at the level of the metaphysis (just distal to the coronoid process) or through the olecranon (olecranon fracture-dislocation). These injuries are often associated with fractures of the radial head and coronoid and injury to the lateral collateral ligament complex. Posterior Monteggia fractures are more challenging to treat, and the results are not as predictable because (1) it can be difficult to obtain solid fixation of the proximal ulna fragment, particularly in patients with osteoporosis; (2) the fracture of the coronoid can be comminuted and difficult to repair; (3) the fracture of the radial head increases the risk of diminished forearm rotation and proximal radioulnar synostosis; and (4) the ulnohumeral joint can be unstable, and this is often not well appreciated. Complications and secondary procedures can be limited by using a plate contoured to wrap around the dorsal surface of the olecranon and proximal ulna to provide more secure fixation of the proximal fragment; by obtaining good exposure and secure fixation of the coronoid; by obtaining stable fixation or replacement of the radial head; and by repairing the lateral collateral ligament when injured.

Radial Fractures

Although textbooks describe isolated fractures of the ulnar diaphysis without proximal or distal radioulnar joint injury (nightstick fractures), isolated radial fractures are often omitted, with classification systems skipping directly to Galeazzi fractures (fracture of radial diaphysis and dislocation of the distal radioulnar joint). A recent article suggests that isolated fractures of the diaphyseal radius are unlikely to be associated with major injury to the distal radioulnar joint (triangular fibrocartilage complex) when the ulnar fracture is greater than 7.5 cm from the radiocarpal joint. It may be unwise to be complacent about the distal radioulnar joint based on the location of the fracture, but what this study supports is the idea that many isolated fractures of the radius occur without major radioulnar ligament injury (Figure 6). After stable anatomic fixation of the radius, the distal radioulnar joint should be evaluated and compared with a preoperative examination of the opposite, uninjured side. In the absence of substantial instability, immediate active mobilization may be safe and worthwhile. If the distal radioulnar joint is unstable there are several treatment options: (1) repair of a large ulnar styloid fracture if present; (2) repair of the triangular fibrocartilage complex; (3) immobilization of the forearm in midsupination; and (4) cross-pinning of the radius and the ulna in midsupination.

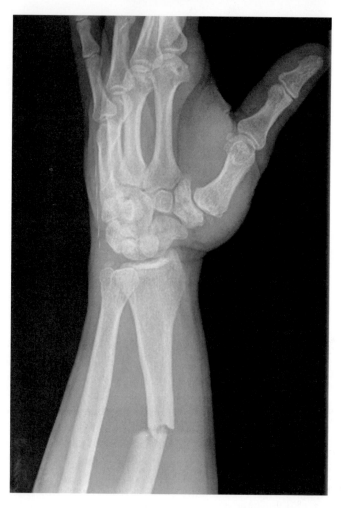

Figure 6 Preoperative radiograph of a patient with a radial diaphysis fracture. Many such fractures do not have associated injury to the distal radioulnar joint and can be managed with early mobilization after plate fixation. Preoperative radiographic alignment and location of the radius fracture can be helpful, but surgeons should always base treatment decisions on a careful evaluation of the distal radioulnar joint after plate fixation. (© Copyright D. Ring, MD & J.B. Jupiter, MD.)

Annotated Bibliography

Distal Humeral Fractures

Frankle MA, Herscovici D Jr, DiPasquale TG, Vasey MB, Sanders RW: A comparison of open reduction and internal fixation and primary total elbow arthroplasty in the treatment of intraarticular distal humerus fractures in women older than age 65. *J Orthop Trauma* 2003;17: 473-480.

The authors of this study retrospectively reviewed 24 patients older than 65 years with bicondylar (C2 or C3) fractures of the distal humerus that were treated with either total elbow arthroplasty (12 patients) or plate and screw fixation (12 patients). At a short-term follow-up of between 2 and 6 years (average just under 4 years), the functional results were somewhat better in the total elbow arthroplasty than the internal fixation group, with an average arc of flexion of 113° versus 100° and an average Mayo Elbow Performance Index of 95 versus 88 points, respectively.

Pajarinen J, Bjorkenheim JM: Operative treatment of type C intercondylar fractures of the distal humerus: Results after a mean follow-up of 2 years in a series of 18 patients. *J Shoulder Elbow Surg* 2002;11:48-52.

In this study, 8 of 18 patients (all of whom were older than 50 years) had an unsatisfactory result after plate and screw fixation of a bicolumnar fracture of the distal humerus. Poor bone quality and open fracture were also associated with inferior results.

Ring D, Jupiter JB, Gulotta L: Articular fractures of the distal part of the humerus. *J Bone Joint Surg Am* 2003; 85:232-238.

In this study, 21 patients with apparent fractures of the capitellum had more complex fractures of the articular surface of the distal humerus. The authors report that fixation with buried screws and wires achieved healing with slight settling of the fracture fragments in two patients and no major osteonecrosis. Ten patients required a second surgical procedure, and five patients had an unsatisfactory functional result related to persistent elbow stiffness.

Ring D, Gulotta L, Chin K, Jupiter JB: Olecranon osteotomy for exposure of fractures and nonunions of the distal humerus. *J Orthop Trauma* 2004;18:446-449.

In this study, 45 patients had an apex distal chevron-shaped olecranon osteotomy repaired with Kirschner wires directed out the anterior ulnar cortex distal to the coronoid process, and bent 180° and impacted into the olecranon proximally with two 22-gauge figure-of-8 stainless steel tension wires. The only failure occurred in a patient who returned to athletic activities too soon. Only six patients (13%) had a subsequent surgical procedure performed specifically to remove the wires.

Schildhauer TA, Nork SE, Mills WJ, Henley MB: Extensor mechanism-sparing paratricipital posterior approach to the distal humerus. *J Orthop Trauma* 2003;17:374-378.

Extra-articular fractures (Opthopaedic Trauma Association [OTA] type A) and simple articular distal humeral fractures with simple or multifragmentary metaphyseal involvement (OTA type C1 and C2) were treated by elevating the triceps off of the back of the humerus and working through the medial and lateral paratricipital windows (an exposure described previously by Allonso-Llamas).

Wilkinson JM, Stanley D: Posterior surgical approaches to the elbow: A comparative anatomic study. *J Shoulder Elbow Surg* 2001;10:380-382.

In this study, the median-exposed articular surface for triceps splitting, triceps reflecting, and olecranon osteotomy approaches was 35%, 46%, and 57%, respectively.

Radial Head Fractures

Liow RY, Cregan A, Nanda R, Montgomery RJ: Early mobilisation for minimally displaced radial head frac-

tures is desirable: A prospective randomised study of two protocols. *Injury* 2002;33:801-806.

In this study, 60 patients with minimally displaced fractures of the radial head were prospectively randomized to undergo either immediate active mobilization or 5 days of splint immobilization. All patients achieved excellent results. Patients treated with immediate mobilization had less pain and better elbow function at 1 week. There were no adverse consequences of immediate mobilization.

Moro JK, Werier J, MacDermid JC, Patterson SD, King GJ: Arthroplasty with a metal radial head for unreconstructible fractures of the radial head. *J Bone Joint Surg Am* 2001;83:1201-1211.

In this study, 25 patients with metal radial head prostheses were evaluated an average of 39 months after injury. The average flexion arc was 132°, the average forearm arc was 146°, the average disabilities of the arm, shoulder, and hand score was 17, and the average Mayo Elbow Performance Index score was 80. There were eight unsatisfactory results related to associated injuries, psychiatric problems, and secondary gain. Asymptomatic lucencies around the stem were the rule because the implant functions as a spacer and is not intended to have a tight fit in the radial neck.

Pomianowski S, Morrey BF, Neale PG, Park MJ, O'Driscoll SW, An KN: Contribution of monoblock and bipolar radial head prostheses to valgus stability of the elbow. *J Bone Joint Surg Am* 2001;83-A:1829-1834.

In this study, three metal radial head prostheses were shown to restore valgus stability in the medial collateral ligament deficient elbow close to the status with an intact radial head.

Ring D, Psychoyios VN, Chin KR, Jupiter JB: Nonunion of nonoperatively treated fractures of the radial head. *Clin Orthop* 2002;398:235-238.

The authors of this study describe five patients with a radial neck nonunion after a minimally displaced radial head fracture. These fractures are usually asymptomatic.

Ring D, Quintero J, Jupiter JB: Open reduction and internal fixation of fractures of the radial head. *J Bone Joint Surg Am* 2002;84:1811-1815.

In this study, 56 patients in whom an intra-articular fracture of the radial head had been treated with open reduction and internal fixation were evaluated at an average of 48 months after injury. The authors report that good results were obtained in all of the patients with isolated partial radial head fractures, in 4 of 15 of those with partial radial head fractures that were part of a complex injury to the elbow or forearm, and in 11 of 12 of those with fracture of the entire head into two or three large fragments. Among patients with fracture of the entire head into greater than three fragments, 13 of 14 had an unsatisfactory result, with three early failures and six nonunions.

Smith AM, Urbanosky LR, Castle JA, Rushing JT, Ruch DS: Radius pull test: Predictor of longitudinal forearm instability. *J Bone Joint Surg Am* 2002;84:1970-1976.

In this sequential cutting study in cadavers, the authors showed that after radial head resection 3 mm of proximal radial migration with longitudinal traction indicated disruption of the interosseous membrane and migration of 6 mm or greater indicated gross longitudinal instability with disruption of all ligamentous structures of the forearm.

Elbow Dislocations

McKee MD, Schemitsch EH, Sala MJ, O'Driscoll SW: The pathoanatomy of lateral ligamentous disruption in complex elbow instability. *J Shoulder Elbow Surg* 2003; 12:391-396.

Six patterns of injury to the lateral collateral ligament injury were observed in 62 patients with a surgically treated dislocation or fracture-dislocation of the elbow (proximal avulsions in 32, bony avulsions of the lateral epicondyle in 5, midsubstance ruptures in 18, ulnar detachments of the lateral collateral ligament in 3, ulnar bony avulsions in 1, and combined patterns in 3). The common extensor origin was also ruptured in 41 patients (66%).

Coronoid Fractures

Ring D, Jupiter JB, Zilberfarb J: Posterior dislocation of the elbow with fractures of the radial head and coronoid. *J Bone Joint Surg Am* 2002;84-A:547-551.

The authors of this article describe 7 of 11 terrible triad elbows that redislocated in a splint after manipulative reduction. Five patients, including four who were treated with resection of the radial head, experienced redislocation after surgical treatment. Only four patients reported satisfactory results, all of whom had retained the radial head and two of whom had lateral collateral ligament repair. The subsequent letters to the editor adds additional perspective to the current concepts regarding the treatment of these injuries.

Olecranon Fractures

Bailey CS, MacDermid J, Patterson SD, King GJ: Outcome of plate fixation of olecranon fractures. *J Orthop Trauma* 2001;15:542-548.

Near normal motion, strength, and disabilities of the arm, shoulder, and hand scores were observed after plate fixation of 25 displaced olecranon fractures. The authors report that 20% of patients requested plate removal.

Hutchinson DT, Horwitz DS, Ha G, Thomas CW, Bachus KN: Cyclic loading of olecranon fracture fixation constructs. *J Bone Joint Surg Am* 2003;85:831-837.

As might be expected based on the size of the implants alone, a large screw limits displacement of an olecranon osteotomy better than Kirschner wires with a tension band wire in biomechanical tests in cadavers. Unfortunately, the authors of this study interpreted their data as disproving the tension band concept (a basic engineering principle that cannot be disproved) and as discouraging immediate active mobilization of the arm (a mainstay of effective treatment and not associated with major problems in prior clinical series).

Karlsson MK, Hasserius R, Besjakov J, Karlsson C, Josefsson PO: Comparison of tension-band and figure-of-eight wiring techniques for treatment of olecranon fractures. *J Shoulder Elbow Surg* 2002;11:377-382.

In a long-term study of olecranon fractures, one subset of patients was treated with tension band wiring and the other was treated with a simple figure-of-8 wire. The authors report that the results were comparable for both groups, with a high rate of hardware removal occurring in both groups after tension band wiring (81% of patients) and after figure-of-8 wiring (43%).

Karlsson MK, Hasserius R, Karlsson C, Besjakov J, Josefsson PO: Fractures of the olecranon: A 15- to 25-year followup of 73 patients. *Clin Orthop* 2002;403:205-212.

In a long-term follow-up of 70 patients who were treated for olecranon fractures, the authors report excellent or good results in 96%, slight loss of elbow flexion and extension and mild or moderate degenerative changes in over 50%. The authors conclude that adequately treated fractures of the olecranon have a favorable long-term outcome.

Diaphyseal Forearm Fractures

Dumont CE, Thalmann R, Macy JC: The effect of rotational malunion of the radius and the ulna on supination and pronation. *J Bone Joint Surg Br* 2002;84:1070-1074.

In this cadaver study, the authors report that substantial rotational malalignment of the radius and/or ulna was necessary before forearm rotation was affected.

Handoll HH, Pearce PK: Interventions for isolated diaphyseal fractures of the ulna in adults. *Cochrane Database Syst Rev* 2004;2:CD000523.

A review of trials was performed to determine the effects of different treatment methods (in adults) for isolated fractures of the ulnar shaft. The authors concluded that there was insufficient evidence from randomized trials to determine the most appropriate treatment method.

Hertel R, Eijer H, Meisser A, Hauke C, Perren SM: Biomechanical and biological considerations relating to the clinical use of the Point Contact-Fixator: Evaluation of the device handling test in the treatment of diaphyseal fractures of the radius and/or ulna. *Injury* 2001;32(suppl 2):B10-B14.

In this study of 83 diaphyseal forearm fractures in 52 patients that were repaired using a Point Contact-Fixator (Synthes, Paoli, PA), 76 bones healed with callus without further intervention. Stripping of the hexagonal slot was reported to be a problem at removal of the implant.

Kasten P, Krefft M, Hesselbach J, Weinberg AM: How does torsional deformity of the radial shaft influence the rotation of the forearm? A biomechanical study. *J Orthop Trauma* 2003;17:57-60.

The authors of this study report that significant loss of forearm rotation was not observed until a minimum of 30° of rotational malunion.

Rettig ME, Raskin KB: Galeazzi fracture-dislocation: A new treatment-oriented classification. *J Hand Surg Am* 2001;26:228-235.

In this review of 40 patients with Galeazzi fracture-dislocations, the authors suggest that more proximal fractures are less likely to have distal radioulnar joint instability. Among 22 fractures in the distal third of the radius (within 7.5 cm of the radiocarpal joint), 12 had intraoperative distal radioulnar joint instability. Among 18 more proximal fractures, only one had intraoperative distal radioulnar joint instability after plating of the radius.

Classic Bibliography

Anderson LD, Sisk D, Tooms RE, Park WI III: Compression-plate fixation in acute diaphyseal fractures of the radius and ulna. *J Bone Joint Surg Am* 1975;57: 287-297.

Beredjiklian PK, Nalbantoglu U, Potter HG, Hotchkiss RN: Prosthetic radial head components and proximal radial morphology: A mismatch. *J Shoulder Elbow Surg* 1999;8:471-475.

Broberg MA, Morrey BF: Results of treatment of fracture-dislocations of the elbow. *Clin Orthop* 1987;216: 109-119.

Chapman MW, Gordon JE, Zissimos AG: Compression plate fixation of acute fractures of the diaphysis of the radius and ulna. *J Bone Joint Surg Am* 1989;71:159-169.

Josefsson PO, Gentz CF, Johnell O, Wendeberg: Dislocations of the elbow and intraarticular fractures. *Clin Orthop* 1989;246:126-130.

Mason ML: Some observations on fractures of the head of the radius with a review of one hundred cases. *Br J Surg* 1959;42:123-132.

McKee MD, Wilson TL, Winston L, Schemitsch EH, Richards RR: Functional outcome following surgical treatment of intra-articular distal humeral fractures through a posterior approach. *J Bone Joint Surg Am* 2000;82: 1701-1707.

Regan W, Morrey BF: Fractures of the coronoid process of the ulna. *J Bone Joint Surg Am* 1989;71:1348-1354.

Ring D, Jupiter JB, Sanders RW, Mast J, Simpson NS: Transolecranon fracture-dislocation of the elbow. *J Orthop Trauma* 1997;11:545-550.

Ring D, Jupiter JB, Simpson NS: Monteggia fractures in adults. *J Bone Joint Surg Am* 1998;80:1733-1744.

Schemitsch EH, Richards RR: The effect of malunion on functional outcome after plate fixation of fractures of both bones of the forearm in adults. *J Bone Joint Surg Am* 1992;74:1068-1078.

Chapter 28

Elbow Reconstruction

Scott P. Steinmann, MD

William B. Geissler, MD

Diagnostic Studies

For evaluation of most elbow disorders, plain radiographs are usually sufficient. Standard views should include AP, lateral, and oblique. Radiographs are often the only imaging study needed in the clinic or emergency department if an arthritic process or a minor fracture is detected. If a more detailed examination is desired, CT is helpful to define an arthritic process, detect loose bodies, or pinpoint the location of heterotopic bone. Occasionally, a suspected radial head fracture will not be seen on plain radiographs but will be confirmed by CT. CT can also be quite helpful for defining the extent of a fracture to help determine a surgical repair strategy.

Fluoroscopy plays a very important role in examination of the elbow. Elbow instability is often subtle and sometimes it can be difficult to determine the pattern of subluxation based solely on the clinical examination. Fluoroscopic examination under anesthesia should be considered a standard first step before many elbow surgical procedures. In the trauma patient obvious fractures may be seen on radiographs but fluoroscopic evaluation under anesthesia may demonstrate any associated ligamentous injuries. Similarly, an occult instability pattern may be detected with fluoroscopic examination under anesthesia in a patient undergoing an elective elbow procedure.

MRI can be helpful in examining a patient with suspected medial or lateral instability. Although MRI cannot be a substitute for a thorough clinical examination, it can detect frank disruption of the collateral ligament and partial tears. Unusual causes of elbow pain such as a glomus tumor or an osteoid osteoma may also be detected by MRI. Occasionally, distal biceps tendinopathy can be seen on MRI, which may correlate with a clinical diagnosis of partial biceps tendon tear.

Arthroscopy

Elbow arthroscopy has become a more common procedure over the past decade. Elbow arthroscopy is technically demanding to perform and requires surgeon experience in advanced arthroscopic techniques. Advantages of arthroscopic treatment of elbow disorders include improved articular visualization and potentially decreased postoperative pain. Patients may also benefit from a decreased morbidity and a faster postoperative recovery. Presently, elbow arthroscopy can be performed for resection of symptomatic plica, removal of loose bodies, synovectomy for inflammatory arthritis, release of capsule in patients with contractures, removal of osteophytes, treatment of osteochondritis dissecans, débridement of lateral epicondylitis, and treatment of elbow fractures. Elbow arthroscopy is difficult because of the smaller joint working space and the unique articular anatomy of the elbow. The risk of injury to neurovascular structures is not insignificant. Contraindications to elbow arthroscopy include significant prior trauma or surgical scarring. Prior surgery is not a contraindication but loss of joint space as a result of prior trauma makes joint visualization very difficult. Previous trauma may also distort the local anatomy, making accurate identification of neurovascular structures difficult. A subluxating ulnar nerve is not a contraindication to arthroscopy, but should be identified before beginning the surgical procedure. Before ulnar nerve transposition can be performed, the nerve's location must be known before a medial portal can be established; an open incision on the medial side or intraoperative ultrasound can be used to identify the nerve.

Arthroscopic Technique

Patients undergoing elbow arthroscopy are typically placed under general anesthesia, which allows for muscle relaxation and permits placing the patient in either a prone position or the lateral decubitus position, which might otherwise not be tolerated by an awake patient (Figures 1 and 2). Regional nerve blocks can be used as anesthesia for elbow surgery; however, any position other than the supine position may be difficult for the patient to maintain. Additionally, if a nerve block has been administered, it is impossible to assess the patient immediately postoperatively for potential nerve injury.

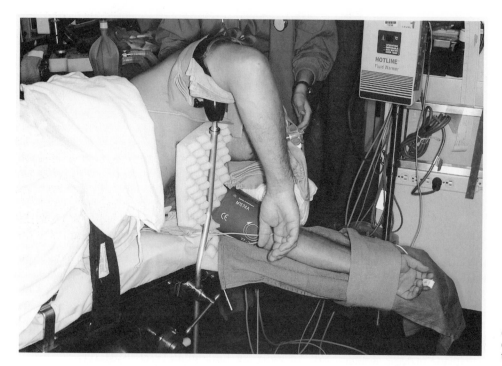

Figure 1 Lateral decubitus position for elbow arthroscopy. A dedicated arm holder is useful for positioning the elbow at the ideal height.

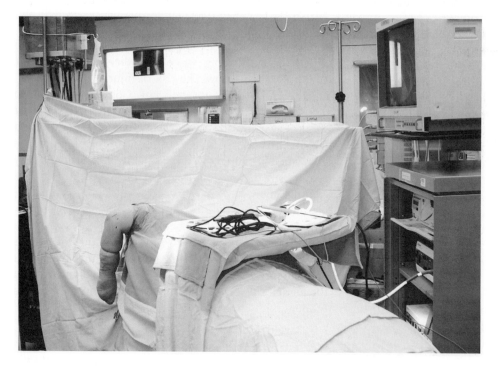

Figure 2 View of elbow arthroscopy after final positioning and draping.

Elbow arthroscopy can be performed in either the supine, prone, or lateral decubitus position.

The lateral decubitus position is fairly easy to maintain and is probably the most popularly used position. At the time of surgery, the ulnar nerve is palpated to be sure of its location and to check that it does not subluxate from the cubital fossa. It is best to mark all portal sites before surgery when the elbow is not distended and palpation of bony landmarks can be done more precisely. Distending the elbow with saline before making the initial starting portal and inflating the tourniquet is extremely helpful. With the elbow joint distended, the major neurovascular structures are positioned further from the starting portal and entry into the joint is also easier.

Once the arthroscope has been successfully placed into the joint, visualization can be maintained by either pressure distention of the capsule or by retraction. Pres-

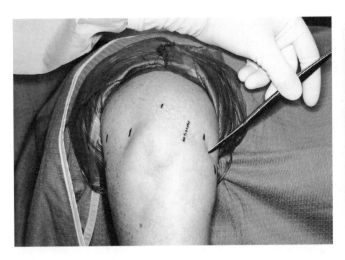

Figure 3 Portals marked with a surgical pen prior to beginning arthroscopy. A long dotted line represents the area of the ulnar nerve. The retractor is placed between anteromedial portals.

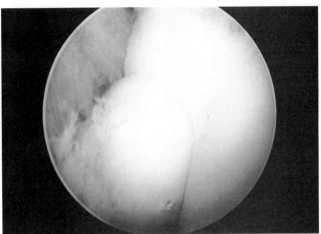

Figure 4 Arthroscopic view of coronoid as viewed from the anterolateral portal.

sure distention works quite well but will eventually lead to significant fluid extravasation during a long arthroscopic procedure. The use of retractors is an alternative to pressure distention. Retractors for elbow arthroscopy are simple lever-type retractors such as a Howarth or a large blunt Steinmann pin. Retractors are placed into the elbow joint via accessory portals, which are typically 2 to 3 cm proximal to the standard arthroscopic viewing portals. By holding the capsule away from the joint, retractors allow adequate visualization with a low-pressure inflow system.

Portal Placement
Safe initial portal entry can be made either from the medial or lateral side of the elbow depending on the preference of the surgeon (Figure 3). The anterolateral portal is often the initial portal placed and is usually placed just anterior to the sulcus between the capitellum and radial head. This is an easily located anatomic area to find in most patients. The radial nerve is in close proximity to this portal. Once the arthroscope has been placed into the joint from the anterolateral portal, the surgeon should be able to visualize the trochlea, coronoid process, coronoid fossa, and the medial aspect of the radial head (Figure 4). After it has been confirmed that the arthroscope is in the elbow joint, then an anteromedial working portal can be established. This maneuver is easiest to perform from an inside-out approach. The arthroscope is removed from the sheath and a blunt trocar placed back in and then gently pushed straight across the joint. With gentle pushing and rotation, the tip of the trocar will begin tenting the skin on the medial side of the elbow. The skin is then incised over the tip of the trocar and the sheath pushed out of the skin. A working cannula can then be placed over the tip of the sheath and pushed back into the joint.

An anteromedial portal may be placed before the anterolateral portal based on the surgeon's preference. The anteromedial portal is placed 2 cm distal and 2 cm anterior to the medial epicondyle. This will penetrate the common flexor origin and the brachialis. The medial antebrachiocutaneous nerve is at risk with its portal, often only several millimeters from the starting position.

The posterolateral portal is an excellent initial viewing portal for the posterior aspect of the elbow. Unlike the anterior portals, where palpation of the median or radial nerve is not possible, establishment of posterior portals should be a safe undertaking once the ulnar nerve is palpated and identified. The posterolateral portal is made lateral and level with the tip of the olecranon with the elbow flexed 90°. The trocar should be aimed at the center of the olecranon fossa. Viewing is often difficult initially posteriorly, because the fat pad normally occupies a large portion of the potential joint space. The direct posterior portal is a good initial working portal. Through this portal loose bodies and osteophytes in the entire olecranon fossa can be removed while viewing from a posterolateral portal. This portal is established 2 cm proximal to the tip of the olecranon at the proximal margin of the olecranon fossa. After creating this portal, a shaver can be placed into the joint and débridement performed. The arthroscope and shaver can be switched back and forth between the direct and the posterolateral portal to enable efficient completion of posterior débridement.

Arthroscopic Treatment of Degenerative Arthritis
Degenerative arthritis is accompanied by osteophyte formation and capsular contraction. In addition to removal of loose bodies, the surgeon should be prepared to remove all impinging osteophytes and to release a potentially tight, thickened capsule. It is the rare patient who has an

isolated loose body, perhaps after an osteochondral injury. After initial joint inspection and removal of all obvious loose bodies, bony work should commence. A shaver or burr can be used to remove osteophytes from the radial and coronoid fossae of the humerus and the tip of the coronoid can be excised. The medial coronoid should also be examined for osteophytes, which may be missed if not positively identified. It is helpful to perform most of the bony work using a burr before completion of the capsulectomy because neurovascular structures are better protected and visualization is improved before muscle or soft tissue impedes the arthroscopic view. Once the osteophytes have been excised, the anterior capsule can be removed. It is often helpful to take the capsule off the humerus as a first step. Care should be taken when excising capsule just anterior to the radial head. The radial nerve is at great risk of injury at this location. Often a small fat pad can be visualized in this area, the radial nerve being just anterior.

Complications

Complications that can arise from elbow arthroscopy include compartment syndrome, septic arthritis, and nerve injury. In a report of 473 elbow arthroscopies, there were four types of minor complications in 50 procedures, including infection, nerve injury, prolonged drainage, and contracture. The most common complication was persistent portal drainage. Neurologic complications were limited to transient nerve palsy. The rate of permanent neurologic injury appears to be higher in the elbow than in the knee or shoulder. The risk of nerve injury is higher in patients with rheumatoid arthritis or in those undergoing a capsular release. Significant nerve injury during elbow arthroscopy has been reported involving the radial, median, and ulnar nerves. The use of retractors is probably the most important factor in preventing nerve injury. In some instances, arthroscopic identification of nerves will allow for safer capsulectomy.

Instability
Pathophysiology

Interest in elbow instability has increased over the past several years as more has been learned about the pathoanatomy of elbow dislocation. There are essentially three patterns of acute elbow instability: (1) posterolateral rotatory, (2) valgus, and (3) varus posteromedial rotatory instability. Posterolateral rotatory instability is the most common mechanism of acute instability and can progress from a simple dislocation to a complex fracture-dislocation (terrible triad). Valgus instability occurs most commonly as a chronic overload problem, particularly in throwers. Varus posteromedial rotatory instability has recently been recognized as a significant pattern of instability, usually associated with a medial coronoid fracture.

Knowledge of the static and dynamic constraints of the elbow is helpful in understanding the progression of acute elbow instability. The three primary static constraints are the ulnohumeral articulation, anterior band of the medial collateral ligament (MCL), and the lateral ulnocollateral ligament (LUCL). The secondary constraints include the radiocapitellar articulation, common flexor and extensor origins, and the capsule. The flexor and extensor muscle groups across the elbow play a major role in creating dynamic instability and in producing compressive forces at the elbow joint. Particularly, the anconeus, because of its origin in the lateral epicondyle and broad insertion on the ulna, is designed to function as a dynamic stabilizer against posterolateral rotatory instability. An elbow will remain stable if the three primary constraints are intact. If the MCL is disrupted, the radial head and coronoid become more critical for stability. If the coronoid is fractured, the radial head becomes the prime stabilizer and must be reconstructed or replaced. Likewise, if the radial head is fractured, stability will be difficult to achieve if the coronoid fracture remains unrepaired.

Posterolateral Rotatory Dislocation

A simple elbow dislocation is usually the result of posterolateral rotatory instability. This injury pattern occurs during a valgus moment to the elbow with simultaneous forearm supination. Progressively the radial head and coronoid rotate under the capitellum and dislocation occurs. The disruption of the soft tissues begins laterally and progresses to the medial side of the elbow (Figure 5). This progressive disruption occurs in a circle pattern simultaneously anteriorly and posteriorly and has been referred to as the Horii circle and is analogous to the Mayfield circle of progressive carpal instability.

Varus Posteromedial Rotatory Dislocation

Similar to posterolateral rotatory instability, varus posteromedial rotary dislocation also occurs during axial loading of the elbow during flexion. A varus moment occurs with internal rotation of the forearm resulting in a fracture of the anteromedial coronoid with disruption of the LUCL. Unlike posterolateral rotatory instability, where dislocation can occur without a fracture, the key to varus posteromedial rotatory dislocation is an anteromedial coronoid fracture (Figure 6).

Recurrent Valgus Instability

Valgus instability can occur as an acute event or after chronic valgus overload. This condition involves a distinctly different pattern of instability as compared with posterolateral rotatory instability. As an acute event it results in rupture of the MCL from a pure valgus load to the elbow. As the injury occurs, the force is transmitted from medial to lateral, potentially resulting in radial

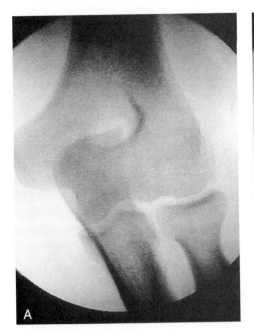
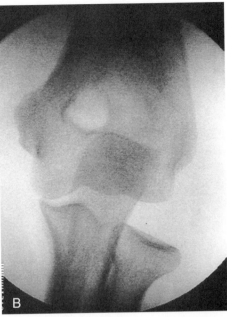

Figure 5 Fluoroscopic examination under anesthesia demonstrating disruption of the lateral collateral ligament and lateral soft-tissue attachments. **A,** Resting position. **B,** Gross lateral instability is seen after varus stress is applied.

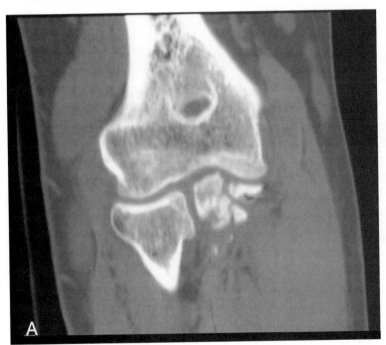
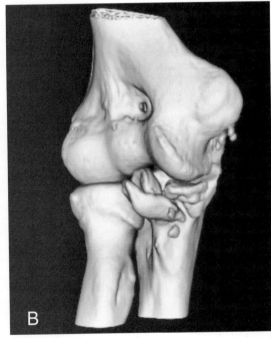

Figure 6 A, CT scan showing varus posteromedial rotatory instability. The comminuted fracture of the coronoid and collapse pattern is best seen on the three-dimensional reconstruction (**B**).

head fracture. If in this situation the radial head is excised, the elbow is at significant risk of remaining permanently unstable in valgus. This injury pattern does not typically result in an acute dislocation. Acute rupture of the MCL may occur as a catastrophic terminal event in high-demand overhead throwing athletes but is usually the result of a chronic valgus overload.

Posterolateral Rotatory Instability
Recurrent instability following simple dislocation of the elbow involves posterolateral rotatory instability in almost every case. The essential lesion is detachment or attenuation of the LUCL. Although both the MCL and LUCL are usually disrupted, the LUCL is at risk of not healing because of repetitive varus stresses applied to

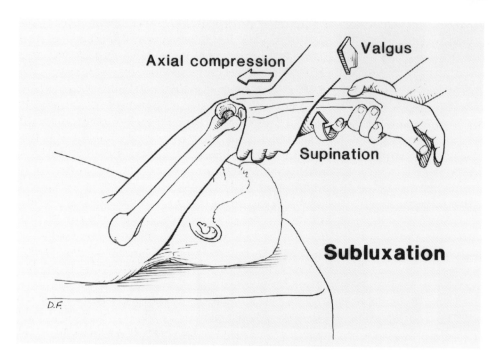

Figure 7 Demonstration of lateral pivot shift test for posterolateral rotatory instability. The test is begun with the elbow extended. The elbow is then placed in supination with a moderate force. As the elbow is flexed to 40° or more a valgus force torque is increasingly applied. Reduction of the ulna and radius together on the humerus occurs suddenly with a palpable visible clunk. The reduction is what is sensed and palpated, not the dislocation.

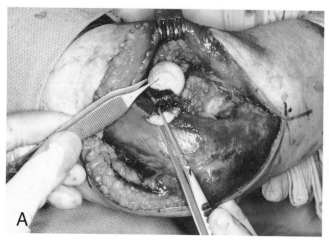
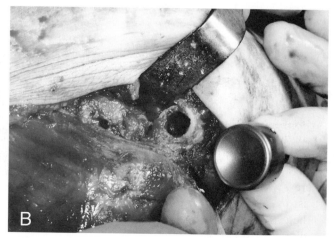

Figure 8 Comminuted radial head fracture. Pieces of the radial head have been removed (**A**). The shaft of the radius is then reamed and the end of the fracture is planed to a level position. The radial head implant is then ready for placement (**B**).

the elbow, caused by the force of gravity when the shoulder is abducted. The typical patient has a history of recurrent painful snapping or locking of the elbow. A careful history would demonstrate that symptoms occur during extension arc of motion with the forearm in supination. Examination for posterolateral rotatory instability is best performed with the patient supine and the affected extremity overhead (Figure 7).

Radial Head Replacement

Radial head replacement is indicated for comminuted fractures of the radial head associated with elbow instability (Figure 8). Routine replacement of comminuted radial head fractures without associated MCL disruption or interosseous membrane disruption has not tradi-

tionally been performed. This viewpoint has begun to change as newer prostheses have been developed and as greater awareness occurs of the accelerated degenerative process that can occur at the ulnohumeral joint after radial head excision even with an initially stable MCL. In long-term studies in which patients were examined after radial head excision, a high percentage of patients developed significant radiographic ulnohumeral arthrosis. Additionally, radial head excision may cause decreased grip strength, wrist pain, and progressive valgus instability.

Elbow Contractures

Most elbow contractures are mild and usually well tolerated. The functional range of motion has been defined as between –30° full extension to 130° flexion. Mild loss of terminal extension is usually well tolerated, but there are certain exceptions. Basketball players with loss of extension typically report that the contracture affects their jump shot; loss of extension affects gymnasts as well. Primary loss of flexion is usually not well tolerated because it often affects the ability to perform common activities of daily life.

The pathogenesis of elbow contractures is poorly understood. Patients with an injured elbow typically will hold the extremity in a flexed position, which minimizes the intra-articular pressure from a joint effusion. A fibrous tissue response occurs as a result of periarticular muscular and capsular tearing. The capsule hypertrophies to a thick contracted structure (normal capsules are transparent and thin). There are severe intrinsic and extrinsic factors involved in an elbow contracture. Intrinsic factors include joint incongruity, loose bodies, synovitis, articular surface ankylosis, and capsular contracture, all of which may be amenable to treatment with arthroscopic elbow contracture release. Extrinsic factors include heterotopic bone formation, myositis ossification, collateral ligament contracture, and muscle contractures, all of which are more amenable to treatment with open elbow contracture release. In many patients, intrinsic and extrinsic factors coexist.

Heterotopic ossification has been shown to occur in 3% of patients with elbow dislocations. It has been documented that the incidence of heterotopic ossification increases to 20% in patients with an elbow dislocation associated with a fracture. Heterotopic ossification occurs in 5% of patients with isolated neuraxis trauma and increases dramatically to 75% to 86% when brain injury is associated with elbow trauma. An increased incidence of heterotopic ossification has also been shown to occur in patients with thermal injuries.

Patients with less than 40° of extension or 105° of flexion are candidates for elbow contracture release. The ulnar nerve is particularly vulnerable to injury and scarring. In patients with preoperative ulnar nerve symptoms and loss of marked flexion of the elbow, neurolysis and transposition of the ulnar nerve should be considered.

The traditional timing of release was to wait at least 1 year after the initial injury. Other previous recommendations included waiting until bone scans became cold and nonreactive and to follow serial alkaline phosphatase levels until a normal range was reached. However, in reality, patients rarely gain motion after 6 months, with the exception of pediatric patients. During this time, the soft-tissue contractures continue to mature. New recommendations have been made that suggest elbow contracture release be considered after 6 months when patients have no significant improvement from physical therapy.

The medial over-the-top release allows decompression to the ulnar nerve in patients with preoperative ulnar nerve symptoms. The lateral approach has been popularized in several studies; this type of release is particularly advantageous in the treatment of patients without preoperative ulnar nerve symptoms. In this approach, the origin of the extensor digitorum communis and extensor carpi radialis brevis is elevated to expose the joint capsule. The joint capsule is then excised. The posterior compartment is slightly more difficult to approach from the lateral side. It is important to approach the posterior compartment by subperiosteally elevating the triceps and working proximal to distal. The key is to approach the olecranon fossa proximally and avoid dissection and involvement of the lateral ulnohumeral complex. The olecranon fossa is débrided, and the tip is excised.

The risk of recurrent heterotopic ossification is low, but some patients may be candidates for postoperative radiation. Although there is significant evidence in the literature to support the use of postoperative radiation in patients with acetabular fractures who have undergone hip replacement, its use in patients with heterotopic ossification of the elbow remains undefined.

One study recently reported the results of 20 patients with complete ankylosis of the elbow caused by heterotopic bone formation who underwent surgical release without severe injury to the central nervous system. In this series, the average arc of ulnar humeral motion was 81° in patients with burns and 94° in patients with ankylosis secondary to trauma. Six of 11 limbs in the burn group and 5 of 9 patients in the trauma group had good results. The authors concluded that surgeons should be aware of the small risk of recurrent heterotopic ossification, mild pain, and recurrent contracture after surgical release. However, they believed the procedure was effective and safe.

Techniques of Elbow Reconstruction

Rheumatoid arthritis, posttraumatic arthritis, and osteoarthritis are the three major types of arthritis that affect the elbow. Pain is the primary complaint of patients with these disorders, although some may also experience stiffness, weakness, and potentially instability. Several treatment options are available, depending on the type and stage of arthritic changes.

Synovectomy

Rheumatoid arthritis is the most frequent type of arthritis that affects the elbow joint. Four stages of rheumatic disease of the elbow have been described based on radiographic and pathologic criteria. In stage I rheumatic disease, synovitis is present, but a normal joint surface has been maintained. In stage II, mild to moderate synovitis is present and evidence of joint space narrowing is seen on radiographs, but the joint contour is still maintained. In stage III, mild to moderate synovitis and mild to moderate alteration of the joint surface are typically present, and there is loss of joint space. In stage IV, mechanical instability with bone on bone articulation and complete joint space destruction is evident on radiographs.

When conservative measures fail to relieve symptoms, arthroscopic or open synovectomy is frequently recommended. The role of radial head excision with synovectomy, however, remains controversial. Good pain relief and preservation of motion have been reported with arthroscopic and open synovectomy.

The commonly described approaches for open synovectomy include extended lateral approach, mediolateral approach, and transolecranon approach. A total synovectomy may be performed using the extended lateral approach with radial head excision. The proximal ulna is displaced medially for adequate medial compartment synovectomy when this approach is selected.

Arthroscopy allows a complete synovectomy to be done without the need for large capsular incisions, which are required for any open approach. The arthroscope with a blunt trocar is introduced into the anterior compartment after it is inflated with approximately 20 mL of sterile lactated Ringer's solution. A proximal anterolateral portal is made using either the inside-out or outside-in technique. The view offered by the more proximal portals allows excellent visualization of both the medial and lateral anterior compartments of the elbow. The goal is to excise the excessive synovitis, taking care not to aggressively cut through the anterior capsule. The arthroscope and shaver will need to be switched between the portals to gain good access for the synovectomy. Once the synovium has been resected, the radiocapitellar articulation is evaluated. If there is significant involvement of the radial head, then radial head excision may be required. A synovectomy of the posterior compartment is then performed.

Open synovectomy of the elbow is an accepted procedure with good results. The published results on this remain consistent. Pain relief is regularly seen in 80% to 90% of patients at 3- to 5-year follow-up. Although recurrence of synovitis is common at 10- to 20-year follow-up, approximately two thirds of patients were satisfied with the results of the procedure. Range of motion will improve in approximately 40% of patients, decrease somewhat in approximately 15%, and the remainder will be unchanged. Arthroscopic synovectomy is a highly demanding procedure. One study of 14 arthroscopic synovectomies revealed an early success rate of 95%. However, at 3-year follow-up, approximately 60% of patients reported satisfaction with the results. One study reported on 46 elbows that underwent arthroscopic synovectomy for the treatment of inflammatory arthritis. All 46 elbows had improved motion and decreased pain. One patient developed a synovial fissula, two patients required repeat synovectomy, and one patient required a total elbow arthroplasty.

Outerbridge-Kashiwagi (Ulnohumeral) Arthroplasty

In patients with primary degenerative arthritis or post-traumatic degenerative arthritis who have pain on terminal flexion and extension, the traditional procedure has been the Outerbridge-Kashiwagi (ulnohumeral) arthroplasty. This procedure may be performed open or arthroscopically. In the open procedure, an incision is made 3 cm proximal to the tip of the olecranon with splitting of the triceps. The tip of the olecranon is excised, and a foramenectomy in the distal humerus can then be made using a 4.5-mm drill bit and then enlarged with a burr. Care must be taken not to involve the medial and lateral columns of the elbow.

This procedure is done arthroscopically through a trocar, and a 4.5-mm drill bit is used to create a foramina in the center of the olecranon fossa. Once the initial foramina has been made with the drill, it is then enlarged by an arthroscopic burr inserted in the posterior central portal. In one report of 12 patients, all had relief of pain and locking at follow-up of 3 to 30 months. A similar experience was reported in 21 patients who underwent débridement and removal of loose bodies in both anterior and posterior compartments. In this group, the average follow-up was 3 years, and 84% noted satisfactory outcomes.

Interposition Arthroplasty

Patients with posttraumatic arthritis may present with stiffness, pain, or a combination of both. Traditionally, total joint arthroplasty has not provided favorable experience in the management of patients with posttraumatic arthritis. In younger patients with posttraumatic arthritis, an interposition arthroplasty is the treatment of choice. If this procedure is performed, the elbow is often protected with an external fixator, which decompresses the joint to decentralize motion while the tissues are healing.

Arthrodesis

The functional use of the hand depends on the elbow. It has been show that approximately 50% loss of elbow motion results in an 80% loss of function to the upper extremity. Additionally, elbow flexion is usually not well tolerated. Arthrodesis of the elbow is not compatible with satisfactory function because range of motion of the elbow is essential for use of the hand. There is no single ideal position for arthrodesis. Indications for arthrodesis include the presence of intractable sepsis and in patients for whom there is no possibility of total elbow reconstruction. Because arthrodesis is primarily a salvage procedure, its use in young men who perform heavy labor is controversial.

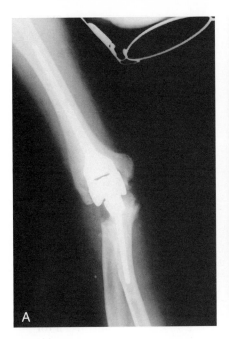

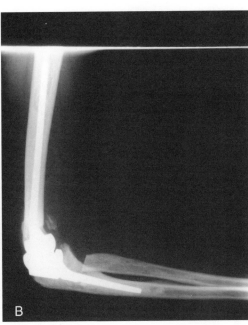

Figure 9 AP **(A)** and lateral **(B)** radiographs of a patient with an unlinked total elbow implant. The patient had good bone stock and competent ligaments. If bone stock or ligaments are found to be of poor quality at the time of surgery, the prosthesis can be converted to a linked implant by exchanging the intra-articular components.

Total Elbow Arthroplasty

Although the results with early elbow prosthesis were initially disappointing, improvements in surgical techniques and implant designs have made total elbow arthroplasty a reliable procedure for many patients with rheumatoid arthritis or osteoarthritis, selected older patients with posttraumatic arthritis, and selected patients with comminuted acute fractures and nonunions.

There are two types of prosthetic joint designs in use: unlinked (previously referred to as nonconstrained) and linked (semiconstrained). Recently, implants have been designed that can be converted intraoperatively from unlinked to linked. Total elbow arthroplasty is contraindicated in patients who are candidates for alternative procedures, such as synovectomy, débridement, and open reduction and internal fixation. Previous infection is a relatively strong contraindication; however, recent studies suggest that total arthroplasty can be successfully performed in selected patients using staged débridements with negative cultures.

The decision to use unlinked or linked arthroplasty depends on the amount of bone destruction, the status of the capsule ligamentous tissues of the elbow joint, and the surgeon's experience. Unlinked designs seek to replicate the axis of motion to the elbow to optimize ligamentous balance and maintain joint stability. Major forces about the elbow are absorbed by the soft tissues and theoretically protect the bone-cement interface. To have sufficient stability, an unlinked arthrodesis requires adequate bone stock and competent ligaments (Figure 9). The loss of continuity of the soft tissues that can be seen after trauma or long-standing rheumatoid arthritis would be a contraindication for an unlinked prosthesis.

Several linked semiconstrained, softly hinged prostheses have been designed for a degree of laxity that permits the soft tissue to absorb some of the stresses that would normally be applied to the prosthesis-bone interface. Static loading conditions of the elbow can result in forces equal to three times body weight, and dynamic loading can equal up to six times body weight. These tremendous forces can ultimately lead to aseptic implant loosening and failure. A linked prosthesis may be used in a patient with bone loss (such as a patient with humeral nonunion or chronic instability) resulting from previous trauma or erosion from advanced rheumatoid arthritis (Figure 10). The stability provided by a linked arthroplasty allows for a complete release of soft tissues, which may lead to more predictable gains in motion.

Various surgical approaches have been described for total elbow arthroplasty. A distal-based triceps flap has been used, particularly for unlinked implants. A standard posterior approach to the elbow is made; then a triangular or rectangular distal-based triceps flap is made. Care is taken to retain the triceps tendon attachment to the olecranon. Dissection is then continued along the lateral side of the olecranon, and the joint is exposed and hinged on the intact medial collateral ligament. The attachment of the medial collateral ligament is preserved. Dissection can then continue proximally along the lateral collateral ligament insertion on the humerus, and release of the anterior capsule can be done to gain more exposure. The tip of the base of the olecranon and radial head may then be excised to gain further exposure for joint arthroplasty. Management of the ulnar nerve is controversial. Most surgeons recommend

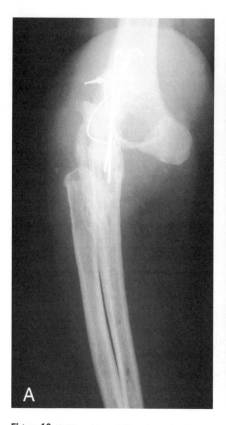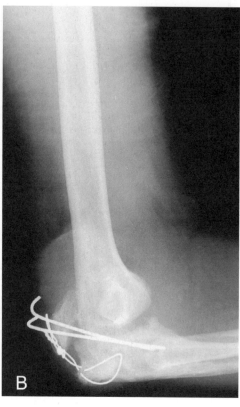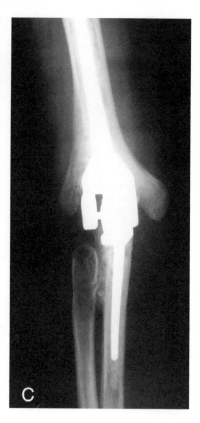

Figure 10 AP **(A)** and lateral **(B)** radiographs of a 68-year-old woman with rheumatoid arthritis and elbow trauma with bone deformity and ligament instability. **C**, AP radiograph after a linked total elbow implant was inserted. The decision to link the elbow was made because of the bone deformity and ligament instability.

identification and protection of the nerve without formal transposition.

A Bryan-Morrey approach is typically used for a linked arthroplasty. The triceps is elevated from medial to lateral off the olecranon in continuity with the anconeus muscle. Before this approach is attempted, the ulnar nerve should be well identified and protected. A long periosteal strip of the triceps off of the olecranon and proximal ulna is made, creating a continuous extensor mechanism sling. The triceps tendon with the long periosteal sleeve is then reattached with sutures through multiple drill holes in the olecranon.

There are numerous published reports of unlinked elbow arthroplasties. Pain relief and restoration by functional arc of motion have been reported in more than 90% of patients. The designers of this implant report excellent results in patients with rheumatoid arthritis, with only a 1.5% incidence of postoperative dislocation and a low incidence of aseptic loosening.

The success of linked total elbow arthroplasty has also been well documented. A series of 58 modified Coonrad semiconstrained total elbow arthroplasties followed for 3.8 years postoperatively yielded a 91% excellent or good result, with 84% of patients having no pain. Similar results were reported with the use of a semiconstrained prosthesis (GSB III Elbow System, Zimmer,

Warsaw, IN), with 91% excellent or good results reported at 4-year follow-up.

In another study, 26 patients underwent either a linked or unlinked total elbow arthroplasty; all procedures were performed by a single surgeon. The authors reported that no significant differences were found in functional performance or progressive radiolucent loosening and concluded that, when properly performed, total elbow arthroplasty with either type of prosthesis yielded satisfactory results.

Recently, linked elbow arthroplasty has been recommended for the treatment of elderly patients with severely comminuted intra-articular fractures of the distal humerus. Additionally, elbow arthroplasty has been recommended for distal humeral nonunions (Figure 11). Under certain conditions, it is standard practice to excise humeral condyles during insertion of the linked total elbow prosthesis. One study recently reviewed the results of condylar resection on forearm, wrist, and hand strength in 32 patients who underwent total elbow arthroplasty. The normal contralateral limb served as the control, and strength values were given as a percentage of the normal side. The humeral condyles were intact in 16 patients and had been resected in the other 16 patients. The authors found no significant difference between the two groups with regard to strength of pronation and supination, wrist extension, or grip strength.

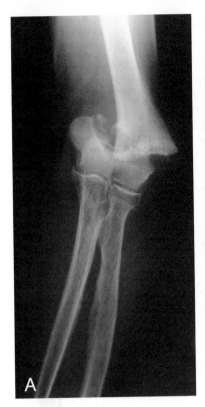

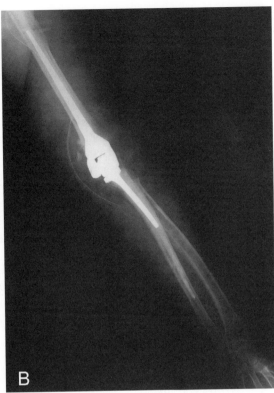

Figure 11 A, AP radiograph of a 75-year-old woman with a 2-year history of a distal humeral nonunion. **B,** AP radiograph after a linked total elbow implant was inserted. For this type of arthroplasty, the distal supracondylar bone fragments are removed, and the patient is started on immediate range-of-motion exercises.

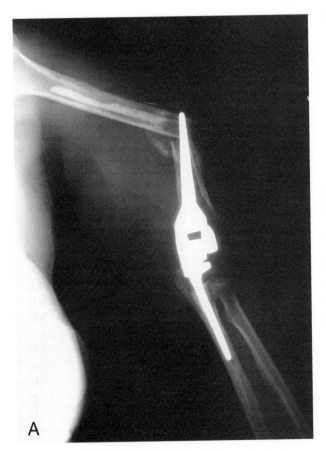

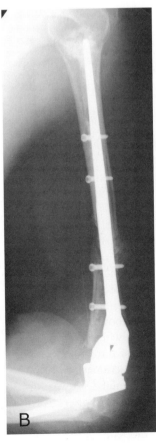

Figure 12 A, AP radiograph of a 72-year-old woman 8 months after undergoing total elbow arthroplasty. The patient fell and thereby sustained the humeral periprosthetic fracture. **B,** AP radiograph showing a custom-made, long-stem humeral component with interlocking screws. Two screws were placed proximal and distal to the fracture .

There was no significant difference between the two groups with regard to Mayo Elbow Performance Scores (79 in the group with intact condyles versus 77 in the group with resection of the condyles).

The most devastating complication of total elbow arthroplasty is infection. Infection rates between 2% to 5% have been reported. Late infections with persistent sepsis despite débridements should be managed by removal of the implant and all cement. Ulnar nerve neuropathy is common after total elbow arthroplasty. Usually, it most often results in transient numbness, which resolves itself. However, residual sensory and motor symptoms are occasionally reported. The nerve may be compressed, and the elbow may be subluxated to replace the components and damaged by retraction or thermal injury from extravasated bone cement. It is important to take care to protect the ulnar nerve during the procedure. Intraoperative fractures of one or both humeral columns may also occur, usually at the MCL column as a result of stress on the MCL during the procedure. Open reduction and internal fixation of the fracture column may be performed either with intramedullary screws or potentially a plate. This also usually involves conversion of an unlinked to a linked component.

Periprosthetic fractures around the elbow have been reported. If minimally displaced, the fracture may be managed nonsurgically with bracing. Displaced or unstable fractures may require surgical intervention. Previous options included plate fixation around the prosthesis or further stabilization with allografts. Recently, the use of custom-made long-stem implants that act as intramedullary rods to cross over the fracture site with interlocking screws has been reported (Figure 12.)

Emerging Concepts

The outcome of total elbow arthroplasty has markedly improved over the past two decades as a result of improved implant designs and surgical techniques. Recent studies have demonstrated that total elbow arthroplasty in patients with an inflammatory arthritis is quite successful. Patients who are difficult to treat, such as those with osteoarthritis and posttraumatic arthritis, remain problematic because implant survival rate has been lower. Opportunities for improvement include advances in implant design and implantation techniques. Titanium, cobalt-chromium, and polyethylene are the most common materials currently used in elbow arthroplasty. Whether ceramic or other materials will improve the longevity of elbow arthroplasty will require further investigations. The optimal stem shape and length for total elbow arthroplasty has yet to be determined. Newer implants that allow the surgeon to decide intraoperatively whether linked or unlinked components may be best for the patient have recently been developed.

Annotated Bibliography

Arthroscopy

Kelly EW, Morrey BF, O'Driscoll SW: Complications of elbow arthroscopy. *J Bone Joint Surg Am* 2001;83:25-34.

A large study of 473 elbow arthroscopies was conducted in 449 patients. A serious complication (joint space infection) occurred in four (0.8%). Minor complications, such as superficial infection, minor contracture, and transcient nerve palsy, occurred after 50 (11%) of the procedures. Although there were no permanent nerve injuries, the risk to neurovascular structures is emphasized, particularly in patients with rheumatoid arthritis.

Steinmann SP: Elbow arthroscopy. *JASSH* 2003;3:199-207.

Review of technique for elbow arthroscopy. This article describes the operating room setup and indications for elbow arthroscopy. Discussion of technique for treatment of different conditions is included.

Instability

Ball CM, Galatz LM, Yamaguchi K: Elbow Instability: Treatment strategies and emerging concepts. *Instr Course Lect* 2002;51:53-61.

A description of biomechanics of elbow instability and relevant anatomy is presented. Treatment of acute and chronic instability is discussed.

Thompson WH, Jobe FW, Yocum LA, Pink MM: Ulnar collateral ligament reconstruction in athletes: Muscle-splitting approach without transposition of the ulnar nerve. *J Shoulder Elbow Surg* 2001;10:152-157.

The technique for MCL reconstruction is reviewed. The authors describe in a large series the step-by-step procedure for ligament reconstruction.

Radial Head Replacement

Moro JK, Werier J, MacDermid JC, Patterson SD, King GJ: Arthroplasty with a metal radial head for unreconstructible fractures of the radial head. *J Bone Joint Surg Am* 2001;83:1201-1211.

Patients treated with a metal radial head arthroplasty had mild to moderate impairment of elbow and wrist function. Use of a metal radial head, however, was found to be safe and effective treatment.

Elbow Contractures

Ring D, Jupiter JB: Operative release of complete ankylosis of the elbow due to heterotopic bone in patients without severe injury of the central nervous system. *J Bone Joint Surg Am* 2003;85:849-857.

The authors found that attempts to regain motion in this class of patients are both worthwhile and safe in their experience with 11 elbows in seven patients.

Techniques of Elbow Reconstruction

King GJ: New frontiers in elbow reconstruction: Total elbow arthroplasty. *Instr Course Lect* 2002;51:43-51.

This article reviews the literature comparing linked and unlinked total elbow arthroplasty and the relative indications for each type of prosthesis.

McKee MD, Pugh DM, Richards RR, Pedersen E, Jones C, Schmitsch EH: Effect of humeral condylar resection on strength and functional outcome after semiconstrained total elbow arthroplasty. *J Bone Joint Surg Am* 2003;85:802-807.

The authors found condylar resection had a minimal, clinically irrelevant effect on forearm, wrist, and hand strength and no significant effect on the Mayo Elbow Performance score following total elbow arthroplasty in 16 patients.

Classic Bibliography

Evans EB: Orthopaedic measures in the treatment of sever burns. *J Bone Joint Surg Am* 1966;48:643-669.

Ewald FC, Simmons ED Jr, Sullivan JA, et al: Capitellocondylar total elbow replacement in rheumatoid arthritis. *J Bone Joint Surg Am* 1993;75:498-507.

Froimson AI: Interposition arthroplasty of the elbow, in Morrey BF (ed): *The Elbow*. New York, NY, Raven Press, 1994, pp 329-342.

Garland DE, Hannscom DA, Keenan MA, et al: Resection of heterotopic ossification in the adult with head trauma. *J Bone Joint Surg Am* 1985;67:1261-1269.

Hastings H II, Cohen MS: Post–traumatic contracture of the elbow: Operative release using a new approach. *Trans ASES* 1996, 13-32.

Hastings H II, Graham TJ: The classification and treatment of heterotopic ossification about the elbow and forearm. *Hand Clin* 1994;10:417-437.

Hedley AK, Mead LP, Hendren DH: The prevention of heterotopic bone formation following total hip arthroplasty using 600 rad in a single dose. *J Arthroplasty* 1989;4:319-325.

Herold N, Schroder HA: Synovectomy and radial head excision in rheumatoid arthritis: Eleven patients followed for 14 years. *Acta Orthop Scand* 1995;66:252-254.

Hotchkiss RN, An Kn, Weiland AJ, et al: Treatment of severe elbow contractures using the concepts of Ilizarov. *61st Annual Meeting Proceedings*. Rosemont, IL, American Academy of Orthopaedic Surgeons, 1994.

Ikeda M, Oka Y: Function after early radial head resection for fracture: A retrospective evaluation of 15 patients followed for 3-18 years. *Acta Orthop Scand* 2000;71:191-194.

Jones GS, Savoie FH: Arthroscopic capsular release of flexion contractures (arthrofibrosis) of the elbow. *Arthroscopy* 1993;9:277-283.

King GJ, Morrey BF, An K-N: Stabilizers of the elbow. *J Shoulder Elbow Surg* 1993;2:165-174.

King GJ, Zarzour ZD, Rath DA, Dunning CE, Patterson SD, Johnson JA: Metallic radial head arthroplasty improves valgus stability of the elbow. *Clin Orthop* 1999;368:114-125.

Kraay MJ, Figgie MP, Inglis AE, et al: Primary semiconstrained total elbow arthroplasty: Survival analysis in 113 consecutive cases. *J Bone Joint Surg Br* 1994;76:636-640.

Lee BP, Morrey BF: Arthroscopic synovectomy of the elbow in rheumatoid arthritis: A prospective study. *J Bone Joint Surg Br* 1997;79:770-772.

Ljung P, Jonsson K, Larsson K, et al: Interposition arthroplasty of the elbow in rheumatoid arthritis. *J Shoulder Elbow Surg* 1996;5:81-85.

Modabber MR, Jupiter JB: Reconstruction for posttraumatic conditions of the elbow joint. *J Bone Joint Surg Am* 1995;77:1431-1446.

Morrey BF: Primary degenerative arthritis of the elbow: Treatment by ulnohumeral arthroplasty. *J Bone Joint Surg Br* 1992;74:409-413.

Morrey BF, Adams RA: Semiconstrained arthroplasty for the treatment of rheumatoid arthritis of the elbow. *J Bone Joint Surg Am* 1992;72:479-490.

Morrey BF, Adams RA, Bryan RS: Total elbow arthroplasty for post-traumatic arthritis of the elbow. *J Bone Joint Surg Br* 1991;73:607-612.

Nestor BJ, O'Driscoll SW, Morrey BF: Ligamentous reconstruction for posterolateral rotatory instability of the elbow. *J Bone Joint Surg Am* 1992;74:1235-1241.

Nowicki KD, Shall LM: Arthroscopic release of a posttraumatic flexion contracture in the elbow: A case report and review of the literature. *Arthroscopy* 1992;8:544-547.

O'Driscoll SW: Arthroscopic treatment for osteoarthritis of the elbow. *Orthop Clin North Am* 1995;26:691-706.

O'Driscoll SW, Morrey BF: Surgical reconstruction of the lateral collateral ligament, in Morrey BF (ed): *Master Techniques in Orthopedic Surgery: The Elbow*. New York, NY, Raven Press, 1994, pp 169-182.

Ogilvie-Harris DJ, Gordon R, MacKay M: Arthroscopic treatment for posterior impingement in degenerative arthritis of the elbow. *Arthroscopy* 1995;11:437-443.

Ring D, Jupiter JB: Fracture-dislocation of the elbow. *J Bone Joint Surg Am* 1998;80:566-580.

Ross G, McDevitt ER, Chronister R, Ove PN: Treatment of simple elbow dislocation using an immediate motion protocol. *Am J Sports Med* 1999;27:308-311.

Rymaszewski L, Glass K, Parikh R: Post-traumatic elbow contracture treated by arthrolysis and continued passive motion under brachial plexus anesthesia. *J Bone Joint Surg Br* 1996;76:S30.

Rymaszewski LA, Mackay I, Amis AA, Miller JH: Long-term effects of excision of the radial head in rheumatoid arthritis. *J Bone Joint Surg Br* 1984;66:109-113.

Savoie FH III, Nunley PD, Field LD: Arthroscopic management of the arthritic elbow: Indications, technique, and results. *J Shoulder Elbow Surg* 1999;8:214-219.

Thal R: Arthritis, in Savoie FH, Field LD (eds): *Arthroscopy of the Elbow*. New York, NY, Churchill Livingstone 1996, pp 103-116.

Tulp NJ, Winia WP: Synovectomy of the elbow in rheumatoid arthritis: Long term results. *J Bone Joint Surg Br* 1989;71:664-666.

Vasen AP, Lacey SH, Keith MW, et al: Functional range of motion of the elbow. *J Hand Surg Am* 1995;20:288-291.

Wright TW, Wong AM, Jaffe R: Functional outcome comparison of semiconstrained and unconstrained total elbow arthroplasties. *J Shoulder Elbow Surg* 2000;9:524-531.

Chapter 29

Wrist and Hand: Trauma

Emily Anne Hattwick, MD, MPH

Edward Diao, MD

Distal Radius Fractures

Distal radius fractures are the most common orthopaedic fractures. These fractures are associated with osteoporosis in the elderly and high-energy trauma in younger patients. Successful treatment outcomes are correlated with accuracy of articular reduction, restoration of normal anatomic relationships, and early efforts at regaining motion in the fingers and wrist.

The mechanism of injury is most commonly an axial load through the hand and wrist. Useful imaging studies include AP, lateral, and oblique radiographs, arthrogram, CT, and MRI. Reconstructed CT studies are helpful in planning for articular reduction of die-punch lesions, and MRI studies identify associated soft-tissue injuries in complex fractures such as to the triangular fibrocartilage complex (TFCC) and scapholunate, and the lunotriquetral ligaments.

Several classification systems describe fracture patterns. Restoration of radial height (average, 13 mm), volar tilt (average, 11°), radial inclination (average, 23°), and articular surface are associated with good outcomes (Figure 1). In extra-articular fractures, radial shortening is associated with the greatest loss of wrist function and incidence of wrist degenerative changes, including changes to the TFCC. Intra-articular fractures with greater than 1 mm of articular incongruity are also associated with early radiocarpal degenerative changes.

Extra-articular Distal Radius Fractures

Extra-articular fractures with minimal displacement can be treated nonsurgically with closed reduction and splinting or casting with the wrist in a neutral position. Studies have shown increased carpal tunnel pressures associated with increasing wrist flexion and extension positions, and extreme flexion or extension should be avoided when immobilizing wrist fractures. Closed reduction and percutaneous pinning relies on either intrafocal manipulation and pinning or manual traction, reduction, and pinning to hold the fracture in appropriate anatomic alignment. A percutaneous or limited incision technique is involved. Anatomic studies confirm the risk of injury to the sensory branch of the radial nerve and the radial artery with percutaneous pinning through the snuffbox. Limited incisions or protective devices such as angiocatheters can be used to protect the distal radial sensory nerve branches from injury. External fixation should be used in unstable fractures to provide distraction at the fracture site and prevent collapse and loss of reduction over time. External fixation relies on ligamentotaxis to maintain a reduction, but excessive traction across the wrist ligaments leads to stiffness and can precipitate complex regional pain syndrome. Clinical range of motion of the fingers intraoperatively along with radiographic evaluation of joint distraction can help avoid overdistraction. The addition of two Kirschner wires to facilitate external fixation has been shown to increase stability of the fracture with digital and forearm motion, in some patterns approaching a 3.5-mm AO plating technique. Bicolumnar plating uses orthogonal plates, which provide greater stability with smaller lower profile plates. This "paperclip" system of plating uses several small incisions to approach the radial, dorsal, and ulnar columns of the distal radius and place plates at 90° to each other. Multiple incisions and increased technical difficulty are disadvantages to this system. Dorsal plating has historically been associated with extensor tendon irritation, plate prominence, and tendon rupture. Newer systems have been developed using lower profile plates with recessed screw heads but there is still a low incidence of tendon irritation and synovitis. Recently, volar plates that are similar in concept to a blade plate have been introduced. These more rigid plates with locking screw or peg constructs have been designed to support the subchondral bone at the articular surface, and even the dorsal articular surface if necessary.

Intra-articular Distal Radius Fractures

Indications for surgical treatment of intra-articular fractures are based on patient age and activity level and include articular step-off and gap greater than 2 mm, oblique volar fractures, die-punch fractures, significant

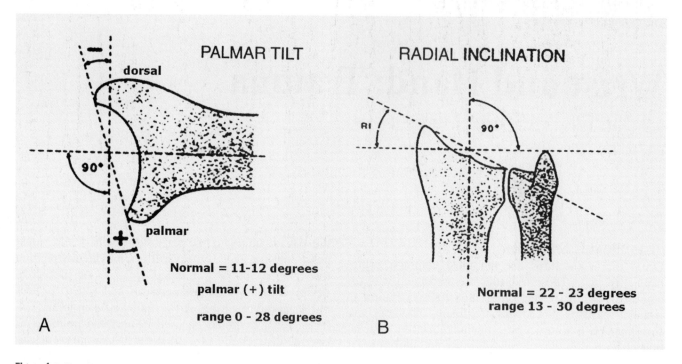

Figure 1 **A**, Normal anatomy of the distal radius on lateral radiograph. Volar or palmar tilt is 11° to 12°. **B**, Normal anatomy of the distal radius on AP radiograph. Radial inclination is 22° to 23° and radial height between the tip of the radial styloid and the ulnar border of the radius is 11° to 13°. *(Reproduced with permission from Jafarnia K, Jupiter J. Distal radius fracture: Anatomy, biomechanics and classification, in Trumble T (ed):* Hand Surgery Update 3. *Rosemont, IL, American Society for Surgery of the Hand, 2003, p 84.)*

dorsal comminution involving more than one third the anteroposterior diameter of the radius, and fractures that lose reduction in the first weeks after injury. Treatment options are similar to those for extra-articular fractures. Closed reduction and percutaneous fixation, external fixation, plating using orthogonal plating, and dorsal or volar plating have been described to restore articular and cortical alignment and relationships. Arthroscopy has been used to assess and improve these described treatment options. A study of 34 intra-articular fractures revealed improved clinical outcomes with arthroscopically-assisted reduction compared with classic open reduction and internal fixation of these fractures. Complex fractures may benefit from bone grafting at the time of surgery. Autograft, allograft, and synthetic grafts all are available, as well as bone cement, which can provide temporary structural support before being absorbed.

At the time of definitive treatment, assessment of distal radioulnar joint (DRUJ) function is critical to ascertain adequate pronation and supination without undue instability. Complications associated with distal radius fractures include malunion, nonunion, extensor pollicis longus rupture, and early degenerative changes. Reconstructive options will be discussed in detail in chapter 30.

Distal Ulna Injuries

When distal radius fractures are displaced more than 1 cm, ulnar-sided injuries such as TFCC tears or ulnar styloid fractures are the rule. Concomitant assessment of the stability of the DRUJ is key to deciding when to repair distal ulna fractures or ligamentous injuries. The ulnar styloid is devoid of ligamentous attachments, but the fovea at the base of the styloid is where the ulnar-sided ligaments of the TFCC attach. Nondisplaced fractures proximal to the ulnar styloid can be treated with cast immobilization. Displaced fractures or bony avulsions of the ligamentous structures in the face of a grossly unstable DRUJ should be repaired. An unstable DRUJ can be defined as an ulnar head that subluxates its full width out of the sigmoid notch with the forearm in a neutral position.

In patients with complex elbow injuries, wrist radiographs should be obtained and a careful clinical examination of the wrist should be performed. In an Essex-Lopresti injury pattern, radial head pathology is coupled with an interosseous membrane injury extending to the DRUJ, creating an unstable relationship between the radius and ulna. Proximal migration of the radius results in secondary DRUJ pathology and ulnocarpal abutment. Following appropriate treatment of the bony pathology (radial head, shaft fracture), pinning the DRUJ

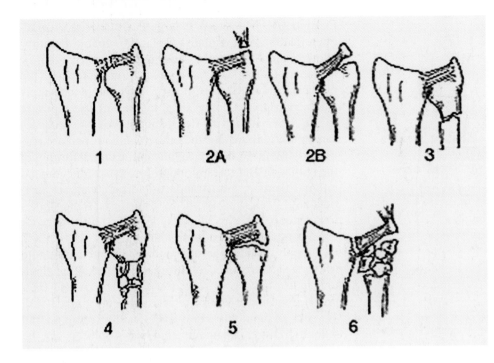

Figure 2 Trumble classification of distal ulna fractures/DRUJ injuries. Type 1 is a disruption or fracture of the fibrocartilage disk of the TFCC. Type 2A is an avulsion of the tip of the ulnar styloid leaving the TFCC intact and stable. Type 2B disrupts the stability of the TFCC with a fracture through the base of the styloid and loss of integrity of the ulnar attachments of the TFCC. Type 3 is a fracture through the metaphyseal/diaphyseal ulna with minimal comminution. Type 4 is a comminuted fracture involving the metaphyseal/diaphyseal region of the ulna. In both types 3 and 4 the articular surfaces of the distal ulna are uninvolved. In type 5, the fracture is near the epiphysis and enters the sigmoid notch disrupting the DRUJ articulation. Type 6 fractures disrupt the TFCC, the DRUJ, and the articular surface of the ulna. (Courtesy of Thomas Trumble, MD.)

for 6 weeks in neutral position may facilitate ligamentous healing. Essex-Lopresti injuries that have been neglected or failed prior treatment may require radial head implant reconstruction.

Indications for fixation of distal ulna fractures includes displaced fractures of the base of the styloid, sigmoid notch fractures, and Galeazzi fracture patterns (Figure 2). Methods of fixation include using a headless screw such as a Herbert screw, wire or suture tension-banding, and excision of the fragment with soft-tissue repair (Figure 3). Repairable TFCC tears can be approached through an open incision or increasingly with arthroscopically-assisted outside-in or the inside-out approaches. More sutures can be placed using the outside-in technique but the dorsal sensory branch of the ulnar nerve is at risk and the carpal ligament repair is more difficult (Figures 4 and 5).

Carpal Fractures

The scaphoid is the most commonly fractured carpal bone. More than half of the bone is covered by articular cartilage. The dorsal surface of the scaphoid has a nonarticular ridge where the dorsal carpal branch of the radial artery enters and provides blood supply to the proximal pole and 80% of the scaphoid. The superficial volar branch of the radial artery supplies the remainder of the blood supply to the scaphoid. The usual mechanism of injury is an axial load across a hyperextended, ulnarly deviated wrist. Pain with resisted pronation, snuffbox tenderness, and scaphoid tuberosity tenderness should raise the suspicion of a scaphoid fracture. Radiographs should include an AP, lateral, and PA view of the scaphoid with the hand in ulnar deviation, and an ob-

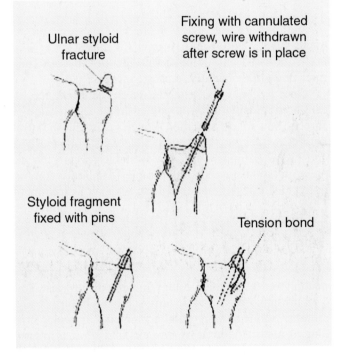

Figure 3 Methods of fixation for unstable distal ulna fractures. (Courtesy of Thomas Trumble, MD.)

lique 45° view with the hand in pronation. Even with normal radiographs, a high level of clinical suspicion should lead to immobilization in a thumb spica splint or cast and reevaluation in 14 to 21 days. Repeat films after 14 to 21 days can reveal an occult scaphoid fracture. Bone scans have an 85% to 93% positive predictive value at 72 hours after injury and have been used when

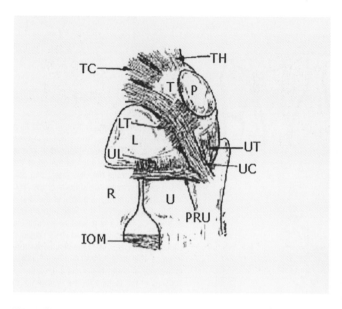

Figure 4 Illustration of the ligaments of the ulnar side of the wrist. PRU = palmar radioulnar; UL= ulnolunate; UC = ulnocapitate; UT = ulnotriquetral; LT = lunotriquetral (palmar region); TC = triquetrocapitate; TH = triquetrohamate; IOM = interosseous membrane; R = radius, U = ulna; L = lunate; T = triquetrum; P = pisiform. (Courtesy of Thomas Trumble, MD.)

radiographs are not revealing and clinical suspicion remains high. Sagittal and coronal CT scans have been used, and MRI allows immediate identification of fractures and later evaluation for osteonecrosis.

Once a scaphoid fracture has been identified, the location and degree of displacement influences treatment choices. Several classification schemes exist but the most helpful in planning treatment is derived from Herbert and Fisher defining a fracture as stable (occult, incomplete, or nondisplaced) or unstable (displaced, comminuted, dislocated, and combined). A delay in treatment of less than 28 days was associated with a 5% nonunion rate in one study, whereas a delay of more than 28 days led to a rate of 45%.

Nonsurgical treatment of stable fractures is with a below-elbow thumb spica cast for 2 to 5 months depending on the location of the fracture: distal waist, 2 to 3 months; midwaist, 3 to 4 months; proximal third, 4 to 5 months. Some authors still recommend 6 weeks in a long arm cast followed by 6 weeks in a short arm cast. Fracture healing can be determined by clinical assessment of the degree of tenderness and with plain radiographs, CT, or MRI. Athletes should not return to play until studies show a healed fracture, although high-level competitors have returned to play in custom casts. In a recent prospective study, the incidence of union of stable fractures treated nonsurgically was 35 of 45 patients.

Displaced fractures more than 1 mm, those with a radiolunate angle greater than 15°, those with an intrascaphoid angle greater than 35°, scaphoid fractures associated with perilunate dislocations, and proximal pole fractures require surgical treatment (Figure 6.) Optimal treatment is with screw fixation. Percutaneous or mini-open fixation of minimally displaced scaphoid fractures allows minimal dissection and preservation of extrinsic ligaments. During a dorsal approach to the scaphoid, the physician should be careful to preserve the blood supply when entering the dorsal ridge by limiting the exposure to the proximal half of the scaphoid. Volar approaches can be useful to expose the entire scaphoid, and are particularly useful to reduce significant flexion deformity of the scaphoid. The rates of union for open reduction and internal fixation, both standard and percutaneous fixation, have been shown to be 89% to 100%; some studies found faster times to union and earlier return to work when compared with nonsurgical treatment.

Lunate dislocations are more common than lunate fractures and are associated with a spectrum of ligamentous injuries in the wrist as described by Mayfield (Figure 7). Avulsion fractures of the lunate are treated with 4 weeks of immobilization and gradual return to full mobility. Larger fragments that are displaced can be treated with screw fixation, but osteonecrosis may result from the injury.

Hamate fractures usually occur from a direct blow such as from a baseball bat or a golf club. The most common presentation is a hook of hamate fracture and is best visualized with a carpal tunnel radiograph. Hamate body and proximal pole fractures are less common. Because these fractures are often difficult to see on plain radiographs, CT scans are helpful in symptomatic patients. Excision of the hook of hamate fragment is the preferred treatment to avoid the sequelae of fracture nonunion and persistent pain. At the time of surgery, releasing Guyon's canal and identification of the ulnar artery and nerve is recommended.

Triquetral avulsion fractures frequently result from a fall on an outstretched hand and can be treated with a brief period of immobilization (as with a wrist sprain) without resultant instability.

Carpal Instability
Scapholunate Instability
Scapholunate injuries are not always recognized acutely and present as a spectrum of injuries involving the scapholunate interval and extrinsic ligaments such as the radioscaphocapitate and scaphotrapezial ligaments. These injuries can be classified as occult (partial scapholunate ligament injury, normal radiographs), dynamic (incompetent or torn scapholunate ligament, bx-abnormal stress radiographs), static or complete scapholunate dissociation (complete tear of scapholunate ligaments and torn extrinsic ligaments, abnormal static radiographs), and dorsal intercalated segment instability (DISI), and scapholunate advanced collapse (SLAC) wrists (chronic patterns frequently with degenerative changes). DISI is a progressive pattern of inter-

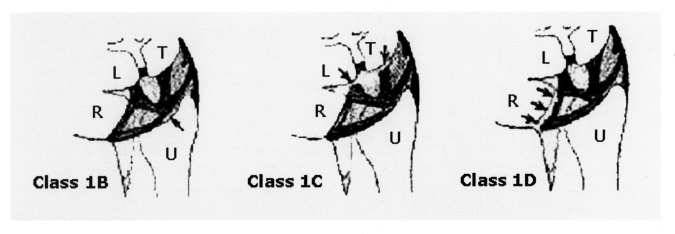

Figure 5 Palmar classification of TFCC injuries. Class 1A injuries involve the horizontal or central portion of the TFCC disk and are treated nonsurgically or with débridement. Class 1B tears represent an avulsion of the peripheral portion of the TFCC from the insertion on the distal ulna. Class 1C tears involve disruption of the ulnocarpal ligaments creating an avulsion of the TFCC from its carpal attachment. Class 1D tears are an avulsion of the TFCC from its radial attachment. (Courtesy of Thomas Trumble, MD.)

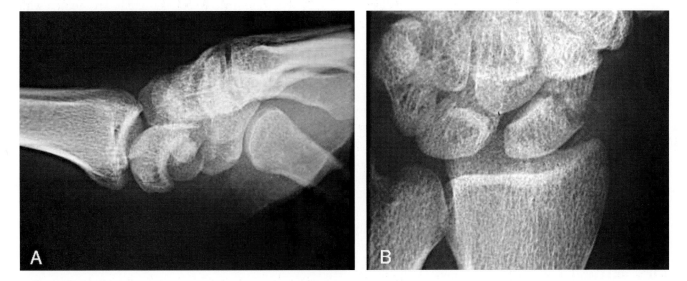

Figure 6 A and **B**, Transscaphoid perilunate carpal dislocation. Note the widened scapholunate interval suggesting a scapholunate ligament tear. (Courtesy of the University of California, San Francisco, CA.)

carpal instability with a dorsiflexed lunate and a volar-flexed scaphoid, frequently caused by a disruption of the scapholunate ligament (Figure 8). Volar intercalated segment instability (VISI) describes the opposite deformity with a volar-flexed lunate, frequently caused by disruption of the lunotriquetral ligament. The abnormal distribution of forces across the midcarpal and radiocarpal joints leads to pain, weakness, and early degenerative changes. SLAC describes a scenario in which the chronic dissociation between the scaphoid and lunate results in wear, sclerosis, and a degenerative arthritis initially involving the radioscaphoid and capitolunate joints (Table 1).

Careful clinical and radiographic examination is important. Common symptoms include difficulty bearing loads across the wrist, symptomatic dysfunction, and abnormal kinematics through the full range of motion.

Tenderness directly over the scapholunate ligament can be expected and a positive scaphoid shift test (Watson test) is helpful but must be compared with the contralateral side to confirm true ligamentous laxity (Figure 9).

Radiographic diastasis of the scapholunate joint greater than 2 mm is associated with a complete tear, although the reliability of this measurement on plain radiographs has been questioned and contralateral comparison views are essential. Neutral PA, clenched fist AP, true lateral, ulnar deviation PA, and fully flexed lateral radiographs provide helpful information. Important radiographic findings include a scapholunate angle greater than 70°, dorsal flexion of the lunate greater than 15° on a neutral lateral radiograph, and the scaphoid ring sign in which the flexed distal pole of the scaphoid projects a ring pattern at the distal scaphoid on the AP projection. MRI studies show poor sensitivity

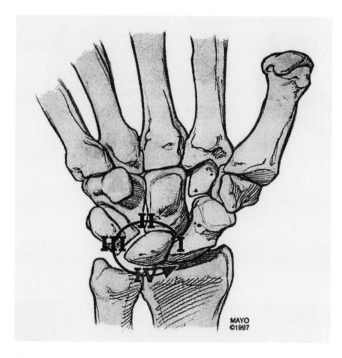

Figure 7 Mayfield's staging of the progression of perilunate injury and instability. Stage I is a scapholunate ligament disruption. Stage II is a disruption of the capitolunate articulation. The lunotriquetral ligament is disrupted in stage III and complete dislocation of the lunate with loss of the short radiolunate ligament occurs in stage IV. *(Reproduced with permission from the Mayo Foundation, Rochester, MN.)*

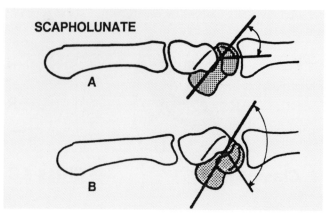

Figure 8 The normal scapholunate angle **(A)** averages 47° with a range of 30° to 60°. An angle greater than 80° **(B)** indicates complete scapholunate dissociation or a displaced scaphoid fracture. *(Reproduced with permission from Garcia-Elias M: Carpal instabilities and dislocations, in Green DP, Hotchkiss RN, Pederson WC (eds): Green's Operative Hand Surgery. Philadelphia, PA, Churchill Livingstone, 1993, p 878.)*

with significant normal variation, but magnetic resonance arthrograms have shown 93% sensitivity for perforations. The most effective test is arthroscopy.

The treatment of scapholunate instability depends on the stage of instability. Occult scapholunate instability without kinematic abnormalities can be treated with arthroscopic or open débridement, and a period of postoperative immobilization. Dynamic instability should be assessed arthroscopically. Incomplete tears are débrided and pinned followed by dorsal capsulodesis. Complete tears require repair or reconstruction of the scapholunate ligament and dorsal capsulodesis. Some authors advocate débridement of the scaphoid and lunate and pinning to promote healing. The more accepted treatment is open repair with sutures through drill holes or suture anchors. Dorsal capsulodesis is recommended. The Blatt capsulodesis describes taking a proximally based capsuloligamentous flap and inserting it into a notch on the dorsal scaphoid distal to the axis of rotation. A distally based flap has been described, and a strip of dorsal intercarpal ligament has been used to control rotatory subluxation of the scaphoid. More recently, ligamentous reconstruction of the scapholunate interval with bone-ligament-bone constructs has been described with limited follow-up (capitate-hamate and cuneonavicular). Some physicians advocate the use of a Herbert bone screw to stabilize the scapholunate joint, but still allow some rotation between these bones. Intercarpal arthrodeses such as scaphotrape-

zial trapezoid and scaphocapitate fusions have better outcomes and successful fusion rates than scapholunate fusions (one seventh of the scapholunate fusion rate in one study), but may require later revisions if progressive arthritic changes occur in the remaining mobile joints.

Lunotriquetral Instability

A sudden twisting injury or forced dorsiflexion of the wrist can result in rupture of the lunotriquetral ligament. This injury can cause lunotriquetral instability, which can manifest as a VISI deformity when associated with damage to extrinsic wrist ligaments. This ligamentous injury can be imaged with PA and radial/ulnar deviation radiographs and magnetic resonance arthrography. Treatment options include acute primary repair, reconstruction of the ligamentous structures with tendon or bone-ligament-bone construct, and dorsal capsulodesis for dynamic instability. Arthrodesis has been advocated, but nonunion can occur. Bone suture anchors now provide excellent alternatives to creating bone tunnels for tendon-based ligamentous reconstruction.

Metacarpal and Phalangeal Fractures

Most metacarpal and phalangeal fractures can be treated nonsurgically with closed reduction, short-term splinting, and early protected range of motion. Indications for surgical treatment include displaced intraarticular fractures, unstable diaphyseal fractures, rotational deformity, open fractures, fractures with associated tendon injuries, and multiple fractures (Figures 10 and 11).

Metacarpal Fractures

In general, metacarpal fractures have apex-dorsal angulation caused by the pull of the intrinsic muscles. Acceptable angulation in metacarpal diaphyseal fractures

Table 1 | Stages of Scapholunate Instability

Stage	Occult	Dynamic	Scapholunate Dissociation	DISI	SLAC
Injured ligaments	Partial SLIL	Incompetent or torn SLIL; partial palmar extrinsics	Complete SLIL, volar or dorsal extrinsics	Complete SLIL, volar extrinsic; secondary Δ's: RL, ST	As in stage IV
Radiographs	Normal	Usually normal	SL gap > 3 mm ± SL angle > 70°	SL angle > 70° SL gap > 3 mm RL angle > 16° CL angle < 15°	I. Styloid DJD II. RS DJD III. CL DJD IV. Pancarpal
Stress radiographs	Normal; Abnormal fluoroscopy	Abnormal	Grossly abnormal	Unnecessary	Unnecessary

DISI, dorsal intercalated segment instability; SLAC, scapholunate advanced collapse; SL, scapholunate; RL, radiolunate; SLIL, scapholunate interosseous ligament; DJD, degenerative joint disease; CL, capitolunate; RS, radioscaphoid; ST, scaphotrapezium

(Courtesy of S Wolfe, MD.)

increases from 15° to 20° in the index and middle metacarpals to 40° to 50° in the ring and small metacarpals. This increase is a result of the increased mobility at the carpometacarpal joint of the fourth and fifth metacarpals at the hamate compared with the more fixed unit of the second and third metacarpals. At these levels, rotational deformity will lead to scissoring of the fingers. Long oblique and spiral diaphyseal fractures of the index and small fingers can be unstable and may need surgical treatment. Kirschner wire fixation minimizes soft-tissue damage and can be used for transverse, longitudinal, or a combination of fixation patterns. Two wires may be required to control rotation. Plate fixation can be used dorsally with early motion to prevent adhesions. Short periods of splinting with early protected motion will help maximize return to full function.

Phalangeal Fractures

Phalangeal fractures may have significant angulation resulting from the opposing pull of intrinsic and extrinsic tendons across fracture sites. Intrinsic structures insert relatively proximally and function as flexors. Extrinsic structures insert relatively distally and function as extensors. Phalangeal fractures consequently tend toward apex-volar angulation. Closed reduction is best accomplished by flexion of the distal fragment to match the volar angulation of the proximal fragment. Stable closed reduction may be limited by these forces, and internal fixation with Kirschner wires or plating may be more reliable in ensuring acceptable bony alignment. Distal phalanx tuft fractures frequently involve the nail bed, and suture repair of the nail bed may be sufficient to reduce the bony fragments and allow a bony or fibrous union. Alternatively, longitudinal pin fixation may be used. Fibrous union of comminuted distal tuft fractures

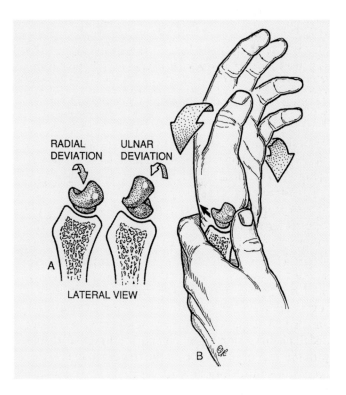

Figure 9 Watson's scaphoid shift test. The thumb is placed on the volar scaphoid tuberosity and pressure applied while moving the hand from ulnar to radial deviation. The scaphoid will move from extension in ulnar deviation to flexion in radial deviation. Palmar pressure on the scaphoid tubercle prevents scaphoid flexion and will produce dorsal subluxation of the scaphoid in a patient with a torn or lax scapholunate ligament producing a painful snap. *(Reproduced with permission from Watson HK, Weinzweig J: Intercarpal arthrodesis, in Green DP, Hotchkiss RN, Pederson WC (eds): Green's Operative Hand Surgery. Philadelphia, PA, Churchill Livingstone, 1993, p 115.)*

usually results in a stable, pain-free digit over time. Flexor digitorum profundus-avulsion fractures can be treated with open reduction and repaired over a button or with suture anchors. Volar fractures of the base of the

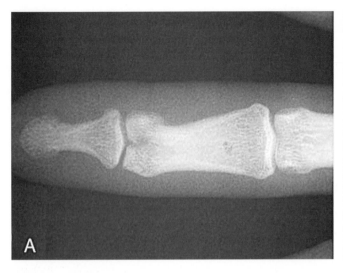

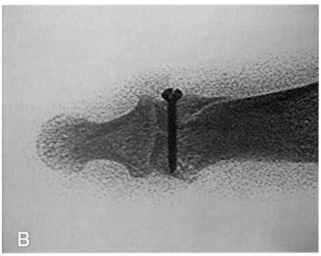

Figure 10 A, Intra-articular condylar fracture of the middle phalanx with 2 mm of displacement. **B**, Limited open reduction and screw fixation of intra-articular condyle fracture.

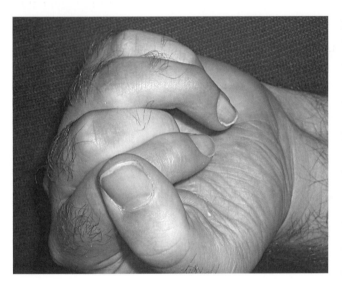

Figure 11 Scissoring of the fingers after index and middle metacarpal fractures prevents the patient from making a composite fist.

distal phalanx should be pinned or they will displace with the pull of the flexor on the fragment.

Thumb Fractures

Fractures of the base of the thumb metacarpal require anatomic reduction and fixation as needed to maintain the reduction. Nondisplaced intra-articular fractures can be treated in a thumb spica cast for 4 weeks. Bennett's fracture-dislocations of the metacarpal from a bony fragment attached to the volar beak ligament are usually unstable from the pull of the abductor pollicis longus on the metacarpal base (Figure 12). The reduction maneuver is traction, pronation, and ulnar pressure over the base of the metacarpal. Kirschner wires can be placed across the fracture, into the adjacent index metacarpal, or from the thumb metacarpal into the tra-

pezium. Screw fixation can be used if the fragment is large enough and early motion can be started. Rolando's fracture, a Y-shaped intra-articular fracture of the base of the thumb, can be treated with closed reduction and Kirschner wires or open reduction and plate and/or screw fixation using small implants. Accurate reduction of the articular surface is important to prevent carpometacarpal arthritis.

Intra-articular Fractures

Proximal interphalangeal (PIP) joint fracture-dislocations result from axial loading of the PIP joint in hyperextension and are difficult to treat. Volar lip fractures involving less than 30% of the articular surface are treated in extension blocking splints to maintain a congruent joint reduction while gradually increasing motion. The articular contour is less important than preserved range of motion in these fractures. Fractures involving more than 30% of the joint surface frequently are unstable and difficult to control. Fixation options include volar plate arthroplasty, open reduction, external fixation, or dynamic traction (Figure 13). Use of osteochondral grafts from sources such as the distal dorsal hamate bone has been described.

Ligament Injuries of the Hand

PIP joint injuries represent the most common ligamentous injuries in the hand. These range from "jamming" the finger to irreducible dislocations and fracture-dislocations. Dorsal dislocations are most common and varying degrees of volar plate, collateral, and accessory collateral ligaments are torn with the injury. The volar plate, soft tissues, and fracture fragments can be interposed between joint surfaces, preventing a concentric reduction. Stable motion is the goal; dynamic traction, extension blocking splints or pins, open reduction, and

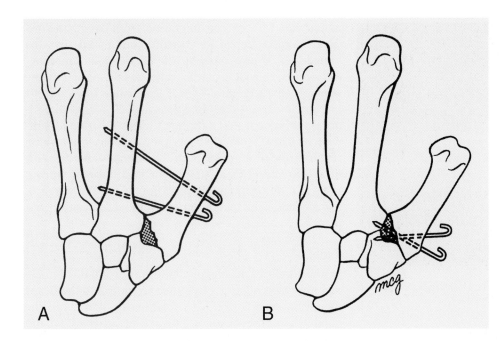

Figure 12 Methods of percutaneous fixation of Bennett's fracture. Kirschner wire fixation into the second metacarpal **(A)** or across the fracture into the trapezium and base of the second metacarpal after closed reduction **(B)**. *(Reproduced with permission from Stern P: Fractures of the metacarpals and phalanges, in Green DP, Hotchkiss RN, Pederson WC (eds): Green's Operative Hand Surgery. Philadelphia, PA, Churchill Livingstone, 1993, p 781.).*

volar plate arthroplasty all are options allowing early motion. Volar dislocations usually result from a rotatory subluxation of the joint on one collateral ligament disrupting the extensor mechanism at the lateral band. The condyle can be entrapped by the stout fibers of the lateral band preventing reduction of the joint. A true volar dislocation can rupture the central slip, changing the treatment to immobilization in extension with gradual increases in flexion.

Metacarpophalangeal (MCP) joint collateral ligament injuries usually involve the radial collateral ligament and are more common in the index and small digits. Examining the finger in full flexion stretches the collateral ligaments. If there is no subluxation, malrotation, or persistent lateral deviation, the injury can be treated conservatively. The joint should be immobilized in 30° of flexion for 3 weeks and then buddy taped to the radial digit for an additional 2 to 3 weeks. Unstable injuries require repair of the ligament with pull-out sutures or suture anchors. Persistent pain and instability may require reconstruction of the radial collateral ligament.

Gamekeeper's Thumb

Ulnar collateral ligament (UCL) injury in the thumb MCP joint is known as gamekeeper's thumb or skier's thumb. The mechanism of acute injury is a radially directed force to the flexed MCP joint of the thumb. Testing the thumb in 30° of flexion isolates the proper collateral ligament, whereas positioning the thumb in extension tests the volar plate and accessory collateral ligament. The lack of a defined end point or 30° of laxity greater than the contralateral thumb in both extension and flexion suggests a complete tear of the ligament.

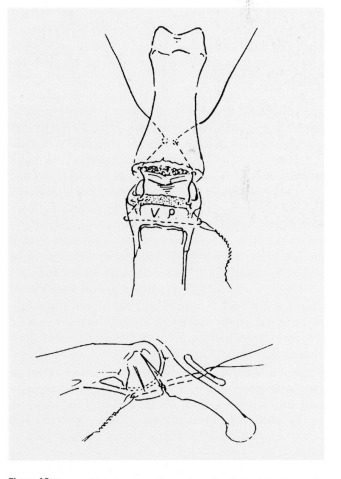

Figure 13 Diagram of Eaton's method of volar plate arthroplasty using suture or wire through the volar plate and a trough in the distal insertion site tied over a button. VP = volar plate. *(Reproduced with permission from Glickel SZ, Barron OA, Eaton RG: Dislocations and ligament injuries in the digits, in Green DP, Hotchkiss RN, Pederson WC (eds): Green's Operative Hand Surgery. Philadelphia, PA, Churchill Livingstone, 1993, p 778.)*

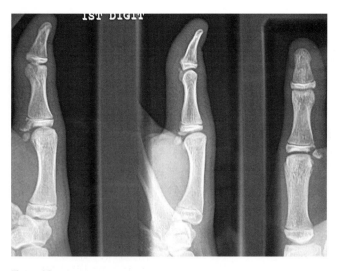

Figure 14 Radiographic views of a physeal gamekeeper's avulsion fracture. Failure of the physis occurs before failure of the collateral ligament.

UCL avulsions can be associated with a small bony fragment, which usually involves minimal articular surface. Distal tears are five times more common than proximal tears. Skeletally immature patients present with bony avulsions more commonly than ligamentous avulsions (Figure 14). The Stener lesion involves complete rupture of the UCL distally with interposition of the adductor aponeurosis. The aponeurosis prevents reapposition of the UCL to the proximal phalanx. Thus, complete ruptures should be surgically repaired primarily, with pull-out sutures or with suture anchors. Partial ruptures, however, can be treated with 4 weeks of immobilization followed by 2 weeks of gradual motion and a total of 3 months of protected activity. Differentiating between partial and complete tears is important in choosing a treatment plan. Ultrasound has been used with moderate reliability, whereas MRI provides the most accurate diagnosis with up to 94% specificity for Stener lesions.

Thumb carpometacarpal dislocations involve rupture of the volar beak ligament and radial collateral ligament. A PA stress radiograph of both thumbs pressed together along their radial borders moves the proximal metacarpal laterally and will show a shift of the metacarpal on the trapezium. The reduction must maintain the metacarpal-trapezial relationship and casting or pinning can be used to hold the reduction. If the metacarpal is unstable, reconstruction of the ligament with flexor carpi radialis or abductor pollicis brevis should be considered.

Flexor Tendon Injuries

Rapid and reliable restoration of function is the goal of flexor tendon surgery. Healing of injured or lacerated tendons has been demonstrated on a biologic basis without significant input from the circulating blood and ele-

ments and without cell migration from exogenous tissues. Tendon repair is clearly influenced by the biomechanical environment. The application of mechanical forces can change the time course of improving strength characteristics as well as change the load displacement curves over time. It is also clear that there is no repair system that can match the strength and stiffness of native uninjured tendons. Advances in tendon repair strive to improve both the strength and the stiffness characteristics at the repair site through innovations of multistrand methods, different configurations of the strands, and recent innovations of nonsuture implants.

Anatomy

In the forearm, the flexor digitorum profundus muscle and musculotendinous structures are dorsal to the flexor digitorum superficialis. This relationship persists in the hand where the flexor digitorum superficialis tendon crosses the palm volar to the flexor digitorum profundus. At the level of the A1 pulley, flexor digitorum superficialis divides and moves dorsal to the flexor digitorum profundus and inserts on the proximal end of the middle phalanx. The flexor digitorum profundus tendon then continues to insert on the proximal end of the distal phalanx.

The course of the flexor tendon system in the hand has been divided into zones used to describe the level of injury and prognosis for repair (Figure 15). Zone I is distal to the insertion of the flexor digitorum superficialis. In the thumb, zone TI is overlying and distal to the interphalangeal joint. Zone II (no-man's land) starts at the distal palmar crease and ends at the flexor digitorum superficialis insertion. Zone TII in the thumb is between the MCP joint and the interphalangeal joint. Zone III is the zone of lumbrical origin and extends from the distal palmar crease to the distal edge of the transverse carpal ligament. Zone TIII refers to the flexor tendons to the thumb as they pass through the thenar region of the hand. Zone IV is the carpal tunnel, and zone V is the distal forearm. The pulley system in the fingers and hand provides a biomechanical advantage for maximal tendon excursion and range of motion. The vascular supply to the flexor tendons dorsally is via the vincula, which contain vessels coursing from intraosseous vessels. The volar flexor tendon receives its blood supply from small vessels in the peritenon.

Flexor Tendon Repair

Increasing the caliber of the suture and increasing the number of strands in the core suture improves overall tendon repair performance in terms of load to failure, gap formation, and cyclic loading strength. At the same time, increasing the number of strands of core suture may increase the work of flexion. This suture method

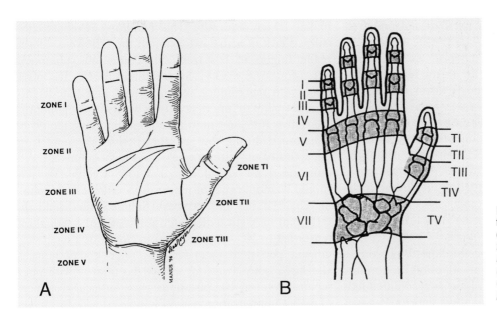

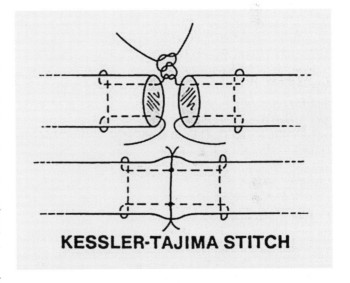

Figure 15 Zones of injury on the flexor surface of the hand (**A**) and the extensor surface of the hand (**B**). *(Reproduced with permission from Strickland JW: Flexor tendon: acute injuries, in Green DP, Hotchkiss RN, Pederson WC (eds): Green's Operative Hand Surgery. Philadelphia, PA, Churchill Livingstone, 1993, p 1856.)*

may translate to a potential increase in adhesion formation in the biologic/clinical setting if efforts are not made for earlier and more aggressive immobilization. Recent studies comparing different suture methods and number of suture strands conclude that a four-strand modified Kessler technique provides a repair that is strong enough to reliably allow immediate controlled active flexion postoperatively (Figure 16).

The strength of a conventional core suture repair can be doubled with the use of simple continuous running suture of 6-0 prolene, when the sutures are placed within the substance of the tendon rather than just the epitenon. Some physicians advocate the placement of peripheral suture first, followed by core suture. This method has been shown to decrease bunching and overlap of the tendon repair site.

Nonsuture techniques have been explored for flexor tendon repair applications. Internal splint repairs have been associated with good mechanical strength, but also excessive work of flexion and tendon necrosis. An internal tendon implant consisting of a corkscrew-like device called Teno-Fix (Ortheon Medical, Winter Park, FL) has recently been approved for use in the United States. This device is introduced into either end of the cut tendon and connected and tensioned by a stainless steel woven cable and crimped beads. Early clinical trials, canine studies, and biomechanical testing suggest that this Teno-Fix device may facilitate early active motion after tendon repair.

Pulley Repair and Reconstruction

If critical pulleys are deficient, loss of flexor tendon function results. The A2 and A4 pulleys are the most significant pulleys and should be preserved at all costs.

KESSLER-TAJIMA STITCH

Figure 16 Modified Kessler suture technique with 4-0 monofilament nylon and 6-0 prolene deep epitendinous suture. *(Reproduced with permission from Strickland JW: Acute injuries, in Green DP, Hotchkiss RN, Pederson WC (eds: Green's Operative Hand Surgery. Philadelphia, PA, Churchill Livingstone, 1993, p 1861.)*

Step-cuts in the pulley make direct repair easier when the pulley needs to be divided. An irreparable pulley can be reconstructed with tendon grafts, retinacular tissues, or processed tissue grafts. A study examining flexor digitorum profundus tendon repair compared work of flexion when A2 pulleys were kept intact, incised, or enlarged. Gliding excursions were reduced in the intact pulley group in comparison with the incised or enlarged pulley groups, and work of flexion increased. This study supports the notion of partial or complete pulley release after tendon repair in improving overall gliding excursion. Preservation of A2 and A4 pulleys, however, prevents flexor bowstringing and maximizes end range of motion.

An antiadhesion barrier gel has been used for prevention of adhesion in Europe for flexor tendon injuries. In one clinical study of zone II flexor tendon repairs, the active PIP joint motion was improved (89.5° compared with 65° in controls). Polyvinyl alcohol shields have been used to decrease tendon adhesions but have also shown an increase in repair site rupture. 5-fluorouracil is also being investigated to reduce peritendinous adhesions; adverse tendon healing effects have not been shown.

Rehabilitation of Flexor Tendon Injuries

Many different protocols have been followed to protect flexor tendon repair but prevent adhesions that ultimately affect motion. Immobilization is recommended for children and patients with cognitive deficits. Passive mobilization, a variant of early passive mobilization, and an active place and hold model of mobilization have been described. The goal, regardless of the protocol chosen, is early motion while protecting the repair sufficiently to allow healing. Current studies are aimed at providing repairs that led to earlier active motion. A recent study used flexor tendon force transducers to show that tenodesis motion requires less force than place and hold motion. A tendon healing study found that breaking strength and cellular activity increased with both early motion and tension. Therefore, current recommendations of four- to eight-strand repairs with a deep epitendinous running suture are directed at earlier active motion.

Extensor Tendon Injuries

The extensor mechanism of the hand is a complex structure that when damaged requires recognition of injury, appropriate repair, and early motion to preserve maximum function. More than 60% of injuries to the extensor mechanism are also associated with bony, joint, or ligamentous injuries. Suture repair of extensor tendon laceration should be with a modified Kessler or modified Bunnell repair using 4-0 synthetic nonabsorbable suture. The extensor tendon excursion is less than the flexor tendon excursion; therefore, preservation of length and prevention of gapping is important to prevent loss of motion. The extensor mechanism, like the flexor system, is divided into zones for discussion of injury and treatment (Figure 15). The even zones are overlying the bones (phalanges, metacarpals, and forearm bones) and the odd zones are overlying the joints (distal interphalangeal [DIP], PIP, and MCP joints, and wrist).

Mallet Finger

Disruption of the extensor tendon at the level of the DIP joint as a tendinous or bony avulsion results in a mallet finger deformity. This condition presents clinically as lack of active extension at the DIP joint. Closed mallet fingers are best treated by continuous splinting in extension for 8 weeks. This treatment is effective in patients with acute injury, and in patients in whom diagnosis and treatment are delayed for weeks or even months.

Active PIP joint motion is important and should be maintained during the splinting period. Weaning from the splint begins after 8 weeks, and night splints are recommended for an additional 4 to 8 weeks. The skin should be monitored for maceration and necrosis; splinting changes may be necessary. Splints should hold the DIP joint in slight hyperextension. A slight residual extensor lag (< 10°) may result from closed treatment. Significant persistent extensor lags, open mallet injuries, and large bony avulsions should be treated with open repair; however, complications from surgical treatment of mallet injuries approach 50%.

Boutonniere Deformity

Disruption of the central slip results in loss of extension at the PIP joint and hyperextension of the DIP joint or a boutonniere deformity. The primary injury is to the central slip, the "jammed" finger. The clinical picture is a result of subluxation of the lateral bands from an extensor position to a flexor position at the PIP joint. Treatment with splinting in extension at the PIP joint allows for DIP joint motion and allows maintenance of normal lateral band length and position.

Surgical indications for an acute boutonniere deformity include a displaced avulsion fracture at the base of the middle phalanx, axial and lateral instability of the PIP joint associated with loss of active or passive extension of the finger, or failed nonsurgical treatment. Passing a suture through the central tendon and securing it to the middle phalanx (with or without the bony fragment) accomplishes primary repair of an avulsion fracture. Dorsal fixation of the lateral bands addresses the soft-tissue boutonniere deformity, and transarticular pin fixation of the PIP joint is often used to secure full extension. If primary repair is not possible, portions of the lateral bands can be sutured together in the dorsal midline to reconstruct the central slip.

Zone V Injuries

The most common injury to the extensor mechanism in zone V is from a "fight bite" sustained through a laceration from a human tooth when striking a blow to the face. This injury occurs with the MCP joint in flexion. Deeper injury to the extensor tendon will be proximal to the skin wound when the fingers are extended. These partial tendon injuries can be treated conservatively. The skin wound, however, should be treated aggressively with thorough wound assessment, cultures, surgical débridement, broad-spectrum intravenous antibiotics, and initial splinting with gradual transition to range-of-motion exercises. Devastating complications including articular damage, septic arthritis, and osteomyelitis can arise from a human bite.

Rupture of a sagittal band can result from a blunt injury to the MCP joint. Most commonly, the radial sagittal band is damaged and the extensor tendon subluxates into the ulnar gutter. This injury presents as lack of full extension at the MCP joint. The tendon can be seen on the ulnar aspect of the MCP joint and passively reduced into a central position. Active flexion produces a painful snap as the tendon dislodges into the ulnar gutter. Nonsurgical treatment of an acute injury can be attempted with the finger splinted in extension for 6 weeks. If this treatment fails or if the diagnosis is delayed, surgical repair is indicated. Primary repair reinforced with an ulnar-based flap of extensor tendon is strong enough to allow early active motion.

Closed rupture of the extensor pollicis longus following a distal radius fracture has become a well-recognized entity. Attritional rupture secondary to irritation from fracture fragments, ischemia, or hemorrhage within the tendon sheath are commonly proposed theories of injury. The patient will present several weeks after fracture with loss of interphalangeal joint extension and weak adduction of the thumb. Nonsurgical treatment is not appropriate and direct surgical repair is often not possible. Free tendon grafting with an intercalated graft or extensor indicis proprius-to-extensor pollicis longus transfer are two common techniques for reconstruction and both are associated with good results.

Rehabilitation of Extensor Tendon Injuries

Static splinting has been the standard with good long-term results following extensor tendon repairs. Recently, early active motion using dynamic splinting has shown better functional results. Immobilization of tendons is associated with adherence of the tendon to surrounding soft tissues, producing loss of both extension and flexion. The immobilized tendon loses strength over time, and aggressive rehabilitation following prolonged immobilization can further attenuate the repair. Controlled motion has been shown to increase tensile strength of tendons, improve gliding properties, increase repair-site DNA, and accelerate changes in the surrounding vascularity.

Dynamic extension splinting allows several millimeters of extensor gliding without placing stress across the repair site. A splint holding the wrist in extension and the MCP joints in 10° to 15° of flexion allows limited motion at the interphalangeal joints both in active flexion and passive extension. Improved outcomes have been shown using dynamic extension splinting for proximal injuries.

Nerve Injury and Repair

Injury

Peripheral nerve injuries can be classified by injury severity. Neurapraxia describes temporary failure of conduction in a nerve usually caused by contusion or stretch in injury. Neurapraxic injuries heal without significant delay or sequelae. Axonotmesis describes a disruption of the nerve fibrils but an intact endoneurium and epineurium. The intact neural tube functions as a conduit to allow nerve healing and regeneration. Nerve regeneration can be followed by an advancing Tinel's sign. A fibroblastic reaction within the nerve sheath can impede nerve growth leading to a neuroma in continuity. These injuries can result from crush or severe stretch mechanisms. A completely lacerated nerve is an example of neurotmesis in which the axons and endoneurial tubes are disrupted. The proximal nerve ending undergoes retrograde degeneration to the next node of Ranvier where a disorganized tangle of regenerating axons forms a neuroma. The distal nerve ending undergoes wallerian degeneration, resulting in an end bulb glioma. These injuries are best treated with surgical repair.

Repair

Nerve regeneration following repair is dependent on the type of injury, location, degree of contamination, residual gap, tension, and many other factors currently being investigated. Studies in animals have identified growth factors such as fibroblast growth factor-1 and insulin-like growth factor that promote nerve regeneration and improve outcomes. Different constructs such as reversed vein entubulation, synthetic tubes, and fibrin glue are being studied to replace nerve grafts. One animal study in rat sciatic nerve found that muscle-enriched vein graft potentiates Schwann cell proliferation and is a promising alternative conduit for nerve grafting. Studies using synthetic conduits have shown favorable functional outcomes for digital nerve repair with a gap of 4 mm or less.

Nerve repair techniques include epineurial suturing, group fascicular repair, and individual fascicular repair. Epineural repair and group fascicular repair are most commonly used and the decision of which method to use is dependent on the level of nerve injury, and the appearance of and the ability to line up the fascicles. No study has shown better results with one repair method over the other, which may result from the difficulty in appropriately matching the fascicles. Sensorimotor mapping can be used intraoperatively to maximize pairing of motor and sensory fascicles. This method requires significant patient cooperation and meticulous repair by the surgeon.

The external epineurium is a layer of connective tissue that can hold a suture better than internal epineurium and perineurium. Tension in the repair, however, must be avoided and nerve grafting should be considered if there is too much stretch to allow approximation of the nerve endings. Early nerve repair of transected nerves should be done within 10 to 14 days. Crushed and contused nerves can be followed over time, and early electromyograms (obtained 2 to 3 weeks after injury) can be compared with later studies (obtained after 6 weeks to 3 months) to identify areas of healing. If there are no changes at 3 months, nerve exploration is indicated. Waiting longer than approximately 18 months leads to intraneural fibrosis and muscle fibrosis that may not be reversible.

Rehabilitation and Results

Postoperative care involves splinting to protect the repair from stress for 2 to 3 weeks followed by gradual range of motion across the repair site. Regeneration occurs at a rate of approximately 1 mm per day. Results of nerve repair are better in the younger patient population, possibly because of more effective cortical reeducation. In patients younger than age 20 years, 75% achieved two-point discrimination of less than 6 mm after digital nerve repair. In adults, only 25% to 50% achieve that level of recovery. Median and ulnar nerve recovery can improve for up to 5 years after repair. The results of median and ulnar nerve repair are better for lesions below the elbow than above. Studies have shown that 29% to 37% of patients regain two-point discrimination less than 12 mm, and 14% to 27% regain functional motor activity. Sensory reeducation is now recognized as an important component in nerve recovery and involves desensitization, motion, and tactile discrimination training. Sensory reeducation has been shown to be more difficult when both the flexor tendon and nerve are repaired. This situation suggests that fine motor control assists sensory interpretation in the fingers.

Fingertip Injuries

These common injuries require careful assessment and treatment to maintain proper coverage and functionality of the finger following injury. Appropriate padding and sensibility must be preserved in the fingertip. Nail bed injuries also need careful treatment to avoid painful and cosmetically unappealing results.

Replantation and Local Flaps

The viability of replanted digits and hands has been shown over many microsurgical centers to be approximately 80%. Revascularized parts have higher success rates because some venous outflow is usually preserved. Replantation should be considered when the amputated part is a thumb, multiple digits, partial hand (through the palm), wrist, forearm, elbow, sharp amputation above the elbow, and individual digits distal to the flexor digitorum superficialis insertion, and almost any

part in a child. Other factors impacting the decision to replant a part are ischemic time, patient age, crush versus sharp injury, and segmental injuries. Warm ischemia time should be less than 6 hours; in digits where there is no muscle, warm ischemia time can be up to 12 hours. The amputated part should either be immersed in saline in a bag or sterile container, or wrapped in saline-soaked gauze and then placed on ice. Replantation with bony stabilization should proceed first, followed by tendon repair, arterial anastomosis, venous anastomosis, nerve repair, and finally careful skin approximation or closure, avoiding tension across neurovascular structures.

Soft-tissue coverage of defects associated with amputations depends on the size of the defect, the required sensibility of that area, and other functional needs. Cutaneous flaps such as a groin flap are useful for covering moderate soft-tissue defects of the hand. The radial forearm flap is a fasciocutaneous flap that can be used either as a pedicled flap or a free flap. Myocutaneous flaps using the rectus abdominis, latissimus dorsi, and gracilis muscles can be taken to provide larger soft-tissue coverage options. In these flaps, the associated nerve can be taken and the flap used for reinnervation and replacement of lost motor function in the extremity.

Infections

Infections in the hand are challenging to treat because of the anatomic spaces in the hand, which can allow organisms to spread quickly from distal points of injury to proximal locations. The areas of the hand that facilitate the spread of infection are the dorsal cutaneous space, thenar and midpalmar spaces, Parona's space, the interdigital web spaces, the tendon sheaths, and articular spaces.

Bacterial Infections

The most common bacterial pathogen in hand infections is *Staphylococcus aureus*. Vancomycin-resistant *S aureus* is increasingly prevalent in community-acquired infections. Many infections begin as cellulitis, which, if recognized early, can be treated with antibiotics, elevation, and immobilization. The fundamental principles of treatment are appropriate antibiotic therapy, adequate débridement and drainage, a period of immobilization and elevation, and early remobilization. Tetanus immunization needs to be up to date. Untreated cellulitis may develop into an abscess, which must be drained before antibiotics will be effective.

A paronychia is an infection involving the nail bed that evolves into an abscess that is easily drained by lifting the paronychial skin off the nail plate. Collar button abscesses are located in the webspace and palmar abscesses usually involve the thenar or hypothenar bursas. Infected wounds overlying the dorsal MCP joint are often a result of contact with teeth or an open mouth. These wounds may involve the extensor mechanism proximal to the wound. Evaluation of the extensor with the hand in a fully flexed fist position may reveal partial tendon laceration and allows appropriate débridement of the involved extensor mechanism. A felon is a fingertip pulp infection that requires surgical drainage to prevent a compartment syndrome and potential necrosis of the entire pulp of the finger.

Purulent flexor tenosynovitis warrants early attention because it is a potentially devastating infection with significant long-term morbidity. This infection involves a penetrating injury or hematogenous seeding inside the flexor sheath. Because the sheath extends across the palm, the infection can easily track into the forearm. Patients with this type of infection will present with Kanavel's signs of a digit resting in flexion, pain with passive extension, pain along the flexor sheath, and fusiform swelling in the digit. The most sensitive sign is pain with passive extension. Flexor tenosynovitis can be treated with irrigation of the flexor sheath once it has been opened. A preferred method of irrigation is to place a 16-gauge catheter in the proximal sheath and a penrose drain in the distal sheath in the finger. Every 2 hours, 50 mL of sterile saline is irrigated through the sheath for 48 hours. Motion should begin within the week to prevent excessive stiffness.

Antibiotic coverage of hand infections should be tailored to the cultured organism. As mentioned, the most common pathogen is *Staphylococcus* but human bite wound infections often contain *Eikenella corrodens* and virulent cat bite infections are caused by *Pasteurella multocida*. Penicillin is the drug of choice for these bite infections.

Necrotizing fasciitis is a severe, rapidly spreading infection that carries mortality rates of 8% to 73%. There are two groups of organisms responsible for this infection. Group one includes anaerobic bacteria such as *Enterobacter* and non-group A streptococci. Group two includes group A streptococci with *S aureus* or *Staphylococcus epidermidis*. Patients may present with wounds from minor trauma that progress rapidly from cellulitis and low-grade fever to multisystem organ failure, coma, and hemodynamic compromise. Patients in the intensive care unit are at increased risk of infection by more unusual pathogens such as *Pseudomonas* and *Acinetobacter*. These patients require multiple antimicrobial agent therapy because of multiagent resistant organisms.

Fungal, Mycobacterial, and Viral Infections

Fungal infections in the hand occur in the paronychium, nail, and skin. Chronic paronychial infections are usually caused by *Candida albicans*. Onychomycosis, or fungal nail bed infection, is commonly caused by dermato-

phytes such as *Trichophyton rubrum*. Superficial skin infections are caused by dermatophytes and *Candida*. These relatively superficial nail and skin infections are treated with topical antifungal agents, with conversion to oral agents when treatment appears ineffective. Granulomatous or mycobacterial infections show a predilection for synovium. They may present in a manner similar to rheumatoid arthritis and frequently involve the wrist. Cultures must be directed toward detecting these slow-growing pathogens. *Mycobacterium tuberculosis, M avium-intracellulare,* and *M marinum* have been described in the hand and may be resistant to multiple chemotherapeutic agents. Herpetic whitlow presents as a clear vesicular lesion on the tip of the finger caused by herpes simplex virus type 1 or type 2. Treatment is nonsurgical and the infection is self-limiting and resolved over 3 to 4 weeks.

Burns

Burns over a large surface area are devastating injuries, resulting in months of hospitalization, multiple procedures, and prolonged wound care. Over 2 million burn injuries are reported to require medical care each year, and approximately 6% result in death, usually from smoke inhalation. Most burn injuries are relatively minor and patients are discharged following outpatient treatment. Of those patients who require hospitalization, approximately 20,000 are admitted directly or by referral to hospitals with special capabilities in the treatment of burn injuries. The average hospital stay is 2 months. Criteria for referral to a burn unit are shown in Table 2.

Burns are classified according to the depth of thermal injury, which in turn guides prognosis and treatment plans. The trend is toward classifying burns as partial thickness, which heal on their own, and full thickness, which require skin grafting.

Partial-thickness burns include first- and second-degree burns. First-degree burns only involve the epidermis and require removal of the source of injury and analgesic care. The skin heals within 1 week and there is no permanent damage.

Second-degree burns destroy the epidermis and involve varying amounts of the dermis. The more superficial second-degree burns heal within 2 weeks and leave little permanent scarring. This injury is usually accompanied by blisters that progress over time. Deep second-degree burns produce more scarring, which increases the time to healing. Healing depends on residual epithelial cells in deep dermal sweat glands and hair follicles. Hypertrophic scarring can lead to prolonged healing and infections so that excision and skin grafting may be considered.

Third-degree or full-thickness burns involve all of the dermis and varying amounts of underlying fat, muscle, and bone. The skin may appear white and waxy and

Table 2 | Burn Unit Referral Criteria: American Burn Association 2000

Burn Injuries That Should Be Referred to a Burn Unit:

Partial-thickness burns greater than 10% total body surface area

Burns that involve the face, hands, feet, genitalia, perineum, or major joints

Third-degree burns in any age group

Electrical burns, including lightning injury

Chemical burns

Inhalation injury

Burn injury in patients with preexisting medical disorders that could complicate management, prolong recovery, or affect mortality

Any patients with burns and concomitant trauma (such as fractures) in which the burn injury poses the greatest risk of morbidity or mortality. In such cases, if the trauma poses the greater immediate risk, the patient may be initially stabilized in a trauma center before being transferred to a burn unit. Physician judgment will be necessary in such situations and should be in concert with the regional medical control plan and triage protocols.

Burned children in hospitals without qualified personnel or equipment for the care of children

Burn injury in patients who will require special social, emotional, or long-term rehabilitative intervention.

the severity of the burn can be underestimated. The skin is without sensation and capillary refill and has a leathery appearance.

The pathology of burns has been divided into zones of injury. The zone of coagulation describes the most damaged tissue with coagulated vessels and no blood supply. The zone of stasis has sluggish blood flow but is impacted by early removal of the thermal or chemical source and appropriate intervention. The zone of hyperemia produces an inflammatory response to the injury via bradykinins and histamine producing capillary leaking, edema, and "third-spacing." This can further decrease perfusion to the zone of stasis.

Rapid loss of intravascular fluid and protein occurs during the first 6 hours after a burn. By 36 to 48 hours, capillary integrity is restored but tissue edema continues as a result of protein loss into the burned area and systemic hypoproteinemia. Fluid management, respiratory care, and electrolyte monitoring are essential initial steps in caring for severe burn injuries. Wound care can then be addressed and many options exist for managing the different types of burn wounds.

Antibiotic coverage is important because the skin's immunoprotective function is lost when burned. Silver sulfadiazide is the most common topical agent for burn wounds but can produce a transient leukopenia when used for large burns. Bacitracin, mafenide, betadine, and gentamicin ointments are also used. Skin substitutes are also available, such as split-thickness porcine xenografts and synthetic grafts. Débridement and autogenous split-

thickness grafting is the most desirable treatment for wounds needing coverage, but large volume burns may not leave enough autograft skin.

Injection Injuries

High-pressure injection of material into the hand can produce significant tissue necrosis, edema, and even compartment syndrome. Injection forces have been reported to be between 3,000 and 12,000 psi. The quantity of material injected is difficult to ascertain, but radiographs are sometimes helpful in identifying how far the material has spread. Injected fluids follow bursal planes and tendon sheaths and create both toxic and inflammatory damage to the tissues around them. Negative prognostic factors are presentation for treatment more than 10 hours after injury, injection pressures greater than 7,000 psi, and injection with oil paint.

The initial presentation may be less impressive than anticipated, but over several hours, the swelling, pain, and loss of function can significantly change, requiring prompt action. Amputation rates have decreased from 48% to 16% because of early irrigation and wide débridement. Antibiotic coverage of Gram positive, Gram negative, and anaerobic organisms is important, and a tetanus shot must be administered if the patient's immunizations are not up to date. Close monitoring and repeat débridements may be needed.

Vascular Injuries

Acute vascular injuries to the hand can occur from blunt or penetrating trauma. Patients can present with gross ischemia, progressive hematoma, acute or delayed thrombosis, compartment syndrome, aneurysm development, and distal embolization. The degree to which collateral supply can compensate for the injury is dependent on surrounding tissue damage, vasomotor control, and systemic disease. Acute arterial injuries that present with gross hypoperfusion are treated as emergencies and interventions to return blood flow to the affected part are urgently undertaken. Arterial reconstruction should be considered for critical arterial injury with impending cell death and for noncritical arterial injuries when there is concern for adequate collateral supply, associated nerve injury, and extensive soft-tissue injury. When the artery has sustained extensive damage, vein grafts can be used to replace the damaged area and do not compromise the ultimate reperfusion results. After perfusion is restored, a compartment syndrome may develop and close observation for signs of increasing compartment pressures is essential.

Annotated Bibliography

Distal Radius Fractures

Boyer MI, Galatz LM, Borrelli J Jr, Axelrod TS, Ricci WM: Intra-articular fractures of the upper extremity:

New concepts in surgical treatment. *Instr Course Lect* 2003;52:591-605.

New techniques of internal fixation, postoperative rehabilitation, and emphasis on functional as well as radiographic outcome have refined the surgical treatment of complex fractures of the glenoid, humeral head, supracondylar and intracondylar humerus, olecranon, radial head, distal radius, and distal radioulnar joint over the past decade. Early stabilization and rehabilitation of these injuries leads to soft-tissue stabilization and facilitates the patient's ability to place the hand in three-dimensional space.

Hanel DP, Jones MD, Trumble TE: Wrist fractures. *Orthop Clin North Am* 2002;33:35-57.

The benefits of a well-reduced and well-healed wrist fracture are predictable. After either closed or open reduction, the integrity of the volar ulnar corner of the radius, articular step-off, metaphyseal comminution, and DRUJ stability should be assessed. Reconstruction of the subluxated or dislocated DRUJ starts with the reduction of the radius, frequently obviating the need to address fractures involving the ulnar head and styloid. Most importantly, the results of treatment reflect surgical decision over the fixation method.

Herzberg G, Forissier D: Acute dorsal trans-scaphoid perilunate fracture-dislocations: Medium-term results. *J Hand Surg Br* 2002;27:498-502.

The purpose of this study was to investigate the medium-term results (mean follow-up, 8 years) of a series of 14 trans-scaphoid dorsal perilunate fracture-dislocations treated surgically at an average of 6 days following injury. Eleven patients underwent open reduction and internal fixation through a dorsal approach. Combined palmar and dorsal approaches were used in three fractures, open reduction and internal fixation in two, and proximal row carpectomy in one. The Mayo Wrist Score revealed five excellent, three good, five fair, and one poor result. The average score was 79% (range, 55% to 95%). All internally fixed scaphoids healed and no lunate or scaphoid fragment osteonecrosis with collapse was observed. Carpal alignment was satisfactory in most patients. Posttraumatic radiologic midcarpal and/or radiocarpal arthritis were almost always observed at follow-up, but this did not correlate with the Mayo Wrist Score.

McCallister WV, Knight J, Kaliappan R, Trumble TE: Central placement of the screw in simulated fractures of the scaphoid waist: A biomechanical study. *J Bone Joint Surg Am* 2003;85:72-77.

Recent reports on internal fixation of acute fractures of the scaphoid waist have demonstrated higher rates of central placement of the screw when cannulated screws were used than when noncannulated screws were used. This cadaveric study was designed to determine whether central placement in the proximal fragment of the scaphoid offers a biomechanical advantage. Central placement of the screw in the proximal fragment of the scaphoid had superior results compared with those using eccentric positioning of the screw. Fixation with

central placement of the screw demonstrated 43% greater stiffness, 113% greater load at 2 mm of displacement, and 39% greater load at failure. Central placement of the screw in the proximal fragment of the scaphoid offers a biomechanical advantage in the internal fixation of an osteotomy of the scaphoid waist. Clinical efforts and techniques that facilitate central placement of the screw in the fixation of fractures of the scaphoid waist should be encouraged.

Polsky MB, Kozin SH, Porter ST, Thoder JJ: Scaphoid fractures: Dorsal versus volar approach. *Orthopedics* 2002;25:817-819.

Twenty-six patients with scaphoid fractures were treated with internal fixation using a cannulated differential pitch compression screw. Sixteen patients underwent a dorsal approach (group 1) and 10 patients a volar approach (group 2). Average time from injury to surgery was 6.6 months (range, 0.3 to 19 months) for group 1 and 8.3 months (range, 0.3 to 24 months) for group 2. The rate of union, determined by radiographs and clinical examination, was 81% in group 1 and 80% in group 2. No significant differences were noted between the groups for dorsiflexion/palmar flexion, radial deviation, grip strength, and pain level.

Skoff HD: Postfracture extensor pollicis longus tenosynovitis and tendon rupture: a scientific study and personal series. *Am J Orthop* 2003;32:245-247.

A review of treatment of 200 consecutive patients with distal radius fractures found that the incidence of rupture of the extensor pollicis longus tendon is 3%. Diagnosis is based on persistent dorsal wrist pain and a positive retroflexion sign. In the prerupture setting, recommended treatments include a third dorsal compartment release with or without an extensor retinacular patch graft. If after an acute rupture primary repair is not possible, a palmaris longus graft or a transfer from the extensor indicis proprius to the extensor pollicis longus tendon can be used in the subacute or chronic setting. Results of all treatments seem to be clinically satisfactory.

Slade JF III, Gutow AP, Geissler WB: Percutaneous internal fixation of scaphoid fractures via an arthroscopically assisted dorsal approach. *J Bone Joint Surg Am* 2002;84(suppl 2):21-36.

In a consecutive series of 27 fractures (17 waist fractures and 10 proximal pole fractures) treated with arthroscopically assisted dorsal percutaneous fixation, CT confirmed 100% union at an average of 12 weeks. Eighteen fractures were treated within 1 month after the injury, and nine were treated more than 1 month after the injury. In this series, the fractures that were treated early (less than 1 month after the injury) healed more quickly than those treated later.

Wigderowitz CA, Cunningham T, Rowley DI, Mole PA, Paterson CR: Peripheral bone mineral density in patients with distal radial fractures. *J Bone Joint Surg Br* 2003;85:423-425.

Fractures of the distal forearm are widely regarded as the result of "fragility." This study examines the extent to which patients with Colles' fractures have osteopenia. Bone mineral density was measured in the contralateral radius of 235 women presenting with Colles' fractures over a period of 2 years. Although women of all ages had low values for ultradistal bone mineral density, the age-matched values were particularly low among premenopausal women age 45 years or younger. This finding did not occur because of the presence of women with early menopause. This large survey confirms and extends the findings from earlier small studies. The authors conclude that it is particularly important to investigate young patients with fractures of the distal forearm to identify those with osteoporosis, to seek an underlying cause, and to consider treatment.

Flexor Tendon Injuries

Angeles JG, Heminger H, Mass DP: Comparative biomechanical performances of 4-strand core suture repairs for zone II flexor tendon lacerations. *J Hand Surg [Am]* 2002;27:508-517.

This study compared four-strand core suture repairs, the modified Becker, modified double Tsuge, Lee, locked cruciate, Robertson, and Strickland suture repairs. Work of flexion and ultimate tensile strength were compared, as well as cyclic loading. The greatest interference for gliding was in the modified Becker repair, and the least in the modified double Tsuge repair. None of these repairs had mean gaps after 1,000 cycles to a 3.9 N pulp pinch load approach the clinically important limit of 3 mm of gap. Ultimate tensile strength was highest in the modified Becker (69.4 ± 8.2N) compared to the modified double Tsuge (60.3 ± 15.3N) and locked cruciate (64.1 ± 16.2N), but this was not statistically significant. These authors stated that ease of performance for the surgeon and less interference with tendon gliding favored the locked cruciate and modified double Tsuge repairs compared with the modified Becker repair.

Boyer MI, Strickland JW, Engles D, Sachar K, Leversedge FJ: Flexor tendon repair and rehabilitation: State of the art in 2002. *Instr Course Lect* 2003;52:137-161.

The application of modern multistrand suture repair techniques as well as postoperative rehabilitation protocols emphasizing the application of intrasynovial repair site excursion has led to a protocol for treatment of intrasynovial flexor tendon lacerations emphasizing a strong initial repair followed by the application of postoperative passive motion rehabilitation. Protocols for the reconstruction of failed initial treatment have likewise undergone modification given new findings on the biologic and clinical behavior of flexor tendon grafts. Currently accepted treatment protocols following flexor tendon repair and reconstruction are based on current clinical and scientific data.

Paillard PJ, Amadio PC, Zhao C, Zobitz ME, An KN: Pulley plasty versus resection of one slip of the flexor digitorum superficialis after repair of both flexor tendons in zone II: A biomechanical study. *J Bone Joint Surg Am* 2002;84:2039-2045.

The effects of two strategies to improve postoperative gliding in a human cadaveric hand were studied. Complete lacerations and repairs were made to the profundus and superficialis tendons at a location where both repair sites would pass beneath the A2 pulley with the proximal interphalangeal joint in 45° of flexion. Pulley plasty and resection of one slip of the flexor digitorum superficialis tendon both significantly decreased gliding resistance compared with repair of both slips ($P < 0.001$). There was no difference in the mean gliding resistance between the pulley plasty and one-slip resection groups. The flexor digitorum superficialis slip was stronger after repair with a Becker suture than after repair with a modified Kessler or a zigzag suture. Both pulley plasty and resection of one slip of the flexor digitorum superficialis reduce gliding resistance after tendon repair in zone II of the hand.

Zhao C, Amadio PC, Zobitz ME, Momose T, Couvreur P, An KN: Effect of synergistic motion on flexor digitorum profundus tendon excursion. *Clin Orthop* 2002; 396:223-230.

The dog model was used to evaluate synergistic motion on the flexor digitorum profundus. Eighty percent of lacerations were created and repaired using 4-0 Ticron modified Kessler core suture with circumferential epitenon running 6-0 nylon suture repairs. Metal markers were placed and then divided into two experimental groups. One group had passive flexion and extension of the digits with the wrist fixed in 45° of flexion; in the second group, dogs received synergistic wrist motion with passive digit flexion combined with wrist extension, and passive digit extension with wrist flexion. Time points were 1, 3, and 6 weeks. At 1, 3, and 6 weeks after surgery, the synergistic motion group was superior in total excursion, extension excursion, flexion excursio, and overall percentage of motion compared with unoperated controls.

Extensor Tendon Injuries

Chester DL, Beale S, Beveridge L, Nancarrow JD, Titley OG: A prospective, controlled, randomized trial comparing early active extension with passive extension using a dynamic splint in the rehabilitation of repaired extensor tendons. *J Hand Surg Br* 2002;27:283-288.

Two methods of rehabilitation were compared after extensor tendon repairs in zones IV through VIII. Nineteen patients followed an early active mobilization program and 17 patients followed a dynamic splinting regimen. Data were collected at 4 weeks and at final follow up (median = 3 months). Extension lag, flexion deficit, and total active motion were measured. At 4 weeks, the patients on a dynamic splinting program had better total active motion; however, there were no significant differences in the two groups at final follow-up.

Nerve Injury and Repair

Bell Krotoski JA: Flexor tendon and peripheral nerve repair. *Hand Surg* 2002;7:83-109.

When peripheral nerve injury is combined with flexor tendon injury, sensibility is directly impaired. There is a loss in the sense of finger or thumb position, pain, temperature, and touch/pressure recognition, in addition to the tendon injury.

Day CS, Buranapanitkit B, Riano FA, et al: Insulin growth factor-1 decreases muscle atrophy following denervation. *Microsurgery* 2002;22:144-151.

The purpose of this study was to evaluate the histologic, immunohistochemical, and electrophysiologic differences between normal, denervated, and insulin-like growth factor-1 denervated muscle over an 8-week period. Denervated mice gastrocnemius muscles demonstrated a decrease in muscle weight, a decrease in myofiber diameter, an absence of muscle regeneration, an early increase in the number of neuromuscular junctions, and a decrease in fast-twitch and maximum tetanic strength compared with normal muscle up to 8 weeks following denervation. Insulin-like growth factor-1 denervated muscle, on the other hand, sustained muscle diameter and muscle weight, maintained a smaller number of neuromuscular junctions, and relatively sustained fast-twitch and maximum tetanic strength compared with normal muscle over 8 weeks. These data suggest that insulin-like growth factor-1 may help prevent muscle atrophy and secondary functional compromise after denervation.

Classic Bibliography

Allen CH: Functional results of primary nerve repair. *Hand Clin* 2000;16:67-72.

Diao E, Hariharan JS, Soejima O, Lotz J: Effect of peripheral suture depth on strength of tendon repairs. *J Hand Surg Am* 1996;21:234-239.

Dunning CE, Lindsay CS, Bicknell RT, Patterson SD, Johnson JA, King GJ: Supplemental pinning improves the stability of external fixation in distal radius fractures during simulated finger and forearm motion. *J Hand Surg Am* 1999;24:992-1000.

Garberman SF, Diao E, Peimer CA: Mallet finger: Results of early versus delayed closed treatment. *J Hand Surg Am* 1994;19:850-852.

Geissler WB, Freeland AE, et al: Intracarpal soft-tissue lesions associated with an intra-articular fracture of the distal end of the radius. *J Bone Joint Surg Am* 1996;78: 357-365.

Gelberman RH, Boyer MI, Brodt MD, Winters SC, Silva MJ: The effect of gap formation at the repair site on the strength and excursion of intrasynovial flexor tendons: An experimental study on the early stages of tendon-healing in dogs. *J Bone Joint Surg Am* 1999;81:975-982.

Lotz JC, Hariharan JS, Diao E: Analytic model to predict the strength of tendon repairs. *J Orthop Res* 1998; 16:399-405.

Okafor B, Mbubaegbu C: Mallet deformity of the finger: Five-year follow-up of conservative treatment. *J Bone Joint Surg Br* 1997;79:544-547.

Rockwell WB, Butler PN, et al: Extensor tendon: Anatomy, injury, and reconstruction. *Plast Reconstr Surg* 2000;106:1592-1603.

Soejima O, Diao E, Lotz JC, Hariharan JS: Comparative mechanical analysis of dorsal versus palmar placement of core suture for flexor tendon repairs. *J Hand Surg Am* 1995;20:801-807.

Strickland JW: Development of flexor tendon surgery: Twenty-five years of progress. *J Hand Surg Am* 2000;25: 214-235.

Toby EB, Butler TE, et al: A comparison of fixation screws for the scaphoid during application of cyclical bending loads. *J Bone Joint Surg Am* 1997;79:1190-1197.

Wolfe SW, Austin G, et al: A biomechanical comparison of different wrist external fixators with and without K-wire augmentation. *J Hand Surg Am* 1999;24:516-524.

Chapter 30

Wrist and Hand Reconstruction

Debra M. Parisi, MD

Thomas E. Trumble, MD

Wrist Imaging

The wrist is a relatively small joint in which multiple bony articulations and soft-tissue structures act synergistically to provide motion while maintaining necessary stability. Several different imaging modalities are available to assist the physician in the diagnosis of wrist pain and/or dysfunction. The interpretation of diagnostic images is often dependent on the technique or skill of the clinician evaluating the results.

Plain radiographs supplemented with stress radiographs should be the first imaging examinations ordered when attempting to determine wrist pathology. Supplemental studies (such as CT, MRI, bone scan, and arthrography) may be used for further assessment of wrist pathology (Table 1).

Prior to the widespread use of diagnostic wrist arthroscopy, triple injection wrist arthrography was the gold standard for diagnosing carpal instability. The radiocarpal, midcarpal, and carpometacarpal (CMC) joints are injected sequentially with radiopaque dye. After each injection, the wrist is brought through a range of motion and then a static or fluoroscopic image is obtained to ensure that the dye has not extravasated into another compartment. If dye has traversed from one compartment to another, the integrity of one or more of the intraosseous wrist ligaments has been compromised. A magnetic resonance arthrogram is frequently used in conjunction with fluoroscopic arthrography to improve the diagnostic accuracy of ligament injuries.

Wrist Arthroscopy

Eleven access portals are currently used to access the entire wrist joint. Radiocarpal portals include the 3-4, 4-5, 6R, 6U, and 1-2 portals. Midcarpal portals include the midcarpal radial, midcarpal ulnar, triquetral hamate, and triscaphe portals. Distal radioulnar portals include the proximal and distal radioulnar joint (DRUJ) portals.

Arthroscopy of the wrist is the most accurate and specific method of diagnosing mechanical wrist pathology. Direct visualization of ligament disruption, abnormal motion, and articular pathology can be directly observed during a diagnostic arthroscopic procedure. Arthroscopy also is useful for diagnosing partial and complete tears of the triangular fibrocartilage complex (TFCC) and chondral lesions.

Arthroscopy also has important therapeutic roles. Arthroscopic débridement of the TFCC or excision of the distal ulna can be combined with diagnostic arthroscopy. The radial styloid also may be resected arthroscopically instead of with an open procedure. Under arthroscopic visualization, the styloid may be resected until the radial attachment of the radioscapholunate ligament is reached. TFCC pathology may also be addressed arthroscopically.

Treatment of a symptomatic wrist ganglion may be achieved by arthroscopic exploration of the wrist before arthroscopic or open resection is performed. The wrist scope is placed in the 4-5 or 6R portal and the camera is then directed toward the presumed ganglion. Alternatively, the scope can be placed in the 3-4 portal through the ganglion. If the stalk of the ganglion is visualized, the surgeon can use a second portal to remove it along with a window of capsule using the arthroscopic shaver, or it may be marked and treated with an open approach. The recurrence rate using the arthroscopic technique may be less than with open techniques.

Wrist arthroscopy also is being used to facilitate the reduction of intra-articular distal radius fractures. In a 1999 study, fractures treated with open reduction and plate and screw fixation or external fixation and percutaneous Kirschner wires were compared with fractures treated with arthroscopically guided reduction, percutaneous Kirschner wires, and external fixation. The strength, range of motion, and radiographic appearance were significantly better in patients in the arthroscopically assisted group after a mean follow-up of 31 months. Arthroscopic evaluation of intra-articular distal radius fractures also has the advantage of providing visualization of the surrounding soft-tissue structures (such as the intracapsular ligaments and the TFCC complex), which facilitates the diagnosis of injuries to these structures and helps in directing additional treatment if needed.

Table 1 | Wrist Imaging

Study	Demonstrates	Recommended to Evaluate for:
CT	Bony anatomy	Fracture, tumor
MRI	Soft-tissue integrity, bone viability/vascularity	Osteonecrosis, TFCC tears, ulnar collateral ligament injuries, occult fractures (scaphoid), tumor
Bone scan	Bone turnover activity	Osteonecrosis, infection
Wrist arthrography	Ligament and cartilage integrity	Ligament injury, TFCC tears

Malunion of Distal Radius Fractures

Malunion following a displaced fracture of the distal metaphysis of the radius impairs the normal function of the radiocarpal joint and the DRUJ. The deformity of a malunited distal radius fracture may result in decreased grip strength and range of motion (including flexion-extension, ulnar-radial deviation, and pronation-supination) and an unacceptable cosmetic deformity. Shortening of the radius relative to the distal end of the ulna, in combination with a rotational deformity of the distal fragment, often results in incongruence and/or instability of the DRUJ.

Patients with a malunited distal radius fracture often report pain and loss of function. Younger patients tend to be more symptomatic with smaller degrees of deformity than older, less active patients. The pain and dysfunction often are related to the prominent distal ulna. A distal ulna resection (the Darrach procedure) has been advocated in the past to treat the deformity and abutment. Currently, the preferred treatment of a symptomatic distal radius malunion is corrective osteotomy to restore the anatomy of the distal radius. If the DRUJ cannot be salvaged, a distal ulna resection with or without a closing wedge osteotomy may be indicated.

Criteria for treating distal radius nonunions with a corrective osteotomy with tricortical bone graft include: (1) a loss of radial height of greater than 4 to 5 mm; (2) a loss of 10° or more or radial inclination; and/or (3) a reversal of the palmar tilt to 15° or more of dorsal angulation or an increase in palmar tilt to 25° or more. A contraindication to corrective osteotomies includes the development of significant traumatic arthritis. The goal of surgery is to correct as much of the deformity as possible in all three planes (Figure 1). Careful preoperative planning using templates made from high-quality radiographs is essential.

Wrist Arthritis Secondary to Trauma

Scapholunate Advanced Collapse

Scapholunate advanced collapse (SLAC) is the most common form of wrist arthritis. It is the predictable outcome of an untreated injury to the scapholunate interosseous and palmar radioscaphoid ligaments. When these ligaments are disrupted, there is a shift in the pressure distribution among the carpal bones during motion and loading. The resulting degenerative changes advance in a predictable fashion and can be divided into four stages (Figure 2). Initially, in stage I, increased contact pressure results in joint space narrowing between the articular surface of the radial styloid and the distal scaphoid. As the disease progresses, the entire articular surface between the scaphoid fossa of the distal radius and the radial curvature degenerates. In stage III, the capitolunate joint becomes involved with joint space narrowing, sclerosis, and cyst formation. Pancarpal arthrosis occurs during stage IV. The radiolunate joint is consistently spared.

If conservative treatment measures fail, surgical treatment to correct the abnormal loads is attempted. With disruption of the scapholunate and palmar radioscaphoid ligaments, the scaphoid rotates into excessive flexion. This situation creates the excessive loading of the radioscaphoid, scapholunate, and capitolunate joints. Once there is evidence of stage I SLAC, ligament reconstruction cannot consistently correct the excessive flexion deformity of the scaphoid. Thus, a radial styloidectomy is the procedure of choice to treat stage I disease.

For wrists with more advanced degenerative arthritis (stage II and stage III), a motion-preserving reconstructive procedure is recommended. Either a capitate-lunate-hamate-triquetrum (four-corner) arthrodesis with scaphoid excision or a proximal row carpectomy may be performed with reliable results. Attempts to limit the fusion to the capitolunate joint to achieve higher postoperative carpal motion have been unsuccessful because of high rates of nonunion.

With proximal row carpectomy, a high percentage of wrist motion and grip strength are maintained. However, pain may persist, and many patients fail to return to work. Conversion to wrist arthrodesis has been required in up to 15% of patients. A carefully performed four-corner fusion with excision of the scaphoid results in a comparative level of patient satisfaction and grip strength relative to proximal row carpectomy. However, patients with four-corner fusions have approximately 15° to 20° less motion than patients with proximal row carpectomy. A four-corner fusion may be preferable after the midcarpal joint has become involved (stage III). After the disease has progressed to stage IV (pancarpal arthritis), total wrist arthrodesis is the treatment of choice.

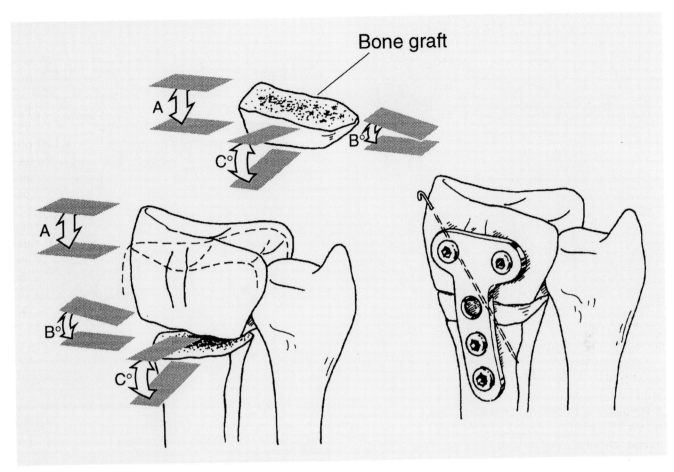

Figure 1 Corrective osteotomy with tricortical bone graft for a distal radius malunion. The osteotomy and graft shape should be designed to correct the radial height (A), radial inclination (B), and palmar tilt (C). *(Reproduced with permission from Trumble TE: Fractures and malunions of the distal radius, in Trumble TE (ed): Principles of Hand Surgery and Therapy. Philadelphia, PA, 2000, p 172.)*

Scaphoid Nonunion Advanced Collapse

Untreated scaphoid nonunions also lead to a predictable progressive pattern of wrist arthrosis, termed scaphoid nonunion advanced collapse (SNAC) (Figure 3). Similar to a wrist with SLAC, degenerative changes first develop in the radial styloid (stage I). In stage II SNAC, there is joint space narrowing of the entire radioscaphoid articulation. In stage III SNAC, the capitate migrates proximally, resulting in a loss of carpal height. As the disease progresses to its final stage (IV), the midcarpal and radiocarpal articulations develop degenerative changes. The radiolunate joint and the articular surface under the proximal fragment of the scaphoid are usually preserved.

As with the treatment of SLAC, various techniques have been described for the treatment of SNAC. The appropriate procedure depends on multiple factors, including the stage of the progression and individual patient factors. In patients with a scaphoid nonunion who have developed degenerative changes of the radial styloid (stage I SNAC), radial styloidectomy in addition to open reduction and internal fixation with bone grafting of the scaphoid is usually successful in halting progression of the arthrosis. If there is evidence of more advanced carpal arthrosis (stage II or greater SNAC), bone grafting will not reliably relieve the patient's symptoms and a salvage procedure is more appropriate (proximal row carpectomy or four-corner fusion).

An option for patients without capitolunate arthrosis is excision of the distal pole of the scaphoid. A recent study suggests that this procedure improves range of motion and increases grip strength in patients with stage II SNAC. Patients who do not have radiocarpal disease may also benefit from either a four-corner fusion and scaphoidectomy (Figure 4) or a proximal row carpectomy.

A proximal row carpectomy is a good procedure to eliminate pain and preserve wrist motion. However, once the progression of arthrosis involves the capitolunate articulation, a proximal row carpectomy is no longer indicated. Therefore, stage III SNAC is most appropriately treated with a four-corner fusion and scaphoidectomy, and stage IV SNAC is best treated with a total wrist arthrodesis.

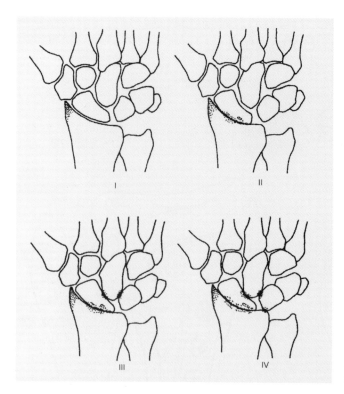

Figure 2 The stages of SLAC. In stage I, there is beaking of the radial styloid. In stage II, there is narrowing and arthrosis of the radioscaphoid joint. In stage III, there is arthrosis between the capitate and the scaphoid and/or lunate as the capitate displaces between the scaphoid and lunate with the carpal collapse. In stage IV, all of the above changes occur along with degeneration of the radiolunate joint. *(Reproduced with permission from Trumble TE, Gardner, GC: Arthritis, in Trumble TE (ed): Principles of Hand Surgery and Therapy. Philadelphia, PA, 2000, p 406.)*

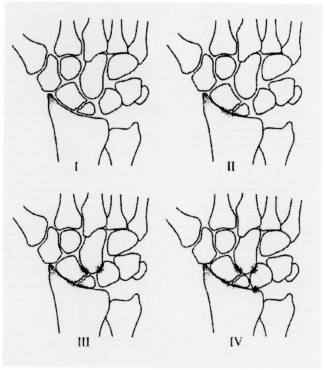

Figure 3 The stages of SNAC. Similar to SLAC, stage I is hallmarked with radial styloid arthritis. In stage II, there is progression of the arthritis to the scaphoid fossa. In stage III, capitolunate arthritis is observed. In stage IV, there is diffuse carpal arthritis with sparing of the lunate fossa. *(Reproduced with permission from Knoll VD, Trumble TE: Scaphoid fractures and nonunions, in Trumble TE (ed): Principles of Hand Surgery and Therapy. Philadelphia, PA, 2000, p 167.)*

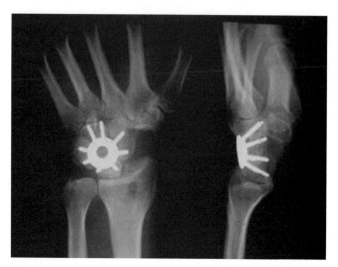

Figure 4 Radiographs showing scaphoidectomy and four-corner fusion using an innovative plate and screw system.

Osteonecrosis of the Carpus

Kienböck's Disease

The etiology of idiopathic lunate osteonecrosis (Kienböck's disease) is not fully understood. Approximately 20% of lunates have only a single vessel as its nutrient supply. An injury to this vessel cannot be compensated for by collateral flow, and the lunate with a single nutrient vessel therefore may be more susceptible to osteonecrosis. The role of ulnar length in the development of Kienböck's disease is still uncertain. When the distal ulna articular surface sits more proximally than the articular surface of the distal radius (ulna negative variance), abnormally increased shear forces across the radiolunate joint may compromise a marginally perfused lunate.

Patients with Kienböck's disease present with an insidious onset of wrist pain that is localized over the middorsum of the wrist. Examination shows only mild tenderness with palpation over the lunate; however, decreased carpal range of motion, particularly in extension, is frequently noted. Plain radiographs may show obvious density changes. MRI has replaced bone scan as the best test to diagnose early stages of Kienböck's disease. It is important to differentiate avascular changes involving the entire lunate consistent with Kienböck's disease and ulnar-sided lunate changes related to impaction syndrome. Intraosseous ganglia also can be mistaken for Kienböck's disease.

Kienböck's disease progresses in a predictable fashion through four radiographically defined stages, which are helpful in guiding treatment (Figure 5) (Table 2). Pa-

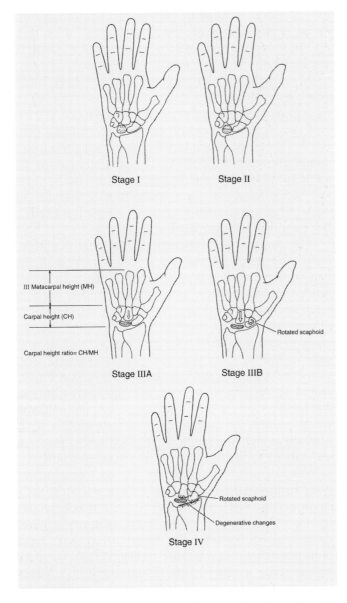

Figure 5 The radiographic stages of Kienböck's disease. *(Reproduced with permission from Allan CH, Trumble TE: Kinebock's disease, in Trumble TE (ed): Principles of Hand Surgery and Therapy. Philadelphia, PA, 2000, pp 441-443.)*

Table 2 | Stages of Kienböck Disease

Stages	Radiographic Findings	Recommended Treatment
I	No findings on plain radiographs, but + bone scan and MRI	Activity modification
2	Lunate sclerosis without collapse	Negative variance: Radial shortening ± vascularized graft to lunate Neutral or positive variance: capitate shortening, ± capitohamate arthrodesis, ± vascularized graft to lunate
3A	Fragmentation and collapse of lunate	Same as stage 2
3B	DISI deformity	Intercarpal arthrodesis (scaphotrapeziotrapezoid or scaphocapitate)
4	Degenerative changes of radiocarpal or midcarpal joint on plain radiographs	Proximal row carpectomy or total wrist arthrodesis

DISI=Dorsal intercalated segmental instability

tients with stage I disease may improve with activity modification and immobilization, and this should be the first line of treatment. If there is no clinical improvement or if the patient advances to stage II disease, surgery may be indicated. Arthroscopic inspection and synovectomy and/or débridement may have a role in the treatment of early Kienböck's disease, particularly because the natural history of untreated Kienböck's disease remains elusive. In patients without a fixed collapse of the lunate and scaphoid rotation (stages I, II, and IIIA), a lunate-salvaging procedure may allow for revascularization of the lunate, maintaining carpal kinematics. In patients with ulnar-negative variance and stage I, II, or IIIA disease, an unloading or joint leveling proce-

dure may be considered. Radial shortening with or without vascularized bone graft to the lunate is the most successful procedure. If the patient with stage I, II, or IIIA disease has ulnar-positive or neutral variance, radial shortening will not decrease the load on the lunate. In this situation, capitate shortening with capitohamate fusion has been shown to successfully decrease the load across the radiolunate articulation.

Stage IIIB Kienböck's disease is characterized by carpal instability with either scaphoid hyperflexion or widening of the scapholunate interval and subsequent migration of the capitate. After the disease has progressed to this stage, simply addressing the load on the lunate does not correct the instability. The scaphoid must be stabilized. This goal can be accomplished by an intercarpal arthrodesis that bridges the midcarpal joint, such as a scaphotrapeziotrapezoid arthrodesis or a scaphocapitate arthrodesis. The goal is to stabilize the scaphoid in a nonrotated position to prevent abnormal kinematics and subsequent degenerative changes in the wrist, while simultaneously transferring some of the radiocarpal load away from the lunate.

Preiser's Disease

Idiopathic osteonecrosis of the scaphoid (Preiser's disease) occurs less frequently than Kienböck's disease. Patients generally report pain at the radial aspect of the wrist. Radiographs at the time of presentation show sclerosis of the involved areas and fragmentation of the

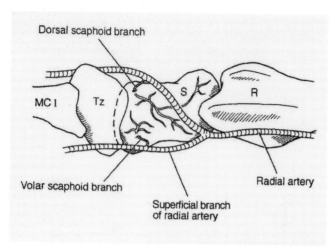

Figure 6 The vascular supply of the scaphoid. MC 1 = first metacarpal, Tz = trapezium, S = scaphoid, R= radius. *(Reproduced with permission from Trumble TE: Fractures and dislocations of the carpus, in Trumble TE (ed): Principles of Hand Surgery and Therapy. Philadelphia, PA, 2000, p 94.)*

proximal articular surface. This disease must not be confused with posttraumatic proximal osteonecrosis. Vascularized bone grafting can be successfully used if fragmentation of the proximal pole has not occurred. A salvage procedure may be required. The most common procedures used to treat Preiser's disease are proximal row carpectomy or scaphoidectomy and four-corner fusion. Recently, arthroscopic inspection and débridement has been described for its treatment.

Capitate Osteonecrosis

Capitate osteonecrosis is a very rare condition. It is usually associated with high-dose steroid use, chemotherapy, or trauma (such as transperilunate transcapitate fracture-dislocations). Surgical treatment options include vascularized grafting, fragment excision with tendon interposition arthroplasty, and four-corner arthrodesis. Most recently, scaphocapitolunate arthrodesis has been used to treat osteonecrosis of the capitate. Osteonecrosis of the other carpal bones is rarely seen.

Scaphoid Nonunion and Osteonecrosis

Osteonecrosis of the proximal pole of the scaphoid is frequently posttraumatic and is associated with nonunion of a proximal pole or scaphoid waist fracture. This condition is unique and should be approached differently than Preiser's disease. Most of the scaphoid is vascularized via a dorsal branch of the radial artery, which perforates the distal third of the dorsal cortex of the scaphoid. Intraosseous blood flow is retrograde, leaving the proximal pole with a tenuous blood supply (Figure 6). The more proximal a scaphoid fracture, the more likely is delayed healing or nonunion and osteonecrosis. Fine-cut (1-mm) sagittal and coronal CT images provide excellent detail of the fracture fragments and can be

used to assess location of the fracture, size of the fragments, extent of collapse, and progression of union (Figure 7). Preoperatively, MRI is a good tool to evaluate the vascularity of the proximal pole (Figure 8).

Many patients with scaphoid fractures have subtle symptoms leading to a delay in diagnosis. It may be months or years before radiographs are taken that reveal the scaphoid nonunion causing the patient's pain. By this time, the scaphoid has usually collapsed into a humpback type of deformity. The proximal pole is extended through the pull of the scapholunate ligament and the influence of the triquetrohamate articulation, while the scaphotrapeziotrapezoid articulation exerts a flexion moment on the distal scaphoid.

The duration of the nonunion influences the probability of surgical success. A scaphoid nonunion of less than 5 years duration is more likely to heal with appropriate surgical treatment than a nonunion that has been untreated for longer than 5 years. Proper resection of all fibrous material, thorough débridement of the sclerotic margins, and adequate bone grafting are necessary to achieve healing of a nonunion. Precise surgical technique and positioning of the implant is critical for obtaining union. The use of a variable-pitch screw enables compression between the two fragments and enhances union results. The placement of a compression screw centrally within the scaphoid fragments also increases the stability of fixation and the likelihood of union.

Vascularized bone grafts are a good treatment option for proximal pole nonunions when osteonecrosis is confirmed by MRI. The vascularized graft is harvested from the dorsal aspect of the distal radius and rotated on a regional pedicle. The radial artery has dorsal branches defined in reference to the extensor compartments. The artery of Zaidemberg (1,2-intercompartmental supraretinacular artery), located between the first and second compartments, is most commonly used (Figure 9).

Triangular Fibrocartilage Complex and the Distal Radioulnar Joint

Anatomy and Biomechanics

The TFCC is composed of the triangular fibrocartilage and its supporting ligaments. The triangular fibrocartilage is a meniscus-like structure with a high proportion of type II collagen in addition to type I collagen. Surrounding the periphery of this structure is the meniscal homolog, a fibrocartilaginous rim that stabilizes the triangular fibrocartilage to the ulnar styloid and the ulnar collateral ligament. This structure has a distinct blood supply that enters from the periphery of the TFCC. The ulnar periphery of the triangular fibrocartilage has the richest blood supply and the best potential for healing (Figure 10).

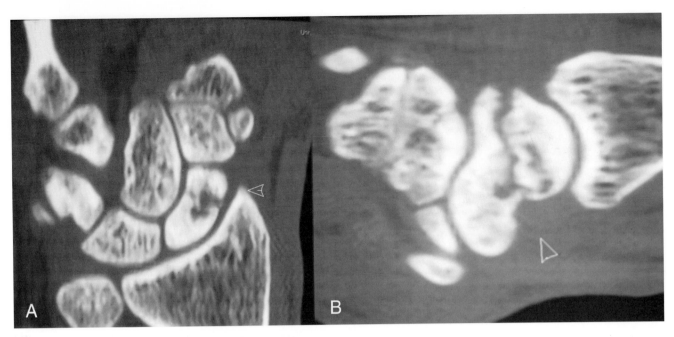

Figure 7 Fine-cut coronal **(A)** and sagittal **(B)** CT images provide excellent detail of fracture fragments (arrowheads) of the scaphoid nonunion. *(Reproduced with permission from Trumble TE, Fractures and dislocations of the carpus, in Trumble TE (ed): Principles of Hand Surgery and Therapy. Philadelphia, PA, 2000, p 102.)*

The TFCC arises from the articular cartilage at the corner of the sigmoid notch of the radius and inserts onto the base of the ulnar styloid and volarly into the ulnocarpal ligament complex formed by the ulnar triquetral ligament and the ulnar lunate ligament. The ligaments and the TFCC, which support the DRUJ and ulnar portion of the carpus, form a three-walled pyramidal structure. The triangular fibrocartilage is the floor of this pyramid. The ligaments forming the walls of this pyramid stabilize the carpus to the triangular fibrocartilage and the ulnar styloid so that they maintain their relationship to the TFCC while rotating around the ulna. The ulnar triquetral ligament and the ulnar lunate ligament form the volar wall of this box. The undersurface of the extensor carpi ulnaris tendon forms the ulnar wall of the box, and the dorsal radial triquetral ligament forms the dorsal wall of this compartment. These structures maintain the relationship between the carpus and the ulna.

In addition to the DRUJ and ulnocarpal ligaments, the TFCC is a key stabilizer of the DRUJ and a stabilizer of the ulnar carpus. The amount of load transferred to the distal ulna from the carpus is directly proportional to the ulnar variance. In neutral ulnar variance, approximately 20% of the load is transmitted via the TFCC. With positive ulnar variance, the load across the TFCC is increased, with a resultant thinning of its central disk. In pronation, the radius moves proximally relative to the ulna, while in supination the radius moves distally. This movement results in a relative positive variance in pronation and a relative negative variance in supination. Thus, a greater load is transferred to the distal ulna from the carpus via the TFCC in pronation than

in supination. In pronation, the radius also moves volarly relative to the ulna, tightening the dorsal ligament fibers of the TFCC. In supination, the radius moves dorsally such that the volar ligament fibers of the TFCC tighten. As these respective ligaments tighten, they help to support the carpus on the distal forearm.

Triangular Fibrocartilage Complex Injuries

TFCC injuries can be classified into two basic categories: type I, traumatic injuries, and type II, degenerative lesions. Traumatic lesions are classified according to the location of the tear within the TFCC; degenerative lesions are associated with positive ulnar variance and often have associated pathology (for example, lunotriquetral ligament attenuation or carpal arthrosis) (Table 3).

Type IA lesions are usually treated with arthroscopic débridement of the unstable portion of the tear that has occurred in the avascular zone. If more than two thirds of the central disk is débrided, the DRUJ becomes unstable. The peripheral 2 mm of the triangular fibrocartilage must be maintained to avoid DRUJ instability.

Chronic type IB lesions can be difficult to diagnose. Examination shows ulnar-sided wrist pain and mild DRUJ instability. Radiographs may demonstrate an ulna styloid fracture or may be normal. Diagnostic arthroscopy reveals that the TFCC has lost its normal tension. Isolated peripheral tears are repaired arthroscopically. If the tear is associated with an ulna styloid fracture and instability, an open reduction with internal fixation of the ulnar styloid fragment or styloidectomy is performed before reattaching the TFCC to the remaining distal ulna. Treatment of this injury consists of ar-

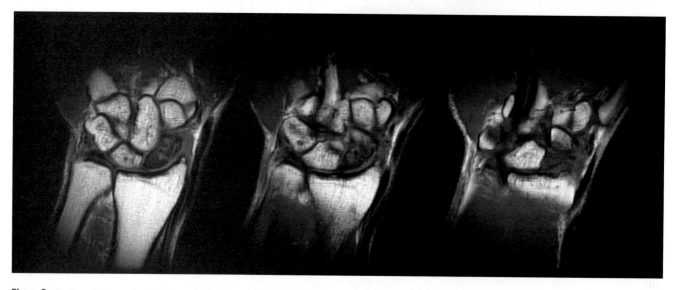

Figure 8 MRI of scaphoid nonunion showing proximal pole avascularity. Each image shows hypoechoic signal in the proximal pole suggestive of avascularity.

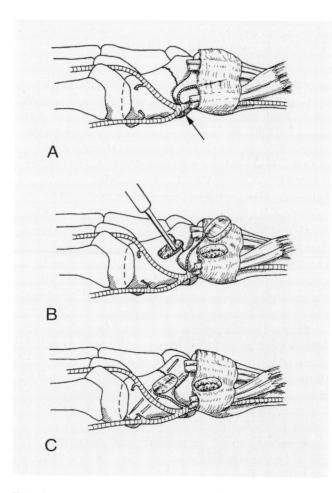

Figure 9 Vascularized bone grafts for the scaphoid are based on the artery of Zaidemberg (1,2-intercompartmental supraretinacular artery). **A,** The 1,2 intermetacarpal artery is shown (arrow). **B,** The vascularized pedicle has been harvested. A burr is used to create a recipient channel for the graft. **C,** Two Kirschner wires are used to stabilize the bone graft. Note the vascularized pedicle. *(Reproduced with permission from Thiru RG, Ferlic DC, Clayton ML, McClure DC: Arterial anatomy of the triangular fibrocartilage of the wrist and its surgical significance. J Hand Surgery [Am] 1986;11:258-263.)*

throscopic or open repair of the TFCC tear. Three or four sutures are placed through the most volar aspect of the tear, which is then tied over the capsule (Figure 11).

The diagnosis of a type IC lesion is made arthroscopically after noting a loss of tension in the ulnar extrinsic ligaments, as well as easy and direct visualization of the pisotriquetral joint. This lesion may be repaired arthroscopically or openly depending on the size of the defect. Type ID lesions are frequently associated with distal radial fractures. This corner of the TFCC has poor vascularity. However, if the articular cartilage of the sigmoid notch is disrupted by fracture, or intraoperatively by the surgeon, healing to vascularized bone readily occurs (Figure 12).

The outcome of TFCC injuries also depends on the chronicity of the tear. Patients with acute tears, which are repaired within 3 months after injury, recover 80% of the grip strength and range of motion as is present on the contralateral side. Subacute injuries (3 months to 1 year) are still amenable to direct repair, but regain less strength and range of motion. Arthroscopic repairs result in greater range of motion, grip strength, and patient satisfaction compared with open repairs. Chronic injuries to the TFCC frequently benefit from ulnar shortening to decrease the load distributed to the distal ulna via the TFCC, with or without débridement of the TFCC.

Degenerative TFCC Lesions (Ulnocarpal Impaction Syndrome)

Type II or degenerative lesions of the TFCC are related to chronic overload of the ulnar side of the wrist. Once symptomatic, chronic ulnar abutment or impaction is progressive and deterioration of the TFCC as well as ulnar-sided articulations occur over time. Abutment may be idiopathic; patients with positive ulnar variance are more susceptible to overload with chronic perforations of their TFCC than patients with neutral or negative ulnar variance (Figure 13). Ulnar impaction also may be secondary to a change in wrist anatomy after a traumatic insult. Malunion of the distal radius with excessive shortening and dorsal tilt, growth arrest after a distal radius physeal fracture, or proximal migration of the radius following a radial head excision may all result in ulnar impaction syndrome.

The progressive degenerative changes of type II TFCC lesions associated with ulnar abutment are classified into five stages: A through E (Table 3). The primary goal of treatment of ulnar impaction is to unload or decompress the ulnar carpus and ulnar head. This decompression can be accomplished by several different techniques: ulnar shortening osteotomy, partial ulnar head resection (wafer procedure), or an ulnar salvage procedure. Type IIA and IIB lesions are early stages in the degenerative process. There is no perforation of the triangular fibrocartilage, and thus, no débridement is necessary, and an open ulnar shortening osteotomy should sufficiently unload the ulnocarpal joint. Type IIC lesions are preferentially treated with an arthroscopic débridement of the perforation. An arthroscopic wafer resection may then be performed through the débrided area of the triangular fibrocartilage. Conversely, an ulnar shortening procedure can be done in addition to the arthroscopic débridement (Figure 14). The major disadvantage of an ulnar shortening procedure is that the ulna may be slow to unite or may even fail to unite. The wafer resection procedure does not have the complications associated with an osteotomy; however, this procedure may accelerate the onset of DRUJ arthritis. Type IID and IIE lesions represent end stages of ulnar impaction syndrome, with arthritic changes and instability. If there is no notable lunotriquetral instability or DRUJ arthrosis, the treatment of choice is ulnar shortening followed by arthroscopic débridement. If there is demonstrable lunotriquetral instability after débriding the TFCC and the frayed lunotriquetral ligament, an ulnar shortening osteotomy is performed. Lunotriquetral stability often improves after the osteotomy because of tightening of the ulnar extrinsic ligaments. If, however, significant lunotriquetral instability persists, the lunotriquetral joint should be percutaneously pinned with two 0.045-inch Kirschner wires. If significant arthritic changes are noted at the DRUJ, an ulnar salvage procedure (such as a modified Darrach, an ulna hemiresection with tendon interposition, or a distal ulna replacement arthroplasty) is a better surgical option.

Instability and Arthritis of the DRUJ

Patients with DRUJ pathology can be divided into three categories: those with instability only, those with arthritis only, and those with both arthritis and instability of the DRUJ. In patients with DRUJ instability, the radius

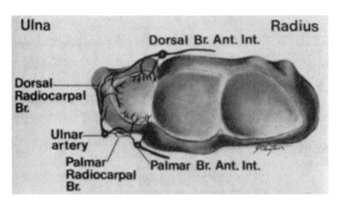

Figure 10 Vascular supply to the TFCC enters via the periphery. Br = branch, Ant = anterior, Int = interosseous. *(Reproduced with permission from Thiru RG, Ferlic DC, Clayton ML, McClure DC: Arterial anatomy of the triangular fibrocartilage of the wrist and its surgical significance. J Hand Surgery [Am] 1986;11:258-263.)*

impinges on the ulna, causing a painful click during attempts to pronate and supinate the wrist. Over time, this impingement can result in degenerative changes within the joint. As degenerative changes develop in the DRUJ, the instability between the ulna and radius may lessen.

DRUJ instability is the result of bone deformity, ligamentous injury, or a combination of the two. In patients with chronic instability without bony deformity, the radioulnar ligaments are usually irreparable. Treatment consists of some type of soft-tissue reconstruction. Reconstruction of the distal radioulnar ligaments can potentially restore stability without substantial loss of motion or strength. Several techniques of reconstruction have been described. A careful evaluation of the patient is necessary, however, because significant joint incongruity and frank arthritis of the DRUJ are contraindications to reconstruction.

A recent study assessed DRUJ ligament reconstruction using a palmaris tendon graft passed through bone tunnels to restore both the volar and dorsal ligaments. Stability was restored in 12 of 14 of patients who underwent this DRUJ ligament reconstruction. These patients returned to full activities and recovered 85% of motion and strength. This procedure was considered effective for restoring DRUJ stability; however, it requires a competent sigmoid notch and did not fully correct associated ulnocarpal instability.

Recently, attempts to manage early DRUJ arthrosis have focused on retaining the ulnar head and altering the contact surface by performing either an ulna shaft shortening osteotomy or débriding osteophytes from the proximal margin of the joint. More traditionally, patients with DRUJ arthritis have been treated by either ulna head resection or distal radioulnar fusions. Patients with stable arthritic joints have classically been treated with excision and careful repair of the surrounding joint capsule (Darrach or modified Darrach procedure).

Table 3 | TFCC Lesions

Traumatic			Degenerative		
Type	Location	Treatment	Type	Character	Treatment
IA	Central tears without instability	Arthroscopic débridement of unstable portion	IIA	Wearing without perforation or chondromalacia	Ulnar shortening
IB	Peripheral tear at the base of the ulnar styloid	Isolated TFCC tear: Arthroscopic repair Associated with ulna styloid fixation: ORIF of ulna styloid and repairing TFCC	IIB	Wearing with chondromalacia of either lunate or ulna	Ulnar shortening
IC	Avulsion from ulnar extrinsic ligaments	Arthroscopic versus open repair	IIC	Perforation of triangular fibrocartilage with lunate chondromalacia	Arthroscopic débridement of TFCC; ulnar shortening or wafer resection
ID	Detachment from sigmoid notch; often associated with distal radius fixation	Arthroscopic versus open repair	IID	Perforation of triangular fibrocartilage, lunate, and/or ulna chondromalacia, LT disruption without instability	Arthroscopic débridement of TFCC and LT ligaments; ulnar shortening If DRUJ arthrosis, modified Darrach or ulna hemiresection
			IIE	Generalized arthritic changes, LT disruption with volar intercalcated segmental instability	Arthroscopic débridement of TFCC and LT ligaments; ulnar shortening If instability persists after shortening, pin LT joint If DRUJ arthrosis, modified Darrach, hemiresection or ulna replacement arthroplasty

ORIF = open reduction and internal fixation; LT = lunotriquetral

Patients with instability associated with arthritis are at increased risk for persistent instability and are best treated with a procedure designed to stabilize the ulna and buffer the distal radioulnar articulation, such as an ulnar hemiresection with tendon interposition. In younger patients, with posttraumatic DRUJ arthritis and an intact TFCC, a Sauvé-Kapandji procedure is an alternative approach described to maintain grip strength. In the Sauvé-Kapandji procedure, the DRUJ is fused and a pseudarthrosis is created proximal to the DRUJ to allow for rotation of the radius around the ulna. The Sauvé-Kapandji procedure is often subject to complications related to an unstable proximal stump.

Distal ulna implant arthroplasty is an attractive alternative for the treatment of DRUJ arthritis and instability (Figure 15). Normal mechanical function and stability of the DRUJ requires an intact ulnar head. A functional ulnar head implant would alleviate impingement and restore near-normal load transmission. Thus, ulnar head replacement may be an alternative to the modified Darrach procedure. In the past, patients with recurrent instability of the ulna caused by excessive proximal excision of the radial head, excessive resection of the distal ulna, or combined radial head excision and distal ulna excision were treated with arthrodesis of the radius and ulna (creation of a one-bone forearm) performed as a salvage procedure. A total DRUJ prosthesis is now available and has many advantages over the one-bone forearm. Currently, there are several designs available for ulnar head implants and total DRUJ prostheses. However, although these devices show promise, there are no long-term clinical studies that clearly delineate the indications for their use.

Degenerative Arthrosis of the Thumb and Fingers

Thumb Carpometacarpal Joint

The CMC joint of the thumb has a biconcave saddle shape, which imparts little intrinsic bony stability. In a recent study, 16 ligaments surrounding the trapeziometacarpal joint were identified. The deep volar (anterior oblique) ligament, which passes from the trapezium to the volar beak of the thumb metacarpal, and the dorsoradial ligament play the most significant role in maintaining CMC stability. The deep volar ligament resists

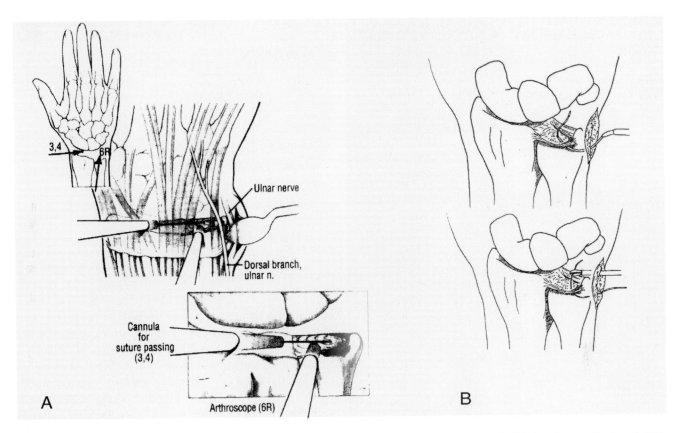

Figure 11 Arthroscopically assisted TFCC repair using the outside-in technique. **A,** Shows the 3-4 and 6R portals used to access the TFCC. A needle is used to pierce the TFCC. **(B)** A suture is threaded through the needle and grasped. The suture is tied to the capsule. *(Reproduced with permission from Trumble TE: Distal radioulnar joint triangular fibrocartilage complex, in Trumble TE (ed): Principles of Hand Surgery and Therapy. Philadelphia, PA, 2000, pp 136-137.)*

the dorsal subluxation force created by pinch. Attenuation of the volar (anterior oblique) ligament allows for dorsoradial subluxation of the metacarpal base and initiates articular cartilage degeneration. Degenerative changes begin volarly and progress dorsally.

Patients with thumb basal joint arthritis can be divided into those with arthritis isolated to the CMC joint (type A), those with arthritis isolated to the scaphotrapeziotrapezoid joint (type B), and those with pantrapezial arthritis (type C). Patients with involvement of the CMC joint can further be divided into those with instability (dorsal subluxation of the metacarpal on the trapezium with or without compensatory metacarpophalangeal joint hyperextension) and those without instability. In patients with metacarpophalangeal joint hyperextension coexisting with dorsal CMC joint subluxation (swan neck thumb), it is critical to correct the metacarpophalangeal joint hyperextension via capsulodesis or arthrodesis to eliminate the long moment arm that continues to exert a dorsally directed force on the CMC joint during pinch activities.

CMC joint arthritis is most commonly treated with excision of the distal half or the entire trapezium with tendon interposition and some form of ligament reconstruction. The flexor carpi radialis can be used to stabilize the joint and serve as the anchovy interpositioned between

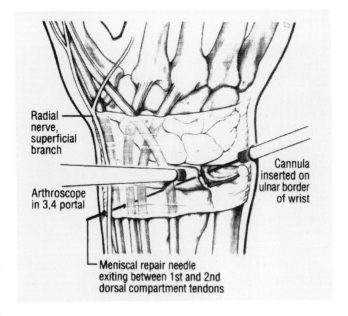

Figure 12 Arthroscopic repair of a TFCC type ID lesion. *(Reproduced with permission from Trumble TE, Gilbert M, Vedder N: Isolated tears of the triangular fibrocartilage: Management by early arthroscopic repair. J Hand Surg [Am] 1997;22:57-65.)*

the scaphoid and the metacarpal (ligament reconstruction tendon interposition); or a slip of the abductor pollicis lon-

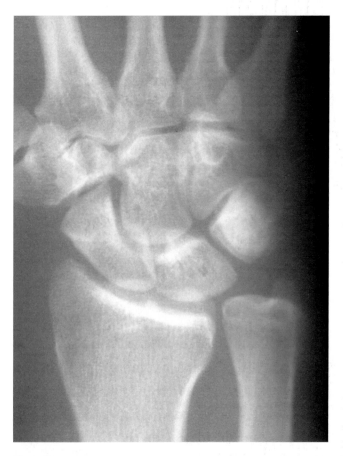

Figure 13 Ulnar impaction syndrome. Radiographic changes are localized to the ulnar aspect of wrist and are associated with ulnar positive variance. *(Reproduced with permission from Conduit DP: Carpal avascular necrosis, Trumble TE (ed): Hand Surgery Update 3: Hand, Elbow, and Shoulder. Rosemont, IL, American Society for Surgery of the Hand, 2003, p 218.)*

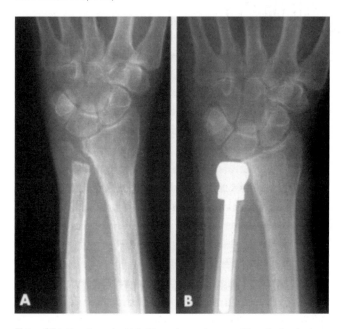

Figure 15 A, PA radiograph of failed Darrach resection caused by radioulnar impingement. **B**, A distal ulna prosthesis (Avanta Orthopaedics, San Diego, CA) restored alignment and stability to the DRUJ. *(Reproduced with permission from Adams BD: Distal radioulnar joint, in Trumble TE (ed): Hand Surgery Update 3: Hand, Elbow, and Shoulder. Rosemont, IL, American Society for Surgery of the Hand, 2003, p 154.)*

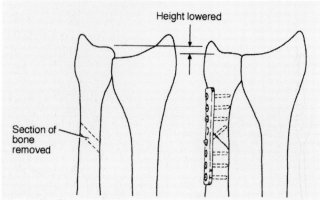

Figure 14 An ulna shortening osteotomy should be performed in patients who have type II TFCC lesions and positive ulnar variance. *(Reproduced with permission from Trumble TE: Distal radioulnar joint and triangular fibrocartilage complex, in Trumble TE (ed): Principles of Hand Surgery and Therapy. Philadelphia, PA, 2000, p 139.)*

gus can also be used as a sling to suspend the metacarpal and recreate a volar beak ligament, after excision of the trapezium (abductor pollicis longus suspensionplasty). Studies have shown that basal joint arthroplasties with a firm interposition graft provide a greater degree of stability than grafts composed of tendon. Thus, an alternative technique is interposition with a costochondral allograft spacer (lifesaver technique). One half of the flexor carpi radialis is harvested and used to stabilize the spacer (Figure 16).

Other options include thumb metacarpal extension osteotomy for patients with early degenerative changes isolated to the volar aspect of the joint and CMC joint arthrodesis in younger patients who require strength and stability. Scaphotrapeziotrapezoid arthritis is a contraindication for CMC joint arthrodesis. Arthroscopic débridement of the CMC joint may also play a role in the treatment of CMC joint arthritis. For patients with an early disease stage, arthroscopic synovectomy and electrothermal shrinkage of the trapeziometacarpal capsule to provide symptomatic relief has been described. For patients with more advanced disease, hemitrapeziectomy and complete trapeziectomy with electrothermal shrinkage of the anterior oblique ligament may be performed arthroscopically.

Metacarpophalangeal Joint Arthrosis

When contemplating treatment of arthrosis of the metacarpophalangeal joint of the thumb, the entire thumb axis must be considered. If the interphalangeal and CMC joints are not diseased, arthrodesis is the procedure of choice. The metacarpophalangeal joint of the thumb is often fused because of instability, pain, and deformity, which impairs pinch.

In patients with rheumatoid arthritis and osteoarthritis, arthroplasty of the thumb metacarpophalangeal joint with newer articulating implants that preserve col-

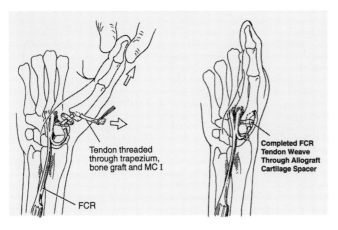
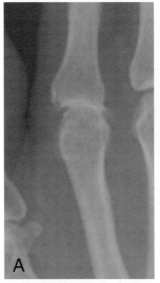
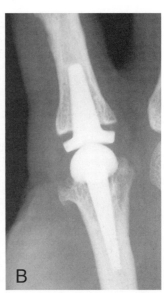

Figure 16 Lifesaver technique of CMC joint arthroplasty. MC I = first metacarpal, FCR = flexor carpi radialis. *(Reproduced with permission from Trumble TE, Garnder GC: Arthritis, in Trumble TE (ed): Principles of Hand Surgery and Therapy. Philadelphia, PA, 2000, p 429.)*

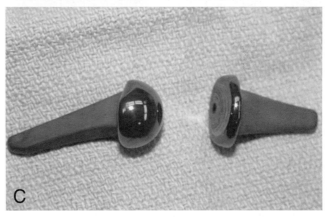

Figure 17 Preoperative (**A**) and postoperative (**B**) AP radiographs of a patient with posttraumatic metacarpophalangeal joint arthritis, treated with a newer, anatomically designed metacarpophalangeal joint arthroplasty **C,** Photograph of implant components. (Ascencion Orthopaedics, Austin, TX.)

lateral ligaments, may be performed in conjunction with fusion of a diseased interphalangeal joint. Arthroplasty of the metacarpophalangeal joint may be preferred to arthrodesis in this clinical scenario because it preserves thumb length, improves position of thumb tip for opposition, and decreases the stress transferred to the CMC joint. However, after arthroplasty, a deficient ulnar collateral ligament and the decreased ability to generate pinch force may ultimately result in failure of the arthroplasty.

Whereas arthrodesis is commonly indicated in the proximal interphalangeal (PIP) and distal interphalangeal joints of the fingers, arthrodesis is very functionally limiting in the metacarpophalangeal joint and is rarely performed. Soft-tissue deformity in the metacarpophalangeal joints caused by rheumatoid arthritis is often severe, which increases the difficulty of obtaining a good result from arthroplasty. If the metacarpophalangeal collateral ligaments are intact, an articulating prosthesis can be used (Figure 17). If the collateral ligaments are deficient, a Silastic spacer is a better implant choice. The status of the PIP joint and the wrist must also be considered when contemplating metacarpophalangeal arthroplasty.

Proximal and Distal Interphalangeal Joints
The PIP joint is the "soul" of the hand and thus there is no good position for arthrodesis. PIP joint arthrodesis (in 40° of flexion for the index finger, 45° of flexion for the middle finger, 50° flexion for the ring finger, and 55° of flexion for the small finger) is a poor secondary option. However, arthrodesis does provide a stable, pain-free digit and is indicated for high-demand patients with PIP joint arthrosis. A significant amount of lateral stress is placed on the PIP joint of the index finger during pinch; therefore, PIP arthrodesis should be considered in all patients with index PIP disease.

Loss of motion of the PIP joint results in the inability to make a fist. Therefore, arthroplasty is a viable alternative when motion of the joint needs to be preserved. Classically, Silastic joint spacers have been used to preserve motion, but these implants are not very durable. Recently, several two-piece prostheses have been anatomically designed specifically for PIP joint arthroplasty. Early results suggest that these prostheses may function better than an arthrodesis. Similar to the effects of rheumatoid arthritis on the metacarpophalangeal joints, rheumatoid disease often causes soft-tissue imbalance of the interphalangeal joints, which must be considered at the time of surgery.

The distal interphalangeal joint is most commonly involved in degenerative osteoarthritic conditions. For patients who do not respond to nonsurgical treatment, surgical options include resection arthroplasty, implant arthroplasty, and arthrodesis. Arthrodesis in 10° to 20° of flexion is the preferred treatment.

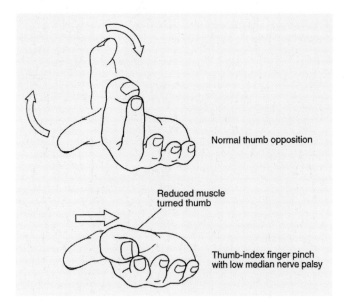

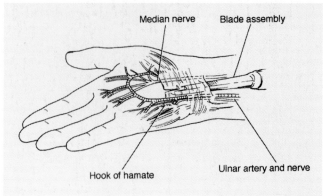

Figure 19 Illustration of endoscopic carpal tunnel release. *(Reproduced with permission from Trumble TE: Compressive neuropathies, in Trumble TE (ed): Principles of Hand Surgery and Therapy. Philadelphia, PA, 2000, p 334.)*

Figure 18 Thumb opposition is a complex motion requiring trapeziometacarpal abduction, flexion, and pronation. *(Reproduced with permission from Trumble TE: Tendon transfers, in Trumble TE (ed): Principles of Hand Surgery and Therapy. Philadelphia, PA, 2000, p 351.)*

Nerve Compression Syndromes

Carpal Tunnel Syndrome

Carpal tunnel syndrome (CTS) is a condition of compression of the median nerve as it traverses the wrist and causes a constellation of related signs and symptoms. Patients often report intermittent or constant numbness or tingling in the median nerve distribution, which may be associated with pain. Night pain that awakens the patient from sleep is also common. In severe cases, there may be denervation of the thenar muscles with resultant weakness and atrophy.

CTS is the most common entrapment neuropathy, occurring in 0.1% to 10% of the general population. Risk factors include obesity, hypothyroidism, diabetes, pregnancy, renal disease, inflammatory arthritis, acromegaly, mucopolysaccharidosis, genetic predisposition, advancing age, smoking, and repetitive or extreme wrist flexion at work. However, in more than 95% of patients, CTS is idiopathic.

CTS is a clinical diagnosis based on history and physical examination and is confirmed by electrodiagnostic studies. Other pathologies (such as cervical radiculopathy, brachial plexopathy, thoracic outlet syndrome, apical lung tumor, pronator syndrome, cubital and ulnar tunnel syndromes, and peripheral neuropathy) may cause hand numbness; these disease processes must be ruled out before making the diagnosis of CTS. A combination of findings in the history and physical examination is more accurate than the same findings in isolation. CTS is accurately diagnosed 86% of the time when night pain, a positive Semmes-Weinstein monofilament test, a positive carpal tunnel compression test (Durkhan's sign), and a

consistent Brigham hand diagram are all present. The probability of having CTS when all of these tests are negative is 0.68%. Electrodiagnostic studies do not add to the diagnostic reliability of this combination of tests.

Electrodiagnostic studies (nerve conduction velocities and electromyography) are used to confirm the clinical diagnosis. A pathologic nerve conduction velocity study includes decreased action potential amplitude, increased distal latency, and a decreased velocity. A distal motor latency of more than 4.5 ms and a sensory latency of more than 3.5 ms is abnormal. Abnormal electromyographic findings include increased insertional activity, fibrillations at rest, positive sharp waves and complex repetitive discharges, and decreased motor unit recruitment.

Nonsurgical treatment of CTS includes activity modification, night splinting, steroid injection into the carpal canal, and oral medication (such as nonsteroidal anti-inflammatory drugs and vitamin B6). Neither nonsteroidal anti-inflammatory drugs nor vitamin B6 has been definitively shown to be effective in isolation. Steroid injection into the carpal tunnel combined with nocturnal splinting has a short-term success rate of 80% in relieving symptoms. However, after 12 to 18 months, only 22% of patients treated with this regimen remain symptom free.

Surgical treatment is indicated for patients who have not responded to nonsurgical treatment and for patients with thenar weakness, atrophy, or electrodiagnostic evidence of denervation (Figure 18). Several well-controlled studies indicate that there is no appreciable benefit of internal neurolysis or epineurotomy. Also, there does not seem to be a role for tenosynovectomy with carpal tunnel release in patients with idiopathic CTS.

Regardless of the technique used, the many anatomic variations in the region of the carpal tunnel demands that care be taken during the procedure. There have been major complications reported in association with all techniques of carpal tunnel release including open, endoscopic, and limited open techniques (with or without specialized instrumentation). Several prospective randomized studies have shown that endoscopic release results in better early patient satisfaction scores and earlier return to work (Figure 19).

The incidence of persistent symptoms after carpal tunnel release range from 1% to 25%. Incomplete transverse carpal ligament release is the most common cause of recurrent symptoms. Transverse and mini-incisions have a higher incidence of incomplete release. Endoscopic carpal tunnel release does not have an increased risk of incomplete release when compared with the traditional open technique. Other causes of recurrent CTS include incorrect diagnosis, double crush phenomena, concomitant peripheral neuropathy, a persistent carpal tunnel space occupying lesion, and iatrogenic median nerve injury.

Pronator Syndrome and Anterior Interosseous Nerve Compression Syndrome

At the level of the elbow, the median nerve has two branches: one branch innervates the pronator teres, flexor carpi radialis, and palmaris longus; the other branch forms the anterior interosseous nerve. In most cases, the median nerve then dives to pass between the superficial and deep heads of the pronator teres. Up to 15% of patients have a Martin-Gruber anastomosis where the intrinsic motor fibers that traveled within the median nerve from the level of the brachial plexus cross over at this level to return to the ulna nerve. At the level of the elbow and proximal forearm, the potential sites of median nerve compression are the supracondylar process, the ligament of Struthers, the bicipital aponeurosis, the lacertus fibrosus, fascia between the two heads of the pronator (most common cause), and under the fascial arch of the flexor digitorum superficialis.

The incidence of both pronator syndrome and anterior interosseous nerve compression syndrome is 100 times less common than CTS. Pronator syndrome is more common in women. Patients generally present with reports of pain in the anterior proximal forearm. Hand numbness, nocturnal paresthesias, and objective neurologic findings are rare. Silent motor weakness is common. Frequently, there is a decrease of nerve conduction across the elbow. Additionally, pronator syndrome can be differentiated from CTS by sensory disturbance in the distribution of the palmar cutaneous branch of the median nerve and a positive proximal Tinel's sign. Specific provocative maneuvers help isolate the site of entrapment. Exacerbation of symptoms with (1) resisted elbow flexion with forearm supination suggests the compression is under the bicipital aponeurosis; (2) resisted forearm pronation with elbow extension

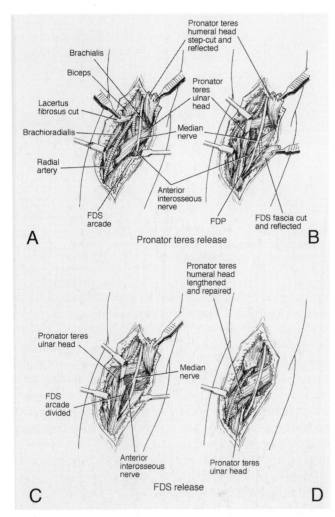

Figure 20 Decompression of the proximal median nerve involves release of the lacertus fibrosus and lengthening the humeral head of the pronator teres (**A** and **B**), and release of the vascular leash proximal to the flexor digitorum sublimis (FDS) and release of the flexor digitorum sublimis fascia (**C** and **D**). FDP = flexor digitorum profundus. *(Reproduced with permission from Trumble TE: Compressive neuropathies, in Trumble TE (ed): Principles of Hand Surgery and Therapy. Philadelphia, PA, 2000, p 339.)*

suggests entrapment between the two heads of the pronator; and (3) resisted long finger PIP joint flexion suggests the nerve is trapped under the origin of the flexor digitorum sublimis. During surgical decompression, all of these sites should be sufficiently released (Figure 20). Pronator syndrome is often associated with medial epicondylitis. Conservative treatment of the epicondylitis often relieves the pronator syndrome as well.

The anterior interosseous nerve is the largest branch of the median nerve, arising 5 to 8 cm distal to the level of the lateral epicondyle. The anterior interosseous nerve is a pure motor branch innervating the flexor pollicis longus, flexor digitorum profundus to the index finger and occasionally the middle finger, and the pronator quadratus. Compression of the anterior interosseous nerve results in weakness or paralysis of one or more of these muscles. If only one muscle is involved, the com-

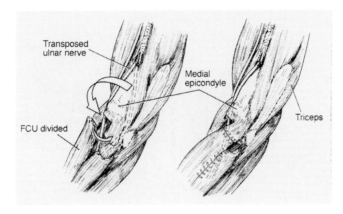

Figure 21 Submuscular transposition of the ulnar nerve. FCU = flexor carpi ulnaris. *(Reproduced with permission from Trumble TE: Compressive neuropathies, in Trumble TE (ed): Principles of Hand Surgery and Therapy. Philadelphia, PA, 2000, p 328.)*

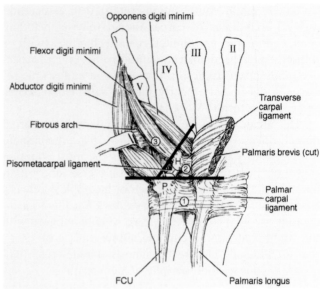

Figure 22 The ulnar tunnel can be divided into three sections. Lesions in zone I (1 in the figure) tend to produce a combined sensory and motor deficit. Lesions in zone II (2) generally produce pure motor deficit. Lesions in zone III (3) usually produce pure sensory deficits. FCU = flexor carpi ulnaris. *(Reproduced with permission from Trumble TE: Compressive neuropathies, in Trumble TE (ed): Principles of Hand Surgery and Therapy. Philadelphia, PA, 2000, p 330.)*

pression may be misdiagnosed as a tendon rupture. The typical symptom, however, is the inability to form an "O" with the thumb and index finger. There also will be changes on the electromyogram recording of the flexor pollicis longus. Parsonage-Turner syndrome (brachial neuritis), which is generally associated with intense pain during its onset, must be differentiated from a mechanical compression. The incidence of true entrapment neuropathy is very low; therefore, surgical decompression should be reserved for patients who have no recovery after 3 months.

Cubital Tunnel Syndrome

Although the incidence of cubital tunnel syndrome is second only to CTS, it is a relatively uncommon disorder. The anatomic structures that can potentially cause constriction of the nerve include the arcade of Struthers (the medial intermuscular septum), the medial head of the triceps, the ligament of the cubital tunnel or Osborne's ligament (the most common cause), the anconeus epitrochlearis (an accessory muscle), and the fascia of the flexor carpi ulnaris. The nerve may subluxate over the medial epicondyle causing chronic irritation. Cubital tunnel syndrome may be associated with prior elbow trauma. A patient may seek treatment many years after an elbow (for example, lateral condyle) fracture with a tardy ulnar nerve palsy. Cubital tunnel syndrome also may be associated with medial epicondylitis. Patients with cubital tunnel syndrome generally present with numbness along the ring and small fingers without involvement of the medial forearm. Elbow flexion exacerbates the symptoms. Nocturnal symptoms are very common because people generally sleep with their elbows flexed.

On examination, patients have a positive Tinel's sign with gentle percussion at the cubital tunnel. Monofilament and two-point testing often detect decreased sensation in the ulnar nerve distribution, including the ul-

nar aspect of the dorsum of the hand. Wartenberg's sign (an abducted small finger) may occur early and indicates intrinsic muscle weakness. In more severe cases, atrophy of the first dorsal interosseous and adductor pollicis with a concomitant Froment's paper sign may be seen. Severe cases may also be associated with clawing of the ulnar digits. Weakness may be masked by a Martin-Gruber anastomosis distal to the level of compression. Nerve conduction velocity studies are very helpful for confirming the diagnosis; when they are negative, nonsurgical management (nocturnal soft splints to prevent hyperflexion of the elbow) should be the mainstay of treatment.

Surgical decompression of all potential sites of entrapment (and possible transposition) is indicated for symptomatic patients with positive nerve conduction velocity studies. Intramuscular transposition may result in recurrent entrapment from perineural scarring. One prospective, randomized study comparing in situ release, subcutaneous transposition, and submuscular transposition did not find any statistically significant difference in outcome. However, the results were slightly better in the patients who underwent a subcutaneous or submuscular transposition (Figure 21). In situ decompression is only indicated for patients with mild symptoms and a nonsubluxating nerve. Submuscular transposition may be favored for patients with a thin layer of subcutaneous fat. Muscle wasting is a poor prognostic sign for surgery because it suggests the presence of irreversible nerve damage. Ideally, surgical intervention should be performed

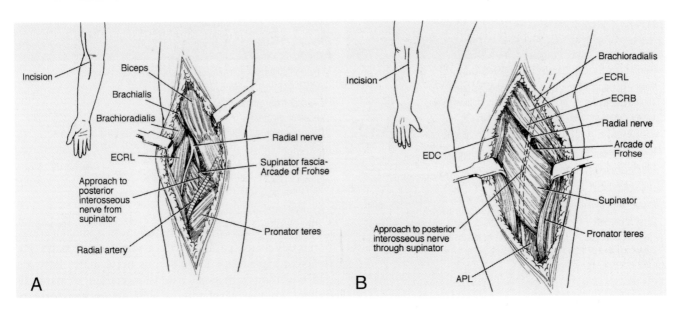

Figure 23 A, The anterior approach (Henry's approach) for decompression of the distal portion of the radial nerve and the posterior interosseous nerve. **B,** The posterior approach (Thompson's approach) for radial nerve decompression. ECRL = extensor carpi radialis longus, ECRB = extensor carpi radialis brevis, EDC = extensor digiti communis, APL = abductor pollicis longus. *(Reproduced with permission from Trumble TE: Compressive neuropathies, in Trumble TE (ed): Principles of Hand Surgery and Therapy. Philadelphia, PA, 2000, p 328.)*

before there is notable atrophy. Patients with milder compression are best treated with night splints.

Ulnar Tunnel Syndrome

Ulnar tunnel syndrome is a rare condition that usually results from the effect of some mass in the ulnar tunnel (Guyon's canal) such as a ganglion from the wrist joint or an aneurysm of the ulnar artery. The ulnar tunnel has been divided into three zones: zone I is proximal to the bifurcation of the ulnar nerve, zone II surrounds the deep motor branch and is dorsal and ulnar, and zone III is palmar and radial, surrounding the superficial palmar branch of the ulnar nerve (Figure 22). The most common cause of compression is different in each zone. Nerve compression in zone I and II is most commonly associated with either ganglia or fractures of the hook of the hamate and ulnar nerve compression in zone III is most frequently the result of a thrombosis or aneurysm of the ulnar artery.

Numbness in the ring and small fingers without involvement of the dorsum of the hand is the most common presenting symptom. Patients also may report pain with flexion or extension and/or weakness of the hand. Atrophy of the ulnar hand intrinsic muscles can occur, especially in the adductor pollicis and the first dorsal interosseous muscle. The Allen test should be performed to rule out ulnar artery pathology. Treatment depends on the underlying pathology. In patients with concomitant CTS, release of the carpal tunnel is often sufficient for decompressing the ulnar nerve. If a ganglion cyst is suspected, surgical exploration and excision is indicated. Fractures of the hook of the hamate are treated with excision. Ulnar artery aneurysm and thrombosis is treated

with resection or grafting, depending on the competency of the palmar arch.

Radial Nerve Entrapment

Compressive lesions of the radial nerve are relatively rare. The five sites for compression of the radial nerve are the fibrous bands near the radiocapitellar joint, a vascular leash proximal to the supinator muscle (leash of Henry), the leading edge of the extensor carpi radialis brevis, the proximal edge of the supinator muscle fascia (arcade of Fröhse), and the distal edge of the supinator fascia. The most common site of compression is at the proximal edge of the supinator muscle. Patients may present with painless weakness of finger or thumb extension (posterior interosseous nerve compression syndrome) or may present with pain mimicking lateral epicondylitis without neurologic deficit (radial tunnel syndrome).

Patients with posterior interosseous nerve compression syndrome generally present with insidious, painless finger extension weakness and radial wrist deviation (the extensor carpi radialis brevis, extensor carpi radialis longus, and supinator are innervated above the arcade of Fröhse and therefore generally not involved). Electrodiagnostic studies will confirm the diagnosis. If there is no improvement after 1 to 3 months of nonsurgical treatment, surgical release of all the potential sites of compression is indicated.

The pain of radial tunnel syndrome generally occurs during lifting, especially with the elbow and wrist in extension. Pain associated with radial tunnel syndrome is more distal than lateral epicondylitis (approximately 4 cm distal to the lateral epicondyle) and may be pro-

Table 4 | Best Combination of Tendon Transfers for Radial Nerve Palsy

Flexor Carpi Radialis Transfer (Starr, Brand, Tsuge)
Wrist extension: PT to extensor carpi radialis brevis
Thumb extension: PL to rerouted extensor pollicis longus
Finger extension: flexor carpi radialis to EDC

Superficialis Transfer (Modified Boyes)
Wrist extension: PT to extensor carpi radialis brevis
Thumb extension: PL to extensor pollicis longus
Finger extension: flexor digitorum sublimis IV to EDC

Flexor Carpi Ulnaris Transfer (Jones)
Wrist extension: PT to extensor carpi radialis brevis
Thumb extension: PL to rerouted extensor pollicis longus
Finger extension: flexor carpi ulnaris to EDC

PT = pronator teres; PL = palmaris longus; EDC = extensor digiti communis

Table 5 | Tendon Transfer for the Treatment of Low Median Nerve Palsy

Four Reliable Opponensplasties (to abductor pollicis brevis)
Flexor digitorum sublimis of ring
Extensor index proprius
Abductor digiti mini
Used in reconstruction of the congenital hypoplastic thumb
Palmaris longus
Used in patients with long standing CTS
Provides greater abduction than opposition

voked with resisted wrist extension or supination when the elbow is in extension, or resisted middle finger extension. Electrodiagnostic tests are generally normal but may show increased latencies in the area of compression during provocative forearm positioning. Electrodiagnostic testing can be very useful in delineating radial tunnel syndrome from the more common lateral epicondylitis for which it is often confused. Injection of an anesthetic into the radial tunnel should produce a posterior interosseous nerve palsy and alleviate pain, confirming the diagnosis. Approaches directed anteriorly (Henry's) or posteriorly (Thompson's) to the mobile wad provide a wider exposure to identify the possible locale of radial nerve compression (Figure 23).

Wartenberg's Disease

Compression of the superficial branch of the radial nerve is known as Wartenberg's disease. Injuries to the superficial branch of the radial sensory nerve have been reported after tight handcuff placement and excessively tight wrist taping. The superficial branch of the radial sensory nerve pierces the deep fascia between the dorsal border of the brachioradialis and the extensor carpi radialis longus muscles and then continues to travel distally in the subcutaneous plane. Direct compression or shear stress can injure this nerve resulting in an annoying neuropathy that is difficult to treat.

Reconstruction for Nerve Paralysis

Radial Nerve Palsy

Depending on the level of nerve damage, patients with radial nerve palsy will have functional limb deficits resulting from the loss of extension of the wrist joint and metacarpophalangeal joints of the fingers, and from loss of extension and radial abduction of the thumb. The inability to actively extend the wrist and to stabilize it for

all hand activities is probably the most significant functional deficit for patients with a radial nerve palsy. Patients with posterior interosseous nerve palsy have radial deviation with wrist extension caused by paralysis of the extensor carpi ulnaris, and unopposed force of the extensor carpi radialis longus and extensor radialis brevis (innervated by the radial nerve proper). Patients with a complete palsy of the radial nerve have a wrist drop in addition to the loss of wrist and finger extension. Insufficient recovery of function after observation for 6 to 12 months is an indication for tendon transfers. Serial examinations and electromyograms are indicated to assess recovery. If there is evidence of recovery of function, continued observation is warranted. Available donor muscles include all of the extrinsic muscles innervated by the median and ulnar nerves. All tendon transfers for radial nerve palsy include transferring the pronator teres to the extensor radialis brevis for wrist extension. Options for restoration of hand function in radial nerve palsy include the flexor carpi radialis transfer, the superficialis transfer, and the flexor carpi ulnaris transfer for finger extension (Table 4).

Median Nerve Palsy

Tendon transfers also may be effective treatment of low median nerve palsy. The major deficit associated with low median nerve palsy is the loss of thumb opposition. Thumb opposition is a complex motion requiring trapeziometacarpal abduction, flexion, and pronation. Lack of pronation is primarily caused by the denervation of the abductor pollicis brevis. The goal of these tendon transfers is to reconstruct the course of the fibers of the abductor pollicis brevis. The vector of the abductor pollicis brevis muscle intersects the pisiform. Tendon transfers that are distal to the pisiform provide more thumb flexion than abduction, and tendon transfers that are proximal to the pisiform provide more thumb abduction than flexion. Table 5 lists transfers commonly used to treat low median nerve palsy.

Additional deficits associated with proximal (high) medial nerve palsies include loss of flexion of the index and long fingers as well as the interphalangeal joint of the thumb. When the ulnar nerve is intact, side-to-side transfers of the index and long finger flexor digitorum profundus to the flexor digitorum profundus of the ring and small fingers, with sufficient tension to restore digital cascade, is a simple and effective procedure. Restoration of thumb interphalangeal joint flexion is achieved by transferring the brachioradialis to the flexor pollicis longus. Occasionally, loss of active forearm rotation from paralysis of the pronator teres and quadratus will require biceps tendon rerouting. Reattaching the distal biceps tendon laterally on the radius can improve active pronation.

Ulnar Nerve Paralysis

Paralysis of the ulnar nerve distal to the innervation of the flexor digitorum profundus results in significant hand deformity and loss of function. With low ulnar nerve palsy, the index and long fingers do not show clawing because the lumbricals to these two fingers are innervated by the median nerve, thus preventing dynamic deformity. Clawing does not occur in high ulnar nerve palsy because the flexor digitorum profundus (as well as the lumbricals) to the small and ring fingers is paralyzed in this injury. Thus, there is no longer unopposed flexion of the interphalangeal joints.

Power pinch restoration can be achieved by an extensor carpi radialis brevis transfer to the adductor pollicis via a palmaris longus tendon graft. One option for restoration of power pinch is transferring the flexor digitorum sublimis of the ring finger to the adductor pollicis. The use of the extensor carpi radialis brevis is an excellent option for restoration of power pinch because wrist extension and power pinch are synergistic.

Transfers to correct an ulnar palsy claw deformity may be static or dynamic. Static transfers act as tenodeses and do not require an innervated muscle. A static distal tenodesis is accomplished by passing a free tendon graft from the ulnar lateral band of the extensor mechanism of the ring finger around the deep transverse metacarpal ligament onto the radial lateral band of the extensor mechanism of the small finger. Dynamic tenodeses consist of tendon transfers (such as flexor digitorum sublimis to intrinsic muscles) that pass palmar to the deep transverse metacarpal ligament, through the lumbrical canals to the radial bands of the extensor mechanism. As the wrist flexes, tension is generated, creating active metacarpophalangeal flexion with interphalangeal extension. The intact ring finger flexor digitorum sublimis, extensor carpi radialis longus, brachioradialis, extensor index proprius, or extensor digiti minimi may be used.

The additional functional loss associated with high ulnar nerve palsy when compared with a more distal lesion is the loss of ring and small finger flexion. Performing a side-to-side tendon transfer between the index and long flexor digitorum profundus to the flexor digitorum profundus of the ring and small fingers can restore this functional deficit.

In treating combined palsies, the surgeon must define what muscle-tendon units are functional, what spare units are available for transfer, and what function is needed. The preferred transfers then can be systematically chosen.

Brachial Plexus Injuries

The etiology of injuries of the brachial plexus can be classified as open penetrating injuries, closed or traction injuries, injuries caused by radiation, and obstetric palsies. Traction injuries are defined by the anatomic location, either supraclavicular or infraclavicular. Supraclavicular injuries are further divided into preganglionic and postganglionic injuries depending on where in the nervous system the avulsion has occurred. Preganglionic lesions occur proximal to the dorsal root ganglion and have a poor prognosis because they are lesions of the central nervous system, which lacks the capacity to regenerate. Postganglionic and infraclavicular lesions have a better prognosis because these are lesions of the peripheral nervous system. Most traction injuries are supraclavicular.

The diagnosis depends on an accurate history and physical examination. MRI can identify root avulsions and the site of injury in postganglionic lesions. Electromyograms and nerve conduction velocity studies may be used to localize lesions of the brachial plexus preoperatively, and to follow their progress postoperatively. Within 3 weeks after an injury, changes will be noted on an electromyogram. Nerve conduction velocity studies with somatosensory evoked potentials can help differentiate preganglionic from postganglionic lesions.

The decision to proceed with surgical intervention is not always straightforward and depends on the nature of the injury. Timing of surgical intervention also is critical; repairs attempted more than 6 months after injury have a poor prognosis. Partial nerve injuries have the best prognosis. Nerve conductions studies should be used to evaluate the patient at 1 month and then at 3 months after the injury. Patients who have persistent deficits (such as lack of elbow flexion) at 3 months without evidence of improvement should be considered for surgical exploration. When the entire plexus is involved, the prognosis is poor, and immediate exploration may be indicated. Nerve grafts and transfers can be performed in an attempt to circumvent nerve root avulsions and restore neurologic function. A common pattern is injury to the upper and middle trunks. This injury pattern can be treated with nerve grafts to the suprascapular, musculocutaneous, axillary, and radial nerves (Figure 24).

The options for surgical reconstruction include neurolysis, primary nerve repair, nerve repair using nerve

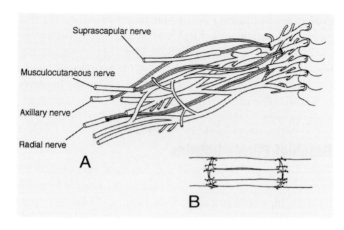

Figure 24 Cable grafts are used to bypass the large zone of scar tissue in the region of the scalene muscle just distal to the brachial plexus roots. Cable grafts are in place in the brachial plexus **(A)**. Close-up view of the cable nerve graft **(B)**. *(Reproduced with permission from Trumble TE: Brachial plexus injuries, in Trumble TE (ed): Principles of Hand Surgery and Therapy. Philadelphia, PA, 2000, p 305.)*

graft, nerve transfers, tendon transfers, free muscle transfers, and arthrodesis and/or tenodesis to stabilize joints. Depending on the injury and the patient, one or more of the techniques may be used in an attempt to improve function. The first priority of reconstruction is to reestablish elbow flexion. Without the ability to position the hand in space, hand function is severely compromised. The second goal is to stabilize the shoulder. Because it is difficult to position the extremity in a patient with a fused shoulder, if a shoulder arthrodesis is indicated, this procedure should be the last step in the series of reconstructive procedures. The next set of objectives includes obtaining and maintaining wrist and digit motion.

The most proximal muscles are more successfully reinnervated after nerve reconstruction, because they require less axonal input and are a shorter distance from the site of injury. After 12 to 18 months without neurologic input, the motor end plates in the muscle completely degenerate and the muscle loses its ability to be successfully reinnervated. The success rate for reinnervation of the muscles innervated by the axillary, suprascapular, and musculocutaneous nerves approaches 70% to 80%. Unfortunately, more distal muscles in the forearm and hand have a much poorer prognosis for reinnervation. Younger patients and patients who receive nerve grafts within the first 3 months after injury have the best prognosis.

A recent study demonstrated reliable deltoid reconstruction for upper arm brachial plexus injury by nerve transfer to the deltoid using the nerve to the long head of the triceps in conjunction with spinal accessory nerve transfer to the suprascapular nerve. The ipsilateral C7 nerve root also may be transferred with or without simultaneous transfer of the spinal accessory nerve to the suprascapular nerve to treat C5 and C6 root avulsions

of the brachial plexus. Good results have also been obtained with ulnar nerve fascicle transfers to the biceps and brachialis branches of the musculocutaneous nerve for improved elbow flexion strength.

Annotated Bibliography

Wrist Imaging

Steinborn M, Schurmann M, Staebler A, et al: MR imaging of ulnocarpal impaction after fracture of the distal radius. *AJR Am J Roentgenol* 2003;181:195-198.

Ulnocarpal impaction is a common finding after distal radius fracture. MRI can detect characteristic bone marrow changes of the lunate early after the trauma. A significant correlation exists between MRI findings and the extent of post-traumatic ulnar variance and pain levels.

Wrist Arthroscopy

Shih JT, Lee HM, Hou YT, Tan CM: Arthroscopically-assisted reduction of intra-articular fractures and soft tissue management of distal radius. *Hand Surg* 2001;6: 127-135.

Arthroscopy was used to help reduce intra-articular fracture of the distal radius and treat soft-tissue injuries in 33 acute patients. The fractures were treated by reduction under arthroscopic control and percutaneous fixation with or without external fixation. The TFCC was torn in 18 of 33 patients (54%). All tears were peripheral and were repaired with arthroscopic procedures. Scapholunate ligament injuries with instability of the scapholunate joint were noted in 6 patients (18%). This injury was treated with scapholunate débridement and stabilization of the joint with Kirschner wires. Four patients (12%) had lunotriquetral ligament injuries; three of these patients were treated with Kirschner wire transfixion. Six patients (18%) had chondral fractures. All 33 patients healed without measurable incongruity of the joint surface and excellent or good results according to the modified Mayo wrist score.

Wrist Arthritis Secondary to Trauma

Cohen MS, Kozin SH: Degenerative arthritis of the wrist: Proximal row carpectomy versus scaphoid excision and four-corner arthrodesis. *J Hand Surg [Am]* 2001;26:94-104.

Two cohort populations of 19 patients from separate institutions who underwent either a scaphoid excision and four-corner arthrodesis or proximal row carpectomy for scapholunate advanced collapse were compared. The results of the study suggest that both proximal row carpectomy and scaphoid excision and the four-corner arthrodesis are motion-preserving options for the treatment of scapholunate advanced collapse. There were minimal subjective or objective differences in short-term follow-up evaluations.

Soejima O, Iida H, Hanamura T, Naito M: Resection of the distal pole of the scaphoid for scaphoid nonunion with radioscaphoid and intercarpal arthritis. *J Hand Surg [Am]* 2003;28:591-596.

Nine patients with recalcitrant scaphoid nonunion and associated degenerative arthritis were treated by resection of the distal scaphoid fragment. At an average follow-up of 28.6 months, these patients had less pain and improved motion and grip strength compared with that found at their preoperative evaluation. Radiographically, neither additional degeneration nor progress of degenerative changes was noted after surgery in eight of nine patients.

Osteonecrosis of the Carpus

Shin AY, Bishop AT: Pedicled vascularized bone grafts for disorders of the carpus: Scaphoid nonunion and Kienböck's disease. *J Am Acad Orthop Surg* 2002;10: 210-216.

The use of reverse-flow pedicled vascularized bone grafts from the dorsal distal radius makes it possible to transfer bone with a preserved circulation and viable osteoclasts and osteoblasts. The resultant primary bone healing without creeping substitution within the dead bone is an alternative to conventional bone grafting. Recent advances in understanding the anatomy and physiology of vascularized pedicled bone grafts have increased their use in treating a variety of carpal maladies such as scaphoid nonunions and Kienböck's disease.

Scaphoid Nonunion and Osteonecrosis

McCallister WV, Knight J, Kaliappan R, Trumble TE: Central placement of the screw in simulated fractures of the scaphoid waist: A biomechanical study. *J Bone Joint Surg Am* 2003;85:72-77.

This cadaveric study was designed to determine whether central placement in the proximal fragment of the scaphoid offers a biomechanical advantage. Eleven matched pairs of scaphoids were removed from fresh cadaveric wrists, osteotomized and fixed with either eccentric or central placement of a Herbert-Whipple cannulated screw. Central placement of the screw in the proximal fragment of the scaphoid had superior results compared with those using eccentric positioning of the screw. Clinical efforts and techniques that facilitate central placement of the screw in the fixation of fractures of the scaphoid waist should be encouraged.

Steinmann SP, Bishop AT, Berger RA: Use of the 1,2 intercompartmental supraretinacular artery as a vascularized pedicle bone graft for difficult scaphoid nonunion. *J Hand Surg [Am]* 2002;27:391-401.

Fourteen patients with established scaphoid nonunion were treated with vascularized pedicle bone grafting. All nonunions healed at a mean of 11.1 weeks. Wrist motion was minimally affected by surgery. Intercarpal and scaphoid angles were improved after surgery, particularly in patients with preoperative humpback deformity who had undergone previous interposition grafting. Vascularized bone grafts are indicated in proximal pole fracture nonunions, in the presence of osteonecrosis, and after conventional grafts. Radiocarpal arthritis, if present before surgery, is a poor prognostic sign.

Trumble TE, Kearny R: *Scaphoid Nonunions.* Orthopaedic Knowledge Online Website. American Academy of Orthopaedic Surgeons. Available at: http://www5.aaos.org/oko/hand_wrist/scaphoid_nonunion/pathophysiology/pathophysiology.cfm. Accessed October 29, 2004.

The pathophysiology, etiology, diagnosis, management options, and surgical procedures commonly used to treat scaphoid nonunions are discussed.

Triangular Fibrocartilage Complex and the Distal Radioulnar Joint

Adams BD, Berger RA: An anatomic reconstruction for the distal radioulnar ligaments fro posttraumatic distal radioulnar joint instability. *J Hand Surg [Am]* 2002;27: 243-251.

Fourteen patients with posttraumatic DRUJ instability were treated with a DRUJ ligament reconstruction using a technique that is anatomic, reproducible, and requires less dissection than other described techniques. All of the patients had joint instability and an irreparable TFCC. Stability was restored and symptoms relieved in 12 of 14 patients. All patients attained nearly full pronation and supination. This procedure is effective for an unstable DRUJ when the articular surfaces are intact and other wrist ligaments are functional. It can be used in conjunction with a distal radius osteotomy.

Cober SR, Trumble TE: Arthroscopic repair of triangular fibrocartilage complex injuries. *Orthop Clin North Am* 2001;32:279-294.

The TFCC is a functionally and anatomically intricate group of structures located at the ulnar aspect of the wrist. Injury to this structure affects the biomechanics of the wrist and makes functional restoration difficult. This article reviews the anatomy, biomechanics, diagnosis, and arthroscopic treatment of TFCC injuries.

Ditano OA, Trumble TE, Tencer AF: Biomechanical function of the distal radioulnar and ulnocarpal wrist ligaments. *J Hand Surg [Am]* 2003;28:622-627.

This study was designed to provide quantitative information about the functions of the ligaments that stabilize the DRUJ. This joint permits the radius to rotate around a nearly fixed ulna allowing supination and pronation of the hand. Understanding their function is important in developing procedures for reconstruction. Using a ligament tension transducer, the tension of six ligaments of the DRUJ was determined in nine cadaver arms in pronation and supination of the hand. In supination of the forearm all ligaments except for the dorsal distal radioulnar ligament had equivalent tensions, indicating their role in stabilizing the joint to this motion. In pronation, ligament tensions generally were lower but were distributed over all six ligaments tested. The dorsal ulnocarpal ligament tension was equivalent in both supination and pronation, unlike the other ligaments that had greater tensions in supination.

Scheker LR, Babb BA, Killion PE: Distal ulnar prosthetic replacement. *Orthop Clin North Am* 2001;32:365-376.

The advantages and disadvantages of four prostheses are discussed and early clinical results of a new design are presented.

Tomaino MM, Weiser RW: Combined arthroscopic TFCC debridement and wafer resection of the distal ulna in wrists with triangular fibrocartilage complex tears and positive ulnar variance. *J Hand Surg [Am]* 2001;26:1047-1052.

TFCC débridement with arthroscopic wafer resection was performed in 12 patients with TFCC tears and positive ulnar variance. Eight patients had complete pain relief; four patients had only minimal residual symptoms. Grip strength improved.

Degenerative Arthrosis of the Thumb and Fingers
Fulton DB, Stern PJ: Trapeziometacarpal joint arthrodesis in primary osteoarthritis: a minimum two-year follow-up. *J Hand Surg [Am]* 2001;26:109-114.

The authors report their retrospective review of 59 trapeziometacarpal arthrodeses with follow-up from 2 to 20 years. Only four nonunions (7%) occurred, and only one of these was symptomatic and required reoperation. Peritrapezial arthrosis was seen in seven patients at the last follow-up.

Nerve Compression Syndromes
Trumble TE, Diao E, Abrams RA, Gilbert-Anderson MM: Single-portal endoscopic carpal tunnel release compared with open release: A prospective, randomized trial. *J Bone Joint Surg Am* 2002;84:1107-1115.

This prospective, randomized, multicenter study compares open carpal tunnel release with single-portal endoscopic carpal tunnel release. The open method was performed in 95 hands in 72 patients, and the endoscopic method was performed in 97 hands in 75 patients. Follow-up evaluations with use of validated outcome instruments and quantitative measurements of grip strength, pinch strength, and hand dexterity were performed at 2, 4, 8, 12, 26, and 52 weeks after the surgery. Complications were identified. The cost of the procedures and the time until return to work were recorded and compared between the groups. During the first 3 months after surgery, the patients treated with the endoscopic method had better validated outcomes, better subjective satisfaction scores, as well as significantly greater grip strength, pinch strength, and hand dexterity. The open technique resulted in greater scar tenderness during the first 3 months after surgery as well as a longer return to work interval. No technical problems with respect to nerve, tendon, or artery injuries were noted in either group. There was no significant difference in the rate of complications or the cost of surgery between the two groups.

Reconstruction of Nerve Paralysis
Fridén J, Lieber RL: Mechanical considerations in the design of surgical reconstructive procedures. *J Biomech* 2002;35:1039-1045.

The principles of muscle-tendon units as they relate to tendon transfers are reiterated. The importance of considering muscle architecture and length-tension relationships when choosing an appropriate donor is discussed. The limitations of excursion relative to connective tissue factors as well as consequences of overstretching musculotendinous units are also delineated. The role of synergism and joint moment arm changes are outlined.

General
Trumble TE (ed): *Hand Surgery Update 3: Hand, Elbow, & Shoulder.* Rosemont, IL, American Society for Surgery of the Hand, 2003.

A comprehensive review of the cutting-edge advances as well as core knowledge in upper extremity surgery is presented.

Trumble TE (ed): *Comprehensive Review for Hand Surgery* [book on CD-ROM]. Rosemont, IL, American Society for Surgery of the Hand, 2003.

An advanced review of the core concepts of hand anatomy, biomechanics, and pathology as well as diagnostic and treatment methods relating to hand surgery are presented.

Classic Bibliography
Almquist EE: Capitate shortening in the treatment of Kienböck's disease. *Hand Clin* 1993;9:505-512.

Berger RA: The ligaments of the wrist. *Hand Clin* 1997; 13:63-82.

Bettinger P, Linsheid R, Berger R, Cooney W, An K: An anatomic study of the stabilizing ligaments of the trapezium and trapeziometacarpal joint. *J Hand Surg [Am]* 1999;24:786-798.

Cooney WP, Linscheid RL, Dobyns JH: Triangular fibrocartilage tears. *J Hand Surg [Am]* 1994;19:143-154.

Doi K, Hattori Y, Otsuka K, Abe Y, Yamamoto H: Intra-articular fractures of the distal aspect of the radius: Arthroscopically assisted reduction compared with open reduction and internal fixation. *J Bone Joint Surg Am* 1999;81:1093-1110.

Feldon P, Terrono AL, Belsky MR: Wafer distal ulna resection for triangular fibrocartilage tears and/or ulna impaction syndrome. *J Hand Surg [Am]* 1992;17:731-737.

Fernandez DL: Malunion of the distal radius: Current approach to management. *Instr Course Lect* 1993;42:99-113.

Gilula LA: Carpal injuries: Analytic approach and case exercises. *AJR Am J Roentgenol* 1979;133:503-517.

Green DP, Hotchkiss RN, Pederson WC (eds): *Green's Operative Hand Surgery*, ed 4. Philadelphia, PA, Churchill Livingston, 1999.

Kirschenbaum D, Schneider LH, Adams DC, Cody RP: Arthroplasty of the metacarpophalangeal joints with use of silicone-rubber implants in patients who have rheumatoid arthritis: Long-term results. *J Bone Joint Surg Am* 1993;75:3-12.

Levinsohn EM, Rosen ID, Palmer AK: Wrist arthrography: Value of the three-compartment injection method. *Radiology* 1991;179:231-239.

Malerich MM, Clifford J, Eaton B, Eaton R, Littler JW: Distal scaphoid resection arthroplasty for the treatment of degenerative arthritis secondary to scaphoid nonunion. *J Hand Surg [Am]* 1999;24:1196-1205.

Szabo RM, Slater RR Jr, Farver TB, Stanton DB, Sharman WK: The value of diagnostic testing in carpal tunnel syndrome. *J Hand Surg [Am]* 1999;24:704-714.

Trumble TE, Gilbert M, Murray LW, Smith J, Rafijah G, McCallister WV: Displaced scaphoid fractures treated with open reduction and internal fixation with a cannulated screw. *J Bone Joint Surg Am* 2000;82:633-641.

Trumble TE, Gilbert M, Vedder N: Ulnar shortening combined with arthroscopic repairs in the delayed management of triangular fibrocartilage complex tears. *J Hand Surg [Am]* 1997;22:807-813.

Trumble TE, Nyland W: Scaphoid Nonunions: Pitfalls and Pearls. *Hand Clin* 2001;17:611-624.

Trumble TE, Rafijah G, Gilbert M, Allan CH, North E, McCallister WV: Thumb trapeziometacarpal joint arthritis: partial trapeziectomy with ligament reconstruction and interposition costochondral allograft. *J Hand Surg [Am]* 2000;25:61-76.

Trumble TE, Shon FG: The physiology of nerve transplantation. *Hand Clin* 2000;16:105-122.

Weiss AP, Weiland AJ, Moore JR, Wilgis EF: Radial shortening for Kienböck's disease. *J Bone Joint Surg Am* 1991;73:384-391.

Section 5

Lower Extremity

Section Editors:
Daniel J. Berry, MD
Steven M. Raikin, MD

Chapter 31

Biomechanics of Gait

Alberto Esquenazi, MD

Introduction

Gait analysis is a useful clinical tool and a recognized medical procedure for evaluating and treating patients with ambulatory impairments. It is challenging for many physicians to achieve a clear understanding of gait analysis data and to meaningfully interpret the clinical applicability of the data to a patient's impairment, disability, or handicap. Familiarity with the complex physiologic interactions of normal gait and movement biomechanics, functional anatomy, normal and abnormal patterns of motor control, and with the technology used for its assessment will contribute to better care for patients with ambulatory difficulties.

Gait can be described as an interplay between the two lower limbs, one in touch with the ground, producing sequential restraint and propulsion, while the other swings freely and carries with it the forward momentum of the body. By the age of 4 to 8 years, most healthy individuals have established a similar manner of walking because of a common, basic anatomic and physiologic makeup. However, because of inherent differences in body proportions, level of coordination, motivation, and other factors, each person's gait pattern is unique. Despite these complexities, gait patterns are highly repeatable both within a subject and between subjects; however, each person has a unique walking style.

The modern quantitative study of human locomotion dates back to the early part of the 19th century with Muybridge's sequential photographs. Inman and associates, from the University of California, refined the simultaneous recording of multiple muscle group activity during normal ambulation and published their findings in a textbook, which has become a classic reference for the field.

Normal Locomotion

Based on the timing of reciprocal floor contacts, the gait cycle can be defined as a single sequence of functions by one limb. Each gait cycle has two basic components—the stance phase, which designates the duration of foot contact with the ground; and the swing phase, which oc-

curs when the foot is in the air for limb advancement. The stance phase can be subdivided into five subphases: initial contact, loading response, midstance, terminal stance, and preswing. The swing phase can be divided into three functional subphases: initial swing, midswing, and terminal swing (Figure 1) (Table 1).

The stance phase can alternately be subdivided into three periods according to floor contact patterns. Both the beginning and the end of the stance phase are the double support period during which both feet are in contact with the floor. Single limb support begins when the opposite foot is lifted for the swing phase. The broad normal distribution of the periods of floor contact during the gait cycle are 40% for the swing phase and 60% for the stance phase (each double support time period accounts for approximately 10% of the stance phase). These ratios apply to individuals with normal gait patterns who are walking at a self-selected, comfortable speed. These proportions will vary greatly with changes in walking velocity. For example, walking more slowly will reduce single limb support time and will increase double limb support time. With increasing cadence (steps per minute), the double limb support period steadily decreases, and disappears during running.

The step period is the time measured from initial contact in one foot to the subsequent occurrence of the same event in the other foot. There are two steps in each stride or gait cycle. The stride period can be defined as the time from initial ground contact of one foot until the next ground contact for the same foot; the stride period is normally equal for left and right strides. Stride length is the distance covered during one stride. The stride period is often normalized to the full gait cycle for the purpose of averaging gait parameters over several strides both within and between subjects. The step period is useful for identifying and measuring asymmetry between the two sides of the body, especially in pathologic conditions. Step length is the distance covered during one step. Side-to-side symmetry of step length and step time is characteristic in individuals with normal gait.

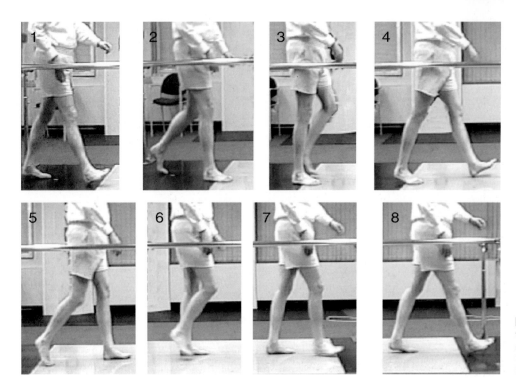

Figure 1 Time-elapsed pictorial depiction of the normal gait cycle with number-coded phases as described in Table 1. Phases of the gait cycle are shown from initial contact to ipsilateral initial contact.

Table 1 | Phases of the Gait Cycle and Reference Points

Stance Phase	Reference Point
Initial contact	1. The instant the foot contacts the ground
Loading response	2. From flatfoot position until the opposite foot is on the ground for swing
Midstance	3. From the time the opposite foot is lifted until the ipsilateral tibia is vertical
Terminal stance	4. From heel rise until the opposite foot contacts the ground (contralateral initial contact)
Preswing	5. From initial contact of the opposite foot and ends with ipsilateral toe-off
Swing Phase	**Reference Point**
Initial swing	6. Begins with lift-off of the foot from the floor and ends when the foot is aligned with the opposite foot
Midswing	7. Begins when the foot is aligned with the opposite foot and ends when the tibia is vertical
Terminal swing	8. Begins when the tibia is vertical and ends when the foot contacts the ground (initial contact)

Under normal conditions, a comfortable walking speed corresponds to the speed at which the energy cost per unit distance is optimal. Energy efficiency is dependent on unrestricted joint mobility and the precise timing and intensity of muscle action. The result of abnormal biomechanics is increased energy cost, usually with a compensatory decrease in walking speed.

The kinematics (geometry of motion without regard to the forces that cause it) of the gait cycle are organized to minimize the movement of the body's center of gravity in both the vertical and horizontal planes, which results in energy-efficient movement. The average total displacement of the center of gravity in a stride is less than 5 cm in individuals with normal gait. Impairments of the gait mechanism can result in decreased energy efficiency caused in part by increased excursions of the center of gravity.

The clearance mechanisms for the swinging limb require specific coordinated events to achieve swing phase limb-length reduction. These include knee flexion in preswing, coordinated hip and knee flexion in the early to midswing phases, and ankle dorsiflexion in the midswing phase. Stabilization of the pelvis is also critical and is achieved by the hip abductors, which control the amount of pelvic drop (tilt) in swing phase. To further ensure limb clearance while optimizing energy efficiency, the stance limb has several mechanisms to provide sufficient clearance for the swinging limb. These include midstance ankle dorsiflexion control (to prevent excessive forward rotation of the tibia through the forces exerted by the ankle plantar flexors), midstance to terminal stance knee extension, and terminal stance heel rise (ankle plantar flexion).

To achieve the most efficient gait while maximizing step length, controlled, coordinated leg movements must occur. For step length to be greatest, the swinging limb must have hip flexion that will occur in coordination with terminal swing knee extension. At the same time the stance limb permits ankle dorsiflexion to control forward progression of the tibia, while knee and hip extension and pelvic tilt and internal rotation take place.

Quantitative Gait Analysis

Visual analysis of gait is routinely done as part of the clinical assessment of patients. This type of analysis does not provide quantitative information and has many limitations because of the complexity and speed of the events that occur during walking, coupled with deviations and possible compensations that occur in pathologic gait. Three primary components of quantitative gait analysis that can be recorded are kinetics (the analysis of forces that produce motion), polyelectromyography (poly-EMG) or dynamic EMG (the analysis of muscle activity), and kinematics (the analysis of motion and the resulting temporal and stride measurements). Gait analysis that is useful in the clinical evaluation of patients and in choosing treatment options must provide measured parameters that correlate with the functional capacity of the patient, supply additional and more relevant information than clinical examination, be accurate and repeatable, and must result from a test that does not alter the natural performance of the patient.

Kinematics

Temporal and Spatial Descriptive Measures

To characterize gait, basic variables concerning the temporal-spatial sequencing of stance and swing phases can be measured (Figure 2). These data can be obtained by measuring the distances and timing involved in the foot-floor contacts. Temporal-spatial footfall patterns are the end product of the total integrated locomotor movement. Techniques to obtain these data include the use of simple ink and paper to foot switches and other more sophisticated measuring systems. By comparing information from the two legs, measures of symmetry can be obtained to determine the extent of unilateral impairment.

Motion Analysis

Kinematic data provide a description of movement without regard to the force generating it (Figure 3). Earlier techniques included photographic and cinematographic analysis. Other techniques include the use of accelerometers and electrogoniometry. Modern systems involve the use of high-speed video recording or specialized optoelectronic apparatus in which passive (such as retroreflective markers) or active optical sources (such as light emitting infrared diodes) are attached to the subject and serve as markers.

In optoelectronic systems, the spatial coordinates of the markers are generated directly by the computer after the system has been calibrated. Kinematic information can be used to provide coordinate data, which can

be processed and displayed as a function of time or as a percent of the stride period. Derived data include joint angles, angular velocities, acceleration, and limb segment rotation.

Kinetics

Kinetic analysis involves study of the forces that develop during walking. Ground reaction forces are generally measured using a triaxial force platform. It is preferred that two platforms, placed adjacent to each other, be used so that the forces transmitted through the contact surface for each foot can be recorded simultaneously and independently. The reaction forces are divided into their orthogonal components, and plotted as a function of time or as a function of the stride time percentage. For comparison to standards, the measured ground reaction forces are often normalized and reported as a percentage of body mass.

Two orthogonal components of force define a time-varying force vector. In some laboratories the vertical/sagittal vector is displayed using laser optics or computer technology in real time and superimposed on the image of the walking subject (Figure 4).

The magnitude of the ground reaction forces and their relationship to anatomic joint centers are the factors that determine moments or torque about a joint, which indicate the direction and magnitude of joint rotation. Internal forces generated by muscles, tendons, and ligaments act to control these external forces.

Electromyographic Activation Patterns in Human Gait

Because of the redundant relationship between muscles about a joint, there is no unique association between a particular joint movement and the pattern of muscle forces giving rise to that movement. In normal locomotion, the gravitational forces are carefully controlled by opposing muscle forces to yield a smooth and energy-efficient movement pattern. The EMG signal can be used as an indication of neurologic control over muscle activation. Superficial muscles can be studied using bipolar surface electrodes. For deep muscles or to differentiate between adjacent muscles, indwelling Teflon-coated wire electrodes are inserted through a hypodermic needle.

EMG timing patterns from a patient can be compared to normative data (including both a mean and standard deviation) to identify deviations from normal EMG patterns (Figure 5). Because EMG patterns are very sensitive to walking velocity, data from a patient walking at a slow speed should not be compared with data from an able-bodied control patient who walks at a higher velocity and with a natural cadence.

A particular muscle may be overactive or underactive during a given segment of the gait cycle. When such

Test Condition   with shoes, no UE assist

Standing Leg Length   (m)   **Left**   0.98   **Right**   0.98   **Stride Time**   1.15   (s)

Velocity   1.29   (m/s)   **Combined Cadence**   104   (steps/min) **Left**   105   **Right**   105

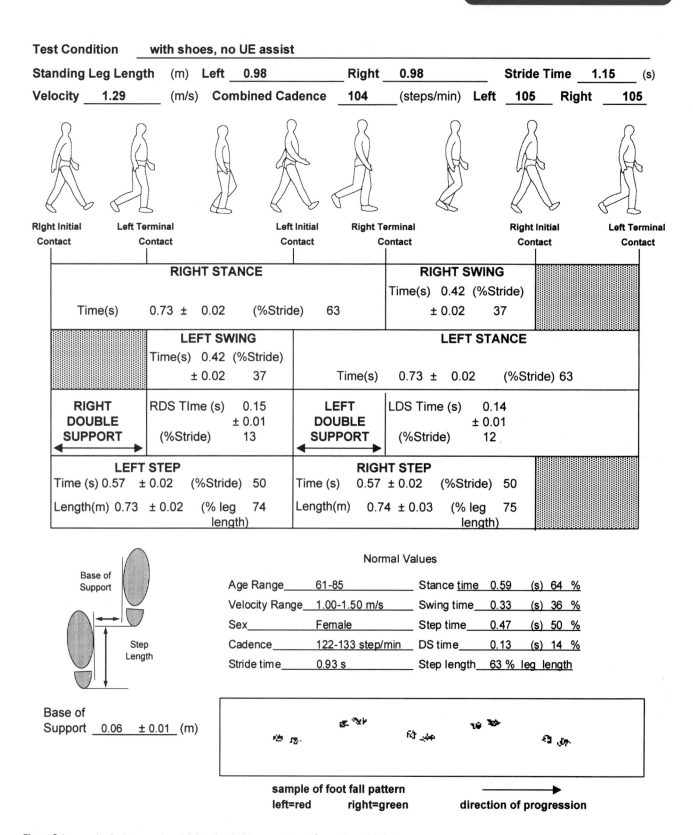

| Right Initial Contact | Left Terminal Contact | | Left Initial Contact | Right Terminal Contact | | Right Initial Contact | Left Terminal Contact |

RIGHT STANCE		RIGHT SWING	
Time(s) 0.73 ± 0.02 (%Stride) 63		Time(s) 0.42 (%Stride) ± 0.02 37	

LEFT SWING		LEFT STANCE
Time(s) 0.42 (%Stride) ± 0.02 37	Time(s) 0.73 ± 0.02 (%Stride) 63	

RIGHT DOUBLE SUPPORT	RDS TIme (s) 0.15 ± 0.01 (%Stride) 13	LEFT DOUBLE SUPPORT	LDS Time (s) 0.14 ± 0.01 (%Stride) 12

LEFT STEP		RIGHT STEP	
Time (s) 0.57 ± 0.02 (%Stride) 50		Time (s) 0.57 ± 0.02 (%Stride) 50	
Length(m) 0.73 ± 0.02 (% leg 74 length)		Length(m) 0.74 ± 0.03 (% leg 75 length)	

Base of Support

Step Length

Base of Support   0.06   ± 0.01   (m)

Normal Values

Age Range	61-85	Stance time	0.59 (s) 64 %
Velocity Range	1.00-1.50 m/s	Swing time	0.33 (s) 36 %
Sex	Female	Step time	0.47 (s) 50 %
Cadence	122-133 step/min	DS time	0.13 (s) 14 %
Stride time	0.93 s	Step length	63 % leg length

sample of foot fall pattern

left=red   right=green   direction of progression

Figure 2 An example of gait temporal-spatial data that depicts measurement of symmetry and timing.

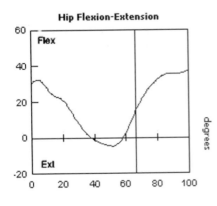

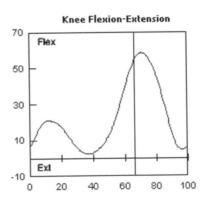

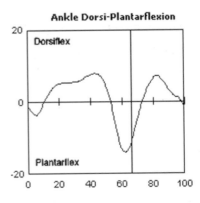

Figure 3 Normal three-dimensional sagittal kinematic gait data obtained with CODA mpx30 motion tracking system (Charnwood Dynamics, Leicestershire, England). Normalized gait cycle; 0 = initial contact, vertical line swing phase, 100 = next initial contact.

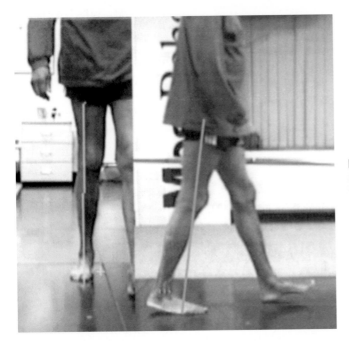

Figure 4 Force line visualization system in the AP and medial lateral views obtained using the DIGIVEC system (BTS, Milan, Italy).

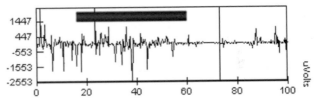

Figure 5 Representative raw EMG data for gastrocnemius during walking. Normalized gait cycle; 0 = initial contact, vertical line swing phase; 100 = next initial contact. Solid horizontal bar represents normative data.

deviations are observed, they should be carefully correlated with the measured kinematics. When interpreting dynamic EMG data, it is important to distinguish between cause and effect. If there is a clinical correlation between the EMG pattern and the observed kinematics, then a fairly confident diagnostic conclusion may be drawn regarding the cause of an observed gait deviation.

Clinical Applications of Gait Analysis

Pathologic gait can result from a variety of clinical conditions that can be classified into three major etiologic categories: structural (musculoskeletal deformities such as limb amputation), joint and soft-tissue pathology (arthritis or soft-tissue contractures), and neurologic disor-

ders (pathology of the peripheral and/or central nervous system). Gait analysis can be used to evaluate the dynamic basis for an observed gait deviation, to objectively assess the impact of various treatment interventions, and to develop objective selection criteria for different treatment options. Instrumented gait analysis and accurate clinical diagnoses can be used to guide specific recommendations regarding surgery, therapeutic exercises, walking aids, and mechanical and electrical orthoses. Examinations can be performed before and after a therapeutic intervention to help assess the effectiveness of the treatment. Such interventions would include surgical reconstruction, application or modification of an orthosis or special shoe, pharmacologic treatments (such as chemodenervation with botulinum toxin), realignment of a prosthetic limb, or the use of a walking aid (such as a cane).

Careful assessment can lead to the development of rational criteria for specific surgical interventions such as tendon releases and transfers. For example, an equinovarus foot posture can result from several distinct dynamic EMG patterns (such as overactivity of the gastrocnemius-soleus complex along with the anterior and/or posterior tibialis) that can best be differentiated with gait analysis and dynamic EMG. In patients with arthritis, data from gait analysis can be used to help se-

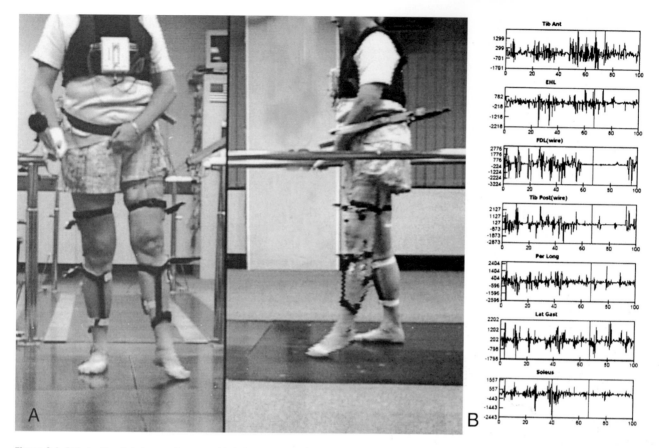

Figure 6 A, Patient with swing phase equinovarus ankle foot posture second to upper motor neuron syndrome. **B,** Dynamic EMG confirms overactive tibialis posterior and gastrocnemius-soleus complex during the swing phase of gait. Normalized gait cycle; 0 = initial contact, vertical line indicates swing phase; 100 = ipsilateral initial contact.

lect patients who would benefit from joint arthroplasty and to assess the impact of such surgery on gait biomechanics. In patients with chronic neurologic impairment, gait analysis together with selective nerve and motor point blocks can be used to differentiate fixed contractures (static deformity) from spasticity and muscle overactivity (dynamic deformity), allowing more appropriate treatment selection.

Pathologic Gait

Functional gait deviations may be applicable to many conditions rather than just to a specific disease. From a functional perspective, gait deficiencies can be categorized based on their timing with respect to the gait cycle. During the stance phase, an abnormal base of support and limb instability may make walking unsteady and energy inefficient, and possibly painful. Inadequate limb clearance and advancement during the swing phase will interfere with balance and energy efficiency.

Abnormal Base of Support

The ankle/foot posture is critical in the interface with the walking surface during the stance phase. Ankle plantar flexion, inversion or eversion, and toe flexion or ex-

tension can all interfere with normal gait. An inadequate base of support can result in instability of the entire body; therefore, the correction of the abnormal ankle/foot posture by conservative, interventional, or surgical methods is essential.

Equinovarus deformity is one of the most common abnormal lower limb postures seen in patients with neurologic disorders. Contact with the ground occurs with the forefoot first (with decreased or absent heel contact), resulting in the weight being borne primarily on the lateral border of the foot, which can produce an unstable base of support. Limited ankle dorsiflexion will prevent forward progression of the tibia over the stationary foot, resulting in knee hyperextension and interference with terminal stance and preswing and loss of the propulsive phase of gait. During the swing phase, there is a sustained plantar-flexed and inverted posture of the foot resulting in difficulty with limb clearance. Results of dynamic poly-EMG show that prolonged activation of the gastrocnemius-soleus complex is the most common cause of sustained plantar flexion. Inversion is the result of the abnormal activities of the tibialis posterior and/or tibialis anterior in combination with long toe flexors and the gastrocnemius-soleus complex group (Figure 6).

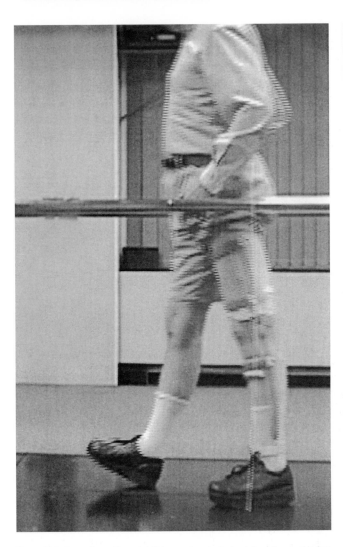

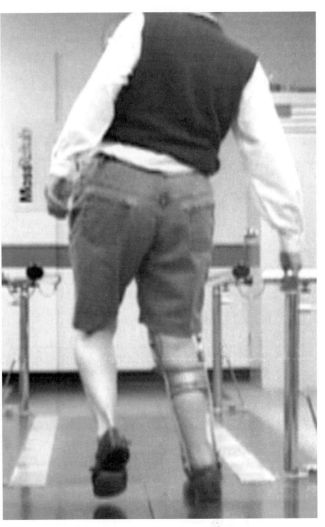

Figure 7 Polio survivor with weak left knee extensors that require a knee ankle-foot orthosis to stabilize the knee joint. Note line of force through the knee joint of the orthotic device.

Figure 8 Patient with insufficient hip abductor musculature that produces a compensated gluteus medius gait. Note lateral trunk lean toward the stance limb.

An abnormal base of support also occurs in foot drop. The use of a mechanical device (such as an ankle-foot orthosis) during the stance and swing phases may help to control the abnormal ankle posture.

Studies have shown that botulinum toxin injected into the hyperactive musculature can provide selective time-limited relief of spasticity. Surgical interventions such as gastrocnemius-soleus complex–soleus lengthening, split tibialis anterior, tendon transfer, and lengthening of the tibialis posterior and of the toe flexors to attain a balanced foot posture may be necessary.

Abnormal Limb Stability

Knee flexion or hyperextension during the early stance phase caused by ligamentous instability, degenerative joint disease, muscle weakness, or flaccidity can make walking unsteady and increase the risk for falling. The patient is unable to control the normal knee flexor mo-

ment that occurs during the early stance phase. This abnormality may be evident in a transfemoral amputee and can interfere with the ability to ambulate or may result in hyperextension of the knee joint as a compensatory mechanism. The dynamic poly-EMG shows shortened or uncoordinated activities of the quadriceps musculature. Occasionally, increased activities of the knee flexors also are found. A shoe with a soft heel, a molded ankle-foot orthosis (set in a few degrees of plantar flexion), or a knee-ankle-foot orthosis with posterior offset knee joints or stance phase stabilization joints all can provide improved knee stability by positioning the ground reaction force anterior to the knee joint center. For the above-the-knee amputee, changes in alignment to improve knee stability, the use of an articulated prosthetic foot, or the use of a mechanical knee lock is required (Figure 7).

Knee hyperextension during the stance phase may occur as the result of spasticity of the ankle plantar flex-

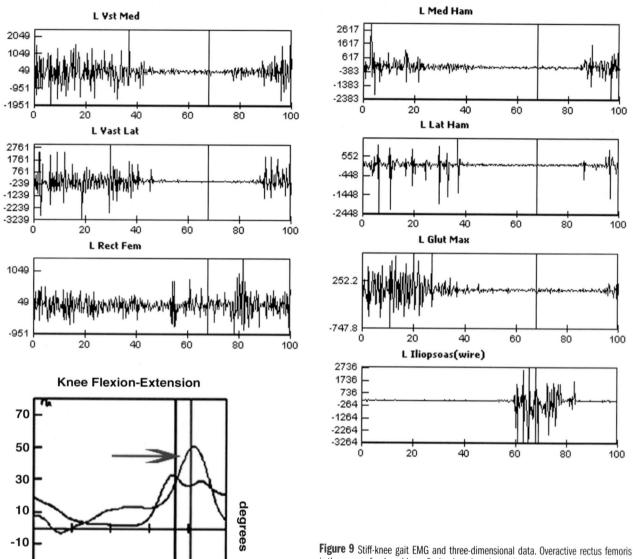

Figure 9 Stiff-knee gait EMG and three-dimensional data. Overactive rectus femoris is the cause of reduced knee flexion in swing phase when compared with normal data. Normalized gait cycle; 0 = initial contact, vertical line indicates swing phase; 100 = ipsilateral initial contact.

ors or knee extensors, a plantar flexion contracture, or as a compensatory mechanism for quadriceps weakness. This abnormal posture of the knee prevents normal forward advancement of the tibia during the stance phase and restricts contralateral limb advancement. Correction of the knee deformity can be achieved by decreasing the ankle plantar flexor or knee extensor spasticity, if present, by the use of selected botulinum toxin injection into the gastrocnemius-soleus complex or by appropriate surgical intervention through gastrocnemius-soleus complex lengthening. Compensation for the ankle deformity can be achieved with the use of a heel lift to accommodate the ankle equinus. The use of a knee-ankle-foot orthosis with offset knee joints and hy-

perextension control is indicated to compensate for knee extensor weakness when present.

Trendelenburg Gait

Insufficient hip abductor musculature or mechanical deficiency of the hip joint caused by pain, degenerative changes, malalignment, or a nerve injury can result in a gluteus medius gait pattern (Figure 8). During the stance phase, the patient will have an exaggerated ipsilateral trunk lean (compensated gluteus medius gait) in an attempt to stabilize the pelvis. Some patients will be unable to compensate and have a pelvic drop of the swinging limb resulting in a noncompensated gluteus medius gait. The use of a cane held by the contralateral hand should result in a marked improvement in this pathologic gait pattern.

Limb Clearance and Advancement

Limb clearance and advancement occurs during the swing phase of gait. When limb clearance is inadequate, limb advancement is compromised. The most common causes of limb clearance difficulties are lack of adequate hip flexion, and inadequate knee flexion and/or ankle dorsiflexion. It is important to recognize that synchronized lower limb motion during the swing phase is essential to produce adequate limb clearance.

Stiff-knee gait pattern can result from orthopaedic intervention intended to provide joint stability or relieve pain (knee fusion) or may be found in patients with spasticity. The patient is unable to flex the knee adequately, creating a large moment of inertia, which increases the energy required to initiate the swing phase of the involved limb. This condition requires the patient to use ipsilateral hip, trunk, and contralateral limb compensatory motions. Even if the ankle-foot system has an appropriate position, early swing toe drag can occur and can be corrected only by increasing hip flexion, increasing the contralateral limb length, or generating knee flexion.

In patients with a spastic stiff knee, a dynamic poly-EMG will show increased activity in the quadriceps muscles as a group. In patients who have had a stroke, preferential activation of the rectus femoris and vastus intermedius with or without hamstrings co-contraction is found (Figure 9). Lack of momentum caused by decreased walking speed can be another possible cause for stiff-knee gait. Quadriceps chemodenervation, selective surgical releases, or tendon transfer may be useful treatments.

In some patients, inadequate hip flexion is also a cause of abnormal limb clearance. This condition effectively prevents physiologic shortening of the limb, producing a swing phase toe drag. Decreased muscle strength or delayed activation of the iliopsoas (as shown with EMG) is a primary cause of this gait deviation. Strengthening of the iliopsoas, if possible, or a contralateral shoe lift to facilitate limb clearance can be used to treat this gait deviation.

Increased hip adduction can interfere with ipsilateral and contralateral limb advancement. Increased activity of the hip adductor musculature or imbalance in strength between the hip abductor and adductor muscle groups is the main cause of this type of abnormal gait. Percutaneous phenolization of the obturator nerve or obturator neurectomy (with or without adductor tenotomy) is the most common treatment.

Incomplete knee extension during the late swing and early stance phases, which result from joint derangement or hamstrings spasticity, is another important gait deviation. This condition interferes with ipsilateral limb advancement as the knee will be flexed and the limb is not able to easily reach the ground. Contralateral limb clearance also will be affected as a decrease in total functional height will occur, requiring increased hip and knee flexion to avoid foot drag. Total knee joint replacement or hamstring release may be useful as a treatment option.

Hip retraction or lack of pelvic rotation affecting the involved limb during the gait cycle may interfere with limb advancement, resulting in a shortened step length because of limited hip motion. Total hip arthroplasty or iliopsoas lengthening may address this gait deviation.

Annotated Bibliography

Al-Zahrani KS, Bakheit AM: A study of the gait characteristics of patients with chronic osteoarthritis of the knee. *Disabil Rehabil* 2002;24:275-280.

The kinematic and kinetic parameters of gait and the pattern of activation of four lower limb muscles were examined during walking at a self-selected pace on level ground in this study. The spatiotemporal parameters of gait were also computed in 58 patients with severe osteoarthritis of the knee and a control group of 25 age-matched healthy people. The patients with osteoarthritis had a significantly reduced walking speed; shorter stride length; a more prolonged stance phase of the gait cycle; less range of motion at the hip, knee and ankle joints; and generated less moments and powers at the ankle and more moments at the knee than the control group. It was concluded that the observed gait abnormalities were caused by instability of the knee joint in the stance phase. This finding may have important clinical implications for the rehabilitation of patients with severe osteoarthritis of the knee.

Esquenazi A, Mayer NH, Keenan MA: Dynamic poly-electromyography, neurolysis, and chemodenervation with botulinum toxin A for assessment and treatment of gait dysfunction. *Adv Neurol* 2001;87:321-331.

This review article describes evaluation techniques using gait analysis and possible treatment options for patients with gait dysfunction resulting from upper motor neuron syndrome. Treatment interventions ranging from focal injections of botulinum toxin to surgery are described.

Fantozzi S, Benedetti MG, Leardini A, et al: Fluoroscopic and gait analysis of the functional performance in stair ascent of two total knee replacement designs. *Gait Posture* 2003;17:225-234.

This article reviews stair ascent kinematics and kinetics of two types of knee joints (mobile bearing or posterior stabilized) using three-dimensional fluoroscopy and gait analysis techniques. Statistical significant correlation was found between knee flexion at foot strike and the position of the midcondylar contact points and between maximum knee adduction moment and corresponding trunk tilt. Results of this study suggested that a combined evaluation technique is more useful than fluoroscopic assessment of the knee alone.

Fuchs S, Tibesku CO, Frisse D, Laass H, Rosenbaum D: Quality of life and gait after unicondylar knee prosthesis are inferior to age-matched control subjects. *Am J Phys Med Rehabil* 2003;82:441-446.

A total of 17 patients were examined at an average follow-up of 21.5 months after implantation of unicondylar sledge knee prostheses. Patients had clinical evaluation, three-dimensional gait analysis, surface EMG investigation of the lower limb, and quality-of-life assessment using the Short Form-36 health questionnaire. Results were compared with a control group of 11 healthy individuals. Significantly poorer results were found for the patient group in the Hospital for Special Surgery score, the Knee Society score, the patella score, and the Visual Analog Scale for pain. Significant differences also were found in the level of physical functioning, role limitation because of physical complications, and the presence of pain. EMG activities during gait were significantly lower in the patient group, except for the rectus femoris and the tibialis anterior. Gait analysis showed a significant difference between the two groups for ground reactive forces and stride length; maximum knee extension and flexion did not vary significantly.

Fuller DA, Keenan MA, Esquenazi A, Whyte J, Mayer N, Fidler-Sheppard R: The impact of instrumented gait analysis on surgical planning: Treatment of spastic equinovarus deformity of the foot and ankle. *Foot Ankle Int* 2002;23:738-743.

This article reports the results of a prospective investigation of the impact of instrumented gait analysis on surgical planning for the treatment of equinovarus foot deformity in patients with spasticity. The patients in the study had instrumented gait analysis and poly-EMG data collection using a standard protocol. The agreement between the surgical plans of two surgeons were compared before and after the gait study. Results showed that instrumented gait analysis can produce higher agreement between surgeons in surgical planning for patients with spastic equinovarus deformity of the foot and ankle.

McGibbon CA, Krebs DE: Compensatory gait mechanics in patients with unilateral knee arthritis. *J Rheumatol* 2002;29:2410-2419.

Ankle, knee, hip, and low back mechanical energy expenditures and compensations during gait were characterized in 13 elderly patients with unilateral knee osteoarthritis and a control group of 10 age-matched healthy people studied during preferred and paced speed gait. Patients with knee osteoarthritis had a lower (but not significantly different) walking speed and step length compared to the control group, and had significantly different joint kinetic profiles.

Schmalz T, Blumentritt S, Jarasch R: Energy expenditure and biomechanical characteristics of lower limb amputee gait: The influence of prosthetic alignment and different prosthetic components. *Gait Posture* 2002;16:255-263.

The influence of different prosthetic alignments and components on oxygen consumption and the important biomechanical characteristics of the normal gait pattern of 15 transtibial and 12 transfemoral amputees was studied. Oxygen consumption while walking on a treadmill was analyzed and biomechanical parameters during walking on even ground at a self-selected speed were defined. It was found that variations of the prosthetic alignment affect the energy consumption of transfemoral amputees more significantly than transtibial amputees. All investigated variations could be clearly characterized by the sagittal moments acting on the joints of the prosthetic limb during gait.

Stevens PM, MacWilliams B, Mohr RA: Gait analysis of stapling for genu valgum. *J Pediatr Orthop* 2004;24:70-74.

This article evaluates the effects of stapling or epiphysiodesis of the distal medial femur as a treatment for correcting genu valgum. Clinical improvement (in appearance, pain, and function) and objective evidence of kinetic and kinematic improvement was shown. Preoperative and postoperative measurements in a series of patients treated for genu valgum were compared to document the benefits of normalizing the mechanical axis. Results indicated that knee and hip angles and knee moments were returned to the normal range (compared with an age-matched control group) for patients treated with surgery.

Classic Bibliography

Esquenazi A, Talaty M: Physical medicine and rehabilitation: The complete approach, in Grabois M, Garrison SJ, Hart KA, Lehmkuhl LD (eds): *Normal and Pathological Gait Analysis.* New York, NY, Blackwell Science, 2000, pp 242-262.

Gage JR: *Gait Analysis in Cerebral Palsy.* New York, NY, Mac Keith Press, 1991.

Inman VT, Ralston HJ, Todd F: *Human Walking.* Baltimore, MD, William & Wilkins, 1981.

Perry J: *Gait Analysis: Normal and Pathological Function.* Thorofare, NJ, Slack Inc, 1992.

Perry J, Waters RL, Perrin T: Electromyographic analysis of equinovarus following stroke. *Clin Orthop* 1978;131:47-53.

Chapter 32

Pelvis and Acetabulum: Trauma

Mark C. Reilly, MD

Pelvic Fractures

Evaluation

Fractures of the pelvic ring frequently result from high-energy injuries. The orthopaedic surgeon should be involved early in the treatment process. Patient evaluation should begin with information from the injury scene, and the patient's hemodynamic stability assessed while en route to the emergency department. A physical examination should identify associated integument, neurologic, urologic, and skeletal injuries. A careful evaluation of the soft tissues surrounding the pelvis should include an evaluation of the perineum for evidence of swelling, laceration, or deformity. The patient should be log rolled to allow for examination of possible open wounds or subcutaneous degloving injuries. Rectal and vaginal examinations are mandatory and may identify lacerations in connection with the pelvic ring injury.

Concomitant urologic injuries are present in approximately 15% of patients with pelvic fractures and are most commonly urinary tract injuries. Physical findings often associated with urethral injury in men are blood at the meatus and a high-riding or excessively mobile prostate. Female patients should be examined for vaginal wall, urethral, or labial lacerations. Hematuria, when present, is an accurate indicator of urologic injury (particularly bladder injuries). A retrograde cystourethrogram should be done on hemodynamically stable male patients with displaced anterior pelvic ring injuries before Foley catheter placement. In female patients, catheter placement may be performed without a urethrogram because the urethra is short and is not often injured. Retroperitoneal bladder ruptures are generally repaired at the time of anterior pelvic ring fixation. If no anterior pelvic ring surgery is performed, these ruptures may be treated nonsurgically. Although controversy exists concerning the treatment of urethral injuries, multiple studies have shown that early endoscopic primary realignment is associated with an acceptably low rate of intraoperative morbidity, stricture formation, impotence, and incontinence.

The trauma AP pelvis radiograph is recommended as an Advanced Trauma Life Support diagnostic adjunct for use in the resuscitation of blunt trauma patients and provides information about the mechanism of injury that may contribute to the initial treatment protocol. However, because most blunt trauma patients also will undergo a CT scan, the utility and cost effectiveness of the trauma AP radiograph as a resuscitative adjunct has been questioned. In one study of awake, alert trauma patients, physical examination was found to be as sensitive as the AP radiograph of the pelvis in identifying unstable pelvic injuries. Another large study found that physical examination alone would not have identified a significant number of unstable pelvic ring injuries.

Definitive radiographic evaluation of a patient with a pelvic ring injury should include the AP radiograph of the pelvis and the 40° caudad (inlet) and 40° cephalad (outlet) projections. The CT scan of the pelvis, usually obtained in conjunction with the trauma abdominal CT scan, should include cuts of 5 mm or less through the posterior pelvic ring. Results from the CT scan will help determine the location and type of posterior pelvic ring injury, identify compression of neurologic elements, and highlight subtle ligamentous or bony injuries that may alter the treatment plan. The lower lumbar spine can be seen and concurrent injuries may be identified.

Classification

Systems based on the anatomic location of the injury, mechanism of injury, or stability of the pelvic ring are used to classify pelvic ring injuries. These classification systems are usually used together. The anatomic classification system helps to identify all of the injured bony and ligamentous structures. The mechanism of injury system aids in fracture pattern recognition and assists in the early resuscitation and treatment of the patient (Figure 1). Determining the stability of the pelvic ring can help in the selection of the most appropriate definitive fixation for the injury.

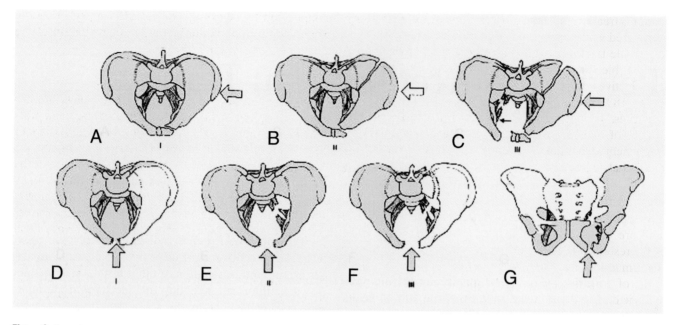

Figure 1 Young-Burgess classification of mechanism of injury. **A**, Lateral compression, grade I. **B**, Lateral compression, grade II. **C**, Lateral compression, grade III. **D**, Anterior-posterior compression, grade I. **E**, Anterior-posterior compression, grade II. **F**, Anterior-posterior compression, grade III. **G**, Vertical shear. *(Reproduced from Tornetta P III: Pelvis and acetabulum: Trauma, in Beaty JH (ed): Orthopaedic Knowledge Update 6. Rosemont, IL, American Academy of Orthopaedic Surgeons, 1999, pp 427-439.)*

Initial Treatment

Resuscitation

Pelvic ring injuries may be associated with significant hemorrhage. The patient's response to resuscitation, which begins during the initial trauma evaluation, will guide the overall treatment plan. Patients with pelvic fractures often will require blood replacement in addition to receiving fluid and crystalloid. Patients presenting in shock (systolic blood pressure less than 90 mm Hg) have mortality rates of up to 10 times of those found in normotensive patients. In one study, the presence of shock on arrival in the emergency department and revised trauma score were determined to be the most useful predictors of mortality and transfusion requirement. The most common direct causes for mortality in patients with pelvic fractures are head and thorax injuries; however, hemorrhage from pelvic fractures may be a significant contributing factor to mortality. Hypothermia and coagulopathy frequently contribute to ongoing blood loss and should be treated aggressively if present. Most pelvic bleeding is venous and can be controlled with mechanical stabilization, prevention of clot disruption, and treatment of coagulopathy.

External Stabilization

If the pelvic ring is mechanically unstable, external immobilization may be indicated. Initial stabilization for transport from the injury site may consist of sandbags, beanbags, or military antishock trousers (MAST). All devices must be removed for the evaluation of the trauma patient. The MAST suit should be deflated gradually to avoid a sudden expansion in intravascular volume and subsequent hypotension.

In the emergency department, external stabilization may be an important factor in patient resuscitation. Circumferential pelvic antishock sheeting or the placement of a pelvic binder is a noninvasive and rapid means for obtaining pelvic stability and has been shown to achieve reduction and stabilization of external rotation-type pelvic fractures. Pelvic sheeting has replaced the application of a resuscitative external fixator in many treatment centers because it avoids the delay required to apply the frame and may be applied earlier in the course of treatment to prevent ongoing hemorrhage. The trauma AP radiograph of the pelvis should be reviewed to determine the fracture pattern (before application of the sheet) to ensure that the injury is not a lateral compression injury, which could be further displaced by such treatment. When used, external fixation pins may be inserted into the medius tubercle portion of the iliac crest or just above the anterior inferior iliac spine. Skeletal traction also may be indicated as an additional method for temporary stabilization, particularly for fractures with cranial displacement.

Angiography

Angiography with selected embolization is useful for patients who are not responding to fluid and blood resuscitation. In one study, it was found that hemorrhage in patients with unstable pelvic fractures usually originated from pelvic sources and was often treatable with embolization. In patients with both pelvic and abdominal sources of bleeding, mortality was lower in the group of patients treated with angiography followed by laparotomy compared with a group first treated with laparotomy.

Stable fracture patterns also may be complicated by arterial bleeding and may be appropriate for treatment by selective embolization. Arterial bleeding can occur in up to 18% of patients with mechanically stable pelvic fractures. In one study however, an intra-abdominal source of bleeding was found in 85% of patients who were hemodynamically unstable but had mechanically stable pelvic fractures.

Definitive Treatment

Most pelvic fractures are mechanically stable injuries and are often caused by a lateral compression mechanism resulting in an anterior impaction fracture of the sacrum and pubic rami fractures. If there is less than 1 cm of posterior pelvic ring displacement and no neurologic deficit, these injuries are appropriate for nonsurgical treatment with progressive mobilization. Repeat radiographs should be obtained after mobilization to ensure that there has been no further displacement. Fractures of the processes of the pelvis, such as anterior superior iliac spine avulsion fractures, do not disrupt the stability of the pelvic ring and are usually treated nonsurgically unless significant displacement is present.

External Fixation

External fixation as definitive treatment is generally only appropriate for rotationally unstable injuries. The most common scenario involves an AP compression injury, which results in an external rotation of one or both hemipelves. The anterior ring usually fails as a symphysis dislocation or less commonly as fractures of the pubic rami. The posterior ring injury is incomplete. In this situation, the external fixator may provide enough anterior stability to allow the anterior injury to heal. In a lateral compression injury, distraction external fixation with external rotation of the injured hemipelvis has been used with success; this treatment is only required if there is neurologic compression or unacceptable deformity. Although it may be used in association with internal fixation for some injuries, external fixation alone is not appropriate for the treatment of unstable posterior pelvic ring injuries. The posterior pelvic ring injury may ultimately heal; however, it will heal in a displaced position and may lead to pelvic obliquity, pain, and long-term disability.

Internal Fixation

Internal fixation is the most biomechanically stable fixation for the pelvic ring. The implants are situated closer to the site of injury than in external fixation and may be optimally located to resist the forces applied to the pelvic ring. Achieving an accurate reduction of the pelvic ring may be a prerequisite to achieving stable fixation. Placement of internal fixation for the pelvis may be complicated by neurologic or vascular injury, infection, wound complications, and nonunion or malunion of the pelvic ring, and loss of reduction.

Anterior Pelvic Ring Injuries

Injuries to the anterior pelvic ring include symphysis dislocations, pubic body fractures, and pubic rami fractures. These injuries may occur alone, in combination, or in association with a posterior pelvic ring injury. All complete dislocations of the symphysis pubis should be stabilized. Displacements of less than 2.5 cm in conjunction with an intact posterior pelvic ring are incomplete injuries and can be considered for nonsurgical treatment. Because radiographs of the injury may not reflect the magnitude of the initial displacement, close follow-up is warranted if nonsurgical treatment is selected. The symphysis dislocation is most effectively and efficiently treated with a single plate applied superiorly through a rectus-splitting Pfannenstiel approach. This procedure may be done in conjunction with an emergent laparotomy or urologic surgery and adds the least amount of additional soft-tissue disruption.

Fractures of the superior pubic ramus rarely require stabilization; even those that occur in association with symphyseal dislocations are usually treated nonsurgically. Poupart's, Cooper's, and the inguinal ligaments combine with the periosteum of the ramus to provide stability for these injuries. It is believed that more than 2 cm of residual distraction or fracture gap of the ramus after treatment of the posterior pelvic injury implies disruption of these soft tissues and fixation may be needed. Fixation may be achieved with open reduction and plate osteosynthesis; intramedullary screw fixation or external fixation also has been used. If the fracture involves the body of the pubis (medial to the pubic tubercle), the supporting tissues mentioned above are all lateral to the site of injury and cannot contribute to stability. Pubic body fractures are generally treated as symphysis dislocations and require reduction and plate fixation.

Posterior Pelvic Ring Injuries

The posterior pelvic ring is the most important component in overall stability and function of the pelvis. The anatomic site of injury will determine the surgical approach and the type of fixation used. Unstable posterior pelvic ring injuries are ilium fractures, sacroiliac (SI) joint dislocations, sacral fractures, or SI joint fracture-dislocations. It is usually best to reduce the posterior pelvic ring injury first, building to the intact portion of the pelvis. This is particularly crucial if there are many sites of pelvic displacement. If there are only two sites of injury within the pelvic ring, reduction of the anterior ring may facilitate reduction of the posterior pelvis in some circumstances; however, beginning treatment with the posterior injury is still recommended.

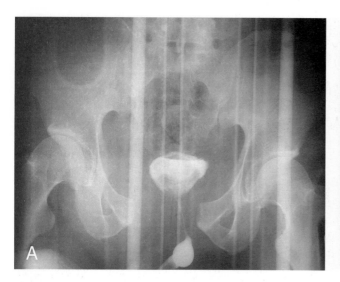
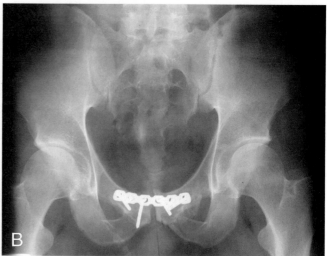

Figure 2 A, Radiograph showing dislocation of the symphysis pubis and incomplete injuries to both SI joints. **B,** Radiograph at 2 years shows maintenance of the reduction of the pelvic ring without evidence of SI joint arthrosis.

Ilium Fractures

Ilium fractures typically propagate from the iliac crest to the greater sciatic notch and are unstable injuries. Although nondisplaced fractures may be treated nonsurgically, displaced fractures require reduction and fixation. A posterior pelvic approach is useful, although some fracture patterns may be treated through the lateral window of the ilioinguinal approach. Fractures that involve only the iliac wing are stable injuries, are often minimally displaced, and can be treated nonsurgically. If significant displacement is present, open reduction and internal fixation may be indicated. These fractures are generally reduced and fixed through the lateral window of the ilioinguinal approach. Iliac wing fractures have a high incidence of local arterial injuries, bowel injury, and soft-tissue degloving. Plate or screw fixation between the tables of the ilium can be useful.

Sacroiliac Joint Dislocations

A complete radiographic evaluation including CT scan is often required to differentiate between incomplete SI joint injuries and complete SI dislocations. The anterior pelvic ring and anterior SI ligaments may be significantly disrupted, whereas the posterior SI ligaments remain intact. These injuries are only rotationally unstable and usually require treatment of only the anterior ring injury (Figure 2). The posterior ring injury will reduce indirectly and be stabilized by the anterior ring fixation. Complete dislocations of the SI joint are vertically unstable injuries and require posterior pelvic ring fixation in addition to anterior ring fixation (Figure 3).

Reduction and fixation of the SI joint may be done either open (through an anterior or posterior approach) or through closed manipulation with percutaneous fixation. The anterior approach to the SI joint allows direct visualization of the cranial aspect of the joint to the pelvic brim, and the ilium can be manipulated through the placement of clamps on the crest or through the interspinous notch. Excessive retraction or retractors placed too medially on the sacrum may cause injury to the L5 nerve root. Fixation is achieved through the use of plates applied with a single screw in the sacrum and with one or two screws placed into the ilium. The use of two plates, oriented at 90° to each other, is recommended. In the obese patient, reduction and fixation through the anterior approach can be very difficult because of the inability to retract the abdominal contents. Fixation also may be compromised if there is a marginal fracture of the sacral lip of the SI joint. This fracture can be identified on the CT scan preoperatively and may preclude stable plate fixation from the anterior approach. Fixation also can be achieved through iliosacral screws placed percutaneously while the patient is supine and while the reduction is assessed and held from the anterior approach.

Reduction and fixation is facilitated by the use of an open reduction done through the posterior pelvic approach with the patient prone. The posterior-inferior SI joint is visualized while the anterior joint is palpated through the greater sciatic notch. Reduction is performed with a combination of clamps placed between the ilium and sacrum. Fixation is achieved with the fluoroscopically guided placement of iliosacral lag screws. The iliosacral screws are inserted through a separate incision with a percutaneous technique; it is rarely possible to insert the screws through the posterior approach incision. If the reduction of the SI joint can be achieved with closed manipulation and traction, the joint may be similarly stabilized with iliosacral lag screws placed with the patient either prone or supine.

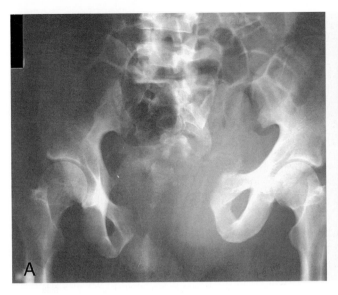
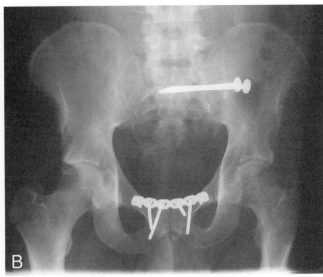

Figure 3 **A,** Patient with dislocation of the symphysis pubis, incomplete injury to the right SI joint, and complete dislocation of the left SI joint. Note the cranial displacement of the left hemipelvis. **B,** Open reduction of the SI joint was performed through a posterior pelvic approach and the joint stabilized with iliosacral screw fixation. Open reduction and internal fixation of the symphysis pubis followed.

Sacroiliac Fracture-Dislocations

SI fracture-dislocations are a combination of an iliac fracture and an SI dislocation. The posterior superior spine and often the posterior iliac crest remain attached to the sacrum by the posterior SI ligaments. The remaining portion of the ilium dislocates from the sacrum as the anterior SI ligaments rupture. Fracture-dislocations, which leave only a small intact iliac fragment, resemble pure SI dislocations and are treated similarly. Fracture-dislocations with a large intact iliac fragment have been termed crescent fractures and may be large enough to maintain the integrity of the posterior SI ligaments. In this situation, interfragmentary fixation of the ilium will restore skeletal stability and the posterior SI ligaments will maintain the reduction of the SI joint. If the fragment is small or the integrity of the posterior SI ligaments cannot be ensured, interfragmentary fixation must be augmented with SI joint fixation. Generally, rami fractures are the type of anterior ring injury seen in association with the SI fracture-dislocation; this injury may be treated nonsurgically if secure posterior fixation is achieved. Closed reduction and percutaneous fixation of SI fracture-dislocations has been reported but has been associated with a significant incidence of fixation failure. Outcome, as measured by patient satisfaction, was acceptable.

Sacral Fractures

Most fractures of the sacrum are minimally displaced and stable. Those associated with lateral compression-type injuries are often impacted and have a negligible incidence of subsequent displacement. Displaced and unstable sacral fractures require reduction and fixation.

Open accurate reduction and internal fixation is recommended, but closed reduction and percutaneous fixation also has been advocated. Open reduction through a posterior pelvic approach allows direct visualization of the fracture site and sacral nerve roots. This approach allows for direct decompression of the nerve roots and visualization of the fracture during fixation to ensure that the fracture is reduced and not overcompressed. Closed manipulation and percutaneous fixation may increase the risk for iatrogenic nerve injury if the fracture is not aligned and is overcompressed. The space available for safe placement of iliosacral screw fixation is increasingly compromised with the increasing magnitude of malreduction. In either open or closed reduction, it is imperative to obtain an accurate reduction to ensure safe fixation.

A subgroup of sacral fractures is the U-shaped fractures in which bilateral transforaminal sacral fractures are connected by a transverse fracture, usually between the second and third sacral segments. This condition represents a complete spinopelvic dissociation and often occurs with a sacral kyphosis and disruption of the cauda equina at the level of the transverse sacral fracture. Percutaneous screw fixation has been used without reduction of the kyphotic deformity; however, reduction of the deformity and fixation with spinopelvic instrumentation is recommended. Late decompression is reserved for patients with neurologic deficits and no evidence of spontaneous recovery. Midline sagittal sacral fractures also have been reported. These fractures are generally vertically stable injuries and are treated with fixation of the anterior ring injury alone and indirect reduction of the sacral fracture.

Open Versus Closed Reduction

Although percutaneous fixation of the pelvic ring has been proposed, the most important factor in the treatment of pelvic ring fractures remains the reduction. The stability of the fracture fixation and the safety of fixation placement has been shown to be compromised with fracture malreduction. In one study, 20% of patients with sacral fractures who were treated with closed reduction and percutaneous iliosacral screws had fixation failures and displacement, and 13% required revision surgery. CT-guided, computer-, fluoroscopic-, and endoscopic-assisted insertion techniques for internal fixation have all been described but only a few of these techniques review the reduction obtained. In one study of closed reductions, 92% of iliac wing and SI fracture-dislocations were reduced to within 1 cm of residual displacement. Fractures may be treated with internal fixation using many different techniques, but successful closed reduction of the pelvic ring remains a challenge.

Closed reduction of the pelvic ring is most successful when applied early in the postinjury period. Open reduction of posterior pelvic ring injuries has been shown to result in accurate reductions but increases the risk of posterior wound complications. Infection rates after open reduction and internal fixation of the posterior pelvic ring are reported to be 4%. Significant posterior soft-tissue injury should be considered a relative contraindication to a formal, open posterior approach.

Iliosacral Screw Fixation

Iliosacral screws are used in the internal fixation of SI dislocations, fracture-dislocations, and sacral fractures. The placement of these screws is technically demanding and requires a thorough knowledge of the three-dimensional anatomy of the posterior pelvic ring. Common bony anatomic variants such as transitional vertebrae and hypoplastic first sacral segments may complicate or preclude the safe placement of iliosacral screws. Screw malposition has been reported to be as high as 13% and may be associated with serious complications. In one study, 8% of patients treated with iliosacral screw fixation had errant screws and neurologic complications. These findings highlight the need for careful screw placement, adequate imaging, fracture reduction, and surgeon familiarity with the procedure. It has been suggested that the increased proprioceptive feedback that is obtained by using an oscillating drill rather than a threaded guide-wire may allow for safer and more accurate screw insertion. Some surgeons recommend the use of electromyogram monitoring during screw insertion. If this device is used, the anode must be located at or beyond the patient's midline.

Outcome

Outcome after pelvic fracture is more a function of the effects of associated injuries than of the pelvic ring injury itself. At long-term follow-up after pelvic fracture, patients reported decreased satisfaction in most of the categories measured by the Medical Outcomes Study Short Form-36. Pain, general health, and physical functioning are typically affected. Clinical results appear to decline with the increasing level of instability caused by the initial injury. In one study, functional and radiographic results were worse and mortality was higher in patients with more unstable fracture patterns. Good and excellent outcomes after rotationally unstable fractures have been reported in up to 96% of patients, whereas up to 70% of patients with vertically unstable fractures reported acceptable results.

Associated neurologic, urologic, and lower extremity injuries are the most common causes of long-term disability, pain, and impaired function. Resolution of neurologic dysfunction has been seen in up to 50% of patients at long-term follow-up, with the L5 nerve root being the least likely to regain normal function.

Sexual dysfunction after pelvic fracture has been noted in women. Dyspareunia was reported in 43% of female patients who had more than 5 mm of residual displacement. In another study of functional outcomes after pelvic fracture, 44% of patients reported significant sexual dysfunction after unstable pelvic injuries. A study of erectile dysfunction after pelvic fracture found that 30% of male patients who were sexually active after pelvic fracture reported some degree of erectile dysfunction; those patients sustaining symphyseal disruptions reported the greatest dissatisfaction. Disruption of the cavernosal nerves has been implicated in this complication.

Urologic injury may result in a significant compromise in patient outcome after pelvic fracture. Urethral stricture, incontinence, and erectile dysfunction may complicate the treatment of urethral injuries, particularly delayed perineal reconstruction. Patients who undergo early endoscopic primary realignment have been shown to have a lower rate of incontinence and impotence when compared with patients who have delayed open repair. Management of concurrent urologic trauma may impact the treatment of the patient's skeletal injury. In up to 35% of patients, orthopaedic treatment was altered because of urologic intervention.

Acetabular Fractures

Acetabular fractures are usually the result of high-energy injuries and are frequently associated with other skeletal, visceral, or abdominal injuries. The position of the hip at the time of injury and the direction of impact will determine the fracture pattern. A detailed patient evaluation is mandatory to identify life-threatening associated injuries,

Elementary Fractures

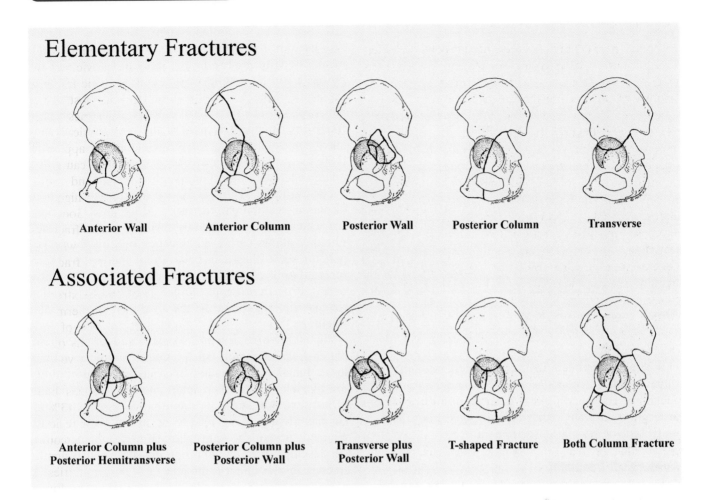

Anterior Wall   Anterior Column   Posterior Wall   Posterior Column   Transverse

Associated Fractures

Anterior Column plus Posterior Hemitransverse   Posterior Column plus Posterior Wall   Transverse plus Posterior Wall   T-shaped Fracture   Both Column Fracture

Figure 4 The classification system of Letournel and Judet. (Courtesy of Joel M. Matta, MD)

complications associated with the acetabular fracture, and other skeletal injuries requiring treatment. Approximately one half of patients with an acetabular fracture will have an injury to another organ system.

Although hemodynamic instability occurs infrequently with isolated fractures of the acetabulum, persistent unexplained blood loss despite resuscitation may be caused by vascular injury. Fractures involving the greater sciatic notch may injure the superior gluteal artery, requiring angiography and selective embolization. Neurologic injury is frequently associated with fractures of the acetabulum and may be present in up to 20% of patients. The peroneal division of the sciatic nerve is the most frequently injured. Closed reduction of associated hip dislocations should be performed as quickly as possible to reduce the risk of osteonecrosis of the femoral head. Persistent subluxation of the hip may be caused by either the fracture displacement or from intra-articular fracture fragments and should be treated with urgent skeletal traction to prevent the head from wearing against the fracture edge or incarcerated fragment. Soft-tissue degloving injuries (Morel-Lavallé lesions) may be initially recognized by a fluid wave on palpation

and may be later recognized by the presence of a fluctuant circumscribed area of cutaneous anesthesia and ecchymosis. These injuries should be treated with débridement and delayed acetabular fixation because of the significant incidence of positive bacterial culture from these lesions.

Diagnosis and Classification

The diagnosis of acetabular fractures begins with appropriately positioned, well-penetrated, plain radiographs. The AP pelvis radiograph and the Judet views (45° obturator and iliac oblique) are needed for accurate interpretation and fracture classification. A CT scan can better define rotational displacements, intra-articular fragments, marginal articular impactions, and associated femoral head injuries. A three-dimensional CT reconstruction may be helpful in understanding the relationships between multiple sites of injury, but is not a replacement for plain radiographs. The classification system of Letournel and Judet, which groups acetabular fractures into five elementary and five associated fracture patterns, is used to classify the fractures (Figure 4). The interobserver and intraobserver reliability of the

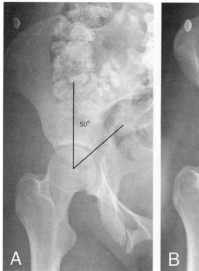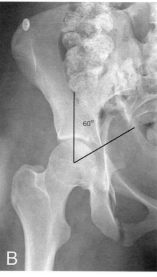

Figure 5 Measurement of the posterior and medial roof arcs as measured on the iliac oblique (**A**) and the AP (**B**) radiographs.

classification has been found to be excellent on the basis of plain radiographs alone; the CT scan did not improve reliability. However, CT has been reported to be more accurate than plain radiographs in measuring the true magnitude of articular displacement.

Nonsurgical Treatment

Fracture displacements of greater than 3 mm are generally treated surgically. Certain fractures, however, may be amenable to nonsurgical treatment. Roof arc measurements are a means of determining fractures with an intact weight-bearing dome, which is defined as having medial, anterior, and posterior roof arcs of greater than 45° as measured on the AP, obturator, and iliac oblique radiographs. Geometric analysis has shown that the cranial 10 mm of the acetabulum on the CT scan corresponds to the area defined as the weight-bearing dome by roof arcs (Figure 5). It has been postulated that fractures that do not involve this dome are unlikely to lead to posttraumatic arthrosis and are candidates for nonsurgical treatment. Prerequisites for nonsurgical treatment of associated acetabulum fractures include both intact roof arc measurements and congruence of the femoral head to the intact acetabulum on nontraction AP and Judet radiographs. Roof arc measurements are not applicable to associated both-column fractures because there is no intact portion of the acetabulum to measure. Instead, perfect secondary congruence of an associated both-column fracture on all three standard radiographs, taken when the patient is out of traction, is necessary for nonsurgical treatment. Although a fracture healed with secondary congruence may have an adequate articular surface, the resultant shortening of the limb and medialization of the hip may not be accept-

able. Secondary congruence alone, therefore, is necessary but not a sufficient criterion for nonsurgical treatment. The criteria also do not apply to fractures of the posterior wall. It is believed that at least 50% to 60% of the width of the posterior wall on the CT scan must be intact for satisfactory clinical outcome after nonsurgical treatment. Smaller fractures of the posterior wall may allow hip subluxation; stress radiographs taken while the patient is under anesthesia may be useful in determining whether surgical intervention is required.

Nonsurgical treatment is also appropriate for nondisplaced acetabulum fractures. Although it has been suggested that percutaneous fixation of nondisplaced fractures allows earlier mobilization of multiply injured patients, some physicians believe that nondisplaced fractures are unlikely to displace even with early mobilization. CT or fluoroscopic-guided percutaneous fixation remains investigational in the treatment of acetabular fractures.

In addition to fracture location and displacement, patient-related factors such as age, preinjury activity level, functional demands, and medical comorbidities must be considered when determining whether a patient is best served by surgical or nonsurgical treatment. Nonsurgical treatment of elderly or infirm patients, with planned subsequent arthroplasty if symptomatic arthritis develops, may be appropriate—particularly if the fracture displacement is minimal.

Surgical Treatment

Open anatomic reduction and internal fixation is the treatment of choice for displaced fractures of the acetabulum. The goal of surgical treatment is to obtain an anatomic reduction of the articular surface while avoiding complications. This treatment restores the contact area between the femoral head and the acetabulum, produces a stable painless joint, and maximizes the potential for long-term survival of the hip (Figure 6). Clinical outcome is correlated with the quality of the articular reduction. The results of perfect reductions (less than 1 mm of residual displacement) are superior to those of imperfect (1 to 3 mm) and poor (greater than 3 mm) reductions at long-term follow-up. Other factors associated with poor outcomes are femoral head injuries and postoperative complications.

Surgical Approach

The choice of surgical approach is determined by the fracture pattern. A single surgical approach is generally selected with the expectation that the fracture reduction and fixation can be completely performed though the one approach. The most commonly used surgical approaches are the Kocher-Langenbeck and the ilioinguinal approaches. The extended iliofemoral approach is an extensile approach developed to allow maximal simultaneous access

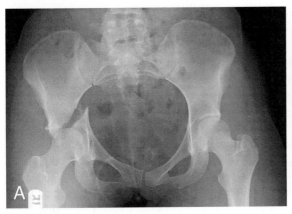
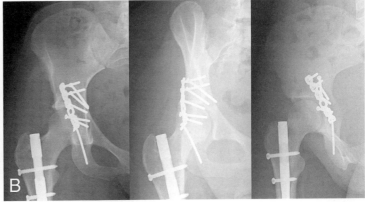

Figure 6   A, Associated transtectal transverse plus posterior wall acetabular fracture in an 18-year-old woman. **B,** AP and Judet radiographs at 3 years after injury. The patient's hip is rated 6,6,6 on the modified D'Aubigne and Postel scale.

to both columns of the acetabulum. It is most often used in associated fracture patterns that are surgically treated more than 21 days after injury or on certain transverse or both-column pattern fractures with complicating features that are not amenable to treatment by either of the two more limited approaches. Modifications of all three approaches have been described; however, long-term clinical outcomes of large numbers of patients are not available for comparison.

Closed reduction and percutaneous screw fixation of acetabular fractures has not been shown to achieve comparable articular reductions when compared with traditional surgery. Because there is a strong correlation between accuracy of reduction and clinical outcome, such techniques should be considered investigational until appropriate results and long-term outcome data are available.

Posterior Wall Fractures

Posterior wall fractures are the most common type of acetabular fracture. Although they account for nearly one third of all acetabular fractures, patients with this type of fracture have a disproportionate number of poor outcomes. Suboptimal outcomes have been reported in up to 32% of patients with these injuries despite perfect reductions in 92% to 100% of the fractures. Risk factors for poor outcome are delay in reduction of associated hip dislocation, age older than 55 years at the time of injury, intra-articular comminution, and osteonecrosis. When postoperative CT is added to the routine evaluation of the posterior wall fracture, however, the association between fracture reduction and clinical outcome is reinforced. The CT scan may be more accurate (particularly in the evaluation of multifragmentary posterior wall fractures) in determining true residual fracture displacement and identifying small articular malreductions. Articular reduction of the posterior wall fracture as measured by CT was found to strongly correlate with long-term outcome.

Complications

The primary complication after fracture of the acetabulum is posttraumatic arthrosis. Although symptomatic arthritis after acetabular fracture is generally treated with arthroplasty, arthrodesis and osteotomy remain viable treatment options. Posttraumatic arthritis is more common after poor articular reductions than after a perfect reduction. Evidence shows that, if arthritis develops after a perfect reduction, the onset is later and the progression slower than arthritis that develops after a poor reduction.

Heterotopic ossification is related to the degree of soft-tissue disruption, from either the injury or the surgical approach. Other factors associated with the formation of heterotopic ossification include head injury, prolonged mechanical ventilation, and male gender. Use of an extensile approach also contributes to the formation of heterotopic ossification and is probably caused by the amount of muscle dissection and elevation from the ilium. Most patients who develop heterotopic ossification after acetabular fracture do not have functional restrictions of their hip motion. Prophylactic treatments for heterotopic ossification include 6 weeks of indomethacin use, single-dose external beam radiotherapy, or a combination of both treatments. In a direct comparison of irradiation with indomethacin use, no difference was shown in the development of heterotopic bone. In the same study, 38% of the patients who were not treated with prophylaxis developed clinically significant heterotopic ossification when compared with 7% in those patients who received some form of prophylaxis. Other prospective randomized studies have failed to confirm the efficacy of indomethacin use compared with no prophylaxis. Because of concerns about the use of irradiation in young adults, prophylaxis with indomethacin is preferred by many physicians. One study, however, showed an increased incidence of long bone nonunion in patients treated with indomethacin for concurrent acetabular or pelvic fractures.

Deep venous thrombosis and pulmonary embolism are common complications after pelvic or acetabular fractures treated without prophylaxis. Chemoprophylaxis with low molecular weight heparin or warfarin sodium may reduce the incidence of thromboembolic disease, particularly in association with mechanical prophylaxis. Duplex ultrasound is typically used preoperatively to identify patients with venous thrombosis, however, it is limited in its ability to detect proximal thrombi. Despite earlier studies that suggested that magnetic resonance venography was more sensitive than ultrasound at detecting proximal thrombi, an evaluation of contrast CT and magnetic resonance venography showed a significant false positive rate in both studies. This finding was confirmed by invasive contrast venography. If thrombi are present, the placement of an inferior vena caval filter is recommended before fracture surgery.

Iatrogenic neurologic injury has been reported in 2% to 15% of patients who were surgically treated for acetabular fractures. Intraoperative neurologic monitoring has been recommended but there is no evidence that the routine use of monitoring lowers the incidence of iatrogenic injury. A direct comparison of monitored and nonmonitored acetabular fracture surgeries used both sensory and motor pathway monitoring but failed to show a difference in the incidence of iatrogenic nerve injury. Most orthopaedic trauma surgeons use prophylaxis to help prevent heterotopic ossification and deep venous thrombosis; however, nerve monitoring is not routinely used.

Annotated Bibliography

Pelvic Fractures

Eastridge BJ, Starr A, Minei JP, O'Keefe GE, Scalea TM: The importance of fracture pattern in giving therapeutic decision-making in patients with hemorrhagic shock and pelvic ring disruptions. *J Trauma* 2002;53:446-451.

In 86 patients with pelvic fracture with persistent hemodynamic instability, abdominal hemorrhage was responsible for hypotension in 85% of stable pelvic fractures. Hemorrhage was from pelvic sources in 59% of patients with unstable fracture patterns. Patients with unstable fracture patterns had a higher mortality (60%) when celiotomy was performed before angiography when compared with patients in which angiography was performed first (25% mortality).

Gonzalez RP, Fried PQ, Bukhalo M: The utility of clinical examination in screening for pelvic fractures in blunt trauma. *J Am Coll Surg* 2002;194:121-125.

In this study, 2,176 trauma patients were evaluated. Ninety-seven patients (4.5%) were diagnosed with a pelvic fracture. Clinical examination was found to be as sensitive as the AP pelvic radiograph at identifying pelvic fracture in the awake, alert trauma patient.

Griffin DR, Starr AJ, Reinert CM, Jones AL, Whitlock S: Vertically unstable pelvic fractures fixed with percutaneous iliosacral screws: Does posterior injury pattern predict fixation failure? *J Orthop Trauma* 2003;17:399-405.

Sixty-two patients were treated with closed reduction and percutaneous iliosacral screw fixation for posterior pelvic ring injuries. Results show that sacral fractures were significantly more likely to displace than other posterior lesions. Twenty percent (6 of 30) of sacral fractures displaced and 67% of those required revision fixation surgery.

Kabak S, Halicik M: Tuncel M Avsarogullari L, Baktir A, Bastruk M: Functional outcome of open reduction and internal fixation for completely unstable pelvic ring fractures (type C): A report of 40 cases. *J Orthop Trauma* 2003;17:555-562.

This study involved 40 patients with type C pelvic fractures. At 1-year follow-up, sexual dysfunction was found in 44% of patients and correlated with anxiety disorder and major or moderate depression. Seventy-two percent of patients had returned to work at their original jobs, and of those who did not, an increased incidence of depression was found. Persistent pelvic pain was reported by 25% of patients.

Mayher BE, Guyton JL, Gingrich JR: Impact of urethral injury management on the treatment and outcome of concurrent pelvic fractures. *Urology* 2001;57:439-442.

In 61 patients with combined pelvic and lower urinary tract injuries, urologic treatment affected the orthopaedic treatment choices in 35% of patients. Long-term suprapubic catheterization precluded surgical treatment in four patients; three had poor results. The authors recommend early endoscopic realignment for urethral injuries and improved communication and cooperation between subspecialty groups.

Miller MT, Pasquale MD, Bromberg WJ, Wasser TE, Cox J: Not so FAST. *J Trauma* 2003;54:52-59.

In this study, 359 patients with blunt abdominal injury were evaluated with focused assessment with sonography for trauma (FAST) and contrast CT of the abdomen and pelvis. FAST resulted in an underdiagnosis of intra-abdominal injury with a false negative rate of 6% (27% of the false negatives required laparotomy). The authors recommended that CT with contrast remain the gold standard for the evaluation of patients with suspected blunt abdominal injury.

Moudouni S, Tazi K, Koutani A, Ibn Attya A, Hachimi M, Lakrissa A: Comparative results of the treatment of post-traumatic rupture of the membranous urethra with endoscopic realignment and surgery. *Prog Urol* 2001;11: 56-61.

In this study, 29 men with urethral injuries had primary endoscopic urethral realignment. At an average follow-up of 5.6 years, improved rates of continence, potency, and stricture formation were found when compared with rates for patients who had delayed open urethroplasty. The authors recommended early realignment as an effective and safe technique.

Pehle B, Nast-Kolb D, Oberbeck R, Waydhas C, Ruchholtz S: Significance of physical examination and radiography of the pelvis during treatment in the shock emergency room. Unfallchirurg 2003;106:642-648.

In this study, 979 blunt trauma patients were evaluated for pelvic instability. Physical examination alone had a sensitivity of 44% and a specificity of 99% for detecting pelvic fracture. Surgically significant pelvic injury could not be reliably ruled out by examination alone.

Reilly MC, Bono CM, Litkouhi B, Sirkin M, Behrens FF: The effect of sacral fracture malreduction on the safe placement of iliosacral screws. *J Orthop Trauma* 2003;17:88-94.

In a cadaveric model of a zone 2 sacral fracture, increasing cranial displacement of the hemipelvis was found to correlate with a decrease in the space available for the safe placement of iliosacral screws. Space available for safe screw placement was insufficient at displacements greater than 1 cm.

Rommens PM, Hessmann MH: Staged reconstruction of pelvic ring disruption: Differences in morbidity, mortality, radiologic results, and functional outcome between B1, B2/B3, and C-type lesions. *J Orthop Trauma* 2002;16:92-98.

A review of functional outcome of 122 patients with surgically treated pelvic ring injuries was done. Mortality was higher in patients with type C injuries than in those with type B (15% versus 5%). Higher rates of anatomic reductions were found in B1 (open-book) injuries than in lateral compression injuries (B2, B3) or C-type injuries. Good or excellent outcomes were obtained in 74% of patients with B1 injuries, 92% with B2/B3 injuries, and 71% of those with C injuries.

Starr AJ, Griffin DR, Reinert CM, et al: Pelvic ring disruptions: Prediction of associated injuries, transfusion requirement, pelvic arteriography, complications, and mortality. *J Orthop Trauma* 2002;16:553-561.

In a review of 325 trauma patients with pelvic ring injury, the presence of shock on arrival in the emergency department was associated with increased mortality, transfusion requirements, and injury severity score. Mortality of patients presenting in shock was 57%. The authors were unable to identify an association between fracture classification and outcome or fracture presence and/or type of associated injuries.

Acetabular Fractures

Beaule PE, Dorey FJ, Matta JM: Letournel classification for acetabular fractures: assessment of interobserver and intraobserver reliability. *J Bone Joint Surg Am* 2003; 85-A:1704-1709.

The intraobserver and interobserver reliability of the Letournel-Judet classification system for acetabular fractures was assessed by surgeons who studied with Letournel, surgeons who specialize in acetabular fracture surgery, and general orthopaedic trauma surgeons. The reliability of the classification was excellent in the first two groups. Use of the CT scan in addition to the plain radiographs did not increase the reliability of the classification system.

Burd TA, Hughes MS, Anglen JO: Heterotopic ossification prophylaxis with indomethacin increase the risk of long-bone nonunion. *J Bone Joint Surg Br* 2003;85:700-705.

Patients receiving indomethacin for heterotopic ossification prophylaxis were compared with those receiving external radiation therapy. The 38 patients receiving indomethacin had a statistically significant increase in the incidence of long bone fracture nonunion compared with the 38 patients receiving external radiation therapy (26% versus 7%). No difference in the efficacy of both methods of prophylaxis was found in the authors' previous study.

Burd TA, Lowry KJ, Anglen JO: Indomethacin compared with localized irradiation for the prevention of heterotopic ossification following surgical treatment of acetabular fractures. *J Bone Joint Surg Am* 2001;83:1783-1788.

In this study, 166 patients were treated surgically for a fracture of the acetabulum. Seventy-eight patients received external beam radiotherapy, 72 received 6 weeks of indomethacin, and 16 patients received no prophylaxis. Grade 3 or 4 heterotopic ossification developed in 7% of the treated groups and 38% of the untreated group. No difference between the two treated groups was identified.

Haidukewych GJ, Scaduto J, Herscovici D Jr, Sanders RW, DiPasquale T: Iatrogenic nerve injury in acetabular fracture surgery: a comparison of monitored and unmonitored procedures. *J Orthop Trauma* 2002;16:297-301.

This article is a retrospective review of acetabular fracture surgery performed with and without somatosensory evoked potential or electromyography nerve monitoring. The use of intraoperative nerve monitoring did not decrease the rate of iatrogenic nerve palsy. Seven of 10 iatrogenic nerve injuries in the monitored group had previously had normal intraoperative monitoring.

Moed BR, Carr SE, Gruson KI, Watson JT, Craig JG: Computed tomographic assessment of fractures of the posterior wall of the acetabulum after operative treatment. *J Bone Joint Surg Am* 2003;85-A:512-522.

In this study, 67 patients with surgically treated posterior wall acetabular fractures were evaluated for radiographic and functional outcome at a mean of 4 years after injury. Use of postoperative CT scanning to document reduction revealed a strong correlation between quality of reduction and functional outcome. Residual displacement after reduction of posterior wall fractures was more accurately determined on the CT scan than on the plain radiographs.

Moed BR: WillsonCarr SE, Watson JT: Results of operative treatment of fractures of the posterior wall of the acetabulum. *J Bone Joint Surg Am* 2002;84-A:752-758.

In the largest published study to date, the authors present the results of surgical treatment of 100 patients with posterior wall acetabular fractures at a mean follow-up of 5 years after injury. Good or excellent results were obtained in 89% of patients. Risk factors for unsatisfactory outcome were a delay in reduction of hip dislocation of greater than 12 hours, age older than 55 years, the presence of intra-articular comminution, and the development of osteonecrosis.

Stover MD, Morgan SJ, Bosse MJ, et al: Prospective comparison of contrast-enhanced computed tomography versus magnetic resonance venography in the detection of occult deep pelvic vein thrombosis in patients with pelvic and acetabular fractures. *J Orthop Trauma* 2002;16:613-621.

A prospective comparison of magnetic resonance venography and CT venography as screening examinations for pelvic deep venous thrombosis was performed. Invasive contrast venography was used as the confirmatory study. The false positive rate for magnetic resonance venography was 100% and for CT venography was 50%. The authors question the use of either test as the sole means of screening for pelvic deep venous thrombosis after pelvic or acetabular fracture.

Classic Bibliography

Bucholz RW: The pathological anatomy of Malgaigne fracture-dislocations of the pelvis. *J Bone Joint Surg Am* 1981;63:400-404.

Copeland CE, Bosse MJ, McCarthy ML, et al: Effect of trauma and pelvic fracture on female genitourinary, sexual, and reproductive function. *J Orthop Trauma* 1997; 11:73-81.

Dalal SA, Burgess AR, Siegal JH, et al: Pelvic fracture in multiple trauma: Classification by mechanism is the key to pattern of organ injury, resuscitative requirements, and outcome. *J Trauma* 1989;29:981-1000.

Kellam JF, McMurtry RY, Paley D, Tile M: The unstable pelvic fracture: Operative treatment. *Orthop Clin North Am* 1987;18:25-41.

Letournel E: Acetabular fracture: Classification and management. *Clin Orthop* 1980;151:81-106.

Letournel E, Judet R: *Fractures of the Acetabulum*, ed 2. Berlin, Germany, Springer-Verlag, 1993.

Matta JM: Fractures of the acetabulum: Accuracy of reduction and clinical results in-patients managed operatively within three weeks after the injury. *J Bone Joint Surg Am* 1996;78:1632-1645.

Matta JM, Anderson LM, Epstein HC, Hendricks P: Fractures of the acetabulum: A retrospective analysis. *Clin Orthop* 1986;205:230-240.

Matta JM, Siebenrock KA: Does indomethacin reduces heterotopic bone formation after operations for acetabular fractures?: A prospective randomized study. *J Bone Joint Surg Br* 1997;79:959-963.

Routt ML Jr, Simonian PT, Mills WJ: Iliosacral screw fixation: Early complications of the percutaneous technique. *J Orthop Trauma* 1997;11:584-589.

Slatis P, Huittinen VM: Double vertical fractures of the pelvis: A report on 163 patients. *Acta Chir Scand* 1972; 138:799-807.

Tornetta P III, Matta JM: Outcome of operatively treated unstable posterior pelvic ring disruptions. *Clin Orthop* 1996;329:186-193.

Chapter 33

Hip: Trauma

George J. Haidukewych, MD

David J. Jacofsky, MD

Introduction

Fractures and dislocations around the hip remain among the most common injuries and are challenging to treat. With the ever-growing elderly population with osteopenic bone, the number of fractures continues to increase proportionately. Additionally, younger patients may sustain various fractures and dislocations around the hip as a result of high-energy trauma; these injuries can threaten the vascularity of the femoral head and the long-term prognosis of the hip joint.

Hip Dislocations

Hip dislocations typically result from high-energy trauma, such as a motor vehicle accident. Associated injuries are common, and have been reported in more than 70% of patients. Hip dislocations are generally classified as either anterior or posterior. A postreduction 3-mm-cut CT scan is mandatory, even if plain films appear normal. Small osteochondral intra-articular fragments and acetabular and proximal femoral fractures must be excluded by CT scan after closed reduction. If closed reduction cannot be achieved, a CT scan obtained before surgery may guide the surgeon in selecting the surgical approach and evaluating appropriate treatment of associated fractures.

Anterior Hip Dislocations

Anterior hip dislocations are extremely rare. They can be subdivided as superior or inferior in relationship to the pubic ramus; however, treatment is the same. The patient may present with the extremity held in an abducted externally rotated figure-of-4 position after a high-energy injury. Femoral head fractures are commonly associated with anterior hip dislocations and can involve impaction or osteochondral injury of the femoral head on the acetabular rim. Closed reduction requires complete muscle relaxation, traction, extension, and gentle internal rotation. If closed reduction is unsuccessful, then open reduction should be performed, usually through an anterior approach. Forceful closed reduction attempts are not recommended because of the possibility of iatrogenic femoral neck or acetabular fracture.

Posterior Hip Dislocations

Posterior hip dislocations account for most hip dislocations (approximately 90%). These injuries are typically caused by an axial force to the flexed hip, such as the hip striking a dashboard. Bone quality and the position of the limb at the time of impact determines whether an associated acetabular fracture or a simple dislocation occurs. Traumatic posterior hip subluxations, without dislocation, have also been reported with the pathognomonic MRI findings of iliofemoral ligament rupture, hemarthrosis, and marginal posterior acetabular wall avulsion fracture. The treatment of isolated posterior dislocations involves emergent closed reduction or, if necessary, open reduction. Open reduction of irreducible posterior dislocations usually proceeds through the Kocher-Langenbeck approach. Identification and careful protection of the sciatic nerve is recommended because it may be tented by the displaced femoral head. Dislocations with associated posterior wall fractures are treated as indicated based on fragment size, displacement, and hip stability. Postreduction treatment of a simple hip dislocation, regardless of direction, involves early mobilization with gait aids as needed for patient comfort. Patients should avoid hyperflexion of the hip for posterior dislocations and extension and external rotation for anterior dislocations.

Complications

A substantial subset of patients will remain persistently symptomatic after treatment of hip dislocation; however, good to excellent results have been reported in about 70% of patients. Posttraumatic arthritis has been reported in more than 15% of patients in several long-term studies. Osteonecrosis of the femoral head can occur in approximately 10% of hip dislocations. The risk of osteonecrosis increases with the presence of an associated fracture of the acetabulum, probably because of the more extensive soft-tissue injury. Osteonecrosis has also been reported to occur after traumatic hip subluxations. Early reduction of simple dislocations and fracture-dislocations has been suggested to lower the rate of osteonecrosis. Sciatic nerve injuries, most commonly associated with posterior dislocations, have been documented in as many as 8% to 19% of patients.

Femoral Head Fractures

Femoral head fractures have been categorized by Pipkin into four types based on location of the fracture fragment in relation to the fovea centralis and presence of associated fractures. Type 1 fractures are inferior to the fovea, type 2 fractures are superior to the fovea, type 3 also involve a femoral neck fracture, and type 4 also involve a fracture of the acetabulum. Patients with type 1, type 2, and type 4 femoral head fractures should undergo emergent closed reduction of the hip dislocation with postreduction CT scanning to evaluate fracture displacement. In general, femoral head fractures are treated based on fragment location, size, displacement, and hip stability. A nondisplaced or minimally displaced Pipkin type 1 fracture can be managed nonsurgically. Simple excision of a small or comminuted displaced Pipkin type 1 fracture can usually be done because this type of fracture is located below the weight-bearing dome of the femoral head; larger fragments may require surgical fixation. Pipkin type 2 fractures require accurate anatomic reduction and stable internal fixation. Titanium countersunk screw fixation is preferred to allow subsequent MRI if needed. The anterior Smith-Peterson approach is generally preferred because it provides improved visualization for reduction and internal fixation and a lower complication rate as compared with a posterior approach. A trochanteric flip approach may be added. Pipkin type 3 fractures are extremely rare and usually occur in younger patients. These fractures should be treated with internal fixation of the femoral neck and femoral head fracture. In older patients with poor bone quality and low functional demands, prosthetic replacement is probably more predictable and is generally preferred. Pipkin type 4 fractures are treated based on the location of the femoral head fracture and the type of associated acetabular fracture. The most common clinical scenario is a posterior wall acetabular fracture associated with a small, displaced, inferior (infrafoveal) femoral head fracture. This combination of injuries may be treated through a Kocher-Langenbeck approach with excision of the inferior femoral head fragment and simultaneous internal fixation of the posterior acetabular wall fracture. A larger (suprafoveal) femoral head fracture in this situation may require an anterior exposure, for femoral head fracture fixation, and a posterior exposure for posterior acetabular wall fixation or the use of an extensile approach.

Hip Fractures
General Considerations and Risk Factors

Although hip fractures typically occur in elderly, osteopenic patients, often after a low-energy fall, these injuries also occur in younger active patients, usually as a result of high-energy trauma. The number of hip fractures that occur annually continues to rise in proportion to the increasing elderly population. Decision making regarding treatment is based on fracture pattern, patient age, associated injuries, and medical comorbidities.

Clinical and Radiographic Evaluation

In the frail, elderly population with multiple medical comorbidities, preoperative medical evaluation and optimization is important, along with attention to associated injuries that often involve the ipsilateral upper extremity. Elderly patients with hip fractures should be brought to surgery as soon as medically optimal; the benefits of early mobilization cannot be overemphasized. In the younger patient population, life-threatening injuries, if present, should be managed first, and then the hip fracture should be treated in an urgent fashion.

Most hip fractures will be evident on AP and lateral radiographs. However, occult or stress fractures of the femoral neck may require additional imaging studies for diagnosis. MRI can be helpful in not only quickly determining whether a fracture is present but also ruling out other potential causes of hip pain, such as pubic ramus fractures or osteonecrosis. MRI can also provide information about fracture location (femoral neck or intertrochanteric) and fracture verticality. Radionuclide bone scanning can also be useful in this setting, especially if symptoms have been present for several days; however, it cannot provide as much information as MRI.

Femoral Neck Fractures
Classification

Multiple classification schemes for femoral neck fractures exist; the Garden classification is the most common. Although the Garden classification comprises four types, most surgeons group these fractures into those that are displaced (stage III and IV) or nondisplaced (stage I and II) because treatment decisions and prognosis are also grouped in this manner. The Orthopaedic Trauma Association classification has also been used. Although more cumbersome, it distinguishes subcapital, transcervical, and basicervical fractures and also takes into account other potentially important variables such as fracture verticality. The Pauwels' classification has divided femoral neck fractures based on increasing amounts of fracture verticality measured from the horizontal as type 1, less than 30°; type 2, 30° to 50°; and type 3, more than 50°. These fractures are believed to behave in biomechanically distinct ways based on the increase in shear forces imparted at the fracture site by

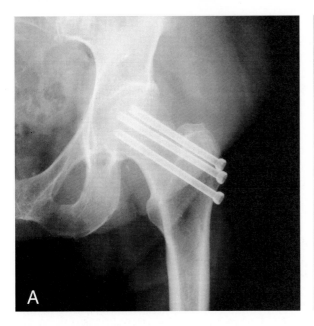 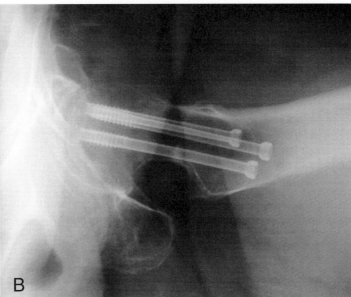

Figure 1 AP view **(A),** and lateral view **(B)** of a valgus impacted femoral neck fracture treated with three cannulated cancellous screws.

increasing degrees of fracture verticality. Some authors have recommended the use of a fixed angle internal fixation device for higher shear angle (more vertical) transcervical and basicervical fractures, and cancellous screws alone for fractures with lower shear angle (more horizontal) transcervical fractures based on this theoretical concern.

Nondisplaced Femoral Neck Fractures

Treatment of nondisplaced fractures is the same regardless of patient age, with internal fixation typically involving multiple parallel cannulated cancellous screws. Nonsurgical treatment is reserved for only the most frail, essentially nonambulatory patients with prohibitive medical comorbidity and minimal discomfort from the injury. Subsequent displacement of nondisplaced or valgus impacted fractures treated nonsurgically has been demonstrated in nearly 40% of patients in a recent series, accompanied by increased rates of osteonecrosis and nonunion. Recent cadaveric data demonstrated superiority of three screws over two screws when used to stabilize subcapital fractures in an inverted triangular configuration. It is important to place the screws near the cortex of the femoral neck to allow host bone to support the shafts of the screws and avoid varus, shortening, and external rotation displacement (Figure 1). Rates of nonunion of less than 5% and osteonecrosis of less than 10% have been reported with this technique. Early postoperative mobilization is encouraged.

Displaced Femoral Neck Fractures: Young Patients

A displaced femoral neck fracture in the young patient should be treated expeditiously. In theory, fracture dis-

placement can kink any vessels that have not been disrupted by the injury. Additionally, intracapsular tamponade can occur because of fracture hematoma that may impede blood flow to the femoral head. Clinical data have documented lower rates of osteonecrosis with early treatment. A gentle closed reduction attempt is reasonable; however, multiple aggressive attempts at closed reduction are not indicated because of potential damage to the remaining femoral head vascularity or potential fracture comminution. If closed reduction is excellent, internal fixation should be performed as fracture pattern (verticality) dictates. If closed reduction cannot be achieved, then open reduction is indicated. No generally accepted guidelines exist on what constitutes an acceptable femoral neck fracture reduction. In general, anatomic reduction is recommended. A slight valgus reduction is acceptable; however, any varus should be avoided. Review of a radiograph of the contralateral hip can assist the surgeon in determining the neck-shaft angle that is anatomic for the patient. Typically the Watson-Jones or Hardinge approaches allow direct visualization of the fracture fragments, anatomic reduction, and internal fixation, usually with multiple parallel cannulated cancellous screws. If the fracture exhibits high verticality and a tendency to shear intraoperatively, screws alone are not recommended and a fixed angle device should be used. In one series, transcervical shear fractures exhibited a high failure rate when treated with screws alone. More data are needed to determine the ideal fixation device for the vertical femoral neck fracture.

The role of capsulotomy in the treatment of femoral neck fractures remains controversial. Original fracture

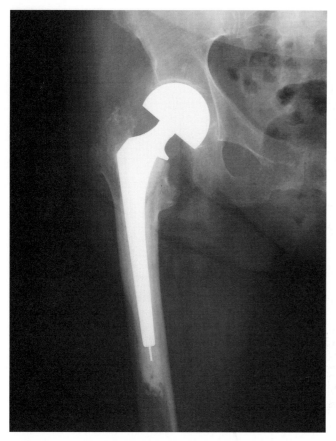

Figure 2 Cemented bipolar hemiarthroplasty.

displacement probably determines the fate of the femoral head. Capsulotomy is recommended because it is relatively simple to perform, exposes the patient to minimal additional risk, and may reduce the intracapsular tamponade effect. In the young patient, efforts are focused on preservation of the femoral head and avoiding arthroplasty at a young age. More data are needed to clearly determine if capsulotomy significantly alters the prognosis for young patients with displaced femoral neck fractures.

Displaced Femoral Neck Fractures: Older Patients

Prosthetic replacement has been favored in the United States for the treatment of displaced femoral neck fractures in older patients because of the challenges of achieving stable proximal fragment fixation in osteopenic bone, the need for a predictable surgery with a low fixation failure rate, and the need for early, full weight-bearing mobilization. A failure rate of nearly 40% has been recently reported in ambulatory elderly patients with displaced femoral neck fractures treated with internal fixation. Fixation failure rates of 30% to 40% have been consistently reported over multiple series over the past few decades. In sharp contrast, multiple series evaluating the outcome of prosthetic replace-

ment in these patients have consistently demonstrated predictable pain relief, functional improvement, and a low revision rate for a patient population that cannot tolerate a prolonged convalescence and multiple surgeries associated with fixation failure. Once prosthetic arthroplasty has been chosen, further controversy surrounds the selection of the type of arthroplasty, unipolar or bipolar, hemiarthroplasty, or total hip arthroplasty, and the type of fixation, cemented or cementless.

Good to excellent results can be expected with either cemented or cementless newer generation arthroplasties. Risks of cementless arthroplasty include femoral fracture, prosthesis subsidence, and anterior thigh pain. Careful attention to accurate prosthetic sizing and appropriate seating on the calcar is essential. Cementation of the prosthesis places the patient at risk for intraoperative death or embolization of marrow content during cementation. This risk may be reduced by canal venting and gentle cement pressurization. The available literature suggests generally better outcomes with cemented arthroplasties. In the nonambulatory patient, when the procedure is performed predominantly for pain control, first-generation cementless (Austin-Moore type) prostheses can be used.

Considerable data exist comparing unipolar with bipolar bearings for elderly patients with displaced femoral neck fractures. Short- to mid-term follow-up studies demonstrate no clear difference in morbidity, mortality, or functional outcome. Longer-term follow-up suggests a lower revision rate for bipolar bearings (Figure 2). This finding is not surprising, because patients who live longer are probably more active, and acetabular erosion is a time-dependent phenomenon. More data are needed to clearly determine the long-term superiority of one design over the other.

Total hip arthroplasty has been classically recommended for patients with displaced fractures and symptomatic ipsilateral degenerative change of the hip. This combination of pathology, however, is very rare. Recent studies have expanded the indications to include active elderly patients with displaced femoral neck fractures and otherwise normal hip joints because of the more predictable pain relief and better function total hip arthroplasty provides, when compared with hemiarthroplasty. The main complication of hip arthroplasty performed in this setting is dislocation, with rates averaging 10% across multiple series. Of those hips that dislocate, approximately 25% have recurrent dislocation. A recent meta-analysis demonstrated a mean dislocation rate approximately seven times greater for total hip arthroplasty compared with hemiarthroplasty in this setting. Considering the large number of patients with displaced femoral neck fractures treated annually, the potential societal and economic impact of such dislocations can be substantial. Use of the anterolateral approach decreases the dislocation rates as does the selective use of

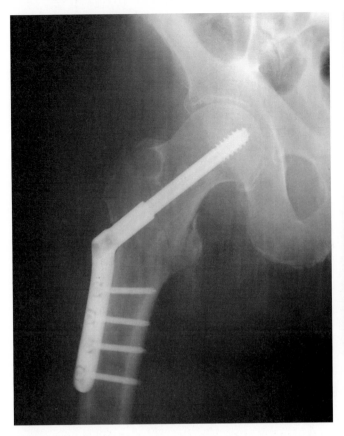

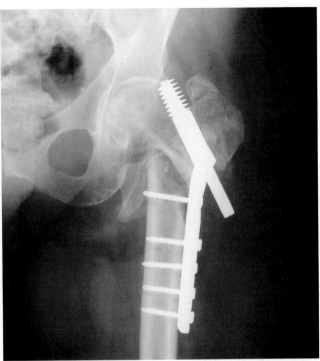

Figure 4 Failed fixation and cut-out of a reverse obliquity fracture treated with a sliding hip screw.

Figure 3 A well-placed sliding hip screw with deep and central position of the lag screw into the femoral head.

larger diameter femoral heads, and should be considered when performing total hip arthroplasty in this setting.

Complications

Nonunion is rare in the younger patient, with most series reporting nonunion rates of less than 10%. Secondary surgeries such as valgus-producing osteotomies are successful in ultimately achieving union, probably because of the excellent bone stock and healing potential in the young patient. Valgus intertrochanteric osteotomies convert the shear forces of a vertical fracture line to compressive forces by increasing fracture horizontality. Nonunion is more common in the older patient, with rates averaging less than 5% for nondisplaced fractures and to over 30% for displaced fractures. Nonunion in the older patient is typically treated with hip arthroplasty.

Rates of posttraumatic osteonecrosis have averaged 10% for nondisplaced fractures and 25% for displaced fractures. Not all patients with osteonecrosis will be symptomatic and require further treatment. The treatment of symptomatic posttraumatic osteonecrosis varies with patient age and osteonecrosis grade.

Intertrochanteric Hip Fractures
Classification

Various classifications for intertrochanteric fractures have been proposed, but none has been widely accepted. Commonly, fractures are described by the number of "parts" and the presence of certain fracture characteristics that indicate greater instability. For example, a large posteromedial fragment, a reverse obliquity configuration, or subtrochanteric extension are commonly considered fracture features that result in more "unstable" fractures. Intertrochanteric fractures are treated similarly regardless of patient age. Choice of internal fixation device should be based on fracture pattern.

Sliding Hip Screw

The most important variables under a surgeon's control when treating an intertrochanteric hip fracture include correct device selection based on fracture pattern, accurate reduction, and placement of the lag screw into the center of the femoral head. Most intertrochanteric fractures can be treated successfully with a sliding hip screw. This device offers the advantages of a simple, predictable surgical technique, and a long clinical history of successful results. An increasing rate of failure and hardware cutout with poor implant placement or poor reduction has been documented. The tip to apex distance has been described as a guide to accurate screw placement, and should be less than 25 mm. Ideally, a center-center position with the lag screw within 1 cm of the

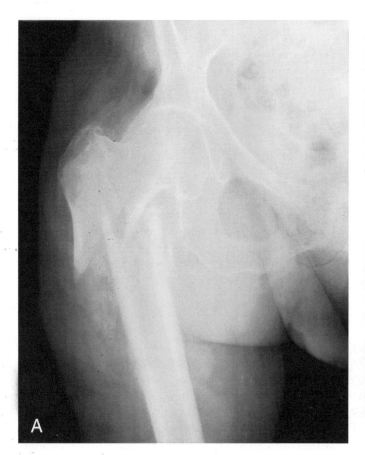

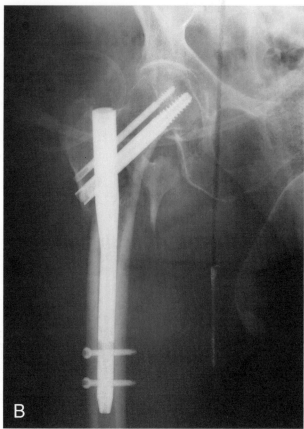

Figure 5 A, Four-part comminuted intertrochanteric fracture with reverse obliquity. **B,** Postoperative view after treatment with an intramedullary hip screw.

subchondral bone on both AP and lateral views is preferred (Figure 3). The sliding hip screw should never be used for fractures with reverse obliquity, because in this situation this device does not allow controlled collapse and fracture compression, but allows shear across the fracture site with medial displacement of the distal fragment, excessive sliding, and eventual lag screw cutout (Figure 4). In one series, a 56% failure rate was noted for reverse obliquity fractures treated with a sliding hip screw. For intertrochanteric fractures with reverse obliquity, either a 95° fixed angle device (such as the 95° dynamic condylar screw and the condylar blade plate) or a cephalomedullary device is recommended. A recent prospective randomized series documented superior outcomes of intramedullary techniques over a 95° dynamic condylar screw (Figure 5).

Studies have compared the results of sliding hip screws with two-hole sideplates to conventional four-hole sideplates for both stable and unstable fractures. No difference in clinical outcomes was noted. The shorter sideplates offer the advantage of less soft-tissue dissection. Newly designed percutaneously applied plates have not demonstrated a clear advantage over traditional open sliding hip screw techniques in early studies.

Intramedullary Devices

Multiple randomized, nonrandomized, prospective, and retrospective studies have compared intramedullary devices with sliding hip screws for the fixation of intertrochanteric fractures. Although the concept of treating these fractures through small incisions and avoiding the usually bloody dissection of the vastus lateralis necessary for sideplate placement is appealing, the literature has not demonstrated the clear advantage of intramedullary devices to justify their routine use. In earlier series that evaluated outdated nail designs, higher complication rates, including iatrogenic femur fractures, were reported. Contemporary intramedullary implant designs have addressed many of these concerns and may allow more minimally invasive fracture management techniques. A recent prospective, randomized series of 400 patients comparing the redesigned gamma nail to a sliding hip screw demonstrated a higher (but not statistically significant) rate of complications with the gamma nail. The authors concluded that the routine use of the gamma nail cannot be recommended. Currently, intramedullary devices may be most suitable for fractures with reverse obliquity or high subtrochanteric or intertrochanteric fractures with subtrochanteric extension. More data are needed to define which fractures derive the most benefit from intramedullary fixation and whether further design refinements will decrease the number of complications noted in earlier series, thereby making intramedullary fixation more widely applicable.

Primary Prosthetic Replacement

The role of primary prosthetic replacement for intertrochanteric fractures remains controversial. The potential advantages of primary prosthetic replacement in the face of an unstable intertrochanteric fracture in a patient with severely osteopenic bone include relatively predictable pain relief, early mobilization, and the fact that revision rates may be lower. The disadvantages include the more extensive nature of the surgical procedure, the frequent necessity to use calcar replacing, long-stem cemented implants in medically frail patients, and the fact that often comminuted, osteopenic trochanteric fragments need to be stabilized with some form of internal fixation. It should be noted from the literature that the overwhelming majority of well-reduced intertrochanteric hip fractures treated with properly selected and accurately implanted internal fixation devices will heal predictably without complication. Additionally, should failure occur, prosthetic replacement for salvage of failed internal fixation has demonstrated excellent durability and predictable pain relief. Prosthetic replacement as the acute treatment of intertrochanteric fractures should be reserved for patients with pathologic fractures as a result of neoplasm, neglected fractures with deformity and poor bone stock precluding internal fixation, or for patients in whom internal fixation attempts have failed. Additionally, prosthetic replacement may be a reasonable therapeutic option for patients with severe ipsilateral symptomatic degenerative joint disease, or certain unfavorable fracture patterns associated with poor bone quality.

Subtrochanteric Fractures

The subtrochanteric area of the femur experiences some of the highest biomechanical stresses in the human body. In general, the subtrochanteric region is considered the anatomic region immediately below the lesser trochanter to the proximal aspect of the femoral isthmus. Various classification systems, including the Russell-Taylor classification, have been proposed based on the location of the fracture relative to the lesser trochanter and the presence of the fracture line extension into the piriformis fossa. More proximal subtrochanteric fractures often involve extension of the fracture line into the piriformis fossa, which influences internal fixation device selection. Multiple fixation methods have been described, including the use of the sliding hip screw, dynamic condylar screw, or angled blade plate for more proximal (high) subtrochanteric fractures, and interlocking cephalomedullary nailing for more distal

(low) subtrochanteric fractures. In general, if the piriformis fossa is intact, a nailing technique is preferred. If the lesser trochanter is intact and the proximal fragment is of sufficient length, then fixation into the femoral head is usually not necessary and a standard antegrade nail with locking into the lesser trochanter is adequate. With shorter proximal fragments without piriformis fossa involvement, cephalomedullary reconstruction nailing with interlocking screw fixation into the femoral head and neck is preferred. A preoperative CT scan may be helpful to evaluate the integrity of the proximal fragment when plain radiographs are difficult to interpret because of factors such as patient size or proximal fragment rotation. If plating techniques are chosen for comminuted fractures, the vascularity of the medial bony fragments should be carefully preserved by avoiding dissection and periosteal stripping in this region. Areas of comminution should be bridged and stable proximal and distal fixation should be obtained while maintaining correct limb alignment, length, and rotation. Such indirect reduction techniques have demonstrated high union rates but are technically demanding. Although plating techniques are associated with potentially lower rates of malalignment, dissection and blood loss can be substantial. Biomechanically, intramedullary fixation of subtrochanteric fractures is generally preferred. Nails provide load-sharing stability that allows early postoperative weight bearing that plated fractures typically cannot tolerate. This condition may be advantageous in multiple trauma patients with other extremity injuries. Nailing short subtrochanteric fractures can be challenging because of the flexed, abducted, and externally rotated position of the proximal fragment. Great care should be taken to avoid varus proximal fragment malalignment, which can occur with conventional antegrade nails placed through a starting point that is too lateral. The use of newer nails designed for entry through the tip of the greater trochanter may facilitate access to the intramedullary canal and result in less potential malalignment for these challenging fractures; however, there are few data to substantiate this speculation.

Pathologic Fractures of the Proximal Femur

Metastatic disease commonly involves the proximal femur, affecting the femoral neck in 50%, subtrochanteric region in 30%, and intertrochanteric region in 20%. Decision making regarding whether some form of prophylactic internal fixation or hip arthroplasty is appropriate is based on the anatomic location of the lesion, size of the lesion, the extent of bony destruction, and anticipated life expectancy of the patient. In general, lesions that cause more than 50% destruction of a cortex or those that present with functional pain should be stabilized. Complete fractures should be treated surgically in all but the most infirm patients. High-quality preoperative radiographs of the acetabulum and entire length of the femur are mandatory to evaluate for ipsilateral lesions. Other sites of bony pain should also be evaluated by plain films and bone scintigraphy. Appropriate preoperative workup in consultation with an oncologist is recommended. A fracture resulting from a solitary pathologic lesion of the proximal femur requires a pathologic tissue diagnosis before internal fixation or prosthetic replacement, even in a patient with a history of cancer. These preoperative studies will help avoid the rare, but potentially disastrous complication of internal fixation of a primary malignancy. If necessary, a CT scan of the proximal femur and the acetabulum can be obtained to further evaluate for proximal lesions. The entire femur should be protected by the internal fixation device, typically a third-generation cephalomedullary nail. Lesion debulking and methacrylate augmentation of the fixation construct may be necessary for larger lesions. If extensive involvement of the proximal femur precludes predictable and durable internal fixation, then prosthetic replacement can provide functional improvement and pain relief in this cohort. Modular, so-called tumor prostheses are available to manage bony deficiency and restore leg length and hip stability. Pathologic fractures of the femoral neck, head, and intertrochanteric region often require treatment with prosthetic replacement. Medical comorbidities are quite common and multidisciplinary management with a medical oncologist, radiation oncologist, or nutritionist is recommended. Postoperative radiation to the entire construct and surgical bed, after the surgical wound has healed, is recommended to minimize the chance of tumor progression and implant failure. Should fixation failure occur, conversion to hip arthroplasty has been shown to predictably improve function and relieve pain; however, these reconstructions are plagued by a high rate of postoperative infection.

Annotated Bibliography

Hip Dislocations and Femoral Head Fractures

Ganz R, Gill TJ, Gautier E, Ganz K, Krugel N, Berlemann U: Surgical dislocation of the adult hip: A technique with full access to the femoral head and acetabulum without the risk of avascular necrosis. *J Bone Joint Surg Br* 2001;83:1119-1124.

The authors describe a safe surgical approach for hip dislocation in 213 hips with no avascular necrosis. This approach, known as the trochanteric flip, is useful for multiple degenerative and traumatic disorders of the hip joint.

Moorman CT III, Warren RF, Hershman EB, et al: Traumatic posterior hip subluxation in American football. *J Bone Joint Surg Am* 2003;85:1190-1196.

The authors discuss the clinical presentation, MRI findings, suggested treatment, and outcomes of eight football play-

ers with traumatic hip subluxation. Two of eight patients developed osteonecrosis and required total hip arthroplasty.

Sahin V, Karakas ES, Aksu S, Atlihan D, Turk CY, Halici M: Traumatic dislocation and fracture-dislocation of the hip: A long term follow-up study. *J Trauma* 2003;54:520-529.

Forty-seven patients with hip dislocation and fracture-dislocation were followed for a mean of 9.6 years. Seventy-one percent had medium to very good results. Sixteen percent developed posttraumatic degenerative joint disease, and 9.6% developed osteonecrosis. Early reduction improved outcomes.

Femoral Neck Fractures

Bartonicek J: Pauwels' classification of femoral neck fractures: Correct interpretation of the original. *J Orthop Trauma 2001*; 15:358-360.

This article discusses Pauwels' classification and gives the correct interpretation of the values.

Bhandari M, Devereaux PJ, Swiontkowski MF, et al: Internal fixation compared with arthroplasty for displaced fractures of the femoral neck: A meta-analysis. *J Bone Joint Surg Am* 2003;85:1673-1681.

The authors evaluated published trials between 1969 and 2002 on the treatment of displaced femoral neck fractures in patients age 65 years or older. Arthroplasty provided a significantly lower rate of revision surgery ($P = 0.0003$) but was associated with greater blood loss, longer surgical time, and a trend toward higher mortality in the first 4 months after surgery (not significant).

Haidukewych GJ, Israel TA, Berry DJ: Long-term survivorship of cemented bipolar hemiarthroplasty for fracture of the femoral neck. *Clin Orthop* 2002;403:118-126.

The results of 212 patients older than age 60 years treated with cemented bipolar hemiarthroplasty are reported. Overall 10-year survivorship free of reoperation for any reason was 94%. Only one patient was revised for acetabular cartilage wear. More than 90% of patients had no or minimal pain at follow-up, and the dislocation rate was less than 2%.

Jain R, Koo M, Kreder HJ, Schemitsch EH, Davey JR, Mahomed NN: Comparison of early and delayed fixation of subcapital hip fractures in patients sixty years of age or less. *J Bone Joint Surg Am* 2002;84:1605-1612.

Delayed treatment of subcapital fractures was associated with a higher rate of osteonecrosis; however, this complication did not significantly affect functional outcome at follow-up.

Keating JF, Masson M, Scott N, et al: Randomized trial of reduction and fixation versus bipolar hemiarthroplasty versus total hip arthroplasty for displaced subcapital fractures in the fit older patient. *70th Annual Meeting Proceedings.*, Rosemont, IL, American Academy of Orthopaedic Surgeons, 2003, p 96.

The authors demonstrate superior functional outcomes for fractures treated with total hip arthroplasty when compared with open reduction and internal fixation or hemiarthroplasty.

Maurer SG, Wright KE, Kummer FJ, Zuckerman JD, Koval KJ: Two or three screws for fixation of femoral neck fractures? *Am J Orthop* 2003;32:438-442.

Three screws demonstrated less fracture displacement than two screws in axial loading in embalmed cadaveric specimens with subcapital osteotomies.

McKinley JC, Robinson CM: Treatment of displaced intracapsular hip fractures with total hip arthroplasty: Comparison of primary arthroplasty with early salvage arthroplasty after failed internal fixation. *J Bone Joint Surg Am* 2002;84:2010-2015.

The authors found better outcomes and fewer complications with primary arthroplasty than when arthroplasty was performed after internal fixation failure in a matched pair case-controlled study.

Ong BC, Maurer SG, Aharonoff GB, Zuckerman JD, Koval KJ: Unipolar versus bipolar hemiarthroplasty: Functional outcome after femoral neck fracture at a minimum of thirty-six months of follow-up. *J Orthop Trauma* 2002;16:317-322.

No difference in functional outcome at midterm follow-up was noted between unipolar and bipolar cemented hemiarthroplasties.

Rogmark C, Carlsson A, Johnell O, Sernbo I: Primary hemiarthroplasty in old patients with displaced femoral neck fracture: A 1-year follow-up of 103 patients aged 80 years or more. *Acta Orthop Scand* 2002;73:605-610.

Treatment with primary hemiarthroplasty showed a lower failure rate than treatment with internal fixation. There was no difference in length of hospital stay or mortality.

Sharif KM, Parker MJ: Austin Moore hemiarthroplasty: Technical aspects and their effects on outcome, in patients with fractures of the neck of femur. *Injury* 2002; 33:419-422.

This retrospective study evaluated radiographic findings with outcomes and revision rates for 243 patients with a mean age of 81 years treated with Austin-Moore hemiarthroplasty. Undersizing of the prosthetic head and poor seating of the prosthesis on the calcar were associated with loosening and residual pain.

Tanaka J, Seki N, Tokimura F, Hayashi Y: Conservative treatment of Garden stage I femoral neck fracture in elderly patients. *Arch Orthop Trauma Surg* 2002;122: 24-28.

Nonsurgical treatment of Garden stage I femoral neck fractures showed a 39% nonunion rate.

Intertrochanteric Hip Fractures

Adams CI, Robinson CM, Court-Brown CM, McQueen MM: Prospective randomized controlled trial of an intramedullary nail versus dynamic screw and plate for intertrochanteric fractures of the femur. *J Orthop Trauma* 2001;15:394-400.

Four hundred patients were randomized for either a sliding hip screw or a gamma nail. The group with the gamma nail had a higher rate of reoperations and complications. The authors concluded that the routine use of an intramedullary device is not recommended.

Haidukewych GJ, Berry DJ: Hip arthroplasty for salvage of failed treatment of intertrochanteric hip fractures. *J Bone Joint Surg Am* 2003;85:899-904.

The durability and predictable functional improvement of hip arthroplasty for failed treatment of intertrochanteric fractures is documented in 60 patients. Long-stem, calcar-replacing prostheses are commonly required. The greater trochanter was a persistent source of discomfort in a substantial subset of patients.

Haidukewych GJ, Israel TA, Berry DJ: Reverse obliquity of fractures of the intertrochanteric region of the femur. *J Bone Joint Surg Am* 2001;83:643-650.

The authors demonstrated a 56% failure rate when the sliding hip screw was used for a reverse obliquity fracture. The 95° blade plate had the lowest failure rate. Few patients were treated with intramedullary fixation during the study period. The authors concluded that the sliding hip screw is contraindicated for reverse obliquity fractures.

Janzig HM, Howben BJ, Brandt SE, et al: The Gotfried Percutaneous Compression Plate versus the Dynamic Hip Screw in the treatment of peritrochanteric hip fractures: Minimal invasive treatment reduces operative time and postoperative pain. *J Trauma* 2002;52:293-298.

One hundred fifteen patients randomized to either the percutaneous compression plate or a sliding hip screw were reviewed. The patients with the percutaneous plate had a lower surgical time and less pain, but more mechanical complications.

Kosygan KP, Mohan R, Newman RJ: The Gotfried percutaneous compression plate compared with the conventional classic hip screw for the fixation of intertrochanteric fractures of the hip. *J Bone Joint Surg Br* 2002; 84:19-22.

One hundred eleven patients were prospectively randomized to the percutaneous compression plate or a sliding hip screw. The percutaneous compression plate was associated with less blood loss and fewer transfusions, but longer surgical time. There was no difference in the number of complications or fracture healing.

Sadowski C, Lubbeke A, Saudan M, Riand N, Stern R, Hoffmeyer P: Treatment of reverse oblique and transverse intertrochanteric fractures with use of an intramedullary nail or a 95 degree screw-plate: A prospective, randomized study. *J Bone Joint Surg Am* 2002;84:372-381.

    Intramedullary fixation demonstrated a lower rate of fixation failure than the 95° dynamic condylar screw.

Subtrochanteric Fractures

Vaidya SV, Dholakia DB, Chatterjee A: The use of a dynamic condylar screw and biologic reduction techniques for subtrochanteric femur fractures. *Injury* 2003;34:123-128.

    Thirty-one patients were treated with indirect reduction techniques. The authors reported a 100% union rate; 6.4% of patients had a malunion.

Classic Bibliography

Alho A, Benterud JG, Solovieva S: Internally fixed femoral neck fractures: Early prediction of failure in 203 elderly patients with displaced fractures. *Acta Orthop Scand* 1999;70:141-144.

Asnis SE, Wanek-Sgaglione L: Intracapsular fractures of the femoral neck: Results of cannulated screw fixation. *J Bone Joint Surg Am* 1994;76:1793-1803.

Barquet A, Francescoli L, Rienzi D, Lopez L: Intertrochanteric-subtrochanteric fractures: Treatment with the long Gamma nail. *J Orthop Trauma* 2000;14:324-328.

Baumgaertner MR, Curtin SL, Lindskog DM, Keggi JM: The value of the tip-apex distance in predicting failure of fixation of peritrochanteric fractures of the hip. *J Bone Joint Surg Am* 1995;77:1058-1064.

Booth KC, Donaldson TK, Dai QG: Femoral neck fracture fixation: A biomechanical study of two cannulated screw placement techniques. *Orthopedics* 1998;21:1173-1176.

Calder SJ, Anderson GH, Jagger C, Harper WM, Gregg PJ: Unipolar or bipolar prosthesis for displaced intracapsular hip fracture in octogenarians: A randomized prospective study. *J Bone Joint Surg Br* 1996;78:391-394.

Chua D, Jaglal SB, Schatzker J: Predictors of early failure of fixation in the treatment of displaced subcapital hip fractures. *J Orthop Trauma* 1998;12:230-234.

Dreinhofer KE, Schwarzkopf SR, Haas NP, et al: Isolated traumatic dislocation of the hip: Long-term results in 50 patients. *J Bone Joint Surg Br* 1994;76:6-12.

Garden RS: Malreduction and avascular necrosis in subcapital fractures of the femur. *J Bone Joint Surg Br* 1971;53:183-197.

Hammer AJ: Nonunion of the subcapital femoral neck fracture. *J Orthop Trauma* 1992;6:73-77.

Kinast C, Bolhofner BR, Mast JW, Ganz R: Subtrochanteric fractures of the femur: Results of treatment with the 95 degree condylar blade plate. *Clin Orthop* 1989;238:122-130.

Koval KJ, Sala DA, Kummer FJ, Zuckerman JD: Postoperative weight-bearing after a fracture of the femoral neck or an intertrochanteric fracture. *J Bone Joint Surg Am* 1998;80:352-356.

Kyle RF, Gustilo RB, Premer RF: Analysis of six hundred and twenty-two intertrochanteric hip fractures. *J Bone Joint Surg Am* 1979;61:216-221.

Lee BP, Berry DJ, Harmsen WS, Sim FH: Total hip arthroplasty for the treatment of an acute fracture of the femoral neck: Long-term results. *J Bone Joint Surg Am* 1998;80:70-75.

Lu-Yao GL, Keller RB, Littenberg B, Wennberg JE: Outcomes after displaced fractures of the femoral neck: A meta-analysis of one hundred and six published reports. *J Bone Joint Surg Am* 1994;76:15-25.

Marchetti ME, Steinberg GG, Coumas JM: Intermediate-term experience of Pipkin fracture-dislocations of the hip. *J Orthop Trauma* 1996;10:455-461.

Maruenda JI, Barrios C, Gomar-Sancho F: Intracapsular hip pressure after femoral neck fracture. *Clin Orthop* 1997;340:172-180.

Parker MJ, Blundell C: Choice of implant for internal fixation of femoral neck fractures: Meta-analysis of 25 randomised trials including 4,925 patients. *Acta Orthop Scand* 1998;69:138-143.

Parker MJ, Pryor GA: Gamma versus DHS nailing for extracapsular femoral fractures: Meta-analysis of ten randomised trials. *Int Orthop* 1996;20:163-168.

Pipkin G: Treatment of grade IV fracture-dislocation of the hip: A review. *J Bone Joint Surg Am* 1957;39:1027-1042.

Robinson CM, Saran D, Annan IH: Intracapsular hip fractures: Results of management adopting a treatment protocol. *Clin Orthop* 1994;302:83-91.

Russell TA, Taylor JC: Subtrochanteric fractures of the femur, in Browner BD, Jupiter JB, Levine AM, Trafton PG (eds): *Skeletal Trauma*, ed. 2. Philadelphia, PA, WB Saunders, 1997.

Sanders R, Regazzoni P: Treatment of subtrochanteric femur fractures using the dynamic condylar screw. *J Orthop Trauma* 1989;3:206-213.

Siebenrock KA, Muller U, Ganz R: Indirect reduction with a condylar blade plate for osteosynthesis of subtrochanteric femoral fractures. *Injury* 1998;29(suppl 3):C7-C15.

Stannard JP, Harris HW, Volgas DA, Alonso JE: Functional outcome of patients with femoral head fractures associated with hip dislocations. *Clin Orthop* 2000;377:44-56.

Stewart MJ, Milford LW: Fracture-dislocation of the hip: An end-result study. *J Bone Joint Surg Am* 1954;36:315-342.

Swiontkowski MF, Thorpe M, Seiler JG, et al: Operative management of displaced femoral head fractures: Case-matched comparison of anterior versus posterior approaches for Pipkin I and Pipkin II fractures. *J Orthop Trauma* 1992;6:437-442.

Thompson VP, Epstein HC: Traumatic dislocation of the hip: A survey of two hundred and four cases covering a period of twenty-one years. *J Bone Joint Surg Am* 1951;33:746-778.

Upadhyay SS, Moulton A, Srikrishnamurthy K: An analysis of the late effects of traumatic posterior dislocation of the hip without fractures. *J Bone Joint Surg Br* 1983;65:150-157.

van Doorn R, Stopert JW: The long Gamma nail in the treatment of 329 subtrochanteric fractures with major extension into the femoral shaft. *Eur J Surg* 2000;166:240-246.

Wiss DA, Brien WW: Subtrochanteric fractures of the femur: Results of treatment by interlocking nailing. *Clin Orthop* 1992;283:231-236.

Chapter 34

Hip, Pelvic Reconstruction, and Arthroplasty

Javad Parvizi, MD, FRCS

James J. Purtill, MD

Scope of Pathology

With the increasing life span of the general population, the incidence of osteoarthritis (OA) of the hip is on the rise. More than 300,000 joint arthroplasties are currently performed annually in the Unites States. By year 2030, this number is expected to exceed 1 million. The two major categories of conditions that give rise to OA of the hip are dysplasia and nondysplasia. Dysplasia, commonly with anterolateral deficiency, may account for up to 40% of OA cases in the United States and over 80% of OA cases in Japan and Italy. In a distinct category of patients, there is no identifiable cause for OA, or so-called idiopathic arthritis. There is emerging evidence that subtle morphologic abnormalities around the hip, resulting in femoroacetabular impingement, may be a contributing factor in many instances.

Clinical Evaluation

The evaluation of a patient with hip pain should begin with a thorough history. It is particularly important to confirm or rule out the hip as the cause of the patient's symptoms. Various intra-abdominal, spinal, and other pathologies may present as hip pain. True hip pain usually presents in the groin, anterior thigh, buttock, or even the knee region. As part of the history, the suitability of the patient for surgical intervention should be determined. Physical examination of the patient includes assessment of gait, limb length, and range of motion, palpation of various regions around the hip, and a complete neurovascular examination. The skin should be examined to ensure no sources of infection exist. Provocative tests such as the impingement test (pain with flexion, adduction, and internal rotation), apprehension test (feeling of the hip popping out of the socket with extension: sign of anterior deficiency), Patrick test (groin pain with hip in figure-of-4 position), and Stinchfield test (pain during resisted straight leg raise) are indicative of hip pathology.

Radiographic Examination

A good quality AP radiograph of the pelvis and AP and lateral radiographs of the hip should be ordered as part of the initial evaluation. The radiographs should be examined for evidence of arthritis, fracture, osteonecrosis, and other morphologic abnormalities that could account for the patient's symptoms. Signs of dysplasia should also be sought (Figure 1).

Subtle signs of dysplasia include isolated anterior acetabular deficiency (often missed), overloading of the rim (os acetabuli or hypertrophic labrum), and rim ossification (double shadow on AP radiograph). An estimate of acetabular version can be determined by defining the outline of the posterior and anterior walls (Figure 2). In a normal anteverted acetabulum the anterior wall lies medial to the posterior wall and does not cross it. Retroversion is characterized by crossover of the anterior and posterior wall markings on a true AP radiograph (coccyx pointing toward the symphysis pubis with a distance of 1 to 2 cm between them).

Functional views with the hip in abduction or adduction should be considered before redirectional osteotomies are performed. Cross-sectional studies may be ordered to define the extent of a particular pathology or confirm its presence. CT is useful for defining bony anatomy and has an invaluable role in the evaluation of pelvic fracture. MRI can be useful for confirmation of osteonecrosis or transient osteoporosis, and when combined with gadolinium arthrogram it is useful for evaluating labral pathology. Imaging of the articular cartilage remains inadequate at present. Patients with dysplasia often have a hypertrophic labrum. Labral tears are common in patients with femoroacetabular impingement (Figure 3).

Femoroacetabular Impingement

The widely accepted theory implicating axial overload for the onset of OA of the hip fails to provide a satisfac-

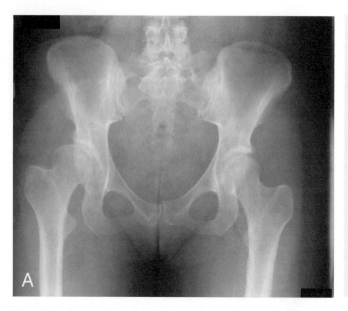

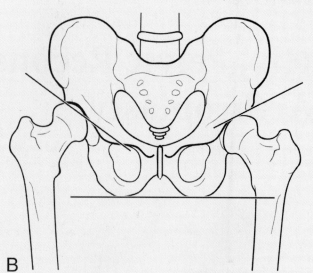

Figure 1 A, AP radiograph of a patient with dysplasia of the right hip. Note the superior inclination of the weight-bearing region (high Tonnis angle), lateralized hip center of rotation, anterolateral deficiency of the femoral head coverage, and coxa valga. **B,** A schematic presentation of the same hip demonstrating the various radiographic measurements that can be used to evaluate dysplasia.

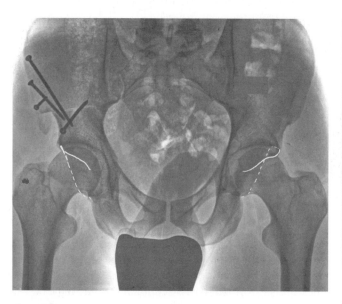

Figure 2 AP radiograph of a patient with bilateral acetabular retroversion is evident by the crossover (Reynolds) sign of the anterior and posterior walls on the left side. The patient has undergone reverse periacetabular osteotomy to correct the retroversion. Note that the anterior and posterior wall marking meet at the point of sourcil and do not cross.

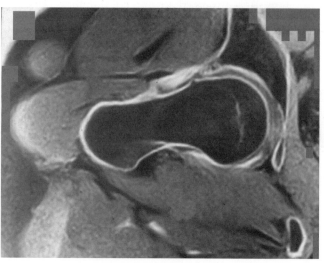

Figure 3 The magnetic resonance arthrogram shows the labral destruction and a secondary ossicle on the femoral neck that resulted from linear contact between the femoral neck and the acetabular rim during flexion (femoroacetabular impingement).

tory explanation for development of arthritis in young patients with apparently normal skeletal structures and intra-articular pressures. Femoroacetabular impingement has been proposed as a possible etiologic mechanism for the development of OA in this patient group. The condition occurs either as a result of morphologic abnormality involving the femur (cam) (Figure 4), the acetabulum (pincer) (Figure 5), or both. Excessive and supraphysiologic demand on the hip may precipitate

symptoms. The abnormal contact between the femoral neck and acetabular rim leads to labral injury, particularly in the anterosuperior zone of the acetabulum (Figure 4). The labral tear as seen on arthroscopy or magnetic resonance arthrogram is frequently accompanied by chondral damage. The typical patient with femoroacetabular impingement is young and has groin pain that is exacerbated by activity or long periods of sitting (such as while driving). Examination of the hip often reveals limitation of motion, particularly internal rotation and abduction in flexion. The impingement test, which is almost always positive, is performed with the patient supine. The

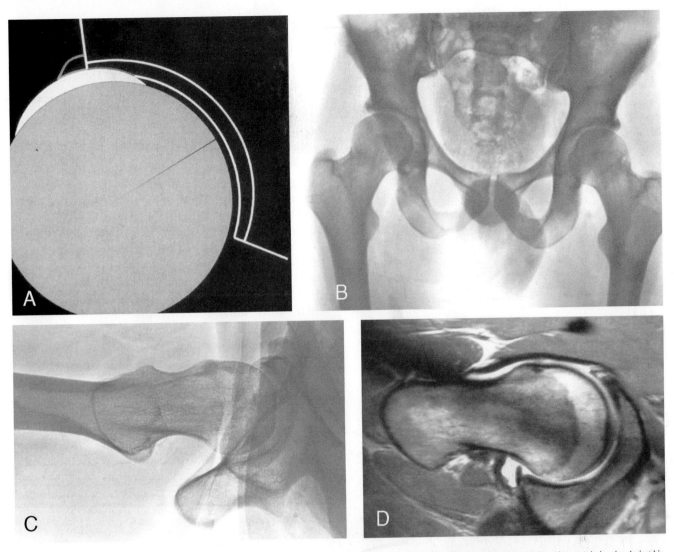

Figure 4 A, Schematic presentation shows the mechanism for cam impingement when nonspherical portion of the femoral head abuts against the acetabular rim during hip flexion. **B,** The AP radiograph appears normal. **C,** The nonspherical femoral head leading to reduced offset at the neck and predisposition to cam-type impingement is visible on the lateral radiograph. **D,** The magnetic resonance arthrogram confirms labral tear and chondral injury resulting from impingement. *(Reproduced with permission from Ganz R, Parvizi J, Beck M, Leunig M, Nötzli H, Siebenrock KA: Femoroacetabular impingement: A cause for osteoarthritis of the hip. Clin Orthop 2003;417:112-120.)*

hip is internally rotated as it is passively flexed to about 90° and adducted. Flexion and adduction lead to the approximation of the femoral neck and the acetabular rim. Forceful additional internal rotation creates a sharp pain when there is a chondral and/or labral lesion.

The radiographs often appear normal at first glance. However, upon detailed review some abnormalities may become apparent. This includes the presence of a bony prominence usually in the anterolateral head and neck junction that is best seen on lateral radiographs (Figure 4, *C*), reduced anterior offset of the femoral neck and head junction, and changes on the acetabular rim such as os acetabuli or double line that are seen with rim ossification. Close scrutiny of the femoral neck may reveal the presence of 'a herniation pit' that is indicative of impingement. Morphologic changes affecting the acetabulum and/or the proximal femur such as retroversion, rel-

ative anterior overcoverage, coxa profunda, protrusio acetabuli, coxa vara, or extreme coxa valga may only become apparent upon systematic examination of the plain radiographs. Magnetic resonance arthrogram using radial sequences is very useful for diagnosis. If conservative treatment is unsuccessful, femoroacetabular impingement can be treated by surgical dislocation of the hip and improvement of femoral head-neck contour. The acetabular rim can also be trimmed. A reverse periacetabular osteotomy may be performed in patients with excessive retroversion and inadequate posterior coverage (posterior rim lies medial to a vertical line drawn through the center of the head).

Hip Arthroscopy

Hip arthroscopy is being used more often for diagnostic as well as therapeutic treatment of intra-articular pa-

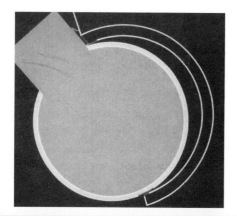

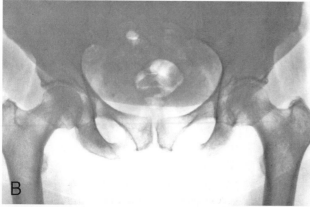

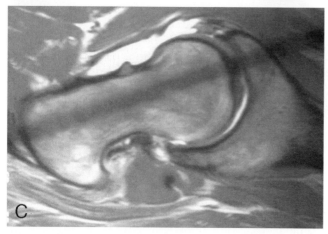

Figure 5 A, Schematic presentation shows the mechanism of pincer impingement that arises from linear contact between the acetabular rim and the femoral head-neck junction. **B,** The femoral head may have normal morphologic features and the impingement is the result of acetabular abnormality (overcoverage, rim ossification, retroversion). **C,** The first structure to fail in this situation is the acetabular labrum as seen on the magnetic resonance arthrogram. The persistent anterior abutment with chronic leverage of the head in the acetabulum may result in chondral injury in the posteroinferior acetabulum. Note the prominence on the femoral neck that is the result of persistent impingement of the neck against deep acetabulum. *(Reproduced with permission from Ganz R, Parvizi J, Beck M, Leunig M, Nötzli H, Siebenrock KA: Femoroacetabular impingement: A cause for osteoarthritis of the hip. Clin Orthop 2003;417:112-120.)*

thology of the hip. Indications include loose bodies, acetabular labral tears, cartilage flaps, and synovitis.

Standard radiographs are unable to adequately detect acetabular labral tears and other subtle intra-

articular hip pathology. MRI as well as magnetic resonance arthrogram of the hip improves diagnostic ability. In addition, hip arthroscopy may be used diagnostically in patients with mechanical symptoms or suspected intra-articular pathology.

Hip arthroscopy may be performed with the patient supine or in a lateral decubitis position. Three portals, anterior, anterolateral, and posterolateral, have been described. Access to the hip joint is accomplished by the use of cannulated trochars. Traction is applied to the leg undergoing surgery with the use of a fracture table. A well-padded peroneal post minimizes risk to the peroneal structures, especially the pudendal nerve. Fluoroscopy is necessary for proper cannula placement.

Acetabular labral tears are the most common indication for hip arthroscopy. These may result from an acute hyperflexion or twisting injury to the hip. In addition to acute injuries, acetabular labral pathology may be associated with early degenerative arthritis. Arthritic changes of the anterosuperior region of the acetabulum may be associated with detachment of the labrum from this region of the joint.

Patients with labral tears typically have intermittent groin pain. Mechanical symptoms such as locking, catching, or clicking are common. Physical examination may demonstrate an increase in groin pain with maximum flexion and internal rotation of the hip. In the absence of significant osteoarthritis, arthroscopic acetabular labral débridement has resulted in relief of mechanical symptoms and a decrease in groin pain in a substantial number of patients. Patients with dysplasia may commonly have labral tears but typically are not ideal candidates for arthroscopic surgery.

Intra-articular loose bodies have a wide range of etiologies including trauma, synovial chondromatosis, and ligamentum teres rupture. Hip arthroscopy provides less invasive access to the loose bodies of the hip joint than standard open techniques. There are several reports of successful removal of intra-articular bullets with hip arthroscopy.

Complications related to hip arthroscopy are rare and occur in fewer than 2% of patients in most large series. Complications include nerve injury (lateral femoral cutaneous, pudendal and femoral), instrument breakage, portal hematoma, septic arthritis, articular cartilage damage, trochanteric bursitis, and extravasation of arthroscopic fluid.

Hip Arthrodesis

Hip arthrodesis traditionally has been considered for the very young patient (especially large male laborers) with severe unilateral hip arthritis. As hip replacement durability has improved and as patients have become aware of the benefits associated with hip replacement, fewer patients are willing to accept arthrodesis. However, satisfactory results in terms of hip pain relief and functional improvement may be expected. Compared with individuals who have not undergone surgery, patients who have undergone arthrodesis of the hip have an approximate increase in energy expenditure during ambulation of 30%.

Abnormal gait resulting from hip fusion causes increased stress on the lumbar spine, and other joints of the lower extremities. Low back pain, ipsilateral knee pain and instability, and contralateral hip arthritis develop in as many as 60% of patients after hip arthrodesis. Pain in the low back or knee typically develops within 25 years of hip fusion and may become disabling over the long term.

Patients with associated contralateral hip, low back, or knee problems may require conversion of the hip fusion to total hip arthroplasty. Patients undergoing ipsilateral knee replacement may gain better knee function if the hip arthrodesis is converted to total hip arthroplasty (THA) before knee replacement. Low back pain may improve after conversion to THA. Because many patients with arthrodesis will eventually require conversion to THA, this eventual possibility should be taken into account during surgery. Suggested surgical techniques include preservation of the abductor musculature, placing the hip in 20° to 25° of flexion, and plate fixation. Because ipsilateral knee and back pain are more common in patients whose hips are fused in abduction, neutral abduction is suggested.

Osteotomy

Osteotomies around the hip are important biologic treatment modalities for patients younger than age 40 to 50 years because they may preserve the host hip joint. For symptomatic patients with structural hip abnormalities and mild or no arthritis, osteotomy may provide long-term pain relief and improve function.

Pelvic Osteotomy

Pelvic osteotomy is indicated for treatment of symptomatic dysplasia in young, active patients. Pelvic osteotomy has traditionally been classified into reconstructive and salvage osteotomy. The latter (shelf and Chiari) does not provide articular cartilage coverage for the femoral head. Salvage osteotomies have been abandoned in favor of THA, except in rare circumstances. Reconstructive osteotomies rely on redirection of the acetabulum to provide better coverage for the femoral head. It is believed that improvement in femoral head coverage halts or retards the progression of the degenerative process in most of these patients. In a recent review of more than 800 patients receiving Ganz or Bernese osteotomy, the procedure failed in 42 patients and THA was required at a mean of 6.8 years after the osteotomy. Function was not affected in the patients who did not

require THA. The results of most pelvic osteotomies have been encouraging. The Bernese osteotomy is preferred by most reconstructive surgeons for treatment of dysplasia in adults because it allows a large degree of correction, permits joint medialization (reducing the joint forces), does not breach the weight-bearing posterior column (allowing early ambulation), does not violate the abductors, and is associated with a relatively low incidence of complications and morbidities.

Femoral Osteotomy

Femoral osteotomy, a once popular option for treatment of dysplasia, has been mostly abandoned in favor of pelvic osteotomy. The current indications for femoral osteotomy include severe deformity of the proximal femur, treatment of femoral neck nonunions in young patients, and patients with osteonecrosis. Varus-producing osteotomy (rotation of the proximal femur into varus) is a valuable option used in isolation or in combination with pelvic osteotomy for treatment of symptomatic coxa valga.

Osteonecrosis of the Femoral Head

The incidence of osteonecrosis is not known with certainty. Osteonecrosis is more common in males and typically affects patients in their late 30s or early 40s. Osteonecrosis of the femoral head is bilateral in approximately 50% of cases.

Symptoms include pain in the groin region that is exacerbated with ambulation and activity. Some patients with early disease may be asymptomatic; therefore, a diagnosis may require a high index of suspicion. MRI or bone scan may show changes in the femoral head before plain radiographs.

Osteonecrosis of the femoral head occurs as a result of altered blood supply to the femoral head, which can result in bone necrosis, subcortical fracture, collapse, and eventual destruction of the hip joint. In some situations, the etiology of vascular compromise is clear (such as hip dislocation or femoral neck fracture with traumatic disruption of the blood vessels). In addition to direct blood flow disruption, other associated causes of osteonecrosis include corticosteroid use, ethanol abuse, and hypercoagulable states. Osteonecrosis is associated with hip trauma in 10% of patients. More than one third of patients have idiopathic osteonecrosis. Patients receiving medical treatment for the virus that causes acquired immunodeficiency syndrome apparently are at risk for osteonecrosis of the hip and other joints.

The widely used classification system for osteonecrosis of the femoral head is a modified version of one proposed by Ficat. In stage zero, osteonecrosis changes of the hip are noted only on MRI in an asymptomatic patient. Stage one osteonecrosis is seen in a symptomatic patient with positive MRI findings but no evidence of abnormalities on plain radiographs. In stage two, radiographs reveal sclerotic bone of the femoral head without subchondral bone collapse. In stage three, subchondral bone collapse (crescent sign) is seen on plain radiographs. In stage four, there is collapse of the femoral head with secondary degenerative changes of the hip joint. Poor prognostic factors for osteonecrosis of the femoral head include high degree of femoral head involvement (greater than 30%) and continued corticosteroid use.

Surgical treatment of osteonecrosis of the femoral head depends on the stage at the time of diagnosis. Stage four is best managed with hip replacement whereas precollapse stages (zero, one, and two) may be initially treated with joint-preserving measures (core decompression or vascularized fibular graft). The treatment of stage three disease in middle-aged and older patients usually is THA; in younger patients, joint-sparing procedures of hemiresurfacing arthroplasty may be considered. In recent years bone grafting of the femoral head by elevating the articular cartilage flap (trapdoor approach) has been attempted for patients with stage two and three disease.

Core decompression involves drilling multiple holes through the avascular portion of the femoral head under fluoroscopic guidance. Vascularized bone grafting, on the other hand, involves the use of a vascularized fibular graft with microsurgical anastomosis to local blood vessels. The vascularized graft is harvested from the central portion of the fibula. It is then inserted through a drill hole into the avascular zone of the femoral head. One recent study noted a survival rate of 67% for postcollapse osteonecrosis of the femoral head treated using this technique.

Total Hip Arthroplasty
Cemented Femoral Component
The best choice for fixation of femoral components continues to be a subject of debate. Several studies have reported excellent mid-term and long-term survivorship with cemented femoral components, particularly with the use of modern cementation techniques. There are a number of important factors that affect the outcome of arthroplasty using a cemented femoral stem. Some of these factors are patient selection, geometry and surface finish of the implant, femoral neck design of the implant, material used for the implant, and surgical technique. Overall, younger patients, who are more active, have an increased risk of cemented femoral component failure than older patients. Men have an approximate twofold higher risk of failure than women. Torsional and axial stability in the cement mantle is an important determinant of the success of cemented femoral components. Numerous designs of femoral stems have been successful in providing stability. Some designs aim to

provide stability without possibility of subsidence (calcar resting stems), whereas others allow controlled subsidence of the stem within the cement mantle over time. Surface finish of the component also contributes to the stability of the stem. The roughened surfaces allow better cement interdigitation and minimize subsidence. The smooth stems, on the other hand, permit taper-slip subsidence. There is conflicting evidence in the literature regarding which type of surface finish will provide better long-term results. One of the primary mechanisms for failure of cemented stems is initiation and propagation of cracks in the cement mantle through preexisting pores. Modern generation cementing techniques with emphasis on porosity reduction, good pressurization of the cement to obtain a uniform cement mantle, and optimal interdigitation into cancellous bone is believed to be a critical determinant of success of cemented femoral components. The long-term performance of cemented femoral stems is likely to be influenced by a combination of these factors.

Cementless Femoral Component
The premise that cement was responsible for the failure of hip arthroplasties led to the development of cementless hip components to decrease the incidence of aseptic loosening following THA. In recent years, there has been a shift toward the use of cementless femoral components in North America, particularly in young patients. Various factors are known to influence the performance of cementless femoral components, such as geometry, surface finish, and the extent of coating. Early clinical studies have shown mixed results for cementless hip femoral components. Some femoral stem designs had high failure rates, whereas others have enjoyed higher rates of success. Durable fixation and a low rate of thigh pain have been reported for different stem designs, including proximally- and extensively-coated stems with different geometries. The value of coating the femoral stem with hydroxyapatite is debatable; it enhanced fixation in one design but has had no influence on the performance of other femoral components.

Cementless Cups
Durable results for porous-coated cups have been reported by various centers. A recent study reported the 15-year outcome of 120 primary THAs performed with a cementless cup in a relatively young patient population. More than half of the patients were still alive after 15 years. No cup was revised for loosening. The linear polyethylene wear was 0.15 mm/yr. Pelvic osteolysis was observed in 6.9% of the surviving patients. The durability of fixation was excellent and was superior to that associated with cups that had been inserted with cement by the same surgeon.

Revision of the Femoral Component

Various factors influence the choice of femoral stem during revision surgery, including the extent of bone loss, age and physical demands of the patient, reason for revision, and status of the femoral canal. Because of a relatively high failure rate, cemented femoral stems are used with decreasing frequency during revision arthroplasty and cemented stems are mostly reserved for the elderly and low-demand patients. Although revision of a failed cementless femoral implant with cement provided pain relief and improved function for most patients, the rate of loosening at the time of intermediate-term follow-up was high. Bone removal at the time of the initial implantation of the cementless stem and bone loss caused by subsequent failure of the cementless implant often left little intramedullary cancellous bone, which may explain the high rate of loosening observed in the first decade after revision. Most surgeons consider cementing of the femoral component (without impaction bone grafting) during revision surgery only if an adequate amount of cancellous bone exists in the canal to allow cement interdigitation. Extraction of a previously cemented femoral component usually leads to the loss of cancellous bone and reduces the fixation of cemented femoral stems under this circumstance. Some surgeons may cement a femoral component into a preexisting, intact, well-fixed cement mantle.

Most of the femoral components used during revision surgery are inserted without cement. Proximally coated monoblock stems have a high failure rate in revision surgery and therefore are rarely used, but modular proximally-coated stems have had a higher success rate. Extensively porous-coated cylindrical stems are used frequently for revision arthroplasty and reportedly are associated with excellent outcome in appropriately selected patients. Ten-year survivorship free of revision for these stems was reported to be 89% in one study. Cylindrical extensively-coated stems have a higher failure rate when used in Paprosky type IIIB or IV defects or with poor cortical bone in the isthmus. Impaction grafting is preferred by some surgeons for these patients. Fluted modular stems that rely on diaphyseal fixation have been popular in Europe and are gaining popularity in North America. However, fluted conical stems may be subject to subsidence. Extended osteotomy may allow better press fit for these stems (Figure 6). In revision surgery, a stem of adequate length should be used. Resistance to torsion progressively increases in association with increasing depth of insertion. A cadaveric study evaluated the rotational stability of two different revision stem designs (plasma sprayed cylindrical stem and fluted cylindrical stems) at varying depths of insertion (20 mm, 40 mm, and 60 mm). There was no difference in rotational stability of the two stems. Importantly, the actual length of bone-implant contact was

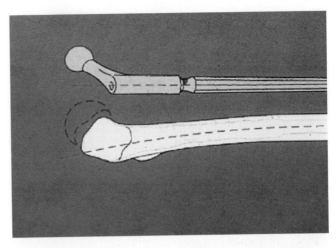

Figure 6 Fluted stems should have 5 to 8 cm of diaphyseal fixation. With the natural curvature of the femur, proper implantation of these stems to obtain the required diaphyseal contact is difficult and may lead to subsidence. Extended femoral osteotomy, with or without transverse reduction osteotomy allows better implantation of these stems.

found to be around 50% of the presumed values at all three depths. Stems with good diaphyseal fixation and poor proximal bone support can fracture (Figure 7).

Revision of the Acetabular Component

Cementless fixation is the preferred technique of acetabular fixation during revision arthroplasty. Excellent mid-term and long-term survivorship free of failure has been reported. Therefore, the use of hemispherical cementless cups is preferred whenever possible. Severe bone loss leading to distortion of acetabular architecture that may in turn compromise fixation, or native bone-to-metal contact that is essential for osseointegration may preclude the use of conventional cementless hemispherical cups. The recent introduction of cups made of the trabecular metal (such as tantalum) possibly with better osseointegration potential has led surgeons to implant these cups when the bone-to-metal contact surface has been small (less than 50% of the surface area). Large or so-called jumbo cementless cups may be used for patients with severe but contained bone defects with an intact acetabular rim. The use of jumbo cups has been reported to result in excellent outcomes, with over 90% survivorship at 10 years, provided that there is sufficient rim and posterior column support. Bone grafting of cavitary or segmental defects is valuable in restoring the bone stock. When placement of an uncemented hemispherical cup is not possible, reconstruction cages may be used, but because of lack of biologic fixation potential, loosening and component fracture occur in some patients.

Isolated liner exchange to address severe wear of polyethylene is an acceptable method of treatment. Some studies of revision surgery for isolated liner exchange have noted a high dislocation rate.

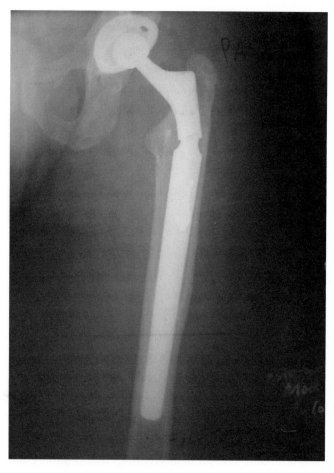

Figure 7 Cantilever failure for cementless stem. The stem is well fixed distally. Because of poor proximal bone support and repeated loading the stem has fractured at the weakest point (neck and body junction).

Infection

Although the management of deep periprosthetic infections has become more successful over the past decade, it is still one of the most challenging complications of joint arthroplasty surgery. The most important issue in management of deep periprosthetic infections is prevention. Prophylactic antibiotic use is likely the most important factor for reducing the incidence of deep infection from 9% 30 years ago to the present rate of between 1% to 2% for primary and 2% to 4% for revision arthroplasty. Antibiotics should be administered 30 minutes before the skin incision and for 24 hours after surgery. However, the orthopaedic community should not rely solely on the use of antibiotics. A clean air environment (vertical laminar flow, body exhaust system, limiting traffic flow and personnel), effective skin preparation (iodine or povidine with alcohol) and draping (use of adhesive iodine), efforts to reduce skin bacteria (shaving, iodine showers, treatment of skin lesions), careful attention to surgical technique, and expeditious execution of the surgery are very important principles. Studies have shown that contamination of instruments

(occurring during set up), suction tips (in 50% of affected patients), splash basins (in 70% of patients), and contamination arising from glove perforations (in 100% of patients after 3 hours) are common.

Treatment options are antibiotic suppression alone, débridement and antibiotics, prosthesis removal with one- or two-staged reimplantation, or resection arthroplasty. Antibiotic suppression without surgery may be indicated for medically infirm patients with susceptible organisms, well-fixed components, and the ability to tolerate oral antibiotics. Antibiotic suppression is contraindicated in patients with resistant organisms. Deep periprosthetic infections presenting within 4 weeks of the initial arthroplasty or a late hematogenous infection presenting with brief history of symptoms such as pain and swelling, or the inciting events that lead to infection may respond to treatment with débridement, retention of the prosthesis, and antibiotics. The success of this procedure depends on host-related factors (immune status, age, soft tissue); organism-related factors (type, susceptibility, response to antibiotics); and surgical factors (interval for presentation before surgery, extent of débridement, soft-tissue coverage). The early success of débridement and antibiotics, in appropriately selected patients, is greater than 70%, but the results deteriorate over time so that by 2 years 56%, and by 5 years only 26% of patients remained infection free in one study. Resection arthroplasty with one-stage or two-stage reimplantation is the treatment of choice for most patients presenting with deep periprosthetic infections. Some authorities advocate removal of the components and insertion of new prosthesis under the same anesthesia (one-stage reimplantation) for patients with low virulence and sensitive organisms, or for patients unable to tolerate multiple procedures. The success (patients who are infection free) of one-stage reimplantation varies between 73% to 92%.

Wear

Wear of the bearing surfaces has become the most important factor limiting the longevity of most hip arthroplasties. Table 1 summarizes the overall advantages and disadvantages of current bearing choices. Age and activity level are among the most important predictors of wear. Increased body mass may have a protective effect on wear as increased body mass index has been associated with reduced activity. The mean number of gait cycles per year as measured with a pedometer is approximately 1.2 million. The mean wear for metal femoral head on conventional polyethylene is 0.14 to 0.2 mm per year. Computerized radiographic wear analysis programs have been developed. These techniques are accurate to a variance in the range of 0.25 to 0.41 mm. Multiple factors can influence the radiographic measurement of polyethylene wear, including the quality of

Table 1 | Bearing Surfaces

Overall Advantages and Disadvantages of Current Bearing Choices

Bearing Combination	Potential Advantages	Potential Disadvantages
Alumina-on-alumina	Usually very low wear High biocompatibility	Sometimes high wear Component fracture Higher cost Technique-sensitive surgery
Cobalt-chromium on cobalt-chromium	Usually very low wear Can self-polish moderate surface scratches	Question of long-term local and systemic reactions to metal debris and/or ions
Ceramic-on-polyethylene	Lower wear of polyethylene than with conventional metal-polyethylene Some additional protection against third body abrasion	Component fracture Difficulty of revision (that is if Morse taper is damaged) Higher cost
Polyethylene sterilized with ethylene oxide or gas plasma	No short-term or long-term oxidation	No cross-linking so does not minimize polyethylene wear
Polyethylene sterilized with gamma in low oxygen	Some cross-linking, some wear reduction	Polyethylene wear not minimized Residual free radicals (long-term oxidation?)
Cross-linked, thermally-stabilized polyethylene	Minimal polyethylene wear rate No short-term or long-term oxidative degradation	Newest of low wear bearing combinations, only early clinical results available Questions remain regarding optimum level and optimum method for thermal stabilization

(Reproduced from McKellop HA: Bear surfaces in total hip replacements: State of the art and future developments. Instr Course Lect 2001;50:165-179.)

the radiographs, polyethylene creep, and the manufacturing tolerances of the shell and the liner. To surmount the problem of wear, various improvements have been achieved.

Highly Cross-Linked Polyethylene

Highly cross-linked polyethylene has demonstrated markedly decreased wear in vitro compared with conventional polyethylene. Retrieval analysis evaluating the microscopic damage to the surfaces did not detect any difference in the quantity or the quality of surface damage between the conventional and the highly cross-linked polyethylene. Multidirectional scratching was the most prevalent pattern of damage on all retrieved liners. Recently, in vivo measurements of highly cross-linked polyethylene are becoming available. In one study, the cross-linked polyethylene was associated with a 65% reduction in the two-dimensional linear wear rate, a 54% reduction in three-dimensional wear rate, and 38% reduction in volumetric wear rate. The mean wear rate for cross-linked polyethylene is 0.07 mm/yr. Early polyethylene wear measurement accuracy is hampered by a "bedding-in" phenomenon (in part, polyethylene creep) over the first 2 years after implantation when femoral head penetration rates are elevated; thereafter, femoral head penetration rates revert to the steady state wear rate.

Ceramic

Ceramic-on-ceramic articulations have been used extensively in Europe. Several series have demonstrated good midterm clinical results with alumina on alumina bearings. The wear rate appears to be very low and risk of ceramic fracture has been markedly reduced compared with early studies. Fractures have not been completely eliminated, however, and the development of improved ceramics continues.

Metal-on-Metal

Because of a relatively high rate of failure, the first generation of metal-on-metal hips were largely supplanted by metal-on-polyethylene prostheses. However, newer generations of metal-on-metal prosthesis have become available and in vitro studies suggest that the metal-on-metal bearing surface has markedly superior wear characteristics to the metal-on-polyethylene surface. Metal-on-metal surfaces do not pose a risk of fracture. The major concern about metal-on-metal prostheses is that they appear to be associated with some elevation of systemic metal ion levels. In theory, elevated ion levels might cause organ toxicity, mutagenicity, and carcinogenicity, but convincing evidence of these effects has not been seen in any clinical studies. Metal-on-metal surfaces have self-healing ability; that is, smaller surface scratches may polish out with time. Surface micropitting, thought to be related to the presence of smaller carbides, has also been observed with some first- and second-generation metal-on-metal prostheses. Although micropitting was not associated with high wear rates, this complication represents an area for potential improvement. Hard-on-hard surfaces (metal-on-metal and ceramic-on-ceramic) probably have better wear characteristics with large femoral heads and these large diameter bearings may also reduce the risk of intra-articular impingement and dislocation. However, any intra-articular impingement with hard-on-hard surfaces can create greater potential problems than with metal-on-polyethylene bearings.

Osteolysis

Improving bearing surfaces and reducing wear particles hopefully will reduce particle-induced periprosthetic osteolysis in the future; currently, osteolysis continues to be a major long-term complication of hip arthroplasty. Osteolysis generally develops and progresses in the absence of clinical symptoms. Hence, close monitoring of hip arthroplasties to detect and treat osteolysis is important. Radiographs underestimate the extent of osteolysis, particularly in the periacetabular region. CT with special software has been used for quantification of pelvis osteolysis. Osteolysis related to particulate debris occurs as a result of phagocytosis of wear debris, which in turn leads to activation of inflammatory cells (macrophages) and ultimately recruitment of osteoclasts. The cytokine OPG/RANKL/RANK is believed to be an important mediator of differentiation of osteoclasts and their interaction with osteoblasts. Osteoprotegerin (OPG) decreases osteoclast differentiation by working through a receptor-ligand interaction (RANKL). Tumor necrosis factor-α, a cytokine released in response to phagocytosis of wear particles, is found to have a role in stimulating osteoclast formation.

Dislocation

In one study, the cumulative risk of any dislocations was 2.2% at 1 year, 3.8% at 10 years, and 6% at 20 years. The 10-year risk was 3.2% for anterolateral approach and 6.8% for posterolateral approach. One third to two thirds of dislocations can be treated by closed reduction without further complications. Dislocation is more common in association with the following factors: posterolateral approach, smaller femoral head size, trochanteric nonunion, obesity, alcoholism, neuromuscular conditions, and revision surgery.

Thromboembolic Disease

The ultimate goal of prophylaxis is to prevent fatal pulmonary embolism. Deep venous thrombosis may also lead to postthrombotic limb syndrome with swelling, ulceration, and extremity pain. The chemical method of prophylaxis is preferred in North America. Coumadin has been shown to be effective in preventing fatal pulmonary embolism. Low molecular weight heparin is also an effective method of prophylaxis but carries a higher rate of bleeding complications according to most studies. Mechanical methods such as pneumatic compression devices have been shown to be effective for reducing the prevalence of thrombosis after THA. These devices are believed to achieve their efficacy by increasing blood flow and localized fibrinolysis (systemic fibrinolysis, once believed to be important, could not be demonstrated by a recent study). Oral anticoagulation agents that do not require serologic monitoring have recently been tested in clinical trails for prevention of deep venous thrombosis following total knee arthroplasty, with promising results.

Periprosthetic Fractures After Total Hip Arthroplasty

Periprosthetic fractures following THA occur in a variety of different clinical situations. They may occur intraoperatively, during the postoperative period, or many years after hip replacement. Periprosthetic fractures may occur as a result of trauma or secondary to late deleterious effects of hip replacement components on the surrounding bone (such as osteolysis or stress shielding).

The incidence of intraoperative periprosthetic fractures after THA is higher using cementless rather than cemented hip replacement components. The location of intraoperative fractures related to cementless components depends on the type of prosthesis used. Wedge-fit, tapered stems tend to cause proximal femur fractures and cylindrical fully porous-coated stems tend to cause a distal split in the femoral shaft.

Several classification systems for periprosthetic femur fractures exist. The Vancouver classification of periprosthetic fractures takes into consideration the stability of the prosthesis as well as the location of the fracture and the quality of the surrounding bone. Type A fractures occur in the trochanteric region. Type B fractures occur around the stem or just below it. Patients in subgroup B1 have a well-fixed stem, in B2 the stem is loose, and in B3 the stem is loose and the proximal bone is of poor quality or severely comminuted. Type C fractures occur well below the prosthesis.

Management of periprosthetic fractures depends on the location of the fracture as well as the quality of bone stock and stability or fixation of the hip arthroplasty components. Type A periprosthetic femur fractures commonly are associated with osteolysis, which may require treatment of the process causing osteolysis. Type B1 periprosthetic fractures almost always are treated surgically, usually with open reduction and internal fixation. Cortical strut allografts, cerclage cables, and locking plates with unicortical screws may be necessary to achieve adequate fixation. Type B2 periprosthetic femur fracture (femoral component is loose) usually are treated with revision of the femoral component and fixation of the fracture fragment. Type B3 periprosthetic fractures require femoral component revision. Usually, either proximal femoral allograft or proximal femoral replacement is necessary. Type C periprosthetic femur fractures usually are treated with open reduction and internal fixation. The hip replacement components can usually be left alone.

Periprosthetic acetabular fractures are less common than femoral fractures. With cementless acetabular components, a tight interference fit is achieved by underreaming the acetabulum. Underreaming by more than 2 mm may create excess stress in acetabular bone, resulting in intraoperative fracture. If acetabular fracture is noted, additional cup fixation with screws may be needed. Osteolysis may result in significant weakening of the retroacetabular bone. Fracture through this weakened bone can cause acute failure of the acetabular component.

Prevention of periprosthetic fractures requires recognition of risk factors. Adequate surgical exposure during primary and revision procedures is necessary. Controlled osteotomy is preferable to damaging weak proximal femoral bone during retraction or implant removal. Special care must be taken when using cementless implants in patients with poor bone stock, such as those with rheumatoid arthritis or severe osteoporosis. Cortical perforations must be bypassed with the implant, structural bone graft, or fracture plate to a sufficient degree to avoid a stress riser. Careful, regular follow-up of arthroplasty patients is necessary to evaluate for failure of implants. Elective revision of failed implants with osteolysis and mechanical failure of components may prevent some periprosthetic fractures.

Annotated Bibliography

Femoroacetabular Impingement
Beck M, Leunig M, Parvizi J, Boutier V, Wyss D, Ganz R: Anterior femoroacetabular impingement: Part II. Midterm results of surgical treatment. *Clin Orthop* 2004; 418:67-73.

The outcome of surgical dislocation and osteoplasty of the femur and the acetabulum in 19 patients with a mean age of 36 years (range, 21 to 52 years) was reported. The follow-up averaged 4.7 years (range, 4 to 5.2 years). Using the Merle d'Aubigne hip score, 13 hips were rated excellent to good. In the hips without subluxation of the head into the acetabular cartilage defect, no additional joint space narrowing occurred. According to this study, surgical dislocation with correction of femoroacetabular impingement yields good results in patients with early degenerative changes not exceeding grade 1 osteoarthrosis.

Ganz R, Gill TJ, Gautier E, et al: Surgical dislocation of the adult hip: A technique with full access to femoral head and acetabulum without the risk of avascular necrosis. *J Bone Joint Surg Br* 2001;83:1119-1124.

The authors describe a novel technique for surgical dislocation of the hip, based on detailed anatomic studies of the blood supply. The approach involves anterior dislocation through a posterior approach with a trochanteric flip osteotomy. The external rotator muscles are not divided and the medial femoral circumflex artery is protected by the intact obturator externus.

Ganz R, Parvizi J, Beck M, Leunig M, Nötzli H, Siebenrock KA: Femoroacetabular impingement: A cause for osteoarthritis of the hip. *Clin Orthop* 2003;417:112-120.

The authors, based on clinical experience with more than 600 surgical dislocations of the hip, allowing in situ inspection of the damage pattern and the dynamic proof of its origin, propose femoroacetabular impingement as a mechanism for the development of early OA for most nondysplastic hips.

Hip Arthroscopy
Clarke MT, Arora A, Villar RN: Hip arthroscopy: complications in 1054 cases. *Clin Orthop* 2003;406:84-88.

Complications in a large series of hip arthroscopies are reviewed.

McCarthy JC, Noble PC, Schuck MR, Wright J, Lee J: The role of labral lesion to development of early degenerative hip disease. *Clin Orthop* 2001;393:25-37.

Arthroscopic findings in a large series of hip arthroscopies are correlated with cadaveric specimens to support the idea that acetabular labral tears and degenerative arthritis are part of a continuum of disease.

Osteonecrosis of the Femoral Head
Berend KR, Gunneson EE, Urbaniak JR: Free vascularized fibular grafting for the treatment of postcollapse osteonecrosis of the femoral head. *J Bone Joint Surg Am* 2003;85:987-993.

A survival rate of 67% is noted for postcollapse osteonecrosis of the femoral head treated with free vascularized fibula grafting.

Total Hip Arthroplasty
Boucher HR, Lynch C, Young AM, Engh CA Jr, Engh C Sr: Dislocation after polyethylene liner exchange in total hip arthoplasty. *J Arthroplasty* 2003;18:654-657.

Twenty-four patients undergoing an isolated polyethylene liner exchange for wear or osteolysis with retention of the acetabular shell and femoral stem were assessed. At a mean 56-month follow-up, six hips (25%) had dislocated. Of these, two underwent repeat surgery for recurrent dislocation; one had three dislocations, one had two dislocations, and two had single dislocations. It was concluded that polyethylene liner exchanges, with or without femoral head exchange for wear or osteolysis, are associated with a high risk of dislocation and possible decrease in function.

Davis CM III, Berry DJ, Harmsen WS: Cemented revision of failed uncemented femoral components of total hip arthroplasty. *J Bone Joint Surg Am* 2003;85:1264-1269.

Forty-eight consecutive hips in which a failed primary cementless femoral component was revised with use of cement at the Mayo Clinic. Rate of loosening at the time of intermediate-term follow-up was higher than that commonly reported after revision of failed cemented implants with use of cement and also was higher than that commonly reported after revision with use of cementless extensively porous-coated implants.

Gaffey JL, Callaghan JJ, Pedersen DR, Goetz DD, Sullivan PM, Johnston RC: Cementless acetabular fixation at fifteen years: A comparison with the same surgeon's results following acetabular fixation with cement. *J Bone Joint Surg Am* 2004;86:257-261.

The outcome of THA using Harris-Galante I cementless acetabular component and cemented femoral stem in 120 patients at 13 to 15 years was evaluated. No acetabular component had been revised because of aseptic loosening, and no acetabular component had migrated. Among the 70 hips with at least 13 years of radiographic follow-up, 5 had pelvic osteolysis and 3 had revision of a well-fixed acetabular component because of pelvic osteolysis secondary to polyethylene wear. The mean linear wear rate was 0.15 mm/yr.

Klapach AS, Callaghan JJ, Goetz DD, Olejniczak JP, Johnston RC: Charnley total hip arthroplasty with use of improved cementing techniques: A minimum twenty-year follow-up study. *J Bone Joint Surg Am* 2001;83:1840-1848.

Of the 91 hips in the 82 patients who were alive at a minimum of 20 years, authors reported five (5%) revisions for aseptic loosening of the femoral component. The rate of failure when radiographic signs of loosening were included was 4.8%. Adequate filling of the femoral canal with cement was found to be associated with improved survival of the femoral component.

Lachiewicz PF, Messick P: Precoated femoral component in primary hybrid total hip arthroplasty: Results at a mean of 10-year follow-up. *J Arthroplasty* 2003;18:1-5.

This study reports the midterm results of a precoated femoral component used in primary hybrid THA. Of an original cohort of 98 hips undergoing THA performed by one surgeon, 75 hips in 65 patients were prospectively followed up for 7 to 12 years. All hips had the same porous-coated acetabular component and a precoated femoral component (with an oval cross-section) implanted using bone cement. There was no femoral component loosening or revision. The authors concluded that if used in this manner in this patient population,

precoating is not detrimental to successful fixation of primary hybrid THA.

Laupacis A, Bourne R, Rorabeck C, Feeny D, Tugwell P, Wong C: Comparison of total hip arthroplasty performed with and without cement: a randomized trial. *J Bone Joint Surg Am* 2002;84:1823-1828.

The study reported the intermediate-term outcome of a prospective, randomized clinical trial in which 250 patients were randomly assigned to receive a hip prosthesis with cement or the same prosthesis designed for insertion without cement. At 6.3-year follow-up, the number of stem revisions in the group that had fixation with cement was significantly higher than that in the group that had fixation without cement ($P < 0.002$).

Parvizi J, Sharkey PF, Hozack WJ, Orzoco F, Bissett GA, Rothman RH: Prospective matched-pair analysis of hydroxyapatite-coated and uncoated femoral stems in total hip arthroplasty: A concise follow-up of a previous report. *J Bone Joint Surg Am* 2004;86:783-786.

This prospective study reporting the results of THA using tapered cementless femoral component with and without hydroxyapatite coating in a matched-pair group of 52 patients noted no difference in osseointegration, revision rate, or radiolucency between the femoral components in each group at 9.8-year follow-up.

Patel JV, Masonis JL, Bourne RB, Rorabeck CH: The fate of cementless jumbo cups in revision hip arthroplasty. *J Arthroplasty* 2003;18:129-133.

This study reported 5-year minimum results of cementless oversized cups used in revision hip arthroplasty, with significant associated bone defects. Forty-three porous-coated jumbo cups were used to treat acetabular defects in revision hip arthroplasty in 42 patients with a mean age of 63 years (range, 25 to 86 years). Morcellized allograft only was used in 27 hips, and bulk allograft was used in 8. At a mean follow-up of 10 years, two acetabular components were revised for aseptic loosening and graft resorption. Dislocation occurred in two hips. A satisfactory 92% Kaplan-Meier shell survival rate was seen at 14 years.

Teloken MA, Bissett G, Hozack WJ, Sharkey PF, Rothman RH: Ten to fifteen-year follow-up after total hip arthroplasty with a tapered cobalt-chromium femoral component (tri-lock) inserted without cement. *J Bone Joint Surg Am* 2002;84:2140-2144.

Excellent 15-year results were reported in a study of 49 patients receieving tapered cobalt-chromium, collarless, proximally-coated tapered stems. No stems were revised for loosening, while two were judged to be loose radiographically. Most importantly, no stem that was judged to be bone-ingrown at 2 years afer surgery progressed to loosening.

Infection

Hanssen AD, Osmon DR: Evaluation of a staging system for infected hip arthroplasty. *Clin Orthop* 2002;403:16-22.

A previously reported staging system for prosthetic joint infection was evaluated in 26 consecutive patients with an infected hip arthroplasty. Six patients were treated by a definitive resection arthroplasty whereas the remaining 20 patients received delayed insertion of another hip arthroplasty. In 4 of the 20 patients (20%) receiving a new prosthesis, reinfection developed. The only common variable among the patients who had reinfection was the use of a massive femoral allograft at reconstruction. The authors concluded that although the concept of a staging system for treatment of an infected hip arthroplasty is promising, the number of patients required to evaluate the use of a staging system will require a multicenter collaborative study.

Wear

Alberton GM, High WA, Morrey BF: Dislocation after revision total hip arthroplasty: An analysis of risk factors and treatment options. *J Bone Joint Surg Am* 2002;84:1788-1792.

Data were obtained from 1,548 revision arthroplasties in 1,405 patients at the Mayo Clinic. The dislocation rate was 7.4%. Larger femoral head and elevated acetabular liners reduced the incidence while trochanteric nonunion was a significant risk factor for subsequent dislocation.

Barrack RL, Cook SD, Patron LP, Salkeld SL, Szuszczewicz E, Whitecloud TS III: Induction of bone ingrowth from acetabular defects to a porous surface with OP-1. *Clin Orthop* 2003;417:41-49.

To evaluate the role osteoinductive bone proteins may play in enhancing bone ingrowth, six canines had bilateral THAs with a cementless press-fit porous-coated acetabular component. The osteogenic protein-treated defects healed more completely than allograft bone-treated or empty defects and achieved a bone density equivalent to the intact acetabulum. Bone ingrowth also occurred to a significantly higher degree in the osteogenic protein group compared with allograft or empty defects, achieving a degree of ingrowth equivalent to the intact acetabulum controls. The osteogenic bone protein was successful in achieving complete defect healing and inducing extensive ingrowth from the defect into the adjacent porous coating.

Berry DJ, Von Knoch M, Schleck CD, Harmsen WS: The cumulative long-term risk of dislocation after primary Charnley total hip arthroplasty. *J Bone Joint Surg Am* 2004;86:9-14.

The cumulative risk of dislocation in 5,459 patients undergoing cemented Charnley hip arthroplasty at one institution was calculated. There were 320 (4.8%) dislocations. The cumulative risk of a first-time dislocation was 1% at 1 month and 1.9% at 1 year and then rose at a constant rate of approximately 1% every 5 years to 7% at 25 years for patients. Multi-

variate analysis revealed that the relative risk of dislocation for female patients (as compared with male patients) was 2.1 and that the relative risk for patients who were 70 years old or older (as compared with those who younger than 70 years old) was 1.3. Three underlying diagnoses, osteonecrosis of the femoral head; acute fracture or nonunion of the proximal part of the femur; and inflammatory arthritis, were associated with a significantly greater risk of dislocation than OA.

Hui AJ, McCalden RW, Martell JM, MacDonald SJ, Bourne RB, Rorabeck CH: Validation of two and three-dimentional radiographic techniques for measuring polyethylene wear after total hip arthroplasty. *J Bone Joint Surg Am* 2003;85:505-511.

This study sought to validate two in vivo radiographic wear measurement techniques by comparing their results with those obtained directly from retrieved specimens. There was good agreement between the wear estimates made with both in vivo techniques and the measurements of the retrieved polyethylene liners made with the coordinate measuring machine. Two-dimensional wear analysis (based on AP radiographs) accounted for most of the polyethylene wear, while one technique of three-dimensional wear analysis demonstrated some additional wear in the lateral plane.

Macaulay W, Westrich G, Sharrock N, et al: Effect of pneumatic compression on fibrinolysis after total hip arthoplasty. *Clin Orthop* 2002;399:168-176.

This prospective randomized clinical trial investigated the possible enhanced systemic fibrinolysis mechanism of venous thrombosis prevention by pneumatic compression after THA in 50 patients. Serum determinations of antigen of tissue plasminogen activator and plasminogen activator inhibitor-1 were done using enzyme-linked immunosorbent assays. The data did not support the enhancement of systemic fibrinolysis mechanism for lowering thromboembolic risk after THA by pneumatic compression devices.

Martell JM, Verner JJ, Incavo SJ: Clinical performance of a highly cross-linked polyethylene at two years in total hip arthoplasty: A randomized prospective trial. *J Arthroplasty* 2003;18:55-59.

The 2-year results for a prospective randomized trial comparing highly cross-linked with standard polyethylene in total hip replacement revealed a significant reduction in two- and three-dimensional linear wear rates (42% and 50%) in the highly cross-linked group ($P = 0.001$ and $P = 0.005$). Forty-six hips were available for radiographic analysis at 2- and 3-year follow-up. Femoral bearings were 28-mm cobalt-chromium, with the polyethylene insert randomly selected at the time of implantation to be highly cross-linked polyethylene or standard polyethylene.

Ulrich-Vinther M, Carmody EE, Goater JJ, Soballe K, O'Keefe RJ, Schartz EM: Recombinant adeno-associated virus-mediated osteoprotegrin gene therapy inhibits wear debris-induced osteolysis. *J Bone Joint Surg Am* 2002;84:1405-1412.

The role of gene therapy using a recombinant adeno-associated viral vector expressing OPG, a natural decoy protein that inhibits osteoclast activation and bone resorption, to inhibit wear debris-induced osteolysis in a mouse calvarial model was investigated. A single intramuscular injection of the vector efficiently tranduced myocytes to produce high levels of OPG. The OPG effectively inhibited wear debris-induced osteoclastogenesis and osteolysis.

Classic Bibliography

Berry DJ, Harmsen WS, Ilstrup D, Lewallen DG, Cabanela ME: Survivorship of uncemented proximally porous-coated femoral components. *Clin Orthop* 1995; 319:168-177.

Callaghan JJ, Brand RA, Pedersen DR: Hip arthrodesis: A long-term follow-up. *J Bone Joint Surg Am* 1985;67: 1328-1335.

Charnley J, Eftekhar N: Postoperative infection in total prosthetic replacement arthroplasty of the hip joint with special reference to the bacterial content of the air in the operating room. *Br J Surg* 1969;56:641-649.

Ganz R, Klaue K, Vinh TS, Mast JW: A new periacetabular osteotomy for the treatment of hip dysplasias: Technique and preliminary results. *Clin Orthop* 1988;232:26-36.

Gie GA, Linder L, Ling RS, Simon JP, Slooff TJ, Timperley AJ: Impacted cancellous allografts and cement for revision total hip arthroplasty. *J Bone Joint Surg Br* 1993;75:14-21.

McDonald DJ, Fitzgerald RH Jr, Ilstrup DM: Two-stage reconstruction of a total hip arthroplasty because of infection. *J Bone Joint Surg Am* 1989;71:828-834.

Mont MA, Carbone JJ, Fairbank AC: Core decompression versus nonoperative management for osteonecrosis of the hip. *Clin Orthop* 1996;324:169-178.

Reynolds D, Lucas J, Klaue K: Retroversion of the acetabulum: A cause of hip pain. *J Bone Joint Surg Br* 1999; 81:281-288.

Rittmeister M, Starker M, Zichner L: Hip and knee replacement after longstanding hip arthrodesis. *Clin Orthop* 2000;371:136-145.

Steinberg ME, Bands RE: ParryS, Hoffman E, Chan T, Hartmean KM: Does lesion size affect the outcome in avascular necrosis? *Clin Orthop* 1999;367:262-271.

Urbaniak JR, Coogan PG, Gunneson EB, Nunley JA: Treatment of osteonecrosis of the femoral head with free vascularized fibular grafting: A long-term follow-up study of one hundred and three hips. *J Bone Joint Surg Am* 1995;77:681-694.

Waters RL, Barnes G, Husserl T, Silver L, Liss R: Comparable energy expenditure after arthrodesis of the hip and ankle. *J Bone Joint Surg Am* 1988;70:1032-1037.

Younger TI, Bradford MS, Magnus RE, Paprosky W: Extended proximal femoral osteotomy: A new technique for femoral revision arthroplasty. *J Arthroplasty* 1995;10:329-338.

Chapter 35

Femur: Trauma

William M. Ricci, MD

Femoral Shaft Fractures

Classification

The Winquist and Hansen classification system for femoral shaft fractures is based on the diameter of bone that is comminuted (Figure 1). Type I fractures have a small area of comminution, with greater than 75% of the diameter of the bone remaining in continuity. Type II fractures have increased comminution, but with at least 50% of the diameter intact. Type III fractures have less than 50% cortical contact. Type IV fractures are defined as having no abutment of the cortices at the level of the fracture to prevent shortening. Type I and II fractures are axially stable, whereas type III and IV fractures are both axially and rotationally unstable. Rotational stability for less comminuted fractures is determined by the amount of comminution and obliquity of the fracture, with more transverse fracture patterns being less rotationally stable. Axially stable fractures are more amenable to earlier weight bearing, especially after intramedullary (IM) nailing.

The AO/Orthopaedic Trauma Association (OTA) classification system is also commonly used, especially for comparative investigations (Figure 2). Fractures of the femoral shaft are designated as "32." Type 32A fractures are simple (without comminution), type 32B are comminuted but maintain some degree of cortical continuity between the proximal and distal shaft fragments, and type 32C fractures have complete loss of continuity between the proximal and distal fragments. Further subtypes represent increasing fracture complexity.

The location of the fracture along the length of the shaft is usually described as being of the proximal, middle, or distal one third. There is some overlap between subtrochanteric fractures and proximal one third shaft fractures. Fractures located within 5 cm of the lesser trochanter are considered to be in the subtrochanteric region.

Evaluation

Fractures of the femur are usually associated with relatively high-energy trauma. Accordingly, patients should be carefully and systematically evaluated for associated injuries. The mechanism of injury should heighten the suspicion for other particular injuries. Motor vehicle crashes, especially those with dashboard impact, have a high incidence of associated knee pathology (up to 60%), including ligamentous injuries, meniscal injuries, and bone contusions. Knee stability should be evaluated with the patient under anesthesia and immediately after bony stabilization. Patients with persistent knee pain should be evaluated for occult internal derangement and bone contusion. Falls from a height can be associated with other injuries that are common after axial loading such as calcaneal fractures and spinal compression fractures. Visceral, chest, and head trauma should always be a consideration in patients with high-energy femoral shaft fractures. Bleeding at the site of the fracture is usually self-limited, but several hundred milliliters of blood can be lost. In patients with bilateral femoral shaft fractures or those with other long bone fractures, the cumulative bleeding associated with these fractures can become clinically significant. These patients should be monitored closely for anemia and hemodynamic changes. Associated neurovascular injury is uncommon, but patients with diminished or asymmetric pulses should be carefully evaluated for this type of injury. Neurologic deficit associated with penetrating trauma may require acute surgical exploration. Although found in only 2.5% to 6% of patients with femoral shaft fractures, associated femoral neck fractures have a high incidence (> 30%) of misdiagnosis. All patients with femoral shaft fractures should have AP and lateral radiographic views of the entire femur and a separate evaluation of the femoral neck with at least AP and lateral radiographic views. CT scans, which are often performed to evaluate the abdomen and pelvis, can be useful to diagnose nondisplaced associated femoral neck fractures and have been advocated as routine screening in patients at high risk.

Treatment

Nonsurgical Treatment

Nonsurgical treatment has a very limited role for adult patients with femoral shaft fractures. Severely debili-

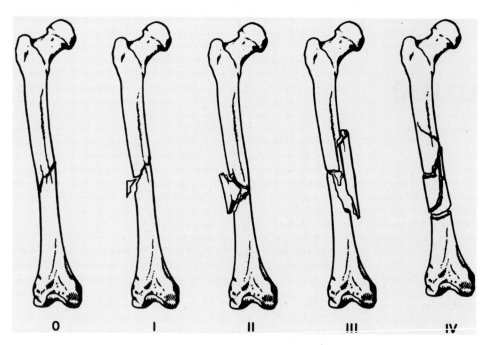

Figure 1 Winquist and Hansen classification of comminuted femoral shaft fractures. *(Reproduced from Poss R (ed): Orthopaedic Knowledge Update 3. Park Ridge, IL, American Academy of Orthopaedic Surgeons, 1990, pp 513-527.)*

tated, nonambulatory patients, including those with paraplegia or those with contraindications to anesthesia, can be treated with skeletal traction for 6 weeks followed by cast-brace application. Skeletal traction is frequently used if a delay in surgical treatment is expected to be greater than 12 to 24 hours. Traction through the distal femur or proximal tibia (provided there are no ligamentous knee injuries) may be used. Distal femoral traction provides improved stability and comfort by avoiding traction through the knee joint.

Intramedullary Nailing

Reamed locked antegrade IM nailing through the piriformis fossa remains the gold standard for treatment of femoral shaft fractures. Healing rates as high as 99% with low complication rates have been achieved with this treatment. Patients with multiple injuries who are treated with early fracture stabilization (within 24 hours) have an improved prognosis, decreased mortality, and fewer pulmonary complications (adult respiratory distress syndrome, fat embolism syndrome, pneumonia, and pulmonary failure). The advantage of early stabilization is therefore magnified in patients with chest trauma. Prospective randomized trials have shown that reamed nail insertion provides better healing rates than nonreamed insertion. Increased IM pressures and fat embolization during the reaming process has made reaming controversial in patients with chest and lung injury. Evidence indicates that the clinical relevance of marrow content embolization during the reaming process is negligible and is outweighed by the benefits of reaming on the healing process. Nonetheless, sharp reamers, proper reamer design, and slow passage of the reamer can decrease IM pressures and fat embolization

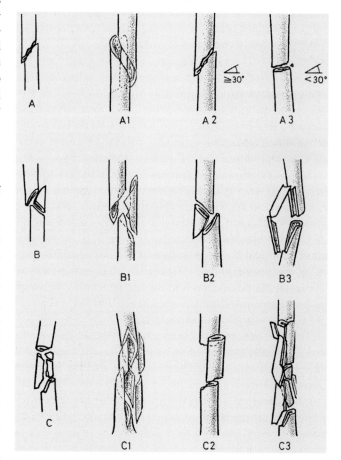

Figure 2 The AO classification of femur fractures. Simple (A), Wedge (B), Complex (C). *(Reproduced with permission from Müller ME, Nazarian S, Koch P, Schatzker J (eds): The Comprehensive Classification of Fractures of Long Bones. Berlin, Germany, Springer-Verlag, 1990.)*

and should be used, especially for patients with associated chest or lung injury.

Supine positioning on a fracture table with skin traction through the distal limb is the most common method for antegrade nailing. Antegrade nailing without traction on a radiolucent table can reduce surgical time and can reduce the incidence of rotational malalignment because it allows for better assessment of the contralateral limb. The lateral decubitus position offers improved access to the piriformis fossa but is associated with higher rates of malalignment. Nail insertion through the tip of the greater trochanter (as introduced by Küntcher) is technically easier than through the piriformis fossa, especially in obese patients. However, varus malalignment and iatrogenic fracture comminution are concerns with the use of this starting point. Implants specifically designed for trochanteric insertion, with a proximal lateral bend, can reduce these risks. Cerclage wire fixation of displaced fragments should be avoided to prevent excessive iatrogenic soft-tissue stripping at the fracture site that can lead to healing complications. Reaming across segmental fracture fragments should be done with great care to avoid spinning and therefore stripping of these fragments.

Retrograde nailing has evolved as a viable alternative to antegrade nailing when the proper technique is used. The insertion site should be in the intracondylar notch approximately 1 cm anterior to the posterior cruciate ligament origin and the nail should be inserted beneath the articular surface. More complications related to the knee have been found after retrograde nailing and more complications related to the hip have been found after antegrade nailing. The relative importance of these complications on functional outcome remains unknown. Knee stiffness and septic arthritis have not been shown to be significant problems after retrograde nailing. Retrograde nailing has the added benefit of improved fracture alignment of distal shaft fractures, decreased surgical time, and decreased blood loss. Current indications for retrograde nailing include the clinical situations in which proximal access to the femur (for antegrade nailing) is either impossible or not desired. Routine use of retrograde nailing for treatment of isolated femoral shaft fractures is limited by the unknown long-term effects on the knee.

External Fixation

External fixation as definitive treatment for acute femoral shaft fractures is limited to the pediatric population. In adults, it can be useful for temporary fixation when IM nailing is not advised, such as in patients with severely contaminated open wounds (especially when repeated access to a contaminated IM canal is indicated) and in patients with associated vascular injury, for whom time constraints preclude IM nailing.

Plating

Because of increased complication rates compared with IM nailing, plate fixation of acute femoral shaft fractures is reserved for pediatric patients and for adults in whom IM nailing is either impossible or undesirable, such as in those with ipsilateral femoral neck and shaft fractures, small IM canals, associated vascular injury, and periprosthetic fractures about IM implants. Minimally invasive methods such as indirect reduction techniques and submuscular plating have been advocated to reduce soft-tissue disruption and maximize healing potential during plating of femoral shaft fractures. Plates with locking screws have theoretic advantages in osteoporotic bone, but the specific benefits and indications of such devices for femoral shaft fractures are yet to be determined.

Special Situations

Open Fractures

Open fractures of the muscle-surrounded femur are much less common (5% to 20%) than those of the subcutaneous tibia. Because of the presence of this large protective soft-tissue envelope, open fractures are often associated with significant soft-tissue trauma. Small skin wounds can disguise more significant deep muscle and periosteal injury. All open fractures of the femoral shaft (except gunshot wounds) should be emergently treated. Wounds should be extended for evaluation of the deep soft tissues. All nonviable soft tissues and bone should be débrided. Serial débridements at 24- to 48-hour intervals are indicated with higher-grade open injuries. Although closure of contaminated wounds should be avoided, there is controversy on whether clean wounds should be left open or closed between serial débridements. Immediate IM nailing of open femoral shaft fractures is indicated except for the most severely injured patients. Provisional external fixation is useful when repeat irrigation and débridement of a contaminated IM canal is necessary. IM nailing can be done when the canal has been sufficiently cleansed. Intravenous antibiotics should be initiated when the patient presents for treatment and should be continued until definitive wound closure takes place. Routine wound culture is not indicated.

Gunshot Fractures

Fractures of the femur resulting from gunshot wounds are technically open fractures; however, they can usually be treated as closed injuries. The entry and exit wounds should be débrided locally at the level of skin and subcutaneous tissue. The deeper tissues do not require formal irrigation and débridement; therefore, fracture stabilization can follow standard treatment protocols for closed fractures. High-velocity gunshot wounds and shotgun blasts at close range are exceptions to this method of treatment because of severe soft-tissue compromise. In these instances, the fractures should be treated like other high-grade open injuries.

Vascular and Nerve Injuries

Femoral shaft fractures associated with either vascular or nerve injury are relatively uncommon (< 1%) and are usually associated with penetrating trauma. Bony stabilization, either definitive or provisional, with attention to obtaining proper limb length should be performed before neurovascular repair. The most expeditious stabilization method is usually external fixation, which can be safely converted to IM nailing within 2 weeks without an increased risk of infection related to pin tracts. Great care should be taken to avoid disruption of the soft-tissue repair during the secondary nailing procedure. Another expeditious alternative is nailing with interlocking deferred until after neurovascular repair.

Compartment Syndrome

Compartment syndrome associated with femoral shaft fracture is uncommon. A heightened index of suspicion should accompany injuries with a crushing mechanism, prolonged compression, vascular injury, systemic hypotension, and coagulopathy. When a clinical diagnosis is made, fasciotomy should be performed emergently. Compartment pressure measurements can be used as an adjunct to clinical diagnosis, especially in obtunded patients.

Obese Patients

It is estimated that approximately 30% to 40% of adults in the United States are obese. Difficulty in obtaining a proper starting point for antegrade nailing in obese patients has been recognized, and is responsible for the increased number of complications when nailing with an entry site through the piriformis fossa is performed. Better results have been obtained with nailing through the tip of the greater trochanter, especially with newer implants that have a proximal lateral bend designed for this insertion site. Patient obesity is a relative indication for retrograde nailing.

Floating Knee (Ipsilateral Associated Tibial Fracture)

Femoral shaft fractures associated with tibial fractures (the floating knee) are usually caused by high-energy injury mechanisms. Good results, similar to those found after high-energy isolated injury, have been obtained with retrograde nailing of the femur followed by antegrade nailing of the tibia through a single anterior knee approach.

Ipsilateral Proximal Femur and Shaft Fractures

Femoral shaft fractures associated with femoral neck or intertrochanteric fractures are challenging injuries to treat. The femoral neck component of such injuries is

the highest priority for optimal, but not necessarily initial, stabilization. Separate treatment with retrograde nailing or plating of the shaft combined with standard fixation of the proximal fracture is associated with the best results. Reduction of these femoral neck fractures can be difficult without an intact shaft. Provisional fixation of the femoral neck before retrograde nailing can be done using guidewires for cannulated screws to help avoid further displacement during retrograde nailing. Control of the shaft component, obtained after locked retrograde nailing, facilitates reduction of the proximal fracture either with manual traction or subsequent placement of the limb in traction on a fracture table. Simultaneous treatment of the proximal and shaft fractures using a single IM device in reconstruction mode is another alternative, but is technically more difficult and is associated with a higher complication rate, especially when applied for an associated femoral neck fracture. Femoral neck fractures, when associated with shaft fractures, are most often vertically oriented and have very little inherent stability. A sliding hip screw construct with a derotation screw may provide improved biomechanics over cannulated lag screws for these fractures. Decompression of the hip capsule has been advocated to decrease the risk of osteonecrosis and formal open reduction of displaced femoral neck fractures is indicated if an anatomic reduction cannot be achieved by closed means.

Complications
Malalignment

Fractures of the middle third of the shaft have a low incidence of angular malalignment (2%), whereas fractures of the proximal and distal thirds of the shaft are at highest risk of malalignment (30% and 10%, respectively). Antegrade nailing can facilitate improved reduction for proximal fractures, and retrograde nailing can be used for distal fractures. All patients should be evaluated for rotational symmetry compared with the uninjured limb before leaving the operating room. When rotational malalignment is identified, immediate correction should be performed.

Delayed Unions and Nonunions

Dynamization for nonunited femoral shaft fractures has been less successful than for tibial fractures and should be reserved for axially stable fracture patterns to avoid limb shortening. Reamed nailing (exchange nailing with the presence of a prior nail) is the treatment of choice for femoral shaft nonunions, particularly in the absence of angular deformity. Nonunion repair with compression plate osteosynthesis with judicious use of autologous bone graft is an effective alternative, especially when exchange nailing has failed or when deformity correction is necessary.

Disability

Pain and functional disability after femoral shaft fracture can occur regardless of the mode of treatment. Antegrade femoral nailing can be associated with hip dysfunction and pain in up to 40% of patients. Heterotopic ossification and prominent implants increase the incidence of these complications. Thorough irrigation of the surgical wound and the use of tissue protectors may reduce heterotopic ossification. Whenever possible, the fixation devices should be countersunk beneath bone to minimize related pain and muscle disfunction. Adequate rehabilitation with attention to abductor, quadriceps, and hamstring strengthening can reduce muscle disfunction. Injury to the patellofemoral articulation can be avoided with retrograde nailing by countersinking the nail beneath the articular surface. Retrograde nails should be locked with at least two distal interlocking bolts, especially for axially unstable fractures, to avoid migration of the nail into the knee joint.

Other Complications

Use of the hemilithotomy position for antegrade femoral nailing increases compartment pressures in the nonoperated leg. Prolonged use of this position should be avoided to prevent contralateral leg compartment syndrome, especially in patients with injury to the contralateral limb. Excessive and prolonged traction against a perineal post should be avoided to minimize the risk of pudendal and sciatic nerve injury from compression and stretch, respectively.

Supracondylar/Intracondylar Femur Fractures
Classification

According to the AO/OTA classification, supracondylar/intracondylar femur fractures are designated as type "33" (Figure 3). Type 33A fractures are extra-articular, type 33B are partially articular (with a portion of the articular surface remaining in continuity with the shaft), and type 33C fractures are completely articular (no part of the articular surface remains in continuity with the shaft). Subtypes of 33A fractures, 33A1 to 33A3 represent increasing comminution of the metaphyseal fracture. Subtypes of 33B fractures represent unicondylar sagittal splits of the lateral femoral condyle (33B1), medial femoral condyle (33B2), or fracture in the frontal plane, the so-called Hoffa fracture (33B3). Subtypes of 33C fractures represent simple articular with simple metaphyseal fractures (33C1), simple articular with comminuted metaphyseal fractures (33C2), and fractures with articular comminution (33C3).

Treatment
Nonsurgical

Nonsurgical treatment may be indicated for nondisplaced extra-articular supracondylar fractures, for pa-

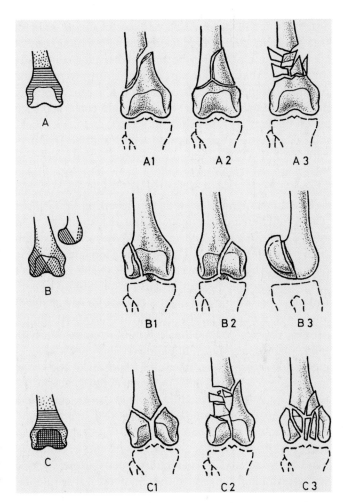

Figure 3 The Müller classification system of supracondylar/intracondylar femur fractures. (*Reproduced with permission from Müller ME, Nazarian S, Koch P, Schatzker J (eds): The Comprehensive Classification of Fractures of Long Bones. Berlin, Germany, Springer-Verlag, 1990.*)

tients who are nonambulatory, or for those who are not candidates for surgery. Long leg casts or cast-braces can be used in such circumstances, but they are associated with poor results when treating displaced fractures in ambulatory patients.

Surgical

Most supracondylar and intracondylar distal femur fractures are amenable to surgical fixation with either plate osteosynthesis or IM nailing. Surgical goals include anatomic reconstruction of the articular surface with restoration of limb length, alignment, and rotation with stable fixation to allow early mobilization and knee range of motion. The more distal the fracture and the more intra-articular involvement, the more amenable such fractures are to plate and screw osteosynthesis. As is true of most articular fractures, the articular reduction and fixation is of paramount importance. After this objective is accomplished, the articular segment is attached to the shaft with attention to proper length, alignment, and rotation. To promote an uneventful union, indirect fracture reduction techniques including percutaneous or submuscular plating can be used. With such minimally invasive techniques, the use of bone grafts, even in the presence of metaphyseal comminution, is not routinely necessary. Plates that offer a fixed-angle construct, such as 95° blade plates, 95° condylar screws, and newer locking plate devices, are indicated when treating fractures with metaphyseal comminution. These constructs minimize the risk of varus collapse seen with traditional nonfixed-angle devices. Blade plates are technically the most demanding, requiring proper insertion in all three planes simultaneously, but they offer the ability to treat very distal fractures. Dynamic condylar screw fixation requires slightly more distal bone for adequate purchase of the condylar screw, but the screw is technically easier to insert than blade plates because of the ability to control plate position in the sagittal plane. The newer fixed-angle plates, designed specifically for the distal femur, provide relative technical ease to insert compared with blade plates and offer multiple distal and proximal locking options. Threads on the outer diameter of the screw head engage and lock into threaded screw holes in the plate. Surgeons using such fixed-angle constructs should be familiar with the unique properties of such systems. Standard nonlocking screws can be used in some of these systems to lag fracture fragments and to compress plate to bone and should be inserted before locking screws. Another alternative to help avoid varus in comminuted metaphyseal fractures is supplemental medial plating. This technique has the disadvantage of requiring increased soft-tissue disruption.

Retrograde IM nailing, with associated screw fixation of simple intra-articular components, also has been successful. The advantage of IM nails for this application is the minimal dissection of the surrounding soft tissues. Newer nail designs with very distal interlocking holes allow nailing of fractures with small (4 to 5 cm) distal fragments. Static distal interlocking with multiple oblique interlocks should be used to enhance stability and reduce the risk of nail migration into the knee. Intra-articular fractures should be treated with appropriate anatomic reduction and stabilization (usually with screws placed such that they do not interfere with subsequent retrograde nailing) before IM nailing. Short, supracondylar nails provide a stress riser at their tip in the diaphyseal portion of the bone and increase the risk of subsequent periprosthetic fracture. Long retrograde nails, therefore, are preferable in most instances.

Special Considerations

Elderly patients with osteopenia and distal femur fractures represent a significant treatment challenge. Polymethylmethacrylate cement can be used to augment screw fixation in the distal fragment segment. The newer

locking plate designs that offer multiple fixed-angle locking screws offer a theoretic advantage in patients with osteopenia. The ideal fixation device and construct in this group of patients remains unproven.

Annotated Bibliography

Femoral Shaft Fractures

Bellabarba C, Ricci WM, Bolhofner BR: Results of indirect reduction and plating of femoral shaft nonunions after intramedullary nailing. *J Orthop Trauma* 2001;15: 254-263.

This article reviews a consecutive study of 23 patients with femoral shaft nonunion after IM nailing. All patients were treated with indirect plating techniques and judicious use of autologous bone graft. Twenty-one of the 23 nonunions healed without further intervention at an average follow-up of 12 weeks.

The Canadian Orthopaedic Trauma Society: Nonunion following intramedullary nailing of the femur with and without reaming. *J Bone Joint Surg Am* 2003;85:2093-2096.

This multicenter, prospective, randomized trial of 224 patients was conducted to compare reamed and nonreamed femoral nailing. Nonunion occurred in 7.5% of patients in the nonreamed group and only 1.7% of patients in the reamed group.

Robinson CM, Alho A, Court-Brown C: *Femur.* London, England, Arnold, 2003.

This is one of four books in a series dedicated to musculoskeletal trauma. It is a contemporary, well-referenced, and complete guide to treating every aspect of femur trauma.

Watson JT, Moed BR: Ipsilateral femoral neck and shaft fractures: Complications and their treatment. *Clin Orthop* 2002;399:78-86.

A retrospective review of 13 patients who had healing complications after surgical treatment of ipsilateral femoral neck and shaft fractures is presented. Lag screw fixation of the neck with reamed IM nailing of the shaft were associated with the fewest complications.

Supracondylar/Intracondylar Femur Fractures

Bellabarba C, Ricci WM, Bolhofner BR: Indirect reduction and plating of distal femoral nonunions. *J Orthop Trauma* 2002;16:287-296.

The results of a prospective study of 20 patients with nonunion of the distal femur are presented. Repair was done with plate fixation using indirect reduction techniques; in 45% of patients, autologous cancellous bone graft was included. All 20 nonunions healed without further intervention at an average follow-up of 14 weeks. The authors concluded that contemporary plating techniques are effective in the treatment of distal femoral nonunions.

Marti A, Fankhauser C, Frenk A, Cordey J, Gasser B: Biomechanical evaluation of the less invasive stabilization system for the internal fixation of distal femur fractures. *J Orthop Trauma* 2001;15:482-487.

This is a biomechanical study using cadaver femurs that compared the Less Invasive Stabilization System (LISS) plate (Synthes USA, Paoli, PA) to conventional condylar buttress plate and dynamic condylar screw plate for fixation of distal femur fractures. The LISS construct had less irreversible deformation and a higher elastic deformation.

Prayson MJ, Datta DK, Marshall MP: Mechanical comparison of endosteal substitution and lateral plate fixation in supracondylar fractures of the femur. *J Orthop Trauma* 2001;15:96-100.

This article presents a review of a biomechanical evaluation using synthetic femur supracondylar fracture model comparing lateral plate fixation to lateral plate fixation with endosteal substitution. Specimens with endosteal substitution showed decreased motion at the fracture site in both torsion and axial loading.

Classic Bibliography

Bhandari M, Guyatt GH, Tong D, Adili A, Shaughnessy SG: Reamed versus nonreamed intramedullary nailing of lower extremity long bone fractures: A systematic overview and meta-analysis. *J Orthop Trauma* 2000;14: 2-9.

Bolhofner BR, Carmen B, Clifford P: The results of open reduction and internal fixation of distal femur fixation using a biologic (indirect) reduction technique. *J Orthop Trauma* 1996;10:372-377.

Brumback RJ, Reilly JP, Poka A, Lakatos RP, Bathon GH, Burgess AR: Intramedullary nailing of femoral shaft fractures: Part 1. Decision-making errors with interlocking fixation. *J Bone Joint Surg Am* 1988;70:1441-1452.

Brumback RJ, Uwagie-Ero S, Lakatos RP, Poka A, Bathon GH, Burgess AR: Intramedullary nailing of femoral shaft fractures: Part II. Fracture-healing with static interlocking fixation. *J Bone Joint Surg Am* 1988;70:1453-1462.

Clatworthy MG, Clark DI, Gray DH, Hardy AE: Reamed versus unreamed femoral nails: A randomized, prospective trial. *J Bone Joint Surg Br* 1998;80:485-489.

Kempf I, Grosse A: Beck G: Closed locked intramedullary nailing: Its application to comminuted fractures of the femur. *J Bone Joint Surg Am* 1985;67:709-720.

Kuntscher G: The intramedullary nailing of fractures. *Clin Orthop* 1968;60:5-12.

Ostrum RF, Agarwal A, Lakatos R, Poka A: Prospective comparison of retrograde and antegrade femoral intramedullary nailing. *J Orthop Trauma* 2000;14:496-501.

Ricci WM, Bellabarba C, Evanoff B, Herscovici D, DiPasquale T, Sanders R: Retrograde versus antegrade nailing of femoral shaft fractures. *J Orthop Trauma* 2001;15:161-169.

Tornetta P, Tiburzi D: Reamed versus nonreamed anterograde femoral nailing. *J Orthop Trauma* 2000;14:15-19.

Winquist RA, Hansen ST, Clawson DK: Closed intramedullary nailing of femoral fractures. *J Bone Joint Surg Am* 1984;66:529-539.

Wolinsky PR, McCarty E, Shyr Y, Johnson K: Reamed intramedullary nailing of the femur: 551 cases. *J Trauma* 1999;46:392-399.

Yang KH, Han DY, Park HW, Kang HJ, Park JH: Fracture of the ipsilateral neck of the femur in shaft nailing: The role of CT in diagnosis. *J Bone Joint Surg Br* 1998;80:673-678.

Chapter 36

Knee and Leg: Bone Trauma

Michael T. Archdeacon, MD, MSE

Patellar Fractures

Mechanism of Injury

Patellar fractures most commonly occur as a result of a direct or indirect trauma to the knee. The direct mechanism involves an impact, typically by a dashboard during a motor vehicle crash or a fall onto the knee. The indirect mechanism results from an abrupt quadriceps contraction, which can result in an avulsion-type fracture of the inferior or superior pole or a transverse patellar fracture. An associated retinaculum injury is common.

Diagnosis

Suspicion for patellar fracture is raised based on the mechanism of injury and the patient's clinical history and physical examination. The ability to extend the knee against gravity can be limited or impossible, and an extensor lag may be noted. It is imperative to confirm that an open fracture or traumatic arthrotomy has not occurred. Confirmation can be achieved with a saline retention test by injecting 30 to 60 mL of saline into the knee and observing extravasation of fluid from the wound. Radiographs including AP and lateral views of the patella usually will show the fracture.

Classification

Fractures are typically classified as transverse, stellate, or vertical. Transverse fractures, classified as displaced or nondisplaced, can be avulsion injuries at either pole, or true fractures occurring anywhere along the length of the patella. Stellate fractures include a spectrum of injury from minimally displaced, multifragment fractures through displaced, comminuted, high-energy injuries. Vertical fractures are believed to occur from direct compression and knee hyperflexion. Finally, a subset of patellar fractures has been reported in patients who have undergone bone-patella-bone autograft donation for anterior cruciate ligament (ACL) reconstruction. It is hypothesized that an accelerated rehabilitation protocol puts the patient at risk for a transverse fracture pattern.

Treatment

Minimally displaced or nondisplaced fractures with an intact extensor mechanism and less than 1 to 2 mm of step-off can generally be treated nonsurgically. Full weight bearing in a long leg cylinder cast or a locked knee brace are reasonable treatment options. Incisions are typically midline longitudinal; however, in large traumatic disruptions, transverse incisions can be incorporated to minimize flap development. Open wounds should be incorporated into the surgical incisions to help prevent flap devascularization. Digital palpation or direct inspection through the traumatic arthrotomy or the fracture planes can facilitate obtaining and assessing the reduction of the joint surface. Maintenance of the length-tension ratio of the extensor mechanism is a secondary goal. Fluoroscopic AP and lateral radiographs of the patella can show articular incongruency.

Fixation techniques include the modified tension band and/or cerclage wire, tension band through cannulated compression screws, or independent lag screws. These techniques can be supplemented with a protective wire around the superior pole of the patella and through a drill hole at the tibia tubercle. For severely comminuted fractures with extensive articular comminution, partial patellectomy may be a reasonable alternative. If patellar tendon advancement is performed, it is critical to reattach the tendon to the remaining central portion of patella to maintain an extensor mechanism that is congruous in the patellofemoral articulation.

The cannulated compression screw technique offers the advantages of a compression screw as well as those of a cerclage wire. Parallel, longitudinal guidewires are passed through the patella and sequentially replaced with cannulated compression screws. Sizes from 3.5 to 6.5 mm can be used. A tension band construct is placed through the cannulated screws and tightened over the anterior surface of the patella. Ideally, the screw is slightly shorter than the length of the patella, which prevents a stress riser in the tension wire at the tip of the screw and allows the tension effect of the wire to fur-

Table 1 | Schatzker Classification of Tibial Plateau Fractures

Type	Characteristics
I	Pure split facture of the lateral plateau
II	Split fracture of the lateral plateau with a depression component
III	Pure depression injuries to the lateral plateau
IV	Medial tibial plateau fracture*
V	Bicondylar fractures, usually the result of a high-energy injury†
VI	Metadiaphyseal dissociation with a unicondylar or bicondylar fracture†

*Commonly associated with a concomitant vascular injury

†Comcomitant injuries including knee dislocations, vascular or neurologic injury, and compartment syndrome are common

ther compress the bony surfaces. The technique is ideal for transverse fractures and useful for comminuted fractures because the screws can be driven in multiple planes and wires can be used to cerclage the multiple fragments.

Postoperatively, patients are treated in a hinged knee brace, which remains locked in extension until the soft-tissue wound heals, typically in 7 to 10 days. If stable internal fixation is achieved, then gentle active-assisted and passive flexion arcs are initiated with wound healing. Active extension is delayed for 6 weeks. When a partial patellectomy has been done or less stable constructs are achieved, the patient is maintained in extension for approximately 6 weeks before initiating flexion arcs.

Complications include loss of fixation and/or reduction, infection, delayed union, malunion, refracture, arthrofibrosis, and extensor lag. Posttraumatic arthritis of the patellofemoral joint can occur.

Tibial Spine Fractures
Classification
Tibial spine or tibial eminence fractures are terms used to describe an injury at the intercondylar region of the tibial plateau. The tuberculum intercondylare mediale is the site of insertion of the ACL. No ligamentous insertions occur on the lateral portion of the tibial eminence. The mechanism of injury for tibial spine fractures is often a simple, low-energy fall onto an outstretched leg. In terms of an avulsion injury, the ACL, although intact, is typically functionally incompetent. Occasionally, the fracture will extend into the weight-bearing portion of the articular surface of the medial tibial plateau.

Type I fractures are nondisplaced, type II fractures are partially displaced or hinged, and type III fractures

are completely displaced. A fourth type, the comminuted tibial eminence fracture, has been described.

Treatment
Surgical intervention has been advised for type III and IV fractures because a high incidence of ACL incompetence has been reported with nonsurgical treatment. An open surgical technique with reduction and internal fixation has been historically advocated. A parapatellar arthrotomy is useful with compression lag-type fixation. The current favored techniques include arthroscopically-assisted and arthroscopic reduction and internal fixation. This technique is accomplished using standard arthroscopic portals with an accessory portal placed high anterolaterally or anteromedially to manipulate the fracture. The fracture is reduced and secured with percutaneous Kirschner wires followed by cannulated screw fixation (with or without a soft-tissue washer). Postoperatively, active-assisted range of motion is initiated immediately in a hinged brace. The patient is allowed to bear weight as tolerated in extension. A rehabilitation protocol, similar to that used for an ACL injury, is followed.

Tibial Plateau Fractures
Mechanism of Injury
Tibial plateau fractures typically have a bimodal age distribution. The spectrum of injury includes high-energy, axial load, or impact injuries with a significant soft-tissue component through low-energy medial-lateral impact injuries to the tibial plateau. The high-energy injuries are more common in the young trauma patient population, and impact injuries are more common in elderly patients with osteopenic bone.

Classification
Tibial plateau fractures have been classified by Schatzker into six types (Table 1). The AO/Orthopaedic Trauma Association classifications are also widely recognized. Type A fractures are extra-articular with increasing severity from subtypes 1 through 3. Type B fractures are unilateral plateau injuries ranging from the pure split injuries through split-depression fractures. Type C injuries are bicondylar injuries increasing in severity from subtypes 1 through 3.

Imaging Evaluation
Imaging studies include orthogonal views of the full-length tibia and oblique views of the knee. CT may delineate the extent of depressed fragments and clarify fracture planes. These studies can be useful for minimally invasive surgical techniques and reduction maneuvers. More recently, MRI of tibial plateau fractures has been advocated. This modality is useful in the diagnosis of associated soft-tissue pathology, including meniscal and ligamentous injuries.

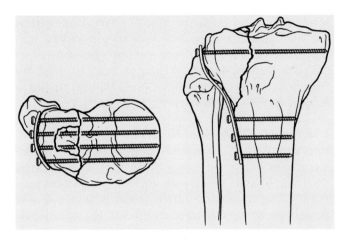

Figure 1 Periarticular tibial plateau fixation with "raft" or subchondral screws. The screws maintain the articular reduction, but offer no stability for the metadiaphyseal component of the injury. *(Reproduced with permission from Karunakar MA, Egol KA, Peindl R, Harrow ME, Bosse MJ, Kellam JF: Split depression tibial plateau fractures: A biomechanical study.* J Orthop Trauma 2002;16:172-177.)

Treatment

Nonsurgical treatment is recommended for low-energy tibial plateau fractures, which are stable to varus-valgus stress, as well as for nonambulatory patients and for those not medically fit for surgery. Nonsurgical treatment is indicated for minimally displaced split fractures or depression injuries with less than 1 cm of depression and is particularly relevant for injuries that occur deep to the meniscal tissue. Treatment should include use of a hinged knee brace and mobilization. Active-assisted and passive range of motion is initiated immediately, and weight bearing is typically delayed for 8 to 12 weeks.

Surgical treatment of closed tibial plateau fractures is indicated based on two criteria. First, the congruency of the joint surface must be evaluated. Although articular congruency should be the goal of treatment, articular displacement up to 10 mm has been accepted. Second, joint stability must be assessed. If instability exists because of depression or condyle subluxation, then surgical intervention should be considered. Additionally, high-energy injuries involving the metadiaphyseal junction or unstable bicondylar fractures should be considered for surgical intervention. Other indications include open fractures, associated neurovascular injuries, compartment syndrome, and floating knee injuries.

A staged treatment protocol has been advocated for high-energy injuries with significant soft-tissue damage. The first step is to ensure immediate stability and ligamentotaxis with spanning external fixation to allow for appropriate preoperative planning. Second, provisional fixation allows the soft-tissue envelope to heal so that future surgical reconstruction can proceed with minimal complications. A high index of suspicion for internal degloving injuries, vascular injuries, and compartment syn-drome is necessary when treating patients with high-energy trauma.

Current surgical treatment strategies include open reduction and internal fixation (ORIF) with adjunctive techniques including limited open reduction, arthroscopically-assisted reduction and fixation, and augmented internal fixation with resorbable bone cements. External fixation including temporary spanning fixators, hybrid and/or fine-wire fixation, and combined limited ORIF are acceptable techniques, particularly for patients with significant soft-tissue injury.

Open Reduction and Internal Fixation

ORIF for tibial plateau fractures has evolved to include implants and techniques that permit adequate periarticular stabilization without extensive exposures and because of advances in soft-tissue injury treatment, including staged reconstruction of high-energy injuries.

Limited ORIF necessitates ligamentotaxis to show which fragments can be reduced without direct surgical intervention or with minimal surgical intervention. Indirect reduction is accomplished with spanning external fixation or a femoral distractor across the knee joint. As major fragments are reduced with ligamentotaxis, articular depression and malreduction can be treated through limited percutaneous wounds or small open incisions. This procedure is guided fluoroscopically or arthroscopically. The use of tamps, elevators, and joystick Kirschner wires can assist in manipulating fragments into acceptable reduction positions. If the articular surface is adequately reduced and the overall alignment of the limb is obtained through ligamentotaxis, periarticular reduction clamps can be used to "close" the unicondylar or bicondylar components onto the elevated articular surface, thus, stabilizing the articular block. "Raft" screws or lag screws are then used across the subchondral region of the plateau (Figure 1).

After the articular surface is restored, the metaphyseal void created by elevating depressed fragments is supported by making a small osteotomy below the articular surface or using a window in the fracture plane to pack the void with autogenous or allogenic bone graft or bone graft substitute. Finally, the restoration of the articular block to the metaphysis-diaphysis is stabilized with a periarticular plate construct.

With the recent advances in locking fixed-angle plates, a single device can be used to stabilize unicondylar and bicondylar injuries and metadiaphyseal injuries. A limited incision into the anterior compartment followed by submuscular dissection allows for percutaneous plating of the proximal tibia. After the submuscular interval has been exposed, a locking, periarticular plate can be passed along the shaft of the tibia, and provisionally secured with fixed-angle screws, wires, or bone clamps. The overall alignment is assessed with fluoroscopy, and if acceptable, locking screws can be placed

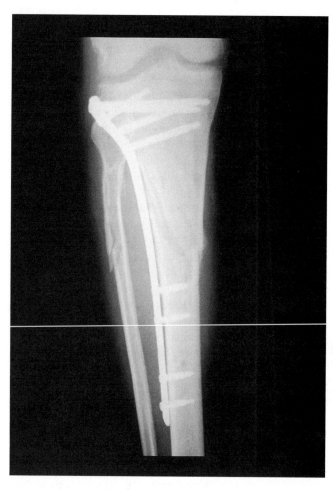

Figure 2 Percutaneous fixation of a bicondylar tibial plateau fracture using a fixed-angle plate-screw construct for metadiaphyseal stability.

throughout the plate. Various available plates have options for locking screws throughout the plate or in the periarticular region. The locking screws or fixed-angle screws are advantageous in the reconstructed subchondral surface and in metadiaphyseal dissociations because these regions are principally susceptible to high shear stress. Additionally, these constructs can maintain the overall alignment of the metadiaphyseal region and the proximal tibia with minimal surgical dissection or trauma (Figure 2).

In patients with high-energy bicondylar fractures, a secondary incision may be required on the posteromedial aspect of the tibial plateau. This type of injury is typically treated with an incision over the posterior compartment, elevating the pes anserine tendons anteriorly and entering the interval between the gastrocnemius and the plateau. This interval allows for manipulation and periarticular clamp placement of the posterior medial fragment. A 3.5-mm dynamic compression plate or a fixed-angle lateral plate for the opposite limb can

be placed in the posterior medial interval to buttress and stabilize these fragments. Patients are treated with immediate active-assisted and passive range-of-motion exercises postoperatively. A hinged brace is used for protection against varus-valgus stress. Weight bearing is delayed for 8 to 12 weeks.

Arthroscopically-Assisted Reduction
Several authors have advocated arthroscopy as an adjunctive technique in the treatment of tibial plateau fractures. Stated advantages include assessment and treatment of associated intra-articular ligamentous and meniscal injuries. A direct assessment of the articular reduction can be obtained with arthroscopy. A potential complication associated with arthroscopically-assisted reduction and fixation of tibial plateau fractures involves the extravasation of arthroscopy fluid through the fracture planes and into the lower extremity compartments. Compartment syndrome has been reported after using this technique. Arthroscopic fluid pumps should not be used or should be kept at low pressure in these circumstances. No studies have shown superior outcomes for tibial plateau fractures treated with adjunctive arthroscopy.

Augmented Internal Fixation
Recent developments in bone graft substitutes have made available calcium phosphate cements and other bone substitutes, which are well suited for the compressive loading environment of the tibial plateau metaphysis. This adjunctive technique involves open or limited internal fixation of the tibial plateau articular surface augmented with calcium phosphate or calcium sulfate bone cements, injected either percutaneously or through surgical wounds to fill metaphyseal voids created with reduction of periarticular fragments. Care must be taken not to allow extravasation of the cement into the joint through articular fractures. Screws must be placed before cement injection or while the cement is in the moldable phase. After the cement cures, screw placement can fracture or crumble the calcium phosphate cements.

External Fixation
External fixation can be used for definitive stabilization of unicondylar, bicondylar, and metadiaphyseal fractures of the tibial plateau. Previously mentioned reduction techniques and limited periarticular fixation can be used in a similar manner for definitive external fixation treatment. Circular fine wire or hybrid external fixation frames are used to associate the articular block to the metadiaphyseal segment rather than using locking, fixed-angle plates. These frames realign the axis of the limb in both the AP and lateral planes and secure fixation of the metadiaphyseal component in patients with high-energy injuries. These external fixation techniques

Table 2 | Open Fracture Classification as Modified by the Lower Extremity Assessment Project

Type	Characteristics
I	Wounds measure less than 1 cm Generally inside-out injuries, low energy, minimal periosteal injury
II	Wounds measure 1 to 10 cm Minimal damage to periosteum and soft tissues
IIIA	A fracture resulting from a high-energy injury with extensive damage to soft tissue, including periosteal stripping (wound size less critical)
IIIB	A fracture resulting from a high-energy injury as with a type IIIA fracture but requiring rotational flap coverage or free-tissue transfer
IIIC	A fracture resulting from a high-energy injury as with a type IIIA or IIIB fracture and resulting in vascular injury requiring repair

are particularly well suited to patients who have fractures with significant soft-tissue injuries.

Tibial Shaft Fractures

Classification

Tibial shaft fractures are classified based on the anatomy of the injury, or by the energy imparted at the time of fracture. The anatomic classification is based on the location and the fracture configuration. Position is defined as proximal, midshaft, or distal. Configuration is classified as simple fractures (such as transverse or spiral fractures) and more extensive patterns (such as butterfly fragments and comminuted fractures). The AO classification advocates a higher level of classification for an increasing severity of injury. Type A fractures are simple fractures that are spiral, oblique, or transverse. Type B fractures result from higher energy dissipation at the level of the injury and are classified as spiral, bending, or fragmented wedges. Complex fractures or type C fractures are multiple spiral fractures, segmental fractures, and highly comminuted fractures.

Open fracture classification is based on the work of Gustilo and Anderson and has been modified in the recent multicenter Lower Extremity Assessment Project study (Table 2).

Mangled Extremity

Recently, several limb salvage indices have been reported in the literature. However, there is no consensus on which index is the most useful, and whether any of these indices are reliable to predict outcomes. The absence of validation of these indices led to the development of the Lower Extremity Assessment Project study

in an attempt to provide criteria for the care of the mangled lower extremity. Analysis of the prospectively collected data revealed that none of the previously developed scoring systems showed any validated clinical utility. Although a high specificity confirmed that limb salvage with low index scores could be predicted, a low sensitivity failed to support any index as a valid predictor of amputation. Currently, no limb salvage index has been statistically confirmed to be reliable in the evaluation and treatment of patients with severely mangled lower extremities. Therefore, current recommendations emphasize early assessment of the extent of injury, along with frank discussions with the patient to explain the potential risks relating to the functional, social, and economic outcomes of limb salvage compared with amputation.

Open Fractures and Soft-Tissue Injury

Care for a patient with an open fracture should include the administration of prophylactic systemic antibiotics in the emergency department. Treatment should consist of a first-generation cephalosporin with the addition of an aminoglycoside for type III open fractures. Penicillin should be administered to patients with massively contaminated wounds when a concern exists for clostridial infection. The regimen is continued for 24 to 72 hours after a clean wound bed has been obtained with surgical débridement. Usually antibiotic coverage is extended for 48 hours after each subsequent surgical procedure. Wound coverage or closure of soft tissues is advocated, ideally within 5 to 7 days after the injury. The use of this protocol results in a 4% to 10% overall infection rate, with a 10% to 20% incidence of deep infection from type III open fractures.

Compartment Syndrome

In 1% to 10% of tibial fractures or lower extremity crush injuries, elevated intracompartmental pressures are known to occur. If an acute compartment syndrome is not treated emergently with surgical decompression, irreversible neurologic damage and myonecrosis will occur. Awareness of the possibility of compartment syndrome is critical and is primarily based on clinical examination. Hallmark symptoms include a tense or increasingly tense lower extremity, incapacitating pain that is not in proportion to the severity of the injury, worsening pain over time, and the most reliable criteria—pain with passive stretch of the ankle or toes. Symptoms of hypesthesia may indicate progressive neurologic injury. The presence of pulses is not a reliable factor for excluding a diagnosis of compartment syndrome.

When clinical examination is not reliable secondary to head injury, intoxication, or sedation, compartment pressure monitoring has been advocated. Criteria include absolute compartmental pressures, with critical values ranging from 30 to 45 mm Hg. A less inconsistent parameter is the absolute difference between the patient's diastolic blood pressure and the intracompartmental pressure. The critical value appears to be at the point when the intracompartmental pressure is within 30 mm Hg of the diastolic pressure.

Compartment syndrome is treated with emergent fasciotomy and decompression of all four compartments of the lower leg. A dual incision medial-lateral technique or single incision lateral technique are acceptable. Incisions approximately 15 to 18 cm in length are required to adequately decompress lower extremity intracompartmental pressure. Postoperative treatment consists of dressing changes followed by delayed primary closure or skin grafting at 3 to 7 days after decompression.

Treatment

Most low-energy tibial shaft fractures can be treated in a closed manner with reduction and application of a long leg cast followed by functional fracture bracing. Parameters accepted for closed treatment vary; however, general recommendations are the presence of less than 1 cm of shortening, less than 5° of angulation in any plane, and rotational deformity limited to 5° after immobilization. Although closed treatment is perfectly acceptable for tibial shaft fractures, caution should be exercised after immobilization with more proximal and distal fractures. These fractures are more difficult to control with functional bracing, and the imposed stability of a periarticular fracture brace may limit the functional range of motion in the adjacent joints.

Plate Fixation

With the widespread use of intramedullary (IM) nailing for tibial fractures, ORIF has been reserved for fractures in the proximal or distal third or fourth of the tibia. The rationale for these recommendations, when using ORIF, include a concern for soft-tissue devitalization, the increased risk of infection in tibial fractures compared with IM nailing, and the disadvantages of a load-bearing device compared with a load-sharing IM nail. However, plate fixation of tibial shaft fractures is still a viable option, particularly in concomitant periarticular fractures for which IM nailing may be very difficult, or in fractures in which an open wound would allow easy access for plating with minimal further dissection. Percutaneous plating techniques, which limit soft-tissue dissection, and fixed-angle locking plates are being used more often. These techniques can provide the theoretical benefits of external fixation with minimal soft-tissue and fracture site disruption and avoidance of the associated IM injury associated with reaming and nailing.

External Fixation

External fixation is an acceptable treatment method for open tibial fractures. Its advantages include minimal soft-tissue disruption, rapid application, and the ability to control difficult fracture patterns in a stable manner. Disadvantages include pin tract infections, delayed union in open fractures, and a higher incidence of malalignment and malunion when compared with IM nailing. The overall risk of infection between external fixation and IM nailing is similar. When significant soft-tissue injury is involved, external fixation is a safe and reliable option. However, in the presence of a healed open fracture wound, exchange of an external fixator for an IM nail is reasonable if this is accomplished within 10 to 14 days of fixator application.

Intramedullary Nailing

Currently, fractures not amenable to closed treatment are most commonly treated with statically locked IM nailing. In open fractures, IM nailing has been shown to be safe and effective with a relatively low risk of infection compared with other treatment modalities. Current data indicate that reamed versus unreamed IM nailing produce no essential difference in infection or nonunion rates. The most reasonable option is the "ream to fit" model in which the IM canal is reamed approximately 1 mm larger than the cortical isthmus of the tibia and a nail one size smaller is placed. Statically locked nailing is advocated; however, in stable shaft fractures for which one segment is controlled through the isthmus of the tibia, dynamic nailing is acceptable.

The indications for tibial nailing have expanded as the interlocking screw configurations have improved and techniques have been developed to treat more proximal and distal fractures. Modalities such as blocking screws and unicortical reduction plates have been advocated as adjunctive techniques in proximal and distal metadiaphyseal fractures treated with IM nails (Figure 3). Additional techniques to prevent malreduction for proximal third tibial fractures include nail placement in the extended position, a slightly more posterior entry portal, a parapatellar arthrotomy, an IM nail with a less acute proximal bend to prevent metadiaphyseal procurvatum deformity, and an external fixator or femoral distractor to maintain reduction during nailing.

Complications

Infection rates following IM nailing of open tibial fractures range from 4% to 20%, with the highest incidence in the type III open fractures. However, aggressive débridement, early stabilization, early prophylactic antibiotics, and meticulous soft-tissue care combined with early coverage all help reduce and maintain a low incidence of infection.

Nonunion has historically been attributed to bone loss, excessive motion at the fracture site, and a tenuous soft-

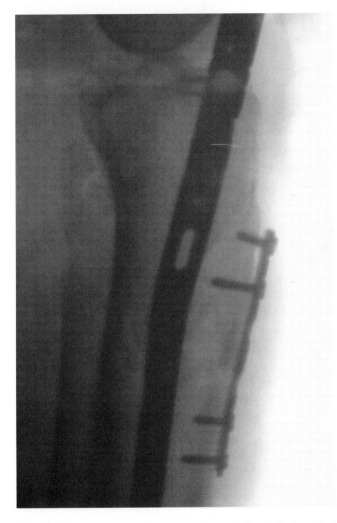

Figure 3 A unicortical reduction plate can be used to maintain reduction in proximal third tibial fractures treated with IM nails.

tissue envelope and/or blood supply. A recent observational study showed that the most reliable predictors of revision for tibial nonunion include an open fracture, a fracture gap after fixation, and a transverse fracture pattern. Recent data also have shown that patients who smoke have a higher risk of nonunion and delayed union. All delayed unions or nonunions in open tibial fractures should be considered as potentially infected. Staged protocols are most reasonable in this situation. Current recommendations for the treatment of tibial nonunions include dynamization by locking screw removal, exchange reamed nailing, compression plate fixation, external fixation with or without fibular osteotomy, posterolateral bone grafting, and/or the use of adjunctive bone stimulators. After 6 to 9 months, dynamization is unlikely to result in union. Other complications include anterior knee pain and failure of fixation. Implant failure generally results from fatigue failure of the locking screws, which can be removed or exchanged if causing painful symptoms.

Annotated Bibliography

Patellar Fractures

Stein DA, Hunt SA, Rosen JE, Sherman OH: The incidence and outcome of patella fractures after anterior cruciate ligament reconstruction. *Arthroscopy* 2002;18: 578-583.

In eight patients, the diagnosis of patellar fractures was made after 618 ACL bone-patellar-bone autograft reconstructions. Five of the injuries were the result of indirect trauma and three were the result of direct injury. All patients regained a full flexion arc. These outcomes were consistent with the remaining population of patients with ACL reconstructions. The authors determined that there were minimal residual sequelae after postoperative patellar fracture following ACL reconstruction.

Tibial Spine Fractures

Osti L, Merlo F, Liu S, Bocchi L: A simple modified arthroscopic procedure for fixation of displaced tibial eminence fractures. *Arthroscopy* 2000;16:379-382.

Ten consecutive adult patients who underwent arthroscopic fixation of displaced tibial spine fractures using an ACL guide to reduce the fracture are described. Arthroscopically placed pins were sequentially replaced with metallic suture wire placed over the tibial eminence and exiting out the anterior cortex of the tibia and tied over a screw. The advantages of this technique include stable fixation, easy device removal, and avoidance of injury to the ACL.

Tibial Plateau Fractures

Hung SS, Chao EK, Chan YS, et al: Arthroscopically assisted osteosynthesis for tibial plateau fractures. *J Trauma* 2003;54:356-363.

Thirty-one patients with tibial plateau fractures had arthroscopically-assisted reduction. More than 50% of the patients had concomitant interarticular injury including 44% with meniscal injuries, 38% ACL injuries, and 20% osteochondral collateral ligament injuries.

Keating JF, Hajducka CL, Harper J: Minimal internal fixation in calcium phosphate cement in the treatment of fractures of the tibial plateau. *J Bone Joint Surg Br* 2003;85:68-73.

Forty-nine lateral tibial plateau fractures were treated with limited ORIF and augmented with subchondral and metaphyseal resorbable calcium phosphate bone cement. Thirty-three of 44 patients were rated as having an excellent reduction at 1-year postoperative follow-up. In seven of the patients, slight loss of reduction (less than 3 mm) was noted; however, it did not require any further action. One infection was found. The authors advocate calcium phosphate bone cement as an adjunctive alternative to bone grafting in tibial plateau fractures.

Lobenhoffer P, Schulze M, Gerich T, Lattermann C, Tscherne H: Closed reduction/percutaneous fixation of tibial plateau fractures: Arthroscopic versus fluoroscopic control of reduction. *J Orthop Trauma* 1999;13:426-431.

Thirty-three patients with unicondylar tibial plateau injuries were reviewed; 10 had arthroscopically assessed reduction. The remaining 23 patients had the reduction judged fluoroscopically. The authors concluded that there was no difference in arthroscopic compared with fluoroscopic assessment of reduction in terms of outcome after limited internal fixation of unicondylar tibial plateau fractures.

Shepherd L, Abdollahi K, Lee J, Vangsness T Jr: The prevalence of soft-tissue injuries in nonoperative tibial plateau fractures as determined by magnetic residence imaging. *J Orthop Trauma* 2002;16:628-631.

Twenty nonsurgically treated tibial plateau fractures were evaluated with MRI; 80% had meniscal tears and 40% had complete ligamentous disruptions. Meniscal injuries were associated with lateral condylar fractures or bicondylar fractures and less with medial condylar fractures. The authors concluded that the use of MRI for tibial plateau fractures can result in the diagnosis of many soft-tissue injuries.

Tibial Shaft Fractures

Bhandari M, Tornetta P III, Sprague S, et al: Predictors of reoperation following operative management of fractures of the tibial shaft. *J Orthop Trauma* 2003;17:353-361.

Two hundred patients with tibial shaft fractures were evaluated for predictors of reoperation within 1 year of the index procedure. Variables that were prognostic for reoperation included an open fracture wound, lack of cortical continuity between the fracture ends after fixation, and a transverse fracture pattern.

Bosse MJ, MacKenzie EJ, Kellam JF, et al: A prospective evaluation of the clinical utility of the lower extremity injury severity scores. *J Bone Joint Surg* 2001;83:3-14.

The Lower Extremity Assessment Project (LEAP Study) was a National Institutes of Health investigation to evaluate limb salvage versus amputation in severe lower extremity injuries. An open fracture classification system was clearly defined by the LEAP authors, so that final grading was determined at the time of definitive closure or amputation. Analysis of prospective data for 556 high-energy, lower extremity injuries revealed that none of the tested limb salvage indices demonstrated any validated clinical utility. Additionally, a high specificity confirmed that limb salvage with low index scores could be predicted, but a low sensitivity failed to support any index as a valid predictor of amputation. Currently, no limb salvage index has been statistically confirmed to be reliable in the evaluation and treatment of patients with severely mangled lower extremities.

Harvey EJ, Agel J, Selznick HS, Chapman JR, Henley MB: Deleterious effect of smoking on healing of open tibia-shaft fractures. *Am J Orthop* 2002;31:518-521.

In this study of 105 patients with 110 open tibial fractures treated with external fixation or IM nailing, smoking was noted to have a deleterious effect on healing. A union rate of 84% occurred in patients who smoked compared with 94% of those who did not smoke. A higher incidence of delayed unions and nonunions occurred in the smoking group compared with the nonsmoking group.

Ricci WM, O'Boyle M, Borrelli J, Bellabarba C, Sanders R: Fractures of the proximal third of the tibial shaft treated with intramedullary nails and blocking screws. *J Orthop Trauma* 2001;15:264-270.

In 12 patients with proximal third tibial shaft fractures treated with IM nailing and blocking screws, the authors concluded that posterior and lateral blocking screws in the proximal fracture reduced procurvatum and valgus malalignment, respectively. These complications are associated with the nailing of proximal third tibial shaft fractures. The authors concluded that blocking screws for proximal third tibial fractures are a useful adjunctive technique to control reduction during IM nailing.

Schmitz MA, Finnegan M, Natarajan R, Champine J: Effect of smoking on tibial shaft fracture healing. *Clin Orthop* 1999;365:184-200.

In a study of 146 tibial fractures treated either surgically or nonsurgically, absolute union rate was not significantly different between smokers and nonsmokers. However, time to union was significantly delayed in patients who smoked with average time to healing at 136 days for nonsmokers and 269 days for smokers. In patients treated nonsurgically, these differences were not significant.

Toivanen JA, Vaisto O, Kannus P, Latvala K, Honkonen SE, Jarvinen J: Anterior knee pain after intramedullary nailing of fractures of the tibial shaft: A prospective, randomized study comparing two different nail-insertion techniques. *J Bone Joint Surg Am* 2002;84-A:580-585.

In this randomized study of 50 patients undergoing either transtendinous or paratendinous tibial nailing, 21 patients in both groups had an average 3-year follow-up. No difference was noted in anterior knee pain with either approach. Knee scoring systems, muscle strength measurements, and functional tests showed no significant difference between the techniques. The authors concluded that there were no significant differences in outcomes for patients treated with the transpatellar versus peritendinous approach for tibial nail insertion.

Classic Bibliography

Bhandari M, Guyatt GH, Tong D, et al: Reamed versus nonreamed intramedullary nailing of lower extremity long bone fractures: A systematic overview and meta-analysis. *J Orthop Trauma* 2000;14:2-9.

Bosse MJ, MacKenzie EJ, Kellam JF, et al: A prospective evaluation of the clinical utility of the lower-extremity injury-severity scores. *J Bone Joint Surg Am* 2001;83:3-14.

Buehler KC, Green J, Woll TS, Duwelius PJ: A technique for intramedullary nailing of proximal third tibia fractures. *J Orthop Trauma* 1997;11:218-223.

Collinge CA, Sanders RW: Percutaneous plating in the lower extremity. *J Am Acad Orthop Surg* 2000;8:211-216.

Finkemeier CG, Schmidt AH, Kyle RF, et al: A prospective randomized study of intramedullary nails inserted with and without reaming for the treatment of open and closed fractures of the tibial shaft. *J Orthop Trauma* 2000;14:187-193.

Gustilo RB, Anderson JT: Prevention of infection in the treatment of one thousand and twenty-five open fractures of long bones: A retrospective and prospective analysis. *J Bone Joint Surg Am* 1976;58:453-458.

Gustilo RB, Mendoza RM, Williams DN: Problems in the management of type III (severe) open fractures. *J Trauma* 1984;24:742-746.

Henley MB, Chapman JR, Agel J, et al: Treatment of type II, IIIA, and IIIB open fractures of the tibial shaft: A prospective comparison of unreamed interlocking intramedullary nails and half-pin external fixators. *J Orthop Trauma* 1998;12:1-7.

Karunakar MA, Egol KA, Peindl R, Harrow ME, Bosse MJ, Kellam JF: Split depression tibial plateau fractures: A biomechanical study. *J Orthop Trauma* 2002;16:172-177.

Keating JF, O'Brien PI, Blachut PA, et al: Reamed interlocking intramedullary nailing of open fractures of the tibia. *Clin Orthop* 1997;338:182-191.

Krettek C, Miclau T, Schandelmaier P, et al: The mechanical effect of blocking screws ("Poller screws") in stabilizing tibia fractures with short proximal or distal fragments after insertion of small-diameter intramedullary nails. *J Orthop Trauma* 1999;13:550-553.

MacKenzie EJ, Bosse MJ, Kellam JF, et al: Characterization of patients with high-energy lower extremity trauma. *J Orthop Trauma* 2000;14:455-466.

Marsh JL, Smith ST, Do TT: External fixation and limited internal fixation for complex fractures of the tibial plateau. *J Bone Joint Surg Am* 1995;77:661-673.

McQueen MM, Gaston P, Court-Brown CM: Acute compartment syndrome: Who is at risk? *J Bone Joint Surg Br* 2000;82:200-203.

Meyers MH, McKeever FM: Fracture of the intercondylar eminence of the tibia. *J Bone Joint Surg Am* 1970;52:1677-1684.

Raiken SM, Landsman JC, Alexander VA, et al: Effect of nicotine on the rate and strength of long bone fracture healing. *Clin Orthop* 1998;353:231-237.

Reynders P, Reynders K, Broos P: Pediatric and adolescent tibial eminence fractures: Arthroscopic cannulated screw fixation. *J Trauma* 2002;53:49-54.

Schatzker J, McBroom R: Tibial plateau fractures: The Toronto experience 1968-1975. *Clin Orthop* 1979;138:94-104.

Sirkin MS, Bono CM, Reilly MC, Behrens FF: Percutaneous methods of tibial plateau fixation. *Clin Orthop* 2000;375:60-68.

Watson JT, Coufal C: Treatment of complex lateral fractures using Ilizarov techniques. *Clin Orthop* 1998;353:97-106.

Welch RD, Zhang H, Bronson DG: Experimental tibial plateau fractures augmented with calcium phosphate cement. *J Bone Joint Surg Am* 2003;85-A:222-231.

Yetkinler DN, McClellan RT, Reindel ES, Carter D, Poser RD: Biomechanical comparison of conventional open reduction internal fixation versus calcium phosphate cement fixation with central depressed tibial plateau fracture. *J Orthop Trauma* 2001;15:197-206.

Chapter 37

Knee and Leg: Soft-Tissue Trauma

Eric C. McCarty, MD

Kurt P. Spindler, MD

Reed Bartz, MD

Collateral Ligament Injury

Injuries to the medial collateral ligament (MCL) occur much more frequently than to the lateral collateral ligament (LCL). The mechanism of MCL injury is a valgus force caused by lateral contact to the knee or lower leg, which either injures the distal femoral physis (in the skeletally immature patient), MCL (in the young to middle-aged adult), or the lateral tibial plateau (in the middle-aged to older adult or senior citizen). Careful physical examination of the knee can confirm the presence of a Salter-Harris injury to the distal physis in the adolescent athlete; pain proximal to the normal insertion of the MCL and, more importantly, pain extending across the femur to the lateral side is common. Radiographs or MRI also can confirm diagnosis. Physical examination determines whether treatment of MCL or LCL sprains is nonsurgical (majority of tears) or surgical (associated with cruciate and/or posteromedial corner tears). Isolated injuries to the MCL are most common, with knee laxity at 20° to 30° of flexion; however, these injuries are stable with the knee in full extension (indicating intact posteromedial capsule). Isolated MCL injuries associated with anterior cruciate ligament (ACL) tears are usually treated nonsurgically at the time of ACL reconstruction. In the relatively rare case of MCL injuries with laxity in full extension, the posteromedial corner is torn and usually one or both cruciates have been torn. In this circumstance, MRI to localize the site of the tear and fully define the associated injuries (especially of the cruciates) is helpful in surgical reconstruction of one or both cruciates and repair of the MCL and posteromedial capsule tears.

Isolated injuries to the LCL are relatively rare but can occur with a contact mechanism that causes a complete ACL rupture.

If laxity is present only in 20° to 30° of flexion, a palpable LCL in the figure-of-4 position is found, and no laxity is present in full extension, then a complete disruption of LCL is not present and the knee can be protected from varus stress with a brace. When significant laxity is present in full extension, then a complete disruption of the LCL with associated posterolateral corner tears with involvement of a cruciate ligament is likely. Primary surgical repair is indicated, usually with cruciate reconstruction. In combined injuries to the LCL and posterolateral corner, MRI can help localize the site of injury (femur versus midsubstance versus fibular head) and identify associated injuries.

Figure 1 outlines the evaluation and treatment approach. Evaluation for growth plate injuries in adolescents, for instability in extension (indicating a posterolateral or medial capsular tear), and for complete cruciate ligament injuries is essential. Isolated injuries documented on physical examination are usually treated nonsurgically with protection from valgus (MCL) and varus (LCL) forces in the healing phase.

Anterior Cruciate Ligament Injury

The physical examination, imaging, timing of surgical reconstruction, and rehabilitation of the ACL have been well defined in the literature. However, there has been intense scientific activity on the choice of autograft, with several randomized clinical trials comparing patellar tendon with hamstrings. New techniques for hamstring fixation have improved stability of the construct and allowed more aggressive rehabilitation.

The most common mechanisms of injury for ACL tears are noncontact (approximately 70%), sports-related (approximately 80%), and recollection of a "pop" (approximately 70%). The overwhelming majority of patients do not return to play in most sports after the injury without surgery. Contact injuries are more likely to involve MCL injuries. Patients injured while jumping have a significant increase in intra-articular injuries. Female athletes have a twofold to fourfold increased risk of ACL tears when participating in the same sports and at the same levels as male athletes.

Physical examination remains the mainstay in diagnosis of ACL (Lachman test) and PCL (posterior drawer test) tears. A positive Lachman test is the absence of a firm end point with or without a perceived in-

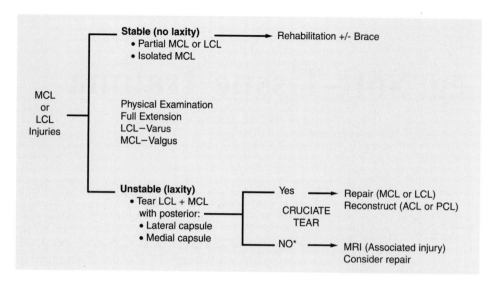

Figure 1 Evaluation and management of collateral ligament injuries. *Rare unilateral collateral (MCL or LCL) tears with instability in extension indicating posterior corner disruption without complete cruciate tear.

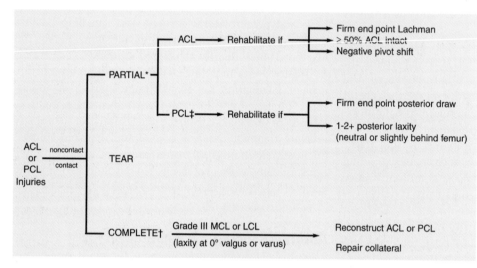

Figure 2 Cruciate ligament injuries in sports. *Partial injuries uncommon in ACL tears but are the majority with PCL tears in sports. †Complete = overwhelming majority of ACL tears but rare for PCL in sports. ‡Follow-up MRI documented return of normal ligament signal on MRI consistent with healing.

crease in excursion. A complete ACL tear is confirmed by a positive pivot shift test. Radiographs are normal in more than 95% of young, active athletes. The rare presence of a tiny fleck of bone on the lateral side at the lateral tibial plateau is indicative of a Segond fracture, which is pathognomonic for an ACL tear. In the middle-aged athlete, radiographs obtained while the patient is standing should be reviewed for evidence of arthritis (narrowing of joint or cartilage space) or evidence of a chronic ACL tear (notch stenosis and tibial spine spurs). MRI is particularly helpful when the diagnosis is in doubt or for identifying clinically relevant pathology, including collateral tears or bucket handle meniscus tears. Figure 2 outlines recommended treatment approaches for a patient whose cruciate ligament is injured during sports activity. Complete posterior cruciate ligament (PCL) tears are extremely uncommon during sports activity (relatively low-velocity mechanism of injury), with the exception of occasional knee dislocations. However, PCL tears involving one or both collateral ligaments are

common during motor vehicle crashes (higher-velocity mechanism of injury) and are discussed in the section on multiple ligament injuries.

Anterior Cruciate Ligament Reconstruction

Patients with partial tears of the ACL or PCL who meet the criteria outlined in Figure 2 can achieve a high level of function and return to sports after rehabilitation. The variables that need to be considered in the decision of whether to reconstruct the ACL-deficient knee without a complete tear of the collateral ligaments or PCL are diagrammed in Figure 3. Key factors to consider include the presence of a repairable meniscus lesion, desired return to competitive sports activity, and involvement in sports activity involving cutting and pivoting. Prerequisites to ACL reconstruction are nearly full range of motion, good quadriceps tone, normal gait, and limited effusion; all are signs that the knee has recovered from acute inflammatory trauma of hemarthrosis and that arthrofibrosis is less likely to develop postoperatively. Al-

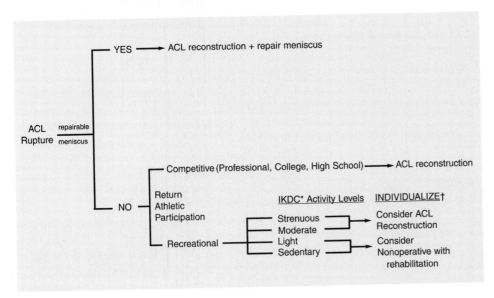

Figure 3 ACL reconstruction decision making. *IKDC = International Knee Documentation Committee consensus classification; strenuous, jumping and pivoting sports; moderate, heavy manual work and skiing; light, light manual work, running; sedentary, activities of daily living. †Individualize based on willingness to change activity levels, occupation, arthritis, other medical conditions.

though the exact type and frequency of supervised rehabilitation for patients undergoing ACL reconstruction has not been determined, monitored rehabilitation by a qualified therapy team immediately after surgery is helpful. Successful home rehabilitation protocols all include preoperative instruction, written materials for patients, regular supervised intervals, and the option for patients to call for advice. Principles of rehabilitation include immediate range-of-motion exercises, early weight bearing, closed chain exercises, safe restoration of quadriceps strength, and an emphasis on proprioceptive training to guide the safe return to sports activity.

There has been debate on the definition of acute versus delayed or chronic ACL reconstruction. As mentioned previously, a prerequisite consideration for ACL reconstruction is restoration of the normal activities of daily living, which indicates that acute inflammatory trauma has subsided and is important in the prevention of postoperative arthrofibrosis. Reinjury to an ACL-deficient knee has been shown to increase the frequency of meniscal tears and articular cartilage injuries, including arthritis. Thus, acute reconstruction can be indicated for patients who have not been reinjured, and delayed or chronic rehabilitation can be indicated for patients experiencing additional episodes of giving way. No exact time frame is recommended. In contrast, some authors believe acute reconstruction should take place within 6 weeks of injury.

A patient with chronic ACL deficiency may have developed medial compartment arthritis, especially if partial medial meniscectomy has been performed. Stiffness and pain are usually the result of arthritis and not instability. Instability from ACL deficiency is associated with giving way or patients describing a "shifting" of the knee. Radiographs should be obtained with the patient standing, and careful evaluation of the patient while walking should be performed. A high tibial osteotomy

(HTO) is indicated if a varus thrust is seen with or without medial arthritis because without correction of mechanical axis, the ACL graft will eventually fail because varus thrusting overstresses the graft. The decision to perform an HTO should be based on the patient's symptoms and the shift of the weight-bearing axis or away from a degenerative medial compartment. If arthritic symptoms are believed to be the predominant complaint, then HTO should be considered before ACL reconstruction. Unless an experienced surgeon is confident that stable fixation of HTO and ACL graft can be achieved so that early motion can begin, staging of these procedures may be more advantageous.

An evidence-based review of ACL ligament surgery shows that the results of randomized clinical trials support the failure of primary repair, and an improved stability and decreased rate of meniscus reinjury after ACL reconstruction. Randomized trials have not shown differences in outcomes using autograft patellar tendon versus hamstring approaches, or arthroscopic surgical techniques (two-incision [rear entry] versus single-incision [endoscopic]). Thus, ACL reconstructions are performed to resume short-term function (2 years), especially for participation in sports activities requiring cutting and pivoting. Whether ACL reconstruction prevents or delays knee osteoarthritis is unknown. Accurate tunnel placement, strong graft choices, solid initial fixation of grafts within the tunnel, and a rational rehabilitation program are factors that have been shown to bring about good to excellent short-term results. Placement of the femoral tunnel within 1 to 3 mm over the top position and tibial tunnel placement behind the intercondylar roof in full extension also are important. Coupling a proven fixation technique with the use of a specific graft and with aggressive rehabilitation seems appropriate. For example, patellar tendon graft with interference screws in young patients allows aggressive rehabilitation. Newer hamstring fixation methods allow similar rehabilitation. Recently, the use of improved aperture fixation at the femoral tunnel with a "cross-pin" and metallic washer at the tibial tunnel have provided improved biomechanical fixation, resulting in adoption of similar rehabilitation protocols as patellar tendon grafts.

Typically, autogenous grafts are harvested from the ipsilateral knee; however, the use of the contralateral patellar tendon for ACL reconstruction has been shown to have good results. Advantages cited are decreased morbidity on the reconstructed knee and faster patient recovery.

Graft sources other than autogenous grafts are often used. Attempts at reproducing the ACL with synthetic grafts was popular in the mid 1980s. Fueled by the desire to decrease donor morbidity and potentially speed rehabilitation, alternative graft sources included three broad categories of synthetic ligament replacements: (1) permanent replacement of the ACL with a prosthesis (for example, the Gore-Tex graft; Gore-Tex, Flagstaff, AZ); (2) use of a stent to augment a biologic graft and protect it during the early postoperative period (for example, the Kennedy ligament augmentation device; 3M, St. Paul, MN); and (3) use of a scaffold for appropriate support for collagen ingrowth to recreate the ligament (for example, the Leeds-Keio polyester device; Yufo Seiki, Tokyo, Japan). These methods were largely abandoned by the mid 1990s because of high rates of complications and failures. Complications included an inflammatory response to the graft and graft wear. Despite these failures, the search for a synthetic graft continues. Two future options are a biologic scaffold and/or a bioengineered prosthesis.

Allograft use for knee ligamentous reconstruction has increased significantly in the past decade. Some of the main reasons cited for the use of allografts include decreased surgical morbidity associated with the graft harvest, a quicker recovery time, smaller incisions, and decreased surgical time. Inherent disadvantages to using allograft tissue include the potential risk of disease transmission, cost, a possibly slower biologic remodeling process, and a theoretic slow chronic immunologic response to the tissue. The allograft tissue provides the collagen scaffold for a process of incorporation of host tissue. The stages of allograft incorporation are similar to those of autograft; however, the remodeling phase of the allograft can be one and a half times as long. The use of allograft tissue for reconstruction of all knee ligaments is becoming more popular. It is appealing for multiligament injuries in which autograft choices may be limited. Some studies have shown good results using allograft tissue for ACL reconstruction, although long-term results are lacking.

Results/Outcomes of Anterior Cruciate Ligament Reconstruction

Overall, the intermediate (5 years) or long-term (10 years or longer) results for ACL reconstruction are not known. Traditional instruments used to judge clinical outcomes following ACL surgery have been anteroposterior stability, nonvalidated activity level scales, and nonvalidated scales combining objective with subjective results into a combined score (International Knee Documenting Committee [IKDC]). Evidence-based medicine has focused on development of validated, questionnaire-based assessment tools, first in knee osteoarthritis with the Western Ontario and McMaster Universities Arthritis Index and with the Medical Outcomes Short Form-36. Sport-specific validated measures of surgical outcome on activity level developed between 1998 and 2001 include the Knee Injury and Osteoarthritis Score and the IKDC questionnaire. The first validated measure of sports activity was developed in 2001. These validated outcome instruments are currently in use by multicenter prospective cohort studies to address clinically relevant questions on putative risk factor assessment for pain, physical function, return to activity level, and global score. The use of these instruments will supplement and provide information not available from smaller stability outcome measures.

Table 1 is a systematic review of nine randomized controlled trials in the literature. All had equal preoperative groups, the same type of rehabilitation, no continuous passive motion, return to sports at approximately 6 months, and follow-up at 2 to 3 years. Several conclusions are evident from these trials. First, 44% (four of nine randomized controlled trials) showed from 0.5° to 3.4° loss of range of motion with patellar tendon reconstruction. Second, 43% (three of seven randomized controlled trials) showed hamstring weakness with hamstring reconstruction. Third, 43% (three of seven randomized controlled trials) of reconstructions using patellar tendons were more stable by KT-1000 [Medmetric, San Diego, CA] arthrometer testing in the 1.0 to 3.4 mm range. Fourth, 89% (eight of nine randomized controlled trials) showed no difference in anterior or patellofemoral pain, but 100% (four of four randomized controlled trials) of the patellar tendon group had more kneeling pain. Fifth, there was no difference in nonvalidated measures of return to preinjury function, Tegner activity level of outcomes by Lysholm, Cincinnati, or original IKDC 1991. Finally, no validated outcome tools previously mentioned were used in the best studies to date on ACL surgery.

Posterior Cruciate Ligament Injury

PCL injuries with or without associated MCL/posteromedial capsular or LCL/posterolateral capsular injuries have been investigated using in vitro biome-

Table 1 | Randomized Controlled Trials Outcomes for ACL Reconstruction: Hamstring Versus Patellar Tendon

	ROM	ISO	KT(n)	Ant Knee Pain	Kneeling Pain	XR	Return Preinjury	Tegner Activity	Lysholm	Cinn	IKDC
O'Neill (1996)	Ns	Ns	Ns (maximum manual)	Ns	–	–	–	–	Ns	–	Ns
Anderson et al (2001)	Ns	Ns	PT 1.0 mm better	Ns	–	Ns	–	–	–	–	PT best
Aune et al (2001)	Ns	↓Ham	Ns	Ns	PT pain	–	–	–	–	Ns	–
Eriksson et al (2001)	↓PT3°	–	–	Ns	PT pain	–	Ns	–	–	Ns	–
Shaieb et al (2002)	↓PT3.4°	–	–	PT > Ham 6 + 24 months	–	–	Ns	–	Ns	–	–
Beynnon et al (2002)	Ns	↓Ham	PT 3.4 mm better	Ns	–	–	–	Ns	–	–	–
Feller and Webster (2003)	↓PT1.5°	↓Ham 7%	PT 1.1 mm better	Ns	PT pain	Ns	Ns	–	–	Ns	Ns
Jansson et al (2003)	↓PT0.5° Ext	Ns	Ns	Ns	–	Ns	Ns	–	Ns	–	Ns
Ejerhed et al (2003)	Ns	Ns	Ns	Ns	PT pain	–	–	Ns	Ns	–	Ns

ROM = range of motion; ISO = isokinetic strength hamstring versus patellar tendon; KT(n) = KT 1000 stability anterior to posterior (n) = Newtons; Ant knee pain = anterior or patellofemoral knee pain; XR = x-rays or radiographs; Cinn = Cincinnati University Knee Rating; IKDC = original subjective and objective scale; PT = patellar tendon; Ham = hamstring; Ns = not significant (*P* >0.05).

chanical studies. Key decision-making criteria in the clinical management include magnitude of trauma (sports activity versus motor vehicle crashes), the degree of posterior laxity in reference to the anterior femur, and associated collateral or ACL tears. The posterior drawer test is performed with the knee flexed and both hands placed around the knee. The joint line is palpated with the thumbs. The degree of laxity is then judged by comparing the posterior tibial translation to the contralateral normal knee with the tibia anterior to the femur. Partial tears to the PCL have an end point and laxity with posterior force with the tibia even or slightly posterior to the femur. Complete tears have no end point to posterior force, even with internal rotation and significant displacement posterior to the femur. Plain radiographs are indicated to rule out bony avulsions, which can be repaired. MRI can be helpful in determining partial versus complete injuries; some fibers have continuity with partial tears. Partial tears are more common in low-velocity injuries (especially from sports activities) and are treated nonsurgically. Patients with partial PCL injuries have shown healing over time on follow-up MRI. It has been shown that 1+ or 2+ (5 to 10 mm) posterior laxity is well tolerated even in the highly competitive athlete. Complete PCL tears are more common from high-velocity injuries resulting from motor vehicle crashes and are often associated with collateral injuries and possible knee dislocation. Figure 2 summarizes treatment approaches to sports-related injuries to the PCL.

When PCL reconstructions are considered, the choice of surgical approach and grafts should be matched. Traditionally a single femoral tunnel approach was used, but several authors have recently proposed the use of two tunnels. A subject of current debate is whether a tibial tunnel with the so-called "killer" curve versus tibial onlay should be used. Tibial onlay requires a bone block and either a patellar tendon or Achilles tendon allograft. If tibial onlay is preferred and autograft tissue is used, then a single femoral tunnel with interference screws is used. An Achilles tendon allograft can be fixed as tibial only and either single or dual tunnels can be used. Reproducible in vitro biomechanical studies have not identified the best approach or graft choice to date; however, research is ongoing. No comparative in vivo animal models or clinical studies have provided a preferred technique. The surgeon should choose the safest, most reproducible approach and technique to improve posterior stability.

Posterolateral Complex Injury

The posterolateral complex includes the biceps tendon, iliotibial band, popliteus tendon, popliteofibular ligament, arcuate ligament, and LCL. The functional and clinical significance of these closely interrelated structures is not yet completely understood. The posterolateral structures act synergistically with the PCL to resist posterior translation and external and varus rotation of the knee. The biceps femoris, a dynamic lateral stabilizer of the knee, inserts on the fibular head. The iliotibial band is an anterolateral stabilizer. The primary function of the popliteus tendon is to externally rotate the femur, unlocking the knee to allow flexion when the knee is loaded. The popliteofibular ligament attaches the popliteus tendon to the posterior fibular head and the anterior lateral femoral condyle, providing resistance to posterior translation and external rotation of the tibia. The arcuate ligament courses from the fibula styloid process to the lateral femoral condyle, with limbs to the popliteus tendon and fascia overlying the popliteus muscle. The LCL is the primary static restraint to varus stress on the knee, and secondary restraint to external rotation of the tibia.

The most common mechanisms of injury to the posterolateral structures are a direct blow to the anteromedial tibia and hyperextension with a varus twisting force.

Physical examination for evaluation of the posterolateral corner include the tibia external rotation test, in which the degree of external rotation of the tibia in relation to the femur of each lower extremity is tested at both 30° and 90° of knee flexion. An increase in external rotation (of at least 10°), found only at 30° of knee flexion, is indicative of an isolated injury to the posterolateral corner. Associated injury to the PCL yields increased external rotation at 90° of flexion. The posterolateral external rotation test is similar to the tibia external rotation test, except a coupled force of posterior translation and external rotation is applied to the knee. The test is positive if posterolateral subluxation of the proximal tibia is noted at 30° of flexion. The reverse pivot-shift test, which is not specific for injury to the posterolateral corner, is performed by applying a valgus stress to the knee while externally rotating the foot and extending the knee from 90° of flexion. A positive test is elicited when a palpable jerk is noted during reduction of the posteriorly subluxated lateral tibia plateau. This test has been reported to be positive in up to 35% of

asymptomatic individuals. The external rotation recurvatum test is performed in a supine patient by grasping the great toes of both feet and lifting both lower limbs off the examining table. Posterolateral corner injury is indicated by recurvatum or varus deformity of the knee and external rotation of the tibia. Other tests for injury to the posterolateral corner include the posterolateral drawer test, adduction stress test, and dynamic posterior shift test.

Plain film radiography may reveal an avulsion fracture of the fibular head from pull of the biceps femoris or LCL. MRI has also proved to be useful for evaluation of these multiligamentous injuries and should include imaging of the entire fibular head.

For partial injuries to the posterolateral corner, including grade I and II instability with a good end point, nonsurgical treatment is recommended. This entails a 3-week period of immobilization with the knee in full extension followed by progressive range-of-motion and strengthening exercises. For acute injuries, primary repair of the posterolateral structures offers the best chance for a successful clinical outcome. Avulsion fractures of the fibular head can be repaired directly. Repair can be augmented with allograft or autogenous tissue. For chronic injuries, various techniques for reconstruction have been recommended with varied clinical results. Graft reconstructions recreating the popliteus tendon and LCL seem to fare the best. Postoperative rehabilitation after surgical treatment of injuries to the posterolateral corner involves protection from external rotation and varus stress with a hinged knee brace for a minimum of 2 months, followed by gradual range-of-motion and strengthening exercises.

Knee Dislocation

Knee dislocation is a devastating injury that usually results from high-energy trauma. Any three-ligament injury should be considered and treated as a knee dislocation. With improvements in surgical technique and instrumentation, the results of surgical treatment have surpassed those of conservative methods and are now the primary form of treatment of the dislocated knee.

Knee dislocation is classified primarily by the direction of the dislocated tibia in relation to the femur (anterior, posterior, medial, lateral, and rotatory). Determining the direction of the dislocation provides information about the likelihood of associated neurovascular injury. Injury to the popliteal artery is more likely with posterior dislocation, whereas injury to the common peroneal nerve is more likely with posterolateral dislocation.

Associated injuries with knee dislocation are common. The incidence of vascular injury with all dislocations has been estimated at 32%. The popliteal artery is injured either by a stretching mechanism secondary to tethering of the vessel at the adductor hiatus or by direct contusion by the posterior tibia plateau. Thrombus formation secondary to intimal damage can occur several days after injury. Decreased pulses or vascular compromise should never be attributed to arterial spasm, and additional investigation is warranted. Injury to the popliteal vein is rare. Injury to the peroneal nerve, or less commonly the tibial nerve, has been estimated to occur in 20% to 30% of knee dislocations. The incidence of associated fractures, usually of the tibia plateau or the distal femur, has been estimated at 60%.

The diagnosis of a dislocated knee is usually obvious; however, it is crucial to remember that a dislocated knee can reduce spontaneously. A spontaneously reduced knee is characterized by gross instability and extensive soft-tissue swelling. With a suspected knee dislocation, immediate evaluation of the vascular status of the involved limb is important because limb ischemia of more than 8 hours duration is likely to result in amputation. Vascular injury has been reported in the presence of normal pulses, Doppler studies, and capillary refill. Repeat neurovascular examination should be performed after any reduction maneuver.

Plain film radiographs should be obtained in two planes to determine the direction and severity of the dislocation, as well as for evaluation for any associated fractures. Slight joint space widening may be indicative of a spontaneously reduced knee dislocation. Plain film radiographs should also be evaluated for avulsion fractures, which may alter the surgical plan. Repeat plain radiographs should be obtained after any reduction maneuver to ensure satisfactory alignment of the joint.

With a suspected arterial injury, immediate arteriography and vascular consultation are warranted. Although arteriograms have been used historically as a screening tool for arterial injury, it is a low yield study in the presence of a normal vascular examination. With no evidence of vascular compromise on physical examination, foregoing an arteriogram and performing regular, detailed neurovascular examinations in an inpatient setting is accepted treatment. If vascular compromise is noted, immediate surgical intervention is indicated. Formal angiography is bypassed to lessen ischemic time.

After the initial survey and acute treatment, MRI is useful for evaluation of ligament and meniscus status, occult fracture, and capsular disruption. MRI gives essential information for preoperative planning for ligament reconstruction, such as the number of allografts that will be needed.

Timely closed reduction is indicated for any dislocated knee. Physical and radiographic examination should be performed immediately after reduction to confirm proper reduction and evaluate postreduction neurovascular status. The presence of the "dimple sign" is indicative of an irreducible posterolateral dislocation,

but it is a contraindication to closed reduction because of the risk of skin necrosis.

Indications for acute surgery after knee dislocation include vascular injury, open fracture, open dislocation, irreducible dislocation, and compartment syndrome. Restoration of vascular integrity takes precedence over other injuries. Open injuries require immediate surgical irrigation and débridement.

Improved surgical techniques and postoperative rehabilitation protocols, and the use of allografts have improved the clinical results for surgical treatment of knee dislocation. Factors to consider in the timing of surgical treatment of knee dislocations include the vascular status of the patient, the presence of open wounds, the success of closed reduction, the stability of the joint after reduction, and the presence of associated injuries.

There has been debate over the timing of surgical procedures after knee dislocation. Two reasons cited for delaying surgery include allowing a period of vascular monitoring and reducing the risk of arthrofibrosis. Multiple ligament injuries may require staged procedures. Posterolateral structures, capsular structures, and avulsion fractures can be repaired acutely. Combined ACL and PCL reconstruction can be performed in delayed fashion with acceptable results. Graft options for ligament reconstruction in the multiligament-injured knee include patellar tendon, hamstring, and quadriceps tendon autografts, and/or allografts. The literature does not support the use of one graft type over another or the use of a particular technique for reconstruction. After combined reconstruction of the cruciate ligaments, the knee has traditionally been kept in extension with no weight bearing for 6 weeks. Postoperative rehabilitation programs after a knee dislocation should allow range-of-motion exercises as soon as the integrity of soft-tissue repair, vascular repair, and ligament reconstruction permit.

Meniscal Injury

The primary function of the meniscus is to evenly distribute the weight-bearing load across the knee joint. The menisci transmit approximately 50% of the load with the knee in extension, and close to 90% of the load at 90° of knee flexion. With flexion past 90°, most of the force is transmitted through the posterior horns. The lateral meniscus has been shown to transmit a greater percentage of the load compared with the medial meniscus.

When meniscal integrity is lost, abnormal articular contact stresses result, leading to potential increased wear of the articular cartilage and early degenerative changes. The more meniscal tissue that is lost, the greater the loss of contact surface area and the greater the increase in peak local contact stresses. Thus, the primary goal of treatment of a meniscal tear is to maintain as much healthy meniscus tissue as possible.

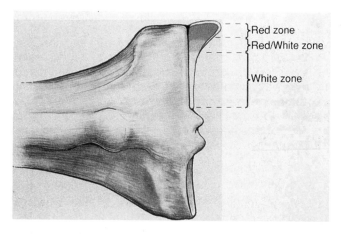

Figure 4 Zone of meniscal vascularity: Red zone = rich in vascular plexus, Red/White zone = transition between vascular zone and avascular zone, White zone = avascular zone. *(Reproduced with permission from Miller, MD, Warner JJP, Harner CD: Meniscal repair, in Fu FH, Harner CD, Vince KG (eds): Knee Surgery. Baltimore, MD, Williams & Wilkins, 1994, p 616.)*

In addition to some biomechanical differences in medial and lateral menisci function, there are several anatomic variances. The medial meniscus is semicircular with disparate insertions, whereas the lateral meniscus is more circular with closely approximated insertions. The medial meniscus is wider posteriorly than anteriorly, whereas the lateral meniscus has posterior and anterior segments that are close to equal in width. The medial meniscus is also more firmly attached to the knee capsule whereas the lateral meniscus is loosely attached.

A key aspect of the meniscal anatomy is its vascularity, which is one of the critical elements in healing of a meniscal repair. The most peripheral 20% to 30% of the medial meniscus and the peripheral 10% to 25% of the lateral meniscus are consistent in vascularity (Figure 4). Branches from the superior, inferior, and lateral geniculate arteries supply this vascular zone. Because of its rich blood supply, this area is commonly referred to as the red zone, and it is an area that has greater healing potential than the inner portions of the meniscus with less or no vascular supply. The inner third of the meniscus is avascular and is referred to as the white zone. This area is nourished by synovial fluid diffusion and repairs usually do not heal well in this zone. The area (middle third) of meniscus between the red and white zones is known as the red/white zone. Because this area does have some blood supply, it has the potential for healing, particularly in the young patient. The area in the posterolateral aspect of the lateral meniscus in front of the popliteus tendon, however, is a watershed area and even its peripheral third is relatively hypovascular.

There are several patterns/types of meniscal tears, each with potential ramifications on healing. Vertical longitudinal tears are common and often can be repaired, especially if located in the peripheral third of the meniscus. If these tears extend in length circumfer-

tially around the meniscus they will become bucket handle tears. Bucket handle tears may become unstable, and the fragment can displace into the knee, causing true locking of the knee. Most bucket handle tears can be repaired and will heal if the fragment is not degenerative and deformed and if the tear is in a vascular area. Radial tears start in the central portion and can propagate toward the periphery. In general, these are not receptive to repair because the circumferential hoop fibers are disrupted and much of the tear is in an avascular zone. Oblique tears often occur at the junction of the posterior and middle thirds of the meniscus and can often be repaired. Flap (parrot beak) tears are meniscal tears that begin as a radial type and then extend circumferentially around a portion of the meniscus. These tears often will have a large flap component that causes significant mechanical symptoms and cannot be repaired. Horizontal tears occur more frequently with age, are often associated with meniscal cysts, and typically are not repairable. Complex tears are also more common in older patients, are typically a combination of the types of tears described previously, and occur in multiple planes. Most often these tears are seen in the posterior horn and are best treated with excision. Tears are sometimes evident in the discoid meniscus. Incidental discoid menisci found at arthroscopy are not treated. If a tear is evident in a classic discoid meniscus, then an excision of the tear is performed with saucerization of the meniscus. Peripheral detachments of the discoid meniscus are repaired.

Some meniscal tears, depending on the symptoms they incur, can be treated nonsurgically. These include (1) longitudinal tears that are stable (displaced < 3 mm) and less than 5 to 8 mm in length; (2) partial tears that are stable; (3) shallow radial tears (< 3 mm in depth); and (4) tears with a favorable natural history, which includes small lateral meniscal tears with a concurrent ACL reconstruction.

A partial meniscectomy is indicated for tears in the avascular (white) zone and radial, oblique, and flap tears. This procedure may also be performed for any tear that has caused significant injury to the body of the meniscus, such as a complex tear, numerous cleavage tears, an alteration in the contour of the meniscal body, or degenerative tears, which may render any repair effort as futile. Injuries to the body of the meniscus may damage the structural integrity of the meniscus and the vascularity may be in doubt. Additionally, it is difficult to hold together degenerative tears with the various meniscal repair techniques. If excision of a meniscal tear is performed, the concept of preserving as much viable meniscal tissue as possible remains applicable. The goal is to remove only a torn, degenerated, or abnormally shaped meniscal fragment and thus perform a partial meniscectomy and not a total meniscectomy. The possible adverse effects a total meniscectomy on the knee joint have been well documented in the literature. The excision of a tear or degenerative tissue will retain functional meniscus. Long-term results after partial meniscectomy seem to indicate satisfactory results, but deterioration of articular cartilage may still occur. Degenerative changes on radiographs and a decrease in function have been shown to occur earlier in patients undergoing partial lateral meniscectomy than in those undergoing partial medical meniscectomy. Additionally, the results of partial meniscectomies are better in patients with acute traumatic tears than in those who have degenerative tears.

If a repair is performed, it is important to consider the numerous factors involved in healing, such as location and vascularity of the tear, the type of the tear, and quality of the meniscal tissue. The stability of the knee is important because repairs are more successful in a stable knee. Also, those repairs concurrently performed with an ACL reconstruction have a higher rate of healing, probably because of the various growth factors in the associated hemarthrosis. Chronicity is also a factor. In general, results of meniscal repair are better acutely after tear (< 8 weeks after injury) than a chronic tear secondary to the potential deterioration of the meniscal tissue with time. Patient age is also a factor. Younger patients have higher healing rates and axial alignment. Those patients with a varus alignment have a lower healing rate for medial repairs.

Meniscal repair can be done by either an open or an arthroscopic technique. Although the open technique has good results, most surgeons now prefer arthroscopic techniques. The traditional gold standard for meniscal repair is the inside-out repair, which is performed with either absorbable or nonabsorbable sutures placed arthroscopically with long needles and retrieved through a small incision on the outside of the capsule. The outside-in technique involves placing a monofilament suture through a spinal needle percutaneously into the knee joint and retrieving it through one of the arthroscopic portals. The all-inside technique is performed through the anterior knee portals and uses numerous devices and variations of techniques to stabilize the meniscus. Most of the devices are absorbable stents, and some are a combination of suture attached to the stent. A cited theoretical advantage to the all-inside technique is a decreased risk of a neurovascular injury that may occur with the use of the needles in the other techniques. All of the meniscal repair techniques have shown reasonable rates of clinical success (73% to 98%) as determined by the absence of symptoms and the patient's return to activities. In studies of second-look arthroscopy, healing rates have ranged from 45% to 91%. Most of the studies on meniscal repair have been retrospective.

Devices and techniques continue to be developed for meniscal repair. Research is focusing more on the bi-

ologic issues of healing and techniques to stimulate or augment that healing. In the past, techniques such as trephination of meniscal tissue, rasping, and fibrin clot have been used to augment the repair of the meniscus. More recently, investigations have targeted growth factors and gene therapy to enhance the healing of the meniscus.

If a total meniscectomy or subtotal meniscectomy previously has been performed, a meniscal substitute is reasonable. Because genetically engineered or other similar biologic replacements are still experimental, a viable option for the meniscectomized knee is a meniscal allograft. Meniscal allografts have been used for over a decade with reasonable results. With proper technique, the grafts have been shown to heal in the peripheral repair site and at its bony insertion. Grafts placed without a bony base, either a plug or block, have been found to have a higher failure rate. A symptomatic patient with lack of a functional meniscus is a candidate for a meniscal allograft. Factors that contribute to the failure of a meniscal allograft and thus are considered contraindications include patients with grade IV chondral changes, ligamentous instability, and knee malalignment.

Patellofemoral Disorders

Patellofemoral pain continues to be an enigma. Conditions causing patellofemoral symptoms include patellofemoral pain syndrome, tracking disorders, instability/dislocation, and chondromalacia.

The initial patient history should determine if the chief symptom is pain or instability. The patient should be questioned about a history of trauma, instability, and activities that initiate or increase symptoms (often ascending or descending stairs). The typical patient with patellofemoral symptoms is a female adolescent or young adult. The onset of anterior knee pain is usually insidious but can be acute. The symptoms of pain are usually worse with activity.

Physical examination must include assessment of lower extremity alignment, quadriceps angle, patellar tracking and mobility, crepitus, patellar apprehension, and specific areas of tenderness.

Standard radiographic evaluation of the knee should include AP, lateral, axial, and long-standing (for alignment) views. The lateral view, which should be obtained with the knee in at least 30° of flexion, is used to assess the position of the patella in relation to the patellar tendon (the Insall-Salvati ratio). The average ratio is 1.02, with a value over 1.2 indicative of patella alta and a value less than 0.8 indicative of patella baja.

Various techniques for axial views of the patellofemoral joint are used to evaluate trochlear morphology and patellar tilt. The Merchant/sunrise view is obtained with the knee flexed 45° and the x-ray tube angled 30° from horizontal. The sulcus and congruence angles are both measured on the Merchant view. Patellar tilt and congruence angles can also be measured using CT midpatellar transverse images with the knee flexed 15°, 30°, and 45°. MRI is useful for the evaluation of articular cartilage status.

Nonsurgical treatment continues to be the primary treatment for patients with a new onset of anterior knee pain. A well-supervised rehabilitation program is augmented by anti-inflammatory medication and local modalities. The goal of the rehabilitation program is to reduce symptoms by emphasizing quadriceps and hamstring stretching, strengthening, and endurance.

As biomechanical studies have shown that patellofemoral contact pressures are lowest between 0° and 30° of knee flexion, closed-chain, short-arc knee extensions performed within a pain-free arc of motion are the mainstay exercises for quadriceps strengthening. Patellar bracing and the McConnell taping technique have been used as an adjunct to a rehabilitation program.

Lateral patellar compression syndrome is characterized by anterior knee pain that increases with patellar loading activities and a patella centered without radiographic tilt. The syndrome has been associated with an increased Q angle (the angle formed by a line drawn from the middle of the tibial tuberosity to the middle of the patella to the anterior-superior iliac spine) and a tight lateral retinaculum. Patients sometimes experience subjective episodes of instability, which are likely caused by quadriceps inhibition. Routine radiographic studies yield little useful information. If nonsurgical treatment fails and the patient has a tight lateral retinaculum, arthroscopic lateral release has yielded successful results in 60% to 91% of patients.

Patellar tilt is similar clinically to lateral patellar compression syndrome with the exception that axial imaging reveals patellar tilt within the trochlear groove. Initial treatment is nonsurgical, followed by arthroscopic lateral release if no improvement is noted. Potential complications following arthroscopic lateral release include hemarthrosis and prolonged quadriceps weakness.

Patellar instability can be classified as subluxation or dislocation. Acute dislocation often occurs with a twisting movement of the knee. Predisposing factors for patellar dislocation include patella alta, generalized ligamentous laxity, lateral femoral condyle hypoplasia, lateral insertion of the patellar tendon, and an increased Q angle. Dislocation results from injury to the medial patellofemoral ligament. The patient may note that the patella initially lies on the lateral aspect of the knee, then relocates with knee extension. There is often an associated hemarthrosis. Physical examination frequently reveals tenderness over the medial retinaculum and the medial femoral epicondyle. MRI is useful for evaluating injury to the medial patellofemoral ligament and assess-

ing for associated injuries, such as osteochondral injuries to the medial facet of the patella or the lateral femoral condyle.

As studies of nonsurgical treatment have reported redislocation rates ranging from 15% to 44%, there has been renewed interest in surgical treatment of patellar dislocation. Surgery is also considered for treatment of associated injuries with an acute patellar dislocation, such as removal, fixation, or débridement of osteochondral injuries. In the young athletic patient, direct repair of the medial patellofemoral ligament to its attachments to the adductor tubercle and vastus medialis obliquus has been advocated. A lateral release can be performed if concomitant patellar tilt is appreciated. For the skeletally mature patient experiencing recurrent episodes of patellar subluxation or recurrent dislocation despite nonsurgical treatment, a distal patellar realignment procedure, such as a Fulkerson or Elmslie-Trillat procedure, should be considered. The Fulkerson procedure is an oblique osteotomy of the tibial tuberosity posterolaterally to anteromedially resulting in an anteromedial transfer of the tuberosity, decreased patellofemoral contact forces, and realignment of the extensor mechanism medially. The Elmslie-Trillat procedure is done by performing the osteotomy laterally to medially, preserving a distal pedicle of the tuberosity and resulting in a medial transfer of the tuberosity.

Patellofemoral chondromalacia continues to be an enigma because studies have shown 9% to 69% of patients with patellofemoral pain have normal cartilage in the patellofemoral joint at the time of arthroscopy. Nonsurgical treatment of patellofemoral chondromalacia consists of activity modification and anti-inflammatory medication to reduce inflammation followed by extensor mechanism strengthening, particularly of the vastus medialis obliquus. Surgical treatment of patellofemoral chondromalacia falls into two categories: (1) treatment aimed at relieving symptoms by decompressing the patellofemoral joint or correcting malalignment, and (2) surgery aimed at directly addressing the chondromalacia. Surgical treatment of patellofemoral chondromalacia secondary to increased compression caused by malalignment or a tight lateral retinaculum includes lateral release and anteromedialization of the tibial tubercle. One study has suggested that release of adhesions in the interval of soft tissue between the anterior proximal tibia and the patellar tendon can decompress the patellofemoral joint. Patellar chondroplasty is used to decrease the mechanical symptoms by using a motorized shaver to smooth or remove regions of cartilage fibrillation or loose flaps. Uniformly successful results with patellar chondroplasty have not been reported. For regions of grade IV chondromalacia, marrow stimulation techniques, such as microfracture or subchondral drilling, have been advocated. Results with marrow stimulation techniques have been unpredictable.

Knee Plica

Three synovial plicae are commonly described: suprapatellar, medial shelf, and infrapatellar. The clinical significance of plicae remains debatable. One hypothesis suggests that these synovial remnants have the potential to undergo an inflammatory process, causing them to become thickened and fibrotic. Repetitive contact between a fibrotic synovial plica and articular cartilage of the knee can lead to cartilage degeneration.

The patient with a pathologic synovial plica reports anteromedial knee pain and often reports an episode of trauma. Other symptoms include swelling, a sense of subpatellar tightness, and tenderness medial to the patella. Physical findings may include a thickened, palpable, tender cord medial to the patella. A palpable snap may be elicited with knee flexion.

Initial treatment of a suspected pathologic plica is nonsurgical, with nonsteroidal anti-inflammatory medication, hamstring and quadriceps stretching and strengthening, and local modalities. Arthroscopy remains the most reliable method for diagnosis of a pathologic synovial plica. Successful results with arthroscopic resection and removal are reliable when a thickened plica is the only pathologic finding in a symptomatic knee.

Extensor Mechanism Disruption

Disruption of the extensor mechanism occurs during a sudden eccentric contraction of the quadriceps muscles with the foot planted and the knee flexed. Disruption usually occurs through the musculotendinous junction of the quadriceps or through a diseased quadriceps or patellar tendon. Early recognition of this injury is crucial because results of early surgical repair of both quadriceps and patellar tendon ruptures are more favorable than late repair or reconstruction.

Patients with extensor mechanism disruption usually present with a history of trauma, pain, swelling, and a loss of extensor function. Physical examination may reveal a palpable defect above the patella with quadriceps rupture and below the patella with patellar tendon rupture. A low-lying patella is associated with quadriceps rupture, whereas a high-riding patella is associated with patellar tendon rupture. Extensor lag is commonly noted.

A lateral plane radiograph is a valuable diagnostic tool for evaluation of extensor mechanism disruption. A patellar fracture needs to be excluded. Patella alta is associated with patellar tendon disruption, whereas patella baja indicates quadriceps disruption. MRI is also useful in identifying the location of the disruption if clinical data are uncertain.

With acute ruptures of the extensor mechanism, direct repair can achieve favorable results. Delay in surgical repair is the factor that most significantly diminishes results of surgical treatment of extensor mechanism disruption secondary to the retraction and contracture of tissue that can occur. Chronic disruption of the extensor mechanism is often associated with soft-tissue retraction, necessitating tendon lengthening or even allograft soft-tissue augmentation.

Advances in Knee Arthroscopy

There are many recent advances in arthroscopic instrumentation and techniques including video and display equipment that use high-definition television cameras for high-definition video display. Images can now be projected onto glasses that the surgeon wears that weigh only 8 oz, thus avoiding the need for large video monitors. New digital capture devices can transfer video sequences from an arthroscopic procedure directly to a digital video disk or picture-archiving and communications system, which can link them directly to the patient's medical records and imaging. The second generation of voice-activated software is now being developed for improved use of hands-free instrumentation. Newer types of arthroscopic instrumentation include new forms of biodegradable implants and improved knotless fixation devices. Research continues with biologic solutions, such as meniscal healing with growth factors and gene therapy. Additionally, bioengineering continues to advance with research involving meniscal, ligamentous, and articular cartilage scaffolds.

Annotated Bibliography

Anterior Cruciate Ligament Injury

Anderson AF, Snyder R, Lipscomb AB, et al: Anterior cruciate ligament reconstruction: A prospective randomized study of three surgical methods. *Am J Sports Med* 2001;29:272-279.

A prospective randomized study was done to ascertain the differences in results of three surgical methods for ACL reconstruction (autogenous bone-patellar tendon-bone graft; semitendinosus and gracilis tendon graft reconstruction with an extra-articular procedure; semitendinosus and gracilis tendon graft reconstruction alone). The authors concluded that ACL reconstruction with a semitendinosus and gracilis patellar tendon autograft may have similar subjective results, but the patellar tendon autograft may provide better long-term stability.

Aune AK, Holm I, Risberg MA, et al: Four-strand hamstring tendon autograft compared with patellar tendon-bone autograft for anterior cruciate ligament reconstruction: A randomized study with two-year follow-up. *Am J Sports Med* 2001;29:722-728.

In this prospective, randomized study, 72 patients with subacute or chronic rupture of the ACL were assigned at random to receive autograft reconstruction with either gracilis and semitendinosus tendon or patellar tendon-bone. Sixty-one patients (32 with hamstring tendon grafts and 29 with patellar tendon grafts) were assessed after 24 months. Anterior knee pain was not significantly different between the two groups, but pain with kneeling was present in the group with patellar tendon reconstructions.

Beynnon BD, Johnson RJ, Fleming BC, et al: Anterior cruciate ligament replacement: Comparison of bone-patellar tendon-bone grafts with two-strand hamstring grafts. A prospective, randomized study. *J Bone Joint Surg Am* 2002;84:1503-1513.

Results from this study indicated that, after 3-year follow-up, ACL replacement with a bone-patellar tendon-bone autograft was superior to replacement with a two-strand semitendinosus-gracilis graft; knee laxity, pivot-shift grade and strength of the knee flexor muscles were improved.

Ejerhed L, Kartus J, Sernert N, et al: Patellar tendon or simitendinosus tendon autografts for anterior cruciate ligament reconstruction: A prospective randomized study with a two-year follow-up. *Am J Sports Med* 2003; 31:19-25.

According to this study, the semitendinosus tendon graft can be considered an equivalent option to the bone-patellar tendon-bone graft for ACL reconstruction.

Eriksson K, Anderberg P, Hamberg, et al: A comparison of quadruple semitendinosus and patellar tendon grafts in reconstruction of the anterior cruciate ligament. *J Bone Joint Surg Br* 2001;83:348-354.

In this randomized study of 164 patients with unilateral instability of the ACL, arthroscopic reconstruction with a patellar tendon graft using interference screw fixation or a quadruple semitendinosus graft using endobutton fixation was done. The authors concluded that medium-term outcomes between the two methods were similar.

Feller JA, Webster KE: A randomized comparison of patellar tendon and hamstring tendon anterior cruciate ligament reconstruction. *Am J Sports Med* 2003;31:564-573.

In this randomized study of 65 patients, patellar tendon and hamstring tendon autografts both resulted in satisfactory functional outcomes; morbidity was increased in the patients who received patellar tendon grafts, and knee laxity and radiographic femoral tunnel widening was increased in the patients who received hamstring tendon.

Jansson KA, Linko E, Sandelin J, et al: A prospective randomized study of patellar versus hamstring tendon autografts for anterior cruciate ligament reconstruction. *Am J Sports Med* 2003;31:12-18.

In this randomized study of 99 patients (89 of whom were available for 2-year follow-up), results were similar for patellar and hamstring tendon autografts for ACL reconstruction.

Peterson RK, Shelton WR, Bomboy AL: Allograft versus autograft patellar tendon anterior cruciate ligament reconstruction: A 5-year follow-up. *Arthroscopy* 2001;17: 9-13.

A prospective nonrandomized study to compare the long-term results of allograft versus autograft central one third bone-patellar tendon-bone reconstruction of the ACL showed no statistically significant differences in the presence of pain, giving way, effusion, Lachman and pivot shift results, or arthrometer measurements.

Shaieb MD, Chang SK, Marumoto JM, Richardson AB: A prospective randomized comparison of patellar tendon versus semitendinosus and gracilis tendon autografts for anterior cruciate ligament reconstruction. *Am J Sports Med* 2002;30:214-220.

In this randomized study, 70 patients with patellar tendon or hamstring tendon autografts for single-incision ACL reconstruction were evaluated at 2-year follow-up. Hamstring tendon autografts performed similarly to patellar tendon grafts; however, more patients who received patellar tendon grafts had patellofemoral pain and loss of motion.

Shelbourne KD: Contralateral patellar tendon autograft for anterior cruciate ligament reconstruction. *Instr Course Lect* 2002;51:325-328.

This article reviews the use and benefits of using the contralateral patellar tendon for ACL reconstruction.

Siebold R, Buelow JU, Bos L, Ellermann A: Primary ACL reconstruction with fresh-frozen patellar versus Achilles tendon allografts. *Arch Orthop Trauma Surg* 2003;123:180-185.

The authors retrospectively evaluated the clinical outcome of 251 fresh-frozen patellar versus Achilles tendon allografts for primary ACL reconstruction with a mean follow-up of 3 years. The authors concluded that satisfactory clinical results can be achieved with the use of allografts for primary ACL reconstruction. They indicated that the Achilles tendon-bone allograft seemed to be advantageous over the bone-tendon-bone allograft for ACL reconstruction because the failure rate was significantly lower.

Posterior Cruciate Ligament Injury

Oakes D, Markolf K, McWilliams J, Young C, McAllister D: A biomechanical comparison of tibial inlay and tibial tunnel posterior cruciate ligament reconstruction techniques: Analysis of graft forces. *J Bone Joint Surg Am* 2002;84:938-944.

This study examines the biomechanics of the tibial tunnel technique compared with the use of a tibial inlay in reconstruction of the PCL.

Posterolateral Complex Injury

Kanamori A, Lee JM, Haemmerle MJ, Vogrin TM, Harner SD: A biomechanical analysis of two reconstructive approaches to the posterolateral corner of the knee. *Knee Surg Sports Traumatol Arthrosc* 2003;11:312-317.

This article reviews a biomechanical study comparing the effects of biceps tenodesis with those of popliteofibular ligament reconstruction. Ten human cadavers were tested intact and in the posterolateral corner-condition, deficient, with each type of reconstruction. The authors concluded that the popliteofibular ligament reconstruction more closely reproduces the primary function of the posterolateral corner compared with the biceps tenodesis.

McGuire DA, Wolchok JC: Posterolateral corner reconstruction. *Arthroscopy* 2003;19:790-793.

This article describes a posterolateral corner reconstruction procedure that uses allograft and interference screw fixation. The authors recommend the use of this procedure in conjunction with PCL reconstruction to restore rotatory and posterior knee instability in the multiligament-injured knee.

Knee Dislocation

Liow RY, McNicholas MJ, Keating JF, Nutton RW: Ligament repair and reconstruction in traumatic dislocation of the knee. *J Bone Joint Surg Br* 2003;85:845-851.

This study compared 8 knee dislocations that were treated acutely (<2 weeks after injury) and 14 dislocations that were treated at least 6 months after injury. Both groups of knees were treated with a combination of repair or reconstruction of all injured ligaments. Although differences were small, the outcome in terms of overall knee function, activity levels, and anterior tibial translation were better for the patients whose knees were reconstructed within 2 weeks of injury.

Shelbourne KD, Carr DR: Combined anterior and posterior cruciate and medial collateral ligament injury: Nonsurgical and delayed surgical treatment. *Instr Course Lect* 2003;52:413-418.

This article reviews management principles of the multiple ligament-injured knee. Four treatment principles are stressed: (1) medial-side injuries can heal with proper nonsurgical treatment; (2) PCL tears with grade II laxity or less can heal with similar long-term results as grade I injuries; therefore, surgery may not be indicated; (3) PCL laxity greater than grade II and a soft end point should be considered for semiacute reconstruction; and (4) ACL injuries in combination with medial or PCL injuries can initially be treated nonsurgically and reconstructed at a later date as symptoms dictate.

Meniscal Injury

Bonneux I, Vandekerckhove B: Arthroscopic partial lateral meniscectomy long-term results in athletes. *Acta Orthop Belg* 2002;68:356-361.

A retrospective case-control study of arthroscopic partial meniscectomy for isolated lesions of the lateral meniscus is presented. An 8-year follow-up on 31 knees found deterioration of results with decreased Tegner scores (7.2 down to 5.7)

and Fairbank changes in 92.9% of the radiographs. The authors noted that the extent of the resection is a significant factor.

McCarty EC, Marx RG, DeHaven KE: Meniscus repair: Considerations in treatment and update of clinical results. *Clin Orthop* 2002;402:122-143.

An updated review of meniscus repair techniques and published results is presented.

Rankin CC, Lintner DM, Noble PC, Paravic V, Greer E: A biomechanical analysis of meniscal repair techniques. *Am J Sports Med* 2002;30:492-497.

Various methods that are used in the repair of meniscal tears were evaluated in bovine meniscus, including a biodegradable meniscal implant without sutures, a suture anchor device, and horizontal and vertical mattress sutures. Suture techniques were stronger at all levels of testing. The ultimate strength of repair was strongest for the vertical sutures (202 ± 7 N) and lowest for the arrow and suture anchor device (95.9 ± 8 N and 99.4 ± 8 N, respectively).

Shelbourne KD, Carr DR: Meniscal repair compared with meniscectomy for bucket-handle medial meniscal tears in anterior cruciate ligament-reconstructed knees. *Am J Sports Med* 2003;31:718-723.

This article presents a retrospective review of 155 patients with isolated bucket handle medial meniscal tears and ACL tears. Outcomes from meniscal repair were not superior to those from partial removal. Patients with repaired degenerative tears had significantly lower subjective scores than those with nondegenerative tears.

Venkatachalam S, Godsiff SP, Harding ML: Review of the clinical results of arthroscopic meniscal repair. *Knee* 2001;8:129-133.

A retrospective review of 62 arthroscopic meniscal repairs is presented. Early repair within 3 months of the tear gave better results (91%) than if performed later (58%). Suture repair alone yielded better results (78%) than meniscal arrows or a suture anchor device (56%). Healing rates of atraumatic meniscal tears were much lower than for traumatic tears (42% versus 73%). The isolated atraumatic medial meniscal tear appeared to heal poorly (33% healing) and was believed to be better treated by meniscectomy.

Patellofemoral Disorders

Aderinto J, Cobb AG: Lateral release for patellofemoral arthritis. *Arthroscopy* 2002;18:399-403.

A retrospective study of 53 patients who underwent lateral retinacular release for symptomatic patellofemoral arthritis is presented. Four patients underwent total knee replacement within 18 months after the lateral release. Of the remaining patients, 80% had a reduction in their preoperative pain, 16% were unchanged, and 4% were worse.

Bizzini M, Childs JD, Piva SR, Delitto A: Systematic review of the quality of randomized controlled trials for patellofemoral pain syndrome. *J Orthop Sports Phys Ther* 2003;33:4-20.

Based on the results of trials exhibiting a sufficient level of quality, treatments that were effective in reducing pain and improving function in patients with patellofemoral pain syndrome included acupuncture, quadriceps strengthening, resistive bracing, and a combination of exercises with patellar taping and biofeedback.

Schneider F, Labs K, Wagner S: Chronic patellofemoral pain syndrome: Alternatives for cases of therapy resistance. *Knee Surg Sports Traumatol Arthrosc* 2001;9:290-295.

The results of a prospective randomized study comparing 20 patients treated with proprioceptive neuromuscular facilitation and 20 patients treated with a special training program using a resistance-controlled knee splint are presented. The knee splint proved more effective than proprioceptive neuromuscular facilitation for treating patellofemoral pain syndrome resistant to conservative therapy.

Knee Plica

Irha E, Vrdoljak J: Medial synovial plica syndrome of the knee: A diagnostic pitfall in adolescent athletes. *J Pediatr Orthop B* 2003;12:44-48.

A prospective study of clinical criteria for the diagnosis of medial plica syndrome is presented. Two physical examination tests that improve the accuracy of the clinical examination for diagnosis of medial plica syndrome are described.

Extensor Mechanism Disruption

Richards DP, Barber FA: Repair of quadriceps tendon ruptures using suture anchors. *Arthroscopy* 2002;18:556-559.

The authors state that this is the first report in the English language literature of a technique using suture anchors to attach the quadriceps tendon to bone.

Classic Bibliography

Ahmad CS, Kwak D, Ateshian GA, Warden WH, Steadman JR, Mow VC: Effects of patellar tendon adhesion to the anterior tibia on knee mechanics. *Am J Sports Med* 1998;26:715-724.

Ahmed AM, Burke DL: In-vitro measurement of static pressure distribution in synovial joints: Part I. Tibial surface of the knee. *J Biomech Eng* 1983;105:216-225.

Andersson C, Odensten M, Gillquist J: Knee function after surgical or nonsurgical treatment of the acute rupture of the anterior cruciate ligament: A randomized study with a long-term followup period. *Clin Orthop* 1991;264:255-263.

Arnoczky SP, Warren RF: Microvasculature of the human meniscus. *Am J Sports Med* 1982;10:90-95.

Burks RT, Metcalf MH, Metcalf RW: Fifteen year follow-up of arthroscopic partial meniscectomy. *Arthroscopy* 1997;13:673-679.

Burks RT, Schaffer JJ: A simplified approach to the tibial attachment of the posterior cruciate ligament. *Clin Orthop* 1990;254:216-219.

Daniel DM, Stone ML, Dobson BE, Fithian DC, Rossman DJ, Kaufman KR: Fate of the ACL-injured patient: A prospective outcome study. *Am J Sports Med* 1994;22:632-644.

Fairbank TJ: Knee joint changes after meniscectomy. *J Bone Joint Surg Br* 1948;30:664-670.

Fulkerson JP: Anteromedialization of the tibial tuberosity for patellofemoral malalignment. *Clin Orthop* 1983;177:176-181.

Fulkerson JP: Patellofemoral pain disorders: Evaluation and management. *J Am Acad Orthop Surg* 1994;2:124-132.

Indelicato PA: Non-operative treatment of complete tears of the medial collateral ligament of the knee. *J Bone Joint Surg Am* 1983;65:323-329.

Maenpaa H, Lehto MU: Patellar dislocation: The long-term results of nonoperative management in 100 patients. *Am J Sports Med* 1997;25:213-217.

O'Neill DB: Arthroscopically assisted reconstruction of the anterior cruciate ligament: A prospective randomized analysis of three techniques. *J Bone Joint Surg Am* 1996;78:803-813.

Seebacher J, Inglis A, Marshall J, Warren R: The structure of the posterolateral aspect of the knee. *J Bone Joint Surg Am* 1982;64:536-541.

Shelbourne KD, Davis TJ, Patel DV: The natural history of acute, isolated, nonoperatively treated posterior cruciate ligament injuries: A prospective study. *Am J Sports Med* 1999;27:276-283.

Tenuta JJ, Arciero RA: Arthroscopic evaluation of meniscal repairs: Factors that effect healing. *Am J Sports Med* 1994;22:797-802.

Veltri DM, Warren RF: Posterolateral instability of the knee. *Instr Course Lect* 1995;44:441-453.

Chapter 38

Knee Reconstruction and Replacement

Mark I. Froimson, MD

Clinical Evaluation

Patients presenting for orthopaedic care of the knee complain primarily of pain and functional decline, marked by difficulty in walking, climbing stairs, and arising from a seated position. In addition, deformity and instability may be contributing symptoms that influence the choice of treatment. A detailed history is essential in determining the impact the knee symptoms have had on quality of life, and should specifically detail the level of impairment. It has been widely recognized that a major source of failure of knee surgery is the inability to live up to unreasonable patient expectations. As a result, it is important for the surgeon to document with specificity the presenting symptoms and objective measures of knee function and performance. Tools that allow for clarification of such patient expectations can help direct care and can provide a baseline against which postintervention outcomes can be compared.

General health assessment questionnaires, including the Western Ontario and McMaster Universities Osteoarthritis Index and the Short Form 36, are being used with increasing frequency to evaluate the impact of knee arthritis and subsequent treatment. These validated measures provide information on the effect of knee procedures on the patient's general sense of well-being and have been shown to offer consistent correlation with clinical outcome measures.

Radiographic Evaluation

Radiographs, including AP, 45° weight-bearing, lateral, and Merchant views, remain the essential diagnostic modality for evaluating the painful knee. Three-joint standing films define the mechanical and anatomic axis of the limb and can assist in surgical planning. Presenting radiographs are often inadequate, and although repeating films can be inefficient and costly, using unsatisfactory imaging studies to plan treatment carries far greater risk. Supine images of the knee, as are routinely obtained in a primary care or emergent setting, can severely underestimate the degree of joint space narrowing and thus the associated cartilage loss.

A second and equally common mistake resulting from poor-quality diagnostic radiographs is the overutilization of more sophisticated and expensive studies. MRI is a sensitive tool in the detection of pathology in the diseased knee, but is not specific for articular cartilage abnormalities, unless certain sequences are requested. Both T1-weighted, fat-suppressed three-dimensional, spoiled gradient-echo technique and T2-weighted fast spin-echo technique are essential to enhance accuracy of detection of articular cartilage lesions. Cartilage has higher signal intensity than fluid on T1 images and a lower intensity on T2 images. Meniscal abnormalities that are readily diagnosed on MRI can be thought to represent the dominant pathology, prompting referral for arthroscopic intervention.

Nonsurgical Care

Many patients with symptomatic knee arthritis will respond to a period of nonsurgical treatment, and most patients expect a major surgical intervention as a final option reserved appropriately for disease and symptoms that are unremitting despite judicious medical management. Although ambulatory aides are often deemed an unacceptable solution for arthritic symptoms, a properly used cane can provide significant functional improvement and pain relief by resting and unloading the joint. A cane can offer a temporary respite from the pain associated with ambulation and can allow for the initiation of other modalities.

The use of braces is also common, but there are few supporting studies to document their efficacy. In addition to the placebo impact of brace wear, nonsupportive sleeves have been thought to provide relative joint unloading by acting as a containment device for the soft tissues, thereby providing a type of hydraulic support.

Joint-Preserving Surgical Procedures
Arthroscopy

The role of arthroscopic surgery in the treatment of knee arthritis has been the subject of considerable controversy. Knee arthroscopy is one of the most commonly

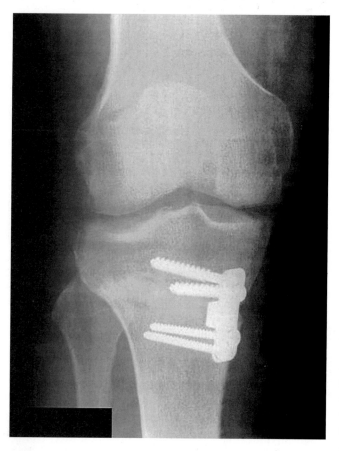

Figure 1 Opening wedge valgus osteotomy of the tibia with plate fixation.

of subsequent knee replacement has been assumed to be negligible, but this has not been adequately studied.

Osteotomy

Malalignment resulting in focal overload of either the medial or lateral compartment of the knee can be successfully managed with osteotomy to restore the mechanical axis of the knee. This strategy has the distinct advantage of joint preservation that is particularly attractive for younger, more active patients. Osteotomy is most likely to succeed when the disease affects predominantly one compartment, and there is therefore healthy tissue onto which to redirect the load. Despite this observation, no advantage has been demonstrated with arthroscopic evaluation of the knee done at the same setting as osteotomy, except to treat mechanically significant lesions. To maintain a joint line perpendicular to the weight-bearing axis, and to avoid joint line obliquity, varus malalignment is most commonly corrected through proximal tibial osteotomy, whereas valgus malalignment is most commonly corrected through supracondylar femoral osteotomy. When the degree of valgus deformity is not severe, and has resulted from proximal tibial deformity such as may occur following tibial plateau fracture, opening wedge varus-producing tibial osteotomy has yielded acceptable results.

Valgus-Producing Tibial Osteotomy

High tibial osteotomy requires careful patient selection and exacting surgical technique. The ideal patient is younger than age 50 years and active, with high functional demands likely to place undesirable stress on an arthroplasty. The procedure works best when performed early enough that symptoms and cartilage loss predominate on the medial side and there is no suggestion of involvement of either of the other two compartments, either clinically or radiographically. Contraindications generally include inflammatory arthritis, poor flexion (< 90°), flexion contracture, ligament instability, and tricompartmental arthritis. The procedure is less successful in smokers and in patients age 60 years or older, when the degree of deformity increases beyond 10° and when the involvement of the remaining compartments increases.

Valgus correction can be achieved by medial lengthening rather than lateral shortening, using either an opening wedge osteotomy and interposition plating or a medial external fixator with gradual distraction. The advantages of correction on the medial side include more anatomic restoration with resultant improvement in ligament stability, and the ability to more finely tune the correction. The main disadvantage of this technique is the risk of nonunion and loss of correction (Figure 1).

performed procedures for the diseased knee because of its ease of application and proven efficacy. Its success in the treatment of the arthritic knee is directly proportional to the degree of mechanical symptoms present preoperatively and inversely proportional to the severity of the underlying arthritis. Although the underlying disease process of cartilage degradation has not been shown to be favorably impacted by arthroscopic intervention, the symptoms associated with the secondary, mechanically significant lesions such as loose bodies, meniscal tears, and unstable cartilaginous flaps can be successfully addressed. Arthroscopic treatment of the arthritic knee is less likely to be effective in the presence of malalignment that causes overloading of the most diseased portion of the knee.

A recent and widely discussed randomized comparison of knee arthroscopy with lavage and sham surgery failed to demonstrate superiority of arthroscopy over sham surgery in a population of men with advanced arthritis. A separate review of arthroscopic débridement performed in a large group of patients older than age 50 years with a variety of diagnoses found that within 3 years, 18% of patients needed total knee arthroplasty (TKA), suggesting overutilization of the index procedure. The effect of previous arthroscopic knee surgery on the results

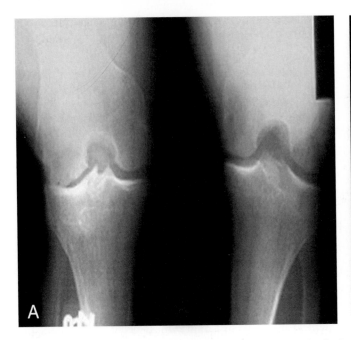
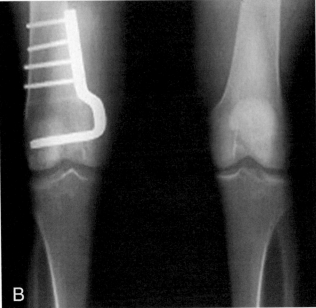

Figure 2 Distal femoral varus osteotomy **(A)**, with medial closing wedge and plate fixation **(B)**.

Varus-Producing Femoral Osteotomy

Valgus deformity may result in isolated lateral compartment disease and symptoms. Younger, active patients with preserved range of motion and no evidence of disease in the remaining compartments are candidates for realignment through varus femoral osteotomy. Ideally, deformity should be less than 15°, without flexion contracture or inflammatory disease. Correction to physiologic valgus (4° to 6°) is obtained through removal of a medial wedge, verified radiographically, and the fragments are rigidly fixed with a blade plate, applied medially (Figure 2).

Total Knee Arthroplasty

Replacement of the knee joint should be viewed as an elective procedure that is indicated when there is evidence of advanced disease resulting in failure of the joint to function satisfactorily. The three key elements considered in the decision to proceed with TKA include debilitating symptoms, failure of such symptoms to respond to less invasive treatment, and medical suitability of the patient to respond to surgery.

Patient and Disease Variables Affecting Outcome

TKA is a very successful procedure, with survivorship exceeding 90% at 10 years, 80% at 15 years, and 75% at 20 years. The probability of the implant surviving at these follow-up intervals can be influenced by patient-related factors including age, gender, and primary diagnosis, and by prosthetic design. Survivorship is adversely impacted in patients younger than 55 years of age, in males, and when the primary diagnosis is osteoarthritis. Patient age of 70 years or older, rheumatoid arthritis, and cemented fixation are factors that increase the long-term survivability of the implant. These factors likely have this effect because of the decreased demand on the implant, rather than specific physiologic factors. In fact, when the impact of specific underlying diseases is examined, unique considerations become apparent.

Obesity

Obesity confers both increased surgical complexity, with risk of improper implantation, and greater demand on the implant. Malalignment in the presence of obesity is not well tolerated, but is more likely caused by difficulties of exposure. Well-aligned, well-fixed implants fare as well in the heavy patient as in the general population. Wound complications are more common and can be minimized with careful surgical technique.

Juvenile Rheumatoid Arthritis

Juvenile rheumatoid arthritis can result in severe joint destruction and the need for reconstructive surgery at a very young age. The level of preoperative function in this group of patients is poor and is generally compromised by coexisting disease of adjacent joints. Altered immune function, along with the impact of disease-modifying agents, result in relatively high rates of infection. Additionally, stiffness remains a problem postoperatively, leading to reoperation in 8% in one study.

Hemophilic Arthropathy

Hemophilic arthropathy develops as a consequence of repeat hemarthrosis secondary to coagulopathy, and most commonly affects the knee. Loss of function and pain are severe, and the advent of adequate management of clotting makes TKA a viable option. These patients are usually relatively young and may have associated immunosuppression caused by human immunodeficiency virus (HIV). Surgery is complicated by high rates of infection, independent of the HIV status of the patient. As a result, the likelihood of survival of implants in these patients is reduced, with at least 10% failing within 5 years. Stiffness and limited functional recovery are also seen with greater frequency, further compromising outcomes.

Osteonecrosis

Osteonecrosis of the knee may occur in younger patients secondary to corticosteroid or alcohol use or in elderly patients as a spontaneous occurrence. Although nonsurgical treatment may be attempted, the majority of patients with this condition ultimately experience joint failure requiring knee arthroplasty. The compromised vascularity of the bone and the potential for significant involvement of large subchondral regions impacts the surgical approach to these patients. Preoperative MRI can assist in determining the amount of periarticular bone involved with disease.

Patellofemoral Arthritis

Isolated patellofemoral arthritis that is recalcitrant to treatment can be successfully managed with TKA in older patients. Functional results are superior to patellectomy or patellofemoral arthroplasty, and are equivalent to TKA done for tricompartmental arthritis. Lateral release is commonly required when preoperative patellar tilt is present. For younger patients with patellofemoral arthritis, nonarthroplasty treatment options may be considered.

Impact of Prior Surgery on Subsequent TKA

TKA may be used to treat posttraumatic arthritis that develops following fixation of tibial plateau fractures. Unique considerations include retained hardware, osseous defects, previous incisions, and a compromised soft-tissue envelope and result in higher complication rates, higher revision rates, and less satisfactory outcomes than primary knee replacements. Previous incisions should be incorporated whenever possible, or the standard incision should be adjusted to maintain an optimal skin bridge. When the ability of the skin to heal is in question, preoperative skin incisions can be useful to confirm healing potential. Hardware can be removed at the time of surgery, but excessive soft-tissue undermining should be avoided to prevent skin necrosis. If hardware is extensive and removal will devascularize the soft tissues, removal may be

staged as a separate procedure. Adjunctive measures such as bone grafting and lateral release are commonly required, and constrained prostheses may be necessary because of impairment of the soft-tissue envelope. Infection is a common complication, and may be heralded by persistent postoperative drainage. Although satisfactory results can be obtained, and pain and function can be substantially improved, patients should be counseled on the compromised outcome expected when TKA arthroplasty is performed following previous fracture fixation.

Prior osteotomy, both high tibial and distal femoral, also can compromise the outcome of a subsequent knee replacement. Osteotomy may result in bone defects or deformity, necessitating bone grafts and/or offset stems. Patella baja is common following tibial osteotomy and can lead to increased tension on the tendon insertion during exposure.

TKA after femoral osteotomy may result in inferior outcomes when compared with primary knee replacement. Ligament instability may occur related to the intra-articular correction of extra-articular deformity and may require use of components with increased constraint. Relative postoperative varus of the femoral component may occur as a result of prior deformity, but its incidence can be reduced with the use of extramedullary alignment verification.

Conversion of a fused knee is a controversial indication for knee arthroplasty and if undertaken can present unique challenges. Although a hinged or constrained prosthesis has typically been recommended, appropriate preservation of the soft-tissue sleeve can allow for successful reconstruction with a standard posterior stabilized design in some patients.

Surgical Technique

Optimal success of TKA can be obtained by accurate restoration of the mechanical axis, good fit and fixation of the implant to host bone, and careful attention to soft-tissue balance. Modern knee systems provide instrumentation that allows for reproducible approaches to prosthesis implantation. Both intramedullary and extramedullary alignment systems have been shown to be accurate, and bone preparation has been facilitated through the use of precise finishing guides that are well fixed to bone and incorporate multiple cuts in one step. Given these tools, attention to soft-tissue balancing has received increased attention as the sometimes overlooked yet essential component of knee replacement success.

The well-functioning knee must be balanced with equal tibiofemoral space in both flexion and extension, producing essentially equal tension in the medial and lateral soft-tissue envelopes following reconstruction. Knees that are too tight exhibit unsatisfactory stiffness, manifested by flexion contracture and/or decreased flexion, depending on whether it is too tight in extension and/or flexion. Excess release can produce functional impairment as a result of instability. Instrumented measures and computer-assisted surgery offer the promise of providing objective data on ligament balance against which subjective surgical experience can be quantified, but to date, such tools have not been validated.

Femoral rotation plays an important role in determining soft-tissue tension and ligament balance in flexion, and has received considerable attention. Because the tibial articular surface is sloped into approximately 3° of varus, an asymmetric resection of the posterior condyles is required to obtain medial and lateral balance of the flexion space at 90°, if the tibia is cut perpendicular to its long axis. Several anatomic references have been proposed to establish the optimum amount of femoral external rotation. Femoral rotation can be determined from one of three femoral axes, or it can be oriented parallel to the tibial cut surface following appropriate soft-tissue releases. The first approach allows femoral preparation to proceed before soft-tissue balancing, whereas the latter approach requires initial tibial resection and soft-tissue balancing. The three femoral referencing axes include a line 3° to 5° externally rotated relative to the posterior femoral condyles, the epicondylar axis, and a line perpendicular to the notch and trochlear axis (Figure 3).

Design Issues

Fixation

TKA has been performed successfully using methylmethacrylate cement for fixation and biologic fixation of the implant to host bone. Whereas cemented fixation can be achieved in nearly all bone types and patient profiles, bone ingrowth around the knee is less predictable. Thus, although loosening can occur with either mode of fixation, early loosening, caused by failure of bone ingrowth, is more common with cementless fixation. Strategies to achieve cementless fixation in the tibia include the use of porous surfaces augmented with pegs, stems, or screws. Micromotion at the screw/ baseplate interface has been implicated as a source of particulate debris, with the screw holes serving as pathways for particle migration. Although successful long-term results have been documented for cementless arthroplasty, higher rates of failure resulting from osteolysis and loosening have been reported. Hybrid fixation, in which the femoral component is inserted without cement and the tibia and patella are cemented, has been proposed as a compromise, but results with this technique have not been consistent. Similarly, cementing only the metaphyseal surface of the tibial component and press fitting the stem or keel has been associated with a higher rate of early implant loosening than full cementation of the tibial component.

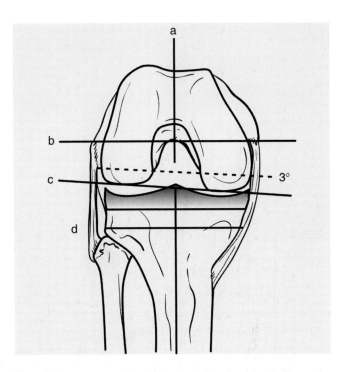

Figure 3 References for femoral rotation: AP axis (a), epicondylar axis (b), posterior condylar axis (c), and tibial cut surface (d).

Posterior Cruciate Ligament

Total knee components have been successfully used that allow for posterior cruciate ligament (PCL) retention, sacrifice, or substitution. Each strategy carries certain advantages and challenges, and there is no consensus regarding which approach provides superior outcomes. Long-term success has been reported with each design.

Proponents of PCL retention describe the potential for more physiologic femoral rollback, accurate joint line restoration, bone preservation, and the proprioceptive role of the ligament as distinct advantages. Because the PCL may play a role in the deformity, some studies advocate limiting its preservation to those knees with minimal angular malalignment and flexion contracture. Balancing of the ligament is advocated, with appropriate recession recommended when the trial components exhibit anterior tibial liftoff (booking open) in flexion. If the PCL is left too tight, it has been shown to result in posterior femoral subluxation, as well as asymmetric posterior polyethylene wear and associated osteolysis. Evidence from fluoroscopic kinematic studies suggests that the PCL, when retained, even in the absence of clinical problems, likely does not function physiologically, and paradoxical anterior femoral sliding rather than posterior rollback can occur in some patients. At the other extreme, overrecessing of the tight PCL can result in late failure with subsequent flexion instability. This latter syndrome is a recently recognized source of TKA failure in patients with well-fixed implants and is characterized by instability, effusion, and pain during

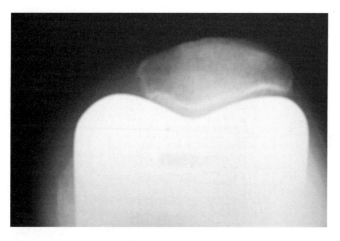

Figure 4 An unresurfaced patella articulating with anatomic femur is shown. The patient is asymptomatic at 10-year follow-up.

weight bearing on the flexed knee. Diagnosis is apparent through clinical examination with demonstrated laxity at 90° of flexion in the unloaded knee.

When the PCL is sacrificed, its function can be substituted for by a cam and post mechanism or by increasing the anterior lip of a conforming tibial polyethylene. Both designs counteract the posterior tibial subluxation resulting from sacrifice of the PCL. Better range of motion has been postulated to occur with the cam and post mechanism because of enforced femoral rollback. These prostheses carry the unique risk of dislocation, a rare complication resulting from collateral ligament laxity, allowing the femoral cam to jump anteriorly over the post. The subluxation height is the amount of laxity required to allow for such clearance. Deep dish tibial components can possess subluxation heights equal to cam and post mechanisms, and because the mechanism is far anterior, the likelihood of dislocation is less.

The cam and post mechanism has been identified recently as an articulation with the potential to produce polyethylene wear debris. One retrieval analysis identified evidence of adhesive and abrasive wear, as well as fatigue, in a wide spectrum of implant designs from several different manufacturers. Kinematic analysis has revealed that anterior impingement of the polyethylene against the femoral component can occur with several designs when the knee hyperextends. When the femoral component is inserted in relative flexion, or there is increased posterior tibial slope, this phenomenon is accentuated. Aseptic loosening and osteolysis have been correlated with post wear and damage and underscore the importance of the design and proper implantation of this type of knee replacement.

Modularity

Modularity has been introduced as a standard design feature of metal-backed tibial components in most total knee systems in current use. The main advantages offered include greater intraoperative flexibility and the potential for simple revision of a worn polyethylene bearing surface without concomitant need to address a well-fixed component. This advance in design has been associated with new problems. Motion between the metal base plate and the polyethylene was an unanticipated consequence of this concept and has been shown to produce polyethylene wear debris associated with osteolysis. Attention has been directed to the role of backside wear, with an attendant redesign of the locking mechanisms. Some designers, recognizing the inability to completely eliminate micromotion, advocate polishing of the tibial base plate to minimize the effects of such motion.

Mobile Bearing Design

An alternative approach is to design the undersurface of the polyethylene insert as an articulating surface, with macromotion expected. By allowing these mobile bearings to rotate, increased articular conformity can be achieved throughout the arc of motion. The theoretical advantage of this design has yet to be demonstrated at long-term follow-up, with equivalent survivorship expected with mobile and fixed bearing designs. Wear and osteolysis have been reported to occur with mobile bearing designs, demonstrating that this phenomenon is clearly multifactorial. As with fixed bearing designs, results with mobile bearing implants are durable well into the second decade. Unique problems include bearing fracture and dislocation, complications that are minimized with appropriate attention to soft-tissue balancing, alignment, and kinematics.

Patellar Resurfacing

Although patellar resurfacing is considered an integral component of TKA for the majority of North American surgeons, the procedure remains controversial and has been the topic of considerable study. Patellar complications remain one of the most common sources of problems after total knee replacement, prompting some surgeons to advocate avoiding this potential by leaving the host patella unresurfaced. Some studies have shown a higher prevalence of anterior knee pain in patients with unresurfaced patellae, whereas other well-designed studies have failed to identify statistically significant differences between the two groups. Certainly, many patients with a native patella articulating with an anatomically designed femoral component will achieve an excellent result (Figure 4). Revision rates have been shown to be either equivalent or higher following knees without patellar resurfacing, although results following such reoperations can vary. Patients with anterior knee pain caused by an unresurfaced patella fare well with secondary resurfacing. Serious complications with a significant adverse impact on the ultimate reconstruction,

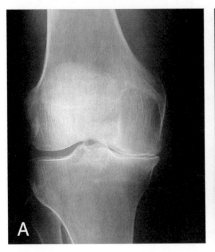
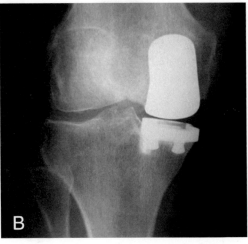
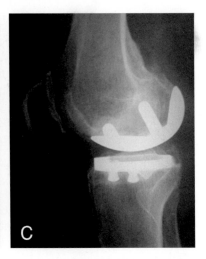

Figure 5 A, Preoperative AP radiograph demonstrating medial compartment arthritis. **B,** Postoperative AP radiograph at 3-year follow-up. **C,** Postoperative lateral radiograph at 3-year follow-up.

such as patella fracture or component loosening, are more common following patella resurfacing and are difficult to treat, often resulting in inferior outcomes. Thus, the consensus has emerged that knees without patellar resurfacing are at a somewhat increased risk for anterior knee pain, but are at a decreased risk for serious patellar complications.

Unicompartmental Arthroplasty

Unicompartmental arthroplasty is an alternative to TKA or osteotomy when the arthritis predominantly affects one compartment of the knee (Figure 5). In such instances, it is possible to resurface the diseased compartment and restore knee alignment that allows for load to be shared between the replaced and unreplaced compartments. Although this procedure lost favor after evidence of inferior survivorship data of several early series, newer techniques and patient demand has driven a resurgence of interest, and survivorship of greater than 90% at 10 years has been documented.

Patient selection and surgical technique are essential elements of a successful outcome. Pain that is well localized to the compartment exhibiting disease responds better to treatment than diffuse or global pain, and although the status of the patellofemoral joint has not been consistently correlated with success, the presence of pain in the lateral or patellofemoral joint preoperatively is a predictor of persistent pain after surgery. Contraindications include inflammatory arthritis, severe fixed deformity, previous opposite compartment meniscectomy, and tricompartmental arthritis. Correction of deformity must allow appropriate load transfer to prevent premature failure, but overcorrection adversely impacts the retained compartment, and also can lead to early failure. Recommended correction of the varus knee has ranged from 1° to 5° of postoperative valgus.

Advantages of unicompartmental arthroplasty may include quicker recovery, fewer short-term complications, and better functional outcome. There is a high rate of short- to mid-term satisfaction, but long-term survivorship has not been comparable to TKA when measured by revision rates.

Failure of a unicompartmental arthroplasty may occur as a result of implant wear, loosening or subsidence, or progression of symptomatic arthritis in the lateral or patellar compartments. Different failure mechanisms may predominate depending on design, with fixed bearing designs exhibiting more component failure and mobile bearing designs failing because of disease progression. Overcorrection may lead to deterioration of the compartment to which load is redirected, whereas undercorrection risks overloading the implant. Patellar impingement against the femoral implant can be symptomatic and lead to revision. Patellar arthritis generally is well tolerated in unicompartmental arthroplasty. Revision of a unicompartmental arthroplasty has been shown to be less complex than revision TKA. Nevertheless, defects in the replaced compartment may necessitate the use of augments, bone grafting, and/or stems.

Newer instrumentation has increased the appeal of the unicompartmental arthroplasty by allowing for small incisions with attendant lower patient morbidity, including less pain and shorter hospital stays. Care must be taken when using a minimally invasive approach to be certain that final implant fixation and alignment, keys to longevity of the construct, are not compromised. The long-term results of these techniques are not yet available, and common sense suggests that the incision size should not be the dominant outcome measure of this technique. Similarly, as this procedure gains popular appeal, its application to younger patients awaits long-term follow-up of success in this population.

Image Guidance

The desire to increase the accuracy of prostheses insertion has led to emerging efforts to use guidance systems to monitor and aid in implantation. Few preliminary data are available on these techniques and no long-term clinical data yet supports the widespread use of such technology.

Complications

Infection

Infection is a devastating problem that is best prevented. Attention to careful surgical technique and soft-tissue handling minimizes would healing problems. Laminar air flow and prophylactic antibiotics have been shown to reduce infection. The impact of dedicated surgical teams and reduced surgical time, while intuitive, are not documented. Immunosuppression, diabetes, smoking, prior surgery, and obesity are known risk factors. Antibiotic-impregnated cement has been shown to lower the incidence of infection and may be considered for high-risk patients. Persistent postoperative drainage is worrisome and should be treated aggressively.

Thromboembolic Disease

In the absence of effective prevention, thromboembolic disease will occur with great frequency following TKA, with historical data suggesting rates as high as 50%. Despite consensus that some form of prophylaxis is recommended in the perioperative management of these patients, controversy remains regarding the optimal prophylaxis regimen. Coumadin and low molecular weight heparin are two agents commonly used to reduce the incidence of thromboembolic disease, and although low molecular weight heparin therapy has been associated with lower rates of venographically documented deep venous thrombosis, (DVT), enthusiasm for its use has been tempered by the higher associated hemorrhagic complications. Early initiation of low molecular weight heparins in the postsurgical period corresponds to reduced rates of DVT but also with higher rates of bleeding. Use of aspirin as a preventive strategy is controversial, with advocates citing no difference in the occurrence of fatal pulmonary embolism, the most serious thromboembolic complication, as rationale for its use. The risk of DVT following TKA is highest in the early postoperative period, suggesting that prolonged prophylaxis is likely unnecessary. Physical modalities including compression stockings, pneumatic compression devices, continuous passive motion machines, and early mobilization are useful adjuncts in the prevention of occurrence, but have not been proven to substitute for pharmacologic prophylaxis. Routine monitoring for clinically silent disease is a widespread practice but has not been shown to be beneficial.

Medial Collateral Ligament Injury

Unanticipated intraoperative disruption of the medial collateral ligament during routine primary TKA has been typically treated with conversion to a prosthesis that provides varus/valgus restraint. Repair or reattachment has been shown to be an equally viable alternative, with a key advantage being the ability to continue with the planned primary knee prosthesis. Following repair, patients wear braces for 6 weeks, but are allowed full range of motion. Knee scores and range of motion at follow-up are equivalent to those of knees without this complication, and revision has not been required.

Extensor Mechanism Failure

Rupture of the patellar tendon is one of the most compromising complications that can occur following knee arthroplasty. Nonsurgical treatment and primary surgical reconstruction have failed to provide a satisfactory solution and are likely to result in significant compromise in functional outcome. Reconstruction with Achilles tendon or extensor mechanism allograft is technically demanding with the potential to salvage this problematic complication. Fresh frozen graft is preferred because of an improved ability of both bone and tendon to incorporate. Secure fixation is essential, with emphasis on a sturdy bone graft, keyholed into a well-prepared tibial bed, augmented by cortical screw fixation. Nonabsorbable suture fixation of the allograft tendon onto a broad base of healthy quadriceps musculature allows reliable incorporation. This reconstructive technique reliably reduces extensor lag and improves active range of motion at short-term follow-up.

Fracture of the patella may occur as a result of compromised circulation, overaggressive resection, maltracking or overt trauma, and may present as an insidious finding or with a sudden change in knee function. The prevalence of this complication is less than 1%, but its occurrence can significantly diminish the function of the knee. It is important to assess three aspects of the injury: whether the patellar component is loose, whether the extensor mechanism is partially or completely disrupted, and the extent of remaining patellar bone. Nonsurgical treatment is successful when the patellar component remains well fixed and the extensor mechanism is not completely dysfunctional. Patients with displacement of the fracture should be carefully assessed for remaining extensor mechanism function, which can be surprisingly satisfactory. A period of nonsurgical care may be preferred, with the possibility of later reconstruction if necessary, given the high incidence of failure and complications with surgical treatment. Surgical treatment is reserved for those patients exhibiting marked extensor mechanism disruption or gross patellar loosening, and generally results in compromised function and high revision rates.

Arthrofibrosis

The stiff total knee is a common source of failure and remains an unsolved problem. The best predictor of postoperative range of motion is preoperative motion. Failure to achieve at least 90° of preoperative motion compromises patient satisfaction. When arthrofibrosis is suspected early, it can be managed with manipulation under epidural anesthesia and aggressive physical therapy. Late treatment of stiffness is less likely to respond to manipulation with increased risk of periprosthetic fracture. Surgical correction often is desired by the unhappy patient, but is unpredictable. Correction of preoperatively identified malalignment, improper positioning, or incorrect component sizing may be successful in selected patients. Lysis of scar tissue, combined with exchange and reduction in polyethylene thickness, although appealing because of its apparent simplicity, has an unacceptably high rate of failure.

Periprosthetic Fracture

Periprosthetic fracture following TKA can occur following minor or substantial trauma and presents a challenge to restoration of knee function. Although the prevalence is low, occurring in less than 2% of patients, treatment of this event carries a high rate of complications. Common risk factors include conditions that create osteoporosis, stress shielding, femoral notching, osteonecrosis, and wear-related osteolysis. Treatment is directed at maintaining alignment and fracture stability, with early range of motion essential to preventing stiffness. In high-risk patients, nonsurgical treatment may be chosen even when immobilization is predicted to result in poor motion or malalignment. Key factors in surgical decision making include fracture displacement, stability of the prosthesis, and quality of the bone.

Failed prostheses demonstrating implant loosening accompanying or predating the fracture necessitates revision arthroplasty. In this setting, associated bone loss may necessitate bulk allograft reconstruction. The implant is cemented to the allograft, with diaphyseal fixation to host bone achieved using long stems. Collateral ligaments are preserved with bone fragments and then fixed to the allograft, but laxity usually necessitates articular constraint.

Displaced fractures associated with well-fixed implants are best treated with reduction and fixation. If the intercondylar notch is open, retrograde intramedullary nailing through a transarticular approach allows fixation without periosteal devascularization. Techniques using fixed angle devices and locked screws are evolving and are effective for treatment of many fractures. Flexible intramedullary nails introduced both medially and laterally offer a less invasive but also a less rigid method of achieving fixation. The key to success under these difficult circumstances is to provide rigid fixation and early motion while minimizing surgical complications.

Revision Total Knee Arthroplasty
Evaluation of Pain

Successful revision of a painful, failed TKA is dependent on an accurate evaluation of the cause of failure. Revision of the painful total knee without specific identification of the source of pain is less likely to result in a pain-free reconstruction and is not recommended. Systematic evaluation of such patients assists in the identification of both intrinsic (knee-related) and extrinsic sources of pain. Failure of the index knee replacement to provide initial pain relief or to alter the character of the pain indicates a second, unrecognized source of knee pain. Despite the widely taught precept that knee pain can originate outside of the knee, patients continue to present to tertiary referral centers with pain in a recently replaced knee whose origin is a diseased hip or lumbar spine. Protocols to evaluate the painful TKA, therefore, generally begin with clinical and radiographic extra-articular assessment. Pain well distal or proximal to the knee suggests referred or radicular involvement. A benign knee examination further raises concern about unrecognized pathology. At times, diagnostic injection of a remote location will be required to show a patient that the problematic knee is not the primary source of pain.

Aspiration is an important component in the evaluation of the suspect knee and should be routinely obtained. When a well-obtained culture is positive it is highly predictive, but failure to recover an organism preoperatively does not exclude infection and may result from suppression because of partial treatment or sampling error. Cell count of the obtained synovial fluid is useful. One recent study suggests that the threshold for a confirmatory result should be reduced from the traditional level of 25,000 white blood cells to a lower value of 2,500 for chronic low-grade prosthetic infection. Repeat aspiration can increase accuracy in problematic cases.

Preoperative Planning

Failure of TKA results in rapid acceleration of symptoms, functional decline, and the need for revision arthroplasty. Several factors, including lower levels of general patient health, decreased soft-tissue integrity, and bone loss encountered during revision arthroplasty, contribute to the increased challenge of obtaining a successful outcome in this setting. Revision knee systems offer a wide array of reconstructive options to restore mechanical integrity to the knee. Despite these advances, complications following revision surgery are much higher than following primary surgery, approaching 25%. Infection, extensor mechanism dysfunction, insta-

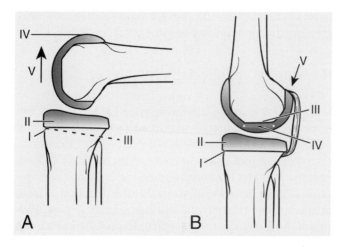

Figure 6 Balancing the flexion and extension spaces in revision surgery. **A,** Factors impacting the flexion space: I, tibial resection level; II, polyethylene thickness; III, tibial slope; IV, AP dimension of the femoral component; V, AP placement of the femoral component. **B,** Factor impacting the extension space. I, tibial resection level; II, polyethylene thickness, III,. distal femoral resection; IV, distal femoral augments; V, posterior capsule.

bility, fixation failure and periprosthetic fracture can all compromise outcome.

Total knee revision can be indicated for gross loosening, fracture, instability, infection, malalignment, wear, osteolysis or extensor mechanism disruption, and knowledge of the specific etiology assists preoperative planning. Appreciation of previous incisions and approaches is essential and will assist in planning for extensile exposure. A midline incision is preferred, but when multiple previous incisions are present, the most lateral incision that permits exposure should be used. Existing implants should be ascertained, and if one or more components remains well fixed, the surgeon must understand the options for incorporating this component into the final construct and/or how best to remove it without sacrificing bone. In addition, assessment should be made of bone damage, remaining bone stock, and extensor mechanism integrity. Collateral ligament integrity will determine the level of constraint required.

Revision surgery demands careful attention to gap balancing and joint line restoration. One useful reference for joint line restoration is its relationship to the fibula on the contralateral knee, generally 1.5 cm proximal to the tip of the fibula. The surgeon should understand the options available to selectively alter either the extension gap, the flexion gap, or both, and the impact such decisions will have on the joint line. Elevation of the joint line results in patellar impingement and reduced quadriceps strength. The flexion gap is impacted by tibial resection level and polyethylene thickness, tibial slope, and by the AP dimension of the femoral implant. The extension gap is also determined by the height of the tibial articular surface, but also by the dis-

tal femoral resection or buildup and the tension of the posterior capsule. Thus, an imbalanced reconstruction usually requires adjustment of the femoral implant position with regard to its distal proximal level or its AP dimension. Adjustment of tibial articular height will result in equal changes in the flexion and extension spaces and is not recommended when an imbalance exists (Figure 6).

Selective Component Retention

Clinically significant polyethylene wear and associated osteolysis is an increasingly common indication for revision TKA. Modular tibial components allow for the isolated replacement of a worn polyethylene insert in those patients with intact prosthesis fixation to bone. Unfortunately, the success of such isolated polyethylene exchanges has not been as high as anticipated. Whether these revisions are performed for instability or wear, the incidence of failure requiring additional surgery is 30% to 40%. Unappreciated malalignment or inadequate soft-tissue balance that may have predisposed the implant to initial wear or instability will remain uncorrected with this approach. Failures present as pain, recurrent instability, recurrent wear, stiffness, or infection. Failure rates are substantially higher than those of routine revision surgery, leading to the recommendation that caution be exercised when considering this strategy. In addition, retrieval analysis has demonstrated that the locking mechanism of modular tibial base plates degrades over time, further raising questions about the advisability of introducing a new insert into such a failing device.

Patellar Failure

Failure of the patellar component is one of the most common indications for revision TKA and can occur alone or in combination with failure of other components. When isolated patellar failure is the indication for revision, a high rate of failure has been recently reported. These poor results are thought to be caused by unrecognized component malalignment, evolving patellar osteonecrosis, and inability to restore bone stock.

Treatment of patellar bone loss that precludes the ability to obtain fixation of a new patellar component traditionally has been with patellectomy or débridement with retention of the patellar bone remnant, both of which lead to extensor lag and weakness caused by loss of patellar height. Bone grafting the residual patellar shell within a soft-tissue pocket secured to the surrounding tissue has been advocated to restore bone stock, improve tracking, and enhance extensor mechanism leverage. Early results in a small group of patients have been encouraging.

Management of Bone Loss

Septic loosening and osteolysis can result in significant bone loss that must be addressed at the time of secondary reconstruction. Preoperative evaluation may underestimate the extent of osteolysis and the need for restoration of bone stock. Defects can be addressed with either metal augments and substitutes or with a variety of bone graft techniques. Contained defects are managed with morcellized allograft and long stem prostheses to offload the periarticular reconstruction. When defects are uncontained, structural allografts are useful, and often essential, tools with which the surgeon should be familiar. Noncircumferential defects can be managed with bulk grafts acting to fill the defect, fixed to host bone with cancellous screws and bypassed with canal filling press fit or cemented stems. Impaction grafting can also be used to restore bone stock around the knee, by converting uncontained defects into contained defects. Metallic mesh is fashioned to restore the missing aspect of the bone and morcellized graft can be impacted into this shell. Preliminary results suggest remodeling and incorporation of bone that is superior to that obtained with bulk graft. Circumferential defects are best treated with allograft prosthesis composites with a step cut junction between allograft and host bone and overlaid, if possible, with a vascularized shell of remnant host bone. Intermediate-term results of structural allograft for complex knee reconstruction are promising, with maintenance of fixation, reliable union at the allograft-host interface and minimal evidence of graft resumption. In one series, repeat revision was required for flexion instability, loosening, or infection in 13% of patients at a mean of 70 months following the index procedure.

Annotated Bibliography

Clinical Evaluation

Mancuso CA, Sculco TP, Wickiewicz TL, et al: Patients' expectations of knee surgery. *J Bone Joint Surg Am* 2001;83:1005-1012.

Patient expectations for anticipated knee surgery include symptom relief and functional improvement. Specific surveys are offered and validated to help surgeons and patients to communicate regarding shared goals of surgery.

Nonsurgical Care

Leopold SS, Redd BB, Warme WJ, Wehrle PA, Pettis PD, Shott S: Corticosteroid compared with hyaluronic acid injections for the treatment of osteoarthritis of the knee: A prospective, randomized trial. *J Bone Joint Surg Am* 2003;85:1197-1203.

A randomized comparison revealed no difference in effectiveness between corticosteroid and hyaluronic acid when measured 6 months following treatment. Women were less likely to respond to treatment.

Joint-Preserving Surgical Procedures

Moseley JB, Petersen NJ, Menke TJ, et al: A controlled trial of arthroscopic surgery for osteoarthritis of the knee. *N Engl J Med* 2002;347:81-88.

This randomized trial of arthroscopic surgery for arthritis failed to demonstrate any measurable advantage of arthroscopic débridement or lavage over placebo surgery with respect to pain in the knee or function when measured 1 or 2 years after treatment

Wai EK, Kreder HJ, Williams JI: Arthroscopic debridement of the knee for osteoarthritis in patients fifty years of age or older: Utilization and outcomes in the province of Ontario. *J Bone Joint Surg Am* 2002;84:17-22.

A review of over 6,000 patients with 3-year follow-up after arthroscopy for arthritis revealed that 18% had undergone total knee replacement. Age was a predictor of subsequent knee replacement, with patients older than 70 years most likely to require additional surgery. These data suggest that arthroscopy is overutilized in elderly patients.

Total Knee Arthroplasty

Argenson JN, Chevrol-Benkeddache Y, Aubaniac JM: Modern unicompartmental knee arthroplasty with cement: A three to ten-year follow-up study. *J Bone Joint Surg Am* 2002;84:2235-2239.

Unicompartmental arthroplasty results in 94% survivorship at 10 years when used for the treatment of unicompartmental noninflammatory tibiofemoral arthritis. Failure can occur as a result of progression of arthritis or polyethylene wear.

Barrack RL, Bertot AJ, Wolfe MW, Waldman DA, Milicic M, Myers L: Patellar resurfacing in total knee arthroplasty: A prospective, randomized, double-blind study with five to seven years of follow-up. *J Bone Joint Surg Am* 2001;83:1376-1381.

No difference in the occurrence of anterior knee pain is seen whether or not the patella was resurfaced, and there were no specific clinical indicators of anterior knee pain.

Mont MA, Rifai A, Baumgarten KM, Sheldon M, Hungerford DS: Total knee arthroplasty for osteonecrosis. *J Bone Joint Surg Am* 2002;84:599-603.

Osteonecrosis can be successfully treated with total knee replacement in a cohort of young patients when cemented fixation and adjunctive stems were used. Survivorship was 97% at a mean of 108 months.

O'Rourke MR, Callaghan JJ, Goetz DD, Sullivan PM, Johnston RC: Osteolysis associated with a cemented modular posterior-cruciate-substituting total knee design: Five to eight-year follow-up. *J Bone Joint Surg Am* 2002;84:1362-1371.

A modular posterior stabilized knee prosthesis demonstrated excellent function at 5- to 8-year follow-up, but osteolysis was present in 16%. No osteolysis was seen when an all polyethylene component was used. Two revisions demonstrated tibial post impingement and backside wear of the polyethylene.

Parvizi J, Lajam CM, Trousdale RT, Shaughnessy WJ, Cabanela ME: Total knee arthroplasty in young patients with juvenile rheumatoid arthritis. *J Bone Joint Surg Am* 2003;85:1090-1094.

TKA in patients with juvenile rheumatoid arthritis can be successful, but poor preoperative function, involvement of multiple joints, and compromised immune system lead to increased rates of postoperative stiffness and infection.

Puloski SKT, McCalden RW, MacDonald SJ, Rorabeck CH, Bourne RB: Tibial post wear in posterior stabilized total knee arthroplasty: An unrecognized source of polyethylene debris. *J Bone Joint Surg Am* 2001;83-A: 390-397.

Retrieval analysis of posterior stabilized knee replacement identified that the tibial post can exhibit significant wear and damage as a result of impingement. This phenomenon was described for several implants and may be related to flexion of the femoral component, or hyperextension of the knee.

Rand JA, Trousdale RT, Ilstrup DM, Harmsen WS: Factors affecting the durability of primary total knee prostheses. *J Bone Joint Surg Am* 2003;85-A:259-265.

Total knee replacement is a successful procedure with long-term durability. Overall, survivorship at 10 years was 91%, 84% at 15 years, and 78% at 20 years. Factors that favorably affect durability were identified and include age over 70 years, rheumatoid arthritis, cemented fixation, female gender, and retention of the PCL.

Saleh KJ, Sherman P, Katkin P, et al: Total knee arthroplasty after open reduction and internal fixation of fractures of the tibial plateau: A minimum five-year follow-up study. *J Bone Joint Surg Am* 2001;83-A:1144-1148.

Prior open reduction and internal fixation of the tibial plateau poses significant challenges for subsequent knee replacement. Wound complications and infection can compromise outcome, and bony defects may dictate reconstruction methods.

Tanzer M, Smith KU, Burnett S: Posterior stabilized versus cruciate retaining total knee arthroplasty: Balancing the gap. *J Arthroplasty* 2002;17:813-819.

A blinded, prospective randomized comparison of these two designs using identical surgical technique reveals no appreciable difference in functional outcome at 2-year follow-up.

Wang JW, Wang CJ: Total knee arthroplasty for arthritis of the knee with extra-articular deformity. *J Bone Joint Surg Am* 2002;84-A:1769-1774.

Extra-articular deformity can be corrected using intra-articular bone resection and ligament balancing when coronal plane deformity is less than 20° in the femur and less than 30° in the tibia.

Complications

Crossett LS, Sinha RK, Sechriest VF, Rubash HE: Reconstruction of a ruptured patellar tendon with Achilles tendon allograft following total knee arthroplasty. *J Bone Joint Surg Am* 2002;84-A:1354-1361.

Rupture of the patellar tendon can be successfully managed by reconstruction using an Achilles tendon allograft. Technical details are critical with proper bone attachment to the tibia and broad soft-tissue repair to the quadriceps. Recurrent failure is minimized with this approach.

Dennis DA: Periprosthetic fractures following total knee arthroplasty. *Instr Course Lect* 2001;50:379-389.

The management of periprosthetic fractures around knee arthroplasty is reviewed. Key determinants of treatment include fracture displacement, bone quality, and status of implant fixation. Closed treatment, open reduction and fixation, and component revision are the primary options.

Leopold SS, McStay C, Flafeta K, Jacobs JJ, Berger RA, Rosenberg AG: Primary repair of intraoperative disruption of the medial collateral ligament during total knee arthroplasty. *J Bone Joint Surg Am* 2001;83-A:86-91.

Following intraoperative injury to the medial collateral ligament, primary repair with use of primary, nonconstrained implants resulted in satisfactory results similar to knees without this occurrence. Conversion to constrained implants was found to be unnecessary.

Ortiguera CJ, Berry DJ: Patellar fracture after total knee arthroplasty. *J Bone Joint Surg Am* 2002;84-A:532-540.

Patellar fracture occurs in less than 1% of cases. Nonsurgical treatment is effective for nondisplaced fractures with intact extensor mechanism. Surgical treatment for displaced fractures or loose patella result in a high rate of complications.

Revision Total Knee Arthroplasty

Babis GC, Trousdale RT, Morrey BF: The effectiveness of isolated tibial insert exchange in revision total knee arthroplasty. *J Bone Joint Surg Am* 2002;84-A:64-68.

Revision knee replacement consisting of isolated exchange of the polyethylene results in a high rate of failure, with 25% requiring rerevision. Preoperative instability resulted in the highest failure rate.

Christensen CP, Crawford JJ, Olin MD, Vail TP: Revision of the stiff total knee arthroplasty. *J Arthroplasty* 2002;17:409-415.

The stiff total knee can be successfully revised with complete exposure and revision of all components, with attention to accepted techniques of gap balancing. All patients in this series had improved motion and satisfactory pain relief and function.

Clatworthy MG, Balance J, Brick GW, Chandler HP, Gross AE: The use of structural allograft for uncontained defects in revision total knee arthroplasty: A minimum five-year review. *J Bone Joint Surg Am* 2001; 83-A:404-411.

Structural allograft used for the treatment of uncontained bone loss around the knee demonstrated a 72% survivorship at 10-year follow-up. Failure occurred as a result of infection or nonunion.

Hansen AD: Bone grafting for severe patellar bone loss during revision knee arthroplasty. *J Bone Joint Surg Am* 2001;83:171-176.

Severe patellar deficiency encountered during revision TKA that precludes reinsertion of a prosthetic component was treated with bone grafting inside a soft-tissue envelope, with improved tracking and restoration of patellar thickness.

Mason JB, Fehring TK, Odum SM, Griffin WL, Nussman DS: The value of white blood cell counts before revision total knee arthroplasty. *J Arthroplasty* 2003;18: 1038-1043.

Analysis of synovial fluid prior to revision TKA is useful in differentiating septic from nonseptic knees. White blood cell counts over 2,500/mm^3 with over 60% polymorphonucleocytes is highly suggestive of infection.

Saleh KJ, Dykes DC, Tweedie RL, Heck DA: Functional outcome after total knee arthroplasty revision: A meta-analysis. *J Arthroplasty* 2002;17:967-977.

In this review of 42 studies on revision arthroplasty, the procedure was shown to be effective in improving knee symptoms and function. Complications occur in 26% of cases and rerevision is necessary in 13% of cases for a variety of reasons including infection, extensor mechanism failure, and loosening.

Sharkey PF, Hozack WJ, Rothman RH, Shastri S, Jacoby SM: Why are total knee arthroplasties failing today? *Clin Orthop* 2002;404:7-13.

The indications for revision arthroplasty were reviewed, and in decreasing order of frequency were: wear, loosening, instability infection, arthrofibrosis, malalignment, and extensor mechanism failure. More than half of all revisions occur within 2 years of implantation because of infection, instability, malalignment, or failure of fixation. Late revision is more commonly a result of wear, implant loosening, or late instability.

Classic Bibliography

Arima J, Whiteside LA, McCarthy DS, White SE: Femoral rotational alignment, based and the anteroposterior axis, in total knee arthroplasty in a valgus knee: A technical note. *J Bone Joint Surg Am* 1995;77:1331-1334.

Blount WP: Don't throw away the cane. *J Bone Joint Surg Am* 2003;85-A:380.

Callaghan JJ, Squire MW, Goetz DD, Sullivan PM, Johnston RC: Cemented rotating-platform total knee replacement: A nine to twelve-year follow-up study. *J Bone Joint Surg Am* 2000;82:705-711.

Cartier P, Sanouiller JL, Grelsamer RP: Unicompartmental knee surgery: 10-year minimum follow-up period. *J Arthroplasty* 1996;11:782-788.

Chandler HP, Tigges RG: The role of allografts in the treatment of periprosthetic femoral fractures. *Instr Course Lect* 1998;47:257-264.

Colizza WA, Insall JN, Scuderi GR: The posterior stabilized total knee prosthesis: Assessment of polyethylene damage and osteolysis after a 10-year minimum follow-up. *J Bone Joint Surg Am* 1995;77:1713-1720.

Coventry MB, Ilstrup DM, Wallrichs SL: Proximal tibial osteotomy: A critical long-term study of eighty-seven cases. *J Bone Joint Surg Am* 1993;75:196-201.

Coyte PC, Hawker G, Croxford R, Wright JG: Rates of revision knee replacement in Ontario, Canada. *J Bone Joint Surg Am* 1999;81:773-782.

Dennis DA, Konistek RD, Stiehl JB, Walker SA, Dennis KN: Range of motion after total knee arthroplasty: The effect of implant design and weight-bearing conditions. *J Arthroplasty* 1998;13:748-752.

Duff GP, Lachiewicz PF, Kelley SS: Aspiration of the knee joint before revision arthroplasty. *Clin Orthop* 1996;331:132-139.

Healy WL, Wasilewski SA, Takei R, Oberlander M: Patellofemoral complications following total knee arthroplasty: Correlation with implant design and patient risk factors. *J Arthroplasty* 1995;10:197-201.

Insall JN, Thompson FM, Brause BD: Two-Staged Reimplantation for the Salvage of Infected Total Knee Arthroplasty. *J Bone Joint Surg Am* 2002;84-A:490.

Murray DW: Goodfellow JW. O'Connor JJ: The Oxford medial unicompartmental arthroplasty: A ten-year survival study. *J Bone Joint Surg Br* 1998;80:983-989.

Naudie D, Bourne RB, Rorabeck CH, Bourne TJ: Survivorship of the high tibial valgus osteotomy: A 10-22-year follow up study. *Clin Orthop* 1999;367:18-27.

Partington PF, Sawhney J, Rorabeck CH, Barrack RL, Moore J: Joint line restoration after revision total knee arthroplasty. *Clin Orthop* 1999;367:165-171.

Ranawat CS, Flynn WF Jr: Saddler S. Hansraj KK, Maynard MJ: Long-term results of the total condylar knee arthroplasty: A 15-year survivorship study. *Clin Orthop* 1993;286:94-102.

Ritter MA, Herbst SA, Keating EM, Faris PM, Meding JB: Long-term survival analysis of a posterior cruciate-retaining total condylar total knee arthroplasty. *Clin Orthop* 1994;309:136-145.

Squire MW, Callaghan JJ, Goetz DD, Sullivan PM, Johnston RC: Unicompartmental knee replacement: A minimum 15-year follow-up study. *Clin Orthop* 1999; 367:61-72.

Stern SH, Insall JN: Posterior stabilized prosthesis: Results after follow-up of nine to twelve years. *J Bone Joint Surg Am* 1992;74:980-986.

Chapter 39

Foot and Ankle Trauma

Richard Marks, MD

Ankle Fractures

Classification

Ankle fractures may be classified by mechanistic or radiographic criteria. The Lauge-Hansen system consists of four hyphenated descriptions of the fracture mechanism (supination-external rotation, supination-adduction, pronation-external rotation, pronation-abduction) (Figure 1). The first word describes the position of the foot at the time of injury; the second word describes the direction of the deforming force, and hence, the foot. All comprise several stages, based on severity. Supination-external rotation injuries are the most common, accounting for approximately 85% of all ankle fractures. The first stage consists of a tear of the anterior capsule and anterior tibiofibular ligament. In stage 2 the injury progresses laterally, resulting in an oblique or spiral fracture of the fibula at the level of the plafond. Stage 3 involves a tear of the posterior capsule or posterior malleolus fracture. Stage 4 consists of a transverse medial malleolus fracture or tear of the deltoid ligament. The pronation-external rotation injury pattern begins medially, with injury to the deltoid ligament or medial malleolus fracture. The second stage is characterized by injury of the posterior malleolus or posterior capsule, whereas the third stage involves a fracture of the fibula above the level of the plafond, with disruption of the syndesmosis. Supination-adduction injuries consist of an anterior talofibular ligamentous tear or an avulsion fracture of the lateral malleolar tip, then advance to an oblique, shear-type fracture of the medial malleolus caused by medial translation of the talus. Pronation-abduction injuries initially place stress on the medial structures, resulting in deltoid ligament failure, or avulsion of the distal tip of the medial malleolus. The second stage involves injury to the posterior complex, and the third stage involves an oblique fracture of the distal fibula caused by shear of the abducted talus.

The Weber/AO classification is based on the level of the fibular fracture (Figure 2). Type A fractures occur distal to the plafond and in more serious injuries involve oblique, shear fractures of the medial malleolus. They correspond to supination-adduction injuries. In type B injuries, the fibular fracture occurs at the level of the plafond, with varying degrees of obliquity and length of the fibular fracture. Medial malleolar avulsion or deltoid ligament disruption is associated with more severe fractures, corresponding to the supination-external rotation and pronation-abduction injuries. Type C fractures occur above the level of the plafond, with varying degrees of syndesmotic involvement, corresponding to the pronation-external rotation pattern. Most type A fractures can be treated with early mobilization; however, if medial malleolar displacement is present, casting or surgical intervention may be required. Type B and C fractures are frequently unstable, requiring surgical stabilization. Neither classification scheme is entirely inclusive or predictive, and the Weber B/AO and supination-external rotation patterns have great variability of fracture presentation. Concomitant syndesmotic involvement with widening of the mortise requires evaluation. The medial clear space should equal the superior clear space. Any inequality of these measurements or an absolute value of greater than 4 mm is indicative of an unstable fracture. Radiographic measurements, however, may be influenced by radiographic rotation or magnification.

Medial Malleolar Fractures

Isolated fractures of the medial malleolus occur with varying degrees of lateral ligamentous involvement. Transverse fractures below the level of the plafond are inherently stable and allow for early weight bearing and mobilization. A transverse fracture at the level of the plafond or an avulsion fracture with suspected medial clear space widening may also involve syndesmotic disruption. The Maisonneuve fracture includes syndesmotic disruption as well as a fracture of the fibular neck. In addition to surgical treatment of the displaced medial malleolar fracture, syndesmotic stabilization is also required. Treatment of oblique fractures at the level of the plafond is dependent on lateral ligamentous involve-

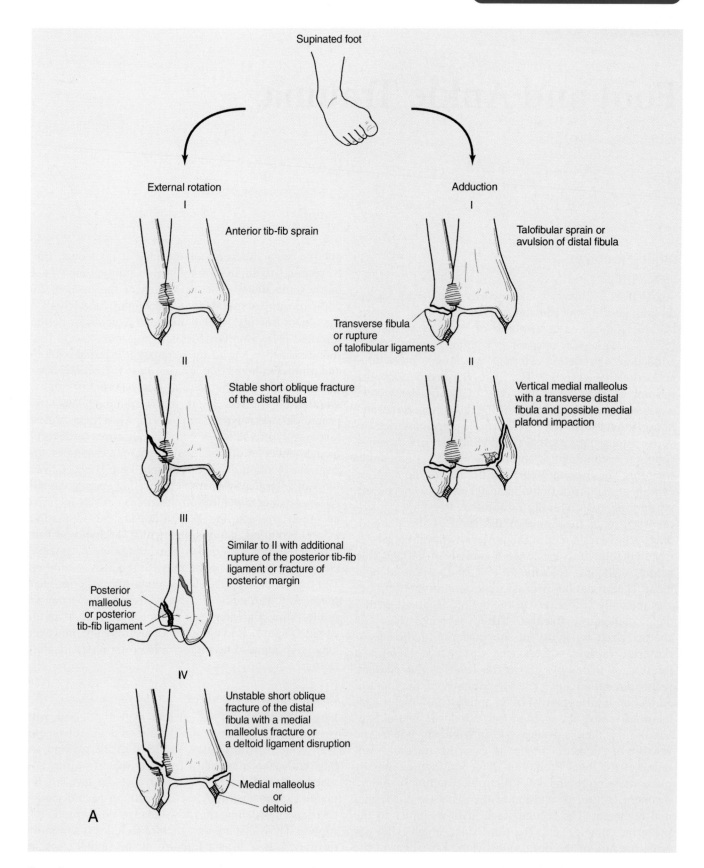

Supinated foot

External rotation
I

Anterior tib-fib sprain

Adduction
I

Talofibular sprain or
avulsion of distal fibula

Transverse fibula
or rupture
of talofibular ligaments

II

Stable short oblique fracture
of the distal fibula

II

Vertical medial malleolus
with a transverse distal
fibula and possible medial
plafond impaction

III

Similar to II with additional
rupture of the posterior tib-fib
ligament or fracture of
posterior margin

Posterior
malleolus
or posterior
tib-fib ligament

IV

Unstable short oblique
fracture of the distal
fibula with a medial
malleolus fracture or
a deltoid ligament disruption

Medial malleolus
or
deltoid

A

Figure 1 A, Schematic diagram and case examples of Lauge-Hansen supination-external rotation and supination-adduction ankle fractures. A supinated foot sustains either an external rotation or adduction force and creates the successive stages of injury shown in the diagram. The supination-external rotation mechanism has four stages of injury, and the supination-adduction mechanism has two stages. tib-fib = tibiofibular *(Reproduced with permission from Marsh JL, Saltzman CL: Ankle fractures, in Bucholz RW, Heckman JD (eds):* Rockwood and Green's Fractures in Adults, *ed 5. Philadelphia, PA, Lippincott Williams & Wilkins, 2001, pp 2001-2090.)*

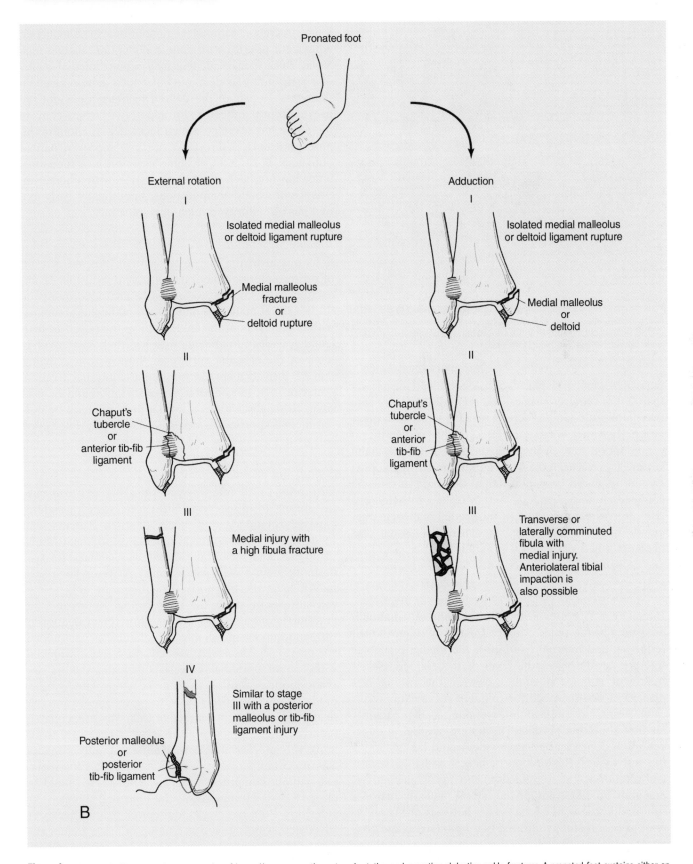

Figure 1 B, Schematic diagram and case examples of Lauge-Hansen pronation-external rotation and pronation-abduction ankle fractures. A pronated foot sustains either an external rotation or abduction force and creates the successive stages of injury shown in the diagram. The pronation-external rotation mechanism has four stages of injury, and the pronation-abduction mechanism has three stages. tib-fib = tibiofibular *(Reproduced with permission from Marsh JL, Saltzman CL: Ankle fractures, in Bucholz RW, Heckman JD (eds): Rockwood and Green's Fractures in Adults, ed 5. Philadelphia, PA, Lippincott Williams & Wilkins, 2001, pp 2001-2090.)*

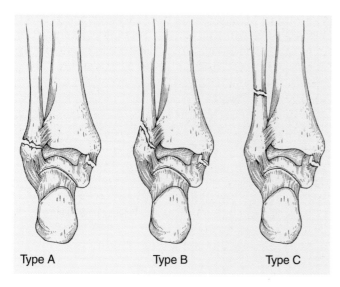

Figure 2 Weber/AO fractures. The staging is completely determined by the level of fibular fracture. Type A occurs below the plafond, whereas type C starts above the plafond. *(Reproduced from Michelson JD: Ankle fractures resulting from rotational injuries. J Am Acad Orthop Surg 2003;11:403-412.)*

ment and medial displacement. Medial shift of greater than 2 mm requires surgical intervention, typically with two parallel 4.0-mm lag screws or a lag screw with derotation Kirschner wire. Poor bone quality or significant comminution may necessitate the use of tension band wiring. If a vertical shear pattern is noted, the screws should be placed perpendicular to the shaft, at times in conjunction with a medial buttress plate to avoid the risk of proximal migration of the medial malleolar fragment. Stress fracture of the medial malleolus has also been described, particularly in patients with a varus heel and repeated adduction moments.

Bimalleolar Fractures

Bimalleolar fractures with displacement or rotational deformity at the time of injury frequently require open reduction and internal fixation. If the medial malleolar fracture occurs below the level of the plafond, closed treatment may be possible; however, the risk of displacement and the need for frequent reevaluation typically results in surgical intervention, if the patient's medical condition permits. The timing of surgical intervention is dependent on ankle edema and the quality of the soft tissues. Restoration of lateral malleolar length and rotation is key to reduction, and any significant lateral shift or shortening of the lateral malleolus can result in alterations of contact characteristics of the ankle joint. A recent study indicated that both lateral and posterior antiglide plating of the lateral malleolus have equivalent clinical and radiographic results, with slightly more peroneal tendon irritation with the antiglide technique. The use of lag screws without plate application has been successfully reported for management of ob-

lique fractures without comminution. In bimalleolar equivalent injuries with deltoid disruption, medial malleolar clear space widening may require medial malleolar arthrotomy to clean out entrapped deltoid ligament remnants. Repair of the deltoid ligament does not improve surgical outcome. Intraoperative arthroscopy of the ankle has revealed a high incidence of chondral injuries; however, arthroscopy has not improved patient outcomes. Postoperative immobilization in a functional brace has not been superior to casting, with a higher incidence of wound complications. Additionally, early motion has not improved functional outcome.

Trimalleolar Fractures

Fractures involving the posterior malleolus are a result of posteroinferior tibiofibular ligament avulsion, or impaction from the talus. Frequently, anatomic reduction of the lateral malleolus and medial malleolus combined with dorsiflexion of the ankle reduces the posterior malleolar fragment. Fragments with less than 25% involvement of the articular surface or those with less than 2 mm of displacement do not require internal fixation. Anterior to posterior percutaneous fixation may be possible, although at times a formal posterolateral or posteromedial approach is necessary to free up interposed soft tissues.

Syndesmotic Complex Injury

Disruption of the inferior syndesmosis ranges from subtle sprain to gross instability seen with pronation-external rotation and Weber C injuries. Patients with tenderness over the medial malleolus, proximal fibula, or interosseous membrane should be evaluated for syndesmotic injury. With subtle injury, MRI or bone scan may help in the diagnosis. Weight-bearing ankle views can sufficiently stress the interosseous membrane and anterior talofibular ligament to allow for evaluation of the syndesmosis and should be obtained as pain allows. As previously discussed, medial clear space widening with loss of tibiofibular overlap indicates deltoid and syndesmotic disruption. In patients with isolated syndesmotic disruption, reduction with percutaneous internal fixation is possible if the medial clear space adequately reduces. If not, a medial arthrotomy is necessary to remove the interposed deltoid ligament. A fully threaded 3.5- or 4.5-mm screw is placed across three or four cortices, without compressive lagging. The screw should be placed 1.5 to 3.0 mm above the joint and directed 30° anteriorly. Both three- and four-cortex fixation has been advocated, with four-cortex fixation offering greater stability, but no study has shown superior results with either method of fixation. Although traditionally the syndesmotic screw is placed with the ankle in a neutral position, the position of the ankle at the time of screw placement does not affect postoperative range of motion. Patients do not bear weight for 8 weeks to allow for sufficient syndesmotic healing, and screws are removed at 3 months to allow for restoration of normal distal fibular motion. Bioabsorbable screws have been shown to have equivalent clinical outcomes compared with metallic screws and avoid the need for screw removal. For Weber B and C injuries, the fibular fracture is rigidly fixed, then the syndesmosis is stressed with external rotation of the talus within the mortise with the ankle in a neutral position. Additionally, the fibula can be grasped with a towel clip, and distal syndesmotic stability evaluated. Typically, fractures less than 4.5 mm above the joint do not require a syndesmotic screw, but this parameter is variable, and intraoperative stressing is advised for all fibular fractures above the level of the joint.

Pilon Fractures

Classification

Tibial pilon fractures occur as a result of either a low-energy rotational mechanism with less comminution and soft-tissue damage or a high-energy injury secondary to vertical compression that can result in significant comminution, chondral damage, and soft-tissue involvement. Foot position at the time of impact can also result in additional injury to the malleoli, talus, and calcaneus. The Ruedi and Allgower classification remains the most commonly used for pilon fractures. Type I fractures are intra-articular with minimal displacement. Type II fractures have significant articular displacement with little comminution, whereas type III fractures have greater comminution and metaphyseal involvement. CT is useful in determining the full extent of the injury and helps with definitive surgical planning.

Treatment

Nonsurgical treatment is possible if articular incongruity is less than 2 mm and is generally reserved for low-energy injuries. Many pilon fractures require surgical intervention, which is performed in stages. The application of an external fixator at the time of injury allows for restoration of length and partial reduction via ligamentotaxis, while minimizing further soft-tissue damage. The fixator may be uniplanar or multiplanar, may cross the ankle and subtalar joints, or be limited to the tibia. Plating of the fibula helps restore length, but is not necessary at the time of initial fixator stabilization. CT is performed after fixator application to better ascertain fracture configuration and can help determine the proper surgical approach to limit soft-tissue stripping. Definitive treatment cannot be undertaken until the soft tissues have healed and swelling has resolved, usually 10 to 21 days after injury. Treatment goals include restoration of articular congruity and reestablishing proper length, rotation, and angulation, while avoiding exces-

sive surgical dissection and soft-tissue stripping. Newer surgical techniques include percutaneous internal fixation, limited open reduction, and subcutaneous plating, thus avoiding soft-tissue healing complications. Care is taken to perform a wound closure free of tension. If a solid construct can be obtained, the external fixator can be removed at the time of definitive treatment; however, this is generally only possible for type I fractures, whereas the higher energy level injuries require a prolonged course of fixator usage, frequently 2 to 3 months, to provide additional stability. If extensive bone loss is encountered, bone grafting at 6 to 8 weeks after injury is performed, with consideration given for the application of a bone stimulator.

Hindfoot Fractures

Talus Fractures

The talus acts as a link between the ankle, subtalar, and transverse tarsal joints. It is devoid of muscle or tendon attachments, and 70% of its surface is covered by articular cartilage for its five weight-bearing surfaces. Its blood supply is limited to the nonarticular surfaces; therefore, vascular compromise may be associated with fractures, particularly those involving the talar neck. Fractures are classified according to anatomic location: body, neck, or head.

Talar Body

Talar body fractures involve the superior articular cartilage and may be classified as coronal, sagittal, or horizontal fractures. These fractures are commonly associated with high-energy ankle fractures. Osteochondral fractures are also associated with ankle fractures, particularly supination-external rotation fracture patterns. Other anatomic locations include fracture of the lateral and posterior processes. Lateral process fractures, also described as snowboarder fractures, are created by forced dorsiflexion and external rotation of the foot. This fracture is commonly missed on initial presentation, but is usually present on plain radiographs of the ankle. CT is helpful to ascertain the extent of the fracture, which may encompass a significant portion of the lateral aspect of the posterior facet. If the fragment size is large and displacement is greater than 2 mm, open reduction and internal fixation is performed. Comminuted fractures may be initially treated with casting or immediate excision with early range of motion. No prospective study has evaluated the superiority of either treatment method. The posterior process consists of posteromedial and posterolateral tubercles. Fractures occur as a result of avulsion of the posterior talotibial and posterior talofibular ligaments, respectively. The posterolateral tubercle is more frequently involved, and because of the close proximity of the flexor hallucis longus tendon in its posterior groove, flexion and extension

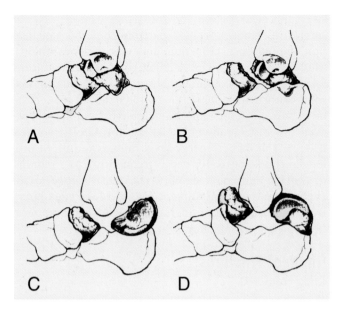

Figure 3 Hawkins classification. **A**, Type I: nondisplaced talar neck fractures. **B**, Type II: displaced talar neck fractures, with subluxation or dislocation of subtalar joint. **C**, Type III: displaced talar neck fractures with associated dislocation of talar body from both subtalar and tibiotalar joints. **D**, Canale and Kelly type IV: displaced talar neck fracture with associated dislocation of talar body from subtalar and tibiotalar joints and dislocation of head/neck fragment from talonavicular joint. *(Reproduced with permission from Sangeorzan BJ: Foot and ankle joint, in Hansen ST Jr, Swiontkowski MF (eds): Orthopaedic Trauma Protocols. New York, NY, Raven Press, 1993, p 350.)*

of the hallux may exacerbate symptoms. Fractures without significant subtalar involvement are initially treated with casting. If subtalar joint involvement is associated with displacement, then surgical reduction is required. Fragment excision is reserved for symptomatic nonunions without significant subtalar joint involvement.

Talar Neck

Talar neck fractures are grouped according to the Hawkins classification (Figure 3). Type I is a nondisplaced fracture. Type II involves subluxation or dislocation of the subtalar joint, and type III involves subluxation or dislocation of the subtalar and ankle joints. Type IV injuries, as described by Canale and Kelly, additionally involve displacement of the talonavicular joint. Type I fractures can be treated with non–weight-bearing casting; however, many surgeons prefer surgical treatment to avoid the risk of late displacement. This fracture pattern is amenable to percutaneous internal fixation from a posterolateral insertion site. Type II, III, and IV fractures require open reduction with internal fixation. Displacement of greater than 1 mm requires surgical care to avoid further vascular and soft-tissue compromise. Irreducible fractures, particularly those with residual subluxation, dislocation, or threatened soft tissues require emergent surgical intervention. Dual anterolateral and anteromedial incisions are usually re-

quired, with osteotomy of the medial malleolus performed if initial exposure is inadequate. Although the strongest screw configuration is from a posterior to anterior direction, crossed screws from an anterior to posterior direction are used for open reductions, whereas the posterior to anterior approach is reserved for those fractures treated in a closed manner. Medial comminution may require bone grafting and medial plating to prevent subsequent varus malunion. Theoretically, titanium screws offer an advantage if postoperative MRI is to be considered for evaluation of postoperative osteonecrosis, which increases in incidence with the severity of the fracture. Hawkins sign represents osteopenia that is seen beneath the subchondral surface of the talar dome and occurs 6 to 8 weeks after the fracture, which is indicative of talar revascularization. If osteonecrosis is suspected, MRI may be useful in making the diagnosis. If the fracture has healed and no cystic changes or collapse are noted, progressive, protected weight bearing can be instituted at 8 weeks, with regular clinical and radiographic reevaluation. Posttraumatic arthrosis of the ankle and/or subtalar joints is present in two thirds of all talar fractures. Fusion procedures may be complicated by varying degrees of osteonecrosis and may require an extended tibiotalocalcaneal arthrodesis. The incidence of osteonecrosis increases with degrees of fracture severity; up to 13% for Hawkins type I fractures, 20% to 50% for Hawkins type II, and 50% to 100% for Hawkins type III. Data are incomplete for Hawkins type IV fractures because of the infrequent presentation of these fractures. The presence of subchondral sclerosis, however, does not dictate the requirement for not bearing weight for prolonged periods. These patients are allowed progressive weight bearing based on symptoms and radiographic appearance of the talus.

Subtalar Dislocation

High-energy mechanisms are responsible for most subtalar dislocations and are frequently associated with open injuries and irreducible dislocation. Overall, the dislocations are closed in approximately 75% of patients, and medial dislocations, with the foot medially displaced relative to the hindfoot, occur 65% of the time. Irreducible dislocations occur in 32% of patients; the peroneal area blocks reduction with medial dislocation, and the posterior tibial and flexor hallucis longus and flexor digitorum longus tendons can block reduction with lateral dislocations. These injuries frequently require emergent open reduction, tendon relocation, and stabilization. Postreduction CT should be performed to fully ascertain the extent of associated injuries, which occur in virtually all patients with subtalar dislocations.

Calcaneal Fractures

The calcaneus is the most frequently fractured tarsal bone, with most fractures occurring as a result of axial loading, such as a fall from a height or during a motor vehicle crash. Given the mechanism of injury, patients should be evaluated for associated injury of the lumbar spine, which occurs in approximately 10% of patients with calcaneal fractures. Axial loading creates an oblique shear fracture caused by impaction of the lateral process of the talus that results in a superomedial fragment that consists of the sustentaculum ("constant" fragment) and a superolateral fragment that has an intra-articular component. In addition to this primary fracture line, a secondary fracture component may be created, based on additional energy imparted and the position of the foot at the time of injury.

Radiographic evaluation should include standard foot views, as well as a Harris axial view, which can provide information concerning shortening and varus angulation of the heel. An AP ankle radiograph may also allow for evaluation of lateral wall extrusion and impingement. Although specialized projections of the subtalar joint have been described (Broden and Isherwood projections), CT imaging provides the most complete, reliable assessment of these fractures.

Fractures may be classified as either extra-articular or intra-articular. Avulsion injuries account for most extra-articular fractures and result in fracture of the anterior process, sustentaculum, or calcaneal tuberosity, which is secondary to avulsion of the Achilles tendon insertion. Occasionally, oblique fractures that do not involve the subtalar joint are seen as well. Surgical indications are detachment of the Achilles tendon insertion, or displacement of greater than 2 mm of the sustentaculum or anterior process.

Intra-articular fractures occur in 75% of patients with calcaneal fractures, and characterization of the degree of displacement and number of posterior facet articular fragments is helpful for treatment recommendations and predictive of treatment outcomes. The Sanders CT classification system is based on the number and location of articular fragments seen on coronal projections (Figure 4). There are four types, based on the number of fragments of the posterior facet, with displacement of greater than 2 mm considered significant. Type I fractures are nondisplaced, regardless of the number of fragments. Types II, III, and IV have corresponding numbers of displaced articular fragments. In addition to displacement of the posterior facet, the surgeon must take into account factors such as shortening and widening of the heel, lateral wall impingement, and peroneal subluxation/dislocation when making surgical decisions. Patient factors, such as overall medical condition, peripheral vascular disease, compromised soft tissues, and a history of smoking also need to be taken

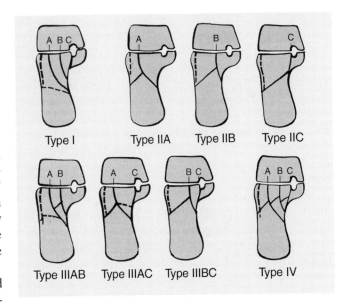

Figure 4 Schematic diagram of Sanders classification. *(Reproduced with permission from Sanders R, Fortin P, Pasquale T, et al: Operative treatment in 120 displaced intra-articular calcaneal fractures: Results using a prognostic computed tomography scan classification. Clin Orthop 1993;290:87-95.)*

into account. Treatment options include no surgery, closed reduction with manipulation with or without limited internal fixation, open reduction with internal fixation, and primary arthrodesis. Nonsurgical treatment is limited to patients with a type I fracture pattern or those with factors or comorbidities that preclude good surgical outcome. The fracture is immobilized until the soft-tissue swelling and fracture blisters resolve, then range-of-motion exercises are instituted. The patient is to refrain from bearing weight for 10 to 12 weeks. Closed reduction and manipulation with or without limited internal fixation can be used for those fractures with mild shortening or lateral impingement, as well as tongue-type fractures that are amenable to this form of treatment. As a result, the late complication of subfibular impingement with peroneal involvement can be avoided and more normal hindfoot anatomy can be restored, while avoiding potential complications associated with open techniques.

Open reduction and internal fixation is indicated for type II and III fractures. Surgery is delayed until swelling subsides, and a "wrinkle" sign is present on the lateral aspect of the heel, usually 10 to 14 days after injury. If a fracture blister is present in the area of the proposed incision, it must resorb and begin to reepithelialize before surgery. The lateral extensile right-angle incision is most commonly used, and although the medial approach has been used successfully, it is typically reserved for fractures with an irreducible medial fragment. A full-thickness flap is created to maintain soft-tissue integrity, and the posterior facet is elevated and reduced. Manipulation of the tuberosity with a Schanz or Steinmann pin can correct shortening and varus angulation and help with reduction of the posterior facet. Following provisional reduction maintained by Kirschner wires, a low profile lateral plate and screws are applied, first stabilizing the posterior facet. Meticulous closure is performed, and the patient is immobilized in a bulky posterior and U splint. Sutures are removed 10 to 14 days after surgery, and if the soft tissues allow, early range of motion is instituted. Patients do not bear weight for 10 weeks, at which time progressive weight bearing is begun.

Primary subtalar arthrodesis combined with open reduction and internal fixation to restore anatomic height, width, and calcaneal pitch is used for type IV fractures. This approach appears to be superior to initial neglect of the fracture followed by delayed subtalar fusion or primary open reduction and internal fixation.

The surgical outcomes of calcaneal fractures correlate with the quality of reduction and number of intra-articular fragments. Two-part fractures are associated with a better outcome than three-part fractures, and four-part fractures have uniformly poor outcomes. The extent of initial injury, initial nonsurgical treatment, and workers' compensation cases are predictors for eventual subtalar fusion. More than half of patients will require a supportive device. Bilateral fractures treated surgically have a worse outcome than unilateral fractures treated surgically, but have a better outcome than those managed nonsurgically. A recent Canadian study has shown comparable results in patients treated surgically and nonsurgically; however, when workers' compensation patients were excluded, those managed surgically had significantly higher satisfaction scores. Complications occur in 18% to 40% of surgical cases. Falls from a height, surgical treatment earlier than 7 days after injury, longer surgical time, and a history of smoking were factors associated with complications.

Neglected displaced fractures often result in a wide, shortened heel, problems with shoe wear, subfibular peroneal impingement, and posttraumatic arthrosis. This may necessitate decompression of the lateral wall of the calcaneus, peroneal relocation, and subtalar distraction arthrodesis to restore proper calcaneal pitch and height.

Midfoot Trauma
Navicular Fractures

The midfoot consists of the navicular, cuboid, the medial, middle, and lateral cuneiforms, as well as the metatarsal-cuneiform articulations. The midfoot has constrained motion because of multiple recessed articulations as well as strong ligamentous and capsular attachments. The navicular articulates with the cuneiforms, cuboid, calcaneus, and talus. Coupled motion between these structures (transverse tarsal joint) provides inversion and eversion of the midfoot and forefoot

relative to the hindfoot. Given the extensive articular surfaces of the navicular, vessels enter from the navicular tuberosity and dorsal and plantar surfaces, with a relatively avascular central portion, which has implications for fracture healing and the development of osteonecrosis.

Fractures can be described as avulsion (chip), tuberosity, or body fractures. Avulsion fractures of the dorsal lip are the most common and occur secondary to a plantar flexion force with varying degrees of inversion or eversion. The patient should be evaluated for associated midfoot or ankle injury. Immobilization is used until symptoms resolve, and for more severe fractures with a larger avulsion fragment and soft-tissue swelling, a non–weight-bearing cast should be used. Delayed excision of fragments is undertaken if they remain symptomatic. If a fragment includes more than 25% of the articular surface, open reduction and internal fixation is indicated to avoid midtarsal subluxation and posttraumatic arthrosis. Navicular tuberosity fractures result from an eversion force applied to the foot, with resultant contraction of the posterior tibial tendon and tension on the superficial deltoid attachment to the navicular. This may also represent a diastasis of the synchondrosis of an accessory navicular. Oblique foot radiographs obtained with the foot in 45° of internal rotation may help identify the fracture, which is differentiated from an accessory bone by the presence of sharp, irregular cleavage lines. Treatment is based on the severity of symptoms; however, given the possible late sequelae of posttraumatic flatfoot deformity, cautious treatment of these injuries is warranted. Injuries with minimal symptoms may be treated with immobilization and weight bearing as tolerated. In more symptomatic injuries with diastasis less than 3 mm, a non–weight-bearing cast is applied for 4 to 6 weeks, followed by gradual mobilization of the foot. Diastasis greater than 3 mm usually requires open reduction and internal fixation, with care taken to repair the posterior tibial tendon and deltoid ligament attachments.

Body fractures of the navicular are the result of direct axial loading, as occurs with a fall from a height. Given the strong ligamentous attachments, this probably requires a plantar flexion/dorsiflexion and rotational moment in addition to axial loading. Three fracture types have been described. Type I is a transverse fracture in the coronal plane, with the dorsal fragment less than 50% of the body, and no angular deformity of the foot. Type II, the most common, is an oblique fracture, from a dorsomedial to plantar lateral direction. The lateral fragment is smaller and often comminuted. There may be an adduction deformity of the foot. Type III fractures occur as a result of axial loading with lateral compression that results in central or lateral comminution and midfoot abduction deformity. The cuboid and anterior calcaneus may also be injured.

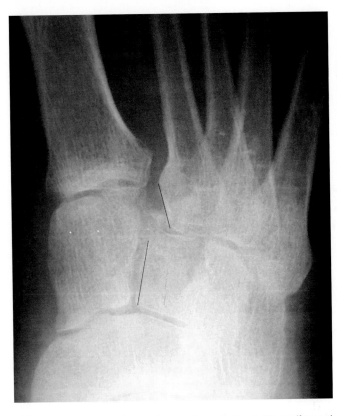

Figure 5 Loss of colinearity between the medial aspect of the middle cuneiform and medial aspects of the second metatarsal base, as denoted by the black lines, is indicative of a Lisfranc injury.

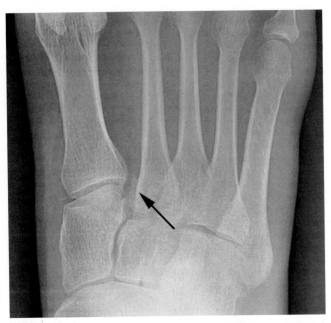

Figure 6 Bony avulsion at the base of the second metatarsal. This "fleck" sign (*arrow*) indicates a Lisfranc injury.

Type I and II nondisplaced fractures may be treated with non–weight-bearing cast immobilization for 6 to 10 weeks. Given the severity of type III fractures, these fractures usually require surgical intervention. Displaced type I fractures are amenable to internal fixation from the dorsal direction via an anteromedial approach. Type II and III fractures may require intraoperative external fixator application to assist with reduction; frequently bone grafting may be necessary for any large lateral defects, and it may be necessary to stabilize the major medial fragment to the cuneiforms to restore normal midfoot alignment. If extensive comminution is present, immediate naviculocuneiform arthrodesis should be considered.

Tarsometatarsal (Lisfranc) Fracture-Dislocations

The Lisfranc joint complex consists of the tarsometatarsal, intermetatarsal, and intertarsal joints. There is inherent osseous stability because of the recessed second metatarsal base between the medial and middle cuneiforms, as well as the cross-sectional trapezoid shape of the first three metatarsals and their corresponding cuneiforms. There are also strong capsuloligamentous attachments, particularly on the plantar aspect of the foot, which provide additional stability. The Lisfranc ligament runs from the base of the second metatarsal to the me-

dial cuneiform. Injuries of the Lisfranc joint complex can result from either direct or indirect mechanisms. Direct injuries result from a dorsally applied force, which will result in plantar displacement of the metatarsals if the force is applied to the metatarsal base or dorsal metatarsal displacement if the force is applied to the cuneiforms. There is a high incidence of associated tarsal fracture, significant soft-tissue destruction, and compartment syndrome. Indirect injuries occur from a combination of axial loading and twisting on an axially loaded, plantar flexed foot. Because of the mechanism of injury, relatively weaker dorsal ligaments, and greater mobility between the first and second metatarsals, displacement is typically dorsal, with diastasis between the first and second metatarsals and their corresponding cuneiforms. AP, internal oblique, and lateral foot radiographs are obtained to evaluate the tarsometatarsal articulations. Normal radiographs include colinearity of the medial aspect of the second metatarsal base and medial cuneiform, the medial aspect of the fourth metatarsal base with the medial aspect of the cuboid, and the medial aspect of the third metatarsal with the lateral cuneiform. Any incongruity is pathologic, as is any dorsal displacement of the metatarsals seen on a lateral radiograph (Figure 5). Diastasis of 2 mm between the medial and middle cuneiforms is considered pathologic. The "fleck" sign represents an avulsion of the Lisfranc ligament off the base of the second metatarsal (Figure 6). If injury is suspected despite normal radiographs, weight-bearing films are obtained once clinically feasible. Stress radiographs, MRI, and CT can also be used to assist in the diagnosis. Lisfranc complex injuries may be classified as total incongruity, partial incongruity, or divergent, but because of tremendous variation in mechanism of injury, there is great variation in radiographic presentation.

Nonsurgical treatment is used for nondisplaced fractures and consists of a non–weight-bearing cast for 8 weeks, followed by gradual weight bearing in a removable boot brace. Surgery is performed for injuries with any displacement seen on radiographs. If anatomic reduction can be obtained by closed means, percutaneous internal fixation is possible, but interposed Lisfranc ligament remnant can frequently block reduction and result in the joint springing open once internal fixation is removed. Therefore, open reduction is frequently necessary through a single or dual longitudinal incision as dictated by the injury pattern. Fixation is achieved with either 3.5- or 4.0-mm screws for the medial (first tarsometatarsal joint) and middle (second, third tarsometatarsal joints) columns and Kirschner wires for the lateral (fourth, fifth tarsometatarsal joints) column. A severe abduction mechanism may result in compression of the cuboid, termed a nutcracker injury. This injury may require lateral plating and bone grafting to avoid residual abduction. Patients should not bear weight for 8 weeks, followed by gradual weight bearing in a removable boot brace. Screws are removed 3 to 4 months after surgery to avoid screw breakage and to allow restoration of sagittal motion at the tarsometatarsal junction. Alternatively, bioabsorbable screws may also be used, obviating the need for additional surgery for screw removal. Immediate complete arthrodesis of the midfoot has poor results, although partial arthrodesis tends to have better results. Late arthrosis is common, even with anatomic reduction. Poor results are associated with nonanatomic reduction, open injury, and extensive comminution.

Metatarsal Fractures

Acute metatarsal fractures may occur as a result of a direct blow, which usually results in a transverse fracture, or as a result of an indirect twisting, or avulsion mechanism. Metatarsal base fractures are associated with midfoot injury, and these fractures carry a high index of suspicion for additional injury. Compartment syndrome can be seen in patients with more severe fractures, particularly those resulting from a direct blow. Nonsurgical treatment is indicated if displacement is less than 3 mm or angulation is less than 10°. Treatment can vary from the use of a postoperative shoe with weight bearing as tolerated for a stable fracture to casting with no weight bearing for an unstable fracture pattern prone to displacement. Surgery is indicated for displacement of greater than 3 to 4 mm or sagittal displacement of greater than 10° because this can lead to either direct overload of a displaced plantar fragment, or transfer metatarsalgia if dorsal displacement is noted. If associ-

ated with a Lisfranc ligamentous injury at the tarsometatarsal junction, surgical stabilization is necessary because of inherent instability. Surgical stabilization may be achieved with Kirschner wires, compression screws, or minifragment plating, as the fracture pattern dictates.

Treatment of fifth metatarsal base fractures is dependent on fracture location. It is helpful to separate fractures of the base of the fifth metatarsal into three types, based on location of the fracture. Type I fractures are true avulsion injuries of the tuberosity, or styloid process, which occur secondary to contraction of the long plantar ligament and peroneus brevis insertion; many are extra-articular. These fractures can typically be treated with a stiff-soled shoe and weight bearing as tolerated once symptoms diminish, with many patients sufficiently asymptomatic after 3 weeks of treatment. If there is a large intra-articular fragment with displacement or if the base fragment has retracted proximally, indicative of peroneus brevis retraction, acute surgical intervention is occasionally necessary. Continued symptoms after nonsurgical treatment are rare and may necessitate removal of the nonunion fragment, with evaluation of the peroneus brevis for possible reattachment directly to bone, or with the use of a suture anchor.

Type II fractures occur at the metaphyseal-diaphyseal junction, approximately 2.5 cm distal to the base. This is a circulatory watershed region that is subject to nonunion secondary to poor blood supply. The acute Jones fracture should be treated with either a non–weight-bearing cast for 6 to 8 weeks, or in a high-performance athlete, with placement of an intramedullary screw, which allows for earlier mobilization. The optimal screw size is largely dependent on the size of the intramedullary canal. One study has shown comparable initial and ultimate failure loads for 4.5- and 5.5-mm partially threaded cannulated screws, whereas another study compared 5.0- and 6.5-mm partially threaded screws and found no difference in bending stiffness, but greater pull-out strength with the 6.5-mm screws. Clinically, failure of fixation has been noted in athletes who returned to full activities before radiographic evidence of complete radiographic union.

Type III fractures occur in the diaphysis and are typically stress fractures. Possible etiologic factors include low arches and associated first metatarsal hypermobility, as well as cavovarus deformities, both of which can result in abnormally high stresses placed on the lateral foot. Altered lateral stresses may also be seen in patients with hereditary sensorimotor neuropathy and diabetic neuropathy. Poor blood supply in this region may also predispose an individual to injury and impair injury healing, resulting in nonunion. Strict adherence to no weight bearing is necessary after a proximal diaphyseal fracture is diagnosed and should be continued until radiographic evidence of fracture healing. Pulsed electromagnetic fields have been shown to accelerate healing. If sclerosis is noted at the fracture site, this indicates circulatory compromise, and surgical intervention is necessary to remove avascular fibrous tissue, combined with intramedullary screw fixation. Cancellous bone grafting may also be necessary. Any contributing structural abnormality should also be addressed.

Complex Regional Pain Syndrome

Complex regional pain syndrome, formerly referred to as reflex sympathetic dystrophy, is a clinical entity that develops after a precipitating traumatic event. It involves dysfunction of the sensory, autonomic, and motor systems and frequently is missed on initial presentation. Patients with acute complex regional pain syndrome describe antecedent trauma, which may be as severe as a crush injury or as nominal as a sprain or twisting injury. The onset of pain may also occur after surgical procedures. In the acute phase, there is an abnormal disproportional painful reaction to a stimulus (hyperpathia), increased sensitivity to a stimulus (allodynia), hyperhidrosis, and cyanosis. Swelling of the foot is typically seen, and radiographs will appear normal. The second phase occurs 2 to 4 months after onset and involves dystrophic and ischemic changes. Hyperpathia and allodynia continue, as does swelling, and hypohydrosis and pallor are experienced. Radiographs typically show demineralization. The third phase is characterized by evidence of joint stiffness, muscular atrophy, and contracture. Swelling may persist, with the skin becoming shiny, dry, and cool. Radiographs show evidence of continued demineralization. This syndrome may also be characterized into complex regional pain syndrome type I, which occurs in a generalized area after a traumatic event, or complex regional pain syndrome type II, which develops in a discrete area secondary to peripheral nerve injury. The diagnosis is assisted by the use of a triple-phase bone scan, which in the delayed phase will show diffuse radionuclide uptake throughout the foot. This procedure is best performed within the first 6 months of the appearance of symptoms. MRI will also show typical marrow edema during this time. Treatment consists of a combination of physical therapy, nerve blocks, and pharmacologic agents, and should be instituted as early as possible. Physical therapy is designed to maximize motion, in combination with desensitization exercises and modalities. Sympathetic nerve blocks are used both for diagnostic and treatment purposes. Failure to respond to a sympathetic block should bring the diagnosis into question. Several pharmacologic agents, including antidepressants, anticonvulsants, and calcium channel blockers have been used for the treatment of complex regional pain syndrome, typically coordinated by a multidisciplinary pain center.

Compartment Syndrome

Acute compartment syndrome develops secondary to local trauma that results in an increase of local tissue interstitial pressure from bleeding and edema from soft-tissue destruction. As a result, vascular occlusion occurs and creates myoneural ischemia. Compartment syndrome has been associated with calcaneal fractures, Lisfranc complex injuries, and crush injuries; however, compartment syndrome should be suspected in any injury mechanism that creates significant swelling. If the ischemic process is left untreated for more than 8 hours, irreversible myoneural necrosis and fibrosis occur; therefore, prompt diagnosis and treatment are of great importance. The diagnosis relies on clinical signs and measurement of compartment pressures. Pain out of proportion to injury severity is a classic sign; however, in the multiply injured patient this symptom is unreliable. Loss of two-point discrimination and light touch is more reliable than loss of sensation, whereas pain is exacerbated with passive dorsiflexion of the toes, which places the intrinsic muscles on stretch. The presence or absence of pulses and capillary refill is unreliable. The compartments of the foot should be measured in patients suspected of having compartment syndrome. Fasciotomy is indicated when the compartment pressures exceed 30 mm Hg or is within 30 mm Hg of the diastolic pressure.

Nine compartments have been described: the medial, lateral, four interosseous, and three central compartments, including the deep central (calcaneal) compartment that contains the quadratus plantae muscle and the posterior tibial neurovascular bundle. Decompression is performed with dual dorsal incisions, which allow for decompression of the first and second interosseous compartments, the medial compartment, and the deep central compartment. The lateral dorsal incision allows for decompression of the two lateral interosseous compartments, the superficial and middle central compartments, and the lateral compartment. A single, medially based fasciotomy has been described, but is technically more difficult to perform. Sometimes the medially based incision may be used in addition to the dorsal approach to adequately ensure decompression of the deep calcaneal compartment. Closure is performed in a delayed fashion, either with primary closure or with split-thickness skin grafts. Exercise-induced compartment syndrome of the foot has been recognized, most commonly affecting the medial compartment, and has been shown to follow the same criteria for diagnosis of chronic exertional compartment syndrome of the leg.

Annotated Bibliography

Ankle and Pilon Fractures

Day GA, Swanson CE, Hulcombe BG: Operative treatment of ankle fractures: A minimum ten-year follow-up. *Foot Ankle Int* 2001;22:102-106.

In this study, 52% of patients with surgically treated bimalleolar fractures had good or excellent results; 24% of patients had a poor outcome.

Dickson KF, Montgomery S, Field J: High energy plafond fractures treated by a spanning external fixator initially and followed by a second stage open reduction internal fixation of the articular surface: Preliminary report. *Injury* 2001;32(suppl 4):SD92-SD98.

This protocol, used to treat patients with highly comminuted fractures, resulted in 81% good or excellent results, a 35% complication rate, and 28% radiographic arthrosis.

Dietrich A, Lill H, Engel T, Schonfelder M, Josten C: Conservative functional treatment of ankle fractures. *Arch Orthop Trauma Surg* 2002;122:165-168.

Ninety percent of patients with an isolated Weber B fracture with less than 1 mm of displacement were treated successfully with a functional brace.

Hasselman CT, Vogt MT, Stone KL, Cauley JA, Conti SF: Foot and ankle fractures in elderly white women: Incidence and risk factors. *J Bone Joint Surg Am* 2003; 85:820-824.

Fibular fractures were the most common ankle fracture (prevalence 57.6%) and occur in younger women with a high body mass index. Fractures of the fifth metatarsal are the most common foot fractures in women with low bone mineral density.

Hovis WD, Kaiser BW, Watson JT, Bucholz RW: Treatment of syndesmotic disruptions of the ankle with bioabsorbable screw fixation. *J Bone Joint Surg Am* 2002; 84:26-31.

Polyevolactic acid screws were used to stabilize syndesmotic disruptions in 33 patients. Twenty-four patients were followed for 34 months after surgery. All patients healed uneventfully, with or without fixation; no patient had osteolysis or inflammation.

Lamontagne J, Blachut PA, Broekhuyse HM; O'Brien PJ, Meek RN: Surgical treatment of a displaced lateral malleolus fracture: The antiglide technique versus lateral plate fixation. *J Orthop Trauma* 2002;16:498-502.

In this study, surgical outcome, complication rate, and requirement for hardware removal was equivalent in the two groups.

Lehtonen H, Jarvinen TL, Honkonen S, Nyman M, Vihtonen K, Jarvinen M: Use of a cast compared with a functional ankle brace after operative treatment of an ankle fracture: A prospective, randomized study. *J Bone Joint Surg Am* 2003;85-A:205-211.

The long-term functional outcome was equivalent between the two groups, with similar fracture healing. The incidence of postoperative wound healing complications was significantly higher with brace treatment.

Loren GJ, Ferkel RD: Arthroscopic assessment of occult intra-articular injury in acute ankle fractures. *Arthroscopy* 2002;18:412-421.

Sixty-three percent of fractures showed chondral injury, more frequently on the medial aspect of the talus. Pronation-external rotation fractures had a higher incidence of injury (70%) than supination-external rotation fractures (46%). Seventy-five percent of fractures with syndesmotic disruption had chondral damage.

Pneumaticos SG, Noble PC, Chatziioannou SN, Trevino SG: The effects of rotation on radiographic evaluation of the tibiofibular syndesmosis. *Foot Ankle Int* 2002;23: 107-111.

Comparisons were made between the tibiofibular clear space, tibiofibular overlap, width of the tibia and fibula, and medial clear space. The width of the tibiofibular clear space did not change with rotation, whereas the other parameters did.

Sinisaari IP, Luthje PM, Mikkonen RH: Ruptured tibiofibular syndesmosis: Comparison study of metallic to bioabsorbable fixation. *Foot Ankle Int* 2002;23:744-748.

Poly-L-lactide bioabsorbable screws showed equivalent results with radiographic measurements, range of motion, and subjective outcome compared with metallic fixation.

Tornetta P III, Creevy W: Lag screw only fixation of the lateral malleolus. *J Orthop Trauma* 2001;15:119-121.

Lag screw only fixation of simple oblique fractures, when compared with plate fixation, resulted in less lateral pain, no palpable hardware (56% plate), fewer shoe wear restrictions, no hardware removal requirements (31% plate), and no loss of fracture reduction.

Tornetta P III, Spoo JE, Reynolds FA, Lee C: Overtightening of the ankle syndesmosis: Is it really possible? *J Bone Joint Surg Am* 2001;83-A:489-492.

There was no difference between the values for maximal dorsiflexion before and after syndesmotic compression in cadaveric specimens fixed with a syndesmotic screw while held in plantar flexion.

Hindfoot Fractures

Bibbo C, Anderson RB, Davis WH: Injury characteristics and the clinical outcome of subtalar dislocations: A clinical and radiographic analysis of 25 cases. *Foot Ankle Int* 2003;24:158-163.

High-energy mechanisms accounted for 68% of subtalar dislocations; 75% of dislocations were closed, 65% were medial dislocations, and 32% of dislocations were irreducible. Radiographic evidence of arthrosis was noted in 89% of ankle and subtalar joints; the subtalar joint was more frequently symptomatic.

Bibbo C, Lin SS, Abidi N, et al: Missed and associated injuries after subtalar dislocation: The role of CT. *Foot Ankle Int* 2001;22:324-328.

In all patients, CT scans identified additional injuries missed on plain radiographs, which altered treatment plans in 44% of patients.

Buckley R, Tough S, McCormack R, et al: Operative compared with nonoperative treatment of displaced intra-articular calcaneal fractures: A prospective, randomized, controlled multicenter trial. *J Bone Joint Surg Am* 2002;84-A:1733-1744.

Equivalent outcomes were noted between the two groups; however, when patients receiving workers' compensation were removed from the comparison, significantly better results were noted with surgical treatment.

Csizy M, Buckley R, Tough S, et al: Displaced intra-articular calcaneal fractures: Variables predicting late subtalar fusion. *J Orthop Trauma* 2003;17:106-112.

Initial injury severity, Bohler angle less than 0, workers' compensation patients, heavy laborers, and those fractures initially treated nonsurgically were factors that were more likely to lead to fusion.

Huefner T, Thermann H, Geerling J, Pape HC, Pohlemann T: Primary subtalar arthrodesis of calcaneal fractures. *Foot Ankle Int* 2001;22:9-14.

Primary fusion for extremely comminuted calcaneal fractures led to good functional outcome.

Ricci WM, Bellabarba C, Sanders R: Transcalcaneal talonavicular dislocation. *J Bone Joint Surg Am* 2002;84-A:557-561.

Dorsal dislocation of the navicular with an associated calcaneal fracture is a severe injury, resulting in severe functional limitations, osteomyelitis, and amputation.

Schulze W, Richter J, Russe O, Ingelfinger P, Muhr G: Surgical treatment of talus fractures: A retrospective study of 80 cases followed for 1-15 years. *Acta Orthop Scand* 2002;73:344-351.

Ankle or subtalar arthrosis was noted in two thirds of fractures. Talar necrosis was noted in 11%; 44% had good or excellent function.

Tennent TD, Calder PR, Salisbury RD, Allen PW, Eastwood DM: The operative management of displaced intra-articular fractures of the calcaneum: A two-centre study using a defined protocol. *Injury* 2001;32:491-496.

A 90% satisfaction rate was noted with surgical treatment. Bilateral injuries resulted in poorer outcome. Delay in operation was associated in a higher infection rate, whereas smoking did not.

Midfoot Trauma

Fulkerson E, Razi A, Tejwani N: Review: Acute compartment syndrome of the foot. *Foot Ankle Int* 2003;24:180-187.

An excellent review of acute foot compartment syndrome is presented.

Glasoe WM, Allen MK, Kepros T, Stonewall L, Ludewig PM: Dorsal first ray mobility in women athletes with a history of stress fracture of the second or third metatarsal. *J Orthop Sports Phys Ther* 2002;32:560-565.

First ray hypermobility is not associated with stress fracture of the second or third metatarsal.

Kelly IP, Glisson RR, Fink C, Easley ME, Nunley JA: Intramedullary screw fixation of Jones fractures. *Foot Ankle Int* 2001;22:585-589.

No significant difference was reported between failure loads of 5.0- and 6.5-mm. screws. Pull-out strength was significantly higher for the 6.5-mm screws.

Korpelainen R, Orava S, Karpakka J, Siira P, Hulkko A: Risk factors for recurrent stress fractures in athletes. *Am J Sports Med* 2001;29:304-310.

Biomechanical factors associated with multiple stress fractures include a high longitudinal arch, forefoot varus, and leg-length inequality. Nearly half of female runners reported menstrual irregularity.

Mollica MB, Duyshart SC: Analysis of pre- and postexercise compartment pressures in the medial compartment of the foot. *Am J Sports Med* 2002;30:268-271.

Normative pressures of the medial foot compartment are comparable to those in the leg. Previous criteria for diagnosis of chronic exertional compartment syndrome of the leg may be used for diagnosis of chronic exertional compartment syndrome of the foot.

Mulier T, Reynders P, Dereymaeker G, Broos P: Severe Lisfrancs injuries: Primary arthrodesis or ORIF? *Foot Ankle Int* 2002;23:902-905.

Primary complete arthrodesis resulted in inferior pain scores, more stiffness, a loss of longitudinal arch, and higher rate of sympathetic dystrophy.

Nunley JA, Vertullo CJ: Classification, investigation and management of midfoot sprains: Lisfranc injuries in the athlete. *Am J Sports Med* 2002;30:871-878.

Primary fusion for extremely comminuted calcaneal fractures led to good functional outcome.

Peicha G, Labovitz J, Seibert FJ, et al: The anatomy of the joint as a risk factor for Lisfranc dislocation and fracture-dislocation: An anatomical and radiological case control study. *J Bone Joint Surg Br* 2002;84:981-985.

A decreased medial depth of the mortise between the medial and middle cuneiforms increases the risk of Lisfranc injury. Lateral depth and second metatarsal length are not risk factors.

Shah SN, Knoblich GO, Lindsey DP, Kreshak J, Yerby SA, Chou LB: Intramedullary screw fixation of proximal fifth metatarsal fractures: A biomechanical study. *Foot Ankle Int* 2001;22:581-584.

Initial failure loads and ultimate failure loads were not significantly different for 4.5- and 5.5-mm cannulated screws.

Teng AL, Pinzur MS, Lomasney L, Mahoney L, Havey R: Functional outcome following anatomic restoration of tarsal-metatarsal fracture-dislocation. *Foot Ankle Int* 2002;23:922-926.

Anatomic reduction of the tarsometatarsal joints correlated with normal gait patterns, yet subjective patient outcomes were less than satisfactory.

Theodorou DJ, Theodorou SJ, Kakitsubata Y, Botte MJ, Resnick D: Fractures of proximal portion of fifth metatarsal bone: Anatomic and imaging evidence of a pathogenesis of avulsion of the planter aponeurosis and the short peroneal muscle tendon. *Radiology* 2003;226:857-865.

Based on plain radiography, CT, and MRI, fracture of the base of the fifth metatarsal are reported to be related to avulsion injury of the plantar aponeurosis and peroneus brevis tendon fibers.

Compartment Syndrome

Fulkerson E, Razi A, Tejwani N: Acute compartment syndrome of the foot. *Foot Ankle Int* 2003;24:180-187.

An excellent review of acute foot compartment syndrome is presented.

Mollica MB, Duyshart SC: Analysis of pre- and postexercise compartment pressures in the medial compartment of the foot. *Am J Sports Med* 2002;30:268-271.

Normative pressures of the medial foot compartment are comparable to those in the leg. Previous criteria for diagnosis of chronic exertional compartment syndrome of the leg may be used for diagnosis of chronic exertional compartment syndrome of the foot.

Classic Bibliography

Al-Mudhaffar M, Prasad CV, Mofidi A: Wound complications following operative fixation of calcaneal fractures. *Injury* 2000;31:461-464.

Benirschke SK, Sangeorzan BJ: Extensive intraarticular fractures of the foot: Surgical management of calcaneal fractures. *Clin Orthop* 1993;292:128-134.

Blotter RH, Connolly E, Wasan A, Chapman MW: Acute complications in the operative treatment of isolated ankle fractures in patients with diabetes mellitus. *Foot Ankle Int* 1999;20:687-694.

Boden SD, Labropolos PA, McCowin P, Lestini WF, Hurwitz SR: Mechanical considerations of the syndesmosis screw: A cadaver study. *J Bone Joint Surg Am* 1989;71:1548-1555.

Canale ST, Kelly FB Jr: Fractures of the neck of the talus: Long-term evaluation of seventy-one cases. *J Bone Joint Surg Am* 1978;60:143-156.

Coughlin MJ: Calcaneal fractures in the industrial patient. *Foot Ankle Int* 2000;21:896-905.

Folk JW, Starr AJ, Early JS: Early wound complications of operative treatment of calcaneus fractures: Analysis of 190 fractures. *J Orthop Trauma* 1999;13:369-372.

Glasgow MT, Naranja RJ Jr, Glasgow SG, Torg JS: Analysis of failed surgical management of fractures of the base of the fifth metatarsal distal to the tuberosity: The Jones fracture. *Foot Ankle Int* 1996;17:449-457.

Gourineni PV, Knuth AE, Nuber GF: Radiographic evaluation of the position of implants in the medial malleolus in relation to the ankle joint space: Anteroposterior compared with mortise radiographs. *J Bone Joint Surg Am* 1999;81:364-369.

Hawkins LG: Fractures of the neck of the talus. *J Bone Joint Surg Am* 1970;52:991-1002.

Kuo RS, Tejwani NC, Digiovanni CW, et al: Outcome after open reduction internal fixation of Lisfranc joint injuries. *J Bone Joint Surg Am* 2000;82:609-618.

Lauge-Hansen N: Fractures of the ankle: II. Combined experimental surgical and experimental-roentgenologic investigations. *Arch Surg* 1950;60:957-986.

Marsh JL, Bonar S, Nepola JV, Decoster TA, Hurwitz SR: Use of an articulated external fixator for fractures of the tibial plafond. *J Bone Joint Surg Am* 1995;77:1498-1509.

O'Malley MJ, Hamilton WG, Munyak J: Fractures of the distal shaft of the fifth metatarsal: Dancer's fracture. *Am J Sports Med* 1996;24:240-243.

Myerson M, Manoli A: Compartment syndromes of the foot after calcaneal fractures. *Clin Orthop* 1993;290:142-150.

Myerson MS: Experimental decompression of the fascial compartments of the foot-basis for fasciotomy in acute compartment syndromes. *Foot Ankle* 1988;8:308-314.

Quill GE Jr: Fractures of the proximal fifth metatarsal. *Orthop Clin North Am* 1995;26:353-361.

Sasse M, Nigg BM, Stefanyshyn DJ: Tibiotalar motion: Effect of fibular displacement and deltoid ligament transaction: In vitro study. *Foot Ankle Int* 1999;20:733-737.

Sanders R, Fortin P, DiPasquale T, Walling A: Operative treatment in 120 displaced intraarticular calcaneal fractures: Results using a prognostic computed tomography scan classification. *Clin Orthop* 1993;290:87-95.

Thordarson DB, Motamed S, Hedman T, Ebramzadeh E, Bakshian S: The effect of fibular malreduction on contact pressures in an ankle fracture malunion model. *J Bone Joint Surg Am* 1997;79:1809-1815.

Thordarson DB, Triffon MJ, Terk MR: Magnetic resonance imaging to detect avascular necrosis after open reduction and internal fixation of talar neck fractures. *Foot Ankle Int* 1996;17:742-747.

Wyrsch B, McFerran MA, McAndrew M, et al: Operative treatment of fractures of the tibial plafond: A randomized, prospective study. *J Bone Joint Surg Am* 1996; 78:1646-1657.

Yablon IG, Heller FG, Shouse L: The key role of the lateral malleolus in displaced fractures of the ankle. *J Bone Joint Surg Am* 1977;59:169-173.

Yamaguchi K, Martin CH, Boden SD, Labropoulos PA: Operative treatment of syndesmotic disruptions without use of a syndesmotic screw: A prospective clinical study. *Foot Ankle Int* 1994;5:407-414.

Zufferey P, Boubaker A, Bischof Delaloye A, So AK, Duvoisin B: Prognostic aspects of scintigraphy and MRI during the first 6 months of reflex sympathetic dystrophy of the distal lower limb: A preliminary prospective study of 4 cases. *J Radiol* 1999;80:373-377.

kle and hindfoot arthritis, several attractive surgical alternatives to ankle arthrodesis that maintain ankle motion continue to show promise. Joint distraction arthroplasty with or without joint débridement involves maintaining 5 mm of ankle joint distraction with thin wire ring fixation. Patients are allowed to bear weight during the 3 months of joint distraction. Early to intermediate results suggest that 75% of patients experienced improvement of symptoms and did not require further surgical management. Fresh tibiotalar "shell" allografts have been used in carefully selected patients. An osteochondral allograft comprising both aspects of the tibiotalar joint replaces the patient's corresponding resected articular surfaces. To optimize the fit of the allograft, total ankle replacement cutting guides are used. Early results are encouraging, but the technique remains experimental. Improved component design and surgical technique for modern-generation total ankle arthroplasty have improved results over those for first-generation implants. Although several different prostheses, each with unique design features, have been introduced worldwide, only the semi-constrained, fixed-bearing Agility ankle (DePuy, Warsaw, IN) has been approved by the US Food and Drug Administration (FDA) (Figure 5). The Agility ankle technique warrants a syndesmotic arthrodesis to increase the surface area and support for the tibial component. The mobile bearing Scandinavian Total Ankle Replacement (Waldemar-Link, Hamburg, Germany) prosthesis affords the advantage of limited bone resection, a resurfacing talar component, and the mobile bearing that reduces constraint and provides modularity to improve soft-tissue balance. As of this writing, the Scandinavian Total Ankle Replacement implant was in clinical trial, awaiting FDA approval. Although techniques for total ankle arthroplasty have been refined, the procedure remains technically demanding. A steep learning curve has been demonstrated for total ankle arthroplasty. As with total hip and total knee arthroplasty, proper alignment and soft-tissue balance are crucial for successful outcome. Current recommendations are for total ankle arthroplasty to be performed by surgeons who have completed special training for this technique, either through fellowship or learning center experience.

Osteochondral Lesions of the Talus

Osteochondral lesions of the ankle are commonly observed anterolaterally and posteromedially on the talar dome. Not all of these lesions are symptomatic and may represent incidental findings. Most osteochondral lesions of the talus are a result of ankle trauma (sprain/fracture), but patients do not always recall a specific traumatic event. Ankle arthroscopy performed simultaneously with open reduction and internal fixation of ankle fractures or in patients with chronic ankle sprains

reveals a high incidence of osteochondral injuries. No clear association between focal osteochondral lesions of the talus and development of diffuse ankle osteoarthritis has been identified. Although radiographs often suggest an osteochondral lesion of the talus, findings may be subtle. Occasionally, a loose body (detached fragment) is evident. MRI is the favored screening tool to identify osteochondral lesions of the talus, and both MRI and CT provide useful information in defining specific characteristics. Although classification schemes for osteochondral lesions of the talus have been developed using both MRI and CT, arthroscopic evaluation is probably most accurate.

Nonsurgical management of symptomatic osteochondral lesions of the talus consists of immobilization and protective weight bearing to promote stabilization of the osteochondral fragment and nonsteroidal anti-inflammatory drugs and/or steroid injection for pain relief/controlling inflammation. Adult patients rarely experience spontaneous healing of osteochondral lesions of the talus, but some authors have recently reported good to excellent results at intermediate-term follow-up with nonsurgical treatment of osteochondral lesions of the talus thought only to respond to surgical intervention. Although arthroscopic débridement and drilling/microfracture remains the standard of surgical care for symptomatic osteochondral lesions of the talus (good to excellent results of 70% to 90% at intermediate follow-up), the concern remains that replacing larger defects with fibrocartilage and not hyaline cartilage may not be a sensible solution. Although cartilage resurfacing procedures, including osteochondral autograft/allograft transfer (mosaicplasty) and autologous chondrocyte transplantation (Carticel procedure), continue to be viewed as salvage procedures, some consideration is being given to applying these techniques as primary surgical treatment of larger osteochondral lesions of the talus, particularly those associated with subchondral cysts (Figure 6). Outcome of osteochondral transfer from the knee to the ankle (osteochondral autograft/allograft transfer and mosaicplasty) have been promising at short- to intermediate-term follow-up, with 88% to 94% good to excellent results for primary and revision surgeries. Autologous chondrocyte transplantation has also proven effective at early follow-up. Cartilage resurfacing in the ankle often warrants medial or lateral malleolar osteotomies to provide adequate access to the osteochondral lesions of the talus. Currently, malleolar osteotomy techniques are being refined and potential local cartilage harvest sites are being identified to decrease the morbidity to the ankle and ipsilateral knee. Lateral defects, particularly those associated with lateral ligamentous instability, may be treated with release and subsequent tightening of the anterior talofibular ligament and calcaneofibular ligament.

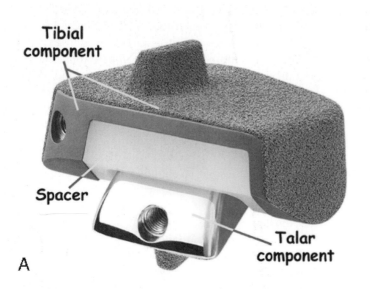

Tibial component

Spacer

Talar component

A

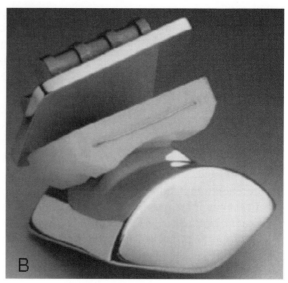

B

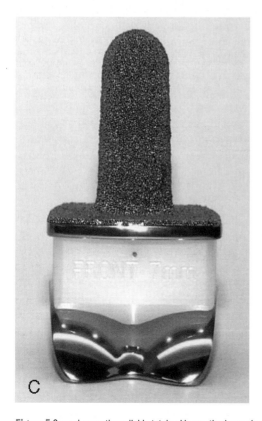

C

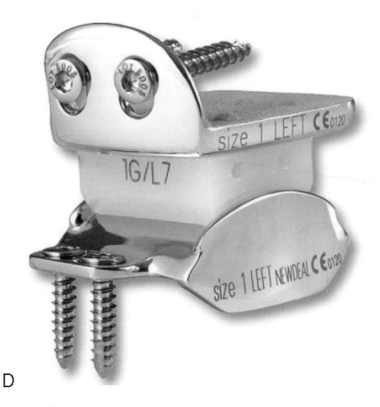

D

Figure 5 Several currently available total ankle prosthesis are shown. **A,** Agility Total Ankle System. (Courtesy of DePuy, Warsaw, IN.) **B,** STAR system. (Courtesy of Waldemar-Link, Hamburg, Germany.) **C,** Buechel-Pappas ankle system. (Courtesy of Endotec, South Orange, NJ.) **D,** Hintegra ankle system. (Courtesy of New Deal, Vienne, France.)

Insertional Achilles Tendinopathy

Insertional Achilles tendinopathy is an enthesopathy of the Achilles tendon insertion that most likely is a result of cumulative trauma/repetitive stress. Although inflammation accompanies this disease process, the primary pathology is tendon degeneration at the Achilles tendon insertion. Patients report pain directly at the junction of the Achilles tendon on the calcaneus with direct pressure and during push-off; swelling at the insertion limits shoe wear with a hard heel counter. Symptoms are exacerbated by walking an incline or during activities that cause dorsiflexion of the ankle. Physical examination will demonstrate an intact Achilles tendon, but often with hyperdorsiflexion of the ankle (secondary to Achilles tendon attenuation). Lateral radiographs demonstrate calcification at the Achilles tendon insertion and frequently a prominent posterior calcaneal tuberosity.

Nonsurgical treatment is successful in most instances, and includes activity modification, use of a cam walker with a posterior heel relief, modalities to diminish associated inflammation, and a heel lift. In approximately 20% to 25% of patients, failure of nonsurgical measures (after at least 6 months) prompts surgical management. Current surgical treatment includes débridement of the Achilles tendon insertion and calcaneal exostectomy. Medial and/or lateral approaches have been described for this procedure, but may not permit adequate débridement of the Achilles tendon insertion. A central approach facilitates such débridement, but necessitates detachment of at least 50% of the Achilles tendon from the calcaneus, and usually requires reattachment of the residual tendon fibers with suture anchors to the residual calcaneus. When the tendon insertion is severely degenerated, necessitating resection of a substantial portion of the insertion, then augmentation with a flexor hallucis longus tendon transfer is recommended. A long flexor hallucis longus tendon harvest (flexor hallucis longus division in the plantar foot) delivers approximately 3 cm more tendon than a short flexor hallucis longus tendon harvest (flexor hallucis longus division at posteromedial ankle).

Acquired Flatfoot Deformity

Posterior tibial tendon dysfunction is the most common etiology for the adult acquired flatfoot deformity. Posterior tibial tendon insufficiency leads to gradual loss of the longitudinal arch, hindfoot valgus, forefoot abduction and forefoot varus/supination. Over time, the deformity may become fixed and even result in deltoid ligament attenuation with resultant valgus talar tilt. This progressive deformity has been categorized into four stages. Clinical evaluation is characterized by pain and tenderness along the posterior tibial tendon and inability to perform a single limb heel rise. In the early stages of the disease, single limb heel rise may be possible but painful; eventually, the heel fails to turn into physiologic varus, and ultimately unsupported single limb heel rise is no longer possible. With advancing disease, subfibular (calcaneofibular) impingement develops with tenderness over the compressed peroneal tendons. In fact, initial medial pain subsides and subfibular lateral foot pain produces the greatest symptoms. Loss of the longitudinal arch, hindfoot valgus, and forefoot abduction (too many toes sign) are evident with progressive posterior tibial tendon attenuation. Radiographic evaluation confirms pes planus alignment. The lateral radiograph demonstrates loss of the longitudinal arch; moderate to severe talonavicular subluxation suggests spring ligament compromise. On the AP radiograph, talar head uncover-

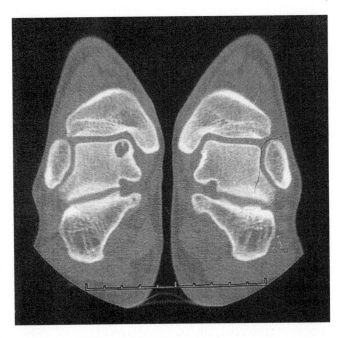

Figure 6 CT scan showing a subchondral cyst of the medial talar dome. Subchondral cysts generally respond poorly to arthroscopic débridement and drilling. Recently developed cartilage repair techniques have shown promise in the primary and secondary surgical treatment of these lesions. *(Reproduced from Scranton PE Jr: Osteochondral lesions of the talus, in Nunley JA, Pfeffer GB, Sanders RW, Trepman E (eds): Advanced Reconstruction Foot and Ankle. Rosemont, IL, American Academy of Orthopaedic Surgeons, 2004, pp 261-266.)*

ing by the navicular demonstrates forefoot abduction. Weight-bearing AP and mortise ankle radiographs must be obtained to detect valgus talar tilt indicative of deltoid ligament attenuation.

Treatment of stage I flatfoot deformity (posterior tibial tendinitis) is nonsurgical with initial immobilization and the administration of nonsteroidal anti-inflammatory drugs, followed by gradual progression to physical therapy and orthotic use. In selected patients, surgical débridement of the posterior tibial tendon sheath may relieve recalcitrant stenosing tenosynovitis. Stage II flatfoot deformity (posterior tibial tendinopathy with flexible hindfoot) can be effectively managed with functional bracing using a University of California at Berkely Laboratory or ankle-foot orthosis. Although bracing supports the foot, it cannot reverse posterior tibial tendinopathy. Surgical management is typically joint sparing with flexor digitorum or flexor hallucis longus tendon transfer combined with either medial displacement calcaneal osteotomy or lateral column lengthening. Medial displacement calcaneal osteotomy is effective in protecting a posterior tibial tendon reconstruction and at least partially restoring longitudinal arch alignment and correcting hindfoot valgus, but proves less effective than lateral column lengthening when deformity is associated forefoot abduction. The medial displacement calcaneal osteotomy generally is associated with high union and low complication rates;

in contrast, lateral column lengthening (either through the anterior calcaneus or calcaneocuboid joint) is associated with a higher complication rate, particularly with regard to nonunion. With proper technique, use of structural autograft and allograft yields equal and favorable results. Associated spring ligament attenuation can usually be corrected with soft-tissue plication; however, larger spring ligament defects represent a greater challenge. The optimal spring ligament reconstruction has yet to be defined. Currently, arthrodesis is usually required to manage large spring ligament tears. Subtalar arthroereisis, a technique traditionally reserved for pediatric patients, has been introduced as an adjunctive procedure in the management of the flexible adult acquired flatfoot deformity; preliminary results and anecdotal experience with this sinus tarsi implant that distracts the subtalar joint show promise. In some patients, a double calcaneal osteotomy (medial displacement calcaneal osteotomy and lateral column lengthening) has proved effective in correcting hindfoot valgus and forefoot abduction when combined with tendon reconstruction. Fixed stage III flatfoot deformity cannot be corrected with joint-sparing procedures and requires realignment through arthrodesis, typically triple arthrodesis. Because posterior tibial tendon dysfunction often is associated with an equinus contracture, correction of deformity requires Achilles tendon lengthening. Traditionally, the Hoke triple cut percutaneous lengthening technique has been used, but anatomic studies demonstrate that the triple cut technique generally fails to follow the orientation of the Achilles tendon fibers. Recently, gastrocnemius-soleus recession has gained popularity as an effective method for Achilles tendon lengthening; although the traditional open technique is most commonly used, interest has been generated for a less invasive endoscopic technique. Stage IV flatfoot deformity remains difficult to treat because an ideal deltoid ligament reconstruction has not been developed. When associated with ankle arthritis, pantalar arthrodesis may be required for severe stage IV disease.

Plantar Fasciitis

The etiology of plantar fasciitis is not fully understood, but the condition is believed to result from cumulative trauma or repetitive stress. Symptoms usually are concentrated at the plantar fascia origin on the plantar medial heel and typically have an insidious onset. Occasionally, plantar heel pain may be associated with a compressive neuropathy of the first branch of the lateral plantar nerve (Baxter's nerve). A heel pain triad has been described with the coexistence of posterior tibial tendon dysfunction, plantar fasciitis, and tarsal tunnel syndrome. Patients typically report start-up pain (heel pain experienced with initial weight bearing after a period of rest) and increasing heel pain after prolonged

standing. The point of maximal tenderness is usually at the plantar fascia origin on the plantar medial heel; tenderness slightly more proximal and medial is suggestive of compressive neuropathy.

Treatment of plantar fasciitis is rarely surgical; traditional treatment with Achilles tendon stretching, night splinting, heel cushion, and nonsteroidal anti-inflammatory drugs continues to be recommended. A prospective, randomized trial suggests that a stretching protocol specific to the plantar fascia may provide advantages over Achilles tendon stretching. Low- and high-energy extracorporeal shock wave therapy are available to treat plantar fasciitis. Prospective randomized studies and meta-analyses demonstrate that both the low- and high-energy devices are safe; however, whether extracorporeal shock wave therapy is effective for recalcitrant plantar fasciitis remains a controversial issue. Surgical treatment is reserved for patients in whom 6 months to 1 year of nonsurgical treatment is unsuccessful. Only the medial third of the plantar fascia should be released; complete release may result in persistent lateral foot pain. Plantar fascia release may be performed with open or endoscopic techniques. Given the overlap of plantar fasciitis and compression neuropathy, open plantar fascia release can be combined with distal tarsal tunnel decompression; good to excellent results can be expected in more than 85% of patients with recalcitrant symptoms who undergo the combined procedure.

Diabetic Foot/Ankle and Charcot Neuroarthropathy

More than 16 million people in the United States have diabetes, and foot problems related to diabetes represent 20% of hospital admissions for diabetics. The lifetime incidence for foot ulceration in diabetic patients is 15%, and 3% to 5% of diabetic patients are amputees. More than 50% of all amputations performed in the United States are for diabetics. Within 3 years of lower extremity amputation, 30% of diabetic patients lose their contralateral leg, and 50% die. Up to half of these amputations are considered preventable. Diabetic risk factors for foot ulceration include neuropathy (sensory, motor, and autonomic), vascular insufficiency, poor glycemic control, malnutrition, and impaired wound healing. Sensory neuropathy (Semmes-Weinstein monofilament < 5.07) leaves patients without protective sensation. Motor neuropathy may lead to joint deformities/contractures that create areas of pressure concentration and difficulties with shoe wear. Autonomic neuropathy results in dry skin with fissures (risk bacterial penetration) and peripheral edema (reduces collateral blood flow/healing potential). Vascular insufficiency (ankle brachial index < 0.45, absolute toe pressures < 50 to 60 mm Hg, transcutaneous oxygen measures < 30 mm Hg) diminishes the patient's ability to heal. Furthermore, poor glycemic control and malnutrition contribute to impaired wound healing mechanisms.

Suspected infection requires further work-up that can be performed by the orthopaedist or in conjunction with an infectious disease specialist. Calluses should be trimmed because they may mask underlying infection. Probing to bone through an ulceration is approximately 80% reliable in diagnosing osteomyelitis. Radiographs demonstrate cortical erosions, but it may take 7 to 14 days before these erosions become radiographically detectable. Therefore, MRI and/or combination technetium bone scan/white blood cell-labeled indium (or gallium) scan may be required to determine if osteomyelitis is present. MRI has high sensitivity, specificity, and accuracy in diagnosing osteomyelitis, but provides poor localization and may in fact overrepresent the area of involvement, thereby leading to overresection of bone. Technetium bone scan is specific only for inflammation but combined with white blood cell-labeled indium scanning the sensitivity, specificity, and accuracy approaches that of MRI. Limitations to technetium bone scanning and white blood cell-labeled indium scanning include poor circulation and prior administration of antibiotics, respectively. The most reliable means of detecting osteomyelitis involves obtaining a deep surgical specimen of infected tissue with the patient refraining from antibiotic administration for at least 48 hours. An abscess is a surgical emergency because this space-occupying lesion will quickly dissect more proximally through potential spaces (such as tendon sheaths) and may create a mass effect on delicate vessels, leading to forefoot ischemia. Typically, the only means of eradicating osteomyelitis in diabetic foot infections is to resect the infected bone. Calcaneal osteomyelitis does not necessitate transtibial amputation; partial calcanectomy followed by appropriate protective bracing in diabetic patients can lead to successful limb salvage.

Most foot ulcers may be treated nonsurgically with proper wound care and appropriate pressure relief. Following satisfactory ulcer débridement, total contact casting remains the gold standard for forefoot/midfoot ulcer management; hindfoot ulcers respond poorly to total contact casting. To better monitor skin and address the ulcer with wound management, improvements have been made to various removable diabetic cam walker boots. The devices have proven at least equally effective in pressure unloading for forefoot and midfoot ulcers as total contact casting. Forefoot ulceration associated with equinus contractures will quickly resolve with Achilles tendon lengthening, particularly if treated in conjunction with total contact casting. Without equinus, percutaneous flexor tenotomies and/or dorsiflexion metatarsal osteotomies may prove beneficial for recalcitrant forefoot ulcers. Exostoses in the midfoot (frequently associated with Charcot neuroarthropathic midfoot collapse) may be excised to effectively unload ulcerated skin.

Charcot Neuroarthropathy

Charcot neuroarthropathy remains a treatment challenge. The exact etiology of Charcot neuroarthropathy is poorly understood, but neurotraumatic and/or neurovascular theories are currently favored. The neurotraumatic theory suggests fracture or fracture-dislocation without protective sensation and a healing response of hypertrophic bone formation in an inherently unstable fracture that has not been stabilized. Conversely, the neurovascular theory suggests nonphysiologic vascular inflow resulting in resorption and subsequent fracture-dislocation.

Eichenholtz staging defines the clinical and radiographic progression of the neuroarthropathy. Stage I is characterized by edema, warmth, erythema, and radiographic evidence of bony acute fracture and/or dislocation (fragmentation); the neuroarthropathy develops during this initial stage. In stage II, the proliferative phase, bony destruction is combined with the fracture/dislocation. Edema and warmth are generally diminished relative to stage I. Progression to stage III is defined by coalescence and remodeling with healing in a foot position resulting from the fracture/dislocation and bony displacement. Typically, patients who were not immobilized and restricted from bearing weight tend to consolidate in a less favorable, nonplantigrade foot position. As for diabetic ulceration/infection, treatment of Charcot neuroarthropathy is improved through patient and physician education. A heightened awareness and appropriate differentiation from osteomyelitis generally can lead to earlier diagnosis, immobilization, and restricted weight bearing. The advantage to identifying the Charcot process early is that progression through the three stages can occur while the foot is maintained in this near anatomic position. If the Charcot process can course through to the consolidation/remodeling phase while avoiding deformity such as arch collapse, outcome may be markedly improved. Unfortunately, the painless Charcot foot often does not prompt immediate medical care and proper diagnosis is frequently delayed. Use of a total contact cast and no weight bearing traditionally have been effective in the management of Charcot neuroarthropathy, but external fixation recently has gained popularity for initial stabilization. Even with deformity following progression to stage III, most Charcot deformities can be managed nonsurgically with total contact inserts, extra-depth shoes, stiffer soles, rocker bottom shoe modification, and bracing above the ankle. Severe deformities may warrant use of a functional total contact cast (such as the Charcot restraining orthotic walker). Some deformities are predisposed to ulceration, infection, and amputation, and brace treatment is not possible. Salvage procedures have been effective. Several classification schemes have been developed to better define deformity patterns and develop treatment algorithms. Although complex, such classification schemes demonstrate good interobserver and intraobserver reliability. It is predicted that such schemes may facilitate treatment strategies. Surgical salvage procedures for ankle, hindfoot, and midfoot Charcot deformity typically require multiplanar realignment osteotomies with arthrodesis and tend to ignore traditional anatomic landmarks. Techniques for internal fixation have been described, but recently developed methods of external fixation for Charcot neuroarthropathy for the diabetic foot and ankle have shown promise. Whereas resolution of ulceration and infection is typically necessary before internal fixation of Charcot deformity, external fixation affords the potential advantage of single-stage resection of the osteomyelitic prominence, ulcer excision, multiplanar realignment osteotomy, and arthrodesis stabilized without implanted hardware.

Salvage procedures may be successful in limb preservation for diabetic patients with ulceration, infection, and/or Charcot neuroarthropathy; however, amputation may remain the only recourse in some situations. If feasible, partial foot amputations provide the advantage of limb support without a prosthesis. However, the patient still may be predisposed to ulceration, and transtibial amputation may be the safest solution.

Annotated Bibliography

Forefoot: Hallux Valgus

Chi TD, Davitt J, Younger A, Holt S: Intra-and interobserver reliability of the distal metatarsal articular angle in adult hallux valgus. *Foot Ankle Int* 2002;23:722-726.

Preoperative and postoperative radiographs of 32 patients undergoing hallux valgus correction using a proximal bony procedure demonstrated a reduction in the DMAA by an average of 3.9°, noted by all observers. However, interobserver reliability of preoperative and postoperative DMAA was poor.

Coetzee JC: Scarf osteotomy for hallux valgus repair: The dark side. *Foot Ankle Int* 2003;24:29-33.

The Scarf osteotomy was performed in 20 consecutive patients, resulting in a high complication rate, limited improvement in the American Orthopaedic Foot and Ankle Society forefoot score, and only a 55% patient satisfaction rate.

Coetzee JC, Resig SG, Kuskowski M, Saleh KJ: The lapidus procedure as salvage after failed surgical treatment of hallux valgus. *J Bone Joint Surg Am* 2003;85-A:60-65.

Twenty-four patients with 26 symptomatic hallux valgus recurrences were selected to undergo the Lapidus procedure. At an average follow-up of 24 months, the average American Orthopaedic Foot and Ankle Society score improved from 47 to 88 points, with average improvements in the hallux valgus angles from 37° to 17° and intermetatarsal angles from 18° to

9°. Complications included three nonunions, all in patients who smoked.

Coughlin MJ, Freund E: The reliability of angular measurements in hallux valgus deformities. *Foot Ankle Int* 2001;22:369-379.

Interobserver and intraobserver reliability within 5° is high for the intermetatarsal angle (97%), good for the hallux valgus angle (86%), and poor for the distal metatarsal articular angle (59%).

Faber FW, Kleinrensink GJ, Mulder PG, Verhaar JA: Mobility of the first tarsometatarsal joint in hallux valgus patients: A radiographic analysis. *Foot Ankle Int* 2001;22:965-969.

Ninety-four feet with symptomatic hallux valgus deformity prompting surgical correction were evaluated clinically and radiographically using the modified Coleman block test. The mean first ray motion was 13° and proved to be significantly greater in the group that demonstrated clinical hypermobility.

Glasoe WM, Allen MK, Saltzman CL: First ray dorsal mobility in relation to hallux valgus deformity and first intermetatarsal angle. *Foot Ankle Int* 2001;22:98-101.

A comparison of 14 hallux valgus patients and asymptomatic controls demonstrated increased mobility in the hallux valgus group. A load-cell device was used to determine the degree of hypermobility.

Kristen KH, Berger C, Stelzig E, Thalhammer E: The SCARF osteotomy for the correction of hallux valgus deformities. *Foot Ankle Int* 2002;23:221-229.

A retrospective analysis of 111 Scarf osteotomies in 89 consecutive patients with moderate to severe hallux valgus revealed an average hallux valgus angle improvement of 19° and intermetatarsal angle improvement of 7°. The average American Orthopaedic Foot and Ankle Society forefoot score improved from 50 to 91 points. Seven patients (6%) experienced a recurrence of deformity and 5% suffered either superficial wound infection, displacement of the distal fragment, or hallux MTP joint stiffness.

Nery C, Barroco R, Ressio C: Biplanar chevron osteotomy. *Foot Ankle Int* 2002;23:792-798.

Fifty-four biplanar distal chevron osteotomies were performed in 32 patients to correct moderate hallux valgus deformity associated with an increased distal metatarsal articular angle. With follow-up of 2 years or longer, the average American Orthopaedic Foot and Ankle Society forefoot score improved from 50 to 90 points, the average hallux valgus angle improved 9°, the intermetatarsal angle improved 4°, and the distal metatarsal articular angle improved from 15° to 5°.

Nyska M, Trnka HJ, Parks BG, Myerson MS: The Ludloff metatarsal osteotomy: Guidelines for optimal correction on a geometric analysis conducted on a sawbone model. *Foot Ankle Int* 2003;24:34-39.

Using a saw bone model, the authors describe technical aspects to achieving desired correction for the modified Ludloff proximal oblique first metatarsal osteotomy for hallux valgus correction.

Forefoot: Hallux Rigidus

Coughlin MJ, Shurnas PS: Hallux rigidus: Demographics, etiology, and radiographic assessment. *Foot Ankle Int* 2003;24:731-743.

This retrospective review of 114 patients treated surgically for hallux rigidus demonstrated that hallux rigidus was associated with hallux valgus interphalangeus, female gender, unilateral disease (history of trauma), and bilateral disease (family history). The condition was not associated with metatarsus primus elevatus, a long first metatarsal, or first ray hypermobility.

Coughlin MJ, Shurnas PS: Hallux rigidus: Grading and long-term results of operative treatment. *J Bone Joint Surg Am* 2003;85-A:2072-2088.

A retrospective review of 114 patients treated surgically for hallux rigidus is presented. Eighty patients (93 feet) had undergone cheilectomy; 30 patients (34 feet) were treated with first MTP joint arthrodesis. Based on 96% of patients available at an average follow-up of 8.9 years, 97% of patients had good or excellent results (American Orthopaedic Foot and Ankle Society forefoot scoring system). Cheilectomy was predictable in lesser grades or first MTP arthritis; arthrodesis was favored for greater degrees of arthritis.

DeFrino PF, Brodsky JW, Pollo FE, et al: First metatarsophalangeal arthrodesis: A clinical, pedobarographic and gait analysis study. *Foot Ankle Int* 2002;23:496-502.

Clinical outcome, dynamic pedobarography (EMED) analysis, and kinematic and kinetic gait analysis were studied in 9 patients (10 feet) who underwent first MTP joint arthrodesis for severe hallux rigidus. The mean American Orthopaedic Foot and Ankle Society score improved from 38 to 90 points, and the EMED analysis demonstrated restoration of the weight-bearing function of the first ray. Kinematic data indicated a shorter step length/loss of ankle plantar flexion and the kinetic data indicated a reduction in ankle power push-off.

Forefoot: Sesamoid Disorders

Allen MA, Casillas MM: The Passive Axial Compression (PAC) test: A new adjunctive provocative maneuver for the clinical diagnosis of hallucal sesamoiditis. *Foot Ankle* 2001;22:345-346.

The authors describe a new provocative test that clinically reproduces the symptoms of sesamoid disorders. The maneuver may be useful in initial diagnosis and monitoring response to treatment of sesamoid problems.

Forefoot: Lesser Toes and Bunionette Deformity

Coughlin MJ, Schenck RC, Shurnas PJ, Bloome DM: Concurrent interdigital neuroma and MTP joint insta-

bility: Long-term results of treatment. *Foot Ankle Int* 2002;23:1018-1025.

Twenty percent (24 of 121 consecutive patients (131 feet and 136 neuromas) were treated for concomitant excision of a second web space neuroma and stabilization of a second MTP joint capsular instability. At an average follow-up of 80 months, 21 feet were available for evaluation. In 15 feet, the procedures were performed simultaneously; in 6 feet, the procedures were staged. Subjective patient satisfaction was high; subjective and objective results were lower in patients with persistent MTP joint instability.

Koti M, Maffulli N: Bunionette. *J Bone Joint Surg Am* 2001;83-A:1076-1082.

This article presents an excellent current review of evaluation and management of bunionette deformity.

Petersen WJ, Lankes JM, Paulsen F, Hassenpflug J: The arterial supply of the lesser metatarsal heads: A vascular injection study in human cadavers. *Foot Ankle Int* 2002; 23:491-495.

Epoxy resin injections performed in cadaveric foot specimens demonstrated an anastomosis of arteries about the lesser metatarsal heads arising from both the dorsalis pedis and posterior tibial arteries. This vascular network is closely associated with the joint capsule. The authors caution that extensive capsular stripping during metatarsal osteotomies may damage this vascular network.

Trnka HJ, Gebhard C, Muhlbauer M, et al: The Weil osteotomy for treatment of dislocated lesser metatarsophalangeal joints: Good outcome in 21 patients with 42 osteotomies. *Acta Orthop Scand* 2002;73:190-194.

A retrospective review of 60 Weil metatarsal osteotomies performed in 31 patients for dislocated lesser MTP joints at an average follow-up of 30 months showed 42 excellent results (21 patients). A major complication was penetrating hardware in 10 patients.

Trnka HJ, Nyska M, Parks BG, Myerson MS: Dorsiflexion contracture after the Weil osteotomy: Results of cadaver study and three-dimensional analysis. *Foot Ankle Int* 2001;22:47-50.

Using both cadaver and saw bone models, the authors demonstrated that the Weil metatarsal osteotomy always creates plantar fragment depression that changes the center of rotation of the MTP joint, causing the interosseous muscles to act more as dorsiflexors than plantar flexors. These findings are believed to be responsible for the high rate of dorsiflexion contractures following Weil metatarsal osteotomies.

Midfoot Arthritis

Berlet GC, Anderson RB: Tendon arthroplasty for basal fourth and fifth metatarsal arthritis. *Foot Ankle Int* 2002; 23:440-446.

At an average follow-up of 25 months, 12 patients undergoing tendon interpositional arthroplasty for fourth and fifth

TMT joint arthritis recalcitrant to nonsurgical treatment were evaluated. In eight patients, the diagnosis was confirmed with preoperative differential injections; six of the eight patients would undergo the procedure again. Outcome, based on the American Orthopaedic Foot and Ankle Society midfoot scale, was most favorable in patients who had a positive response to a preoperative differential injection.

Keiserman LS, Cassandra J, Amis JA: The Piano Key Test: A clinical sign for the identification of subtle tarsometatarsal pathology. *Foot Ankle Int* 2003;24:437-438.

The authors describe a simple test to identify and isolate TMT synovitis and/or arthritis.

Hindfoot and Ankle: Ankle/Subtalar Instability

Jeys LM, Harris NJ: Ankle stabilization with hamstring autograft: A new technique using interference screws. *Foot Ankle Int* 2003;24:677-679.

An anatomic reconstruction of the lateral ankle ligaments is described using bioabsorbable interference screw fixation of a hamstring autograft.

Keefe DT, Haddad SL: Subtalar instability: Etiology, diagnosis, and treatment. *Foot Ankle Clin* 2002;7:577-609.

The authors present a comprehensive review of the current state of the art for the evaluation and treatment of subtalar joint instability.

Krips R, Brandsson S, Swensson C, et al: Anatomical reconstruction and Evans tenodesis of the lateral ligaments of the ankle: Clinical and radiological findings after followup for 15-30 years. *J Bone Joint Surg Br* 2002; 84:232-236.

This retrospective review compares 54 patients undergoing an anatomic reconstruction of the lateral ankle ligaments and 45 patients treated with an Evans tenodesis for lateral ankle instability. The study demonstrated that the functional outcome of the Evans tenodesis deteriorated more rapidly than the anatomic reconstruction. Good to excellent results were noted in 43 patients in the anatomic reconstruction group and 15 in the Evans tenodesis group.

Pijnenburg AC, Bogaard K, Krips R, et al: Operative and functional treatment of rupture of the lateral ligament of the ankle: A randomized, prospective trial. *J Bone Joint Surg Br* 2003;85:525-530.

The authors prospectively randomized 370 patients with a rupture of at least one lateral ankle ligament to undergo either functional or surgical treatment. At a median follow-up of 8 years, 86% of patients were available for evaluation with the Povacz score and anterior drawer testing. Surgical treatment gave better long-term outcome with regard to residual pain, recurrent sprains (22% versus 34%), and stability (anterior drawer positive, 30% versus 54%).

Sabonghy EP, Wood RM, Ambrorse CG, McGarvey WC, Clanton TO: Tendon transfer fixation: Comparing a tendon to tendon technique versus bioabsorbable interference. Fit screw fixation. *Foot Ankle Int* 2003;24:260-262.

In 10 paired fresh cadaver specimens, load to failure was greater using bioabsorbable tendon fixation when compared with traditional fixation techniques. However, the authors supported the use of bioabsorbable screw as the mean fixation strength provides physiologic strength at the tendon-bone interface.

Van Bergeyk AB, Younger A, Carson B: CT Analysis of hindfoot alignment in chronic lateral ankle instability. *Foot Ankle Int* 2002;23:37-42.

The authors compared simulated weight-bearing hindfoot CT scans of 14 ankles with chronic ankle instability to 12 controls in a prospective case control format. Patients with ankle instability had statistically significantly greater hindfoot varus based on the radiographic parameters evaluated. The authors suggested that although a valgus-producing calcaneal osteotomy is not routinely indicated, it may have a role in selected patients who fail to respond to isolated lateral ankle ligament reconstruction.

Hindfoot and Ankle: Ankle Arthritis

Anderson T, Montgomery F, Carlsson A: Uncemented STAR total ankle prostheses: Three- to eight-year follow-up of fifty-one consecutive ankles. *J Bone Joint Surg Am* 2003;85-A:1321-1329.

Fifty-one consecutive cementless mobile-bearing Scandinavian Total Ankle Replacement ankle procedures were evaluated at intermediate follow-up. The median Kofoed score improved from 39 to 70 points at the time of follow-up. Twelve ankles had to be revised (seven loosening, two bearing fracture, three other complications) and eight other ankles had radiographic signs of loosening. Median range of motion was the same preoperatively and postoperatively. With revision as the end point, the estimated 5-year survival was 70%.

Buechel FF, Buechel FF Jr, Pappas MJ: Ten-year evaluation of cementless Buechel-Pappas meniscal bearing total ankle replacement. *Foot Ankle Int* 2003;24:462-472.

Fifty cementless Buechel-Pappas mobile-bearing total ankle replacements in 49 patients were evaluated. Good to excellent results were observed in 88% of patients. Postoperative range of motion was similar to preoperative motion. Revision was required in 4% of patients. Cumulative survivorship (using revision as an end point) was 94% at 10 years.

Coester LM, Saltzman CL, Leupold J, Pontarelli W: Long-term results following ankle arthrodesis for posttraumatic arthritis. *J Bone Joint Surg Am* 2001;83-A:219-236.

At a mean follow-up of 22 years, 23 patients who had a successful isolated ankle arthrodesis for posttraumatic tibiotalar arthritis were evaluated. Most patients had substantial, accelerated arthritic changes in the ipsilateral foot that often limited function when compared with the contralateral foot. Osteoarthritis did not develop more frequently in the ipsilateral knee or contralateral foot.

Coull R, Raffiq T, James LE, Stephens MM: Open treatment of anterior impingement of the ankle. *J Bone Joint Surg Br* 2003;85:550-553.

The outcome for the open treatment of anterior ankle impingement was evaluated at a mean follow-up of 7.3 years in 23 patients. The Ogilvie-Harris score improved in all patients. Ankle dorsiflexion did not return to normal, but symptomatic relief allowed 79% of patients to return to athletic activity at the same level. Two patients with preoperative joint space narrowing had a poor result.

Donley BG, Ward DM: Implantable electrical stimulation in high-risk hindfoot fusions. *Foot Ankle Int* 2002; 23:13-18.

The authors report a single surgeon's experience with 13 implantable bone stimulators used as an adjunct for ankle/hindfoot arthrodeses performed in patients with increased risk for nonunion. At an average follow-up of 25 months, 92% of patients achieved successful fusion. The subcutaneous device was bothersome to eight patients.

Fuchs S, Sandmann C, Skwara A, et al: Quality of life 20 years after arthrodesis of the ankle: A study of adjacent joints. *J Bone Joint Surg Br* 2003;85:994-998.

Retrospective, long-term follow-up of 18 successful ankle arthrodeses (17 patients) demonstrated significant deficits of functional outcome, limitations of activities of daily living, and radiographic changes in adjacent foot articulations, based on the Olerud Molander Ankle score, radiographic evaluation, and the Medical Outcomes Study Short Form-36 outcomes instrument.

Ishikawa SN, Murphy GA, Richardson EG: The effect of cigarette smoking on hindfoot fusions. *Foot Ankle Int* 2002;23:996-998.

In a group of 160 patients who had hindfoot fusions, smokers had a significantly higher nonunion rate than nonsmokers (19% versus 7%). The relative risk of nonunion was 2.7 times higher for smokers than nonsmokers. No statistically significant difference was noted in the rate of infection or delayed wound healing between the groups.

Kim CW, Jamali A, Tontz W Jr, et al: Treatment of posttraumatic ankle arthrosis with bipolar tibiotalar osteochondral shell allografts. *Foot Ankle Int* 2002;23:1091-1102.

Seven patients undergoing fresh tibiotalar osteochondral shell allografts for posttraumatic ankle arthrosis were evaluated at an average follow-up of 12 years. The ankle scores increased from 25 to 43 points; the Medical Outcomes Study 12-Item Short Form scores increased from 30 to 38 (physical) and

46 to 53 (mental). Four of seven patients reported good to excellent results; follow-up radiographs revealed joint space narrowing, osteophytes, and sclerosis even in patients with excellent clinical status. There was a 42% failure rate. Improvements in technique may lead to a more favorable outcome.

Marijnissen AC, Van Roermund PM, Van Melkebeek J, Lafeber FP: Clinical benefit of joint distraction in the treatment of ankle osteoarthritis. *Foot Ankle Clin* 2003; 8:335-346.

The authors describe their technique and results with distraction arthroplasty for ankle osteoarthritis.

Myerson MS, Mroczek K: Perioperative complications of total ankle arthroplasty. *Foot Ankle Int* 2003;24:17-21.

This retrospective review of a single surgeon's experience with 50 consecutive total ankle replacements compares the first 25 with the second 25 procedures. The distinct improvement in component position and fewer complications in the second group suggest that a learning curve exists in performance of total ankle arthroplasty.

Saltzman CL, Amendola A, Anderson R, et al: Surgeon training and complications in total ankle arthroplasty. *Foot Ankle Int* 2003;24:514-518.

The first 10 total ankle replacements of nine orthopaedic foot and ankle surgeons were reviewed. No method of training (observing inventor, hands-on surgical training course, foot and ankle fellowship) had a statistically demonstrable positive impact on preparing surgeons for total ankle replacement.

Thomas RH, Daniels TR: Current concepts review: Ankle arthritis. *J Bone Joint Surg Am* 2003;85-A:923-936.

The authors present a review of the current standards for evaluation and treatment of ankle arthritis.

Wood PL, Deakin S: Total ankle replacement: The results in 200 ankles. *J Bone Joint Surg Br* 2003;85:334-341.

At a mean follow-up of 46 months, the authors reviewed the results in 200 mobile-bearing cementless Scandinavian Total Ankle Replacements. The cumulative survival rate at 5 years was 93%, with decision for revision used as an end point. Most frequent complications were delayed wound healing and malleolar fracture. A complication requiring further surgery developed in 8 ankles, and 14 ankles were either revised or converted to arthrodesis.

Hindfoot and Ankle: Osteochondral Lesions of the Talus

Al Shaikh RA, Chou LB, Mann JA, et al: Autologous osteochondral grafting for talar cartilage defects. *Foot Ankle Int* 2002;23:381-389.

At an average follow-up of 16 months, 19 osteochondral lesions of the talus treated with osteochondral autograft transfer system from the ipsilateral knee trochlear border were evaluated. All patients had failed to respond to nonsurgical measures and 68% had failed to respond to débridement/ excision. The average size of the lesions before the autologous osteochondral grafting procedure was 10 mm × 12 mm. Fourteen patients required malleolar osteotomy (13 medial, 1 lateral). The average postoperative American Orthopaedic Foot and Ankle Society score at follow-up was 91; the average Lysholm knee score was 97.

Hangody L, Kish G, Modis L, et al: Mosaicplasty for the treatment of osteochondritis dissecans of the talus: Two to seven year results in 36 patients. *Foot Ankle Int* 2001; 22:552-558.

Intermediate follow-up of a single surgeon's experience with 36 osteochondral lesions of the talus treated using the mosaicplasty technique he invented demonstrated 94% good to excellent results (Hannover scoring system for ankle function). Osteochondral plugs were transferred from the ipsilateral knee; no long-term donor site morbidity was observed.

Hintermann B, Boss A, Schafer D: Arthroscopic findings in patients with chronic ankle instability. *Am J Sports Med* 2002;30:402-409.

Based on a cohort of 148 patients with symptomatic chronic ankle instability undergoing ankle arthroscopy, 66% of ankles with lateral ligament instability and 98% with deltoid ligament injuries were noted to have associated cartilage damage, respectively.

Peterson L, Brittberg M, Lindahl A: Autologous chondrocyte transplantation of the ankle. *Foot Ankle Clin* 2003;8:291-303.

The inventors of autologous chondrocyte transplantation (Carticel procedure) present their experience with this technique in the management of osteochondral lesions of the talus.

Sammarco GJ, Makwana MK: Treatment of talar osteochondral lesions using local osteochondral graft. *Foot Ankle Int* 2002;23:693-698.

The authors describe a technique for local osteochondral transfer in the management of osteochondral talar dome lesions; the graft was harvested from the medial or lateral talar articular facet. Exposure to the defect was facilitated through a replaceable bone block removed from the anterior tibial plafond. In 12 patients with an average follow-up of 25 months, the average American Orthopaedic Foot and Ankle Society score improved from 64 to 91 points. No complications were reported.

Schafer D, Boss A, Hintermann B: Accuracy of arthroscopic assessment of anterior ankle cartilage lesions. *Foot Ankle Int* 2003;24:317-320.

The authors demonstrated that iatrogenically created talar dome defects were overestimated and underestimated when evaluated arthroscopically in 10 cadaver specimens. These findings have implications should cartilage repair procedures be planned based on arthroscopic sizing of osteochondral defects of the talar dome.

Shearer C, Loomer R, Clement D: Nonoperataively managed stage V osteochondral talar lesions. *Foot Ankle Int* 2002;23:651-654.

Based on nonsurgical treatment of 25 osteochondral lesions of the talus associated with subchondral cysts, the authors suggested that (1) most lesions remain radiographically stable, (2) nonsurgical management is a viable option for stage V osteochondral lesions with little risk of developing significant osteoarthritis, (3) the general course of stage V lesions is benign in most patients, and (4) the development of mild radiographic changes of osteoarthritis does not correlate with outcome. However, the authors acknowledged that lesions that increase significantly in size correlate with poor outcome.

Schimmer RC, Dick W, Hintermann B: The role of ankle arthroscopy in the treatment strategies of osteochondritis dissecans lesions of the talus. *Foot Ankle Int* 2001;22: 895-900.

The authors report that arthroscopy represents a helpful diagnostic tool in assessing extent and, in particular, stability and integrity of the osteochondral talar defect. They recommend that arthroscopy be performed in all patients with osteochondral lesions of the talus to define the treatment strategy.

Schuman L, Struijs PA, Van Dijk CN: Arthroscopic treatment for osteochondral defects of the talus: Results at followup at 2 to 11 years. *J Bone Joint Surg Br* 2002; 84:364-368.

Thirty-eight patients who had been treated with arthroscopic débridement and drilling for osteochondral lesions of the talus were evaluated at a mean follow-up of 4.8 years. Twenty-two patients underwent a primary procedure, and 16 had failed previous surgery. Good to excellent results were found in 86% of the primary procedures and 75% of revision cases.

Scranton PE Jr, McDermott JE: Treatment of Type V osteochondral lesions of the talus with ipsilateral knee osteochondral autografts. *Foot Ankle Int* 2001;22:380-384.

Ten consecutive patients who had osteochondral lesions of the talus were treated with osteochondral autograft transplantation and were evaluated at short-term follow-up. All lesions were associated with subchondral cysts. These preliminary results suggest significant improvement in all 10 patients, with an average increase in the American Orthopaedic Foot and Ankle Society ankle/hindfoot score of 27 points.

Thordarson DB, Bains R, Shepherd LE: The role of ankle arthroscopy on the surgical management of ankle fractures. *Foot Ankle Int* 2001;22:123-125.

Nineteen patients with surgical treatment of their unstable ankle fractures were prospectively randomized to include or not include ankle arthroscopy. Eight of nine patients randomized to the arthroscopy group had articular damage that prompted arthroscopic treatment. At an average follow-up of 21 months, no difference was noted in the Medical Outcomes Study Short Form-36 Health Survey or lower extremity scores between the two groups.

Hindfoot and Ankle: Insertional Achilles Tendinopathy

Calder JD, Saxby TS: Surgical treatment of insertional Achilles tendinosis. *Foot Ankle Int* 2003;24:119-121.

A chart review of 49 open débridements of insertional Achilles tendinosis in which less than 50% of the tendon was excised suggested that early mobilization does not predispose to postsurgical rupture. At a minimum follow-up of 6 months, only two failures were noted: one patient with psoriatic arthritis and another who had bilateral simultaneous procedures.

Den Hartog BD: Flexor hallucis longus transfer for chronic Achilles tendinosis. *Foot Ankle Int* 2003;24:233-237.

Twenty-nine tendons (26 patients) undergoing reconstruction for chronic Achilles tendinosis using a flexor hallucis longus augmentation were evaluated at an average follow-up of 3 years. Time to maximum improvement was 8.2 months. The average American Orthopaedic Foot and Ankle Society ankle-hindfoot score improved from 42 to 90 points. No patient had a clinically significant functional deficit of the hallux.

McGarvey WC, Palumbo RC, Baxter DE, Leibman BD: Insertional Achilles tendinosis: Surgical treatment through a central tendon splitting approach. *Foot Ankle Int* 2002;23:19-25.

Twenty-two patients with insertional Achilles tendinosis were treated through a central tendon splitting approach with tendon débridement, retrocalcaneal bursectomy, and partial calcanectomy. This approach revealed that the disease process was isolated to the central tendon insertion in 21 of the patients. At an average follow-up of 33 months, 82% of patients were satisfied with the surgery, 77% would have the surgery again, but only 59% were completely pain free and could return to unlimited activities.

Tashjian RZ, Hur J, Sullivan RJ, et al: Flexor hallucis longus transfer for repair of chronic achilles tendinopathy. *Foot Ankle Int* 2003;24:673-676.

Using 14 fresh-frozen cadaver lower limbs, a short flexor hallucis longus tendon harvest (posteromedial ankle incision) was compared with a long (traditional) flexor hallucis longus tendon harvest (second medial midfoot incision). The short flexor hallucis longus tendon harvest yielded an average tendon length of 5.2 cm; the long flexor hallucis longus harvest yielded and average tendon length of 8.1 cm.

Hindfoot and Ankle: Acquired Flatfoot Defromity

Choi K, Lee S, Otis JC, Deland JT: Anatomical reconstruction of the spring ligament using peroneus longus tendon graft. *Foot Ankle Int* 2003;24:430-436.

Using a cadaver foot-ankle flatfoot model comparing three methods of spring ligament reconstruction using the peroneus longus tendon, it was shown that a superomedial/plantar passage of tendon through the calcaneus and navicular was most effective.

Coetzee JC, Hansen ST: Surgical management of severe deformity resulting from posterior tibial tendon dysfunction. *Foot Ankle Int* 2001;22:944-949.

A retrospective review of 12 feet in 11 patients undergoing major hindfoot corrective surgery with an extended triple arthrodesis for severe acquired pes planovalgus deformity demonstrated a statistically significant improvement in the average American Orthopaedic Foot and Ankle Society hindfoot score (30 to 74) and radiographic parameters. Despite multiple complications (wound problems, delayed unions) requiring revision surgery, the extensive procedure provided a justifiable improvement in patients' quality of life.

Guyton GP, Jeng C, Krieger LE, Mann RA: Flexor digitorum longus transfer and medial displacement calcaneal osteotomy for posterior tibial tendon dysfunction: A middle-term clinical follow-up. *Foot Ankle Int* 2001; 22:627-632.

At an average follow-up of 32 months, 26 patients undergoing flexor digitorum longus tendon transfer with medial displacement calcaneal osteotomy for stage II posterior tibial tendon dysfunction were evaluated. Only 16 patients were evaluated by physical examination for the follow-up evaluation. The average American Orthopaedic Foot and Ankle Society hindfoot pain subscale score was 35 of 40 and the American Orthopaedic Foot and Ankle Society functional score was 27 of 28. Three failures included two early failures of fixation of the flexor digitorum longus tendon and one failure at approximately 6 years during pregnancy.

Louden KW, Ambrose CG, Beaty SG, et al: Tendon transfer fixation in the foot and ankle: Biomechanical study evaluating two sizes of pilot holes for bioabsorbable screws. *Foot Ankle Int* 2003;24:67-72.

Bioabsorbable screw fixation for tendon transfer procedures, including flexor digitorum longus or flexor hallucis longus transfer to the navicular for correction of posterior tibial tendon insufficiency, is being used with greater frequency in foot and ankle surgery. This biomechanical study performed in cadaver specimens demonstrates that initial pull-out strength for 5- or 7-mm screws exceeds the requisite strength for tendon transfer to the navicular. The 7-mm screw diameter with pilot holes of 5.5 mm or 6.5 mm may be preferable given the average flexor digitorum longus or flexor hallucis longus tendon diameter approaching 5 mm.

Malicky ES, Crary JL, Houghton MJ, Agel J, Hansen ST Jr, Sangeorzan BJ: Talocalcaneal and subfibular impingement in symptomatic flatfoot in adults. *J Bone Joint Surg Am* 2002;84-A:2005-2009.

Nineteen patients with symptomatic acquired flatfoot deformity were evaluated with simulated weight-bearing CT analysis of the hindfoot and compared with a control group. In the study group, sinus tarsi impingement was noted in 92% and subfibular impingement was observed in 66% versus 0 and 5% in the control group, respectively.

Moseir-LaClair S, Pomeroy G, Manoli A: Intermediate follow-up of the double osteotomy and tendon transfer procedure for stage II posterior tibial tendon insufficiency. *Foot Ankle Int* 2001;22:283-291.

Twenty-six patients with 28 acquired pes planovalgus feet (Johnson stage II) were managed with flexor digitorum longus transfer, Achilles tendon lengthening, and a double calcaneal osteotomy (medial displacement and lateral column lengthening). At a mean follow-up of 5 years, the mean American Orthopaedic Foot and Ankle Society ankle-hindfoot score was 90. All osteotomies united and average radiographic parameters remained improved at follow-up. Fourteen percent of patients demonstrated radiographic signs of calcaneocuboid arthritis.

Sammarco GJ, Hockenbury RT: Treatment of stage II posterior tibial tendon dysfunction with flexor hallucis longus transfer and medial displacement calcaneal osteotomy. *Foot Ankle Int* 2001;22: 305-312.

At an average follow-up of 18 months, 17 patients who had undergone medial displacement calcaneal osteotomy and flexor hallucis longus tendon reconstruction for stage II posterior tibial tendon reconstruction were evaluated. The average American Orthopaedic Foot and Ankle Society hindfoot score improved from 62 to 84 points. Despite radiographic assessment demonstrating that there was no statistically significant improvement in the medial longitudinal arch in the study group, good to excellent results were reported in most patients.

Tashjian RZ, Appel AJ, Banerjee R, DiGiovanni CW: Endoscopic gastocnemius recession: evaluation in a cadaver model. *Foot Ankle Int* 2003;24: 607-613.

Endoscopic gastrocnemius recession was evaluated in 15 cadaver specimens. The sural nerve was definitively visualized in 33% of the procedures and an average of 83% of the gastrocnemius aponeurosis was transected. Improvement in mean ankle dorsiflexion with the knee flexed was 20°.

Thomas RL, Wells BC, Garrison RL, Prada SA: Preliminary results comparing two methods of lateral column lengthening. *Foot Ankle Int* 2001;22:107-119.

At a minimum follow-up of at least 1 year, 10 Evans opening wedge osteotomies were compared with 17 calcaneocuboid distraction arthrodeses, both of which were performed with structural iliac crest autograft and flexor digitorum longus

transfer for posterior tibial tendon dysfunction. American Orthopaedic Foot and Ankle Society hindfoot scores and radiographic parameters were significantly improved for both groups. The complication rate (reported for 34 feet) was high for both groups; the rate of nonunion (12%) and delayed union (18%) was considerable for the calcaneocuboid distraction arthrodesis group.

Viladot R, Pons M, Alvarez F, Omana J: Subtalar arthroereisis for posterior tibial tendon dysfunction: A preliminary report. *Foot Ankle Int* 2003;24:600-606.

Twenty-one patients with stage II flexible posterior tibial tendon dysfunction were treated with flexor digitorum longus augmentation or flexor hallucis longus tendon transfer and subtalar arthroereisis (sinus tarsi implant). Nineteen patients reviewed at an average 27-month follow-up had an average improvement in the American Orthopaedic Foot and Ankle Society score from 47 to 82 points. Two patients required removal of the implant secondary to pain.

Wacker JT, Hennessy MS, Saxby TS: Calcaneal osteotomy and transfer of the tendon of flexor digitorum longus for stage-II dysfunction of tibialis posterior: Three-to five-year results. *J Bone Joint Surg Br* 2002;84: 54-58.

At mean follow-up of 51 months, 44 patients treated with flexor digitorum longus transfer and medial displacement calcaneal osteotomy had an average improvement in the American Orthopaedic Foot and Ankle Society hindfoot score from 49 to 88 points. The outcome was good to excellent in 43 patients for pain and function, and good to excellent in 36 patients for alignment. No poor results were observed.

Hindfoot and Ankle: Plantar Fasciitis

DiGiovanni BF, Nawoczenski DA, Lintal ME, et al: Tissue specific plantar fascia-stretching exercise enhances outcomes in patients with chronic heel pain. *J Bone Joint Surg Am* 2003;85-A:1270-1277.

One hundred one patients with chronic plantar fasciitis were randomized to undergo either plantar fascia tissue– or traditional Achilles tendon–stretching regimen. Greater improvement was observed in the plantar fascia–stretching program with regard to pain, activity limitation, and patient satisfaction.

Haake M, Buch M, Schoellner C, Goebel F: Extracorporeal shock wave therapy for plantar fasciitis: Randomized controlled multicentre trial. *BMJ* 2003;327:75.

This multicenter study of 272 patients with chronic plantar fasciitis compared extracorporeal shock wave therapy with a placebo group. The success rate at 12 weeks was 34% in the shock wave therapy group and 30% in the placebo group. The authors concluded that extracorporeal shock wave therapy is ineffective in treating chronic plantar fasciitis.

Labib SA, Gould JS, Rodriguez-del-Rio FA, Lyman S: Heel Pain Triad (HPT): The combination of plantar fasciitis, posterior tibial tendon dysfunction and tarsal tunnel syndrome. *Foot Ankle Int* 2002;23:212-220.

Fourteen patients were surgically treated for a combination of plantar fasciitis, posterior tibial tendon dysfunction, and tarsal tunnel syndrome. At a mean follow-up of 17 months, a marked improvement was noted in 88% of patients for pain, activity level, walking distance, walking surface, and limp.

Rompe JD, Schoellner C, Nafe B: Evaluation of low-energy extracorporeal shock-wave application for treatment of chronic plantar fasciitis. *J Bone Joint Surg Am* 2002;84-A:335-341.

This prospective, randomized, controlled trial of 112 patients with chronic plantar fasciitis compared three applications of 1,000 low-energy shock wave impulses (group I) to three applications of 10 low-energy shock wave impulses (group II). At 6 months, the rate of good to excellent results was significantly better (47%) in group I than in group II. By 5 years, 13% of patients in group I and 58% in group II had undergone surgical plantar fascia release. The authors concluded that treatment with 1,000 impulses of low-energy shock waves may be an effective therapy for plantar fasciitis and may help patients avoid surgery.

Speed CA, Nichols D, Wies J, et al: Extracorporeal shock wave therapy for plantar fasciitis: A double blind randomized controlled trial. *J Orthop Res* 2003;21:937-940.

This double-blind randomized controlled trial compared active therapy (moderate-dose shock wave therapy) to sham therapy for 88 patients with plantar fasciitis of at least 3 months duration. Over a 6-month period, both groups showed significant improvement, but no statistically significant differences were observed in any outcome measures.

Watson TS, Anderson RB, Davis WH, Kiebzak GM: Distal tarsal tunnel release with plantar fasciotomy for chronic heel pain: An outcome analysis. *Foot Ankle Int* 2002;23:530-537.

Seventy-five patients (80 heels) with an average of 20 months of nonsurgical treatment underwent distal tarsal tunnel release with a partial plantar fasciotomy. Eighty-eight percent of patients had good to excellent results at final follow-up; 52% of patients required in excess of 6 months to reach maximum medical improvement. In the 44 patients (46 heels) who responded to a Medical Outcomes Study Short Form-36 and foot function index questionnaire, 91% were somewhat to very satisfied with their outcomes.

Hindfoot and Ankle: Diabetic Foot/Ankle and Charcot Neuroarthropathy

Bollinger M, Thordarson DB: Partial calcanectomy: An alternative to below knee amputation. *Foot Ankle Int* 2002;23:927-932.

At an average follow-up of 27 months, 22 patients with nonhealing heel wounds were treated with partial calcanectomy. Wounds healed in all patients; none required subsequent transtibial amputation. Twelve patients had delayed wound healing, and 11 additional procedures were performed on the heels of 9 patients.

Cooper PS: Application of external fixators for management of Charcot deformities of the foot and ankle. *Foot Ankle Clin* 2002;7:207-254.

A single surgeon's experience with external fixation for the management of infected and noninfected Charcot neuropathic deformities of the foot and ankle is presented.

Guyton GP, Saltzman CL: The diabetic foot: Basic mechanism of disease. *Instr Course Lect* 2002;51:169-181.

The authors present a review of the pertinent basic science, evaluation, and current state of the art in the management of diabetic foot problems.

Mueller MJ, Sinacore DR, Hastings MK, et al: Effect of Achilles tendon lengthening on neuropathic plantar ulcers. *J Bone Joint Surg Am* 2003;85-A:1436-1445.

Sixty-four patients with neuropathic ulcers were randomized to receive total contact casting alone or combined with percutaneous Achilles tendon lengthening. Eighty-eight percent of the ulcers in the total contact cast group and 100% in the Achilles tendon lengthening group healed after a mean duration of 41 days and 58 days, respectively. The risk for ulcer recurrence was 75% less at 7 months and 52% less at 2 years in the Achilles tendon lengthening group than in the isolated total contact cast group.

Classic Bibliography

Berndt A, Hardy M: Transchondral fractures (osteochondritis dissicans) of the talus. *J Bone Joint Surg Am* 1959;41:988.

Brostrom L: Sprained ankles: V. Treatment and prognosis in recent ligament ruptures. *Acta Chir Scand* 1966;132:537-550.

Brostrom L: Sprained ankles: VI. Surgical treatment of "chronic" ligament ruptures. *Acta Chir Scand* 1966;132:551-565.

Coughlin MJ, Carlson RE: Treatment of hallux valgus with an increased distal metatarsal articular angle: Evaluation of double and triple first ray osteotomies. *Foot Ankle Int* 1999;20:771-776.

Gould N, Seligson D, Gassman J: Early and late repair of lateral ligament of the ankle. *Foot Ankle* 1980;1:84-89.

Hattrup SJ, Johnson KA: Subjective results of hallux rigidus following treatment with cheilectomy. *Clin Orthop* 1988;226:182-191.

Hepple S, Winson IG, Glew D: Osteochondral lesions of the talus: A revised classification. *Foot Ankle Int* 1999; 20:789-793.

Johnson KA, Strom DA: Tibialis posterior tendon dysfunction. *Clin Orthop* 1989;239:196-206.

Kumai T, Takakura Y, Higashiyama I, Tamai S: Arthroscopic drilling for the treatment of osteochondral lesions of the talus. *J Bone Joint Surg Am* 1999;81:1229-1235.

Mann RA, Clanton TO: Hallux rigidus: Treatment by cheilectomy. *J Bone Joint Surg Am* 1988;70:400-406.

Mann RA, Rudicel S, Graves SC: Repair of hallux valgus with a distal soft-tissue procedure and proximal metatarsal osteotomy. A long-term follow-up. *J Bone Joint Surg Am* 1992;74:124-129.

Myerson MS, Henderson MR, Saxby T, Short KW: Management of midfoot diabetic neuroarthropathy. *Foot Ankle Int* 1994;15:233-241.

Papa J, Myerson M, Girard P: Salvage, with arthrodesis, in intractable diabetic neuropathic arthropathy of the foot and ankle. *J Bone Joint Surg Am* 1993;75:1056-1066.

Pell RF, Myerson MS, Schon LC: Clinical outcome after primary triple arthrodesis. *J Bone Joint Surg Am* 2000; 82:47-57.

Sangeorzan BJ, Hansen ST Jr: Modified Lapidus procedure for hallux valgus. *Foot Ankle* 1989;9:262-266.

Toolan BC, Sangeorzan BJ, Hansen ST: Complex reconstruction for the treatment of dorsolateral peritalar subluxation of the foot: Early results after distraction arthrodesis of the calcaneocuboid joint in conjunction with stabilization of, and transfer of the flexor digitorum longus tendon to, the midfoot to treat acquired pes planovalgus in adults. *J Bone Joint Surg Am* 1999;81:1545-1560.

Section 6

Spine

Section Editor:
Jeffrey S. Fischgrund, MD

Chapter 41

Adult Spine Trauma

David H. Kim, MD

Steven Zeiller, MD

Alan S. Hilibrand, MD

Cervical Spine Trauma
Clinical Evaluation

The initial evaluation and management of patients with spinal injuries is usually initiated in the field by paramedical personnel. These injuries are frequently the result of high-energy trauma, and patients may require rapid evaluation and resuscitation according to the guidelines established by the American College of Surgeons. Treatment of potential spinal injury begins at the accident scene with proper immobilization using a rigid cervical collar, tape, or straps to secure the patient's neck, and transport on a firm spine board with lateral support devices. In the setting of sports-related injuries, a helmet and shoulder pads should be left on until arrival at the hospital where experienced personnel can perform simultaneous removal of both in controlled fashion.

During the primary survey, protection of the spine and spinal cord is the important management principle. It should be assumed that all trauma patients have a cervical spine injury until proven otherwise, especially those with altered mental status or following blunt head or neck trauma. Inadequate initial stabilization can contribute to further neurologic deterioration in a patient with an acute spinal cord injury and significantly worsen eventual outcome. It has been estimated that 3% to 25% of spinal cord injuries may occur after the initial traumatic episode during early management or transport. While securing an airway, excessive head and neck movement should be avoided and manual in-line immobilization of the head and neck should be maintained whenever immobilization devices are removed. Over the past 30 years, significant improvements in the survival and outcome of patients with spinal cord injuries have been observed, primarily because of improved initial management and rapid delivery by emergency services.

Although the initial neurologic evaluation only assesses the patient's level of alertness and consciousness, a more thorough assessment of neurologic status and potential spinal injury is performed during the second-ary survey. Absence of a neurologic deficit is not sufficient to exclude such an injury, and a hard cervical collar should be applied until the cervical spine has been formally cleared and patients are considered with reasonable certainty to be stable and free of significant injury. Motorcyclists in particular have a higher incidence of thoracic spinal injuries, and evidence of blunt chest trauma should lead to further evaluation of the thoracic spine. Abdominal ecchymoses or abrasions from lap belt injury are associated with flexion-distraction injury of the thoracolumbar spine. Extremity fractures may distract the emergency personnel from identification of a spinal injury requiring treatment. Every multiple trauma patient should undergo visual inspection of the back. A thorough neurologic examination including sensorimotor function and level of consciousness is the final component of the secondary survey. Any neurologic deficit suggests the possibility of an injury to the spinal axis.

Patients with ankylosing spondylitis or diffuse idiopathic skeletal hyperostosis represent a special subpopulation for which extra vigilance is required. Spinal involvement with these conditions, particularly ankylosing spondylitis, appears to increase the risk of fracture, and patients reporting neck or back pain after even relatively minor trauma should be considered for supplemental evaluation with CT. Nondisplaced fractures commonly occur in this setting, most frequently through an ankylosed disk space, and carry a high rate of delayed or missed diagnosis. These fractures are typically unstable and can lead to spinal cord injury if not stabilized appropriately.

A variety of clinical grading systems have been developed for assessing and reporting neurologic status in spinal cord injury patients. The Frankel scale has been supplanted in clinical use by the American Spinal Injury Association (ASIA) scale (Figure 1). This scale was first introduced in 1984 and has undergone revisions in 1989, 1992, and most recently in 1996. The most recent version includes separate motor and sensory scores as well as a general impairment scale and incorporates the functional independence measure, a tool that assesses the functional effect of spinal cord injury. The motor score

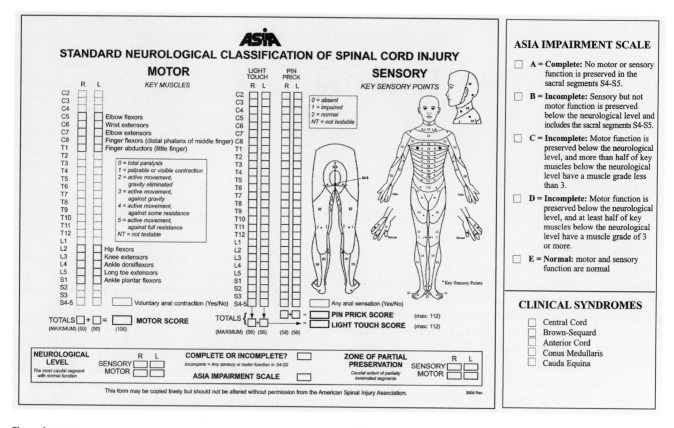

Figure 1 ASIA form for standard neurologic classification of spinal cord injury. *(Reproduced from the American Spinal Injury Association.)*

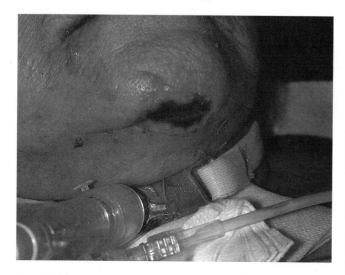

Figure 2 Photograph showing submandibular full-thickness skin necrosis from hard collar immobilization in an elderly multiple trauma patient.

has been shown to correlate with potential for functional improvement and performance during rehabilitation.

The optimal algorithm for cervical spine clearance in trauma patients remains one of the most controversial areas in spinal trauma care. Prolonged cervical collar immobilization in multiple trauma patients is known to

be associated with numerous potential complications including an increased risk of aspiration, limitation of respiratory function, development of decubitus ulcers in the occipital and submandibular areas, and possible increases in intracranial pressure (Figure 2). Moreover, collars limit access for devices such as endotracheal tubes and central lines. Therefore, several strategies have been developed to allow for rapid collar removal in patients for whom continued immobilization is unnecessary.

Results from various studies have defined practice standards in treating the asymptomatic trauma patient. Cervical spine radiographs are not required in trauma patients without neck pain or tenderness who are awake, alert, not intoxicated, and have no distracting injuries. This standard of care is supported by class I evidence from at least nine large prospective studies involving almost 40,000 patients.

In contrast to the low incidence of spinal injury in asymptomatic patients, there is a 2% to 6% incidence of significant cervical spine injury requiring treatment in patients who present with neck pain. It is generally agreed that symptomatic trauma patients with neck pain, tenderness, neurologic deficit, altered mental status, or distracting injuries require radiographic evaluation of the cervical spine before collar removal. Based on available class I evidence, a practice standard has also been suggested for radiographic evaluation of the cervical spine in symptomatic trauma patients. Specifically, a cervical spine series consisting of AP and lateral views in addition to open-mouth odontoid views is recommended. Supplemental CT examination is recommended to provide more detail of inadequately visualized levels. The most common reason for missing a significant injury appears to be inadequate visualization of the injured level, most frequently the occipitoatlantoaxial region or cervicothoracic junction. However, even with adequate plain radiographic visualization, it has been estimated that this three-view series will miss 15% to 17% of injuries.

Following initial plain radiographs and possibly a CT scan, multiple options for determining safe collar removal in symptomatic patients have been proposed. The negative predictive value of a three-view series and CT is greater than 99%, and in certain instances supplemental CT evaluation may be sufficient. However, despite the absence of apparent osseous injury, instability can exist from spinal soft-tissue disruption of ligaments, facet capsules, and disk tissue. MRI is exquisitely sensitive for acute soft-tissue injury and may be an option, but the incidence of MRI abnormalities has been shown to be between 25% to 40%, suggesting that MRI may be oversensitive. Moreover, MRI is only reliable for identifying soft-tissue injury within 48 hours of the traumatic event.

Flexion-extension radiographs are frequently obtained to rule out significant instability. In awake and alert patients, active flexion-extension radiographs are safe, and no significant complications have been reported. The negative predictive value of plain films in conjunction with flexion-extension views is in excess of 99%.

The most controversy surrounds cervical spine clearance in the obtunded patient. Again, MRI has been suggested as an adjunctive test but may be of limited usefulness because of the lack of correlation between MRI findings and clinically significant injury. Passive flexion-extension manipulation of the cervical spine under fluoroscopy has been advocated by several investigators. However, there is a theoretic risk of causing iatrogenic spinal cord injury to these patients because of unrecognized disk herniation. It has been suggested that many obtunded patients are at low risk for any significant injury and can be cleared on the basis of plain radiographs and CT. Proposed high-risk criteria indicating the need for further evaluation include high-velocity motor vehicle accidents (> 35 mph), any fall from a height of more than 10 feet, closed-head injuries, neurologic deficits referable to the cervical spine, and pelvis or extremity fractures.

Anatomy of the Cervical Spine

The cervical spine includes seven vertebrae. The rostral two vertebrae, the atlas (C1) and axis (C2), have distinct morphology and biomechanical characteristics. The third through sixth vertebrae (C3-C6) are considered typical cervical vertebrae with small cylindrical bodies and short bifid spinous processes. The seventh cervical vertebra (C7) is a transitional vertebra between the cervical and thoracic spinal regions and has a large nonbifid spinous process known as the vertebra prominens.

The atlas is a ring containing two articular lateral masses with neither a body nor spinous process (Figure 3). Incomplete formation of the posterior ring is relatively common as a developmental variation and does not represent a traumatic injury. The axis contains the odontoid process or dens, which articulates with the anterior arch of the axis against which it is stabilized by the transverse ligament (Figure 4).

Morphology of the subaxial cervical spine from C3 to C6 is relatively consistent. The articular processes are located at the junction of the laminae and pedicles and form pillars referred to as the lateral masses (Figure 5). The vertebral bodies are predominantly cancellous bone surrounded by thin cortical bone. Superior end plates are concave in the coronal plane and convex in the sagittal plane, whereas the matching inferior end plates are convex in the coronal plane and concave in the sagittal plane. The uncinate processes are osseous projections off the posterolateral surfaces of the superior end plates. Their articulation with the convex inferolateral surface of the more rostral vertebra comprises the joints of Luschka.

The posterior facet joints caudal to C2 are encapsulated synovial joints with overlying hyaline cartilage and containing small menisci. The facet joint angle approximates 45° in the sagittal plane. The transverse processes of each cervical vertebra contain a vascular foramen. The vertebral artery typically passes anterior to the transverse processes of C7 before entering the spine at the C6 vascular foramen. An accessory vertebral vein typically occupies the C7 foramen. At C1, the vertebral arteries pass through a foramen, and then turn posteromedially around the superior articular process before entering the foramen magnum and joining to form the basilar artery. An anomalous course for the vertebral artery is present 3% of the time and most commonly involves medial deviation toward the vertebral body at its midpoint. The incidence of unilateral absence or hypoplasia of the vertebral artery is 5% to 10%. Arterial supply of the anterior two thirds of the cervical spinal cord derives from a single anterior spinal artery, which is fed by segmental arteries derived from the vertebral arteries. Paired posterior spinal arteries derived from either the vertebral arteries or the posterior inferior cerebellar artery supply the posterior one third of the cord. Branches of the vertebral arteries provide a robust blood supply for individual vertebra. Odontoid nonunions were previously attributed to inadequate arterial perfusion; however, recent anatomic studies have revealed an extensive arterial arcade surrounding the odontoid

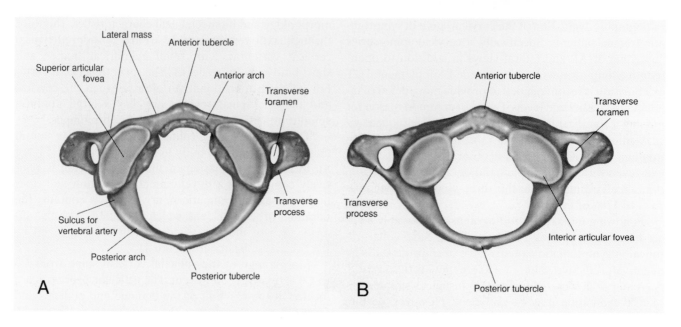

Figure 3 Illustrations of the osseous anatomy of the first cervical vertebra (C1; atlas). **A,** Cranial view of the atlas. **B,** Caudal view of the atlas. *(Reproduced with permission from Heller JG, Pedlow FX Jr: Anatomy of the cervical spine, in Clark CR (ed): The Cervical Spine, ed 3. Philadelphia, PA, Lippincott-Raven, 1998, pp 3-36.)*

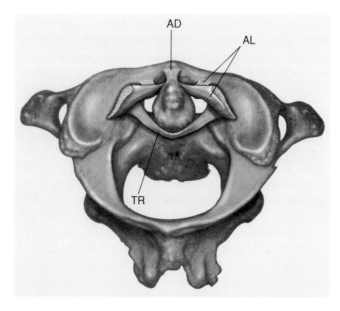

Figure 4 Illustration of the ligamentous stabilizers of the atlantoaxial segment showing the relationship among the transverse (TR), alar (AL), and atlantodens (AD) ligaments. *(Reproduced with permission from Heller JG, Pedlow FX Jr: Anatomy of the cervical spine, in Clark CR (ed): The Cervical Spine, ed 3. Philadelphia, PA, Lippincott-Raven, 1998, pp 3-36.)*

process supplied by anterior and posterior ascending branches of the vertebral arteries and pharyngeal branches from the external carotid arteries. Venous drainage from the cervical spine occurs through pairs of external veins traveling with these major supplying arteries as well as through an internal epidural plexus of valveless sinuses, both of which drain into the superior vena cava and azygos vein.

The central opening in each cervical vertebra is known as the vertebral canal, which in continuity with the vertebral canal of adjacent vertebrae constitutes the spinal canal containing the spinal cord. The average sagittal diameter of the spinal canal averages 23 mm at C1 and decreases progressively to 15 mm at C7. Nerve root pairs exit the canal at each level through the intervertebral foramen formed by notches on the inferior and superior aspects of adjacent pedicles. The anterior border of the foramen is formed by the posterolateral uncovertebral joint and intervertebral disk, whereas the posterior border is formed by the caudal superior articular facet. Each nerve root normally occupies one third of the cross-sectional area of the foramen. The C3 through C8 nerve roots exit anterior to the facet joints in contrast to the C2 nerve roots, which exit posterior to the C1-2 facet joint. The spinal nerves pass posterior to the vertebral artery at approximately the middle of the corresponding lateral mass. Ventral rami of C1 to C4 make up the cervical plexus and provide innervation to the cervical strap muscles and the diaphragm. Ventral rami of C5 to C8 along with T1 make up the brachial plexus. The sympathetic chain lies bilaterally in proximity to the carotid sheath between the longus capitis and longus colli muscles.

Stability of the cervical spine is highly dependent on the integrity of the intervertebral ligaments and disks. The osseous anatomy of the occipitocervical junction provides little inherent stability. Instead, the anterior and posterior atlanto-occipital membranes and the articular capsules provide most of the stability to the craniocervical junction (Figure 6). The atlantoaxial joint provides 50% of overall cervical rotation, with stability

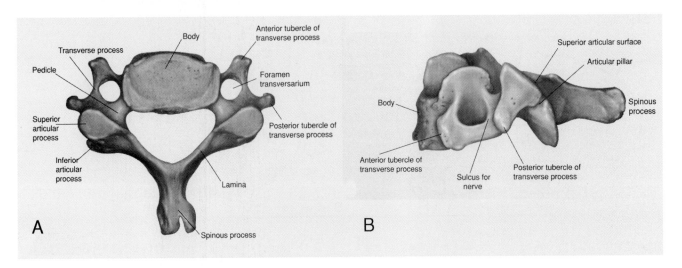

Figure 5 Cranial **(A)** and lateral **(B)** illustrations of the osseous anatomy of the subaxial cervical spine. *(Reproduced with permission from Heller JG, Pedlow FX Jr: Anatomy of the cervical spine, in Clark CR (ed): The Cervical Spine, ed 3. Philadelphia, PA, Lippincott-Raven, 1998, pp 3-36.)*

again provided largely by specific ligamentous structures. In the horizontal plane, the transverse ligament is the primary stabilizer, whereas the apical ligament and the paired alar ligaments constitute secondary stabilizers (Figure 4). In the subaxial spine, the anterior and posterior longitudinal ligaments and intervertebral disk provide significant resistance to shear forces. Posteriorly, the ligamentum nuchae, interspinous ligaments, and ligamentum flavum comprise the posterior ligamentous complex and provide primary resistance against flexion distraction forces.

The cervical spinal cord is ovoid in shape. It is narrower in the sagittal plane and has an expansion between C3 and C6 to provide innervation to the upper extremities. The white matter of the spinal cord exists in the periphery and contains bundles of myelinated axonal tracts that are divided into three discernable columns (Figure 7). The posterior columns conduct ascending proprioceptive, vibratory, and tactile signals from the ipsilateral side of the body. The lateral columns contain the lateral spinothalamic tracts, which conduct ascending pain and thermal signals for the contralateral side, as well as the lateral corticospinal tracts, which conduct 85% of descending voluntary motor signals for the ipsilateral side of the body. The anterior columns contain the anterior spinothalamic tracts, which conduct ascending light touch signals from the contralateral side, as well as the anterior corticospinal tracts, which conduct descending signals underlying fine motor control. Recent evidence suggests that the previously reported highly organized laminar structure of the white matter tracts probably does not exist.

Cervical Spinal Instability

The concept of spinal instability is vague and controversial but remains central to clinical decision making in

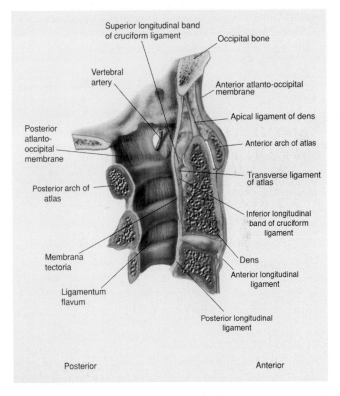

Figure 6 Illustration of the local anatomy of the occipitocervical junction. *(Reproduced with permission from Heller JG, Pedlow FX Jr: Anatomy of the cervical spine, in Clark CR (ed): The Cervical Spine, ed 3. Philadelphia, PA, Lippincott-Raven, 1998, pp 3-36.)*

spinal trauma care. The classic definition by White and Panjabi describes instability as the loss of ability of the spine under physiologic loads to maintain its pattern of displacement so that there is no initial or additional neurologic deficit, no major deformity, and no incapacitating pain. This definition is elegant, but unfortunately

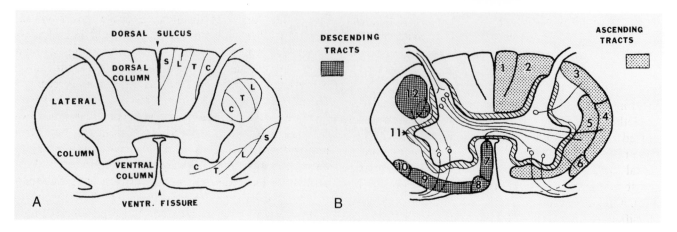

Figure 7 Illustrations of the cross-sectional anatomy of the cervical spinal cord. **A**, S = sacral; L = lumbar; T = thoracic; C = cervical. **B**, 1 = fasciculus gracilis; 2 = fasciculus cuneatus; 3 = dorsal spinocerebellar tract; 4 = ventral spinocerebellar tract; 5 = lateral spinothalamic tract; 6 = spinoolivary tract; 7 = ventral corticospinal tract; 8 = tectospinal tract; 9 = vestibulospinal tract; 10 = olivospinal tract; 11 = propriospinal tract; 12 = lateral corticospinal tract. *(Reproduced with permission from Heller JG, Pedlow FX Jr: Anatomy of the cervical spine, in Clark CR (ed): The Cervical Spine, ed 3. Philadelphia, PA, Lippincott-Raven, 1998, pp 3-36.)*

Table 1 | Criteria for Identifying Instability at the Occipito-cervical Junction

> 8°	Axial rotation C0-C1 to one side
> 1 mm	C0-C1 translation
> 7 mm	Overhang C1-C2 (total right and left)
> 45°	Axial rotation C1-C2 to one side
> 4 mm	C1-C2 translation
< 13 mm	Posterior body C2 to posterior ring C1
	Avulsed transverse ligament

(Adapted with permission from White AA, Panjabi MM: Clinical Biomechanics of the Spine, ed 2. Philadelphia, PA, Lippincott Williams & Wilkins, 1990.)

Table 2 | Checklist for the Diagnosis of Clinical Instability in the Middle and Lower Cervical Spine

Element	Point Value
Anterior elements destroyed or unable to function	2
Posterior elements destroyed or unable to function	2
Positive stretch test	2
Radiographic criteria	4
A. Flexion/extension radiographs	
a. Sagittal plane translation > 3.5 mm or 20% (2 points)	
b. Sagittal plane rotation > 20° (2 points)	
or	
B. Resting radiographs	
a. Sagittal plane displacement > 3.5 mm or 20% (2 points)	
b. Relative sagittal plane angulation > 11° (2 points)	
Abnormal disk narrowing	1
Developmentally narrow spinal canal	1
1. Sagittal diameter < 13 mm	
or	
2. Pavlov's ratio < 0.8 mm	
Spinal cord damage	2
Nerve root damage	1
Dangerous loading anticipated	1
Total (5 points or more = unstable)	

(Adapted with permission from White AA, Panjabi MM: Clinical Biomechanics of the Spine, ed 2. Philadelphia, PA, Lippincott Williams & Wilkins, 1990.)

it is difficult to translate directly into clinical practice. Based predominantly on data from cadaveric studies, more specific criteria have been suggested for identifying instability at the occipitocervical junction (Table 1) and in the subaxial cervical spine (Table 2).

Occipital Condyle Fracture

Diagnosis of occipital condyle fractures has increased in frequency because of greater use of CT evaluation of the cervical spine in trauma patients. Sensitivity of plain radiography for diagnosis is as low as 3%. Occipital condyle fractures should be considered a marker for potentially lethal trauma, with an 11% mortality rate from associated injuries. The rate of associated cervical spine injury at an additional level is 31%. According to the most commonly used classification system for occipital condyle fractures developed by Anderson and Montesano, type I fractures (3% of fractures) are comminuted fractures resulting from axial load, type II fractures (22%) involve extension of a basilar skull fracture into the condyle, and type III fractures (75%) are avulsion

fractures and should raise clinical suspicion for an underlying occipitocervical dissociation. Cranial nerve palsies may develop days to weeks after injury and most frequently affect cranial nerves IX, X, and XI or result in visual disturbance. Treatment of occipital condyle fractures requires ruling out occipitocervical dissociation, particularly in patients with type III fractures, followed by external immobilization in a cervical orthosis.

Occipitocervical Dissociation

Most instances of traumatic occipitocervical dissociation are lethal, with approximately 100 cases having been reported in the literature. Survivors may demonstrate a wide range of neurologic injuries ranging from complete spinal cord lesions to isolated cranial nerve palsies (most commonly affecting cranial nerves VI, X, and XII). Occipitocervical dissociation injuries have been classified as anterior type I, longitudinal type II, or posterior type III.

Diagnosis of this condition can be challenging because of the poorly visualized osseous detail on plain radiographs of this region. The most frequently described measurement is the Powers ratio, which divides the basion to posterior arch distance by the anterior arch to opisthion distance. A ratio greater than 1 suggests possible anterior dissociation. Other measurements considered suggestive of injury include a basion to odontoid distance greater than 10 mm, posterior mandible to anterior atlas distance greater than 13 mm, and posterior mandible to odontoid distance greater than 20 mm. The Harris basion-axial interval–basion-dental interval method measures distance from the basion to a line drawn tangentially to the posterior border of C2 (a distance greater than 12 mm or less than 4 mm is abnormal) as well as the distance from the basion to the odontoid (greater than 12 mm is abnormal) and is considered by some to be the most sensitive measurement. Overall, the sensitivity of plain radiographs for occipitocervical dissociation is approximately 57%. The sensitivity of CT and MRI has been estimated to be 84% and 86%, respectively, and one or both of these adjunctive studies is recommended for patients with suspected occipitocervical dissociation injuries.

Use of traction is associated with a 10% rate of neurologic deterioration and should be avoided in patients with these injuries. In patients with survivable injuries, an instrumented occipitocervical fusion is recommended. Different techniques of fixation have been described, including occipital and cervical wiring, wire mesh and methylmethacrylate, and occipitocervical plating. More recently, modular occipital plates have been developed that can be rigidly locked to longitudinal rods placed across the subaxial cervical spine (Figure 8).

Atlas Fractures

Fractures of the atlas constitute approximately 7% of cervical spine fractures. Jefferson fractures are bilateral fractures of the anterior and posterior arches resulting from an axial load (Figure 9). Long-term stability depends on the mechanism of injury and subsequent heal-

ing of the transverse ligament. Because data from cadaveric studies indicate that a combined lateral mass displacement in excess of 7 mm strongly suggests ligament disruption, an 18% radiographic magnification factor has been incorporated, resulting in an increase in the measurement to 8.1 mm. However, with improvements in MRI technology, it has become a more sensitive means of detecting a ligamentous injury than plain radiographs. Two types of transverse ligament injury have been described. Midsubstance ruptures (type I injuries) are least likely to heal, and early surgical treatment with C1-2 fusion may be necessary. Type II injuries involve an avulsion fracture of the ligamentous insertion. Because of higher rates of healing, an initial attempt at external immobilization using a halo vest is a reasonable treatment option in these patients.

In general, most isolated anterior or posterior arch fractures and lateral mass and transverse process fractures of the atlas can be treated conservatively with 6 to 12 weeks of external immobilization. Burst fractures involving both anterior and posterior arches with an intact transverse ligament are considered stable injuries that should also be treated with external immobilization. Disruption of the transverse ligament introduces the option of early surgical fusion, typically involving a posterior C1-2 fusion. Multiple procedures have been described, including various wiring techniques and screw-rod constructs. C1-2 transarticular screw placement is the most stable form of fixation currently in general use and obviates the need for postoperative halo immobilization required with C1-2 wiring techniques.

Axis Fractures

Odontoid fractures are the most common type of axis fracture and have been classified by Anderson and D'Alonzo as type I avulsion fractures of the tip, type II fractures through the waist of the odontoid process, or type III fractures extending into the C2 vertebral body. Nearly all odontoid fractures will require some form of treatment.

Type I fractures can be treated with an external orthosis once the possibility of an associated occipitocervical dissociation has been excluded. Type III fractures have been reported to have a sufficiently high healing rate with rigid external immobilization in a halo vest. Treatment of type II fractures is controversial and depends largely on specific patient and fracture characteristics. Elderly patients tolerate halo vest immobilization poorly, demonstrate decreased healing rates, and should be considered for early C1-2 surgical fusion. Elderly debilitated patients who are at increased risk of medical complications from surgical treatment can be treated with an external orthosis for 6 to 12 weeks with the understanding that successful fusion is unlikely to occur. In most patients, a fibrous nonunion develops

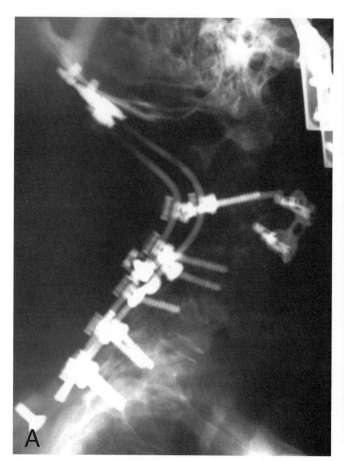
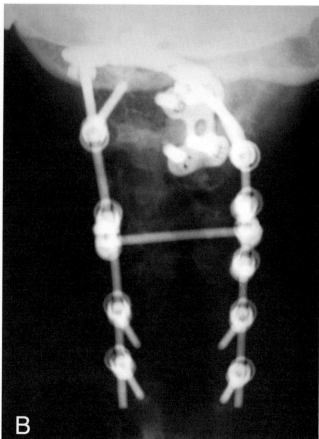

Figure 8 Lateral (**A**) and AP (**B**) radiographs of occipitocervical segmental fixation implants (DePuy AcroMed Summit system, Raynham, MA).

that provides sufficient stability for routine daily activities. Nevertheless, these patients should be informed that they remain at risk for spinal cord injury in the event of a fall or motor vehicle accident.

In younger, healthy patients with a type II fracture, specific fracture characteristics assume increased significance. Nondisplaced fractures diagnosed early should be treated with halo vest immobilization for 6 to 12 weeks. Risk factors for nonunion include fracture comminution, displacement of more than 6 mm, posterior displacement, delay in diagnosis, and patient age greater than 50 years. Early surgical treatment is an option for patients with any of these risk factors. Surgical treatment should also be considered for fractures in which reduction cannot be achieved or maintained.

Anterior odontoid screw osteosynthesis using a single screw placed with lag technique is an option for treating both type II and type III noncomminuted fractures. For the best results using this technique, the fracture should be diagnosed early, reduction must be possible, and patient body habitus must allow achievement of proper intraoperative screw trajectory (Figure 10). In addition, odontoid fracture obliquity should run from anterosuperior to posteroinferior. Otherwise, surgical treatment may involve any of several methods for ac-

complishing a posterior C1-2 fusion. Traditional sublaminar wiring techniques (Gallie and Brooks fusions) are being supplemented or replaced by more rigid fixation methods such as C1-2 transarticular screws and C1 lateral mass and C2 pedicle screw-rod constructs (Figure 11). These more rigid fixation techniques provide the surgeon with the opportunity to avoid postoperative halo vest immobilization.

Traumatic Spondylolisthesis of the Axis

This injury is characterized by bilateral fractures of the pars interarticularis and is also known as a hangman's fracture, although recent efforts have been made to replace this term with traumatic spondylolisthesis of the axis. Most injuries of this type that occur in the United States are the result of motor vehicle accidents, and the forces involved are likely a combination of hyperextension, compression, and rebound flexion. The currently popular classification scheme is Levine and Edwards' modification of previous systems described by Effendi and Francis and is based on mechanism of injury (Figure 12). Type I fractures result from axial compression and hyperextension and demonstrate less than 3 mm displacement and no angulation. Type II fractures result

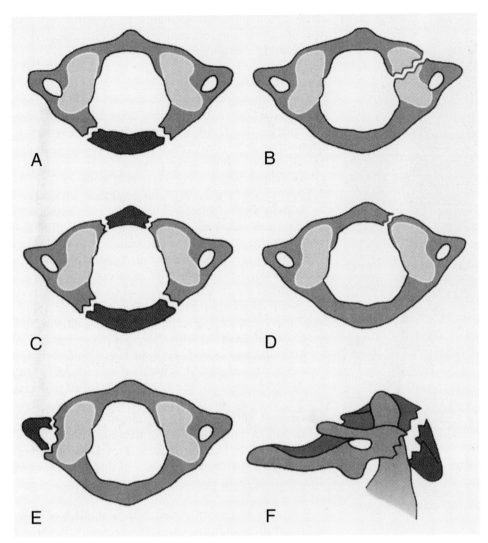

Figure 9 Illustrations of common atlas fracture patterns. **A,** posterior arch fracture. **B,** Lateral mass fracture. **C,** Classic burst (Jefferson fracture). **D,** Unilateral anterior arch fracture. **E,** Transverse process fracture. **F,** Anterior arch avulsion fracture. *(Reproduced with permission from Klein GR, Vaccaro AR: Cervical spine trauma: Upper and lower, in Vaccaro AR, Betz RR, Zeidman SM (eds): Principles and Practice of Spine Surgery. Philadelphia, PA, Mosby, 2003, pp 441-462.)*

from hyperextension and axial load followed by rebound flexion and demonstrate translation of greater than 3 mm as well as angulation. Type IIA fractures are characterized by angulation without significant translation and result from a flexion-distraction injury. Identification of this fracture type is important because application of traction may cause further fracture displacement and should be avoided. Type III fractures are essentially type I pars fractures associated with injury to the C2-3 facet joints, most commonly bilateral facet dislocation. These fractures are thought to result from flexion-distraction followed by hyperextension. A type IA fracture pattern was recently added to this classification system to describe asymmetric fracture lines with minimal translation and no angulation. This fracture is thought to result from hyperextension with a component of lateral bending forces.

Most patients with traumatic spondylolisthesis of the axis can be successfully treated with 6 to 12 weeks of external immobilization in a cervical orthosis or halo vest. Data from a recent cadaveric study have suggested that up to 5 mm of displacement can occur without disruption of posterior ligaments or the C2-3 disk. Suggested indications for surgical treatment include type II fractures with severe angulation, type III fractures with disruption of the C2-3 disk, or inability to achieve or maintain fracture reduction. All type III fractures associated with facet dislocation require open reduction and fusion. Surgical options include anterior C2-3 interbody fusion, posterior C1-3 fusion, or bilateral C2 pars screw osteosynthesis.

Fractures and Dislocations of the Subaxial Spine

The most commonly used classification system for subaxial spine injuries is the system developed by Allen and associates. Six distinct phylogenies were described based on mechanism of injury, with each phylogeny being subdivided into stages of progressive severity. The three commonly observed categories are compressive flexion, distractive flexion, and compressive extension. Vertical compression is observed less commonly, and the two least common categories are distractive extension and lateral flexion.

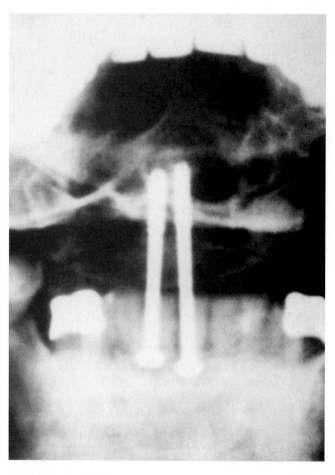

Figure 10 Odontoid radiograph of anterior odontoid screw fixation. *(Reproduced with permission from Klein GR, Vaccaro AR: Cervical spine trauma: Upper and lower, in Vaccaro AR, Betz RR, Zeidman SM (eds): Principles and Practice of Spine Surgery. Philadelphia, PA, Mosby, 2003, pp 441-462.)*

Compression and Burst Fractures

Compression fractures are defined by compressive failure of the anterior half of the vertebral body (anterior column) without disruption of the posterior body cortex and without retropulsion into the spinal canal. Patients are typically neurologically intact, and in the absence of significant deformity or instability, most fractures can be treated with external immobilization for 6 to 12 weeks.

Burst fractures are characterized by compressive failure of the vertebral body with fracture extension through the posterior body cortex and some degree of bone retropulsion into the spinal canal. Burst fractures have a significantly higher rate of instability when compared with compression fractures and are frequently associated with spinal cord injury. A burst fracture in the presence of either complete or incomplete spinal cord injury will typically require surgical decompression and stabilization. In most patients with burst fractures, surgical decompression can be best achieved through an anterior approach with corpectomy of the involved level(s). Interbody fusion with anterior plate fixation may be insufficient to stabilize these fractures in the setting

of disrupted posterior elements. In patients with this type of injury, supplemental posterior instrumented fusion should be considered.

Facet Dislocations

Patients with cervical facet dislocations should undergo timely reduction of their injuries upon diagnosis. Classically, plain radiographic evidence of vertebral body subluxation of 25% has been reported to suggest a unilateral facet dislocation, whereas vertebral body subluxation of 50% has been reported to suggest a bilateral dislocation (Figure 13). Unilateral facet dislocations are commonly associated with a monoradiculopathy that improves following application of traction. Bilateral facet dislocations are often associated with significant spinal cord injuries. Awake and alert patients can safely undergo closed reduction with progressive application of axial traction forces. It is crucial that these patients be closely monitored with serial neurologic examinations and plain radiographic assessment following the placement of each additional weight. Development of new or worsening neurologic deficits is an indication to cease attempts at closed reduction, and an MRI scan should be obtained to rule out herniated disk material. Overall, as many as 26% of patients with cervical facet dislocations will fail attempted closed reduction, with higher failure rates observed for patients with unilateral facet dislocations. Although 50% of patients with facet dislocations will demonstrate signs of disk disruption on MRI, most of these signs are of uncertain clinical significance.

Following successful closed reduction, surgical stabilization of these injuries is typically necessary. In the absence of a traumatic disk herniation, posterior instrumented fusion is recommended. However, various treatment options are available for associated disk herniation. After successful closed reduction, an MRI scan of the cervical spine should be obtained to rule out the presence of associated disk herniation. Anterior diskectomy and fusion with anterior plating has been reported to be successful, although associated with kyphotic deformity in some instances. For this reason, patients with persistent kyphosis following closed reduction who have anterior compression from disk material may require anterior decompression and grafting with a concomitant posterior stabilization.

Failure of closed reduction mandates open reduction and instrumented cervical fusion. A preoperative MRI scan is required to rule out the presence of a herniated disk, which, if present, indicates the need for anterior diskectomy and fusion. A unilateral facet dislocation can often be reduced anteriorly using vertebral body Caspar pins. This technique involves maintaining distraction across these pins followed by rotation of the proximal pin toward the side of the dislocated facet joint. Alternatively, for unilateral or bilateral disloca-

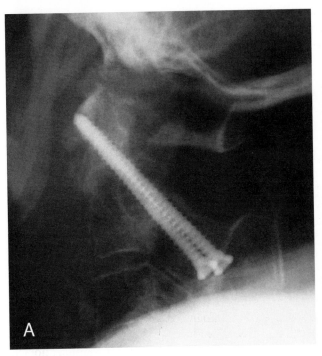

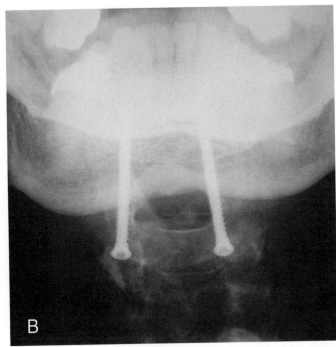

Figure 11 Lateral **(A)** and AP **(B)** radiographs showing C1-2 transarticular screw fixation.

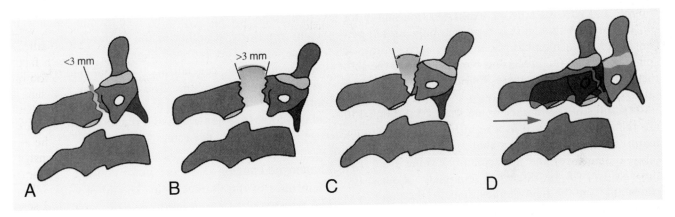

Figure 12 Illustrations of types of traumatic spondylolisthesis of the axis using the Levine and Edwards modification of the Effendi classification system. **A,** Type I. **B,** Type II. **C,** Type IIA. **D,** Type III. *(Reproduced with permission from Klein GR, Vaccaro AR: Cervical spine trauma: Upper and lower, in Vaccaro AR, Betz RR, Zeidman SM (eds): Principles and Practice of Spine Surgery. Philadelphia, PA, Mosby, 2003, pp 441-462.)*

tions associated with a significant disk herniation, an anti-kickout plate can be used to avoid the need for a second anterior stage of the surgery. Following anterior diskectomy and placement of an interbody graft, the plate is fixed only to the superior body. Open reduction can then be performed posteriorly with the plate maintaining position of the graft.

Unilateral facet fractures are the most frequently missed significant cervical spine injuries on plain radiographs. These injuries may reduce in the supine position during initial trauma evaluation. Subtle subluxations or rotational malalignment visualized on plain radiographs should prompt further study with CT. The superior facet is more frequently fractured. Fractures without signifi-

cant kyphosis or subluxations can be considered for nonsurgical treatment with 6 to 12 weeks of external immobilization in a halo vest or cervical orthosis. Kyphotic deformity, significant subluxations, or radiculopathy should be considered for open reduction and posterior instrumented stabilization. Bilateral facet fractures and lateral mass dissociations are typically unstable injuries and may be treated with anterior or posterior instrumented fusion.

Thoracic Spine Trauma

Thoracic spine fractures represent approximately 16% of fractures involving the thoracic and lumbar spine. These injuries typically result from high-energy blunt

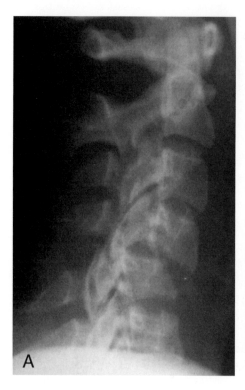

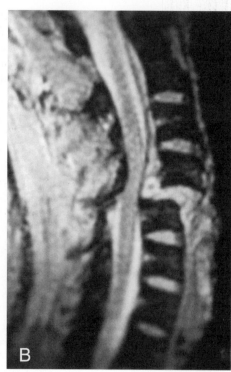

Figure 13 Bilateral cervical spinal facet dislocations. **A,** Plain radiograph demonstrates 50% subluxation of C4 on C5. **B,** T2-weighted MRI scan reveals large posteriorly extruded disk fragment at the level of injury. The patient underwent an anterior decompression and anterior open reduction and instrumented fusion. *(Reproduced with permission from Klein GR, Vaccaro AR: Cervical spine trauma: Upper and lower, in Vaccaro AR, Betz RR, Zeidman SM (eds): Principles and Practice of Spine Surgery. Philadelphia, PA, Mosby, 2003, pp 441-462.)*

trauma, and patients must be evaluated thoroughly for other injuries. Although they represent only a small percentage of thoracolumbar fractures, the narrow thoracic spinal canal and the precarious blood supply to the thoracic spinal cord make these injuries potentially devastating.

Fractures of the thoracic spine from T2 through T10 are relatively infrequent as a result of unique anatomic features of the thoracic spine that provide enhanced stability. Fractures of the thoracolumbar spine from T11 through L2 will be discussed separately because the transition from the rigid thoracic spine to the more flexible lumbar spine creates a transition zone that is susceptible to injury.

Biomechanics

The thoracic spine has several unique anatomic features that provide it with more stability than either the cervical or lumbar spine. Each thoracic vertebra has articulations with and ligamentous attachments to the adjacent ribs at both the transverse process and the vertebral body that increase rigidity. In addition, the ribs articulate with the sternum, which provides another point of fixation and thereby limits thoracic motion. The facets of the thoracic spine are oriented in the coronal plane, with the lamina and spinous processes arranged in a shingled fashion, which reduces the amount of extension of the thoracic spine. The intervertebral disks of the thoracic spine are very thin, which provides increased stiffness and more rotational stability. The vertebral bodies are asymmetric in height from anterior to posterior. The

vertebral bodies are typically 1 to 2 mm smaller in height anteriorly, resulting in the kyphosis seen in the thoracic spine. The kyphotic alignment of the thoracic spine results in the concentration of axial load transmission in the anterior column. The apex of the kyphosis is normally over T6 through T8, where maximal anterior column forces are generated and fractures within the rib cage are most likely to occur.

Diagnostic Imaging

Plain films of the thoracic spine should provide an initial assessment of any fracture as well as its impact on overall sagittal alignment. It is of paramount importance to evaluate the entire spine once a fracture is identified because concomitant spinal fractures can be present in up to 20% of patients. CT scans should be obtained in patients with fractures on plain films, in any multiple trauma patient with lower extremity neurologic deficits, and for any patients with inadequate plain films. The axial images will help evaluate the vertebral body fracture anatomy, pedicle anatomy, and presence of bony retropulsion. Coronal and sagittal reconstructions may reveal fractures missed in the axial plane, and they provide a better appreciation of the fracture anatomy. MRI can be useful in evaluating the soft tissues of the spine. The anterior and posterior ligamentous complexes can be evaluated for injury as well as spinal cord encroachment by either disk or osseous material. In addition, the spinal cord can be evaluated for the presence of edema or hemorrhage.

Classification systems for spinal fractures have been difficult to standardize because of the complex loads that are applied to result in these injuries. A comprehensive classification system has been proposed for thoracic and lumbar fractures based on their radiographic morphology. Three basic forces—compression, distraction, and rotation—were found to be responsible for the injuries and are labeled A, B, and C, respectively. In addition, each group is subdivided into three subgroups. The severity of the injury increases from group A to group C. Because describing every variant in this system is beyond the scope of this text, only the classic examples from each group will be discussed.

Compression Fractures

In its purest form, a compression fracture results from an axial load applied to the spine. The anterior column of the spine (vertebral body and disk) is involved without involvement of the middle column (posterior vertebral cortex and posterior longitudinal ligament). Radiographs will demonstrate a wedge-shaped defect in the vertebral body that results in varying degrees of kyphosis. Neurologically intact patients with less than 30° of kyphosis and less than 50% loss of vertebral body height can be treated with a hyperextension orthosis. Patients with more than 30° of kyphosis or more than 50% loss of vertebral body height can also be treated nonsurgically, but must be watched carefully for possible failure of the posterior ligamentous structures. These patients are more likely to develop a kyphotic deformity, and close radiographic and clinical follow-up is warranted. In patients with fractures above T6, a cervical extension on the thoracolumbosacral orthosis should be used for better control.

Burst Fractures

Burst fractures also result from an axial load and are inherently unstable because of the involvement of the anterior and middle columns of the spine. Radiographs will typically demonstrate a widening of the pedicles at the affected vertebral body and a varying degree of bony retropulsion into the canal. Treatment of these injuries must be based on consideration of neurologic status, sagittal alignment, and the integrity of the posterior ligamentous structures. Patients who are neurologically intact with less than 30° of kyphosis and less than 50% loss of vertebral body height can be managed in a thoracolumbosacral orthosis. Patients with more than 30° of kyphosis and more than 50% loss of vertebral body height with failure of the posterior column should be considered for a posterior stabilization procedure.

Patients with incomplete neurologic deficits and radiographic evidence of spinal cord compression may benefit from an acute anterior decompression and stabilization. However, the benefit of early versus delayed decompression and stabilization of these injuries has yet to be demonstrated in the scientific literature. Patients who have a complete neurologic injury are typically stabilized posteriorly in a nonemergent fashion to facilitate earlier rehabilitation.

Flexion-Distraction Injuries

Flexion-distraction injuries result from a flexion moment that is combined with a fulcrum located at varying distances from the anterior portion of the vertebral column. The resulting injury can involve bone, ligament, or a combination of bone and ligament. When the fulcrum is located adjacent to the vertebral body, the anterior column will fail in compression and the middle and posterior columns will fail in tension. As the fulcrum moves more anterior, the deforming forces become purely distractive and all three columns will fail in tension. Patients with pure ligamentous and combined bony and ligamentous injuries should undergo a posterior stabilization procedure because of involvement of all three columns and the poor healing properties of ligaments. Typically, these injuries can be treated with short-segment posterior compression constructs. Patients with a purely bony injury can undergo reduction in extension and can be treated in a thoracolumbosacral orthosis because of the healing properties of bone. They should be assessed for nonunion and deformity progression.

Fracture-Dislocations

Fracture-dislocations are common injuries in the thoracic spine because of the significant forces acting on a rigid portion of the spine. Up to 90% of these injuries are associated with a spinal cord injury, most commonly complete (ASIA impairment scale category A). Because all three spinal columns are involved, these fractures are very unstable. In patients with complete neurologic injury, a posterior stabilization procedure can be performed once their clinical condition is optimized. This will allow for early mobilization and help minimize the morbidity and mortality associated with these injuries.

Thoracic Pedicle Screws

The use of thoracic pedicle screws has become more widespread based on numerous reports of safe placement techniques and success in clinical practice. Pedicle screws offer several advantages over traditional hook and rod constructs. The pedicle is the strongest bony attachment to the vertebra and provides excellent purchase, even in osteoporotic bone. Pedicle screws provide fixation of all three spinal columns, which provides for better sagittal and coronal stability. This increased stability can decrease the number of levels included in a fusion construct.

The thoracic pedicles are the narrowest in the T4-6 region and become progressively larger toward the lum-

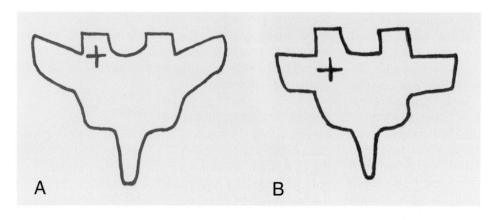

Figure 14 A, From the levels T3 through T10, the entrance point to cannulate the pedicle can be determined by using the intersection point between a line drawn from the superior border of the transverse process and a line drawn from the midpoint of the cephalad facet. **B,** At the levels of T11-12, the entrance point to cannulate the pedicle can be determined by using the intersection point between a line drawn from the middle of the transverse process and a line drawn from the midpoint of the cephalad facet.

bar spine. Preoperative planning with CT is critical in evaluating the diameter of the pedicles to ensure they can accommodate instrumentation. Pedicle screws can be placed with the assistance of fluoroscopy or by using anatomic landmarks. One method that has been described for screw placement between T3 and T10 uses the intersection of a vertical line through the middle of the cephalad articular surface and a horizontal line at the superior border of the transverse process (Figure 14, *A*). At the T11 and T12 levels, the horizontal line should be made from the middle of the transverse process (Figure 14, *B*).

The complications of thoracic pedicle screw placement can be devastating. Injuries to the spinal cord, nerve roots, esophagus, and major blood vessels have all been reported. Thorough preoperative planning with axial CT that documents the diameter and length of the pedicle as well as the angle of insertion and intraoperative neurophysiologic monitoring are important for avoiding complications.

Thoracolumbar Junction Trauma

Biomechanics

Injuries to the thoracolumbar junction (T11 through L2) are usually the result of significant blunt trauma. These injuries represent approximately 50% of all thoracic and lumbar fractures. This increased incidence of fractures to the thoracolumbar junction is the result of its location at the transition point between the rigid thoracic rib cage and the more mobile lumbar spine. In addition, the sagittal alignment of the spine changes from kyphosis to lordosis, which more evenly distributes stress on the anterior and middle columns. The facet alignment changes from a coronal orientation in the thoracic spine to a sagittal alignment in the lumbar spine, allowing for greater flexion and extension motion. Also, the intervertebral disks are taller than in the thoracic spine, decreasing anterior column stiffness.

The indications for surgical management of thoracolumbar fractures remain controversial. Central to defining the need for surgical management is the determi-

nation of fracture stability. A two-column model of the spine was proposed in which it was hypothesized that injuries with involvement of the posterior column are associated with instability. Denis proposed a three-column concept that stressed the importance of the newly defined middle column, which comprises the posterior 50% of the vertebral body and disk along with the posterior longitudinal ligament (Figure 15). Based on biomechanical data, Denis proposed that an isolated posterior ligamentous complex injury was not sufficient to produce instability and that concomitant involvement of the middle column resulted in instability in flexion. However, the integrity of the posterior ligamentous complex (supraspinous and interspinous ligaments) is a crucial factor in determining stability because posterior column disruption in conjunction with involvement of the anterior and middle columns creates instability and increases the risk of posttraumatic kyphosis.

Treatment

The treatment of most patients with thoracolumbar fractures is nonsurgical. Patients who are neurologically intact with less than 25° kyphosis, less than 50% loss of vertebral body height, and less than 50% of canal occlusion and an intact posterior longitudinal ligament are the best candidates for nonsurgical treatment. Depending on the severity of the collapse, these patients may be managed with hyperextension body casting and/or a thoracolumbosacral orthosis for 3 months. Regular clinical and radiographic follow-up of these patients is important to rule out the development of progressive kyphosis or neurologic deficits.

Surgical treatment should be reserved for patients with unstable fracture patterns and/or neurologic deficits. For patients with incomplete neurologic injuries and spinal cord compression, anterior decompression and stabilization is typically required. The anterior procedure may need to be performed in conjunction with a posterior stabilization procedure in patients with posterior column involvement. Early stabilization of patients

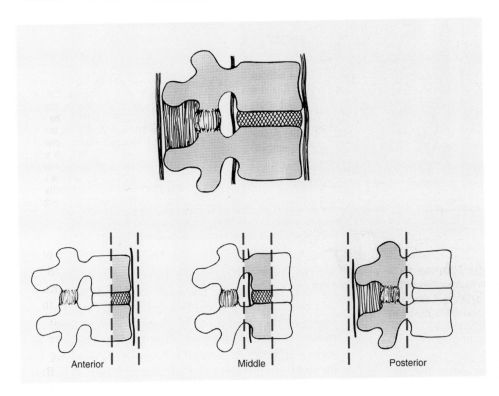

Figure 15 Denis' three-column model of the spine. *(Reproduced with permission from Garfin SR, Blair B, Eismont FJ, Abitol JJ: Thoracic and upper lumbar spine injuries, in Browner BD, Jupiter JB, Levine AM, Trafton PG, Lampert R (eds): Skeletal Trauma: Fractures, Dislocations, Ligamentous Injuries, ed 2. Philadelphia, PA, WB Saunders, 1997, pp 947-1034.)*

with neurologic injuries will allow for early mobilization and rehabilitation placement.

Patients with unstable burst fractures that include failure of the posterior column should undergo an initial posterior stabilization procedure. Posterior instrumentation on a lordosing frame can help restore the normal sagittal alignment of the thoracolumbar spine and will assist in the reduction via ligamentotaxis of the retropulsed fragment. However, patients with excessively comminuted vertebral body fractures may be candidates for a staged anterior procedure.

Recently, prospective studies have compared patients with stable burst fractures of the thoracolumbar junction treated surgically and nonsurgically with regard to pain, spinal canal compromise, and residual kyphosis. In patients with mild to moderate initial kyphosis, much of the sagittal correction gained surgically is lost over time, approaching the final segmental kyphosis seen for these fractures in the nonsurgical treatment group. In addition, residual kyphosis has not been a reliable predictor of chronic pain. Similarly, the degree of spinal canal encroachment has also not been associated with injury to neural structures over the long term. Canal remodeling is to be expected, and up to 50% of the canal can be restored. The degree of remodeling has been reported to be similar in groups of patients treated surgically or nonsurgically.

Lower Lumbar Spine Trauma
Biomechanics

Fractures of the lower lumbar spine (L3-L5) are less common than in the thoracolumbar region. The lower lumbar spine is the lordotic alignment in the sagittal plane, which results in a weight-bearing axis that falls through the middle and posterior columns, making this anatomic region more intrinsically stable. Such fractures are unlikely to progress into a kyphotic deformity. In addition, the facets of the lumbar spine are oriented in the sagittal plane, which can accommodate greater flexion-extension bending moments. Finally, the lumbosacral junction can withstand large forces transmitted across it.

Because the load-bearing axis is more posterior, compression fractures are much less common than burst fractures in the lower lumbar spine. For the anterior column to fail, a significant flexion moment must be applied. However, these large flexion moments are typically neutralized by the increased ability of the lumbar spine to accommodate loads in the sagittal plane. If a compression fracture is detected, suspicion should be high for a concomitant posterior ligamentous injury, especially in the setting of more than 50% loss of vertebral body height.

Burst fractures are the most common fracture pattern seen in the lower lumbar spine. Most of these injuries occur with the spine in a neutral position, resulting in axial loading of both anterior and middle columns of the spine. As with burst fractures in other parts of the spine, a variable amount of bone may be retropulsed

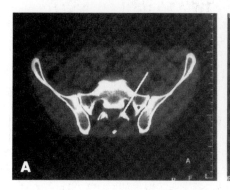
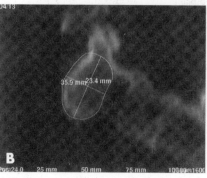
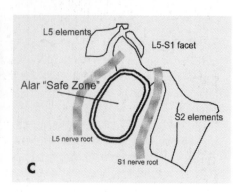

Figure 16 A, An axial CT scan demonstrates the narrowest portion along the sacral pedicle. **B,** Sagittal view of the narrowest portion of the sacral ala with height and width dimensions. **C,** Drawing demonstrating the adjacent bony structures and the L5 and S1 nerve roots. *(Reproduced with permission from Noojin FK, Malkani AL, Haikal L, Lundquist C: Cross-sectional geometry of the sacral ala for safe insertion of iliosacral lag screws: A computed tomography model. J Orthop Trauma 2000;14:31-35.)*

into the spinal canal. However, the incidence of significant and/or permanent neurologic sequelae from these injuries is much lower than elsewhere in the spinal column; the spinal cord ends above this level, and the nerve roots of the cauda equina are more tolerant of compression than the spinal cord.

Flexion-distraction injuries account for less than 10% of lumbar spine fractures. They are most commonly seen at L2, L3, or L4 and are typically the result of the increased stability imparted at the level of L5 to the pelvis via the iliolumbar ligaments. The large flexion moments cause flexion of the upper lumbar segments, whereas the lower segments are stabilized. As a result, the posterior elements fail in tension from the distractive forces.

Treatment

Most patients with lower lumbar fractures can be treated conservatively with external immobilization, a short course of bed rest, and a custom-molded thoracolumbosacral orthosis. A single leg spica attachment may be necessary for fractures of L4 and L5 to allow for control of the pelvis and immobilization of the lumbosacral junction. Patients should wear a brace for approximately 8 to 12 weeks and undergo regular clinical and radiographic follow-up.

Patients who have a cauda equina syndrome or significant neurologic deficit with canal compromise should be considered for surgical treatment. Such patients will typically have near-complete canal occlusion from bony fragments and should undergo decompression and a posterior stabilizing procedure using pedicle screws. The decompression can usually be performed posteriorly via a laminectomy. If a posterior decompression is going to be performed in a patient with a neurologic deficit, evaluation for the presence of a laminar fracture should be sought. Case reports have described herniated nerve root entrapment within the laminar fracture site.

The length of the fusion in the lower lumbar spine typically involves the fractured level and the cephalad and caudad levels. If the fracture involves the L5 level, fusion to the sacrum will be necessary, and attention to the maintenance of the normal lordotic sagittal alignment is important. Isolated injuries of the posterior ligamentous complex may be addressed with a single-level compression construct using screws or hooks. Patients with these injuries may also require a course of postoperative immobilization in a thoracolumbosacral orthosis, which possibly includes leg extension.

Sacral Spine Trauma

Biomechanics

Sacral fractures are usually the result of high-energy trauma and occur in isolation in fewer than 5% of patients. As a result, a thorough evaluation of the pelvis and spine should be undertaken for associated fractures. Sacral fractures are generally classified according to the direction of the fracture line. Fractures may be vertical, transverse, or oblique, although vertical fractures are the most common. Denis' classification system divides the sacrum into three zones. Zone 1 spans the sacral ala to the lateral border of the neural foramen. Zone 2 represents the neural foramen. Zone 3 involves the central sacrum and canal.

Sacral injuries commonly are associated with sacral root deficits. Because of the relative kyphosis of the sacrum, the sacral nerve roots are tethered and restricted within long bony tunnels and therefore not much motion is allowed. These two anatomic factors predispose the neural structures to injury. In addition, the direction of the fracture line and type of fracture determine the likelihood of a neurologic injury. Neurologic injuries of the lower sacral roots (S2-S4) are often missed because only L5 and S1 can be evaluated by manual muscle testing. Perianal sensory changes should be sought in patients with this type of injury. In the Denis classification system, zone 1 vertical injuries have a 5.9% incidence of neural injury. If there is a neural injury, it is usually an injury to the L5 nerve root or the sciatic nerve. Zone 2 fractures have an incidence of 28.4% of neural injury. The nerve injuries are commonly unilateral in nature. This is important because patients with unilateral sacral root injuries usually have normal bowel and bladder function. Zone 3 injuries have a 50% incidence of neurologic injuries, and most of these patients will have bilateral sacral root involvement with bowel, bladder, and sexual dysfunction.

Treatment

Indications for surgical management of sacral fractures include bowel and bladder dysfunction in the setting of an unstable fracture with substantial coronal or sagittal deformity. Vertical fractures can typically be treated with posterior sacroiliac plating or percutaneously placed sacroiliac screws. Placement of percutaneous sacroiliac screws can be technically demanding, and the L5 and S1 nerve roots are at risk during the procedure (Figure 16). If this technique is used to treat a zone 2 injury, the screw should not be loaded in compression to avoid neural injury. Patients who have displaced transverse or oblique fractures may undergo bilateral plating. Neural decompression via laminectomy may be indicated in patients with neurologic deficits and canal compromise, and recovery of bowel and bladder function may be seen. In patients without neurologic injury who have minimally displaced fractures, bracing is only necessary in the setting of fractures, which extend to or above the level of the sacroiliac joint.

Annotated Bibliography

Cervical Spine Trauma

Blake WED, Stillman BC, Eizenberg N, Briggs C, McMeeken JM: The position of the spine in the recovery position: An experimental comparison between the lateral recovery position and the modified HAINES position. *Resuscitation* 2002;53:289-297.

This study identifies a new patient recovery position, the modified HAINES position, in which the patient is in the lateral position with the head lying on the fully abducted dependent arm and both legs are drawn up, with hips and knees flexed. This position results in a more neutral position of the spine compared with the traditional lateral recovery position and may be preferable to the lateral recovery position during resuscitation of trauma patients.

Fisher CG, Dvorak MFS, Leith J, Wing PC: Comparison of outcomes for unstable lower cervical flexion teardrop fractures managed with halo thoracic vest versus anterior corpectomy and plating. *Spine* 2002;27:160-166.

This retrospective cohort study of 45 patients with cervical flexion teardrop fractures indicates that anterior cervical plating is a safe and effective treatment of this patient population and may be superior to halo vest immobilization in terms of

restoring and maintaining sagittal alignment and minimizing the rate of treatment failures.

Guidelines for management of acute cervical spinal injuries. *Neurosurgery* 2002;50(suppl 3):S1-S179.

Under the sponsorship of the American Association of Neurologic Surgeons and the Congress of Neurologic Surgeons, a computerized English-language literature search was performed covering the preceding 25 years. Studies involving cervical spinal trauma were reviewed and critically evaluated. Results were organized and presented in several topical sections designed to provide reasonable standards, guidelines, and options for care of patients with acute cervical spinal injuries.

Peris MD, Donaldson WF, Towers J, Blanc R, Muzzonigro TS: Helmet and shoulder pad removal in suspected cervical spine injury. *Spine* 2002;27:995-999.

This fluoroscopic study supports the efficacy of the current protocol used by the National Athletic Trainers' Association that uses four individuals for the safe removal of the helmet and shoulder pads from an injured football player with minimal cervical motion.

Vaccaro AR, Madigan L, Bauerle WB, Blescia BS, Cotler JM: Early halo immobilization of displaced traumatic spondylolisthesis of the axis. *Spine* 2002;27:2229-2233.

This retrospective study of 31 patients with traumatic spondylolisthesis of the axis confirms that early halo immobilization after traction reduction is a safe and effective form of treatment in this patient population. Patients with type II fractures angled greater than or equal to 12° may require more extended periods of traction.

Thoracic Spine Trauma/Thoracolumbar Junction Trauma/Lower Lumbar Spine Trauma

Finkelstein J, Wai E, Jackson S, Ahn H, Brighton-Knight M: Single-level fixation of flexion distraction injuries. *J Spinal Disord Tech* 2003;16:236-242.

This prospective study evaluated 17 patients with flexion-distraction injuries of the thoracic and lumbar spine. The patients had an average follow-up of 17.6 months and were treated with single-level posterior fixation. The average preoperative kyphosis was 10.1°, which was corrected to a postoperative lordosis of 0.9°. The mean Oswestry score was 11.5 and 88% of the patients reported having only minimal disabilities.

Wood K, Butterman G, Mehbod A, Garvey T, Jhanjee R, Sechriest V: Operative compared with nonoperative treatment of a thoracolumbar burst fracture without neurological deficit: A prospective, randomized study. *J Bone Joint Surg Am* 2003;85:773-781.

This prospective randomized trial evaluated 47 consecutive patients with a thoracolumbar fracture without neurologic deficit for a minimum 2-year follow-up. The group of patients that underwent surgical treatment had a mean preoperative and postoperative kyphosis of 10.1° and 13°, respectively. The group of patients that underwent nonsurgical treatment had a mean preoperative and postoperative kyphosis of 11.3° and 13.8°, respectively. No difference was found between groups with respect to return to work. The average pain scores were similar for both groups. The authors concluded that surgical treatment provided no long-term advantage compared with nonsurgical treatment.

Yue J, Sossan A, Selgrath C, et al: The treatment of unstable thoracic spine fractures with transpedicular screw instrumentation: A 3-year consecutive series. *Spine* 2002; 27:2782-2787.

This study evaluated 32 patients in a 3-year consecutive prospective experience of using pedicle screw fixation to treat unstable thoracic spine injuries. Fracture healing was noted to take place at an average of 4.8 months. Two-hundred fifty-two pedicle screws were placed without any intraoperative complications. The Gardner segmental kyphotic deformity angle preoperative mean was 15.9° and the mean postoperative angle was 10.6° (which was significant). All neurologically intact patients reported very good to good results with regard to pain, activity, function, employment, and satisfaction.

Sacral Spine Trauma

Noojin F, Malkani A, Haikal L, Lundquist C, Voor M: Cross-sectional geometry of the sacral ala for safe insertion of iliosacral lag screws: A computed tomography model. *J Orthop Trauma* 2000;14:31-35.

This study evaluated 13 adult patients with intact pelves in a trauma setting to determine the geometry of the sacral ala for placement of iliosacral screws. Each patient had CT scans of the pelvis with sagittal reconstructions. The narrowest portion of the sacral ala was determined, and height, width, and slope of the geometric center were calculated. The mean width of the sacral ala was 28.05 mm, the mean height was 27.76 mm, and the sacral slope ranged from 25° to 65°. The authors concluded that despite individual variability there is room for two screws to be placed in the sacral ala safely.

Classic Bibliography

Allen BL Jr, Ferguson RL, Lehman TR, O'Brien RP: A mechanistic classification of closed, indirect fractures and dislocations of the lower cervical spine. *Spine* 1982; 7:1-27.

Bohlmann HH: Acute fractures and dislocations of the cervical spine: An analysis of three hundred hospitalized patients and review of the literature. *J Bone Joint Surg Am* 1979;61:1119-1142.

Clark CR, White AA III: Fractures of the dens: A multicenter study. *J Bone Joint Surg Am* 1985;67:1340-1348.

Denis F: Instability as defined by the three-column spine concept in acute spinal trauma. *Clin Orthop* 1984; 189:65-76.

Denis F, Davis S, Comfort T: Sacral fractures: An important problem. Retrospective analysis of 236 cases. *Clin Orthop* 1988;227:67-81.

Hoffman JR, Mower WR, Wolfson AB, Todd KH, Zucker MI: Validity of a set of clinical criteria to rule out injury to the cervical spine in patients with blunt trauma: National Emergency X-Radiography Utilization Study Group. *N Engl J Med* 2000;343:94-99.

Levine AM, Edwards CC: The management of traumatic spondylolisthesis of the axis. *J Bone Joint Surg Am* 1985;67:217-226.

Magerl F, Aebi M, Gertzbein SD, Harms J, Nazarian S: A comprehensive classification of thoracic and lumbar injuries. *Eur Spine J* 1994;3:184-201.

Mestdagh H, Letendart J, Sensey JJ, Duquennoy A: Treatment of fractures of the posterior axial arch: Results of 41 cases. *Rev Chir Orthop Reparatrice Appar Mot* 1984;70:21-28.

Schiff DCM, Parke WW: The arterial supply of the odontoid process. *J Bone Joint Surg Am* 1973;55:1450.

Spence KF, Decker S, Sell KW: Bursting atlantal fracture associated with rupture of the transverse ligament. *J Bone Joint Surg Am* 1970;52:543-549.

Vaccaro AR, Rizzolo SJ, Allardyce TJ, et al: Placement of pedicle screws in the thoracic spine: Part I. Morphometric analysis of thoracic vertebra. *J Bone Joint Surg Am* 1995;8:1193-1199.

Vaccaro AR, Rizzolo SJ, Balderston RA, et al: Placement of pedicle screws in the thoracic spine: Part II. An anatomic and radiographic assessment. *J Bone Joint Surg Am* 1995;8:1200-1205.

Chapter 42

Cervical Disk Disease

Jonathan N. Grauer, MD

John M. Beiner, MD

Todd J. Albert, MD

Introduction

Cervical disk disease is a degenerative process that is often encountered in the aging patient. Although a patient can occasionally identify a single inciting traumatic event, more often no specific trauma is identified. Disk degeneration is thought to be initiated by microtrauma, causing a change in the proteoglycan and collagen content of the nucleus, loss of water content, and ultimately altered biomechanics. Patients may have disk herniation ("soft disk") through an annular tear or loss of disk height, causing bulging past the borders of the vertebral end plates. Osteophyte ("hard disk") formation can contribute to narrowing of the neural foramen, central canal stenosis, and eventually compression of the neural elements. In most of these patients, these events are asymptomatic, even in the presence of advanced radiographic changes.

Symptoms of such disk degeneration can be insidious or acute in onset. Once foraminal or central stenosis has developed, minor injuries have the potential to cause local neural irritation and reaction. This can occur at the level of the root (radiculopathy) or the spinal cord (myelopathy). If there is compression of the nerve roots and spinal cord, both radiculopathy and myelopathy may result (know as radiculomyelopathy).

Pathophysiology and Examination

The pathophysiology of degenerative cervical disease involves the disk, zygapophyseal facet joints, uncovertebral joints of Luschka, posterior longitudinal ligament, and the ligamentum flavum. As the disk loses water content and the proteoglycan content changes, it becomes less able to support load. With progressive degeneration, there is decreased disk height, which is associated with loss of the normal cervical lordosis and the transfer of load to the facet and uncovertebral joints. Osteocartilaginous overgrowth may then occur in accordance with Wolff's law to stabilize the lax segment and increased loads.

With loss of segment height, the ligamentum flavum can become redundant, further contributing to the loss of area available for the spinal cord. Radiculopathy develops as exiting nerve roots become irritated or compressed. This radiculopathy can be caused by either a soft disk herniation, or more commonly it is secondary to a chronic irritation from the uncovertebral or facet joints in the patient with gradual onset of degenerative changes.

Symptoms of radiculopathy include pain, paresthesias, or weakness with or without associated neck pain. Objective signs of a radiculopathy include hyporeflexia in the biceps (C5), brachioradialis (C6), or triceps (C7), weakness or atrophy of the innervated muscle group, or pain or paresthesias in a dermatomal fashion (Figures 1 and 2). Provocative maneuvers such as Spurling's test can exacerbate such symptoms.

The first seven cervical nerve roots originate and exit above their named vertebrae and the eighth cervical root originates and exits below the C7 vertebra. In contrast to the lumbar spine, because the nerves in the cervical spine exit the spinal canal relatively orthogonally at or below the level of the disk space, disk pathology generally affects the exiting nerve at that segment. For example, C6-7 disk pathology will generally affect the C7 nerve root (Figure 3). However, cervical nerve roots exhibit a higher degree of overlap than seen in the thoracolumbar spine, and therefore symptom patterns may fail to localize to a specific nerve root in some patients.

The nerve roots most commonly affected by cervical disk disease are C5, C6, and C7 because the associated motion segments have the most flexion and extension in the subaxial spine and are thus associated with the greatest incidence of spondylosis. In addition, the watershed area of blood supply to the cervical spinal cord and nerve roots makes those nerve roots most susceptible to ischemic injury.

Cervical spondylotic myelopathy involves central rather than foraminal stenosis. This myelopathy is most typically caused by the combination of disk bulging and uncovertebral hypertrophy with vertebral end plate osteophytes (the disk-osteophyte complex) in conjunction with ligamentum flavum hypertrophy/redundancy and

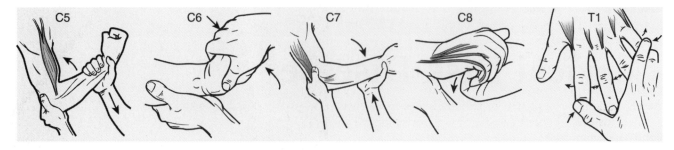

Figure 1 Upper extremity motor testing for the cervical spine. Note there is dual innervation of some of these muscles.

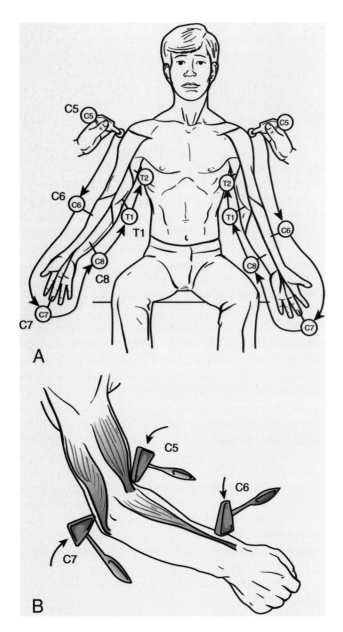

Figure 2 Upper extremity sensory **(A)** and reflex **(B)** examination for the cervical spine.

facet arthrosis. These changes lead to mechanical compression of the spinal cord that can be static or dynamic (such as with neck extension). Anterior pathology may also exert compression on the anterior spinal arteries, which can in turn contribute to ischemia of the spinal cord. Because such insults to the spinal cord occur very slowly, a large degree of central canal stenosis (down to a cross-sectional area of 17 mm^2) can generally be tolerated relatively well.

Myelopathy is most commonly manifested as clumsiness (loss of fine motor skills), ataxia, and spasticity. Specific symptoms may include dropping of objects, changes in handwriting, and restlessness in the legs and can progress to include loss of bowel or bladder control. The physical examination for myelopathy should include testing for pathologic hyperreflexia below the level of spinal cord compression, the presence of Hoffman and Babinski reflexes, and difficulty with tandem gait. Clinicians must have a high level of suspicion for this condition and be vigilant in their evaluation for associated signs and symptoms. Additionally, differential diagnoses such as multiple sclerosis, anterior horn disease, and central nervous system tumors may be considered.

Because radiculopathy and myelopathy are both caused by some of the same underlying pathology, it is not uncommon to see patients with spondylotic radiculomyelopathy. There will often be a combination of the signs and symptoms described for each independent pathology. Hyporeflexia is common in the upper extremities where nerve roots are compressed and hyperreflexia is usually present in the lower extremities below the level of spinal cord compression.

Cervical spondylosis may also be associated with neck pain. In addition to radicular pain, felt in a myotomal nerve root distribution, patients can feel pain or discomfort in a referred sclerotomal distribution corresponding to the embryologic origin of individual nerve roots. Pain can be referred to the occiput, interscapular region, or shoulders. The natural history of cervical disk disease helps dictate treatment guidelines. In more than 75% of patients, symptoms of radiculopathy improve with conservative treatment, including physical therapy, anti-inflammatory medication, and activity modification. Soft disk herniations can resorb or shrink, and inflammation around a compressed nerve root can resolve. In contrast, cervical myelopathy has a less predictable course. Several studies have reported a gradual stepwise progression of the disease, with variable intervals during which patients' symptoms remained quiescent. Most studies, however, demonstrated a slowly worsening clinical picture.

Imaging Studies

Plain radiographs are appropriate in the evaluation of neck pain, cervical radiculopathy, and cervical myelography. Such series include AP and lateral films to assess overall spinal alignment and level of spondylosis, as well as to rule out other structural lesions and deformity.

Flexion and extension radiographs can be used to assess angular or translational instability and demonstrate whether a patient can achieve normal lordosis. Oblique radiographs better visualize the neural foramen and facets and can facilitate visualization of the cervicothoracic junction. A swimmer's view allows for visualization of the cervicothoracic junction, if not otherwise possible, by limiting the obstructions imposed by the shoulders. Other views such as the open mouth odontoid radiograph are generally not needed for degenerative conditions.

Plain radiographs are often all that is needed to initiate conservative treatment. However, if concerns are raised, or if a patient's symptoms persist beyond appropriate conservative treatments, advanced imaging may be indicated. MRI is the axial imaging modality of choice for the cervical spine, allowing visualization of the soft tissues including disks, spinal cord, nerve roots, and ligaments. Sagittal imaging provides a good overview of the levels of cord compression and central disk pathology. However, sagittal imaging can give the false impression of cervical kyphosis if the head of the patient if flexed during the imaging study. Parasagittal imaging can provide information about lateral disk herniations and foraminal narrowing. Axial imaging refines information about cord or root compression and allows for visualization of other surrounding structures such as the vertebral artery or muscles.

CT can be used to define the bony anatomy of the cervical spine. However, as the relationship to the neural elements must be inferred, the use of CT is best combined with an intrathecal injection of a contrast medium for imaging of degenerative conditions (myelography). The contrast medium is injected into the thecal sac via a C1-C2 puncture and allowed to diffuse caudally, or via a lumbar puncture and allowed to diffuse proximally with the patient in the Trendelenburg position. This allows precise visualization of the neural elements, with filling voids present at sites of neural compression. Al-

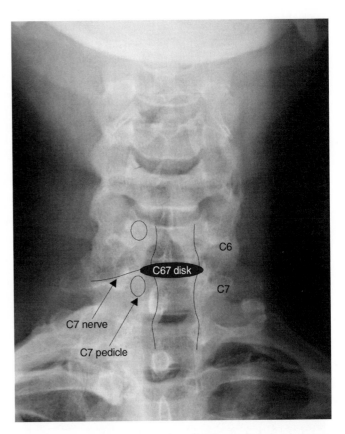

Figure 3 The C7 nerve root exits the thecal sac above the C7 pedicle and is most likely to be affected by pathology at the C6-7 interspace.

though much of this information can be obtained with noninvasive MRI, myelography is particularly useful for patients who cannot have an MRI secondary to implanted devices such as pacemakers. In other patients, myelography can be useful if the results of MRI are inconclusive, such as with dynamic compression of the neural elements that cannot be demonstrated with static imaging. Flexion-extension radiographs following myelography can reveal this dynamic compression.

Diskography has been used to evaluate cervical disk degeneration. The procedure is performed via an anterior approach in a trajectory similar to that used for the standard anterior cervical approach. Once needles are in place in the intervertebral disks, fluid can be injected and the distribution and pain provocation can be studied. However, the validity and usefulness of this procedure is controversial. The risks of this procedure include esophageal puncture and potential mediastinal or disk space infection.

Electrodiagnostic Studies

In most patients, the history and clinical examination can reliably identify the presence and level of nerve root or spinal cord pathology. Combined with radiography and advanced imaging modalities, accuracy rates

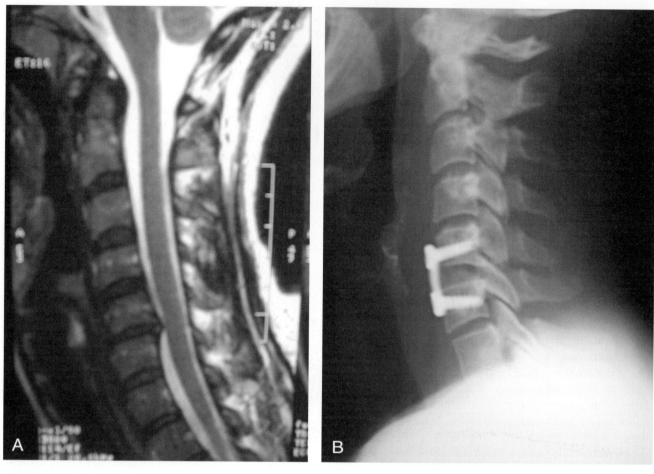

Figure 4 Preoperative sagittal MRI (**A**) and postoperative lateral radiograph (**B**) of a patient with persistent C6 radicular symptoms who underwent anterior cervical diskectomy and fusion with autograft and instrumentation.

are even higher. In some patients, however, the radiation of arm pain or symptoms such as paresthesias cannot be localized to a specific spinal level. In other patients, clinical examination may not correlate with imaging studies or root symptoms may not be adequately differentiated from more distal nerve compression. In these patients, electromyogram and/or nerve conduction velocity studies may be useful to differentiate acute or chronic radiculopathy from more distal compressive neuropathies such as carpal tunnel syndrome or cubital tunnel compression, which may mimic cervical root compression.

Nonsurgical Care

Management of neck pain and cervical radiculopathy should start with conservative, nonsurgical measures, including physical therapy, traction, activity modification, and certain medications.

With physical therapy, extremes of motion are generally not an important objective. Rather, physical therapy should emphasize isometric exercises to build tone and control for debilitated muscles and limit the shear forces

experienced by the spine. Traction may be useful for radicular symptoms and should generally be done with some degree of flexion to open the neural foramen. Although modalities often are useful at the time of application, they are not believed to provide lasting relief.

These therapeutic interventions may break the cycle of irritation and splinting, allowing the reestablishment of painless range of motion. Therapy should then focus on neuromuscular control and active range-of-motion and stabilization exercises. Finally, general aerobic conditioning should be added.

Medical management generally consists of nonsteroidal anti-inflammatory drugs. These drugs can help control the inflammatory factors that are often responsible for acute symptoms. Oral steroids can be considered for significant exacerbations of symptoms, but potential adverse effects must be considered. The role of narcotics in such degenerative processes is limited. Narcotics should be reserved for acute injuries or exacerbations, and they should only be used for a limited period. Narcotics should clearly be avoided for chronic pain.

Selective nerve root blocks and epidural steroid injections can be beneficial both diagnostically and therapeutically. Relatively high concentrations of steroids can be achieved while limiting potential systemic adverse effects. Nevertheless, the risks associated with injections into an already stenotic canal or neural foramen have led to questions about their usefulness.

The role of conservative care in the management of cervical spondylotic myelopathy is more controversial. It appears that early myelopathy may not always follow the pattern of progressive neurologic deterioration, and therefore a close observational treatment may be indicated. Many surgeons believe, however, that once signs or symptoms of myelopathy develop, surgical decompression is indicated to optimize neurologic recovery and abate progression. Radiographic evidence of spinal cord compression is not a surgical indication unto itself because many patients will not have correlating symptoms or examinations.

Surgical Indications

Axial neck pain from degenerative disk disease is rarely an indication for surgical intervention. In patients who have been resistant to conservative measures, success rates of surgical fusion for axial neck pain have generally only been in the 60% to 70% range. This may be related to an incomplete understanding of the associated pain generators and potential painful foci at other cervical levels, posterior facets, or nonspinal sources.

In recent years, clinical trials of cervical disk replacements have begun in the United States. Goals of this technology are to allow decompression or removal of a degenerative disk while preserving motion. However, the role and long-term outcome of such implants have not yet been defined.

In contrast to axial neck pain, radiculopathy responds well to a variety of surgical treatments. When an appropriate course of nonsurgical management has failed, and radiculopathy persists, the surgeon can offer greater than 90% success rates with surgical intervention. Clinically significant myelopathy is generally believed to be an indication for surgical intervention.

Surgical Treatment Options for Radiculopathy and Myelopathy

The type of surgical procedure advocated for cervical arthrosis is dictated by the location and extent of the pathology. There are also situations in which similar pathology can be addressed in several ways, with roughly similar results.

Anterior decompression can be performed, as initially described in the classic study by Smith and Robinson. When there is a central disk herniation, significant uncovertebral spurring, or central canal stenosis, anterior decompression is the most direct means of decompressing the neural elements. Transverse incisions are made for one, two, or arguably three levels, and oblique

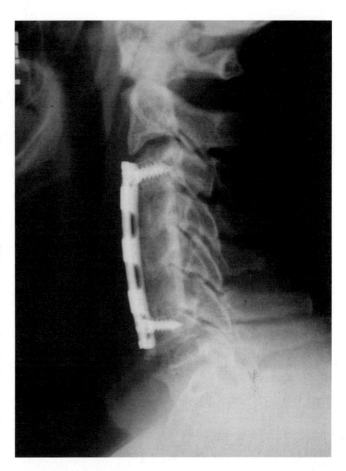

Figure 5 When a patient has cord compression behind the vertebral bodies as well as at the disk spaces, corpectomy should be considered as shown in this radiograph, with a C4 and C5 corpectomy, allograft strut graft, and anterior instrumentation.

incisions may be necessary for longer exposures. The level of incision can be guided by anatomic landmarks. For example, the carotid tubercle, which can be palpated percutaneously, is the lateral process of C6. The cricoid cartilage is approximately at the C6 level, and the thyroid cartilage at the C4-C5 level. The anterior approach is carried down medial to the sternocleidomastoid and carotid sheath and lateral to the trachea and esophagus. This provides exposure to the anterior aspect of the cervical spine. The longus coli are then elevated to allow access to the entire disk space.

Once a diskectomy is carried back to the posterior disk space, the posterior osteophytes can be taken down with or without the associated posterior longitudinal ligament. This scenario may be associated with more immediate and complete relief of symptoms, more complete foraminal decompression, and better identification of extruded disk fragments. Some authors have found that taking down the posterior osteophytes and posterior longitudinal ligament is not always necessary and that disk height restoration and fusion (with its associated elimination of motion) may be adequate and associated with lesser bleeding and surgical times.

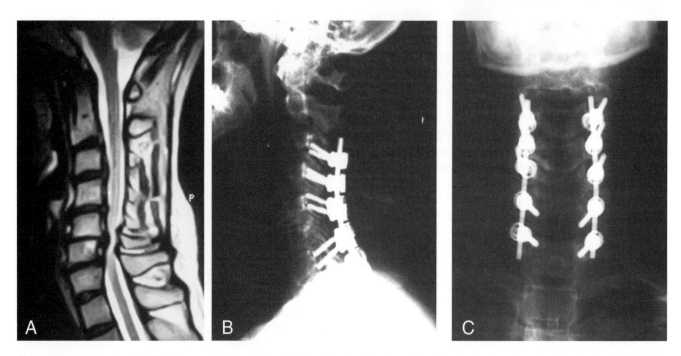

Figure 6 Preoperative sagittal MRI (**A**) and postoperative lateral (**B**) and AP (**C**) radiographs of a patient with multilevel cervical stenosis and myelopathy who was treated with posterior decompression and fusion.

Once the diskectomy and decompression have been achieved, interbody fusion is performed by decorticating the end plates and inserting a bone graft. This has traditionally been iliac crest autograft. However, according to a recent study, allograft has been shown to afford almost identical fusion rates for single-level procedures without the donor site morbidity associated with autograft. This phenomenon does not appear to be as true for multilevel procedures or in the presence of factors that inhibit fusion such as smoking. Diskectomy without fusion has largely been abandoned because of its association with kyphotic collapse, neck pain, and potential for recurrent foraminal narrowing.

Plate fixation can be added to potentially increase the rate of union, limit kyphotic collapse, and minimize the need for external cervical orthoses (Figure 4). Many types of plates exist. All current plate systems lock the screw to the plate to prevent screw backout. Some systems allow for variable angle screw insertions to facilitate implantation. Others systems allow for settling of the screws within the plate (dynamic plates) to allow the graft to be better loaded. Although plates are now routinely used by many surgeons, the justification for this is uncertain given the high fusion rate in single-level noninstrumented fusions. The potential benefits of plating must be contrasted with the expense and the potential, but limited, risks of implantation.

With larger procedures such as multilevel diskectomy, corpectomy, or partial corpectomy, recent studies have indicated that strut grafting is a good surgical alternative. With this technique, central compression behind the vertebral bodies can be addressed. It also offers fewer surfaces to fuse compared with multiple interbody grafts, potentially increasing fusion rates (Figure 5). Bone graft can be autograft, structural allograft (potentially filled with local corpectomy bone), or synthetic cages. As constructs grow in length to corpectomies of two or more vertebral bodies, consideration should be given to supplementation with posterior stabilization. However, it is generally believed that lordosis can be restored and maintained better with multiple interbody grafts.

Alternatively, if there is purely foraminal stenosis and radiculopathy from a soft disk or hypertrophied facet or uncovertebral joint, posterior laminoforaminotomy may be considered. This procedure allows decompression without fusion, and destabilization is avoided as long as the surgeon avoids total facetectomy unilaterally or partial facetectomy bilaterally. Because the disk, which is often thought to be the pain generator for axial pain, is not directly addressed, posterior laminaforaminotomy is not a good treatment option if axial pain is a large component of a patient's symptoms. This approach avoids the dangers of anterior dissection, such as recurrent laryngeal nerve palsy, and preserves the motion segment. However, central pathology cannot be addressed because the spinal cord cannot be retracted to allow access to the region. Furthermore, disadvantages lie in the muscle dissection and facet capsule disruption inherent in the procedure.

Myelopathy can be treated from posterior as well as anterior approaches. The choice of approach depends on

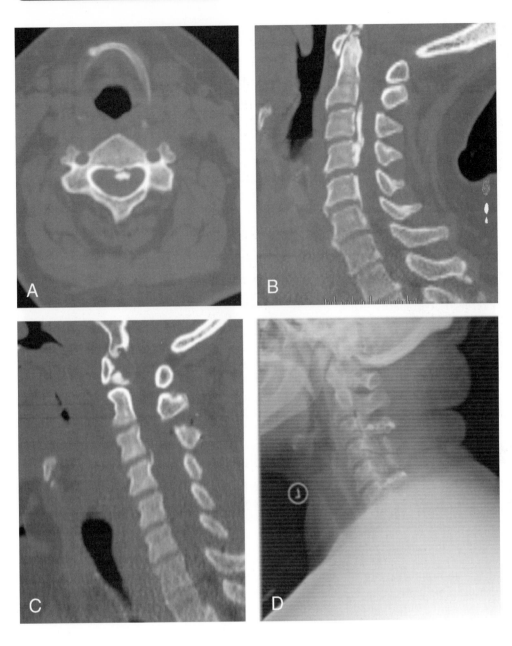

Figure 7 **A** and **B,** Imaging studies of a patient with multilevel cervical stenosis and ossification of the posterior longitudinal ligament who presented with myelopathy. Treatment was laminaplasty at C3-C6 with plate fixation (**C** and **D**). Note the increase in canal diameter between preoperative (**B**) and postoperative (**C**) CT reconstructions.

factors including the site of compression (anterior spurs/ ossification of the posterior longitudinal ligament versus posterior ligamentum flavum hypertrophy/redundancy), overall spinal alignment, and number of levels involved. The anterior approach allows removal of anterior cord compression, but this must often involve removal of the vertebral body if compression is in this region.

Posterior decompression in the form of laminectomy has previously been the standard procedure, but was associated with postlaminectomy kyphosis in a large percentage of patients. Posterior cervical fusion is thus now generally performed with a laminectomy to restore and maintain cervical lordosis and allow the spinal cord to float away from any anterior compressive pathology (Figure 6). Posterior fixation can be achieved with lateral mass

screws at C3-C6 and pedicle screws at C2, C7, and below. The disadvantages of this technique include the morbidity of muscle dissection from a posterior cervical approach and the associated loss of motion.

As an alternative to fusion, laminaplasty was developed in Japan for the treatment of cervical myelopathy associated with ossification of the posterior longitudinal ligament. Laminaplasty involves hinging open the lamina at multiple levels, affecting decompression. Such openings can be held with sutures, instrumentation, and/or structural bone grafts. The goal of the procedure is to decompress without adding the complications inherent to fusion. Outcome studies support these goals, but potential adverse effects include increased axial neck pain and loss of motion (Figure 7).

Fusion procedures may be associated with accelerated degenerative changes adjacent to the fused segments. This phenomenon may be alleviated with laminaplasty as opposed to decompression and fusion. In addition, disk arthroplasty may help limit the incidence of adjacent level disease in the cervical spine, but this has not yet been conclusively demonstrated.

Annotated Bibliography

Bryan VE: Cervical motion segment replacement. *Eur Spine J* 2002;11:S92-S97.

Cervical disk arthroplasty is being developed as an alternative to fusion procedures. The possibility of limiting adjacent level degeneration is one of the potential benefits.

Edwards CC, Heller JG, Murakami H: Corpectomy versus laminoplasty for multilevel cervical myelopathy: An independent matched-cohort analysis. *Spine* 2002;27:1168-1175.

In this study, corpectomy and laminaplasty were found to arrest myelopathic progression and offer the potential for neurologic recovery. However, this study suggested that the laminaplasty group had less pain at follow-up than the multilevel corpectomy group.

Fouyas IP, Statham PFX, Sandercock PA: Cochrane review of the role of surgery in cervical spondylotic radiculomyelopathy. *Spine* 2002;27:736-747.

In this critical review of the literature, it was difficult to draw reliable conclusions about the risk/benefit balance for cervical spine surgery for spondylotic radiculopathy or myelopathy.

Hilibrand AS, Fye MA, Emery SE, Palumbo MA, Bohlman HH: Increased rate of arthrodesis with strut grafting after multilevel anterior cervical decompression. *Spine* 2002;27:146-151.

A higher rate of fusion was seen after corpectomy and strut grafting than after multilevel diskectomy and interbody grafting. This therefore suggests that strut grafting should be considered in patients requiring surgical attention at multiple disk spaces even if there is not compression behind the vertebral body.

Malloy KM, Hilibrand AS: Autograft versus allograft in degenerative cervical disease. *Clin Orthop* 2002;394:27-38.

Although allograft is the gold standard bone grafting material, high fusion rates have been observed when allograft is used, especially for single-level cases in nonsmokers. This offers the potential of eliminating the morbidity associated with the harvest of autograft.

Patel CK, Fischgrund J: Complications of anterior cervical spine surgery. *Instr Course Lect* 2003;52:465-469.

This article presents a review of the potential complications associated with anterior cervical spine surgery for which the incidence is relatively low.

Sampath P, Bendebba M, Davis JD, Ducker TB: Outcome of patients treated for cervical myelopathy: A prospective, multicenter study with independent clinical review. *Spine* 2000;25:670-676.

Authors of this multicenter study of patients with cervical myelopathy concluded that patients treated with surgery appear to do better than those treated nonsurgically.

Classic Bibliography

Bohlman HH, Emery SE, Goodfellow DB, Jones PK: Robinson anterior cervical discectomy and arthrodesis for cervical radiculopathy. *J Bone Joint Surg Am* 1993; 75:1298-1307.

Herkowitz HN: A comparison of anterior cervical fusion, cervical laminectomy, and cervical laminoplasty for the surgical management of multiple level spondylotic radiculoparhy. *Spine* 1988;13:774-780.

Smith GW, Robinson RA: The treatment of certain cervical-spine disorders by anterior removal of the intervertebral disc and interbody fusion. *J Bone Joint Surg Am* 1958;40:607-624.

Chapter 43

Thoracic Disk Disease

Chetan K. Patel, MD

Introduction

Symptomatic thoracic disk disease is relatively uncommon compared with disk disease in the cervical and lumbar regions, with an estimated incidence of between 1 in 10,000 and 1 in 1 million persons. The occurrence of symptomatic thoracic disk herniation is greatest between the fourth and sixth decade of life, with a peak incidence in the fifth decade. Diagnosis can be difficult because of a variety of clinical presentations. Widespread availability and use of MRI has aided in the diagnosis of symptomatic thoracic disk herniations (Figure 1). However, one MRI study documented thoracic degenerative changes in 73% of asymptomatic individuals, with 37% showing a disk herniation.

Anatomy and Biomechanics

The thoracic spine, a relatively rigid structure, is stabilized by the rib cage. Thoracic facets are generally oriented vertically, which allows lateral bending and rotation while limiting flexion and extension. These anatomic and biomechanical properties would be expected to decrease the potential of injury to the thoracic intervertebral disk. This is confirmed clinically by the observation that less than 1% of symptomatic disk herniations occur in the thoracic spine.

When a thoracic disk herniation occurs, biomechanical studies have shown the mechanism to be a combination of torsion and bending load. Several anatomic factors are suspected in the pathogenesis of neurologic compromise in thoracic disk herniations. Kyphosis of the thoracic spine places the spinal cord directly on the posterior longitudinal ligament and the posterior aspect of the vertebrae and disks. Additionally, the vascular supply to the thoracic spine is much more tenuous than that of the cervical and lumbar spine, especially from T4 through T9. Although the size of the spinal cord is smaller in the thoracic spine than in the cervical spine, the cord to canal ratio is actually higher because of the smaller size of the thoracic spinal canal. These factors together explain how the thoracic spinal cord is vulnerable to injury.

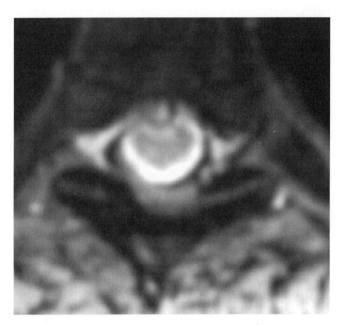

Figure 1 Axial MRI scan demonstrating a thoracic herniated nucleus pulposus.

Etiology

Between 33% and 50% of patients report a history of trauma or significant physical exertion before the onset of symptoms. However, the role of trauma as the cause of thoracic disk herniations is controversial. Most authors favor degenerative processes as the major cause of disk herniations. This theory is supported by the common findings of disk degeneration at the level of herniation and the higher incidence of herniations in the lower thoracic spine where greater degenerative changes have been reported. End plate changes consistent with Scheuermann's disease are seen more often in symptomatic patients than in those who are asymptomatic, suggesting an association between Scheuermann's disease and symptomatic herniated thoracic disks.

Clinical Presentation

The clinical presentation of patients with thoracic disk disease is variable, and the differential diagnosis for tho-

...hy is extensive. The differ-
...cic herniated nucleus pul-
...disk disease, cervical and
...posus, intercostal neural-
...rophic lateral sclerosis,
...s, metabolic bone disor-
...ster, and diseases of the
...ding aneurysm. A thor-
...ation are the best tools
...diagnosis and treatment of patients
... thoracic disk disease.

Symptoms of thoracic disk herniations occur in one of three distinct patterns—axial, radicular, or myelopathic. Axial pain usually presents in the mid- to lower thoracic regions, worsens with activity, and improves with rest. Radicular symptoms typically arise from a lateral disk herniation impinging on a nerve root and producing symptoms that follow the course of that nerve root. Most commonly, pain and paresthesias are reported starting in the back and radiating anteriorly in a band-like pattern in the distribution of the more caudal nerve root. Thoracic dermatomes can be roughly identified by the following landmarks: T4 at the nipple line, T7 at the xiphoid process, T10 at the umbilicus, and T12 at the inguinal crease. If any skin lesions are noted in a dermatomal pattern, herpes zoster may be the underlying cause. Although motor testing is difficult in this region, the patient can do a partial sit-up to help identify an asymmetric contraction of the segmentally innervated rectus abdominis.

Myelopathy may also be the presentation of a thoracic disk herniation when there is significant spinal cord compression. The presentation can vary from subtle sensory changes to obvious paraparesis and bowel and bladder dysfunction. In addition to the motor and sensory examination, attention should focus on upper motor neuron signs such as lower extremity hyperreflexia, clonus, Babinski sign, wide-based gait, and superficial abdominal reflexes. The Romberg sign can help detect subtle changes in proprioception. The results of an upper extremity neurologic examination should be normal in addition to the patient exhibiting a negative Hoffmann sign.

Diagnostic Imaging

Plain radiographs should be obtained first. In addition to being used to assess overall alignment, the plain radiographs should be scrutinized for degenerative changes, calcification in the disk space or in the canal, fractures, and tumors. Intradiskal calcification is noted in 45% to 71% of patients with symptomatic thoracic herniated disks compared with 10% of asymptomatic individuals.

MRI is the diagnostic modality of choice in further evaluation of these patients because it is noninvasive

and highly sensitive. However, as mentioned previously, the findings should be interpreted in the context of clinical findings because of the high percentage of abnormal MRI findings in asymptomatic individuals. A CT myelogram is also highly sensitive, but this modality is invasive and should be reserved for patients who cannot undergo MRI. Diskography is controversial but can be considered in patients with axial pain, multilevel disease, and no neurologic findings. At this time, no outcome studies exist that demonstrate a correlation between diskography results and surgical outcomes.

Nonsurgical Treatment

To decide on the best treatment course for thoracic disk disease, its natural history must first be understood. Asymptomatic patients with abnormal MRI findings were noted to remain asymptomatic at a follow-up of more than 26 months. Children with painful calcified thoracic disks improve spontaneously with resorption of calcification; however, these children should be closely followed because a few instances of neurologic deficit requiring surgical intervention have been reported in this population. In adults, the natural history of acute thoracic disk herniations without neurologic deficit is benign. Most patients can be treated with activity modification, anti-inflammatory medications, exercise, and with bracing in rare occasions. Most patients are expected to return to their normal activities, including vigorous sports and work. In patients with radicular symptoms, corticosteroid injections of intercostal nerves should be considered when other modalities do not provide adequate pain relief.

Surgical Treatment

Indications for surgery include progressive neurologic deficit, myelopathy, and pain refractory to conservative treatment. The herniated thoracic disk can be accessed using the posterior, posterolateral, lateral, or anterior approach (Figure 2).

Laminectomy and the transpedicular approach are posterior approaches. The surgical approach of choice was once straight posterior laminectomy and disk excision. However, because this approach was associated with significant risk of neurologic deterioration, it has been largely abandoned. The transpedicular approach was developed to allow less retraction of the spinal cord by removing the pedicle and facet joint. Although this approach is well suited for the treatment of a lateral disk herniation, a central or paramedial disk herniation is difficult to excise using this approach because of poor visualization. Removal of the pedicle and facet joint complex may lead to instability and postoperative pain.

The posterolateral approach is also known as a costotransversectomy. In this approach, the posteromedial portion of the ipsilateral rib along with the transverse process,

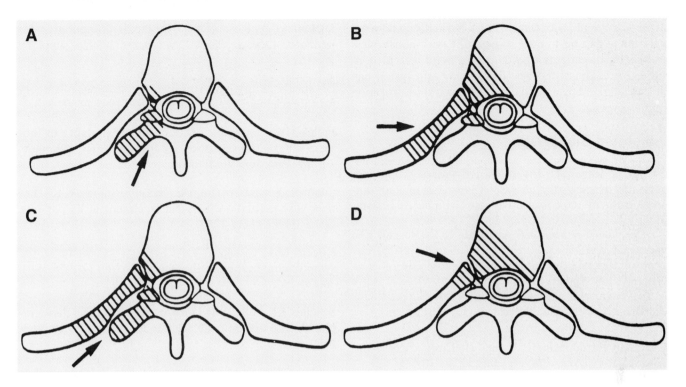

Figure 2 Illustration of four surgical approaches to the thoracic disk pathology: transpedicular **(A)**, extracavitary **(B)**, costotransversectomy **(C)**, and transthoracic **(D)**. *(Reproduced from Wood KB, Mehbad A: Thoracic disk herniation, in Koval KJ (ed): Orthopaedic Knowledge Update 7. Rosemont, IL, American Academy of Orthopaedic Surgeons, pp 621-625.)*

a portion of the pedicle, and the posterosuperior vertebral body are removed. This allows gentle removal of the disk fragment without manipulating the cord. This approach can be used for multiple levels and allows resection of paramedian as well as lateral disks. Visualization of central disks is poor with this approach, and it does involve a generous amount of bone resection and significant disruption of the paraspinal musculature.

The lateral extracavitary approach, another extrapleural approach, is a modification of the lateral thoracotomy approach that involves resection of the posteromedial rib in addition to the transverse process, pedicle, facet, and posterosuperior portion of the vertebral bodies. Midline access is less than optimal, and a large amount of bone resection and disruption of paraspinal musculature can lead to postoperative pain.

The anterior approaches include thoracotomy and video-assisted thoracoscopic surgery (VATS). Anterior approach via a thoracotomy was first reported in 1969 and since then has gained wide popularity. This approach allows excellent visualization of midline and lateral pathology from T5 through T12. Multilevel access is also readily available. The base of the rib articulating with the body and a portion of the pedicle are removed, followed by a partial diskectomy. Using a burr, a trough is created into which disk material can be pulled forward to decompress the canal and remove the herniated fragment. Fusion can easily be added to the diskectomy

with the available exposure. Many authors have reported good visualization and excellent results with this technique. The drawbacks of this technique include the possibility of pneumothorax, pulmonary contusion, atelectasis, pneumonia, and the need for a postoperative chest tube.

VATS was first reported in 1993 as a minimally invasive procedure that can minimize the morbidity of an open thoracotomy and allow excellent visualization of the anterior approach. One of the main disadvantages of this technique is the steep learning curve to attain the high level of technical skills required for the procedure. Calcified protrusions can be adherent to or penetrate through the dura and can be difficult to treat via VATS. Two-year follow-up data are now available and suggest that VATS is effective in a select group of patients.

The role of fusion in thoracic disk surgery is controversial. Relative indications for fusion include multilevel diskectomy, Scheuermann's disease, and bony resection that removes a large portion of the vertebral body or the pedicle facet complex. The resected rib often provides sufficient autologous bone graft material without the need for added morbidity from harvesting a graft. A small fibular allograft augmented with local autograft can also be used. Instrumentation is generally not used because the rib cage provides a protective splinting effect. If deformity correction is desired in multilevel cases, instrumentation should be considered.

Most patients with thoracic disk herniation and axial pain alone can be treated successfully with nonsurgical treatment. In patients who do not respond well to nonsurgical treatment, thoracic diskectomy and fusion can be considered; however, the role of surgical intervention is controversial.

Annotated Bibliography

Anand N, Regan JJ: Video-assisted thoracoscopic surgery for thoracic disc disease: Classification and outcome study of 100 consecutive cases with a 2-year minimum follow-up period. *Spine* 2002;27:871-879.

The authors present their experience of 100 patients who underwent VATS for the treatment of thoracic disk herniations with at least a 2-year follow up. This prospective, nonrandomized study supports the conclusions that VATS is effective in a select group of patients, it is a reasonably safe procedure, and satisfactory outcomes are achieved for most patients.

Oskouian RJ, Johnsin JP, Regan JJ: Thoracoscopic microdiscectomy. *Neurosurgery* 2002;50:103-109.

The authors of this article present a detailed description of a technique for thoracic diskectomy via thoracoscopy.

Classic Bibliography

Arce CA, Dohrmann GJ: Herniated thoracic disks. *Neurol Clin* 1985;3:383-392.

Awwad EE, Martin DS, Smith KR Jr, Baker BK: Asymptomatic versus symptomatic herniated thoracic discs: Their frequency and characteristics as detected by computed tomography after myelography. *Neurosurgery* 1991;28:180-186.

Bohlmann HH, Zdeblick TA: Anterior excision of herniated thoracic discs. *J Bone Joint Surg Am* 1988;70:1038-1047.

Brown CW, Deffer PA Jr, Akmakjian J, Donalson DH, Brugman JL: The natural history of thoracic disc herniation. *Spine* 1992;17(suppl 6):S97-S102.

Currier BL, Eismont FJ, Green BA: Transthoracic disc excision and fusion for herniated thoracic discs. *Spine* 1994;19:323-328.

Dickman CA, Rosenthal D, Regan JJ: Reoperation for herniated thoracic discs. *J Neurosurg* 1999;91(suppl 2):157-162.

Fessler RG, Sturgill M: Review: complications of surgery for thoracic disc disease. *Surg Neurol* 1998;49:609-618.

Fidler MW, Goedhart ZD: Excision of prolapse of thoracic intervertebral disc: A transthoracic technique. *J Bone Joint Surg Br* 1984;66:518-522.

Otani K, Yoshida M, Fujii E, Nakai S, Shibasaki K: Thoracic disc herniation: Surgical treatment in 23 patients. *Spine* 1988;13:1262-1267.

Rogers MA, Crockard HA: Surgical treatment of the symptomatic herniated thoracic disk. *Clin Orthop* 1994;300:70-78.

Schellas KP, Pollei SR, Dorwart RH: Thoracic discography: A safe and reliable technique. *Spine* 1994;19:2103-2109.

Simpson JM, Silveri CP, Simeone FA, Balderston RA, An HS: Thoracic disc herniation: Re-evaluation of the posterior approach using a modified costotransversectomy. *Spine* 1993;18:1872-1877.

Vanichkachorn JS, Vaccaro AR: Thoracic disk disease: Diagnosis and treatment. *J Am Acad Orthop Surg* 2000;8:159-169.

Wood KB, Blair JM, Aepple DM, et al: The natural history of asymptomatic thoracic disc herniations. *Spine* 1997;22:525-530.

Wood KB, Garvey TA, Gundry C, Heithoff KB: Magnetic resonance imaging of the thoracic spine: Evaluation of asymptomatic individuals. *J Bone Joint Surg Am* 1995;77:1631-1638.

Wood KB, Schellhas KP, Garvey TA, Aeppli D: Thoracic discography in healthy individuals: A controlled prospective study of magnetic resonance imaging and discography in asymptomatic and symptomatic individuals. *Spine* 1999;24:1548-1555.

Chapter 44

Lumbar Degenerative Disorders

Raj D. Rao, MD

Kenny S. David, MD

Introduction

Low back pain accounts for more than 15 million patient visits to the physician's office per year in the United States, second only to the number of patient visits for respiratory infections. Complaints of back pain begin around age 35 years and increase in prevalence up to age 50 years in men and age 60 years in women. The overall point prevalence of back pain in the United States is estimated to be 18%. The annual cost for managing back pain is approximately $50 billion, the bulk of which is spent on an estimated 1% of the patients. The three most common lumbar degenerative disorders are lumbar spinal stenosis, lumbar disk herniation, and discogenic low back pain.

Lumbar Spinal Stenosis

Lumbar spinal stenosis is a reduction in the dimensions of the central or lateral lumbar spinal canal that occurs most frequently as a result of chronic degenerative changes at the lumbar motion segment (Table 1). Patients with lumbar spinal stenosis have back pain associated with neurogenic claudication and/or radicular pain.

Pathoanatomy

Absolute stenosis is defined as a decrease in the midsagittal lumbar canal diameter of less than 10 mm, whereas 10 to 13 mm represents relative stenosis. The normal cross-sectional area of the lumbar canal is 150 to 200 mm^2, and a decrease to less than 100 mm^2 is a more reliable indicator of the combined effects of central and lateral lumbar stenosis. Central stenosis results from congenitally short pedicles, diffuse posterior protrusion of the degenerative disk, and infolding of the ligamentum flavum.

The lateral portion of the lumbar canal is divided into three zones: the lateral recess, foraminal zone, and extraforaminal zone (Figure 1). The most common pathology in the lateral recess is bony overgrowth of the superior articular process caused by degenerative facet joint arthrosis. The foraminal zone lies distal to the pedicle and ventral to the pars interarticularis and contains portions of the ventral nerve root, dorsal root ganglion, and nerve root. Stenosis in this region is commonly the result of cartilaginous overgrowth or osteophytes arising from the anterior-inferior aspect of a pars defect, foraminal disk or end plate protrusion, or superior-inferior compression between two pedicles as a result of loss of disk height. Foraminal height normally ranges from 20 to 23 mm, and anterior-posterior depth ranges from 8 to 10 mm in the upper foramen. A foraminal height of less than 15 mm and a posterior disk height of less than 4 mm are associated with nerve root compression in 80% of patients. The lumbar nerve roots lie in the upper foramen and occupy approximately 30% of the available foraminal area. Evidence of obliteration of perineural fat on radiographic images is an early indicator of foraminal stenosis. The extraforaminal zone is lateral to the intervertebral foramen and contains the exiting root.

Alteration of lumbar canal dimensions with trunk posture results in dynamic stenosis. Extension of the lumbar spine leads to reduced interlaminar space and buckling of the ligamentum flavum, which can result in spinal stenosis. Foraminal height and width decrease by 14% to 18% in extension. Foraminal area decreases by 20% during extension. CT studies show that the cross-sectional area of the foramen increases by 12% in flexion, and that nerve root compression is least in flexion and highest in extension.

Pathophysiology

The development of symptoms in a subset of these patients can be explained by the pathophysiologic changes that occur concurrently with the morphologic changes of stenosis. In animals, 50% constriction of the cauda equina results in major changes in cortical evoked potentials and mild motor weakness. These findings generally resolve by 2 months despite persistent compression. With constriction to 75%, motor and sensory deficits are more profound and show only slight recovery at 2 months. Claudication and neurologic symptoms may initially result from venous distension in the nerve roots and dorsal root ganglion. Obstruction of microcircula-

Table 1 | Etiologic Classification of Lumbar Spinal Stenosis

Congenital/Developmental

Chondrodystrophy-achondroplasia

Congenital small spinal canal with short vertebral pedicles

Congenital cysts from the dura/arachnoid narrowing an otherwise normal canal

Osteoporosis

Acquired

Degenerative

  Central canal/lateral recess/foraminal zone

  Degenerative spondylolisthesis

  Degenerative scoliosis

Inflammatory arthritis

Ankylosing spondylitis

Rheumatoid arthritis

Pseudogout

Spondylolytic

Iatrogenic

  Postdiskectomy/laminectomy/fusion

  Postchemonucleolysis

Vertebral fractures

  Traumatic

  Pathologic

Spinal infections with abscess bone collapse

Miscellaneous

  Paget's disease

  Fluorosis

  Acromegaly

  Diffuse idiopathic skeletal hyperostosis

  Pseudogout

  Oxalosis

Combined

Degenerative changes superimposed on a developmentally narrow canal

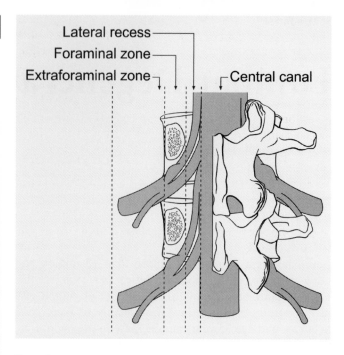

Figure 1 Illustration of lateral recess stenosis in which the superior articular process impinges on the traversing lumbar nerve root. The coronal section shows the relative positions of the central canal, lateral recess, foraminal zone, and extraforaminal zone.

damage. Compression at multiple sites may explain development of symptoms in some patients. Animal studies have shown that single-level compression of 10 mm Hg had marginal effect on nerve function, whereas two-level compression caused significant reduction in blood flow of the cauda equina.

At the cellular level, bone morphogenetic proteins are related to chondrogenesis within the aging disk. The migration of these factors from the region of the vertebral end plates to fibrous cells within the anulus fibrosus may contribute to osteophyte formation and the bone overgrowth seen in the degenerative spine.

Clinical Features

Classically, patients have back, buttock, or posterior leg pain that gets worse with standing and walking. Leg symptoms may also be described as cramps, burning pain, or weakness. Flexion of the trunk alleviates symptoms, and extension aggravates the symptoms. Leaning on a cart helps, primarily because of the flexed posture of the trunk in this position. Sleeping is comfortable in the fetal position. The limitations in activity and stooped forward posture are commonly attributed to age, and many patients learn to work within their limitations. Autonomic sphincter dysfunction manifests as recurrent urinary tract infection associated with an atonic bladder, incontinence, or retention, and occurs in up to 10% of patients with advanced degrees of stenosis.

Claudication manifests as diffuse buttock and/or leg pain, nonspecific paresthesias, or radicular symptoms

tion at the site of constriction, nerve root fibrosis, and wallerian degeneration of the motor root and posterior spinal tracts contribute to subsequent neurologic manifestations. The same general rules appear to apply to the human lumbar canal, with significant symptoms appearing when the stenosis is greater than 75%. Claudication symptoms from lumbar spinal stenosis occur in 90% of patients who have a cross-sectional spinal canal area less than 100 mm².

In animal studies, the rate of onset of compression plays a role in the pathophysiology of stenosis. Rapid onset (0.05 to 0.10 s) compression causes more damage than insidious onset (20 s) pressure. The compressive lesion results in greater mechanical deformation at the edge of nerve root, a phenomenon referred to as the edge effect. Histologic examination of edge segments has revealed significant microvascular and neural tissue that commence with walking for varying distances. Unlike vascular disease, the claudication distance with symptomatic spinal stenosis may vary considerably and is relieved by sitting and not by standing. Activities performed with the trunk flexed, such as cycling or walking uphill, are performed more easily. The exertion-induced symptoms of spinal stenosis can be accurately reproduced using a treadmill, providing a method for preoperative and postoperative quantification of symptoms.

The manifestations of central and lateral canal stenosis are not easily distinguished. Unilateral radicular pain from foraminal stenosis is worsened by extension to the painful side (Kemp sign). Paresthetic and dysesthetic symptoms may be an indicator of dorsal root ganglion entrapment in the foramen. Unlike disk herniations, radicular pain from stenosis is typically not aggravated by Valsalva maneuvers or accompanied by a positive straight leg raising sign.

Management

Nonsurgical therapy with anti-inflammatory agents, analgesics, activity modification, exercises, and soft braces may help patients with exacerbations of pain but seldom achieve sustained improvement. Epidural steroid injections or selective nerve root injections result in substantial relief of radicular pain and may obviate the need for surgery over the short term in a subset of patients. Ideally, the injections are performed at the level of the symptomatic nerve root through a fluoroscopically directed transforaminal technique. One to three injections are typically performed, with 1-to 2-week intervals between injections.

Patients with persistent lower extremity symptoms from lumbar spinal stenosis are generally offered surgical decompression. The physician should make clear that the aim of surgery is to relieve current disability rather than prevent future complications. There is no conclusive evidence that disability from spinal stenosis worsens over time. Less frequent indications for surgery include progressive neurologic deficit or cauda equina syndrome.

The optimal surgical approach combines maximal thecal sac and nerve root decompression and preserves stability. The facet joints, capsule, intervertebral disk, and interspinous ligaments are important lumbar spine stabilizers. In typical degenerative lumbar spinal stenosis, maximal compression of the thecal sac occurs at the level of the disk. Decompression of a single level is achieved by resection of approximately 50% of the cephalad and caudad laminae and the intervening ligamentum flavum. After creation of a central trough, the decompression is extended laterally to the medial wall of the pedicle bilaterally to ensure that the traversing nerve root is free of pressure. Greater than 50% excision of the bilateral facets or unilateral complete facetectomy can result in iatrogenic instability and may require fusion.

There are no guidelines on whether adjacent levels with lesser degrees of stenosis should be included in the decompression. The benefits of a greater decompression of the neural elements need to be weighed against the potential morbidity of a longer operation. In general, a level with mild stenosis may be excluded if radicular symptoms corresponding to that level are absent. Decompressing too few levels may be a source of persistent symptoms postoperatively. Somatosensory-evoked potential techniques may serve as a guide to the extent of decompression in the future.

The anulus fibrosus is left intact when possible, resecting only free fragments or extruded segments of the disk that result in neural impingement. Diffuse bulging of the disk is unlikely to result in continued neural compression in patients who have undergone a wide laminectomy with bilateral partial facetectomy.

Based on the existing literature, a fusion should be considered following decompressive laminectomy in (1) patients who have stenosis with degenerative spondylolisthesis; (2) when radiographic criteria for instability exist preoperatively; (3) when more than a combined 50% of the bilateral facet joints are resected as part of the decompression; and (4) when decompression is performed in a patient with a flexible or progressive degenerative scoliosis.

The precise role of instrumentation in lumbar spinal stenosis is currently unclear. The aims of pedicle screw instrumentation in spinal stenosis surgery include deformity correction, immediate stabilization of an unstable spine, improvement in fusion rates, and faster mobilization of patients. The advantages of instrumentation need to be weighed against the potential morbidity of extending the surgical procedure. A randomized prospective study showed that the addition of instrumentation to lumbar decompression and posterolateral arthrodesis for degenerative spondylolisthesis with stenosis resulted in improved fusion rates, but it did not improve the overall clinical outcome of patients.

Alternative Surgical Techniques

Several limited approaches have been proposed as alternatives to the traditional decompressive laminectomy and partial facetectomy. The rationale for these approaches involves decreased patient morbidity and faster rehabilitation with a more limited operation, limiting the surgery to the pathologic area (the bony and soft-tissue pathology in most patients with degenerative stenosis is at the level of the interlaminar window and can be adequately addressed through an interlaminar fenestration or laminotomy), decreased postoperative radiographic listhesis, reduced scarring posterior to the thecal sac and root, awareness that paraspinal muscle atrophy with wide exposure may be a source of postoperative back pain, and limited surgical destabilization, which potentially obviates the need for fusion. The benefits of these approaches need to be weighed against their limitations, which include a higher incidence of nerve root injury and dural tears, bone regrowth potentially compromising the result, the need for technically demanding procedures and longer surgical times, the fact that most of these procedures do not address central stenosis, and the lack of long-term clinical efficacy studies.

A unilateral hemilaminectomy or laminotomy may be indicated in a patient with one-sided symptoms from lateral stenosis and no significant central stenosis. Simultaneous diskectomy should be performed if there is residual bulging of the disk, especially when the patient has good disk height. Bilateral or multilevel laminotomy may be considered in patients with degenerative stenosis at multiple levels. Myelography in these patients usually shows an hourglass compression of the thecal sac at several levels, with spacious intervening areas. The procedure differs from the traditional multilevel laminectomy by leaving the spinous processes and interspinous ligaments intact. In unilateral laminotomy with bilateral decompression, an ipsilateral laminotomy and decompression is followed by decompression of the contralateral side by angling the microscope or endoscope across the top of the dural sac. Resection of the contralateral ligamentum flavum allows good exposure of the contralateral side.

Prognosis and Outcomes

There is little published information regarding the true natural history of lumbar spinal stenosis. Studies that include nonsurgical treatment show that about 15% to 20% of patients improve, 15% to 20% get worse, and 60% to 70% remain unchanged. Surgery appears to improve short-term outcomes in patients with severe stenosis. In one study, 52% of nonsurgically treated patients showed improvement at 4-year follow-up compared with 70% of surgically treated patients. Patients undergoing surgical treatment generally had more severe degrees of stenosis and were more symptomatic than the nonsurgically managed group.

Appropriate patient selection and thorough decompression result in good long-term results following decompressive lumbar laminectomy with or without fusion. A meta-analysis of the surgical treatment of spinal stenosis found that the average proportion of good to excellent results in 74 studies was 64%. There were no consistent predictors of clinical outcome, but younger age, greater severity and duration of symptoms, previous back surgery, multilevel involvement, coexisting medical morbidity, and litigation issues were associated with poorer outcome. The presence of bladder symptoms

preoperatively may be a negative prognostic indicator. The results in general deteriorate over a 5- to 10-year period, with increasing back pain, claudication, and rates of revision surgery. Mortality in these elderly patients is 0.6% to 1.0% following surgery.

The rates of lumbar fusion vary considerably across geographic regions and specialties, suggesting uncertainty among surgeons on the indications for fusion following decompressive laminectomy. In a multicenter study of patient selection and outcomes following decompressive laminectomy, instrumented and noninstrumented fusion in patients with degenerative spinal stenosis, the major predictor of the decision to perform arthrodesis was found to be the individual surgeon. Other factors associated with this decision were the presence of more than 5 mm of spondylolisthesis, younger age, female patients, scoliosis greater than 15°, patients with greater severity of back pain, and fewer levels decompressed. The authors reported significantly greater relief of back pain after 6 and 24 months in the noninstrumented arthrodesis group. The decreased satisfaction in the instrumented arthrodesis group at these earlier stages cannot be well explained, but it may be related to pain associated with the instrumentation itself. The increased likelihood of a successful arthrodesis with instrumentation may result in improved results in this group over a longer period. Hospital costs were highest in patients who underwent instrumented arthrodesis.

Lumbar Disk Herniation
Pathoanatomy

A disk herniation is a localized displacement of disk material beyond the limits of the intervertebral space. The disk material can be nucleus pulposus, cartilage, anulus fibrosus, fragments of apophyseal bone, or any combination of these materials. A herniated disk should be distinguished from a disk bulge, which is a diffuse symmetric outpouching of the anulus fibrosus associated with varying degrees of disk degeneration. A true herniation may either be a protrusion, extrusion, or sequestration (Figure 2). The base of a protrusion is wider than any diameter of the displaced material. In an extrusion, the diameter of the displaced material in at least one plane is greater than the width at its base. If a displaced fragment loses all continuity with the parent disk, it is termed a sequestration, and is prone to migrate within the spinal canal. The relationship of the herniated nuclear material to the surrounding anulus fibrosus and the overlying posterior longitudinal ligament defines its containment. A herniation completely enveloped by anulus fibrosus, posterior longitudinal ligament, or both is termed a contained herniation. Nuclear material that escapes through the annular periphery and rests beneath the posterior longitudinal ligament has been referred to as subligamentous.

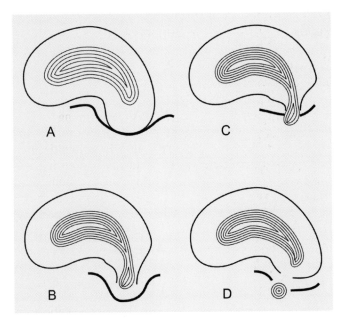

Figure 2 Illustration of four morphologic types of disk herniations: contained disk protrusion **(A)**, noncontained subligamentous disk extrusion **(B)**, noncontained transligamentous disk extrusion **(C)**, and noncontained disk sequestration **(D)**.

The geographic relationship of the herniated nucleus to the circumference of the anulus fibrosus and the intervertebral foramen is used to classify herniations as central, paracentral, foraminal, or extraforaminal. Paracentral herniations are the most common pattern encountered in clinical practice. They are caused by the weaker posterolateral portion of the posterior longitudinal ligament overlying this segment of the anulus fibrosus. Posterolateral herniations compress the lower exiting root (for example, the L5 root at L4-5 level), whereas the more lateral and extraforaminal herniations are more likely to compress the upper root (for example, the L4 root at L4-5 level). Axillary and shoulder descriptions refer to the position of the herniated disk with respect to the origin of the nerve root from the thecal sac.

Pathophysiology

Several pathophysiologic events occur in the nucleus pulposus and adjacent areas that act in concert to produce radicular symptoms. Tumor necrosis factor-α (TNF-α) may be a key component of this process in that it exerts its effect by sensitizing the nerve root to produce pain in the presence of a mechanically deforming force. Local accumulation of sodium ion channels and spontaneous axonal activity may be pathways through which TNF-α acts.

The effects of mechanical deformation are compounded by chemical sensitization of the nerve root. When diskectomy is performed using local anesthetic in human subjects, light mechanical stimulation of nerve roots not exposed to nucleus pulposus have been noted to induce mild local discomfort. Stimulation of a root exposed to nucleus pulposus reproduced sciatic pain in the leg. Epidural application of extracts of nucleus pulposus in animal models when combined with mild deformation of the nerve root and dorsal root ganglion resulted in increased tissue edema, fibrosis in and around nerve root, demyelination of axons, and Schwann cell hypertrophy.

Inflammatory cytokines such as interleukin-1β, interleukin-6, prostaglandin-E2, and phospholipase A2 are found in significant concentrations in the nerve root and dorsal root ganglion, suggesting they play a role in the inflammatory process. The presence of these agents incites vascular changes around the nerve root and also has a direct effect on the blood-nerve barrier, promoting intraneural edema and reducing neuronal perfusion. Interactions between nerve growth factors at the nerve root and dorsal root ganglion may play a role in the central modulation of spinal pain.

Clinical Features

Lumbar disk herniation is the most common cause of radicular pain in the adult working population, with an estimated 2.8 million herniations (1% of the general population) occurring annually. Ninety-five percent of these herniations involve the L4-5 or L5-S1 lumbar disk spaces, and most patients are between the ages of 20 and 50 years. Patients typically present with back pain and sharp, stabbing leg pain accompanied by a feeling of numbness or tingling in a specific dermatomal distribution. One study reports a dermatomal sensitivity and specificity of 74% and 18% for paresthesias from lumbar disk herniation. Referred (sclerotomal) pain in the buttock or posterior thigh arises from stimulation of muscles, ligaments, periosteum, and other structures of mesodermal origin and does not go beyond the knee. Symptoms are aggravated by activities and maneuvers that raise the intra-abdominal and intradiskal pressure, such as coughing, sneezing, and sitting.

Motor, sensory, and reflex evaluation corresponding to the lumbar roots should be specifically evaluated (Figure 3). The straight leg raising test is a clinical maneuver that demonstrates limited excursion of inflamed lumbosacral nerve roots. In lumbar disk herniation, the test is sensitive (true positive in 72% to 97% of patients) but not specific (false positive in 11% to 66% of patients). In contrast, the crossed straight leg raising test has a lower sensitivity (true positive in 23% to 42% of patients) but much higher specificity (false positive in 85% to 100% of patients). There is minimal movement in the sciatic nerve or roots during the first 20° to 30° of straight leg raising; most tension in the roots develops at 35° to 70° of elevation.

Large lumbar disk herniations may result in a cauda equina syndrome, characterized by bilateral leg pain,

Motor   Reflex   Sensory

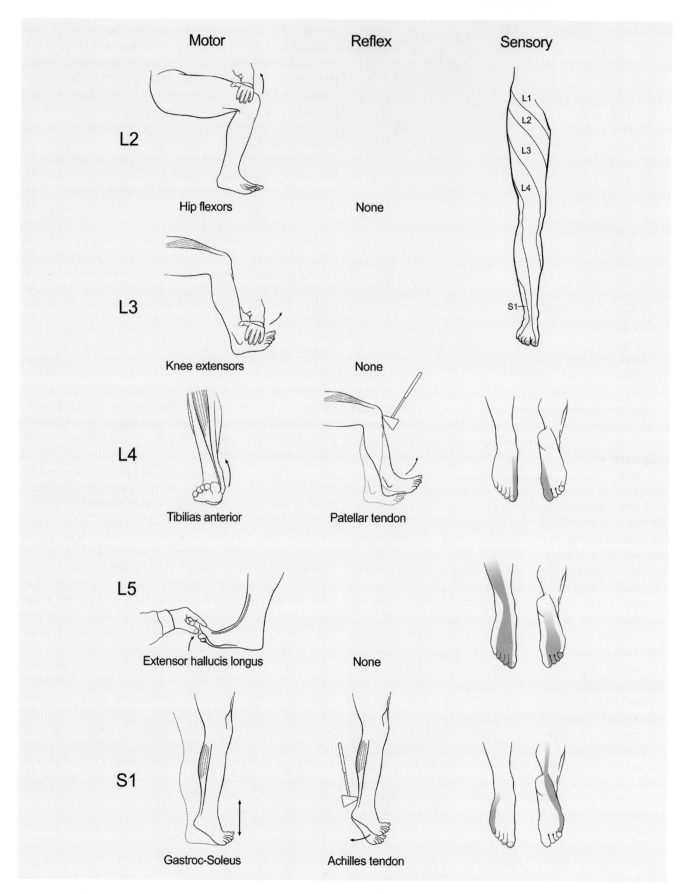

L2 — Hip flexors — None

L3 — Knee extensors — None

L4 — Tibilias anterior — Patellar tendon

L5 — Extensor hallucis longus — None

S1 — Gastroc-Soleus — Achilles tendon

Figure 3 Illustration of the motor, reflex, and sensory radicular findings in various types of lumbar disk herniation.

lower limb weakness, saddle anesthesia, and bowel/bladder changes. One percent to 10% of all patients undergoing surgery for lumbar disk herniation have symptoms of cauda equina syndrome. The incidence may be higher when patients with subtle urinary symptoms are included. Pain varies substantially in patients, and it is modified and influenced by several factors including individual cultural and psychologic factors, sleep deprivation, and secondary gain. Evaluation of the patient should include a skillful appraisal of these issues.

Management

Nonsurgical measures including activity modification, anti-inflammatory agents, physical therapy modalities, exercises, spinal manipulation, corsets, epidural injections, and nerve root blocks result in good resolution of symptoms in most patients. It is unclear whether any of these treatment options actually alters the natural history of disease.

Foraminal epidural steroid injections accurately administered under fluoroscopic control may help in combating the chemical mediators of pain and inflammation associated with disk herniations. A positive response is usually indicated by a reduction of leg pain by more than 50%. The steroid load generally precludes more than three to four injections over a 1-year period. The most important application of these injections may be in shortening the pain-control phase of treatment, which allows early reconditioning to begin.

Persistent intractable pain following nonsurgical treatment during a minimum 6-week period is the most frequent indication for surgery. There is some evidence that results of surgery deteriorate when nonsurgical care exceeds 12 months. Imaging studies must correlate with the symptoms and neurologic findings. The presence of a nerve tension sign improves the likelihood of a good postoperative result.

Other factors that influence the decision to proceed with surgery include disk herniation into a stenotic canal, which may lead to recurrent or persistent symptoms; inability of patients to comply with the dictates of a conservative therapy regimen; and the number of sciatica episodes experienced by a patient. Among patients experiencing a second episode of sciatica, 90% will improve but 50% will have a recurrence of symptoms. The incidence of future episodes of sciatica rises to almost 100% in patients who have experienced three prior episodes. Absolute indications for surgery in lumbar disk herniation are bladder and bowel involvement and progressive neurologic deficit.

A laminotomy and diskectomy (microdiskectomy) is the gold standard for surgical treatment of a posterolateral lumbar disk herniation. This treatment is frequently performed as an outpatient or short-stay procedure using an operating microscope or surgical loupes with a headlight and a small posterior midline incision centered on the disk space. Surgeons must be aware of the anatomic peculiarities of the upper lumbar canal when treating patients with high lumbar disk herniations. Anatomic peculiarities include smaller interlaminar spaces, greater coverage of the disk space by the lamina of the superior vertebra, proximity to the conus medullaris, a smaller spinal canal with a higher volume of nerve tissue, and a more horizontal orientation of the upper lumbar nerve roots. An extraforaminal disk herniation is ideally accessed through the Wiltse paraspinal approach, which preserves motion segment stability by avoiding injury to the lamina and facet joints. Injury to the dorsal root ganglion with postoperative dysesthesias is a potential complication when treating patients with this form of disk herniation. Endoscopic and other percutaneous techniques for disk decompression are discussed in chapter 50.

Prognosis and Outcome Following Intervention

Lumbar disk herniation is a self-limiting disease in most patients. Eighty percent to 90% of patients obtain satisfactory resolution of symptoms with nonsurgical treatment. Imaging studies that monitor the changes in size of nonsurgically treated disk herniations have shown a progressive decrease in the size of herniations over time. Large extrusions have a greater likelihood of total resorption; they are phagocytosed by cells attracted by the disk-incited inflammatory response or from desiccation and atrophy secondary to loss of nutrient supply.

Nonsurgical treatments will likely result in favorable outcomes when the duration of sciatica is less than 6 months, the patient is younger, and there is no litigation involved. The results of surgical treatment are better in patients with large anterior-posterior herniated disk length and in patients who have a greater compromise of the canal area by the disk herniation. Patients who have an extruded or sequestered fragment with a minimal fissure in the anulus fibrosus or those who have a detached fragment lying beneath an intact anulus fibrosus are likely to do better following surgery than those who have an extruded disk with a large or massive annular defect or those who have an intact anulus fibrosus and no detached fragment beneath the anulus fibrosus.

The likelihood of recovery of neurologic deficit is independent of surgical intervention, and patients with neurologic deficit but no pain do not require surgery. Surgery is considered in some patients with painless motor deficits when there is functional weakness in a major muscle group or in those with significant motor deficits and no return of function after 6 weeks. Recovery of motor deficit is the general rule, although in some patients complete recovery may take a long time. Long-term studies have shown that 30% of patients will continue to have sensory deficits despite resolution of pain.

This finding is consistent with the fact that sensory fibers are the most vulnerable to compression (they are affected first and recover last).

One prospective controlled study compared outcomes of surgical and nonsurgical treatment in a group of patients with lumbar radicular pain and concordant myelograms. Surgery was superior to nonsurgical treatment at 1-year follow-up and continued to be slightly better at 4-year follow-up. Outcomes were similar in both groups at 10-year follow-up. Approximately 60% of both groups of patients were symptom free at 10-year follow-up, although clinical recovery occurred earlier in the surgically treated group. In another 5-year follow-up study, 56% of nonsurgically managed patients reported symptomatic improvement compared with 70% of surgically treated patients.

Long-term success rates following open diskectomy are between 76% and 93%. In a study of 63 patients 10 years after interlaminar fenestration and diskectomy, 75% of patients reported some back pain, but only 13% reported severe back pain. Younger patients with preoperative degenerative changes at the disk had a higher incidence of back pain. Sensory disturbances were present in 81% of patients preoperatively, but in only 31% of patients at final follow-up. Motor deficits were present in 76% of patients preoperatively, and in 14% of patients at 10-year follow-up. A complete foot drop was present in four patients preoperatively and this symptom did not improve after surgery. The straight leg raising test was negative in 97% of patients at the 10-year follow-up. Mild preoperative urinary disturbances in four patients resolved completely.

Special Situations

Recurrent Herniation and Reoperation
Recurrent herniations at the same level occur in approximately 5% of surgically treated patients at 5-year follow-up and can be ipsilateral or, less frequently, contralateral. Survival analysis or rates of revision are a better measure of surgical success. A recent large population-based study from Finland analyzed the risk of reoperations after lumbar diskectomy. Fourteen percent of a total of 35,309 patients in the study group underwent a second procedure during the 10-year period of the study. The second procedure was diskectomy in 63% of patients, decompression in 23%, and fusion in 14%. Among the patients who underwent a second procedure, there was a 25% cumulative risk of needing a third spinal surgical procedure within the next 10 years. A pain-free interval of more than 1 year was associated with a lower risk of revision.

Disk Herniation in the Elderly
Disk herniation in elderly patients commonly occurs in the setting of spinal stenosis or spondylolisthesis. Disk herniations in patients in this age group are more frequent in the upper lumbar spine. Nerve root tension signs such as the straight leg raising test are commonly negative in elderly patients. This may be secondary to reduced resting tension in the nerve roots as a result of reduced disk height from the degenerative process or reduced limb length from degenerative hip and knee changes. Chronic fibrosis of the roots from compromised microcirculation may contribute to the severity of the radicular pain. Histologically, the herniated disk fragment primarily contains sections of anulus fibrosus. Spontaneous resorption and improvement is less likely to occur.

Disk Herniation in Young Patients
Pediatric disk herniations constitute 1% to 3% of all instances of lumbar disk herniation. Previous trauma and vertebral column abnormalities such as congenital stenosis or transitional vertebrae may increase the likelihood of herniation. The clinical presentation is similar to that for adults, with back pain and nerve tension signs being frequently reported; neurologic deficits in these patients is typically uncommon. The herniation is frequently an avulsed fragment of the ring apophysis of the vertebral body. In children and adolescents who have persistent symptoms despite nonsurgical treatment, surgery usually results in good relief of symptoms. A unilateral hemilaminectomy with partial diskectomy is sufficient treatment for most patients. A bilateral laminectomy is occasionally necessary when the avulsed apophysis fragment is large.

Discogenic Low Back Pain
Discogenic pain refers to pain originating from a degenerative lumbar disk, which is characterized by axial low back pain without associated radicular findings, spinal deformity, or instability. The controversy surrounding discogenic low back pain primarily exists because degenerative changes at the disks are ubiquitous, yet symptoms arise in only a few patients; multiple additional anatomic sources of low back pain exist (Table 2); the diagnosis of discogenic low back pain is made primarily with provocative diskography, which is controversial in itself; it is unclear whether the treatment options for discogenic low back pain are superior to the natural history of the disorder over the long term. Notwithstanding these issues, the degenerative lumbar disk is being increasingly recognized as a valid source of axial low back pain.

Pathoanatomy and Pathophysiology
As the disk ages, several chemical and mechanical changes occur within it, which result in a continuum of changes that can be observed using radiographic imaging. Type II collagen in the nucleus pulposus and anulus

Table 2 | Differential Diagnosis of Low Back Pain

Spinal Causes
Trauma
  Fractures
  Musculoligamentous injury
  Fracture in pathologic bone
Infections
  Diskitis, osteomyelitis
  Epidural abscess
Inflammatory
  Seronegative spondyloarthropathy
  Rheumatoid arthritis
Tumors
  Primary – arising from bone or marrow elements
  Metastatic
Degenerative conditions
  Spinal stenosis
  Spondylolisthesis
  Scoliosis
  Discogenic low back pain
Miscellaneous
  Paget's disease
  Arachnoiditis
  Sickle cell disease
Extraspinal Causes
Visceral origin
  Urinary system-kidney stones, pyelonephritis
  Reproductive system (endometriosis, retroverted uterus, ectopic pregnancy)
  Gastrointestinal tract (duodenal ulcers, pancreatitis, biliary colic)
  Abdominal aortic aneurysm
  Retroperitoneal tumors
Musculoskeletal origin
  Myofascial pain
  Hip arthrosis
  Sacroiliac joint pathology
Miscellaneous causes
  Psychogenic
  Central pain syndromes

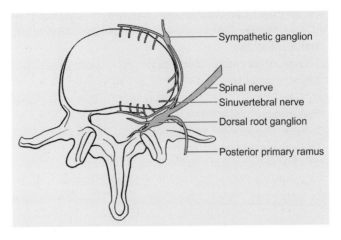

Figure 4 Illustration of the axial lumbar vertebra showing the origin, course, and structures innervated by the sinuvertebral nerve.

fibrosus is increasingly replaced by type I collagen, chondroitin sulfate is replaced by keratan sulfate, and there is increasing dissociation between the collagen and proteoglycans within the disk. The resulting loss in hydrostatic properties of the disk leads to altered load transmission, with asymmetric and abnormal stresses being transmitted from the vertebral end plate to the periphery of the anulus fibrosus. Radial tears develop within the anulus fibrosus, with subsequent fissuring and ingrowth of granulation tissue. As the process continues, the disk loses height, and the vertebral bodies come closer to each other. Laxity in the peripheral attachments of the anulus fibrosus and the facet joint capsules may allow motion or displacement between the vertebral bodies. Increased load transfer at the facet joints and vertebral end plates results in degenerative changes at both these sites.

Nerve fibers and nerve endings found in the peripheral portions of the disk offer a possible mechanism by which lumbar disks act as pain generators. The disk is innervated by the sinuvertebral nerve, which is formed by branches from the ventral nerve root and sympathetic plexus (Figure 4). Once formed, the nerve turns back into the intervertebral foramen along the posterior aspect of the disk, supplying portions of the anulus fibrosus, posterior longitudinal ligament, periosteum of the vertebral body and pedicle, and adjacent epidural veins. The free nerve endings in the peripheral anulus fibrosus are immunoreactive for several pain-related neuropeptides—substance P, calcitonin gene-related peptide, and vasoactive intestinal peptide. In degenerative disks, nerve endings penetrate deep into the anulus fibrosus and even into nucleus pulposus. The free nerve endings that penetrate deep into the disk are also immunoreactive for substance P.

Chemical factors may help explain why pain develops in a subset of patients with degenerative changes. Mechanical deformation of the anulus fibrosus stimulates both mechanoreceptors as well as nociceptors by lowering their firing thresholds. Inflammatory mediators eluted by the disk (phospholipase A2, interleukin-1, and matrix metalloproteinases) may play a role in the sensitization of pain receptors. Phospholipase A2 also stimulates the dorsal root ganglion, which can serve as another pathway for axial pain generation.

Mechanoreceptors and nociceptors in the facet joint capsules and synovium may play an accessory role in the symptoms of discogenic pain. The number of these receptors in the facet joints falls during the weeks fol-

Table 3 | Radiographic Criteria for Lumbar Spine Instability

Resting radiographs

1. Sagittal displacement > 4.5 mm or 15%
2. Relative sagittal plane angulation > 22°

or

Flexion-extension radiographs

1. Sagittal displacement > 4.5 mm or 15%
2. Relative sagittal plane rotation
   > 15° at L1-2, L2-3, L3-4
   > 20° at L4-5
   > 25° at L5/S1

(Reproduced with permission from Posner I, White AA III, Edwards WT, Hayes WC: A biomechanical analysis of the clinical stability of the lumbar and lumbosacral spine. Spine 1982;7:374-389.)

lowing interbody fusion in animals, suggesting that appropriate stabilization of the disk space reduces nociception from the facets. Vertebral end plates and the underlying cancellous bone have an increased density of sensory nerves in patients with degenerative disk disease, thereby providing another pathway for pain generation.

Clinical Features

Clinically, discogenic pain is characterized by axial low back pain without associated radicular pain, nerve tension signs, spinal deformity, or instability. The pain is generally deep, aching, and exacerbated by sitting, bending, and axial loading. Symptoms are predominantly mechanical, and rest may provide relief. There may be a history of prior injury to the spine such as a fall, lifting with outstretched arms, or sudden twisting that resulted in back pain. Instead of getting better, the pain gradually gets worse. Referred pain may radiate in a sclerotomal fashion to the sacroiliac joints, buttocks, or posterior thighs, and occasionally into the inguinal region with involvement of the L5-S1 disk. Greater degrees of back pain appear to be associated with a more distal pattern of pain referral.

Traditional instability of a motion segment is a recognized cause of low back pain. This instability is diagnosed radiographically by intervertebral translation or angulation, using criteria put forth by White and Panjabi (Table 3). Patients frequently have mechanical back pain related to posture or motion but no apparent radiographic instability. These patients may have a painful arc of motion during forward bending or extension or report a sense of shifting of their trunk with certain postures. Micromotion at the intervertebral segment may play a role in the pathogenesis of pain in these patients. There are currently no reliable methods of verifying

small degrees of instability, but intraoperative measurements of motion may provide more information in the future.

Diagnostic Testing

Patients with discogenic low back pain typically have MRI scans showing a degenerative disk without significant stenosis or herniation and concordant provocative diskography. Patients who have normal MRI scans correlate highly with negative lumbar diskograms, and such patients should be presumed to have a nondiscogenic cause of low back pain. Degenerative changes are interpreted with caution in older patients because of the ubiquitous nature of these changes in asymptomatic older patients. Patients who have obvious radiographic instability or multilevel severe degenerative disk and facet joint changes cannot be categorized as having diskogenic back pain. It is helpful to categorize patients into two groups: those who have radiographic evidence of loss of disk height and those who do not.

Patients With Loss of Disk Height

In patients with loss of disk height, plain radiographs show a decrease in disk height, which is often associated with vertebral end plate sclerosis or mild facet joint arthrosis. MRI will usually show a greater degree of degenerative changes at the disk. There is loss of disk height often associated with bulging of the posterior anulus fibrosus into the canal, some infolding of the ligamentum flavum, minor degrees of canal and foraminal stenosis, and abnormal signals at the vertebral end plate.

Provocative diskography is used to confirm the diagnosis of discogenic low back pain when surgery is being considered. The procedure is performed using fluoroscopic control with the patient awake. Several criteria must be met for a diskogram to be considered positive. There must be a concordant pain response from the patient, evidence of abnormal disk morphology on fluoroscopy and postdiskography CT examination, and negative control levels in the lumbar spine. Some authors report that low-pressure pain responses suggest a chemical pathway for pain generation and have better outcomes following fusion.

Although complications from the procedure are uncommon, diskography continues to be controversial. Positive diskograms have been found in up to 25% of patients who were only mildly symptomatic, which raises the risk of overdiagnosing discogenic disease. When using strict criteria, including low-pressure injection and a normal control disk, positive results may be as low as 30% in patients with chronic low back pain. Normal psychologic profiles have been reported in about 20% of patients with chronic low back pain who are candidates for diskography.

Patients Without Loss of Disk Height

Plain radiographs in patients without evidence of loss of disk height generally do not show any significant changes. Disk height is maintained, and there are no facet joint nor end plate changes. MRI typically shows mild changes such as desiccated disks with low signal on T2-weighted imaging or annular tears.

Prognosis

The natural history of acute low back pain is generally excellent. Ninety percent of patients will go on to complete pain relief within 2 to 6 weeks. In patients who have chronic pain, one study found that 40% of patients could be diagnosed as having discogenic back pain with positive diskograms at L4-L5 or L5-S1. There is limited information on the natural history of confirmed discogenic low back pain. One study found 68% of patients improved, 24% worsened, and 8% remained unchanged over a 5-year period.

Management

Anti-inflammatory, analgesic, and antispasmolytic medications are effective in the management of acute back pain, although their usefulness in managing chronic back pain is unclear. Gastrointestinal toxicity and renal impairment are concerns with the use of these drugs, especially in the elderly population. Flexible or rigid spinal supports may reduce lumbar mobility and decrease intradiskal pressure in certain positions of lumbar flexion. A program of physical therapy should be directed at ergonomic instruction, stretching maneuvers, and isometric stabilization exercises. Nonimpact type exercise such as swimming or cycling is recommended. Other measures used with varying degrees of success include acupuncture, hydrotherapy, ultrasound, biofeedback, electrical stimulation, manipulation, massage, and psychotherapy. Intradiskal electrothermal therapy has been proposed as an option in the management of discogenic back pain (see chapter 50).

Lumbar fusion is the surgical procedure of choice for the treatment of discogenic low back pain in patients who have intractable pain after an aggressive nonsurgical management program, MRI findings of disk degeneration, and concordant diskography at one or two levels. Disk excision or other disk decompression procedures are not recommended for these patients.

The fusion approach may be posterior, anterior, or both. Instrumentation is generally used with posterior fusion, and implants or bone graft are used with interbody fusion. Successful fusion is obtained in 60% to 90% of patients who undergo a posterior procedure, but clinical outcomes are satisfactory in only 40% to 70%. Even with posterior instrumentation, there is some motion across the disk space that may account for persistent symptoms in some patients. Residual symptoms in other patients may be associated with approach-related muscle denervation and necrosis or disruption of the adjacent facet joints. Posterior lumbar interbody fusion or transforaminal interbody fusion can allow posterior decompression and concurrent anterior column stabilization, while avoiding the morbidity of a separate anterior operation. The drawbacks include limitations on the size of the anterior graft or implant, nerve root injury, epidural fibrosis and chronic radiculitis, and potential instability from resection of the facet joints needed for exposure.

Anterior lumbar interbody fusion (ALIF) has several theoretic benefits in the treatment of discogenic low back pain. It can remove pain fibers and receptors from the anulus fibrosus and nucleus pulposus, eliminate motion across disk, restore disk height and indirectly decompress foramen, and enable surgeons to avoid posterior muscle disruption during the approach. Fusion rates are high, varying from 80% to 96% of patients. The disadvantages of the anterior approach are the risks of major vessel injury and, in males, retrograde ejaculation and impotence. Laparoscopic ALIF techniques require a skilled general surgeon for the approach and are more likely to be successful at the L5-S1 interspace. The type of anterior structural support used in ALIF surgery has received much attention. Autologous cancellous bone shows high fusion rates, but migration and collapse have been drawbacks. Threaded cages or machined allografts are being increasingly used with interbody fusion, with the aim of reducing the morbidity associated with bone graft harvest. Bone morphogenetic protein used within threaded interbody cages in ALIF shows high fusion rates and relief of back pain similar to autograft over the short term.

Annotated Bibliography

Lumbar Spinal Stenosis

Atlas SJ, Keller RB, Robson D, Deyo RA, Singer DE: Surgical and nonsurgical management of lumbar spinal stenosis: 4-year outcomes from the Maine Lumbar Spine Study. *Spine* 2000;25:556-562.

A cohort of 119 patients underwent either surgical or nonsurgical treatment and were followed for 4 years. Seventy percent of surgically treated patients and 52% of nonsurgically treated patients reported improvement in symptoms. The authors report that the relative benefits of surgery diminished over time but remained superior to those of nonsurgically treated patients.

Fischgrund JS, Mackay M, Herkowitz HN, Brower R, Montgomery D, Kurz LT: Degenerative lumbar spondylolisthesis with spinal stenosis: A prospective, randomized study comparing decompressive laminectomy and arthrodesis with and without spinal instrumentation. *Spine* 1997;22:2807-2812.

This randomized study showed that fusion rates were superior in instrumented patients undergoing single level surgery, but overall clinical improvement was identical in instrumented and noninstrumented groups.

Iguchi T, Kurihara A, Nakayama J, Sato K, Kurosaka M, Yamasaki K: Minimum 10-year outcome of decompressive laminectomy for degenerative lumbar spinal stenosis. *Spine* 2000;25:1754-1759.

In this study, decompressive laminectomies without fusion in patients older than 60 years were shown to produce long-term satisfactory results in more than half of the patients. The authors concluded that the presence of sagittal rotation of more than 10° in patients needing multiple laminectomies may be related to deterioration of outcome.

Katz JN, Lipson SJ, Lew RA, et al: Lumbar laminectomy alone or with instrumented or noninstrumented arthrodesis in degenerative lumbar spinal stenosis: Patient selection, costs, and surgical outcomes. *Spine* 1997;22:1123-1131.

The authors of this study report that adding arthrodesis to decompression for spinal stenosis depends primarily on surgeon preference and that noninstrumented fusions produce superior relief of back pain, whereas instrumentation adds substantial costs to the treatment.

Rao RD, Wang M, Singhal P, McGrady LM, Rao S: Intradiscal pressure and kinematic behavior of lumbar spine after bilateral laminotomy and laminectomy. *Spine J* 2002;2:320-326.

This article presents a biomechanical analysis of bilateral laminotomy as an alternative to wide laminectomy in the decompression of patients with lumbar spinal stenosis.

Lumbar Disk Herniation

Atlas SJ, Keller RB, Chang Y, Deyo RA, Singer DE: Surgical and nonsurgical management of sciatica secondary to a lumbar disc herniation: Five-year outcomes from the Maine Lumbar Spine Study. *Spine* 2001;26:1179-1187.

A 5-year follow-up of 402 patients showed that 70% of surgically treated patients and 56% of nonsurgically treated patients reported improvement in their predominant symptoms. Patients with moderate or severe symptoms did better after surgery than after nonsurgical care.

Carragee EJ, Han MY, Suen PW, Kim D: Clinical outcomes after lumbar discectomy for sciatica: The effects of fragment type and annular competence. *J Bone Joint Surg Am* 2003;85:102-108.

This prospective study correlated intraoperative morphologic patterns of disk herniation with outcomes following surgical intervention, with particular reference to reherniation, reoperation rates, and the incidence of persistent symptoms.

Osterman H, Sund R, Seitsalo S, Keskimaki I: Risk of multiple reoperations after lumbar discectomy: A population-based study. *Spine* 2003;28:621-627.

This 11-year review of 35,309 patients who underwent diskectomy showed that 14% had at least one more operation, whereas 2.3% had two or more operations. Sixty-three percent of the second operations were diskectomies, 14% were fusions, and 23% were decompressions.

Yorimitsu E, Chiba K, Toyama Y, Hirabayashi K: Long-term outcomes of standard discectomy for lumbar disc herniation. *Spine* 2001;26:652-657.

In this study, 74% of patients who underwent lumbar diskectomy reported some back pain at 10 years, although disabling pain was reported in only 12.7%. Decreased disk height was associated with more disability, whereas recurrent herniations were more common in those with preserved disk height.

Discogenic Low Back Pain

Fritzell P, Hagg O, Wessberg P: Nordwall Anders, Swedish Lumbar Spine Study Group: Lumbar fusion versus nonsurgical treatment for chronic low back pain. *Spine* 2001;26:2521-2534.

This randomized controlled multicenter study showed that lumbar fusion in a carefully selected group of patients with severe chronic low back pain decreases pain and disability more than nonsurgical treatment.

Riew KD, Yin Y, Gilula L, Bridwell KH, Lenke LG, Lauryssen CC, Goette K: The effect of nerve-root injections on the need for operative treatment of lumbar radicular pain: A prospective, randomized, controlled, double-blind study. *J Bone Joint Surg Am* 2000;82:1589-1593.

This prospective study demonstrated the efficacy of selective nerve root injections of corticosteroid in patients with lumbar radiculopathy. Twenty of 28 patients who received injection of bupivacaine and betamethasone declined surgery over a 13- to 28-month period after receiving one to four injections, whereas the remainder of the patients eventually underwent surgery.

Classic Bibliography

Abumi K, Panjabi MM, Kramer KM, Duranceau J, Oxland T, Crisco JJ: Biomechanical evaluation of lumbar spinal stability after graded facetectomies. *Spine* 1990;15:1142-1147.

Bogduk N, Tynan W, Wilson AS: The nerve supply to the human lumbar intervertebral discs. *J Anat* 1981;132:39-56.

Freemont AJ, Peacock TE, Goupille P, Hoyland JA, O'Brien J, Jayson MI: Nerve ingrowth into diseased intervertebral disc in chronic back pain. *Lancet* 1997;350:178-181.

Herkowitz HN, Kurz LT: Degenerative lumbar spondylolisthesis with spinal stenosis: A prospective study comparing decompression with decompression and intertransverse process arthrodesis. *J Bone Joint Surg Am* 1991;73:802-808.

Kuslich SD, Ulstrom CL, Michael CJ: The tissue origin of low back pain and sciatica: A report of pain response to tissue stimulation during operations on the lumbar spine using local anesthesia. *Orthop Clin North Am* 1991;22:181-187.

Mixter WJ, Barr JS: Rupture of the intervertebral disc with involvement of the spinal canal. *N Engl J Med* 1934;211:210-215.

Turner JA, Ersek M: Herron L, Deyo R: Surgery for lumbar spinal stenosis: Attempted meta-analysis of the literature. *Spine* 1992;17:1-8.

Weber H: Lumbar disc herniation: A controlled, prospective study with 10 years of observation. *Spine* 1983;8:131-140.

Chapter 45

Spondylolysis-Spondylolisthesis

Thomas J. Puschak, MD

Rick C. Sasso, MD

Introduction

Spondylolysis refers to a bony defect in the pars interarticularis, which is the isthmus or bony bridge that connects the superior and inferior articular facets of the posterior neural arch. Spondylolysis can occur unilaterally or bilaterally and is an acquired condition because it has never been reported at birth. Spondylolysis is more common in males and occurs in approximately 6% of the general population. A higher prevalence (up to 53%) is seen in Eskimo populations. Also, athletes who participate in sports that repeatedly cause the spine to be hyperextended, such as gymnastics, football, and wrestling, may have an increased predisposition to developing spondylolysis. Spondylolysis occurs most often at L5, with decreasing incidence at the more cranial lumbar levels. Several factors have been implicated in the etiology of spondylolysis; however, the primary lesion is believed to be a stress fracture of the pars interarticularis that remains unhealed. This theory is supported by the fact that there are no reported instances of spondylolysis in patients who have never walked. There also seems to be a genetic predisposition for spondylolysis because relatives of index cases have a greater than fourfold increased incidence.

Spondylolisthesis refers to the translation of a vertebral body on the caudal vertebra. This translation can be anterior, lateral, or posterior. The term comes from the Latin roots *spondy*, which means "the spine," and *olisthesis*, which means "a slipping." Spondylolisthesis most often occurs in the lower lumbar spine. Several different forms of spondylolisthesis exist and can be classified by severity of slip, etiology, and potential for progression.

Classification Systems

Meyerding

The Meyerding classification system is a radiographic system based on the severity of vertebral slippage. Slips are classified as grade 1 through grade 4 based on the percentage of translation of the cranial vertebra on the caudal vertebra. The superior end plate of the caudal vertebra is divided into quarters, and the percentage of slippage is recorded. Grade 1 is 0 to 25% slippage (Figure 1), grade 2 is 26% to 50%, grade 3 is 51% to 75% (Figure 2), and grade 4 is 76% to 100% (Figure 3). Slippage of 100% or more is referred to as spondyloptosis. This classification system is frequently used because it is simple and reliable.

Wiltse and Associates

The Wiltse and associates classification system is based on anatomic etiology and classically consists of five types of spondylolisthesis, although iatrogenic postoperative instability is sometimes included as a sixth type. Type 1 slips are dysplastic or congenital. These occur at the lumbosacral junction as a result of incomplete or inadequate development of the facet joints and superior sacral end plate. Facets are often sagittally oriented and the superior end plate of S1 is rounded or domed, which predisposes patients to slippage. The intact pars interarticularis usually limits slippage to approximately 30%. Spondyloptosis can occur, and patients with higher-grade slips of this type can develop significant neurologic symptoms from severe stenosis resulting from an intact pars interarticularis. Type 2 slips are referred to as lytic or isthmic because they are secondary to defects of the pars interarticularis. There are three subtypes in this category: a pars defect, an elongated pars (possibly caused by repeated fracture and healing of the pars), and an acute pars fracture. Type 3 slips are degenerative and occur as a result of the incompetence of arthritic facet joints in the degenerative lumbar spine. Degenerative spondylolisthesis can occur with or without spinal stenosis. Type 4 slips are caused by traumatic injuries to the posterior neural arch in areas other than the pars interarticularis and lead to a destabilization of the facet joints. Type 5 slips are caused by pathologic destabilization of the spine from tumors, infection, and other systemic diseases.

Marchetti and Bartolozzi

The system described by Marchetti and Bartolozzi attempts to classify spondylolisthesis based on anatomic

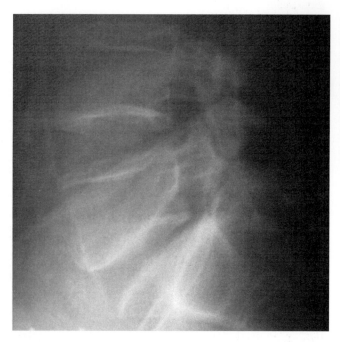

Figure 1 Lateral radiograph showing a Meyerding grade 1 slip.

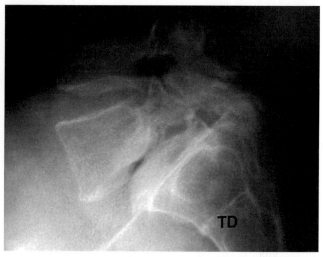

Figure 2 Lateral radiograph showing a Meyerding grade 3 slip. Dysplastic features such as a trapezoidal L5 body and rounded sacral dome are often seen in slips that progress beyond Meyerding grade 2.

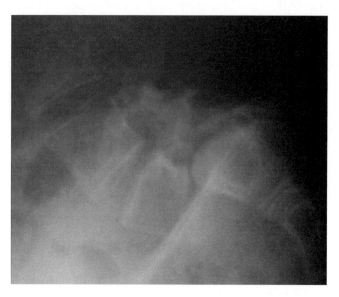

Figure 3 Lateral radiograph showing a Meyerding grade 4 slip. As in Figure 2, significant dysplastic features are present.

etiology and prognostic factors. Slips are divided into two main categories: developmental and acquired. Developmental spondylolisthesis is categorized as either high dysplastic or low dysplastic. Dysplastic features of the anterior and posterior elements, which lead to instability, characterize developmental slips. Posteriorly, the pars interarticularis, laminae, or facets may be incompetent; anteriorly, the L5 body tends to be trapezoidal and oriented toward the floor and the S1 superior end plate tends to be rounded. Low dysplastic slips tend to have less profound dysplastic features than high dysplastic

slips, and therefore, they have less potential for slip progression.

Acquired spondylolisthesis occurs as a result of acquired pathology, such as pars defects, trauma, degenerative facets, pathologic instability, and iatrogenic injury. The main difference between the developmental and acquired categories is that the basic spinal architecture is developed normally in the acquired group and therefore has more potential stability or less potential for progression of slippage.

Diagnostic Imaging
Plain Radiographs
Initial assessment should at least consist of standing AP and lateral radiographs. The standing position may accentuate existing translational deformity. Spondylolisthesis can be missed on supine lateral films up to 20% of the time because of reduction of the deformity when the patient is in the supine position. Standing films may also accentuate angular deformities better than those obtained with the patient supine. Pars interarticularis defects and other defects of the posterior arch such as spina bifida occulta may be identified on AP views. In patients with high-grade slips with significant angulation of the cephalad vertebra, a Napoleon's hat sign may be seen on AP views (Figure 4). A standard AP view may not be helpful for visualization of the pedicles and other surgical anatomy in patients with high-grade slips. In these patients, a Ferguson view (AP radiograph angled 30° cephalad) will yield a true AP view of the lumbosacral junction.

Although pars interarticularis defects are usually identifiable on lateral films, right and left oblique radiographs may help in the diagnosis of subtle pars defects not readily seen on AP or lateral views.

Dynamic flexion-extension lateral radiographs can be helpful in assessing translational stability. Patients with bilateral pars interarticularis defects as well as those with arthritic degenerative facets (especially sagittally oriented facets) may elicit significant translational motion on flexion-extension radiographs that is not evident on standing lateral films. The difficulty in interpreting dynamic radiographs is that there is no clear consensus on the definition of normal translational motion. Traditionally, the definition of instability is greater than 3 mm of translation on flexion-extension views. Several clinical studies have reported large variations in translational motion in asymptomatic individuals. Also, the reliability of dynamic studies is questionable because the quality of the study depends on the effort of the individual. Dynamic radiographs can be valuable diagnostic tools when used in conjunction with other data, but they should not be used as the sole criteria for treatment.

Computed Tomography

CT scans are useful in the diagnosis of occult pars interarticularis defects. Thin section cuts (1 to 2 mm) should be obtained because larger axial sections may miss the defects. Sagittal reconstruction technology is also helpful because pars interarticularis defects may be difficult to see on axial images. These defects often lie in a similar plane to the axial cuts. Pars interarticularis defects tend to lie more dorsal and posterior to the facet joints on the axial images and are often associated with significant bony and cartilaginous overgrowth. In the degenerative spine, axial CT images allow assessment of the orientation of facet joints (coronal or sagittal) to help determine the relative stability of a segment after decompression. CT scans are also helpful in assessing surgical bony anatomy, such as pedicle size and orientation.

Myelograms in conjunction with CT scans are helpful in assessment of the neuroanatomy. Although central and lateral recess stenosis is easily identified, foraminal stenosis may be missed because the compression occurs lateral to the root sleeve beyond the extent of the myelogram dye.

Magnetic Resonance Imaging

MRI scans are not often helpful in identifying spondylitic defects. They are most helpful in the evaluation of the neuroanatomy and disks. Central and lateral recess stenosis caused by facet hypertrophy, overgrown pars interarticularis defects, and translational offset is easily seen. Also, sagittal images allow accurate assessment of the nerve root in the foramina.

MRI scans can evaluate the status of the intervertebral disks at the affected and adjacent levels. Normal disks appear bright on T2-weighted images because of good hydration, and they appear dark when degeneration (relative dehydration) is present. Reactive bony

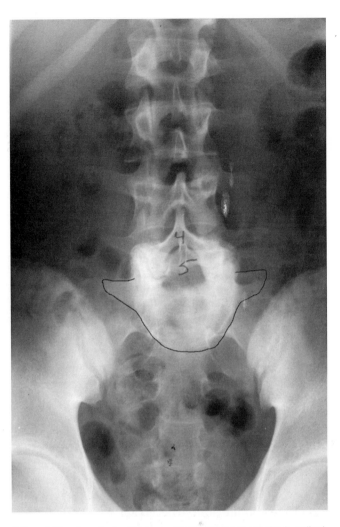

Figure 4 AP radiograph of a high-grade slip. The Napoleon's hat sign is outlined. Severe angulation of the L5 body allows an end-on axial projection on AP views.

end plate changes are also signs of disk degeneration. Often disks adjacent to slips may be radiographically normal, but they elicit significant degenerative changes on MRI, which must be considered during surgical planning. Although knowing the status of the adjacent disk is important, there are no conclusive findings that warrant routinely incorporating the adjacent degenerative level in patients with spondylolisthesis.

Nuclear Medicine Studies

Technetium bone scans have been historically popular in the diagnosis of spondylolysis. These scans are used to determine the acuteness of a pars injury, with positive scans suggesting a more acute injury and greater potential for healing with bracing or conservative care. Negative scans indicate an old or chronic defect with little healing potential. Recently, single photon emission CT has been shown to be more specific and sensitive in detecting radiographically occult pars defects than technetium scans.

Degenerative Spondylolisthesis

Pathogenesis/Pathoanatomy

Degenerative spondylolisthesis tends to occur in patients older than 60 years. It is more prevalent in women and more common in African Americans than Caucasians. It occurs five to six times more frequently at L4-5 than at L3-4 or L5-S1. The average amount of anterior slippage is 15% to 33%. Hormonal influence may contribute to the development of degenerative spondylolisthesis. The increased incidence in women with a history of pregnancy may be the result of increased ligamentous and joint laxity in conjunction with a large flexion moment on the lumbar spine.

The role of facet joint orientation has also been investigated as a potential cause of degenerative spondylolisthesis. Several authors have shown a positive correlation between sagittally oriented facet joints and a predisposition for spondylolisthesis. A bilateral facet angle greater than 45° at L4-5 has been shown to result in a 25-fold increased incidence of degenerative spondylolisthesis. The L5-S1 facet joint tends to be oriented more in the coronal plane, offering greater resistance to anterior translational forces. This orientation may explain the greater incidence of degenerative spondylolisthesis at L4-5 than at L5-S1.

Degenerative changes in the intervertebral disk combined with hormonal factors and facet orientation can lead to intersegmental instability. Disk space collapse leads to buckling of the ligamentum flavum and altered stress loading of the facet joints. Ligamentous laxity and remodeling of the facet joints create a hypermobile segment, which leads to spondylolisthesis. The hypertrophy and buckling of ligamentum flavum combined with bony translational offset lead to central canal stenosis. Hypertrophy of the facet joints creates lateral recess and foraminal stenosis. Facet cysts, often associated with advanced degenerative facet arthrosis, can add to the degree of nerve root compromise in the lateral recess.

Natural History

Few data are available regarding the natural history of degenerative spondylolisthesis. Severe disk space narrowing has been shown to be associated with a lower likelihood of progression of slippage. In a study following patients with degenerative spondylolisthesis who were treated nonsurgically over 10 years, 76% of patients without neurologic symptoms remained symptom free. Eighty-six percent of patients with lower extremity complaints saw an initial improvement in symptoms; however, 37% had redevelopment of symptoms. Eighty-three percent of patients presenting with neurologic symptoms who refused surgical treatment eventually experienced a deterioration of symptoms. Although degenerative spondylolisthesis symptoms tend to be intermittent, complete resolution of symptoms is not likely.

Clinical Presentation

Patients with degenerative spondylolisthesis initially report low back pain secondary to the degenerative changes in the spine. These are usually mechanical complaints worsened with activity and improved with rest. With time, neurogenic back pain may develop in which pain is exacerbated with prolonged standing or walking and improved with sitting and flexion. The back pain tends to be located in the lower lumbar and buttock region and is often described as an aching, burning, or pulling sensation.

As nerve compression progresses, lower extremity symptoms increase. Leg pain may be unilateral or bilateral and neuroclaudicatory or radicular in nature. Symptoms tend to be worsened in an upright or extended posture and improved with sitting and flexion. The L5 root is most commonly affected; however, in patients with instability and foraminal stenosis, the L4 roots are also involved. Reflexes are often diminished or absent, and sensation may be anywhere from normal to severely impaired. Bladder dysfunction only occurs in 3% to 4% of patients.

Peripheral neuropathy must be considered in patients with a history of diabetes and stocking glove pattern dysesthesias. Other diagnoses that can mimic spinal stenosis symptoms are cervical myelopathy and primary hip disease with anterior thigh pain.

Nonsurgical Management

Most patients with degenerative spondylolisthesis will respond to nonsurgical treatment. Initial treatment is focused on the mechanical back pain and consists of a short rest period, administration of nonsteroidal anti-inflammatory drugs, a short course of oral analgesics, and passive physical therapy modalities. Once the acute pain phase is controlled, active physical therapy can be instituted for trunk stabilization and aerobic conditioning. Avoidance of hyperextension activities is recommended to limit recurrence of acute episodes.

Similarly, leg symptoms from spinal stenosis can be managed with rest, nonsteroidal anti-inflammatory drugs, and oral analgesics. Oral steroids and injectable steroids in the form of epidural steroid injections or selective nerve root blocks may also be used. Despite being somewhat controversial and lacking significant prospective data proving their efficacy, epidural steroid injections are widely used and are often effective (if only in temporizing lower extremity symptoms).

Surgical Management

The main goals of surgery are pain reduction, restoration of function, and preservation of neurologic function. The most common indication for surgery is persistent incapacitating claudication and radicular leg pain, which significantly compromises function, and the failure of 6 to 12 weeks of nonsurgical therapy to relieve symptoms. Absolute indications for surgery include progressive and evolving motor deficits and cauda equina syndrome. Surgical intervention should address the two components of degenerative spondylolisthesis—spinal stenosis and instability.

The management of spinal stenosis includes laminectomy or laminotomy with partial or total facetectomy. Depending on symptoms, decompression may be unilateral or bilateral. All regions of compression must be addressed because incomplete decompression of the lateral recess and stenosis can lead to persistent symptoms and poor outcome. Outcomes of decompression without fusion in the face of degenerative spondylolisthesis are mixed. Several studies show significant improvement in leg symptoms initially; however, up to 33% of patients had severe worsening of back and leg symptoms by 5 years, with nearly 25% requiring reoperation for the treatment of recurrence of stenosis and/or progression of instability. In one study, more than half of the patients with decompression alone were unable to walk more than two blocks after 3 to 6 years, and 25% of patients were very dissatisfied with the treatment outcome.

Several studies have addressed the role of arthrodesis in addition to decompression for the treatment of degenerative spondylolisthesis. In a prospective randomized study comparing decompression alone to decompression with posterolateral noninstrumented fusion, at 3-year follow-up 96% of the patients who underwent decompression alone had radiographic slip progression compared with 28% of those in the arthrodesis group. Despite a pseudarthrosis rate of 36%, 96% of patients in the arthrodesis group had good or excellent results compared with 44% of those who underwent decompression alone.

Numerous studies have also assessed the effects of using instrumentation in conjunction with arthrodesis. A randomized prospective study comparing single-level laminectomy and posterolateral fusion with and without transpedicular fixation showed that the addition of instrumentation significantly improves fusion rates. Despite the significant difference in fusion rates, in 83% of patients in the instrumented group versus 45% of those in the noninstrumented group, there was no significant difference in clinical outcomes, with 78% to 85% of those in both groups reporting good and excellent results. Several other authors have reported an improvement in both fusion rates and clinical outcomes when comparing instrumented and noninstrumented fusions for the treatment of patients with degenerative spondylolisthesis.

When surgical treatment is indicated, a thorough decompression is mandatory, and the addition of arthrodesis improves intermediate- and long-term outcomes. The addition of instrumentation increases fusion rates, but it

has not been shown to consistently improve outcome over noninstrumented arthrodesis. No known randomized prospective data have been published to date regarding the role of interbody fusion in the treatment of degenerative spondylolisthesis.

Acquired Isthmic Spondylolisthesis in Adults
Pathogenesis/Pathoanatomy
The primary lesion responsible for isthmic or lytic spondylolisthesis is a defect of the pars interarticularis. Several etiologies for this defect have been proposed, including acute or chronic traumatic injuries. Congenital abnormalities can contribute to instability as well. There are several types of pars defects: chronic stress fractures, elongated pars from healing of multiple stress fractures over time, and acute pars fractures. These lesions are acquired, not congenital, and result from repeated microtrauma of the pars as it is loaded in extension. Isthmic spondylolisthesis occurs at L5-S1 in 82% of patients compared with 11% at L4-5 and 0.5% at L3-4 and L2-3. Forces in the lumbar spine are greatest at the lumbosacral junction and likely are the reason for the high prevalence of pars defects at L5-S1.

Natural History
Relatively few patients with spondylolysis will acquire spondylolisthesis. Those who do typically have some associated dysplastic features such that the true incidence of acquired isthmic spondylolisthesis may be much less. Many patients who eventually acquire spondylolisthesis are asymptomatic. True acquired slips are almost always grade I or II and rarely progress beyond grade I or II severity unless there is dysplasia present. Isthmic spondylolisthesis that progresses beyond Meyerding grade II almost always is associated with dysplasia as well.

Progression of isthmic spondylolisthesis is most common in the adolescent population. Significant increase in slippage in adulthood is uncommon. In contrast to the L5-S1 isthmic slip, lesions at L4-5 or other more cranial levels may remain unstable into the third and fourth decades of life, with progression of translation and increase in back and leg symptoms. An isthmic lesion at L4-5 is less stiff in sagittal rotation and shear translation than a lesion at L5-S1. Overloading a lesion at L4-5 may lead to premature translational wear of the disk, contribute to the inherent instability of the segment, and may be the reason why previously asymptomatic isthmic slips at L4-5 progress later in adulthood.

Clinical Presentation
The most common presenting symptom is low back pain. Patients often have a long history of periodic self-limited low back pain episodes that vary in intensity and/or duration. Neurologic deficits are infrequent be-

cause slips rarely progress beyond grade II and the relative detachment of the posterior arch prevents significant central canal stenosis. Patients may present with unilateral or bilateral radiculopathy. Radicular symptoms may be caused by nerve root irritation from the reactive tissue around the pars defect combined with the micromotion of the unstable posterior arch. Additionally, significant foraminal stenosis may occur as a result of loss of sagittal foraminal height from the translation and degeneration of the intervertebral disk. Typically, the exiting nerve root (L5) is most affected for an L5-S1 isthmic spondylolisthesis.

Nonsurgical Treatment

Most patients with acquired isthmic spondylolisthesis will respond to nonsurgical management. Medical treatment should follow similar guidelines for nonspecific low back pain. Oral anti-inflammatory drugs may reduce acute pain and improve function. Long-term use of these drugs should be avoided if possible because of potential renal and gastrointestinal adverse effects. Narcotic pain medication, muscle relaxers, and other controlled substances should be used with extreme caution and definitely should be avoided in long-term treatment.

There are no known studies that address the role of injections in the facet joints or pars defects in patients with isthmic spondylolisthesis. Injection of local anesthetic and corticosteroid into the facets or pars defects may have therapeutic effects. However, diagnostic information from these injections is at best difficult to interpret because the pars defects often communicate with the facet joints, causing an uncontrolled extravasation of steroid and local anesthetic. In patients with radicular symptoms, selective nerve blocks or epidural steroid injections may be used for diagnostic and therapeutic purposes. No prospective studies have yet been conducted that address the effectiveness of these injections in isthmic spondylolisthesis.

The use of external bracing in the treatment of patients with acquired isthmic spondylolisthesis has been reported. In addition, patients may benefit from initial rest in the acute phase followed by physical therapy that is focused on strengthening of the abdominal and lumbosacral muscles. Physical therapy has been shown to decrease pain and functional disability. Once the acute pain is resolved, the focus of physical therapy is on hamstring stretching, pelvic tilts, and abdominal and pelvic stabilizer strengthening for approximately 6 months.

Surgical Treatment

Failure of conservative management (persistence of pain, progression of neurologic symptoms, or progression of slippage) is an indication for surgical treatment. Numerous approaches to surgical reconstruction have been used. These approaches include anterior interbody fusion, posterolateral fusion with and without instrumentation, anterior-posterior procedures, and posterior interbody procedures.

Posterolateral fusion is commonly used to treat patients with isthmic spondylolisthesis. Midline dissection is performed laterally over the facet joints and transverse processes and sacral alae. Abundant lateral bone graft leads to stabilization of the segment by intertransverse process fusion. A Gill laminectomy may be done in conjunction with the posterior fusion. Removal of the loose lamina and inflammatory pars defect allows decompression of the nerve roots, direct visualization of the pedicles for hardware placement, and potentially removes part of the inflammatory back pain generator. In addition, the laminectomy bone may be processed for bone graft. Although the roles of instrumentation and decompression with posterolateral fusion remain controversial, Gill decompression without fusion is not recommended. Potential complications of the posterior approach include infection, dural tear, nerve root injury, hematoma, and pedicle fracture.

Anterior lumbar interbody fusion (ALIF) can be successfully used to treat isthmic spondylolisthesis even when radicular symptoms are present. Although the direct decompression of nerves is difficult, indirect decompression can be obtained by foraminal distraction. A transabdominal retroperitoneal approach is usually used to minimize the risk to abdominal viscera. Caudal to the iliac vessels, cautery should be used sparingly to decrease the risk of injuring the presacral nerves, which may result in retrograde ejaculation and sexual dysfunction. The anterior approach allows for an aggressive diskectomy with good removal of cartilage from the vertebral end plates and increase of the fusion surface area. Additionally, anterior grafts provide excellent anterior column support and may aid in partial reduction of the slip as well as restoration of disk space height. The choice of graft material is generally based on surgeon preference and includes autologous iliac crest, structural allograft, and various metallic cages packed with autogenous cancellous graft. This method of anterior diskectomy and interbody fusion cannot be done in patients with high-grade spondylolisthesis because of the presence of significant translational and angular deformity. Risks of the anterior approach include wound infection, vascular injury, deep venous thrombosis, pulmonary embolism, sympathetic chain injury, retrograde ejaculation, and ventral hernia.

Stand-alone ALIF reconstruction for patients with isthmic spondylolisthesis works best for those with a Meyerding grade 1 slip. Several clinical studies have shown adequate results with good and excellent results ranging from 87% to 94% at 2 years. One study reported that 75% of patients had excellent and 20% had satisfactory results at 10-year follow-up. The fusion rates in these studies did not correlate with clinical outcome. Some patients had good clinical improvement despite eventually having a pseudarthrosis. Persistent leg pain may occur as a result of inadequate indirect foraminal decompression. Patients may also have persistent low back pain because of the pain fibers present in the inflammatory tissue of the pars interarticularis defect, which is not removed with an isolated anterior approach. Nociceptive pain fibers are histologically present in the pars interarticularis defect.

Circumferential (360°) fusion can be accomplished by a combined anterior-posterior fusion or by a posterolateral fusion combined with a posterior lumbar interbody fusion (PLIF) or transforaminal lumbar interbody fusion. Both techniques provide anterior column support, foraminal distraction, posterior stabilization, arthrodesis, and the ability to perform a Gill laminectomy decompression if indicated. Three series have shown excellent success with circumferential procedures when compared with other approaches alone. In one study, posterolateral fusion alone was compared with posterolateral fusion combined with posterior lumbar interbody fusion. Outcomes were comparable when good and excellent results were grouped together (95% and 97%, respectively). However, the circumferential group had 75% excellent results compared with 45% in the posterolateral fusion group. Several other studies have shown higher fusion rates for circumferential fusions when compared with anterior or posterior fusions alone. Specific risks related to circumferential fusions include increased surgical time, more blood loss, and potentially longer hospital stays.

Developmental Spondylolisthesis

Developmental spondylolisthesis was formerly referred to as congenital spondylolisthesis. Current thought is that the defects and slip are not present at birth but develop over time. Unlike acquired isthmic spondylolisthesis, the pars fractures are thought to develop as a result of the slippage rather than causing the slip. The dysplastic nature of this type of spondylolisthesis often leads to the development of high-grade slips. Developmental spondylolisthesis is the most common type of slip seen in children, and as such will be covered in greater detail in chapter 66. The focus of this section will be on the treatment of high-grade spondylolisthesis in adults.

Pathomechanics/Pathogenesis

Developmental spondylolisthesis is categorized as either high dysplastic or low dysplastic slips based on radiographic findings. Radiographic findings include deficiencies of the posterior arch, a trapezoidal L5 body, rounded sacral dome, incompetent L5-S1 disk, and poorly formed facet articulations. Severe lumbosacral kyphosis with verticalization of the sacrum and hyper-

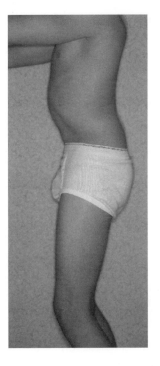

Figure 5 Preoperative photograph of a patient with a high-grade slip. Note the crouching posture caused by severe hamstring tightness. Upper lumbar hyperlordosis is also seen.

lordosis of the upper lumbar spine usually develops. This type of slip has the highest risk for malignant progression. Patients with this type of slip and an intact pars interarticularis must be observed closely because they may develop cauda equina syndrome as the slip progresses.

Low dysplastic slips also tend to occur at the lumbosacral junction. This type of slip is characterized by dysplastic changes in the posterior elements with relatively normal anatomy anteriorly. These slips are less likely to progress given the increased stability of the relatively normal anterior structures. A vertical sacrum and hyperlordosis are not traditionally seen in patients with low dysplastic slips.

Clinical Presentation

Most developmental spondylolisthesis presents in adolescence during the growth spurt. The disease course of patients with low dysplastic slips may progress slowly; consequently, these patients may not present until early adulthood. Traditionally, patients present with severe acute low back pain without neurologic findings. Some patients present in a listhetic crisis (severe back pain, hamstring spasm, and various neurologic deficits). Patients walk with a crouched gait because of severe hamstring tightness (Figure 5). Compensatory upper lumbar hyperlordosis often creates a significant abdominal crease (Figure 6). Neurologic symptoms range from isolated radiculopathy resulting from the stretch of exiting nerve roots to cauda equina syndrome in patients with high-grade slips and intact posterior arches. Because these slips usually occur at the lumbosacral junction, the

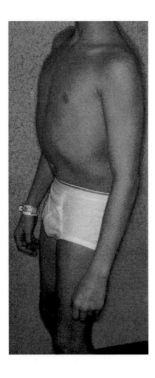

Figure 6 Photograph of a patient with the combination of severe lumbosacral kyphosis with compensatory upper lumbar hyperlordosis, which typically creates a prominent abdominal crease in patients with high-grade spondylolisthesis.

L5 nerve roots are most commonly affected. Some adults with high-grade slips may have subtle bowel and bladder neurologic symptoms resulting from the slow progression of slip over time and may warrant urologic evaluation.

Treatment Algorithm
Treatment recommendations are based on the type of slip (high dysplastic slips versus low dysplastic slips), patient age, neurologic status, slip severity, and the patient's symptoms.

In Situ Fusion
Posterior in situ fusion has been a widely recommended surgical treatment for patients with spondylolisthesis because of the low rates of neurologic injury and high rates of clinical success. Several techniques have been used for in situ fusion, including posterior, posterolateral, anterior interbody, and posterior interbody fusion—all of which can be done with or without instrumentation. In situ fusion with decompression has been shown to provide good results when neurologic symptoms are present preoperatively. Other studies show that in situ fusion without decompression can be effective in treating back pain and radicular symptoms. In one study in which eight high-grade slips were treated with in situ fusion without decompression, all patients achieved fusion and had good resolution of their back and radicular symptoms. In the presence of progressing neurologic deficits or cauda equina symptoms, decompression should be performed in addition to fusion. In the absence of these neurologic symptoms, in situ fusion

without decompression may be considered.

The indication for instrumentation is not well defined. Good clinical results with noninstrumented in situ fusion have been reported in several studies; however, postoperative slip progression has been reported even after successful arthrodesis. The addition of instrumentation may help increase fusion rates and decrease the risk for postoperative slip progression; however, this has not been definitively proven. One randomized prospective study comparing in situ fusions with and without instrumentation found that at 2-year follow-up there was no significant difference in fusion rates and that pain and functional disability were similar in the two groups.

The addition of interbody fusion may help increase fusion rates and minimize progression of slippage postoperatively. The traditional ALIF and PLIF techniques described earlier are not possible in patients with high-grade slips when in situ fusion is performed because of the presence of significant translational and angular deformities. Interbody fusion using fibular struts placed across the L5-S1 disk space through the bodies of L5 and S1 has been described (Figure 7). This technique was first reported with the grafts placed from posterior to anterior after a wide posterior decompression and then augmented with a posterolateral fusion. Patients were followed for 2 to 12 years, and all patients achieved fusion and had significant or complete resolution of preoperative neurologic deficits. This technique has also been described with placement of the grafts from an anterior approach with similar results. No difference in outcomes has been reported when comparing allograft and autogenous fibula.

Reduction
The indications for reduction of spondylolisthesis are extremely controversial, and there are currently no widely accepted reduction guidelines. Reduction of the translational displacement and slip angle may occur independently, either partially or fully. The argument for reduction is to restore sagittal alignment, reduce lumbosacral kyphosis and translation, and restore the normal lumbosacral biomechanics.

The main detraction of using reduction in the treatment of patients with high-grade slips is the risk of significant associated complications. Neurologic complications include L5 and S1 nerve root injuries, paresis, paralysis, cauda equina syndrome, sensory deficits, bowel/bladder dysfunction, and sexual dysfunction. Other complications include nonunion, hardware failure, sacral fracture, dural tear, graft resorption, loss of fixation, and prolonged immobilization or bed rest secondary to unstable fixation. Reported rates of neurologic deficits range from 8% to 30% after reduction of high-grade slips. Although most of these deficits are transitory, permanent deficits have been reported. High

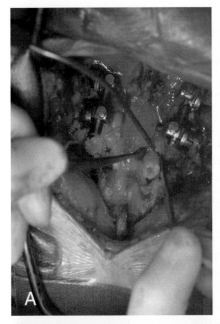

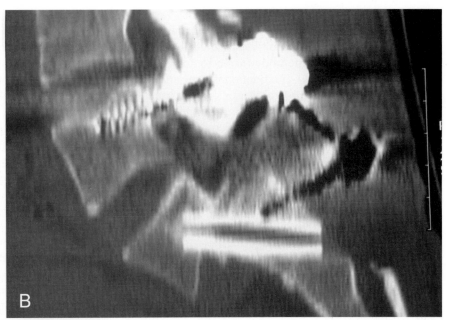

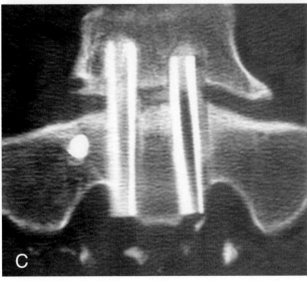

Figure 7 A, Intraoperative photograph of the placement of a transsacral fibula posterior interbody graft. The cauda equina is protected with nerve root retractors as the graft is placed across the L5-S1 disk space through the sacrum and L5 body from a posterior approach. **B,** Postoperative sagittal reconstruction CT scan of a transsacral fibular graft. **C,** Axial CT scan of transsacral fibular grafts in which the grafts are placed bilaterally and purchase in both the S1 and L5 bodies is seen on the same CT cut because of the severity of the slip.

rates of pseudarthrosis, progression of slippage, and hardware failure have also been reported after reduction and posterolateral instrumented fusion. One study reported implant failure in five of six patients who had an isolated posterolateral instrumented fusion following reduction. The addition of anterior interbody fusion after reduction and posterolateral instrumented fusion has been shown to decrease these complications.

Recent improvements in spinal instrumentation have increased the interest in the use of open reduction to treat patients with spondylolisthesis. Several techniques have been described. One technique involves pedicle screw instrumentation from L4 to S1 or S2. A wide decompression is performed so that the nerve roots are directly visualized during reduction. Distraction and poste-

rior translation forces are used to gradually reduce the slip. In the past, repeated wake-up tests were used during the reduction. Electrophysiologic monitoring (somatosensory-evoked potentials, electromyograms, and motor-evoked potentials) should be used with this procedure.

High rates of implant failure and loss of reduction have been reported when reduction is performed and only posterior instrumented fusion is used for stabilization. The reduction of the spondylolisthesis normalizes the shear forces at the lumbosacral junction; however, an anterior column defect is also created by the reduction. Posterior instrumentation may fatigue and fail, resulting in loss of reduction. Posterior distraction forces do not adequately resist shear, and compression forces applied through posterior instrumentation may result in foraminal stenosis. The best way to biomechanically resist these shear forces is by providing anterior column support in the form of interbody fusion to augment the posterior instrumentation. If reduction is near anatomic, traditional ALIF or PLIF procedures can be used for anterior column support, depending on surgeon preference. Several studies have reported decreased nonunion rates when either ALIF or PLIF procedures were combined with posterior instrumented open reduction. In the treatment of patients with high-grade spondylolisthesis the benefits of reduction must be weighed against the significant potential complications and these issues should be discussed with the patient and family in great detail.

Annotated Bibliography

Bartolozzi P, Sandri A, Cassini M, Ricci M: One-stage posterior decompression-stabilization and transsacral interbody fusion after partial reduction for severe L5-S1 spondylolisthesis. *Spine* 2003;28:1135-1141.

This retrospective study suggests that posterior decompression with partial reduction and stabilization with pedicle screw fixation and titanium cage transsacral interbody fusion is a safe and effective treatment for patients with high-grade spondylolisthesis.

Beutler WJ, Frederickson MD, Murtland A, Sweeney MA, Grant WD, Baker D: The natural history of spondylolysis and spondylolisthesis: 45-year follow-up evaluation. *Spine* 2003;28:1027-1035.

This is a prospective study of the natural history of spondylolysis and spondylolisthesis over 45 years. The authors report that patients with pars defects follow a clinical course similar to the general population and that slip progression markedly slows with each decade.

Hanson DS, Bridwell KH, Rhee JM, Lenke LG: Correlation of pelvic incidence with low- and high-grade isthmic spondylolisthesis. *Spine* 2002;27:2026-2029.

This study shows that pelvic incidence is significantly higher in low- and high-grade slips compared with control groups. Pelvic incidence also has a significant correlation with Meyerding-Newman scores.

Hanson DS, Bridwell KH, Rhee JM, Lenke LG: Dowel fibular strut grafts for high-grade dysplastic isthmic spondylolisthesis. *Spine* 2002;27:1982-1988.

This study shows that fibular strut grafting is a safe and effective method for treating patients with partially reduced high-grade slips. The authors found no significant difference between the use of allograft and autograft.

La Rosa G, Conti A, Cacciola F, et al: Pedicle screw fixation for isthmic spondylolisthesis: Does posterior lumbar interbody fusion improve outcome over posterolateral fusion? *J Neurosurg* 2003;99(suppl 2):143-150.

Addition of a PLIF procedure to posterolateral instrumented fusion in patients with isthmic spondylolisthesis improves slip correction and maintenance of reduction over posterolateral instrumented fusion alone. The authors report no difference in fusion rates or functional and neurologic outcome.

Natarajan RN, Garretson RB III, Biyani A, Lim TH, Andersson GBJ, An HS: Effects of slip severity and loading directions on the stability of isthmic spondylolisthesis: A finite element model study. *Spine* 2003;28:1103-1112.

This study shows that the stiffness of a spondylolisthetic motion segment decreases with increasing slip progression. The authors also report that lateral bending and torsion cause the most resultant motion.

Classic Bibliography

Boos N, Marchesi D, Zuber K, Aebi M: Treatment of severe spondylolisthesis by reduction and pedicular fixation: A 4-6 year follow up study. *Spine* 1993;18:1655-1661.

Bradford DS, Boachie-Adjei O: Treatment of severe spondylolisthesis by anterior and posterior reduction and stabilization: A long-term follow-up study. *J Bone Joint Surg Am* 1990;72:1060-1066.

Carragee EJ: Single-level posterolateral fusion, with or without posterior decompression, for the treatment of isthmic spondylolisthesis in adults. *J Bone Joint Surg Am* 1997;79:1175-1180.

Fischgrund JS, Mackay M, Herkowitz HN, Brower R, Montgomery DM, Kurz LT: Degenerative lumbar spondylolisthesis with spinal stenosis: A prospective, randomized study comparing decompressive laminectomy and arthrodesis with and without spinal instrumentation. *Spine* 1997;22:2807-2812.

Herkowitz HN, Kurz LT: Degenerative spondylolisthesis with spinal stenosis: A prospective study comparing decompression with decompression and intertransverse arthrodesis. *J Bone Joint Surg Am* 1991;73:802-808.

Katz JN, Lipson SJ, Chang LC, Levine SA, Fossel AH, Liang MH: Seven- to 10-year outcome of decompressive surgery for degenerative lumbar spinal stenosis. *Spine* 1996;21:92-98.

Marchetti PG, Bartolozzi P: Classification of spondylolisthesis as a guideline for treatment, in Bridwell KH, DeWald RL (eds): *Textbook of Spinal Surgery*. Philadelphia, PA, Lippincott-Raven, 1997, pp 1211-1254.

Smith MD, Bohlman HH: Spondylolisthesis treated by a single-stage operation combining decompression with in situ posterolateral and anterior fusion: An analysis of eleven patients who had long-term follow-up. *J Bone Joint Surg Am* 1990;72:415-421.

Suk S, Lee C, Kim WJ, Lee JH, Cho KJ, Kim HG: Adding posterior lumbar interbody fusion to pedicle screw fixation and posterolateral fusion after decompression in spondylolotic spondylolisthesis. *Spine* 1997;22:210-219.

Wiltse LL, Newman PH, Macnab I: Classification of spondylolysis and spondylolisthesis. *Clin Orthop* 1976;117:23-29.

Chapter 46

Adult Spinal Deformity

Bobby K-B Tay, MD

Introduction

The evaluation and management of adult patients with spinal deformity has undergone a rapid evolution in the past decade. Increasing knowledge about the natural history of adult spinal deformity and the biologic events that mediate the processes of spinal fusion have provided the spinal surgeon with a greater ability to evaluate and treat these complex disorders. Despite these advances, evaluation and optimal treatment of adult spinal deformity remains a significant challenge. In addition, the increasing number of technical options available to the spinal surgeon as well as the many spinal instrumentation systems available today have not made management of adult spinal deformity any less challenging.

It is now well established that untreated scoliosis in the adult is not a benign condition. Common associations include painful, degenerative, spinal osteoarthritis; progressive deformity; spinal stenosis with radiculopathy; muscle fatigue from coronal and sagittal plane imbalance; and poor cosmesis. Accurate determination of pain, impairment in the quality of life, and cosmetic effects of deformity are difficult to measure and compare among groups of patients. These factors, when weighed against the increased complication rate of surgical treatment, makes the decision to operate as important or more important than the technique and expertise with which the procedure is performed.

Prevalence and Natural History

Adult spinal deformity can arise as a sequela of untreated adolescent idiopathic scoliosis, failed surgical or nonsurgical treatment, or de novo spinal deformity developing in the adult. The latter can be caused by degenerative changes of the spinal column leading to instability and deformity, by iatrogenic instability after decompressive procedures for spinal stenosis and radiculopathy, and possibly by metabolic bone diseases such as osteoporosis. The prevalence of scoliosis in adults has been reported to range from 1.4% to 20%.

Clearly, scoliosis can continue to progress after skeletal maturity and into late adulthood. Large thoracic curves (> 60°) show the greatest risk for progression. In a large cohort of patients with adolescent idiopathic scoliosis that was followed for more than 40 years, 68% of patients had progression of their curvature after skeletal maturity. Thoracic curves greater than 50° progressed an average of 1° per year. Thoracolumbar curves progressed about 0.5° per year and lumbar curves progressed 0.24° per year. Thoracic curves less than 30° tended not to progress.

Patients with degenerative scoliosis exhibited a higher rate of curve progression, which on average was about 3.3° per year. The prevalence of lumbar scoliosis in adult patients with low back pain was estimated to be about 7.5%. The prevalence increased with age and included 15% of patients with low back pain who were older than 60 years. Risk factors for curve progression include the presence of a curvature greater than 30°, apical rotation greater than 33%, more than 6 mm of lateral listhesis, and poor seating of L5 on S1.

In contrast to adolescent patients with scoliosis who are usually asymptomatic, adult patients with scoliosis often report back pain. In a recent European study involving 16,394 adolescents and their parents, the lifetime prevalence of low back pain was 50.9% for boys and 69.3% for girls with scoliosis as an independent risk factor. Other smaller but better designed studies have demonstrated that patients with scoliosis have a higher incidence of back pain than age- and sex-matched controls. In general, the overall incidence of pain ranges from 40% to 90%, and the overall prevalence of painful deformity ranges from 60% to 80%. The etiology of the pain is multifactorial. It can arise from muscle fatigue on the convexity of the curvature, trunk imbalance, facet arthropathy on the concavity of the curvature, and degenerative disk disease. Back pain is more common in patients with lumbar curves and in patients with thoracolumbar and lumbar curves exceeding 45° with apical rotation and coronal imbalance. Although the incidence of back pain in patients with adult scoliosis is similar to that in the general population, many studies suggest that back pain in patients with scoliosis is greater and more persistent. In addition to back pain, adult patients are more likely to experience symptoms of spinal stenosis and radiculopathy from osteoarthritis of the spine, rotatory subluxations, anterior listhesis, and lateral listhesis of the vertebral bodies that result in stretching and/or impingement of nerve roots. Again, neurogenic symptoms are more common in patients with lumbar curvatures. However, paresis or paraplegia from untreated scoliosis has not been reported.

Decreased vital capacity and other parameters of pulmonary function may occur in patients with severe thoracic curves (> 60°), especially in the presence of thoracic lordosis that effectively decreases the anterior-posterior chest diameter. In one study, up to 35% of patients with thoracic curves reported cardiopulmonary symptoms. However, significant alterations in vital capacity as a result of restrictive lung disease have not been observed until the curve magnitude exceeds 90° to 100°. In addition, there is no evidence to suggest that an adult patient with previously normal pulmonary function after skeletal maturity will experience deterioration in pulmonary function with progression of the curvature without a preexisting history of smoking or some other pulmonary disease.

Finally, the psychologic impact of chronic pain and deformity must be considered. In a world where appearance and health become increasingly important for social acceptance and well-being, the inability of individuals to function at the level of their peers because of pain or deformity can create a huge psychologic burden. The influence of spinal deformity on psychologic well-being has not been determined in the adult population. Small series of patients with adult scoliosis have been reported to show a significant negative impact of the spinal deformity on patients' perception of health.

Patient Assessment
History and Physical Examination
A complete history followed by a careful physical examination (including a complete neurologic examination) is essential in a patient with adult spinal deformity. The importance of social and family history and occupational history cannot be overstated. Depression, substance abuse, and chronic smoking in patients with adult spinal deformity can result in a less than ideal outcome after major spinal reconstructive surgery. Overall, the evaluation of the adult with scoliosis is much more difficult than that of adolescents because the usual criteria for surgical treatment are more difficult to interpret. In addition, the surgical treatment of scoliosis in adults carries a higher rate of complications and involves a longer recovery period than in adolescents. Proper patient selection is critical for achieving a successful result.

Imaging Studies
Standard PA and lateral full-length spine radiographs are an essential part of the evaluation process. Long cassette 14- × 36-inch weight-bearing scoliosis radiographs are necessary to fully assess the extent of the primary curvature as well as any compensatory curves that may exist. The weight-bearing radiographs also allow physicians to evaluate both coronal and sagittal plane balance. If surgery is contemplated, lateral supine bending films are obtained to assess the flexibility of secondary curvatures. Occasionally, flexion and extension views are helpful to determine lumbar spine flexibility and the presence of sagittal plane instability. These views have been sufficient in most patients for preoperative planning. Traction views may be helpful for assessing severe deformities, but in deformities less than 60°, bending films provide a better assessment of curve flexibility. A fulcrum bending view (in which the PA radiograph is taken with the patient in the lateral decubitus position with the apex of the curvature over a large bolster) or a push-prone radiograph (in which the pelvis of the prone patient is stabilized while the surgeon applies lateral pressure to the major curve) can help access thoracic curve flexibility.

In general, curve magnitude and patient age are the main predictors of curve flexibility. Every 10° increase in curve magnitude over 40° results in a 10% decrease in curve flexibility. Every 10-year increase in age decreases the flexibility of the structural curve by 5% and the lumbosacral fractional curve by 10%.

MRI is reserved to evaluate rapidly progressive curves and to determine the cause of any neurologic abnormalities on physical examination. Myelography is helpful for evaluating the neural elements in patients with severe rotational deformity and in those with metal implants that may obscure the clarity of MRI scans. Diskography has been recommended by some authors as a means of evaluating discogenic pain. This is especially relevant in the evaluation of patients with low back pain and lumbar scoliosis to help determine the distal extent of fusion, especially in patients with disk degeneration and axial low back pain. A positive diskogram in a patient with a degenerated disk below the anticipated fusion levels would be a relative indication to extend the fusion to encompass the involved degenerated disk. However, there are no prospective studies to confirm or refute the efficacy of this rationale because the results of provocative diskograms seem to depend to a great extent on the interpretation and the technique of the examiner.

Preoperative pulmonary function testing is useful for patients with thoracic curves exceeding 70°, patients with a history of pulmonary disease (chronic smokers), and patients who will require thoracoplasty. Adults who undergo thoracoplasty experience a 27% decline in pulmonary function by 3 months postoperatively, which, in contrast to adolescents, does not improve appreciably after 2-year follow-up. Thus, an adult patient with borderline pulmonary function may not tolerate thoracoplasty or thoracotomy.

Treatment

Nonsurgical Treatment

The initial treatment of patients with back pain and scoliosis should not differ from the treatment of patients with mechanical back pain in the absence of deformity. A relative indication for nonsurgical treatment includes patients who physically cannot tolerate the amount of surgery necessary to properly address their pain, deformity, and neurologic dysfunction. A physical therapy program should be instituted to improve aerobic capacity, strengthen muscles, and improve flexibility and joint motion. Although local heat application, analgesics, and bracing all may aid in the amelioration of symptoms, they do not prevent curve progression. Corticosteroid injections in the form of nerve root blocks, facet injections, and epidural steroid injections may be of considerable value in the arsenal of conservative management of adult spinal deformity. In patients who are not surgical candidates, spinal bracing during ambulation may provide some symptomatic relief to improve functionality.

Surgical Treatment

The indications for surgery in the adult patient with scoliosis include thoracic curve greater than 50° to 60°, with chronic pain that is unrelieved by conservative management; significant loss of pulmonary function not attributable to underlying pulmonary disease; documented curve progression with coronal or sagittal plane imbalance; symptomatic deformity that is unacceptable to the patient; and lumbar curvature with associated back or radicular pain or symptoms of spinal stenosis.

Adult patients have a greater risk of experiencing surgical complications than adolescents. Major complications include pseudarthrosis in 5% to 27% of patients, residual pain in 5% to 15%, neurologic injury in 1% to 5%, infection in 0.5% to 5%, and thromboembolism in 1% to 20%.

To avoid the detrimental effects of prolonged immobilization, surgical procedures should be designed to provide maximum stability and thus allow early mobilization with minimal external support. Combined procedures are preferable to staged procedures if this is technically and physiologically feasible. Combined anterior-posterior spinal reconstructive surgery has a lower infection rate than staged procedures as a result of patient malnutrition at the time of the posterior procedure.

Normalization of nutritional status does not occur until 6 to 12 weeks after the index procedure. If surgical procedures need to be staged, the use of hyperalimentation or enteral nutritional supplementation between stages is recommended to help decrease complications, which can result from malnutrition. Use of sequential compression devices or foot pumps to minimize the risk of deep venous thrombosis, mobilization with the assistance of physical therapy, and aggressive respiratory therapy should be routine. Other useful adjuncts to surgery include an autologous blood exchange program, the use of the Cell Saver autologous blood recovery system (Haemonetics, Braintree, MA) at the time of surgery, carefully monitored intraoperative hypotension, routine neurologic monitoring, and an experienced anesthesia staff that can manage the blood loss and fluid shifts that occur during complex spinal reconstruction. Finally, redosing of antibiotics every 4 hours or after 1,500 mL of blood loss to maintain the antibiotic concentration above the minimum inhibitory concentration is recommended.

It is important to remember that the amount of correction obtained in the adult patient is secondary to the achievement of coronal and sagittal plane balance. Thoracic rib prominence is best corrected with thoracoplasty rather than with overcorrection of the thoracic curve. The choice of fixation used to achieve correction and balance is extremely important because osteoporosis is often present in the adult patient. Segmental fixation provides improved purchase in weakened bone and creates a large area for force transmission in the correction of deformity.

The use of thoracic pedicle screws in the treatment of traumatic conditions of the spinal column has become more popular as experience with the technique increases. The primary benefit of pedicle screw fixation is the ability to shorten the length of fusion across the injured level while still having significant three-dimensional control over the spinal deformity to be able to reduce it. Pedicle screw fixation may also provide a more secure anchor at the cephalad extent of the fusion compared with that provided by hooks. The use of transpedicular fixation in the thoracic spine is still controversial because the presence of deformity makes insertion of screws more difficult and hazardous. In addition, in the presence of osteoporosis, the spinal lamina is often the most secure point of fixation. In such instances, excellent correction of thoracic curves can be obtained with a combination of laminar hooks and sublaminar wires. In contrast to adolescent scoliosis, adult curvatures tend to be less flexible and adult patients tend to have osteoporosis and less healing potential. Thus, pedicle screw fixation alone does not substitute for appropriate anterior column releases and fusion.

Intraoperative somatosensory-evoked potential and motor-evoked potential monitoring are especially helpful when there is a possibility of extensive blood loss, hypotension, significant deformity correction, and stiff curvatures. When this type of monitoring is not available, a wake-up test should be performed after instrumentation and correction of the curvatures. Combined somatosensory-evoked potential and motor-evoked potential monitoring is superior to single modality techniques in the assessment of real-time root and spinal cord function. With the development of intercostal muscle and rectus abdominis intraoperative electromyographic monitoring, thoracic pedicle screws can be tested to minimize the risk of perforation into the spinal canal or the neural foramen.

Before any surgical procedure, both surgeon and patient must have realistic expectations for the outcome of the operation. Most studies report a 69% to 95% reduction in the severity of pain and a 30% to 40% correction of deformity.

In general, the approach to the surgical treatment of adult spinal deformity is based on accepted methods of choosing fusion levels, placement of instrumentation, and curve reduction techniques that were derived from experience in the treatment of adolescent spinal deformities. These techniques are then modified to take into consideration the various challenges presented by adult patients. These surgical challenges include the presence of spinal stenosis, stiffer deformities, sagittal plane imbalance, less potential for healing, osteoporosis, the need to extend the fusion to the sacrum because of stiff fractional curvatures in the lower lumbar spine or the presence of spinal stenosis, and discogenic pain. In addition, an anatomic correction of the spinal deformity is not often achieved or warranted in the adult patient. The goal of surgical correction is to obtain a balanced spine in the sagittal and coronal planes.

Fusion levels are often determined from the weight-bearing PA radiographs, with modifications determined by lateral bending and weight-bearing lateral radiographs. Some general guidelines exist. All of the structural curves should be included in the fusion. The end vertebra of the fusion should be within the Harrington stable zone and should be neutrally rotated when the deformity corrects on lateral bending. The first unfused disk space at the caudal end of the fusion should be flexible on lateral bending. The fusion should not be stopped within the apex of the thoracic kyphosis or adjacent to a kyphotic motion segment.

Curves less than 60° to 70° on the Cobb measurement without significant coronal or sagittal plane decompensation can be treated effectively using a single posterior approach. In patients with this type of spinal deformity, radical facetectomies and osteotomies of ankylosed segments will allow sufficient mobility to achieve curve correction and balance. Curvatures greater than 70° are often associated with coronal and sagittal plane decompensation. These deformities are best treated with a combined anterior-posterior approach. Anterior releases and fusions of the most structural portions of the curvature followed by posterior releases and osteotomies with or without rib resections will, in most patients, allow sufficient mobility of the de-

formity to obtain a balanced correction of the curvature. Curvatures that exceed 90° to 100° are often associated with rigid ankylosis of the spine and severe coronal imbalance. In patients with this degree of deformity, a three-stage posterior-anterior-posterior procedure or a vertebral resection procedure is required to gain sufficient spinal mobility and to gain sufficient curve correction to obtain spinal balance.

Patients with spinal stenosis should have decompression of the stenotic levels before instrumentation and correction of the curvatures. Patients with severe lumbar spinal stenosis who also have decompensation in the sagittal plane can be treated with staged posterior and anterior surgery. In these patients, decompression of the stenotic levels should be performed before restoration of sagittal balance. Restoration of lordosis in these patients before decompression of the stenotic levels may result in a neurologic deficit.

Once the spinal deformity is corrected with the appropriate release and instrumentation, a meticulous spinal fusion with bone grafting should be performed. Autogenous graft from the local fusion bed and the iliac crest are placed over the decorticated posterior elements.

Degenerative Lumbar Scoliosis

Degenerative lumbar scoliosis can result from untreated idiopathic scoliosis, but it more frequently occurs independently as a sequela of the aging process in combination with osteoporosis. Many patients with degenerative lumbar scoliosis have a combination of both mechanical back pain and spinal stenosis. Patients may also present with radiculopathy because the neural foramen are narrowed at the concavity of the spinal deformity. Fortunately, most of these patients are well balanced in the sagittal and coronal planes despite the magnitude of the curvature, and their main symptoms are the result of neural compression. Decompression of the stenotic spinal canal and neural foramen often results in significant improvement in pain and function in these patients. Unless the decompressed segments are severely ankylosed, these levels should be fused to prevent progression of the scoliosis (Figure 1). The entire deformity does not need to be included in the fusion as long as the patient is balanced in the sagittal and coronal planes. However, fusion levels should be chosen so as not to end the fusion at a listhetic level, the apex of the curvature, or a kyphotic segment. If instrumentation is used and the patient still has lumbar lordosis, mild distraction between the pedicle screws at the concavity of the curvature helps to enlarge and stabilize the neuroforamen.

Patients with long fusions to the sacrum should also have selective anterior fusion at the L4-5 and L5-S1 segments, with structural grafting to maximize fusion rates and decrease the possibility of failure of the sacral screws.

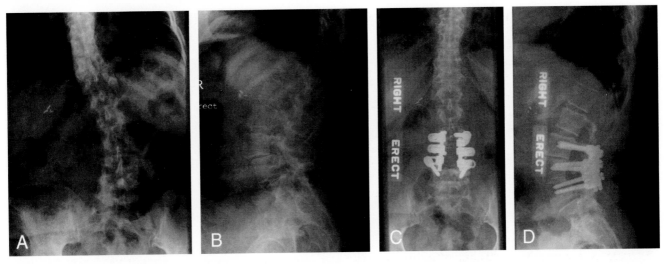

Figure 1 PA **(A)** and lateral **(B)** weight-bearing radiographs of the lumbar spine of a 50-year-old woman with degenerative scoliosis and spinal stenosis who was treated with lumbar laminectomy radical facetectomies, instrumentation with correction of scoliosis, and spinal fusion. Postoperative PA **(C)** and lateral **(D)** weight-bearing radiographs of the same patient after decompression and fusion.

In general, arthrodesis to the sacrum for idiopathic scoliosis should be avoided if possible. Long fusions to the sacrum are associated with a higher rate of pseudarthrosis, fixed sagittal deformity, instrumentation failure, and limited function. Indications to extend the fusion to the sacrum include lumbosacral pain secondary to degenerative disk disease below a lumbar curvature when a decision has been made to correct the lumbar curve, an unbalanced lumbosacral curvature with lumbar scoliosis for which balance in the lumbosacral curve is not achieved (as assessed using appropriate side bending radiographs), and the presence of substantial degeneration of the motion segments of L4-5 and L5-S1 anteriorly and posteriorly. In selected patients with a fixed lumbosacral fractional curve, fusion to the sacrum can be avoided by an end plate osteotomy at L4 or L5 (with concave osteophyte excision) to make the end vertebra horizontal, reduce the fractional curve, and create a stable end vertebra above the pelvis.

When performing long fusions to the sacrum in adults, a combined approach is recommended to maximize the fusion rate, reestablish lumbar lordosis, and prevent implant failure across the lumbosacral junction. Two-stage surgery is preferable with the anterior diskectomies and fusion, with structural grafts or cages performed first followed by posterior fusion and instrumentation.

Many techniques are available to secure fixation across the lumbosacral junction. These include sacral screws placed in a bicortical fashion, sacral screws with intrasacral rods, iliac wing screws, Galveston technique, and convergent and divergent sacral screws. Bicortical sacral screw fixation with structural anterior fusion at L5-S1 appears to be an adequate anchor for most long fusions to the sacrum. In patients with poor bone stock

or in those in whom previously placed sacral screws have failed, iliac fixation is usually necessary. In the adult patient, Luque-Galveston fixation is associated with a high rate of pseudarthrosis (30% to 40%). Although iliac fixation with iliac screws is biomechanically strong, iliac screws can be prominent in very thin individuals (Figure 2).

Salvage Procedures in Adult Patients

The indications for revision scoliosis surgery in the adult include painful pseudarthrosis, progressive deformity from pseudarthrosis or inadequate fusion levels, flatback syndrome from distraction implants across the lumbar spine, symptomatic adjacent segment degeneration or vertebral body fracture, and unacceptable residual deformity.

The goals of surgery are the same as in primary surgery—to obtain a solid arthrodesis, achieve three-dimensional spinal balance, and provide rigid internal fixation. The management of pseudarthrosis in the adult patient with scoliosis depends on the level of the pseudarthrosis, the presence or absence of deformity, the security of preexisting fixation, and especially the presence or absence of pain. A painful pseudarthrosis associated with progressive deformity and loss of fixation is a clear indication for spinal revision surgery via a combined approach. However, thoracic pseudarthrosis that is not associated with deformity or loss of fixation can be adequately managed by single-stage anterior and posterior repair with copious autogenous bone grafting.

Adult patients may present with curve progression above or below a previous fusion that was done in childhood or adolescence. This condition may be secondary to crankshaft phenomenon or the primary fusion being too short. For minor degrees of deformity in young

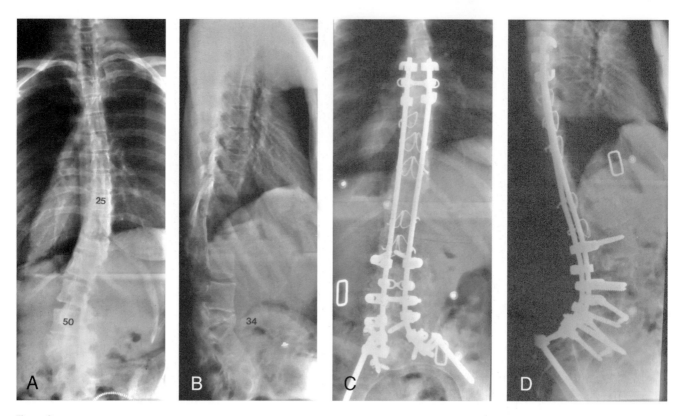

Figure 2 Preoperative PA **(A)** and lateral **(B)** weight-bearing radiographs of an adult patient with scoliosis who was treated with staged anterior and posterior fusion with posterior fixation to the pelvis using iliac screw fixation. Postoperative PA **(C)** and lateral **(D)** weight-bearing radiographs of the same patient.

adults with good bone stock, extension of the fusion to include the involved segments and reinstrumentation are sufficient treatment. However, in patients with a fixed deformity with coronal or sagittal imbalance, especially in the presence of osteopenia, a combined approach is preferable.

Disk degeneration may develop below a fusion and require salvage reconstruction. If there is isolated spinal stenosis, decompression alone is usually sufficient. If the patient has a vertebral insufficiency fracture below the fusion, extension of the fusion and instrumentation is necessary.

Loss of lumbar lordosis occurs gradually with aging. Iatrogenic loss of lumbar lordosis is typically caused by the use of distraction implants across the lumbar spine. Some patients who undergo salvage procedures experience loss of lumbar lordosis secondary to sagittal plane imbalance. In these patients, the primary goal of the index procedure was coronal plane correction. These patients are best treated with a combined surgical procedure. For patients with a solid arthrodesis, a pedicle subtraction osteotomy with vertebral body decancellation using the posterior approach and rigid internal fixation can provide up to 30° to 40° of sagittal plane correction. This procedure is particularly useful in patients with combined anterior and posterior fusion who still have flat-back deformity (Figure 3). A poorer clinical

result is associated with increasing patient comorbidities, thoracic pseudarthrosis, and adjacent segment breakdown caudad to the fusion. To restore lumbar lordosis in patients with multiple pseudarthrosis or fusions that are not intact to the sacrum, a combined approach is preferable. This may be performed as a first-stage posterior procedure with osteotomies and instrumentation to the sacrum followed by anterior interbody fusion with structural allograft or vice versa (Figure 4). For severe, rigid, unbalanced deformity, a spinal shortening procedure such as a vertebral body resection is necessary.

Postoperatively, adult patients are mobilized within 24 to 48 hours depending on pain tolerance and overall general condition. Then the patient is given intravenous narcotic medication via a patient-controlled pump until oral pain medication is tolerated. The use of postoperative anti-inflammatory agents such as ketorolac is contraindicated because the fusion rate is adversely affected. Perioperative antibiotics can be continued for 36 to 48 hours. Antiembolic stockings and sequential compression devices are used to minimize the incidence of venous thrombosis until the patients are ambulatory. Anticoagulation is not performed routinely, but it may be considered in high-risk patients and in patients with a preexisting history of thromboembolic disease. In patients with a history of pulmonary embolism, a vena

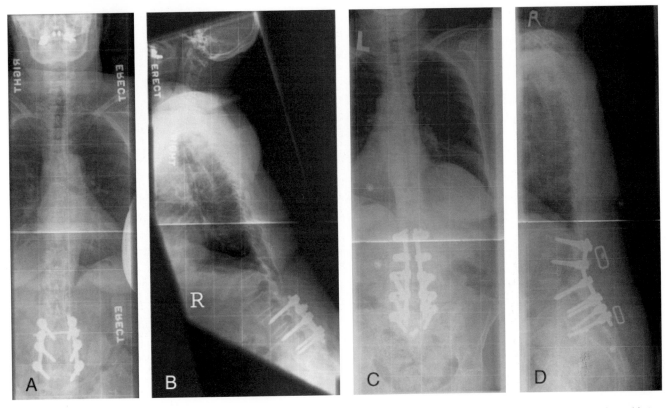

Figure 3 PA **(A)** and lateral **(B)** full-length weight-bearing radiographs of a 56-year-old woman with lumbar flat-back syndrome following lumbar decompression and instrumented fusion. The patient had severe sagittal plane decompensation and recurrent spinal stenosis with back pain and bilateral buttock and leg radiculopathy. Note that the lateral radiograph demonstrates evidence of severe sagittal plane decompensation. Postoperative PA **(C)** and lateral **(D)** full-length weight-bearing radiographs of the same patient after revision laminectomy and transpedicular wedge resection at L3 with restoration of sagittal balance.

cava filter may be considered before surgical intervention. The patients are fitted with a lightweight plastic orthosis within 5 to 7 days of surgery and are instructed to wear the brace full time, except when in bed and for hygiene.

Controversial Issues in Managing Adult Patients With Scoliosis

The absolute indications for combined surgery versus posterior fusion and instrumentation alone are unclear. Combined surgery allows for better correction and reestablishment of physiologic lumbar lordosis through the use of anterior structural grafting, and it increases the probability of successful fusion. In patients with complex deformities involving the lumbar spine in which fusion across the lumbosacral junction is necessary to achieve spinal balance, combined procedures are preferable because 15% to 20% of patients who undergo posterior instrumentation and fusion have pseudarthrosis, even when the stiffer third-generation instrumentation systems are used.

Thoracoplasty is a useful adjunct in treating patients with spinal deformity. Thoracoplasty reduces rib prominence by 71% compared with only a 17% reduction in control subjects. Rib resection also provides a good

source of bone graft. It is well known that pulmonary function can deteriorate after thoracotomy and thoracoplasty. These procedures should be used with extreme caution in patients with severely compromised pulmonary function. Unlike adolescents, adult patients with scoliosis do not recover lost pulmonary function, even at 2-year follow-up.

Results and Complications

The results of surgical correction of spinal deformity in adults have improved significantly over the past decade. The rate of complications ranges from 12% to 23% of patients. Pseudarthrosis rates have varied between 5% to 27% of patients, with higher rates of pseudarthrosis occurring after revision surgery and after using nonsegmental posterior implants in distraction mode. Pain in these patients is seldom totally alleviated by surgical correction. However, reports of residual pain after complex spinal reconstructive surgery vary between 5% and 25% of patients. Approximately 61% of patients report improved sleep patterns after surgical treatment, and 57% are able to return to work. Mortality remains low in patients who undergo complex spinal reconstructive surgery, but it is not insignificant (< 1% to 5% of patients). Overall, patient outcomes as assessed by the

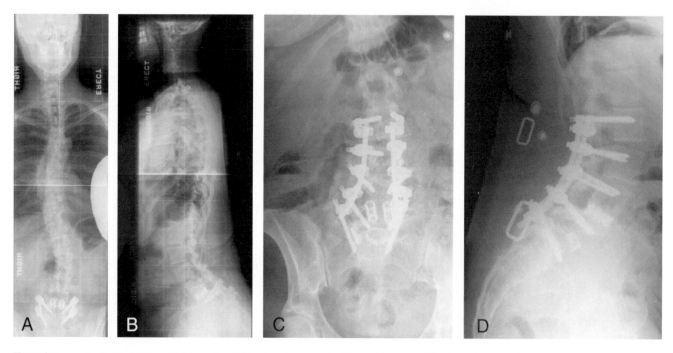

Figure 4 Preoperative PA **(A)** and lateral **(B)** full-length weight-bearing radiographs of a 50-year-old woman with flat-back syndrome and pseudarthrosis after posterior lumbar interbody fusion with threaded cages at L4-5 and instrumented posterolateral fusion at L5-S1. Note that the lateral radiograph shows evidence of significant sagittal plane decompensation. Postoperative PA **(C)** and lateral **(D)** radiographs of the same patient after multiple level Smith-Peterson osteotomies and instrumented fusion and repair of pseudarthrosis. Note that the postoperative lateral radiograph shows evidence of restoration of lumbar lordosis.

Medical Outcomes Study Short Form 36-Item Health Survey (SF-36) and the American Academy of Orthopaedic Surgeons' Modems Instrument are significantly associated with radiographic correction of the lumbar lordosis to greater than 25° and coronal plumb alignment to within 2.5 cm. Patients with primary degenerative lumbar scoliosis as well as those who have had long fusions to L4, L5, or the sacrum have improved gait parameters (both speed and endurance) after spinal decompression and fusion, with restoration of coronal and sagittal balance. Outcomes assessment in this challenging group of patients is necessary to determine the impact of deformity correction on the patients' quality of life and daily function. The Modified Scoliosis Research Society Outcomes Instrument for Adult Deformity, the Oswestry Disability Index, and the SF-36 are the most commonly used validated outcomes questionnaires for adult patients undergoing spinal deformity surgery.

Neurologic injury occurs in fewer than 1% to 5% of patients who undergo surgical treatment for spinal deformities. Significant risk factors for major intraoperative neurologic deficits include combined anterior and posterior surgery and hyperkyphosis. Delayed postoperative paraplegia is another devastating complication after extensive spinal reconstructive surgery, and it can occur several hours after the completion of the procedure. This phenomenon has been attributed to ischemia of the spinal cord from postoperative hypovolemia, mechanical tension of spinal blood vessels on the concavity

of the curve, and preexisting atherosclerosis. Thus, proper postoperative volume support and vigilance are essential. Loss of vision as a complication of spinal reconstructive surgery is a rare but often permanent event that can occur as the result of ischemic optic neuropathy, retinal artery occlusion, or cerebral ischemia. The incidence of pulmonary embolism varies from 1% to 20% of patients, depending on the series. Air embolism can occur in patients with patent foramen ovale. However, only a few isolated instances of this complication have been reported. Flail chest can occur with overaggressive thoracoplasty, especially in revision situations.

Infection is a relatively rare event in patients who undergo surgery for spinal deformities; it occurs in between 1% and 8% of patients. In addition, infection after anterior surgery alone occurs in about 1% of patients. However, the sequelae of deep postoperative infection are substantial, with up to 38% to 64% of patients having pseudarthrosis at 37-month follow-up. Delayed infections can occur more than 2 years postoperatively, typically with low virulent organisms.

If coronal and sagittal balance is achieved and maintained with a solid fusion, the outcomes are generally excellent. Pulmonary improvement after correction of spinal deformity is unlikely to occur in the adult and the use of thoracoplasty may actually reduce pulmonary function. The correction of curvature varies from 30% to 60% and depends on the nature and flexibility of the patient's preoperative curve and the technique used for correction. Despite these relatively modest gains, satisfaction with surgical correction is generally high and can reach up to 90% of patients.

Annotated Bibliography

Prevalence and Natural History

Kovacs FM, Gestoso M, Gil del Real MT, Lopez J, Mufraggi N, Mendez JI: Risks factors for non-specific low back pain in school children and their parents: A population based study. *Pain* 2003;103:259-268.

In this European study involving 16,394 adolescents and their parents, the lifetime prevalence of low back pain was 50.9% for males and 69.3% for females. Scoliosis was an independent risk factor.

Schwab F, Dubey A, Pagala M, et al: Adult scoliosis: A health assessment analysis by SF-36. *Spine* 2003;28:602-606.

This prospective self-assessment of a consecutive series of adult patients with scoliosis showed that scoliosis has a significant impact on patients' perception of health.

Weinstein SL, Dolan LA, Spratt KF, Peterson KK, Spoonamore MJ, Ponseti IV: Health and function of patients with untreated idiopathic scoliosis: A 50-year natural history study. *JAMA* 2003;289:559-567.

This prospective cohort analysis of 117 untreated patients with idiopathic scoliosis followed over a 50-year span showed a greater incidence for back pain and cosmetic deformity in patients with scoliosis compared with 62 control patients. Patients with thoracic curves greater than 80° were more likely to report shortness of breath, suggesting a deterioration of pulmonary function in this subgroup.

Patient Assessment

Davis BJ, Gadgil A, Trivedi J: Ahmed el NB: Traction radiography performed under general anesthetic: A new technique for assessing idiopathic scoliosis curves. *Spine* 2004;29:2466-2470.

Traction radiographs taken with the patient under general anesthesia allow a better assessment of curve flexibility than standard supine bending radiographs. This finding may obviate the need for anterior release and fusion in select patients. Comparison to fulcrum bending radiographs was not performed in this study.

Treatment

Ali R, Boachie-Adjei O, Rawlins BA: Functional and radiographic outcomes after surgery for adult scoliosis using third-generation instrumentation techniques. *Spine* 2003;28:1163-1169.

This retrospective radiographic and chart review of 28 patients with adult scoliosis treated with primary corrective surgery showed significant clinical and radiographic improvements using third-generation spinal implants.

Suk S, Kim WJ, Lee SM, et al: Thoracic pedicle screw fixation in spinal deformities: Are they really safe? *Spine* 2001;26:2049-2057.

In this study, 4,604 thoracic pedicle screws were placed in the treatment of adult patients with spinal deformity; the authors report an overall rate of screw malposition of 1.5%. Most thoracic pedicle screws were placed inferior or lateral to the pedicle. Screw-related complications occurred in 0.8% of patients. Deformity correction was 69.9% for patients with coronal plane deformities and 47° for those with kyphosis.

Voos K, Boachie-Adeji O, Rawlins BA: Multiple vertebral osteotomies in the treatment of rigid adult spinal deformities. *Spine* 2001;26:526-533.

This retrospective chart and radiographic review of 27 consecutive adult patients with spinal deformity demonstrated the efficacy of multiple vertebral osteotomies in the management of rigid adult spinal deformities. The authors reported that the average scoliosis correction for these patients was 40% and the average correction in sagittal balance was 6.5 cm.

Degenerative Lumbar Scoliosis

Berven S, Hu SS, Deverin V: Lumbar end plate osteotomy in adult patients with scoliosis. *Clin Orthop* 2003; 411:70-76.

The authors of this study discuss a technique of end plate osteotomy and concave osteophyte excision in adults with fixed lumbosacral fractional curves that avoids extension of fusion to the sacrum.

Bridwell KH, Edwards CC II, Lenke LG: The pros and cons to saving the L5-S1 motion segment in a long scoliosis fusion construct. *Spine* 2003;28:S234-S242.

This article presents a review of the literature and the authors' personal experiences concerning the advantages and disadvantages of extending a long scoliosis fusion to the sacrum. The subject is controversial and no good studies exist that definitively answer the question.

Tribus CB: Degenerative lumbar scoliosis: Evaluation and management. *J Am Acad Orthop Surg* 2003;11:174-183.

This article presents a review of evaluation and treatment of degenerative scoliosis.

Salvage Procedures in Adult Patients

Berven SH, Deviren V, Smith JA, Hu SH, Bradford DS: Management of fixed sagittal plane deformity: Outcome of combined anterior and posterior surgery. *Spine* 2003; 28:1710-1715.

Twenty-five patients with fixed sagittal imbalances were treated with combined anterior-posterior fusion. This study showed that combined surgery is an effective method to treat fixed sagittal deformity. Patients with preoperative hypolordosis (relative flat-back syndrome) who had good restoration of lumbar lordosis and sagittal plane balance had the best outcomes.

Bridwell K, Lewis S, Lenke LG, et al: Pedicle subtraction osteotomy for the treatment of fixed sagittal imbalance. *J Bone Joint Surg Am* 2003;85-A:454-463.

In this study, 27 consecutive patients with fixed sagittal imbalance and treated with pedicle subtraction osteotomy were evaluated using Oswestry and Modified Scoliosis Research Society Outcomes Instrument for Adult Deformity questionnaires. The authors report that pedicle subtraction osteotomy is an effective procedure in this group of patients, with significant improvements in overall Oswestry scores and decreased pain scores. A poorer clinical result was associated with increasing patient comorbidities, pseudarthrosis in the thoracic spine, and subsequent breakdown caudad to the fusion.

Results and Complications

Eck KR, Bridwell KH, Ungacta FF, et al: Complications and results of long adult deformity fusions down to L4, L5, and the sacrum. *Spine* 2001;26:E182-E192.

The authors of this study report the outcomes and complication rates of patients treated surgically for adult lumbar scoliosis at an average 5-year follow-up (minimum 2-year follow-up). They report that patients with fusions short of the sacrum who developed distal spinal degeneration had worse outcomes that those patients with fusion to the sacrum.

Emami A, Deverin V, Berven S, et al: Outcome and complications of long fusions to the sacrum in adult spinal deformity. *Spine* 2002;27:776-786.

This is a retrospective study of 54 adult patients with spinal deformities who were treated with different techniques to achieve long fusion to the sacrum. All patients had combined anterior and posterior reconstruction with a minimum 2-year follow-up. The authors report a 34% pseudarthrosis rate in patients who had Luque-Galveston fixation compared with bicortical sacral screw and iliac screw fixation.

Lapp MA, Bridwell KH, Lenke LG, et al: Long-term complications in adult deformity patients having combined surgery: A comparison of primary to revision patients. *Spine* 2001;26:973-983.

This outcomes analysis compares the complication rates of primary surgery and revision surgery in 44 consecutive patients who underwent combined procedures for correction of adult spinal deformity with a minimum 2-year follow-up. The results demonstrated similar rates of minor complications (22% to 23% of patients). The primary surgery group had a higher rate of major complications and a significantly higher rate of pseudarthrosis compared with the revision surgery group.

Parsch D, Gaertner V, Brocai DR, Carstens C: The effect of spinal fusion on the long-term outcome of idiopathic scoliosis: A case control study. *J Bone Joint Surg Br* 2001;83:1133-1136.

In this study, 68 patients with scoliosis (34 treated and 34 untreated) compared with age- and sex-matched controls were evaluated for severity of back pain and overall function. Functional scores for patients with scoliosis were lower than those for the control group. Frequency and severity of back pain scores were lower in patients treated with fusion than in the patients with untreated scoliosis.

Classic Bibliography

Albert TJ, Purtill J, Mesa J, McIntosh T, Balderston RA: Health outcome assessment before and after adult deformity surgery: A prospective study. *Spine* 1995;20:2002-2005.

Ascani E, Bartolozzi P, Logroscino CA, et al: Natural history of untreated idiopathic scoliosis after skeletal maturity. *Spine* 1986;11:784-789.

Boachie-Adjei O, Bradford DS: Vertebral column resection and arthrodesis for complex spinal deformities. *J Spinal Disord* 1991;4:193-202.

Bradford DS, Tribus CB: Vertebral column resection for the treatment of rigid coronal decompensation. *Spine* 1997;22:1590-1599.

Collis DK, Ponseti IV: Long-term follow-up of patients with idiopathic scoliosis not treated surgically. *J Bone Joint Surg Am* 1969;51:425-445.

Dickson JH, Mirkovic S, Noble PC, Nalty T, Erwin WD: Results of operative treatment of idiopathic scoliosis in adults. *J Bone Joint Surg Am* 1995;77:513-523.

Goldberg MS, Mayo NE, Poitras B, Scott S, Hanley J: The Ste-Justine Adolescent Idiopathic Scoliosis Cohort Study: Part II. Perception of health, self and body image, and participation in physical activities. *Spine* 1994;19:1562-1572.

Hu SS, Fontaine F, Kelly B, Bradford DS: Nutritional depletion in staged spinal reconstructive surgery: The effect of total parenteral nutrition. *Spine* 1998;23:1401-1405.

Hu SS, Holly EA, Lele C, et al: Patient outcomes after spinal reconstructive surgery in patients > or = 40 years of age. *J Spinal Disord* 1996;9:460-469.

Jackson RP, Simmons EH, Stripinis D: Incidence and severity of back pain in adult idiopathic scoliosis. *Spine* 1983;8:749-756.

Lenke LG, Bridwell KH, Blanke K, Baldus C: Analysis of pulmonary function and chest cage dimension changes after thoracoplasty in idiopathic scoliosis. *Spine* 1995;20:1343-1350.

Nachemson A: Adult scoliosis and back pain. *Spine* 1979;4:513-517.

Thomasen E: Vertebral osteotomy for correction of kyphosis in ankylosing spondylitis. *Clin Orthop* 1985;194: 142-152.

Vanderpool DW, James JI, Wynne-Davies R: Scoliosis in the elderly. *J Bone Joint Surg Am* 1969;51:446-455.

Weinstein SL, Ponseti IV: Curve progression in idiopathic scoliosis. *J Bone Joint Surg Am* 1983;65:447-455.

Chapter 47

Spinal Infections

Eric S. Wieser, MD

Jeffrey C. Wang, MD

Introduction

Historically, patients with spinal infections experienced poor results with high morbidity and mortality rates. Medical innovations over the past several decades, including the improvement of antimicrobial chemotherapy, powerful laboratory and imaging techniques, and advancements in surgical techniques have significantly improved the outcomes of patients with spinal infections. Earlier detection of vertebral osteomyelitis and diskitis through increased clinician awareness and the use of advanced imaging modalities are crucial in limiting or avoiding complications associated with progressive spinal infection such as epidural abscess, structural deformities, chronic osteomyelitis, paralysis, sepsis, and death.

Pyogenic Vertebral Osteomyelitis

Epidemiology and Pathogenesis

The demographic features of patients with vertebral osteomyelitis have changed over the past years because of medical advances and the aging of the population. Vertebral osteomyelitis affects approximately 2% to 7% of all patients with pyogenic osteomyelitis in developed countries. Despite an overall decrease in the incidence of tuberculous spondylitis, the incidence of pyogenic vertebral osteomyelitis appears to have increased. This increase is probably related to the growth in the elderly and immunocompromised populations, increases in the number of invasive medical procedures, and an increase in intravenous drug use. Risk factors for pyogenic vertebral osteomyelitis that have recently been described in the literature are listed in Table 1.

Several theories exist regarding the mechanism of bacterial seeding of the spine. Pyogenic vertebral osteomyelitis is a bacterial infection with several possible sources including direct inoculation, contiguous spread from local infection, or hematogenous seeding. Direct inoculation can occur after penetrating trauma, open spinal fracture, and following percutaneous or open spinal procedures (such as diskography, diskectomy, chemonucleolysis, or any other diagnostic or therapeutic

injection). Contiguous spread of infection to the spine is most commonly associated with retropharyngeal and retroperitoneal abscesses. Any condition that causes a transient bacteremia may ultimately lead to hematogenous vertebral osteomyelitis.

The pathogenesis of spinal infection in children differs significantly from that of adults because of the differences in the vascular anatomy of the vertebrae and intervertebral disks. Isolated diskitis primarily occurs in children and vertebral osteomyelitis is common in adulthood. In children, vascularity extends through the cartilaginous growth plate into the nucleus pulposus, allowing direct deposition of bacterial emboli into the center of the disk. However, in adults, blood vessels reach only to the anulus fibrosus, limiting deposition of bacteria to the vertebral body metaphysis and end plate.

Hematogenous seeding of the vertebrae is described by two major theories. First, Batson described retrograde flow through the valveless vertebral venous plexus within the vertebral metaphyseal region where bacterial seeding could occur under increased abdominal pressure. This theory was refuted with another theory that proposed that bacteria can become wedged in the end metaphyseal arteriole loops. Infection spreads after the microorganisms are lodged in the low-flow vascular loops in the metaphysis and at the end plates. After the infection is established near the end plate of one vertebral body, it can penetrate through the end plate into the adjoining disk. The avascular disk material is destroyed by bacterial enzymes, allowing the infection to spread to the adjacent vertebral body. Posterior spinal arteries have abundant anastomoses about the disk, which probably contributes to the spread of the infection from one level to the next.

Staphylococcus aureus remains the most common organism cultured from pyogenic vertebral osteomyelitis and is found in 50% to 65% of culture positive cases. *S aureus* accounts for more than 80% of pediatric spinal infections. There also has been an increase in the number of gram-negative bacillus spinal infections over the past decade. The genitourinary tract, respiratory tract, and soft-tissue infections are often the source of these

Table 1	Risk Factors for Pyogenic Vertebral Osteomyelitis

Male sex
Intravenous drug abuse
Diabetes mellitus
Urinary tract infection
Respiratory tract infection
Recent genitourinary procedure
Previous spinal procedure
Morbid obesity
Alcohol abuse
Human immunodeficiency virus/acquired immunodeficiency syndrome
Malignancy
Corticosteroid use
Penetrating trauma

Table 2	Risk Factors for Neurologic Deterioration With Vertebral Osteomyelitis

Diabetes mellitus
Rheumatoid arthritis
Systemic corticosteroid use
Advanced age
Cephalad level of infection (high thoracic or cervical)
Staphylococcal infection

gram-negative infections. *Escherichia coli, Pseudomonas,* and *Proteus* infections often occur after genitourinary infections or procedures. *Pseudomonas* infections are also often seen in intravenous drug users. From intestinal flora, *Salmonella* can cause vertebral osteomyelitis in children with sickle cell disease. *Enterococcus, Propionobacterium acnes, Streptococcus viridans, Staphylococcus epidermidis* and diphtheroids have all been causative organisms of pyogenic vertebral osteomyelitis.

Clinical Characteristics

The clinical presentation of vertebral osteomyelitis is highly variable depending on the location of infection, the virulence of the organism, and the immunocompetency of the host. Pyogenic infections of the spine occur 50% of the time in the lumbar spine followed by approximately 40% in the thoracic spine, and only about 10% of the time in the cervical spine. Fever and constitutional symptoms are present in approximately 50% of the affected population. Weight loss is common but rarely recognized by the patient.

Approximately 90% of patients with pyogenic infections will have back or neck pain that is often quite severe and insidious in onset, which accounts for the frequent delay in diagnosis. Because the pain is often present at rest and at night, there is concern for the differential diagnosis of potential malignancy. Muscle spasms often are associated with neck or back pain. Torticollis and dysphagia often accompany fever as the only symptoms of cervical infection. Lumbar infection can lead to loss of lumbar lordosis, hamstring tightness, hip flexion contracture, or a positive straight leg raising test.

Neurologic deficits are present in about 10% of patients secondary to nerve root or spinal cord compression, especially with cervical or thoracic level disease. Patients may report radicular pain, motor nerve root paresis, and paralysis. Risk factors predisposing patients

to paralysis include diabetes, rheumatoid arthritis, systemic steroid use, increasing age, *Staphylococcus* infection, and a more cephalad level of infection. The risk factors for neurologic deterioration with vertebral osteomyelitis are summarized in Table 2.

Laboratory Evaluation

Laboratory studies often support the diagnosis of infection but remain nonspecific. The white blood cell count is elevated in about 50% of patients. The erythrocyte sedimentation rate (ESR) is a much more sensitive test and is elevated in more than 90% of patients; however, its specificity for infection is poor. All patients should have a C-reactive protein (CRP) test, which is slightly more sensitive and specific than the ESR. The CRP is also elevated sooner than the ESR. Both tests are helpful in following the course of treatment of the infection. However, each of these markers of inflammation will be elevated following an invasive procedure without any infection present. A substantial decrease in the ESR and CRP suggests an adequate response to treatment.

The definitive diagnosis of spinal pyogenic osteomyelitis requires identification of the organism through either a positive blood culture with confirmatory clinical and imaging features or from a biopsy and culture of the infected site. Blood and urine cultures should be done on all patients before the administration of any antibiotics. Blood cultures have been reported to be positive in 25% to 60% of patients. A positive urine culture does not necessarily confirm the diagnosis because a different organism may be identified at the time of vertebral biopsy. In general, it is appropriate to delay antibiotics until all cultures have been obtained; however, if the patient is septic or critically ill, antibiotics should be initiated immediately.

Biopsy of the infected site is often necessary to identify the infecting organism and exclude other potential etiologies. Spinal biopsies may be performed percutaneously using fluoroscopy or more accurately with CT. A second closed biopsy is recommended if the diagnosis is not confirmed after the first attempt. CT-guided biopsy provides the best results, with positive cultures in 68% to 86% of patients. Open biopsy is indicated when needle biopsy fails to identify the organism. Minimally invasive techniques such as endoscopic or thoracoscopic approaches may be considered when appropriate. Open biopsies yield positive results in more than 80% of patients. All biopsy specimens should be sent for Gram stain, acid-fast and potassium hydroxide staining, and cultures (including aerobic, anaerobic, mycobacterium, fungi, and atypical mycobacterium). All cultures should be retained to allow for the growth of mycobacterium and low virulence organisms. Especially with low-virulence and indolent bacteria, polymerase chain reaction has facilitated earlier identification of the infecting organism. Caution is needed to avoid cross contamination with the use of polymerase chain reaction. Specimens also should routinely be sent for histologic analysis to rule out malignancy.

Malnutrition is often coincident with spinal infection; therefore, an evaluation of the patient's nutritional status is crucial in determining appropriate nutritional therapy as a part of treatment. Laboratory measures such as serum albumin level less than 3 g/dL, a serum transferrin level of less than 150 ug/dL, and an absolute lymphocyte count less than 800/mL suggest severe malnutrition, which should be addressed as part of the treatment of the vertebral osteomyelitis.

Radiographic Evaluation

Imaging studies lag behind the clinical course of pyogenic vertebral osteomyelitis but are vital in localizing and determining the extent of involvement of the infection and for assessing the response to treatment. Plain radiographs can show subtle paravertebral soft-tissue swelling in the first few days of infection. After 7 to 10 days, disk space narrowing can be observed. After several weeks, radiographs show frank erosion and destruction of the vertebral end plates and anterior vertebrae with extension into the central portion of the vertebral body. The disk space continues to collapse and vertebral compression and paraspinal mass are noted. CT scans show paravertebral soft-tissue masses and, most importantly, define the extent of bony involvement of the infection. CT scans show the anatomy in detail and can be used to guide percutaneous drainage or biopsy and for preoperative planning.

Radionuclide studies also are useful in evaluating spinal infections and can be positive before the development of radiographic changes. Technetium Tc 99m bone scintigraphy is more than 90% sensitive, but it lacks specificity for infection. Scans that combine technetium Tc 99m with gallium 67 increase both the sensitivity and specificity for identifying infection. Indium 111-labeled leukocyte scans are not recommended for vertebral osteomyelitis because of poor sensitivity (17%). Gallium scans may be used to follow treatment response because they begin to normalize during the recovery phase. MRI with gadolinium contrast has become the imaging mo-

dality of choice for the diagnosis of spinal infections. MRI has a sensitivity of 96% and specificity of 93% for the diagnosis of vertebral osteomyelitis. On T1-weighted images, the affected vertebral body and disk both show low signal intensity with loss of distinction at their margins, secondary to the marrow edema and decreased fat content. In contrast, on T2-weighted images, the vertebral body has increased signal intensity secondary to the increase in water content associated with the inflammation and edema. On gadolinium-enhanced T1-weighted images, abscess collections show abnormal rim enhancement, whereas areas of active inflammation in the vertebral body and disk are enhanced.

Treatment

The goals for treatment of spinal infections include establishing a diagnosis and identifying the organism, eliminating the infection, preventing or improving neurologic involvement, and maintaining spinal stability. As with other illnesses, nutritional repletion and optimization of medical comorbidities are crucial to eradication of the infection.

Treatment of vertebral osteomyelitis usually entails a trial of nonsurgical treatment with spinal immobilization, early ambulation, proper nutritional support, and intravenous antibiotics followed by oral antibiotics (specific for the organism cultured). If the offending organism cannot be identified even after biopsy, empiric parenteral antibiotics should be administered. Parenteral antibiotics are generally recommended for 4 to 6 weeks to prevent high failure rates of nonsurgical treatment in patients with pyogenic infections. Patients are converted to oral antibiotics after signs of clinical improvement, normalization of the ESR and CRP levels, or resolution of the infection on imaging studies.

Immobilization of the affected area helps prevent deformity and aids in pain relief. The application of a rigid contact brace is effective in the lumbar region. A rigid cervicothoracic orthosis or halo is often required for cervical osteomyelitis. Serial laboratory tests (CRP and ESR) should be followed to monitor response to treatment. Approximately 75% of patients respond to nonsurgical treatment with resolution of pain and often spontaneous fusion.

Surgical intervention is warranted to obtain a tissue diagnosis after failed percutaneous needle biopsies, to address neurologic deficit secondary to compression, to treat spinal instability or significant deformity, to drain infectious foci causing sepsis, or for failure of nonsurgical medical treatment alone. Nonsurgical treatment is often unsuccessful in elderly and immunocompromised patients, who then require surgical management. The location of the infection and the goals of the surgery dictate the intervention performed. If the surgery is intended to obtain a specimen for diagnosis, then an

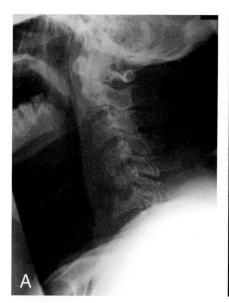 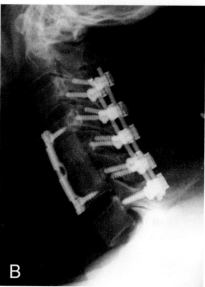 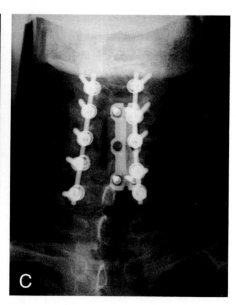

Figure 1 Imaging studies of an 80-year-old man with a 3-month history of increasing neck pain and recent onset of fever. **A,** A lateral radiograph shows collapse of the C5 vertebral body and end plate erosion of C4 and C6 with segmental kyphosis secondary to pyogenic vertebral osteomyelitis. The patient was treated with anterior débridement and corpectomy of C5, with partial corpectomy of C4 and C6, and with allograft fibula strut graft. This treatment was followed by posterior stabilization with C3-7 lateral mass fixation and iliac crest bone graft. Postoperative lateral **(B)** and AP **(C)** radiographs.

anterior or posterior transpedicular biopsy (possibly using minimally invasive techniques) is appropriate.

The anterior approach is preferred for the treatment of vertebral osteomyelitis because it permits débridement of the infected bone and tissue, decompression of the neural elements, drainage of an epidural abscess, and stabilization of adjacent spinal segments. Posterior infections are exceedingly rare but are amenable to a posterior approach for débridement. Cultures should always be obtained intraoperatively and thorough irrigation and débridement of all infected and necrotic tissue is required. The anterior débridement inevitably leaves a bony void, which often requires stabilization of the anterior column with interbody arthrodesis and posterior stabilization (Figure 1). If a kyphotic deformity is present, it can be reduced and maintained with appropriate interbody graft placement. Autogenous tricortical iliac crest, rib, or fibular strut grafting (vascularized or nonvascularized) has proven safe and effective in the presence of acute infection. Freeze-dried allografts are being used with successful results, but autogenous sources are preferred because of better incorporation. In the presence of a severe kyphotic deformity or when a multilevel anterior construct is required, the addition of posterior fusion with instrumentation is recommended to adequately stabilize the spine (Figure 2). The procedure can be performed concomitantly or in a staged manner. A recent study showed superior deformity correction with anterior titanium mesh cages filled with autograft followed by posterior instrumentation.

Spinal Epidural Abscess
Epidemiology and Pathogenesis
There has been an increased incidence of spinal epidural abscess over the past decade. The reported incidence of the disease, however, is only 1.2 per 10,000 hospital admissions. Patients are most often age 60 years or older; men and women are equally affected. Factors that contribute to the relative increased incidence of epidural abscess include an increase in intravenous drug use, an increase in the number of immunocompromised hosts secondary to malignancy or human immunodeficiency virus and/or acquired immunodeficiency syndrome, and an increase in the number of invasive spinal operations and procedures (such as epidural anesthesia, spinal injections, and diskography).

A spinal epidural abscess is a collection of pus or inflammatory granulation tissue between the dura mater and the surrounding epidural adipose tissue. The presence of a spinal epidural abscess is typically associated with a coexistent vertebral osteomyelitis or diskitis. Contiguous spread of pathogens from adjacent disk or bone is the most common route of infection. However, hematogenous seeding of bacteria into the epidural space occurs rarely. Recently, studies have documented spinal epidural abscess after direct inoculation during spinal procedures. The causative organism remains *S aureus* in more than 60% of patients. Gram-negative rods account for approximately 18% of infections. *Pseudomonas* is commonly found in intravenous drug users.

Epidural abscesses are found in the cervical spine in approximately 14% of patients, and most are found an-

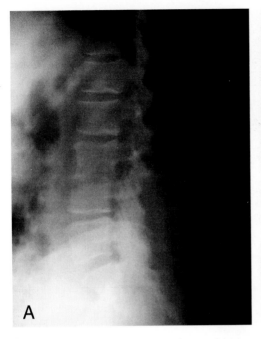
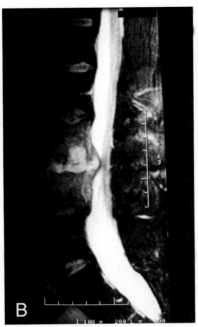
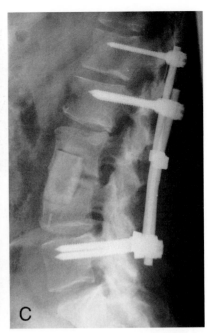

Figure 2 Imaging studies of a 60-year-old man who had worsening back pain for 2 months. **A,** Lateral radiograph of the lumbar spine shows complete loss of disk space at L3-4 and end plate erosions of the L3 and L4 vertebrae. **B,** T2-fat suppressed MRI scan of the lumbar spine shows L3-4 diskitis and associated pyogenic vertebral osteomyelitis. **C,** The patient was treated with anterior débridement with interbody fusion using allograft strut followed by posterior fusion with instrumentation.

teriorly. The majority of spinal epidural abscesses are found in the thoracic (51%) and lumbar (35%) spine. Most of these infections are posterior unless contiguous with vertebral osteomyelitis. Three to four spinal segments are usually involved, but the entire spinal column is at risk.

Initially, there is an inflammatory reaction in the epidural fat that progresses to suppuration, necrosis, and fibrosis in the epidural space. The pathogenesis of the neurologic manifestations is related either to direct compression of the neural elements or to compromise of the intrinsic circulation of the spinal cord.

Clinical Characteristics and Diagnosis

Intractable back or neck pain is the most common symptom in patients with a spinal epidural abscess. However, the clinical presentation of a patient with an epidural abscess can be highly variable; this variability leads to frequent misdiagnosis on initial presentation. Most patients with an acute spinal epidural abscess have fever, back pain, and spinal tenderness; however, these outward signs may be absent if the disease is chronic. If treatment is not initiated early, the back pain is followed by radicular pain, weakness, paralysis, and even frank sepsis. The immune status of the host and the virulence of the offending pathogen dictate the timing and severity of the progression of the infection. If the abscess penetrates the dura, a subdural abscess or meningitis may occur.

Patients with an acute epidural abscess usually have more systemic illness than those patients with vertebral osteomyelitis. Laboratory evaluation shows leukocytosis (mean, 22,000 cells/mm^3), elevated ESR (mean, 86.3 mm in 1 hour), and an elevated CRP. Plain radiographs are usually normal unless contiguous vertebral osteomyelitis or diskitis has been present long enough for the radiographic findings to be positive. CT scans have a poor sensitivity for epidural abscess. MRI with gadolinium contrast is the imaging modality of choice for the diagnosis and evaluation of spinal epidural abscess. The exact location and extent of the abscess, the amount of neurologic compression, and the presence and severity of contiguous infection can all be evaluated with MRI. Pus in the epidural space will enhance with gadolinium, whereas the cerebrospinal fluid will show low signal intensity on T1-weighted images. Biopsy of the adjacent disk, vertebral body, or surrounding tissue provides the definitive diagnosis of spinal epidural abscess and identification of the offending organism.

Treatment and Prognosis

Historically, the presence of spinal epidural abscess has been regarded as a medical and surgical emergency. The objectives of treatment of epidural abscesses are eradication of infection, prevention or improvement of neurologic sequelae, and preservation of spinal stability. Nonsurgical treatment of a spinal epidural abscess is only indicated in patients who are neurologically stable or are unsuitable surgical candidates because of medical

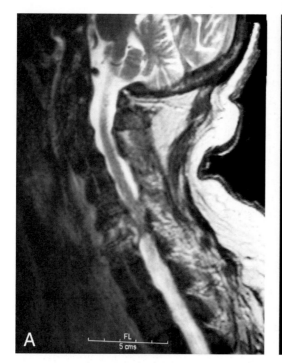

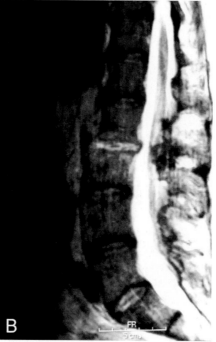

Figure 3 Imaging studies fof a 65-year-old man who developed cervical pyogenic osteomyelitis with associated epidural abscess and neurologic deficits with concomitant lumbar diskitis. **A,** Sagittal T2-weighted MRI scan of the cervical spine shows increased signal intensity throughout the C6 and C7 vertebral bodies with associated diskitis and epidural abscess causing anterior mass effect on the spinal cord. **B,** Sagittal T2-weighted image of lumbar spine shows signal enhancement of L2-3 disk and end plates consistent with diskitis and early pyogenic vertebral osteomyelitis.

comorbidities. A recent study showed that nonsurgical treatment of spinal epidural abscess is possible if no neurologic compromise has occurred. A new or progressive neurologic deterioration warrants immediate change from nonsurgical to surgical treatment.

Surgical intervention is the current treatment for most patients with spinal epidural abscess. The surgical approach and technique depend on the location and extent of the infection. Because the location is usually posterior, a decompressive laminectomy over the involved levels generally is the treatment of choice. Wide decompression with facetectomy is not usually required for adequate débridement and should be avoided because iatrogenic spinal instability may result. If anterior vertebral osteomyelitis or diskitis is present, combined anterior and posterior débridement may be necessary (Figure 3). Reconstruction of the anterior column with structural graft or instrumentation may be required if significant bony destruction has occurred. Posterior fusion with instrumentation often is preferred when acute infection is present after anterior débridement. Parenteral antibiotics are chosen based on the culture and sensitivity results, and are continued for 2 to 4 weeks after adequate surgical débridement. If vertebral osteomyelitis is present, parenteral antibiotics should be administered for at least 6 weeks.

Spinal epidural abscesses continue to have significant morbidity and mortality as a result of diagnostic delay. Recent literature reports that early diagnosis remains the most essential factor in preventing devastating outcomes. A recent retrospective study found that factors associated with improved outcome of patients

with spinal epidural abscess included younger age, less than 50% thecal sac compression, lumbosacral location, the presence of pustular abscesses as opposed to granulation tissue, and shorter duration of symptoms.

Nonpyogenic Vertebral Osteomyelitis

Nonpyogenic or granulomatous infections of the spine may be caused by fungi, atypical bacteria, or spirochetes. These infections are grouped together because, although the lesions resulting from these causes are not common, when they occur they have a similar clinical and histologic presentation. Most spinal infections in patients in the United States are pyogenic; however, with the increased number of immunocompromised hosts, more nonpyogenic infections have emerged in the past decade. The pathophysiology of granulomatous spinal infection differs from that of pyogenic infections. By far, the most common granulomatous disease of the spine is caused by *Mycobacterium tuberculosis*. Tuberculous spondylitis (Pott's disease) is the most extensively researched disease in this group of infections.

Epidemiology and Pathogenesis

Although tuberculosis (TB) is endemic in many developing countries, it was nearly eradicated in the United States. Nevertheless, there has been a resurgence of TB infection in the past decade, with the disease often occurring in immunocompromised patients and with resistant strains of the organism. The human immunodeficiency virus and acquired immunodeficiency syndrome epidemic is a major cause of the increase in TB infection in the United States. Ten percent of patients infected with TB will develop musculoskeletal infection, but 50% of these patients will have spinal involvement.

Hematogenous seeding from the respiratory or genitourinary tract is the usual mode of spread of infection to the spine. Local spread by direct extension is also possible. Most active cases of spinal TB in adults are actually reactivations of quiescent lesions from previous infection.

The three major types of spinal involvement of vertebral TB describe the pattern of bony involvement. The most common form is the peridiskal type, which begins with infection in the metaphyseal area that spreads under the anterior longitudinal ligament and later involves the adjacent vertebral bodies. In contrast to pyogenic infection, the disk is relatively resistant to infection and is often preserved until late in the infection process despite extensive bony destruction. With the anterior type, infection spreads beneath the anterior longitudinal ligament and may involve several vertebral levels, causing anterior erosions on the involved vertebral bodies. Central type infections often are mistaken for tumors because they remain isolated to one vertebra and often cause collapse and deformity. Isolated posterior element involvement has been described but is exceedingly rare.

The pathologic findings in tuberculous spondylitis differ in several respects from pyogenic vertebral osteomyelitis. The disk is relatively resistant to infection by TB. In addition, the development of the infection takes a longer period of time, and more deformity is typically observed at the time of presentation. Large paraspinal abscesses are more common with tuberculous infections. The thoracic spine is the most common location for spinal TB followed by lumbar involvement. The cervical spine is rarely involved.

Other etiologies of granulomatous infection are also increasing in incidence with the increasing number of immunocompromised hosts. Atypical bacteria such as *Actinomyces israelii*, *Nocardia asteroids*, and *Brucella* species also cause chronic granulomatous infection. *Treponema pallidum*, the organism responsible for syphilis, causes gummatous lesions in the spine, which are syphilitic granulomas representing the local reaction of the tissues to the organism and its products. Fungal infections of the spine are uncommon and often have a significant delay in diagnosis. *Coccidioides immitis*, *Blastomyces dermatitidis*, *Cryptococcus neoformans*, *Candida* species, and *Aspergillosis* are all responsible for fungal infections of the spine. In a recent study of patients with fungal spinal infections, the *Candida* species were the most common fungal pathogens.

Clinical Presentation and Evaluation

The onset of symptoms with tuberculous spondylitis is typically more insidious than with a pyogenic infection. Patients usually report pain in the spine and constitu-

tional symptoms of chronic illness including intermittent fever, malaise, night sweats, and weight loss. Neurologic deficit is present in 10% to 47% of patients with Pott's disease. Deformity at the time of diagnosis is more common in TB infection than in pyogenic spinal infection.

Laboratory studies are helpful but nonspecific. The white blood cell count often is not elevated. The ESR is usually elevated but may be normal in up to 25% of patients. Purified protein derivative skin tests typically are positive, which suggests either active or previous disease. False negative results are possible because of anergy, which could result from any condition that compromises host immunity. A chest radiograph should be obtained in all patients to rule out active lung involvement.

Plain radiographs are useful in diagnosis, but they will vary in appearance depending on the pathologic type and chronicity of the infection. After several weeks of infection, radiographs show vertebral end plate lucency and loss of cortical margins. Soft-tissue swelling and expansion across two to three spinal segments follow. Eventually, the classic pattern of disk space destruction with lucency and compression of adjacent vertebral bodies is seen, followed by further collapse into a kyphotic deformity.

Nuclear medicine studies with a combination of technetium and gallium nuclear scans have been shown to have the highest sensitivity for detecting infection. CT scans are beneficial in evaluating the extent of bony destruction and in surgical planning. However, the preferred imaging study for the diagnosis of tuberculous and fungal infections remains MRI with gadolinium contrast. MRI helps to differentiate metastatic disease from vertebral osteomyelitis; the lack of disk space involvement is seen with MRI only with metastatic disease.

Definitive diagnosis requires a positive biopsy with culture of the organism. Studies have shown that CT-guided biopsy with cultures and staining allows identification of the organism. Mycobacteria are acid-fast bacilli and may take up to 10 weeks to grow in culture. Polymerase chain reaction has been used for fast identification of mycobacteria with a sensitivity of 95% and accuracy of 93%.

Treatment

Nonpyogenic vertebral osteomyelitis is usually treated with chemotherapy directed at the offending pathogen. Additionally, an external immobilization device may be used for pain control and prevention of deformity. Tuberculous spondylitis is treated with isoniazid, rifampin, and pyrazinamide for 9 to 18 months depending on response to treatment. Ethambutol or streptomycin is usually added to the regimen for at least part of the treatment. It is recommended that an infectious disease

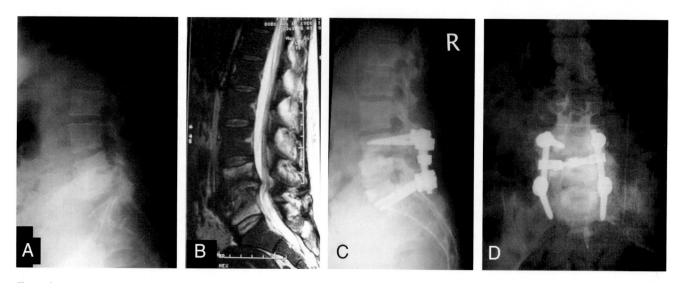

Figure 4 Imaging studies of a 48-year-old woman who presented with a 6-month history of severe low back pain. **A,** Plain radiograph shows evidence of chronic pyogenic vertebral osteomyelitis of L4-5 with sclerosis and apparent autofusion consistent with the duration of symptoms. **B,** Sagittal T2-weighted MRI shows continued enhancement of L4 and L5 vertebral bodies as well as diskitis at L5-S1. AP **(C)** and lateral **(D)** postoperative radiographs of the patient who was treated with anterior débridement and interbody fusion of L4-L5 and L5-S1, with femoral ring allografts followed by posterior fusion with instrumentation.

consultation be done in conjunction with the chemotherapy regimen because of varying regional resistance patterns. Amphotericin B and ketoconazole provide the mainstay for the treatment of most fungal infections. Brucellosis is typically treated with tetracycline and streptomycin. *Nocardia* infections are treated with sulfonamides, whereas actinomycosis is still treated with penicillin.

The surgical indications for treatment of nonpyogenic spinal infections are neurologic deficits, failure of response to nonsurgical treatment after 3 to 6 months, the need for tissue for diagnosis, spinal instability, progressive kyphotic deformity, and/or recurrence of the disease. Surgical options include anterior débridement and strut graft alone or with posterior instrumentation and fusion (Figure 4), or posterior débridement without anterior surgery done only for isolated posterior disease. If a laminectomy were performed for isolated posterior arch disease or posterior epidural abscess, then a supplemental fusion would be recommended. Anterior débridement and reconstruction at the site of pathology has shown the best long-term neurologic and structural results. Graft choice is dependent on surgeon preference. Autogenous and allograft strut grafts are acceptable with good results. A recent study showed that anterior spinal instrumentation with structural allograft fibula could be used after proper anterior débridement of tuberculous spondylitis with a 96% fusion rate and no recurrence of infection. Patients did not require external support in the postoperative period. Another study, using fresh frozen femoral allografts and stabilization with a single-rod construct after anterior débridement, showed excellent results with incorporation of the allografts between 12 and 18 months. These studies suggest that anterior instrumentation reduces kyphotic deformity without increasing the risk of disease recurrence. In patients with neurologic deficit, earlier débridement led to a faster and better neurologic recovery. There is a direct correlation between duration of preoperative symptoms and neurologic recovery.

Postoperative Spinal Infections

An increase in the incidence of postoperative infections has been documented in the past decade. Postoperative infections result from inoculation during the index procedure or by hematogenous seeding of the surgical site. Lumbar diskectomy performed with the use of prophylactic antibiotics carries a 0.7% incidence of infection. The use of the operating microscope for diskectomy increases that rate to 1.4%. Studies have shown that lumbar fusion with instrumentation has an estimated incidence of postoperative infection of 6%. A recent retrospective review showed a wound infection rate of 10% in trauma patients who underwent fusion for thoracolumbar fractures. The authors concluded that the overall risk of infection is higher in the trauma patient than in the elective surgery population and that those patients with complete neurologic deficit are at a greater risk of infection. Another recent study showed that late pain at the surgical site appearing 12 to 20 months after scoliosis surgery with posterior instrumentation is most often attributable to a subacute low-grade implant infection.

Prophylactic antibiotics have been shown in several studies to significantly reduce the incidence of postoperative infections. Prophylactic antibiotics should reach peak concentrations quickly and cover *S aureus* and *S epidermidis*. Cefazolin, a first-generation cephalospo-

Table 3 | Risk Factors for Developing Postoperative Infections

Advanced age
Obesity
Diabetes mellitus
Smoking
Immunocompromised host
Length of preoperative hospitalization
Myelodysplasia
Revision surgery
Increased surgical time
Spinal instrumentation
Bone graft
Methylmethacrylate
Arthrodesis
Trauma

rin, has good *Staphylococcus* coverage and should be administered at least 20 minutes before surgery. To prevent resistance, vancomycin should be used for prophylaxis only in patients at high risk for methicillin-resistant *S aureus*. Risk factors for postoperative spinal infections are listed in Table 3.

Clinical presentation of postoperative infections depends on timing and the depth of the infection. In the immediate postoperative period, patients with superficial wound infections may have pain, fever, tenderness, erythema, and drainage from the incision site. Diagnosis of deep wound infections is more difficult because complete onset may be delayed, with only constitutional symptoms and a well healed surgical incision. Laboratory values including leukocyte count, ESR, and CRP are often elevated. The acute phase reactants are normally elevated in the immediate postoperative period. The ESR remains elevated for up to 6 weeks, whereas the CRP normalizes in approximately 2 weeks. *S aureus* is cultured in about 60% of wound infections.

Aggressive surgical intervention is generally recommended for postoperative infections. Administration of antibiotics should be delayed until intraoperative superficial and deep cultures are obtained. Aggressive débridement followed by copious irrigation is recommended. Wound closure over closed suction drains is required unless the wound is packed open for repeat débridements. Recent studies advocate the use of antibiotic beads, especially in the presence of hardware. Unless the fusion is solid, most surgeons retain the instrumentation and bone graft. If significant soft-tissue necrosis or dead space is present, plastic surgical techniques including musculocutaneous flaps may be necessary. For patients with soft-tissue and wound infections, 10 to 14 days of antibiotics are sufficient. Parenteral an-

tibiotics taken for 6 weeks are required for patients with deep infection, bony involvement, or retained hardware.

Annotated Bibliography

Pyogenic Vertebral Osteomyelitis

Hee HT, Majd ME, Holt RT, Pienkowski D: Better treatment of vertebral osteomyelitis using posterior stabilization and titanium mesh cages. *J Spinal Disord Tech* 2002;15:149-156.

The authors evaluated the efficacy of using titanium mesh cages anteriorly and posterior instrumentation after anterior débridement in the surgical treatment of vertebral osteomyelitis. Patients treated with cages had better sagittal and coronal correction.

Schimmer RC, Jeanneret C, Nunley PD, Jeanneret B: Osteomyelitis of the cervical spine: A potentially dramatic disease. *J Spinal Disord Tech* 2002;15:110-117.

A retrospective review of 15 patients treated for osteomyelitis of the cervical spine is presented. Good results were achieved by early and aggressive surgical intervention.

Spinal Epidural Abscess

Tang HJ, Lin HJ, Liu YC, Li CM: Spinal epidural abscess: Experience with 46 patients and evaluation of prognostic factors. *J Infect* 2002;45:76-81.

This article reviewed 46 patients treated for spinal epidural abscess with emphasis on defining clinical characteristics, treatment options, and evaluation of prognostic factors.

Nonpyogenic Vertebral Osteomyelitis

Frazier DD, Campbell DR, Garvey TA, Wiesel S, Bohlman HH, Eismont FJ: Fungal infections of the spine: Report of eleven patients with long-term follow-up. *J Bone Joint Surg Am* 2001;83:560-565.

This article presents a retrospective review of 11 patients treated for spinal osteomyelitis caused by a fungus. The authors describe delay in treatment and diagnosis as important factors in poor outcomes. They recommend performing fungal cultures whenever a spinal infection is suspected.

Govender S: The outcome of allografts and anterior instrumentation in spinal tuberculosis. *Clin Orthop* 2002; 398:50-59.

This article presents a review of 41 patients with neurologic deficits caused by spinal TB who were treated with radical anterior decompression with reconstruction of the anterior column with fresh-frozen femoral ring allograft and stabilized with a single-rod screw instrumentation construct.

Ozdemir HM, Us AK, Ogun T: The role of anterior spinal instrumentation and allograft fibula for the treatment of pott disease. *Spine* 2003;28:474-479.

The authors retrospectively reviewed 28 patients with multilevel spinal TB who had anterior débridement, decompression, and fusion with anterior spinal instrumentation and fibular allograft. A 96% fusion rate with no graft complications was recorded.

Postoperative Spinal Infections

Kothari NA, Pelchovitz DJ, Meyer JS: Imaging of musculoskeletal infections. *Radiol Clin North Am* 2001;39: 653-671.

This article reviews the epidemiology, pathophysiology, and the clinical and imaging presentations of musculosketetal infections of all types. Discussion is presented on the imaging characteristics of plain radiographs, CT scans, MRI, and nuclear studies for various spinal infections.

Rechtine GR, Bono PL, Cahill D, Bolesta MJ, Chrin AM: Postoperative wound infection after instrumentation of thoracic and lumbar fractures. *J Orthop Trauma* 2001;15:566-569.

Twelve of 117 patients (10%) with thoracolumbar fractures who had surgical intervention developed postoperative wound infections. The authors observed that the overall risk of infection is higher in trauma patients especially those with neurologic deficit.

Tay BK, Deckey J, Hu SS: Spinal Infections. *J Am Acad Orthop Surg* 2002;10:188-197.

A thorough review of the literature and a concise description of current methods of diagnosis, laboratory assessment, imaging, and treatment of spinal infections in both children and adults are presented.

Vaccaro AR, Harris BM, Madigan L: Spinal infections, pyogenic osteomyelitis, and epidural abscess, in Vaccaro A, Betz R, Zeidman S (eds): *Principles and Practice of Spine Surgery*. Philadelphia, PA, Mosby, 2003, pp 165-174.

This chapter presents a current comprehensive review of spinal infections.

Classic Bibliography

An HS, Vaccaro AR, Dolinskas CA, Colter JM, Balderston RA, Bauerle WB: Differentiation between spinal tumors and infections with magnetic resonance imaging. *Spine* 1991;16(suppl 8):S334-S338.

Carragee EJ: Pyogenic vertebral osteomyelitis. *J Bone Joint Surg Am* 1997;79:874-880.

Currier BL, Eismont FJ: Infections of the spine, in Herkowitz HN, Garfin GR, Balderston RA, Eismont FJ, Ball GR, Wiesel SW (eds): *The Spine*. Philadelphia, PA, WB Saunders, 1999, pp 1207-1258.

Eismont FJ, Bohlman HH, Soni PL, Goldberg VM, Freehafer AA: Pyogenic and fungal vertebral osteomyelitis with paralysis. *J Bone Joint Surg Am* 1983;65:19-29.

Emery SE, Chan DP, Woodward HR: Treatment of hematogenous pyogenic vertebral osteomyelitis with anterior debridement and primary bone grafting. *Spine* 1989; 14:284-291.

Heggeness MH, Esses SI, Errico T, et al: Late infection of spinal instrumentation by hematogenous seeding. *Spine* 1993;18:492-496.

Moon MS: Tuberculosis of the spine: Controversies and a new challenge. *Spine* 1997;22:1791-1797.

Rezai AR, Woo HH, Errico TJ, Cooper PR: Contemporary management of spinal osteomyelitis. *Neurosurgery* 1999;44:1018-1026.

Thalgott JS, Cotler HB, Sasso RC, LaRocca H, Gardner V: Postoperative infections in spinal implants classification and analysis: A multicenter study. *Spine* 1991;16: 981-984.

Wheeler D, Keiser P, Rigamont D, Keay S: Medical management of spinal epidural abscesses: Case report and review. *Clin Infect Dis* 1992;15:22-27.

Yilmaz C, Selek HY, Gurkan I, Erdemli B, Korkusu Z: Anterior instrumentation for the treatment of spinal tuberculosis. *J Bone Joint Surg Am* 1999;81:1261-1267.

Chapter 48

Tumors of the Spine

Gurvinder S. Deol, MD

Rex Haydon, MD, PhD

Frank M. Phillips, MD

Introduction

Primary and metastatic tumors of the spine encompass a wide spectrum of disease processes requiring many different treatment algorithms. The treatment of spinal tumors has evolved over the course of the past decade with the advent of improved diagnosis, staging, and nonsurgical and surgical treatment.

Primary Tumors

Primary tumors of the spine account for 2% to 5% of all spinal neoplasms, with metastatic tumors accounting for most spinal tumors. Within the group of primary tumors, benign tumors are far more common than malignant tumors.

Benign Tumors

Osteoid Osteoma

Osteoid osteomas are probably the most common primary benign vertebral tumors, and they are usually diagnosed during the first three decades of life, with a peak incidence at age 15 years. Ten percent to 25% of all osteoid osteomas occur in the spine, and nearly 70% of painful juvenile scoliotic deformities are associated with osteoid osteomas that typically occur at the apex of the concavity of the curve as a cortically based nidus of osteoid-producing cells surrounded by a dense halo of sclerosis, which may be the only radiographic sign at diagnosis. Histologically, the lesion manifests as a nidus of highly vascular osteoid-producing spindle cells surrounded by dense sclerotic bone. Pain is the most common presenting symptom and is characteristically worse at night and relieved by treatment with nonsteroidal anti-inflammatory drugs (NSAIDs). On plain radiographs, the overlying bony structures often obscure the appearance of osteoid osteoma, making additional imaging studies necessary. The most sensitive study for osteoid osteoma is the bone scan, which targets the rapid bone turnover, a hallmark of this lesion. Increased uptake of technetium Tc 99m occurs in the area of the lesion, often surrounded by a zone of diminished uptake, creating a distinctive target sign. Although bone scans represent perhaps the most sensitive test for osteoid osteoma, a CT scan is the most specific. Treatment of this disorder includes both medical and surgical options. Pain associated with osteoid osteoma, as a rule, responds to treatment with NSAIDs. Given the usually self-limited nature of osteoid osteoma, NSAIDs and observation are the initial treatment. In patients in whom NSAIDs are either not tolerated or are contraindicated or in patients whose osteoid osteoma is associated with progressive scoliotic deformities, more aggressive therapies can be considered. Excision of the lesions results in reliable pain relief, and most associated scoliotic deformities improve. Good short-term results with percutaneous radiofrequency ablation of osteoid osteoma have been reported.

Osteoblastoma

Histologically, osteoblastomas are often indistinguishable from osteoid osteomas except for their size, but the clinical features and natural history of these two disorders have notable differences. Spine involvement is even more commonly associated with osteoblastoma, accounting for approximately 40% of instances; lesions typically localize to the posterior elements in 55% of patients. The most common presenting symptom in patients with osteoblastoma is focal pain, which is less responsive to NSAIDs than the pain associated with osteoid osteoma. The pain is more typically activity-related. Cortical expansion can result in impingement of neural elements. Painful scoliotic deformities can also occur in the setting of osteoblastoma; however, this is much less common than with osteoid osteoma. Osteoblastomas are more readily detected on plain radiographs because of their larger size (> 2 cm), and their propensity to cause cortical expansion. The internal characteristics of osteoblastomas can be variable, but ossification is the predominant pattern, which is consistent with its osteoblastic origin. Osteoblastoma is a slowly progressive lesion that does not normally respond to conservative management. Surgical resection of the lesion is therefore indicated; however, local recurrences occur in 10% to 15% of patients, and the recurrence rate can be as high as 50% in patients with high-grade subtypes of osteoblastoma. Debate exists regarding the adequacy of curettage in the treatment of osteoblastoma, and it has yet to be determined whether marginal resection results in a lower risk of recurrence. Surgical treatment (simple curettage or resection) should be planned based on the location of the lesion, concomitant symptoms, and risk of morbidity. Malignant transformation of osteoblastomas has been documented.

Giant Cell Tumor

Giant cell tumors can range in behavior from slowly growing, relatively innocuous tumors to locally aggressive tumors that metastasize. The spine is a relatively common site for giant cell tumors, comprising between 5% and 10% of all instances of giant cell tumor. Unlike their appendicular counterparts, however, there is often a significant delay between the onset of symptoms in the spine and the diagnosis. Pain and radiculopathy are the most common presenting symptoms, and they have often been present for several months before the patient's initial contact with a physician. Spinal giant cell tumors are most commonly diagnosed during the third and fourth decades of life, and they occur at a slightly more frequent rate in women. Within the axial skeleton, the sacrum is the most common region affected, and lesions are typically found in the vertebral body. Plain films generally demonstrate a well-demarcated, radiolucent lesion with a variable amount of cortical expansion and local remodeling. Even in the most aggressive instances of giant cell tumor, a thin shell of cortical bone will usually remain at the periphery of the lesion, which helps distinguish it from a malignant bone tumor. Giant cell tumors involving the spine are typically treated by curettage. En bloc surgical resection is considered to be the optimal treatment of this disorder and appears to reduce the rate of local recurrence. In the spine, the proximity of vital structures to the lesion, as well as the considerable morbidity associated with this approach has limited the use of en bloc resections. Spinal giant cell tumors have a considerably poorer prognosis than those in the appendicular skeleton, with recurrence rates reaching almost 80% in grade III giant cell tumors. Furthermore, metastasis occurs in just under 10% of patients.

Chondroblastoma

Chondroblastoma of the spine is extremely rare, and published articles regarding spinal chondroblastoma are mostly limited to case reports. Nonetheless, most patients with this disorder have been diagnosed during the second or third decade of life. Radiographic evaluation of spinal chondroblastomas generally reveals a well-demarcated radiolucent lesion. Evidence of internal matrix calcification may be apparent on plain radiographs or CT scans; however, this is not a universal finding in all patients with chondroblastoma. Because of the lim-

ited number of patients with this disorder, it is difficult to define a clear predilection for either the anterior or posterior spinal elements; however, it has been reported that most spinal chondroblastomas occur in the posterior elements. Chondroblastomas usually contain numerous osteoclast-like giant cells; matrix calcification, when present, often has a distinctive chicken-wire appearance, which is a histologic hallmark of this lesion. Cellular atypia can vary from moderate to high, which is believed to reflect the spectrum of behavior of chondroblastoma from slowly progressive local growth to aggressive local growth and metastatic spread. Treatment of these lesions consists predominantly of curettage or excision; however, it is not clear whether this treatment is effective in the spine, given the limited number of patients with spinal chondroblastomas. The recurrence rate for chondroblastomas of the spine is likewise unclear.

Osteochondroma

Spinal osteochondromas account for less than 10% of all osteochondromas. They usually arise from the posterior elements. Typically, they are slow-growing masses and rarely cause mechanical or compressive symptoms. They are therefore largely observed unless they begin to cause problems such as persistent pain or radiculopathy. If this occurs, these tumors can be resected. The rate of recurrence after resection in adults is low, and in skeletally immature patients it is imperative to resect the cartilage cap to prevent recurrence. Malignant transformation to chondrosarcomas has been reported and occurs more commonly in patients with multiple hereditary exostoses. These lesions tend to be low grade and respond well to local wide resection.

Langerhans Cell Histiocytosis

This condition, more commonly known as eosinophilic granuloma, represents a usually benign, self-limiting process that usually causes focal areas of well-demarcated bone resorption, which in the spine gives rise to the classic vertebra plana sign. The underlying etiology of this disorder is unknown, and it usually affects individuals during the first and second decades of life, with a 2:1 predilection for males. The spine is involved in 10% to 15% of patients, but the condition more commonly affects the skull and flat bones of the pelvis, rib cage, and shoulder. Although most instances of this disorder are self-limiting and resolve on their own, surgical intervention may be indicated in patients with progressive kyphosis or neurologic symptoms. Low-dose radiation therapy has also shown to be effective in patients who are not amenable to resection. It is important to be aware of two systemic disease processes associated with eosinophilic granuloma: Hand-Schüller-Christian disease and Letterer-Siwe disease. Both of these disease processes involve multifocal lesions along with other systemic manifestations.

Aneurysmal Bone Cyst

Aneurysmal bone cysts involve the spine in 10% to 30% of patients, and they are most commonly found in the posterior elements of the thoracolumbar spine. They can occur at any age but are most common during the first two decades of life. Unique to aneurysmal bone cysts is their ability to involve multilevel adjacent spinal segments. Radiographically, aneurysmal bone cysts cause cortical expansion and thinning, and have a characteristic "bubbly" appearance created by multiple cavernous chambers. MRI is needed to detect smaller aneurysmal bone cysts, and fluid/fluid levels, which represent old areas of hemorrhage, are almost pathognomonic for aneurysmal bone cysts. Treatment includes curettage, wide local excision, embolization, and sometimes radiation. The rate of local recurrence has been estimated to be between 15% and 30% of patients; recurrence is treated by repeat curettage.

Hemangioma

Hemangiomas of the spine represent the most common tumor of the spine and are usually identified as an incidental finding. At autopsy, 11% of individuals are reported to have hemangiomas. These occur as singular lesions in approximately two thirds of individuals, and the lesions are characterized radiographically by vertical trabecular striations resembling a honeycomb that most commonly involve the vertebral body, with the thoracic spine being the most commonly affected. Plain radiographs can be sufficient to diagnose those lesions that involve greater than 30% to 40% of the vertebral body; however, CT or MRI may be more helpful in detecting the presence of more subtle lesions. Neurologic symptoms may occur as a result of neural compression caused by cortical expansion or soft-tissue extension beyond the vertebral body. Hemangiomas are radiosensitive, and low-dose radiation has been shown to be effective as a treatment of symptomatic lesions, as has embolization via angiography. In those instances where pathologic fracture or deformity results in instability or neurologic compromise, surgical resection and stabilization may be indicated. Vertebral cement augmentation procedures (vertebroplasty and kyphoplasty) have also been successfully used to treat hemangiomas.

Malignant Tumors

Osteosarcoma

Osteosarcoma of the spine carries with it an especially bleak prognosis. Osteosarcoma of the spine accounts for approximately 2% of all osteosarcomas throughout the body, and 3% to 14% of malignant tumors involving the spine. Most tumors arise in the lumbosacral region and involve the vertebral body in up to 90% of patients. As an entity, osteosarcoma includes any malignant spindle tumor that produces osteoid; however, this encompasses a variety of histologic subtypes. Treatment and prognosis are, therefore, dependent on appropriate histologic diagnosis. There is a bimodal distribution in the age of presentation of patients with osteosarcomas involving the spine; a young patient population (age 10 to 25 years) typically has the more classic type of osteosarcoma, whereas patients older than 50 years typically have secondary osteosarcomas. When viewed collectively, osteosarcoma of the spine has a generally poorer prognosis and occurs in older age groups when compared with appendicular osteosarcoma. The primary lesion can be either radiolucent or radiodense, with prominent periosteal reaction and usually soft-tissue extension. The internal characteristics of the lesion demonstrate ossification consistent with the degree of osteoid production. Numerous histologic subtypes of osteosarcoma exist that are designated by location (central, parosteal, and periosteal), grade (low versus high), predominant cell type (osteoblastic, chondroblastic, and fibroblastic), or etiology (radiation-induced, and Paget's sarcoma). With the exception of low-grade lesions such as parosteal osteosarcomas, patients with osteosarcoma of the spine receive preoperative chemotherapy followed by surgical resection and usually adjuvant therapy. As with other malignant lesions of the spine, wide resections or even marginal resections are often not possible, making radiation therapy and adjuvant chemotherapy necessary to treat the residual disease. Estimation of the outcome in patients with osteosarcoma of the spine has been hampered by its relative rarity. Metastasis at diagnosis, large size, sacral location, and intralesional resections are associated with adverse outcomes.

Chondrosarcoma

After chordomas, chondrosarcoma is the most common primary malignant tumor of bone in the spine, accounting for approximately 7% to 12% of all spine tumors. Chondrosarcomas occur more commonly in men than women and later in life, with the average age at diagnosis being 45 years. Chondrosarcoma can vary considerably in its behavior, and it is generally described according to grades I through III, with each grade corresponding to an increasing tendency for metastasis and, therefore, a poorer prognosis. Plain films typically demonstrate a centrally based destructive lesion with calcification. In patients with low-grade chondrosarcoma, the lesion can cause scalloping of the bony cortex or cortical expansion. In patients with high-grade chondrosarcoma, the tumor can erode through the cortex and form a large extraosseous mass, also containing diffuse areas of calcification. Identification of the grade of the tumor is essential to determine prognosis, and it is based primarily on the cellularity of the tumor and pleomorphism of the tumor cells. Such information is also useful to determine the usefulness of adjuvant treatments such as radiation therapy. The treatment of chondrosarcoma is complicated by its lack of response to conventional chemotherapy and/or radiation therapy. No known clinical trials have demonstrated any survival benefit among patients receiving chemotherapy, and the use of radiation in this patient population is controversial. Surgical excision, therefore, is the mainstay of treatment of chondrosarcoma. As a result, the survival rate of patients with chondrosarcoma is closely associated with adequate lesion excision and clean margins. Median survival in patients with chondrosarcoma of the spine is approximately 6 years.

Ewing's Sarcoma

Ewing's sarcoma of the spine is a relatively rare entity, accounting for only 8% of a large reported series of patients with Ewing's sarcoma. It is actually more common for this tumor to metastasize to the spine from other locations than it is for it to originate in the spine as a primary tumor. Its clinical features are similar to those for all patients with Ewing's sarcoma; it most commonly arises during the second decade of life, and it affects males more frequently than females. The most common presenting symptom among patients with Ewing's sarcoma is pain, often in the sacrococcygeal area. Although instances of Ewing's sarcoma involving the cervical spine have been reported, they are extremely rare. Osseous findings in patients with Ewing's sarcoma can be extremely subtle. Plain radiographs can, therefore, appear normal, often belying a large soft-tissue mass. In this respect, CT or MRI may be far more informative in defining tumor extent. In patients with Ewing's sarcoma, these imaging modalities can demonstrate evidence of a large mass originating in the vertebral body, with variable amounts of internal mineralization. C-reactive protein levels and erythrocyte sedimentation rates are often elevated, and can therefore be useful adjuncts for the diagnosis of Ewing's sarcoma. Histologically, Ewing's sarcomas are composed of sheets of small blue cells, occasionally forming pseudorosettes around areas of necrosis. Nearly all Ewing's sarcomas possess a characteristic t11:22 chromosomal translocation. Although the treatment of patients with Ewing's sarcoma has varied considerably, the condition currently is treated using a combination of chemotherapy, surgical resection, and radiation therapy, each of which is effective against this tumor individually. The use of adjuvant treatments is especially critical given the difficulty of performing wide resection in the spine.

Chordoma

Chordomas are the most common nonhematogenous primary malignant tumors of the spine, and, unlike other malignant tumors discussed, they do not normally occur outside of the spine. They account for 1% to 4% of all primary bone tumors, with 20% of those occurring in the spine. Originating from remnants of the notochord, chordomas typically involve either the sacrococcygeal or sphenooccipital regions of the axial skeleton. The average age at diagnosis is 56 years; however, these tumors can occur in almost any age group. Clinical presentation is often subtle, with a gradual onset of neurologic symptoms including pain, numbness, motor weakness, incontinence, and constipation. Chordomas are slowly growing lesions and are often quite large when initially discovered. When located in the sacrum, the mass usually protrudes anteriorly, thereby preventing the lesion from causing a noticeable external mass. On radiographic evaluation, the bone from which the tumor arises may demonstrate noticeable changes, but the most impressive feature of chordomas is the large soft-tissue mass. Unless a significant amount of internal calcification is present, the soft-tissue component can be missed or underestimated on the basis of plain radiographs; therefore, either CT or MRI is required for definitive evaluation. On MRI chordomas are lobulated masses with a distinctly myxoid (mucoid) consistency. Because they are generally slow-growing tumors, they are associated with a pseudocapsule. The histologic appearance of chordomas can vary from relatively cellular masses to fluid-filled cysts. Classically, they are composed of chords of physaliphorous cells that are organized into lobules. Similar to chondrosarcoma, chordomas demonstrate a poor response to both radiotherapy and chemotherapy. Surgical excision with wide margins, therefore, offers the only significant possibility of cure in these patients. The average 10-year survival rate among patients with sacral chordomas is 20% to 40%, usually because of recurrence and direct spread of the tumor. The reported rate of metastasis varies widely in different series, ranging from 10% to 27% for sacral lesions; however, this rarely represents the cause of death in patients with chordomas.

Multiple Myeloma

Multiple myeloma and its solitary counterpart, plasmacytoma, are both B-cell lymphoproliferative diseases. Solitary plasmacytoma often progresses to multiple myeloma. Multiple myeloma is the most common primary malignancy of bone and the spine. Patients often present with pain from spontaneous vertebral compression fractures. Multiple punched-out lesions on a lateral skull radiograph are a classic finding, and this warrants a skeletal survey which may reveal other lesions. Bone scans are classically negative because of the lack of local bone reaction, and the diagnosis is confirmed with the presence of a monoclonal spike with serum electrophoresis. Chemotherapy and radiation therapy have long been the mainstays of treatment of this condition.

With advances in chemotherapeutic treatments, patients with multiple myeloma often live longer than patients with bone metastases from other malignancies.

This has prompted a more aggressive approach in the treatment of myeloma affecting the spine to improve quality of life. Radiation may be quite effective in treating spinal cord compression from epidural tumor. In patients with vertebral collapse with neurologic symptoms or advanced kyphosis, surgery may be indicated. Even with more advanced disease, surgical decompression and reconstruction may be warranted, and the outcomes from a recent study seem to favor this approach in carefully selected patients. Similarly, in patients with myeloma and pathologic vertebral compression fractures, kyphoplasty has been shown to result in improved quality of life as well as correction of vertebral deformity.

Metastatic Tumors

Because the spine is the most common site of skeletal involvement of metastatic disease, metastases account for most tumors surgically encountered in the spine. Approximately 50% of these tumors arise from carcinoma (lung or breast), lymphoma, or myeloma. In regard to the solid tumor primaries, breast, lung, and prostate are the most common, followed by renal, thyroid, gastrointestinal, and rarely primary soft-tissue sarcomas. Breast, prostate, and renal metastases are more likely to be seen by the spine surgeon than either pulmonary or gastrointestinal tumors because of longer patient survival rates.

The most common and usually the first symptom of spinal metastases is that of localized pain, which may occur at night and awaken patients from sleep. Patients may also present with radicular or myelopathic symptoms. If a suspected metastatic spinal lesion is found, a search for the primary tumor as well as for other sites of metastatic disease must be made. This workup may identify other lesions that are more accessible for biopsy than the spine. The type of tumor often dictates the treatment; however, the goals of treatment include decreasing the tumor burden, relief of pain, prevention and reversal of neurologic deficits, and preserving or restoring spinal stability. The modes of treatment will be discussed later in the chapter.

Spinal Cord Tumors

Tumors of the spinal cord are divided into three categories: extradural, intradural-extramedullary, and intramedullary.

Extradural tumors are very uncommon. The most common malignancy in the epidural space is lymphoma, with most being spread from the vertebral body or paraspinous nodes; however, a small number do arise primarily from the epidural space. Excision and posterior neural decompression is usually the treatment of choice for extradural tumors. Ten percent of neurofibromas are extradural. They usually arise from a spinal nerve root, and because malignant degeneration is pos-sible, excision is indicated. Although epidural lipomas are uncommon, they are a well-documented entity and can cause cord compression. Lipomatosis, especially when steroid-induced, is another possible diagnosis in patients with extradural tumors. Extradural tumors can initially be observed using MRI, but excision is recommended in patients with any progressive neurologic deficits. Epidural hemangioma and meningioma are both rare.

Intradural-extramedullary tumors make up approximately 85% of intradural tumors and largely consist of neurofibromas, meningiomas, and ependymomas. The two predominant intramedullary tumors are astrocytoma (high and low grade) and ependymomas, with hemangiomas and lipomas being exceedingly rare. As with extradural neurofibromas, the intradural counterpart also arises from the nerve roots, usually the dorsal sensory roots. The so-called "dumbbell" tumor is an intradural neurofibroma that is following the nerve root through the foramen. Again, complete excision is the treatment of choice. Meningiomas are usually found in the anterolateral canal and should be excised when identified. Ependymomas usually arise from within the cord and should be excised; however, extramedullary ependymomas can arise from the tip of the conus at its junction with the filum terminale. Astrocytomas are intramedullary and should be excised. High-grade astrocytomas have no visible margin and are usually debulked followed by neoadjuvant chemotherapy. Patients with high-grade astrocytomas have a bleak prognosis.

Diagnosis and Evaluation

The most common presenting symptom among patients with tumors of the spine is pain, which is reported by more than 80% of patients at initial visit. Typically, tumors with a more rapid onset of pain reflect more aggressive tumors, whereas benign or more slowly growing tumors may be characterized by gradually increasing pain spanning several months to years, with sudden increases in pain suggesting pathologic fracture. Neurologic compromise can also be a presenting symptom because of compression of either nerve roots or the spinal cord. Depending on the precise location and size of the tumor, neurologic symptoms can range from subtle motor or sensory deficits to paraplegia. Other presenting symptoms such as spinal deformity are considerably less common. A careful history should also include constitutional symptoms such as weight loss, fevers and chills, and lethargy as well as a complete medical history, including any personal history or family history of malignancy.

Radiographic evaluation generally begins with plain films, with notation of the location of the lesion, any soft-tissue extension, the zone of transition, and internal characteristics. For tumors involving the spine, certain

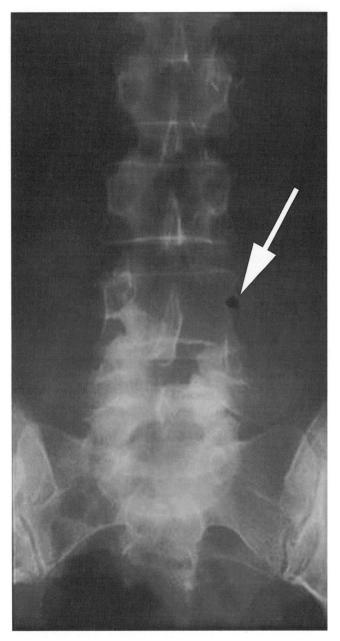

Figure 1 AP radiograph demonstrating the winking owl sign in which the right-sided pedicle has been destroyed by tumor, so that the pedicle ring is absent (*arrow*).

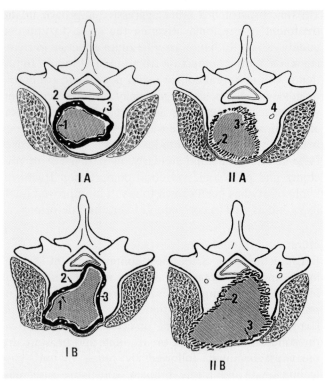

Figure 2 Enneking's oncologic stages (IA, IIA, IB, and IIB) of malignant tumors to the spine. 1 = tumor capsule, 2 = pseudocapsule, 3 = tumor with pseudocapsule, 4 = skip metastases. (*Reproduced with permission from Boriani S, Biagini R, DeJure F: Bone tumors of the spine and epidural cord compression: Treatment options. Semin Spine Surg 1995;7:317-322.*)

classic radiographic signs have been described, such as the winking owl sign, in which the pedicle has been eroded by an expanding tumor (Figure 1), or vertebra plana, in which there is vertebral body collapse. Although these signs are considered to be classic radiographic signs for spinal lesions, they are typically seen only after considerable bony destruction has occurred. Advanced imaging studies are mandatory in any evaluation of spinal tumors. MRI provides not only unparalleled soft-tissue detail, but it also evaluates the neural elements. MRI can reveal important tissue characteristics of the tumor, such as density, vascular perfusion and

necrosis, and extent of marrow involvement. When the lesion is primarily bony, CT provides excellent detail and is a valuable tool for preoperative planning. For patients with malignant tumors or metastatic disease, staging studies should also include a chest radiograph, chest, abdominal, and pelvic CT, and bone scan. Finally, before beginning any definitive treatment, a pathologic diagnosis should be obtained by performing a biopsy, either CT-guided or open, depending on the location and size of the lesion.

Staging systems attempt to predict outcome among patients with benign and malignant tumors by using clinical variables such as the histologic grade of the tumor, local behavior, and metastatic spread. In bone and soft-tissue sarcomas, staging systems have also been designed as preoperative aides to define the surgical planning for optimal local control. For benign tumors of bone, the Enneking system is commonly used and divides tumors into one of three categories: inactive, active, and aggressive. To address malignant bone lesions, Enneking developed a surgical staging system based on the grade of the tumor, intracompartmental or extracompartmental status, and metastatic disease (Figure 2). Although this staging system has been adopted for the staging of pelvic and extremity tumors, it has proved to be less useful in the treatment of spinal tumors. A staging system for spinal tumors was developed based on the lesion's location and local extension (Figure 3). The vertebral body is divided into twelve sectors similar to a clockface, and the tumor location is plotted according to this grid. Furthermore, five layers are described, beginning with the paraspinal soft tissues peripherally to the intradural space centrally. The system is primarily descriptive, and it can therefore be for the staging of both benign and malignant tumors. The Harrington staging system has been applied to metastatic spinal tumors (Figure 4).

Nonsurgical Treatment

The management of patients with benign primary tumors includes close clinical and radiographic observation. Bracing has a limited role in treatment, but it may provide some symptomatic relief of pain. Specific strategies for certain tumors have been discussed individually. Surgical excision should be considered when the patient has evidence of neurologic deficit, tumor progression, progressive deformity, or pain.

In patients with malignancies, chemotherapy plays an important role in treating tumors such as osteosarcoma, Ewing's sarcoma, and lymphoma for which chemotherapeutic regimens have proved to be systemically effective. Chemotherapy can be used both preoperatively and postoperatively as an adjuvant agent, and in some patients, it can even be used as a primary treatment to reduce tumor burden. Stem cell and bone marrow salvage is allowing higher doses of chemotherapy to be administered for longer periods, which in turn is more lethal to tumors. Radiation therapy, as with chemotherapy, can be used either as an adjuvant or primary treatment. Patients with radiosensitive tumors (lung, prostate, breast) who present early with metastatic disease without spinal instability or dense neurologic compromise can be managed with radiation therapy. In patients with higher tumor load requiring surgical intervention, external beam irradiation can be used as an adjuvant therapy either preoperatively or postoperatively. Recent advances in radiosurgery allow the delivery of a single, large dose of radiation (proton beam) to a localized tumor using a stereotactic approach, resulting in precise delivery to the target. This may be useful in the treatment of chordomas, recurrent tumors, or sarcomas without clear resection margins.

Surgical Treatment

The primary goals of surgery in patients with spinal tumors are to reduce pain, to preserve or restore neurologic function, and to establish spinal column structural integrity. Less commonly, excision of the tumor in an attempt at a cure is performed. In patients with tumors that do not respond to radiotherapy and chemotherapy, earlier surgery to prevent impending vertebral collapse

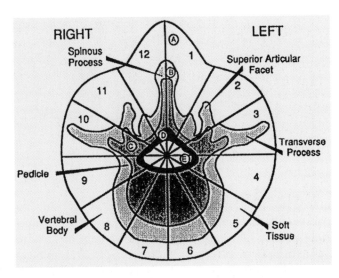

Figure 3 Proposed system of surgical staging of spine tumors, defining the extent of the tumor. A = extraosseous soft tissues, B = intraosseous (superficial), C = intraosseous (deep), D = extraosseous (extradural), E = extraosseous (intradural), and M = metastasis. Numbers 1 through 12 represent location of tumor. *(Reproduced with permission from Boriani S, Weinstein JN, Biagini R: Primary bone tumors of the spine. Spine 1997;22:1036-1044.)*

and/or neurologic deterioration may be considered. Specific treatment considerations for the various types of spinal tumors have been discussed. In patients with highly vascular tumors such as renal cell carcinoma, preoperative tumor embolization may help reduce intraoperative bleeding. In general, the location and extent of the tumor dictate the approach (anterior, posterior, or combined), and the extent of destabilization caused by the decompression or removal of tumor then determines the method of restabilization and reconstruction of the spine. The immediate proximity of vital structures (particularly the neural elements) to the tumor often precludes wide surgical excision, and spinal tumors are invariably treated with intralesional surgery. Such surgeries are therefore palliative, and are performed in an attempt to improve the quality of the patient's life.

Spinal Stability

The definition of spinal instability in the setting of vertebral destruction by tumor remains elusive. Unlike long bones, the spine may continue to exhibit a degree of load bearing without catastrophic failure after fracture, so that the concept of patients being at risk for pathologic fracture is not as intuitive for those with tumor-related spinal instability. Although various criteria for spinal stability in the face of spinal tumors have been reported, they have not been particularly useful in predicting which patients may benefit from spinal surgery before the development of profound instability or neurologic deficit.

Varied grading systems and parameters have been devised to determine when surgical intervention is re-

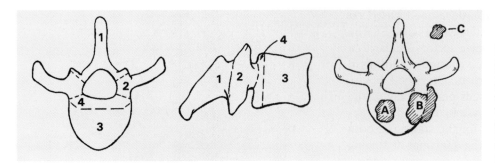

Figure 4 Illustration of Harrington's classification of spinal metastases. Numbers 1 through 4 represent the anatomic location of tumor. A = tumor confined to the vertebra; B = tumor extends beyond the vertebra; C = distant metastases. *(Reproduced from Beaty JH (ed):* Orthopaedic Knowledge Update 6. *Rosemont, IL, American Academy of Orthopaedic Surgeons, 1999, pp 723-736.)*

quired to treat impending instability as a result of pathologic vertebral replacement. In the thoracic spine, 50% to 60% of vertebral body involvement or 25% to 30% of body involvement with costovertebral involvement have been suggested as criteria for impending collapse. In the lumbar spine the suggested criteria for impending collapse are 35% to 40% of body involvement alone or 25% of body involvement with pedicle or posterior body involvement. Even when adhering to these guidelines, each patient should be assessed individually, taking tumor load, type, location, and prognosis of the patient into account. More recently, finite element models have shown that tumor size, magnitude of spinal loading, and bone density are predictive of the initiation of burst fractures in metastatically affected vertebrae and that pedicle involvement and disk degeneration are less important.

Radiation Treatment

In patients with spinal tumors causing neural compression, treating physicians are required to weigh the relative advantages of initiating treatment with radiation therapy against primary surgical decompression. If the tumor is radiosensitive and neural progression is gradual, radiotherapy may be the initial treatment of choice. Patients with limited ambulatory function as a result of tumor causing neural compression have a 60% chance of improvement after undergoing radiation treatment. Patients who have lost sphincter function have less than a 40% chance of regaining function after radiation treatment. When spinal radiation is ineffective in improving neurologic deficits, subsequent surgical decompression is fraught with complications. Operating through a radiated field will increase the risk of wound nonhealing and surgical site infections. In some patients, radiation injury to the skin in the surgical field may prevent or delay surgical intervention. In addition, the potential advantages of initiating radiation treatments after surgical resection (when the tumor volume has been significantly reduced) must be considered.

Surgical Approach

Performing an anterior and posterior surgery when either approach alone would suffice exposes the patient to unnecessary risks, morbidity, and a prolonged recovery. In patients for whom posterior stability is maintained, reconstructing the anterior spinal column with anterior surgery only after tumor removal may be all that is necessary. The corollary to this is that performing "too little" surgery does the patient a similar disservice. In patients with significant comorbidities and reduced life expectancy, it is tempting to perform a lesser procedure. If however the patient does not leave the operating room with effective neural decompression and spinal stability, the likelihood of early or late failure is great. Having to return a patient to surgery after a failed initial surgical procedure is an extremely undesirable and potentially avoidable situation.

In general, the site of the lesion dictates the surgical approach. When the vertebral body is involved and neural compression is anterior, an anterior approach will allow for tumor resection and direct decompression of the neural elements. Anterior reconstruction, usually involving a strut spanning the excised level or levels is required to restore spinal stability. The involved segments are typically further stabilized with rigid anterior instrumentation. If the morbidity of an anterior approach is prohibitive, vertebral body excision and anterior neural decompression may be accomplished through a posterolateral approach involving removal of the pedicles so that the vertebral body can be accessed lateral to the dura. A posterior approach is also preferred when the tumor involves the posterior elements (Figure 5). The posterior approach will also allow for multilevel posterior segmental fixation to stabilize the spine, whereas anterior approaches tend to allow for stabilization of fewer segments. If both the vertebral body and posterior elements of the spine are involved, posterior instrumentation in addition to anterior decompression-reconstruction will be necessary to stabilize the involved spine (Figure 6). Isolated laminectomy has a small role in the treatment of spinal tumors.

Optimal timing of treatments such as chemotherapy and radiation therapy after spinal surgery remains poorly defined. These treatments will interfere with wound healing as well as with bone graft incorporation and fusion. Animal research suggests that radiation therapy should be delayed for 6 weeks after spinal recon-

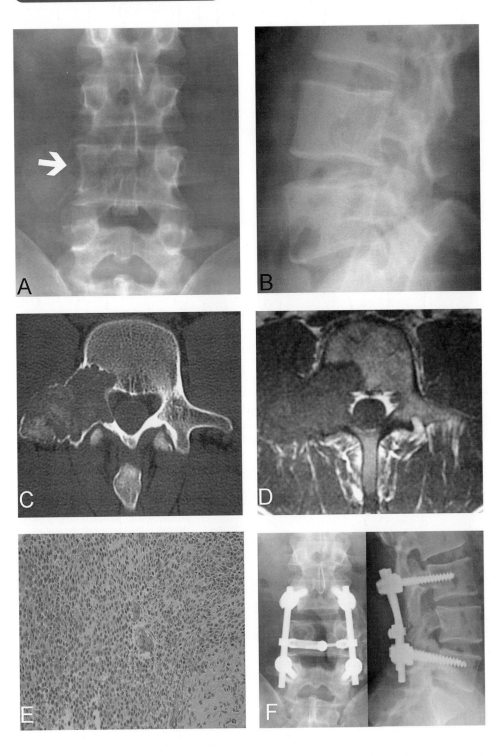

Figure 5 AP (**A**) and lateral (**B**) radiographs of a 29-year-old man with a 2-year history of slowly progressive low back pain; the pain occasionally radiated to the right thigh, but no paresthesias nor weakness was reported. The AP radiograph is significant for a classic winking owl sign at the right pedicle of L4 (*arrow*). **C,** A subsequent CT scan reveals an expansile lesion involving the right pedicle and transverse process of L4 that contains a limited amount of intralesional mineralization. **D,** MRI further demonstrates the extent of the lesion and suggests that the lesion may be compressing the L3 nerve root. No central compression was present. Clinical history and imaging suggested a benign lesion, although a precise diagnosis was not possible. Osteoblastoma was considered to be the most likely diagnosis. **E,** Histologic analysis of the pathology specimen contained polygonal chondroblasts with numerous giant cells, indicating that the lesion was, in reality, a chondroblastoma. **F,** Postoperative AP and lateral radiographs show that an excision was performed with posterior instrumented L3-L5 fusion.

struction involving arthrodesis to permit the critical early phases of bone graft revascularization. Obviously, decisions regarding the timing of adjuvant treatments need to be made by taking into account the likely course of the patient's underlying malignancy.

En Bloc Tumor Resection
Surgery for spinal tumors typically involves intralesional excision with debulking followed by adjuvant therapy.

This has been reported to provide palliation in many series; however, the recurrence rates have been quite high. This has prompted interest in en bloc spondylectomy for the treatment of patients with solitary metastases or intracompartmental primary malignant tumors. In case reports, en bloc resection or total spondylectomy has been suggested to decrease recurrence and improve survival. En bloc spondylectomy usually involves removal of the posterior elements and osteotomy of the pedicles, followed by posterior stabilization with pedicle fixation

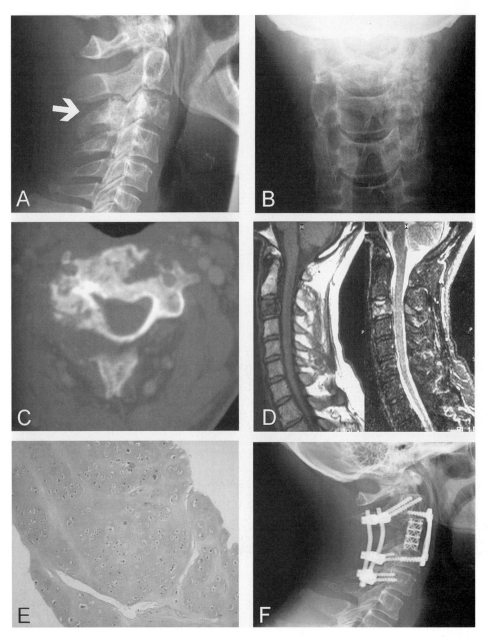

Figure 6 AP **(A)** and lateral **(B)** radiographs of a 44-year-old man with a several-month history of progressive neck pain, no radicular symptoms, and no upper motor neuron signs at presentation demonstrate a lesion (*arrow*) involving the body and posterior elements of the C3 vertebra with soft-tissue extension. **C,** Axial CT demonstrates the mass and suggests that it contains mineralized matrix. **D,** MRI further delineates the extent of the tumor and reveals that there is no spinal cord compression. The patient underwent a CT-directed biopsy of the C3 mass, and the results of histologic analysis **(E)** were most consistent with the presence of a low-grade chondrosarcoma. Because wide resection was not possible because of the proximity of the mass to both vertebral arteries and the spinal cord, the patient underwent preoperative radiotherapy, followed by a front-back resection of C3 with an anterior cage/C2-C4 plate and C2-C5 posterior instrumentation. Intraoperative radiotherapy was administered to the anterior dura, and the patient underwent proton radiotherapy postoperatively. **F,** Postoperative radiograph.

one to two levels above and below the resected level. This is followed by the en bloc removal of the vertebral body and reconstruction of the anterior column, which can be accomplished either through the same posterior surgical approach or through a separate anterior approach.

Metastatic Disease

Diffuse metastatic disease still poses a significant challenge for the spinal surgeon, and the combination of debulking, intralesional excision, and spinal reconstruction is the mainstay of treatment. The surgical approach is either anterior, posterior, or both, depending on the location of the tumor. Even though surgery is palliative, it can enhance a patient's quality of life by relieving se-

vere pain and preventing neurologic impairment, including retention of bowel and bladder control. Recent studies have demonstrated that in appropriately selected patients, surgical management is able to positively affect the overall quality of life in those with spinal metastases.

Vertebral Augmentation

Vertebroplasty and kyphoplasty have shown promise in the treatment of patients with multiple myeloma or spinal metastases. These percutaneous modalities have been widely used for the treatment of benign osteoporotic fractures and are increasingly being used to treat pathologic compression fractures caused by metastatic disease and vertebral body pain secondary to tumor infiltration. The indications for these techniques include refractory pain without neurologic compromise. The posterior vertebral body wall must be intact to prevent extravasation of cement into the spinal canal. Short-term results appear promising, with good and rapid relief of pain, improved function, and even restoration of vertebral body height with kyphoplasty in some patients. Most reported complications in patients who have undergone vertebroplasty have been the result of extravertebral cement extravasation. This risk is higher when treating patients with metastatic as opposed to osteoporotic vertebral fractures. Kyphoplasty, which involves the creation of an intravertebral cavity with a balloon tamp, has a lower risk of extravertebral cement extravasation than vertebroplasty. Although these minimally invasive treatments may not impact the prognosis or the disease process, they can provide substantial and immediate pain relief with a reported low risk of complications.

Annotated Bibliography

Primary Tumors

Abe E, Koboyashi T, Murai H, et al: Total spondylectomy for primary malignant, aggressive benign and solitary metastatic bone tumors of the thoracolumbar spine. *J Spinal Disord* 2001;14:237-246.

Fourteen patients with malignant or aggressive benign vertebral tumors of the thoracolumbar spine underwent total spondylectomy. Pain relief was achieved in all 14 patients, and no serious complications occurred. Local recurrence was found in three patients at a mean follow-up of 3.2 years. Total spondylectomy appears to be an effective method for controlling local recurrence without major complications.

Durr HR, Wegener B, Krodel A, Muller PE, Jansson V, Refior HJ: Multiple myeloma: Surgery of the spine. Retrospective analysis of 27 patients. *Spine* 2002;27:320-324.

This is a report on the clinical course of 27 consecutive patients who were surgically treated for solitary or multiple myeloma of the spine. Life quality, reported to be 48% before surgery, improved to 59% 1 month after surgery and to 73% in 24 survivors after 1 year. The authors concluded that surgical treatment of myeloma of the spine seemed to be an effective method of treatment with respect to neurologic function and life quality in selected patients.

Ghanem I, Collet LM, Kharrat K, et al: Percutaneous radiofrequency coagulation of osteoid osteoma in children and adolescents. *J Pediatr Orthop B* 2003;12:244-252.

In this study, 23 patients who underwent percutaneous radiofrequency coagulation for osteoid osteoma were retrospectively reviewed. Pain disappeared immediately after the procedure in 21 patients. At an average of 3.5-year follow-up, all patients were pain free.

Nonsurgical Treatment

Ryu S, Fang YF, Rock J, et al: Image-guided and intensity-modulated radiosurgery for patients with spinal metastasis. *Cancer* 2003;97:2013-2018.

In this study, 10 patients with spinal metastasis were treated with image-guided and intensity-modulated radiosurgery. The authors reported that the most patients had pain relief within 2 to 4 weeks of treatment.

Surgical Treatment

Dudeney S, Lieberman IH, Reinhardt MK, Hussein M: Kyphoplasty in the treatment of osteolytic vertebral compression fractures as a result of multiple myeloma. *J Clin Oncol* 2002;20:2382-2387.

Fifty-five consecutive kyphoplasties were prospectively evaluated in 18 patients. Mean follow-up was 7.4 months, and there was significant improvement in Short Form-36 scores for bodily pain, physical function, vitality, and social function.

Fourney DR, Schomer DF, Nader R, et al: Percutaneous vertebroplasty and kyphoplasty for painful vertebral body fractures in cancer patients. *J Neurosurg* 2003;98:21-30.

In this study, 97 procedures (65 vertebroplasty and 32 kyphoplasty) were performed in 56 patients with myeloma and primary malignances. The authors report that 84% of patients experienced complete pain relief at a median follow-up of 4.5 months.

Krepler P, Windhager R, Bretschneider W, et al: Total vertebrectomy for primary malignant tumors of the spine. *J Bone Joint Surg Br* 2002;84:712-715.

Vertebrectomy was performed on seven patients, with a mean follow-up of 52 months. In five patients, a wide resection was achieved. The authors conclude that vertebrectomy seems to be an appropriate procedure for the treatment of primary lesions of the spine.

Sundaresan N, Rothman A, Manhart K, Kelliher K: Surgery for solitary metastases of the spine, rationale and results of treatment. *Spine* 2002;27:1802-1806.

This is a retrospective review of 80 consecutive patients with solitary sites of spine involvement from solid tumors. The overall median length of survival after surgery was 30 months. Complete surgical excision before irradiation was recommended to increase the prospects of palliation and possible cure.

Wai EK, Finkelstein JA, Tangente RP, et al: Quality of life in surgical treatment of metastatic spine disease. *Spine* 2003;28:508-512.

In this study, 25 consecutive patients undergoing surgery for spinal metastases were prospectively evaluated. After surgery, the largest improvement was with pain, but there were also improvements with tiredness, nausea, anxiety, drowsiness, appetite, and well-being.

Whyne CM, Hu SS, Lotz JC: Burst fracture in the metastatically involved spine: Development, validation, and parametric analysis of a three-dimensional poroelastic finite-element model. *Spine* 2003;28:652-660.

A finite-element study and in vitro experimental validation was performed for an investigation of features that contribute to burst fracture risk. The authors report that the principal factors affecting the initiation of fracture were tumor size, magnitude of spinal loading, and bone density.

Classic Bibliography

Bohlman HH, Sachs BL, Carter JR, Riley L, Robinson RA: Primary neoplasms of the cervical spine. *J Bone Joint Surg Am* 1986;68:483-494.

Boriani S, Biagini R, De Iure F, et al: En bloc resections of bone tumors of the thoracolumbar spine: A preliminary report of 29 patients. *Spine* 1996;21:1927-1931.

Galasko CS, Norris HE, Crank S: Spinal instability secondary to metastatic cancer. *J Bone Joint Surg Am* 2000;82:570-594.

Hart RA, Boriani S, Biagini R, Currier B, Weinstein JN: A system for surgical staging and management of spine tumors: A clinical outcome study of giant cell tumors of the spine. *Spine* 1997;22:1773-1783.

Harrington KD: The use of methylmethacrylate for vertebral-body replacement and anterior stabilization of pathologic fracture-dislocations of the spine due to metastatic malignant disease. *J Bone Joint Surg Am* 1981;63:36-46.

Harrington KD: Anterior decompression and stabilization of the spine as a treatment for vertebral collapse and spinal cord compression from metastatic malignancy. *Clin Orthop* 1988;233:177-197.

Hekster RE, Luyendijk W, Tan TI: Spinal cord compression caused by vertebral haemangioma relieved by percutaneous catheter embolisation. *Neuroradiology* 1972;3:160-164.

Kostuik JP, Errico TJ, Gleason TF, Errico CC: Spinal stabilization of vertebral column tumors. *Spine* 1988;13:250-256.

Marsh BW, Bonfiglio M, Brady LP, Enneking WF: Benign osteoblastoma: Range of manifestations. *J Bone Joint Surg Am* 1975;57:1-9.

Pettine KA, Klassen RA: Osteoid osteoma and osteoblastoma of the spine. *J Bone Joint Surg Am* 1986;68:354-361.

Samson IR, Springfield DS, Suit HD, Mankin HJ: Operative treatment of sacrococcygeal chordoma: A review of twenty-one cases. *J Bone Joint Surg Am* 1993;75:1476-1484.

Shives TC, Dahlin DC, Sim FH, Pritchard DJ, Earle JD: Osteosarcoma of the spine. *J Bone Joint Surg Am* 1986;68:660-668.

Stener B: Complete removal of vertebra for extirpation of tumors: A 20 year experience. *Clin Orthop* 1989;245:72-82.

Sundaresan N, Galicich JH, Lane JM, et al: Treatment of neoplastic epidural cord compression by vertebral body resection and stabilization. *J Neurosurg* 1985;63:676-684.

Sundaresan N, Steinberger AA, Moore F, et al: Indications and results of combined anterior-posterior approaches for spine tumor surgery. *J Neurosurg* 1996;85:438-446.

Yuh WT, Quets JP, Lee HJ, et al: Anatomic distribution of metastases in the vertebral body and modes of hematogenous spread. *Spine* 1996;21:2243-2250.

Chapter 49

Spondyloarthropathy

Tushar Patel, MD

Mark J. Romness, MD

Introduction

Many inflammatory diseases are known to occur in the musculoskeletal system, but the primary inflammatory conditions that affect the spine, in descending prevalence, are rheumatoid arthritis, ankylosing spondylitis, and juvenile rheumatoid arthritis. These three inflammatory conditions alone are estimated to affect over 3 million patients in the United States. Juvenile rheumatoid arthritis is discussed in chapter 21.

Rheumatoid Arthritis

Definition

Rheumatoid arthritis is a systemic autoimmune disease of unknown etiology that causes progressive joint swelling, pain, and stiffness secondary to synovitis. The onset of symptoms usually occurs between 20 and 45 years of age. Seventy percent of patients with rheumatoid arthritis are female. A genetic component continues to be supported but is not well defined. A positive rheumatoid factor is present in approximately 85% of patients, but is not specific for rheumatoid arthritis and can be present in normal individuals and in other medical conditions. A positive rheumatoid factor is clinically associated with more severe symptoms, including extra-articular manifestations and a more aggressive disease course. Patients with rheumatoid arthritis who have a negative rheumatoid factor may eventually convert to a positive rheumatoid factor and follow a similar clinical progression as patients who are initially positive. Severe spinal involvement is primarily cervical in patients with rheumatoid arthritis, and up to 85% of patients with rheumatoid arthritis develop cervical radiographic changes within 10 years of disease onset. Lumbar problems are less significant, but low back pain was present in 40% and radiographic evidence of lumbar pathology was found in 57% of 106 patients with rheumatoid arthritis. The primary spinal deformities in rheumatoid arthritis are atlantoaxial subluxation, superior migration of the odontoid, and subaxial subluxation (Figure 1). All of these conditions can lead to neurologic impairment. Superior migration of the odontoid is also known as basilar invagination, cranial settling, and atlantoaxial impaction.

Natural History

The progressive nature of rheumatoid arthritis is well known, as is the variable expression of the disease in different patients. Several studies have attempted to cor-

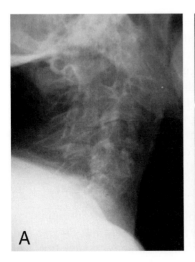

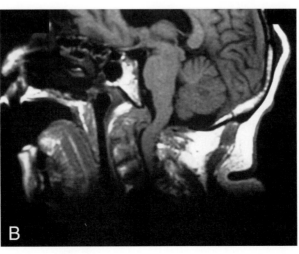

Figure 1 Lateral radiograph (**A**) and corresponding sagittal MRI (**B**) showing the combined manifestations of cranial settling, atlantoaxial subluxation, and subaxial subluxation.

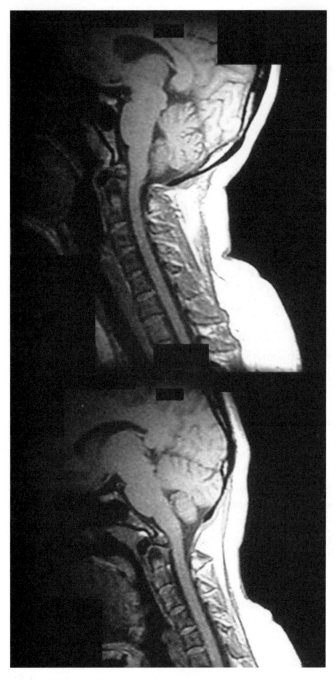

Figure 2 Dynamic flexion-extension MRI panels showing evidence of dynamic cord compression at the occipitocervical junction.

relate serologic tests and radiographic changes with cervical progression. Rheumatoid factor-positive serology, more extensive peripheral joint involvement, male gender, and corticosteroid use are factors that have been linked to greater cervical involvement. Cervical myelopathy has been associated with progression to bed confinement or death within an average of 35 months if untreated in patients with rheumatoid arthritis and extensive mutilating-type changes of the peripheral joints. In 21 untreated patients with rheumatoid arthritis

myelopathy secondary to irreducible atlantoaxial subluxation, all were confined to bed within 3 years and died within 8 years.

Imaging
Plain Radiographs
Plain radiographs remain the standard modality to diagnose, classify, and monitor spinal arthropathy. Plain images provide cost-effective screening for skeletal changes. Early radiographic changes including the presence of osteophytes and disk space narrowing may not be symptomatic. Flexion and extension lateral views are used to define stability between the spinal segments and are the primary method to assess the cervical spine for the primary spinal deformities that occur in rheumatoid arthritis. The use of select digital imaging and software allows electronic measurements such as the atlanto-dens interval.

Magnetic Resonance Imaging
MRI provides information on soft tissues and structural bone details not seen with conventional radiography. Tomographic representation clarifies anatomic structures, and the use of gadolinium enhancement has been shown to increase the sensitivity of diagnosis and to help in determining the extent of the disease. Dynamic studies are possible with MRI (Figure 2), but when dynamic MRI and plain flexion-extension films were compared in 23 patients with rheumatoid arthritis, the magnitude of atlantoaxial subluxation was less with MRI in all patients; MRI was not able to detect atlantoaxial subluxation that was seen in four patients using radiography. MRI is required for evaluation of neurologic structures and is the standard method for evaluation of superior migration of the odontoid. Correlation of cord compression or impingement at the atlantoaxial level on initial MRI and development of subarachnoid space encroachment on sequential MRI scans have both been shown to be predictive of neurologic deterioration.

CT Myelogram and Bone Scan
The use of CT myelograms is beneficial for unique situations such as for patients who had previous surgery and who have ferromagnetic implants in the area to be imaged, or for those who are not candidates for MRI because of cochlear implants, pacemakers, or neurostimulators. Nuclear imaging is a sensitive screening tool for identifying occult fractures in patients with rheumatoid arthritis. The advantage over MRI is the ability to image the whole body efficiently and cost-effectively.

Bone Density Studies
Osteoporosis is common in most forms of spinal arthropathy. Contributing factors include the disease process itself, genetics, limitations in activity, nutrition, and

treatments such as the use of corticosteroids. However, the presence of osteoporosis is not limited to patients with severe disease or those treated with corticosteroids. Bone density studies quantitate the extent of osteoporosis and help determine whether treatment is indicated.

Indications for Surgery

Neurologic impairment is the most urgent indication for surgery in patients with spinal arthropathy. Impairment can be determined by history, clinical examination, electrodiagnostic studies, or MRI. Because progression of myelopathy is the natural history in rheumatoid arthritis, any myelopathic findings should be considered a surgical indication.

Pain and instability often are associated with neurologic involvement, except in patients with gradual displacement over time. Pain alone is a subjective indication; instability without neurologic deficit has specific parameters to warrant surgery. These parameters include posterior atlanto-dens interval of 14 mm or less in flexion on plain radiographs for atlantoaxial subluxation and MRI findings of cord diameter of less than 6 mm in flexion, cervicomedullary angle of less than 135°, and 13 mm or less of space available for the spinal cord. Superior migration of the odontoid alone is not an indication for surgery and documentation of neurologic impingement or myelopathy on flexion MRI or by examination should be documented before surgery is recommended.

Spinal fractures in patients with rheumatoid arthritis usually require fixation, and fixation needs to compensate for the often-associated osteoporosis and accompanying deformity. This may require fusion and instrumentation of more levels than would ordinarily be considered for patients with normal bone quality.

Surgical Treatment

Decompression

Myelopathy may require decompression if the deformity is fixed, but reduction of the deformity may preserve bony areas for fusion healing. Solid fusion prevents spinal cord irritation and has been shown to relieve myelopathy. Anterior transoral decompression was previously recommended for spinal cord compression, but the only current indication for transoral decompression is the presence of cranial nerve deficits.

Arthrodesis

Arthrodesis is the treatment of choice for either primary instability resulting from inflammatory process or secondary instability caused by late manifestations of pseudarthrosis or sterile spondylodiskitis. Fusion to the occiput is indicated when adequate fixation at C1 is not possible or when there is instability at the occiput–C1 junction.

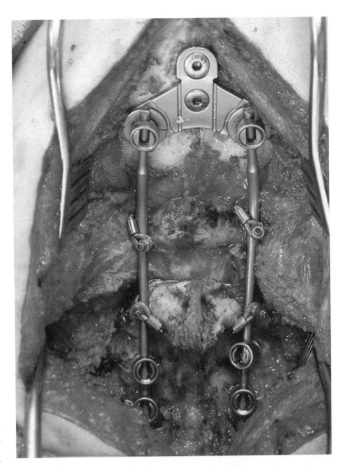

Figure 3 An example of posterior occiputocervical fusion construct.

Instrumentation

Wire fixation is extensively used for stabilization in the cervical spine and has been described in the literature. Additional methods for instrumentation of the cervical spine have been recently described. At the occipital area, cranial bolts placed using the inside-outside technique and connected to plates and lateral mass screws were used for 21 patients with rheumatoid arthritis; results showed no instrument failures and significantly reduced pain scores. Cadaver studies have shown increased axial rotation stiffness with rod and screw fixation (Figure 3) compared with plate and screw or loop and cable constructs, and better restoration of sagittal plane balance and maintenance of correction.

The use of screws throughout the spine has increased treatment options. Transarticular C1-2 fixation, and more recently, segmental fixation of C1 to C2 using polyaxial screws inserted into the lateral masses of C1, has replaced the requirement of fusion from the occiput to C2 (or lower) in most instances when C1 laminectomy is performed. The technique of placing screws into the lateral mass of C1 increases the risks of bleeding from the venous plexus accompanying the dorsal ramus of the C2 nerve root as well as direct injury to the root, but affords additional safety compared with the use of transarticular screws because the path of the vertebral artery is avoided.

Surgical Outcomes

The benefits of surgical intervention have been well documented and recent outcomes studies have supported this treatment option. For irreducible atlantoaxial instability with myelopathy in patients with rheumatoid arthritis, C1 laminectomy and fusion with rectangular rod fixation from the occiput to C2 (16 patients) to C3 (2 patients) or to C4 (1 patient) led to 68% improvement of at least one Ranawat class and 5- and 10-year survival rates of 84% and 37%, respectively. Without surgery, 21 matched patients were all bedridden within 3 years and died within 8 years. Similar neurologic improvements were noted in 67% of patients (37 of 55) with occipital neuralgia, myelopathy, or both treated with various procedures. Mortality at 2 years was 27% and resulted mainly from nonsurgery-related causes.

Patients with inflammatory spondylitis often have multiple comorbid medical conditions that contribute significantly to management and potential complications. Involvement of the temporomandibular joint may interfere with intubation, and peripheral joint contractures can make surgical positioning and rehabilitation more challenging. Osteoporosis impairs fixation potential, and many authors recommend the use of orthotic devices after surgery if osteoporosis is present. Poor skin quality, impaired healing, and dental problems increase the risk of infection. Despite all the potential risks, careful patient preparation and planning combined with up-to-date skilled care can improve function and survival.

Ankylosing Spondylitis

Definition

Ankylosing spondylitis is the prototype disease of seronegative spondyloarthropathies—a family of arthritic conditions not associated with positive rheumatoid factor serology. Other related conditions are reactive arthritis (Reiter's syndrome), spondylitic forms of psoriatic arthritis and inflammatory bowel disease (Crohn's disease), juvenile spondyloarthropathy, and undifferentiated spondyloarthropathy. Disease onset typically occurs between the ages of 20 and 30 years. Males are more commonly affected, and symptoms in females are usually milder and harder to diagnose. Early symptoms of ankylosing spondylitis are commonly overlooked in young adults as simply "back pain," but awareness of early findings such as lumbar stiffness and decreased lordosis may lead to a correct diagnosis. Positive HLA-B27 assay is present in 80% to 98% of patients with ankylosing spondylitis versus 8% of the general population. Spinal involvement is primarily lumbar at onset

and spreads cephalad. Neck pain caused by spontaneous anterior atlantoaxial subluxation has been reported as an initial symptom. One study showed that 49% of patients (89 of 181) with ankylosing spondylitis had radiographic changes, but atlantoaxial subluxation was present in 2% to 20% of patients with ankylosing spondylitis compared with 16% to 25% of adult patients with rheumatoid arthritis; superior migration of the odontoid has not been reported with ankylosing spondylitis alone.

Natural History

The natural history of ankylosing spondylitis is progressive loss of posture and mobility. The rate of progression is variable. Mild spinal changes in ankylosing spondylitis occur first, with squaring of the lumbar bodies and syndesmophytes. More severe involvement leads to changes characteristic of so-called "bamboo spine." Spinal deformity in ankylosing spondylitis develops secondary to limitation of motion at ankylosed areas or increased motion at nonankylosed areas. Pain can develop at remaining motion segments but resolves once that segment is ankylosed. Ankylosis in a relatively kyphotic position occurs at the cervical, thoracic, and lumbar spine, but etiology for kyphosis has not been defined.

With long rigid spinal segments and focused areas of osteoporosis, fractures are common even with minimal trauma and can cause significant morbidity and mortality. Mortality can occur from initial injury, fracture treatment, or epidural hematomas that can develop up to weeks after injury. Recent articles on trauma have emphasized the importance of strict neck immobilization for patients with ankylosing spondylitis, even in those who have experienced mild low-energy injuries.

Imaging

Plain Radiographs

Plain radiographs may provide clues for the initial diagnosis of ankylosing spondylitis. Classic changes at the sacroiliac joints may not be identified initially, but initial presentation with thoracic spine changes in a female patient has been reported. Spondylodiskitis (also known as Andersson lesions) is a destructive diskovertebral lesion occurring in ankylosing spondylitis that usually occurs at the thoracolumbar junction. Both inflammatory and noninflammatory types of destructive lesions occur. The inflammatory type is defined radiologically as a reduced disk space with a defect of vertebral bodies and dense cancellous bone sclerosis. The noninflammatory type is associated with a fracture through an ankylosed disk or a pseudarthrosis. Lateral flexion and extension views of the cervical, thoracic, and lumbar spine are essential to identifying instability and ankylosis in patients with ankylosing spondylitis.

Computed Tomography and Magnetic Resonance Imaging

Excellent evaluation of the sacroiliac joints is possible with CT. Sacroiliac joint space narrowing, erosions, and sclerosis are all classically seen on the axial views without reconstruction or contrast. Canal stenosis secondary to the combined effects of kyphosis and ankylosis is well defined with MRI. Contrast gives better definition of which structures are involved and if spinal cord pathology is present.

Bone Scan

The presence of activity in the sacroiliac joints and in the spinal column on bone scans may help with the diagnosis of ankylosing spondylitis. Nuclear imaging is an effective screening tool to identify occult fractures in ankylosing spondylitis and should be considered early in the assessment of patients with this disease who sustain even minor trauma. There have been reports of devastating complications from undiagnosed fractures.

Bone Density Studies

A decrease in bone density has been shown to be related to persistent systemic inflammation in patients with ankylosing spondylitis. Spinal density measured by dual-energy x-ray absorptiometry (DEXA) increases as ankylosis progresses; therefore, DEXA hip measurements or quantitative CT should be used.

Surgical Indications

Neurologic compromise may be less obvious in patients with ankylosing spondylitis than in those with rheumatoid arthritis. A recent meta-analysis of 52 articles discussing 86 patients with ankylosing spondylitis and cauda equina syndrome showed that nearly all patients had sensory, motor, or reflex deficits on examination and 30% had previous prostate surgery without improvement for incontinence. Compensations in gait caused by spinal ankylosis may mask the true myelopathic contribution to gait. As myelopathy is associated with rheumatoid arthritis, any myelopathic findings should be considered a surgical indication.

There are no specific indications for correction of chin on chest deformity from cervical kyphosis; however, commonly accepted indications for surgical intervention include the inability to perform the activities of daily living (including those related to personal hygiene). Correction of thoracolumbar kyphosis was recommended if the global kyphosis was greater than 50°, or in patients with less severe kyphosis in whom nonsurgical management of symptomatic spondylodiskitis was unsuccessful.

Fractures associated with ankylosing spondylitis often are associated with neurologic deficit that rarely resolves but can improve with surgery. In 11 patients with ankylosing spondylitis and fractures, 6 had neurologic deficits; 3 of 6 patients had improved neurologic function with surgery. Most fractures are unstable because the ankylosis forms a rigid column that does not follow the same three-column criteria of Denis for stability as seen in normal spines. The rigid columns act as long level arms concentrating forces (such as motion) at the fracture site. Epidural hematomas commonly produce neurologic impairment because of the confined rigid canal. Surgery for unstable fractures and epidural hematomas is required and combined anterior and posterior approaches and extended fixation must be considered. Only minor nonstructural fractures should be considered stable fractures that can be treated nonsurgically in patients with ankylosing spondylitis.

Surgical Treatment

Decompression

Emergency decompression is indicated for epidural hematomas. Laminectomy is required for cauda equina syndrome in patients with ankylosing spondylitis. A study found that 55 patients who had nonsurgical treatment showed no improvement of sensory, bowel, or bladder deficit; only 2 of these patients had motor improvement.

Osteotomy

Extension osteotomy to correct kyphosis at both the cervicothoracic junction and lumbar spine is well described in patients with ankylosing spondylitis. Cervical deformity is best corrected with osteotomy between C7 and T1, which is the widest area of the cervical canal and is caudal to the vertebral artery entry at C6. Cervical osteotomies above C7 are rarely required and have a higher risk of complications.

Thoracic kyphosis is best treated with extension osteotomy at or below L2. Thoracic osteotomies are rarely indicated. Patients who have osteotomy at L4 may have difficulty sitting on the floor; however, the procedure may need to be considered if two osteotomies are being performed. Two levels of osteotomy are recommended for deformity greater than 70° and should be separated by one or two levels to distribute the amount of anterior angulation and distraction.

Arthrodesis and Instrumentation

Arthrodesis is required for fractures and after kyphectomy. Fusion rates are similar to those seen in the normal spine. Modifications to the standard techniques of instrumentation may be necessary because of the obliteration of bony landmarks that ordinarily serve as reference points.

Surgical Outcomes

Correction of kyphosis by posterior subtraction osteotomy has previously been described and reported. In a recent large series, 92 osteotomies were done in 78 patients with mean correction of 34.5% per osteotomy level; the maximum correction attained was 100°. Neither deaths nor vascular complications were noted compared with previously reported mortality of up to 10% with anterior opening wedge osteotomy. Loss of correction occurred in only two patients. Patients reported outcome as excellent (83%) or good (15%); one patient outcome was not reported.

Annotated Bibliography

Ahn NU, Ahn UM, Nallamshetty L, et al: Cauda equina syndrome in ankylosing spondylitis (the CES-AS syndrome): Meta-analysis of outcomes after medical and surgical treatments. *J Spinal Disord* 2001;14:427-433.

A case report of acute onset of cauda equina syndrome associated with ankylosing spondylitis is presented and a review of 52 articles with 86 patients is evaluated regarding treatment outcome. Onset of symptoms was found to be gradual. Only 22% of the patients had radicular symptoms, yet nearly all patients had some neurologic deficit on physical examination. Thirty percent of the male patients had undergone prostatectomy for misdiagnosed prostatic hypertrophy. Improvement of sensory, bowel, and bladder dysfunction was not noted with nonsurgical treatment, but in 6 of the 15 patients who had surgery, some form of improvement was shown. Neurologic deficit progressed much less in the surgically treated group.

Chen IH, Chien JT, Yu TC: Transpedicular wedge osteotomy for correction of thoracolumbar kyphosis in ankylosing spondylitis: Experience with 78 patients. *Spine* 2001;26:E354-E360.

A retrospective study of a single surgeon's experience is evaluated. Modifications to Thomasen's original description for closing wedge osteotomy are included. With a mean follow-up of 3.8 years, excellent results were noted in 83% of patients and good results in 15%. Only two patients had a loss of correction within the osteotomy segment. Average correction of the osteotomy was 34.5°.

Chou LW, Lo SF, Kao MJ, Jim YF, Cho DY: Ankylosing spondylitis manifested by spontaneous anterior atlantoaxial subluxation. *Am J Phys Med Rehabil* 2002;81:952-955.

A case report of spontaneous anterior atlantoaxial subluxation is presented. There was no history of trauma or back pain and no alteration of bowel or bladder function. Examination revealed severe cervical but only mild lumbar spine mobility limitations. The patient underwent C1 laminectomy and occiput to C2 fusion and fixation and had almost complete resolution of his neurologic symptoms.

Kawaguchi Y, Matsuno H, Kanamori M, Ishihara H, Ohmori K, Kimura T: Radiologic findings of the lumbar spine in patients with rheumatoid arthritis, and a review of pathologic mechanisms. *J Spinal Disord Tech* 2003;16: 38-43.

In this study, 106 patients were evaluated by questionnaire and lumbar spine radiographs. A scoring system was used for the radiographs and consensus of significant changes by three observers was required. Low back pain was noted by 40% of the patients and was believed to be severe by 3%. Leg pain and leg numbness were noted in 18% and 14%, respectively. Significant radiologic findings were noted in 57% of patients. In order of frequency, these findings were disk space narrowing, postural anomaly, olisthesis, end of plate erosion, and facet erosion. End plate erosion correlated closest to clinical symptoms.

Kurugoglu S, Mihmanli I, Kanberoglu K, Kanberoglu A: Destructive diskovertebral lesions in ankylosing spondylitis: Appearance on magnetic resonance imaging. *South Med J* 2001;94:837-841.

A case report of an 18-year-old woman with initial complaints of back and chest pain is presented. The patient had no restriction in motion or neurologic symptoms. Diskovertebral lesions were found diffusely throughout the spine. Involvement of the sacroiliac joint was found 6 months later by nuclear scintigraphy and CT scan. HLA-B27 was positive.

Laiho K, Soini I, Kautiainen H, Kauppi M: Can we rely on magnetic resonance imaging when evaluating unstable atlantoaxial subluxation? *Ann Rheum Dis* 2003;62: 254-256.

Twenty-two patients with rheumatoid arthritis and one patient with juvenile idiopathic arthritis were evaluated for neck pain. Evaluation included flexion and extension lateral cervical spine radiographs and functional cervical spine MRI. The magnitude of anterior atlantoaxial subluxation in flexion was greater in all patients measured by radiography than by MRI. Seventeen percent of the flexion MRI scans did not show subluxation that was seen by radiography.

Matsunaga S, Sakou T, Onishi T, et al: Prognosis of patients with upper cervical lesions caused by rheumatoid arthritis: Comparison of occipitocervical fusion between c1 laminectomy and nonsurgical management. *Spine* 2003;28:1581-1587.

Treatment of myelopathy secondary to irreducible atlantoaxial dislocation was compared between 19 patients undergoing C1 laminectomy with occipital cervical fusion and instrumentation and 21 matched patients who were treated nonsurgically. All patients were followed until their deaths, which averaged 9.7 years in the surgically treated patients and 4.2 years in the nonsurgically treated patients. Pain improved with all patients following surgery and neural improvement of one or more Ranawat levels was found in 68% with worsening in only 5%. The 10-year survival rate with surgery was 37% and 0% without surgery.

Reijnierse M, Dijkmans BA, Hansen B, et al: Neurologic dysfunction in patients with rheumatoid arthritis of the cervical spine: Predictive value of clinical, radiographic and MR imaging parameters. *Eur Radiol* 2001;11:467-473.

Forty-six patients with rheumatoid arthritis for at least 5 years were followed annually with examination, radiographs, and MRI to correlate neurologic dysfunction with diagnostic changes. All patients had a second examination and eight had five sequential examinations. Subjective muscle weakness was the only symptom associated with neurologic dysfunction. No significant radiographic abnormalities could be statistically correlated to neurologic dysfunction. The only MRI abnormality that was statistically significant was decreased subarachnoid space along the entire cervical spine, which was a subjective interpretation.

Sandhu FA, Pait TG, Benzel E, Henderson FC: Occipitocervical fusion for rheumatoid arthritis using the inside-outside stabilization technique. *Spine* 2003;28:414-419.

The technique using cranial bolts for occipital cervical stabilization is described, and the results in 21 patients who underwent a stabilization and fusion are presented. No implant complications or failures occurred. Ranawat neurologic level improved in 62% of the patients. There was no decline in neurologic level immediately following surgery or during the follow-up period that averaged 25.5 months.

van Asselt KM, Lems WF, Bongartz EB, et al: Outcome of cervical spine surgery in patients with rheumatoid arthritis. *Ann Rheum Dis* 2001;60:448-452.

Various types of cervical fusion in patients with rheumatoid arthritis and cervical myelopathy and/or occipital neuralgia were followed for 2 years. Mortality at 2 years was 27% because of a variety of reasons. Of the surviving patients, 73% had neurologic improvement at 3 months and 67% had an improved neurologic level at 2 years.

Classic Bibliography

Boden SD, Dodge LD, Bohlman HH, Rechtine GD: Rhematoid arthritis of the cervical spine: A long term analysis with predictors of paralysis and recovery. *J Bone Joint Surg Am* 1993;75:1282-1297.

Conaty JP, Mongan ES: Cervical fusion in rheumatoid arthritis. *J Bone Joint Surg Am* 1981;63:1218-1227.

Crockard HA: Surgical management of cervical rheumatoid problems. *Spine* 1995;20:2584-2590.

Lipson SJ: Rheumatoid arthritis in the cervical spine. *Clin Orthop* 1989;239:121-127.

Morizono Y, Sakou T, Kawaida H: Upper cervical involvement in rheumatoid arthritis. *Spine* 1987;12:721-725.

Neva MH, Kauppi MJ, Kautiainen H, et al: Combination drug therapy retards the development of rheumatoid atlantoaxial subluxations. *Arthritis Rheum* 2000;43:2397-2401.

Rana NA: Natural history of atlanto-axial subluxation in rheumatoid arthritis. *Spine* 1989;14:1054-1056.

Ranawat CS, O'Leary P, Pellicci P, Tsairis P, Marchisello P, Dorr L: Cervical spine fusion in rheumatoid arthritis. *J Bone Joint Surg Am* 1979;61:1003-1010.

Santavirta S, Slatis P, Kankaanpaa U, Sandelin J, Laasonen E: Treatment of the cervical spine in rheumatoid arthritis. *J Bone Joint Surg Am* 1988;70:658-667.

Thomasen E: Vertebral osteotomy for correction of kyphosis in ankylosing spondylitis. *Clin Orthop* 1985;194:142-152.

Chapter 50

Endoscopic and Minimally Invasive Spine Surgery

Eeric Truumees, MD

Introduction

Minimally invasive and endoscopic spine surgery does not refer to a single technique, but rather to a set of tools in a continuum of less morbid approaches to the treatment of spine problems. These tools continue to emerge and will ultimately include injection techniques (epidural injections, diskography, and facet and nerve root blocks), percutaneous therapeutic modalities (intradiskal electrothermal therapy [IDET], vertebroplasty, and kyphoplasty), true endoscopic procedures (endoscopic diskectomies, endoscopic lumbar fusions, and endoscopic transthoracic procedures), image-guided surgery, bone substitutes and enhancers, nuclear replacement, and injection of growth factors.

There is no clear delineation between traditional and minimally invasive spine surgery. Minimally invasive approaches reflect a trend in orthopaedic surgery to closely target the pathology during a given therapeutic intervention while minimizing damage to the surrounding tissues. Typically, these techniques represent new ways to perform traditional surgical procedures, such as instrumentation and fusion. Occasionally, newer surgical interventions are introduced, such as percutaneous vertebral body polymethylmethacrylate augmentation.

Surgical indications are not changed by the way in which the procedure is done. In considering the role of minimally invasive spine surgery as part of a continuum of spine care, it is useful to remember that the most minimally invasive modality remains nonsurgical care. Nonsurgical treatment is appropriate and effective for most patients with degenerative conditions of the spine, especially those with axial pain in the absence of neurologic dysfunction. For newer technologies, surgical indications are evolving.

These newer surgical technologies can be categorized by the spectrum of invasiveness each requires—from truly percutaneous, to endoscopic, to mini-open. Spinal endoscopy refers to the use of an endoscope and light source for visualization and magnification through small percutaneous portals. Conceptually, endoscopy is an attractive treatment option because the spinal column lies centrally in the body. Open surgical approaches involve significant soft-tissue dissection, which affects risk, recovery, and long-term function. Endoscopically assisted and mini-open approaches rely on advances in surgical lighting, corridor retractors, and image guidance during standard operations with standard instruments to perform spine surgery with less fascial plane violation and dead space creation.

Most thoracic and lumbar spine procedures are performed posteriorly. Posterior approaches offer relatively direct access to the bony elements and the spinal canal. However, canal exposure may result in symptomatic epidural fibrosis. The dissection and retraction of the paraspinal muscles may lead to dead space formation and extensor muscle disruption. Such disruption has been referred to as fusion disease, which may be associated with early fatigability and other long-term symptoms. Less invasive posterior techniques may allow for less disruption of the posterior musculature and a smaller laminotomy.

Anterior fusion procedures have become more common in the treatment of symptomatic lumbar disk degeneration, spinal deformity correction, and the ablation of tumors and infections. Traditional anterior approaches may require large incisions, rib resections, and division of major muscle groups. Several endoscopic approaches, including transthoracic, transperitoneal, and retroperitoneal approaches, have been described in an effort to limit the morbidity associated with anterior surgical approaches.

Percutaneous Disk Procedures
Percutaneous Diskectomy Techniques

Over time, various radiographically guided procedures have been developed as both diagnostic and therapeutic interventions that can significantly limit perioperative risk and morbidity. Chymopapain, a proteolytic enzyme obtained from a papaya extract, has been used as a percutaneous treatment modality for disk herniations. The enzyme hydrolyzes the nuclear bulge and thereby decreases nerve root pressure. However, it does not affect

Table 1 | Fractures Less Likely to Improve With Standard Medical Management

Fractures of thoracolumbar junction (T11-L2)
Bursting fracture patterns
Wedge compression fractures with > 30° of sagittal angulation
Vacuum shadow in fractured body (ischemic necrosis of bone)
Progressive collapse seen in office follow-up

extruded or sequestered fragments. Although good results continue to be published in the world literature, chymopapain injection has fallen out of favor in North America because of complications, including anaphylaxis and transverse myelitis.

Several percutaneous techniques of microdiskectomy have been developed as well. In the 1970s, instrumentation was developed to access the disk space percutaneously from a posterolateral approach. These procedures were believed to debulk the central disk, thereby indirectly reducing nerve root irritation and nociceptor stimulation of the anulus fibrosus. Modifications of the procedure allowed direct visualization through an arthroscope. Like chymopapain injections, these techniques, which continue to be performed at some institutions, are reserved for patients with contained herniations and bulges. Studies comparing automated percutaneous diskectomy with open microdiskectomy usually demonstrate better results with open microdiskectomy.

Endoscopic diskectomy is performed in a manner nearly identical to open diskectomy, with the exception that the surgical instruments are passed through a tubular retractor. With these systems, a transmuscular rather than subperiosteal approach is undertaken because it is theorized that the smaller incisions will result in reduced postoperative pain and improved mobilization.

Potential disadvantages with these techniques include limited visualization, a long learning curve during which complications are more frequent, the risk of inadequate exposure or incomplete decompression, the risk of vessel or nerve root damage, limits in the ability to treat lateral recess and foraminal stenosis, and difficulty accessing the L5-S1 disk space from a far lateral approach in some patients (especially male patients with a narrow pelvis).

Intradiskal Electrothermal Therapy

Given the mixed outcomes of fusion surgery when treating patients with discogenic back pain, newer modalities such as thermal energy have been applied to the disk. IDET is conceptually based on the conversion of radiofrequency energy into thermal energy. With fluoroscopic guidance, a catheter probe is steered along the posterior annular wall. Once in place, the tissues are heated to 65°

for 17 minutes. Possible goals include collagen fibril shrinkage to stabilize the motion segment or destruction of nociceptive fibers.

The published indications for IDET include more than 6 months of discogenic pain, more than 3 months of failed medical treatment and physical therapy, concordant diskography, maintenance of at least 50% residual disk height, and the absence of neurocompressive pathology.

Initial outcomes reports have been highly varied. A designer series of 25 consecutive patients reported a 2-point difference in pain scores at an average follow-up of 7 months. Improvements in the Medical Outcomes Study Short Form 36-Item (SF-36) scores for physical function and body pain subscales were noted in 72% of patients. No complications were reported. A recent update, also by the product's designers, found that improvements increased from 1- to 2-year follow-up. These and other IDET articles have been criticized for the relatively low hurdle (for example, 2 points on the visual analog scale) that was used to determine significance. Others argue that in the absence of significant complications, IDET remains a viable modality in a small number of patients. Yet, complications have been reported, including diskitis and cauda equina syndrome.

Recent basic studies questioned the ability of the IDET probe to affect collagen denaturation or nociceptive fibers. One biomechanical study showed an increase in motion at the treated segment, raising the possibility of long-term destabilization. A recent MRI study found no change in the appearance of the high-intensity zone in degenerated disks after IDET.

Vertebral Body Augmentation (Vertebroplasty and Kyphoplasty)

In the United States, approximately 700,000 osteoporotic vertebral compression fractures occur each year. Traditionally, these fractures were thought to heal uneventfully with few, if any, sequelae. However, compression fractures represent a serious and growing health care problem worldwide. Long-term sequelae of vertebral compression fractures are common and include pain, deformity, pulmonary decline, gastrointestinal disturbance, gait and functional decline, and increased mortality. Population studies report that significant functional impairment can occur among people with vertebral compression fractures who do not seek medical attention.

The pain associated with a given vertebral compression fracture is highly variable. Of those patients presenting to physicians with pain after a vertebral compression fracture, many respond to treatment with narcotic pain medications and bracing. In some patients, bracing is not well tolerated or it does not immobilize the fracture adequately (Table 1). It has been estimated

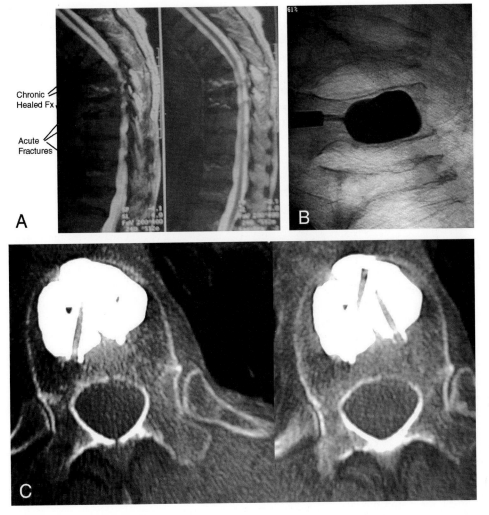

Figure 1 A, Preoperative T2-weighted MRI study demonstrating several osteoporotic fractures. The healed fracture has a normal marrow signal, whereas the acute fracture demonstrates increased signal (marrow edema). **B,** A lateral fluoroscopic image of the same patient undergoing kyphoplasty with balloon reduction of the fracture. **C,** Postoperative axial CT scans of the treated level show evidence of a well-contained cement mantle.

that each year approximately 150,000 patients with compression fractures require hospitalization with protracted periods of bed rest and administration of intravenous narcotics. In elderly patients, osteoporosis with bed rest is associated with an additional 4% loss of bone mineral density.

On plain radiographs, vertebral compression fractures have different configurations. In the thoracic spine, fractures often have a wedge appearance caused by kyphotic loading. In the lumbar spine, central end plate cupping of lordotic lumbar bodies is seen. These levels are also more likely to demonstrate a bursting pattern. It may be difficult to distinguish fracture age using plain radiographs alone. A sclerotic band below the end plate may represent healing or merely compressed trabeculae. Comparison with older films (even a recent chest radiograph) may help. MRI has a high sensitivity for fracture acuity, which is reflected by peri–end-plate edema and is typically seen as an increased signal on T2-weighted or short T1 inversion recovery images (Figure 1). T1-weighted signal intensity is usually diminished. MRI is also used to assess fracture architec-

ture and possible instrument trajectories. In patients who are unable to undergo MRI, a bone scan may estimate fracture acuity. A CT scan will provide similar morphologic information, particularly when sagittal reconstructions are ordered.

Vertebroplasty involves a unilateral or bilateral percutaneous approach to the vertebral body. Various needle and applicator systems are available through which liquid polymethylmethacrylate bone cement is introduced into the vertebral body. The early clinical results of vertebroplasty suggest that it is effective in decreasing pain in most patients. However, the mechanism of pain relief is controversial. Patient groups responding well to these techniques typically have mechanical incompetence of their vertebral body. Polymethylmethacrylate bone cement restores the load-bearing capacity of the vertebral body. This restoration of stiffness is thought to provide pain relief. A degree of postural reduction is also possible in some fractures treated with vertebroplasty.

Kyphoplasty extends the vertebroplasty concept. During this procedure, a bilateral approach to the verte-

Table 2 | Precautions and Contraindications to Kyphoplasty and Vertebroplasty

Neurologic symptoms
Young patients*
Pregnancy
High-velocity fractures
Fractures pedicles or facets
Burst fracture with retropulsed bone
Medical issues†
Allergy to devices
Allergy to contrast medium
Bleeding disorders
Severe cardiopulmonary difficulties
Technically not feasible
Vertebra plana
Multiple painful vertebral bodies
Level above T5
Neoplasm
Osteoblastic metastasis
Patients with significant long-term survivability
Primary spinal neoplasm
Severe cortical destruction
Local spinal infection

*Age range varies; caution in patients younger than 65 years
†Severe pulmonary problems precluding prone positioning because of vertebral size or imaging problems

Table 3 | Applications for Video-Assisted Thoracic Spinal Surgery

Infection
Biopsy
Débridement
Drainage of abscess
Tumor
Biopsy
Tumor excision
Corpectomy and grafting
Degenerative disease
Excision of herniated thoracic disk
Trauma
Corpectomy
Cancellous bone grafting
Deformity
Anterior releases for scoliosis or kyphosis
Anterior fusion and instrumentation
Hemivertebra excision
Internal thoracoplasty

Table 4 | Contraindications to Thoracoscopic Spine Surgery

Inability to tolerate one-lung ventilation
Severe or acute respiratory insufficiency
High airway pressures with positive pressure ventilation
Pleural symphysis
Bullous lung pathology
Empyema (relative)
Previous thoracotomy (relative)
Previous tube thoracostomy (relative)
Narrow anterior posterior chest diameter (relative)

bral body is made through 1-cm incisions. Cannulas allow introduction of balloon tamponades. Sequential inflation of these tamponades creates a void in the cancellous bone of the vertebral body and attempts to reduce the deformity. The balloon tamponades are then removed. Another theoretic advantage is that viscous polymethylmethacrylate bone cement can be introduced into the void for a more controlled fill.

Vertebral body augmentation should be considered in patients who are bedridden because of pain or in those whose pain does not begin to decline after several weeks of nonsurgical care. Results are best for patients with focal, intense, deep pain in the midline. Usually, pain worsens with activity and is relieved when recumbent. The contraindications of vertebral body augmentation are listed in Table 2.

Vertebral body augmentation procedures are usually well tolerated. Good to excellent short-term pain relief has been reported in more than 80% of patients. Complications typically occur in association with polymethylmethacrylate bone cement extravasation and can lead to canal compromise or pulmonary embolism. These complications appear to be more common among patients who undergo vertebroplasty. Additional reduction is possible with kyphoplasty, but it may be variable as a function of fracture age.

Endoscopic and Mini-Open Procedures
Thoracic Spine

Most endoscopic spine surgery is directed anteriorly where larger incisions and postthoracotomy pain may be avoided. Video-assisted thoracic spinal surgery has the same indications and goals as open thoracotomy (Tables 3 and 4).

Many of these techniques are technically demanding and are only performed in select centers worldwide. Before attempting thoracoscopic approaches to the spine, the surgeon must be thoroughly familiar with open anterior spinal anatomy and have considerable animal laboratory and proctored surgical experience. The largest early experience with video-assisted thoracic surgery has been in patients undergoing treatment for spinal deformities. A thoracoscope can be used to assist anterior release surgery in patients with large kyphotic or scoliotic deformities. The advantages and disadvantages of thoracoscopic surgery are listed in Table 5.

Thoracoscopic spinal surgery requires a fluoroscopic table and selective double lumen endotracheal intubation. Surgery proceeds in stages, beginning with the selection of access sites. The sixth intercostal space at the midaxillary line gives an unobstructed view of the entire hemithorax. The rib cage and chest wall form a rigid open space in which to work. Unlike laparoscopy, carbon dioxide insufflation is not required during thoracoscopic spinal surgery.

Instruments are centered at the level of the pathology. The lung may require retraction with an endoscopic fan retractor or strategically placed sponges. Once the level of the pathology has been identified, the parietal pleura is incised. The parietal pleura is bluntly dissected proximally, distally, and anteriorly to expose as much of the vertebral margins as necessary.

After the anulus fibrosus is incised with cautery, the disk and cartilage end plates are removed to bleeding bone with long pituitaries, Cobb elevators, and curets. For patients undergoing kyphosis correction, the anterior longitudinal ligament and opposite side of the anulus fibrosus is incised. In patients undergoing releases for the treatment of scoliosis, it is mandatory to incise the posterolateral corner of the disk spaces in the concavity of the curve. Morcellized rib or iliac crest graft can be delivered by a funnel or a structural graft (femoral ring allograft or cage) delivered through an enlarged portal.

In certain patients, a thoracoscopic release, with the patient in the prone position, may be done concurrently with open posterior stabilization. Similarly, internal thoracoplasty may also be performed concurrently or as an independent procedure. Rib resections are planned as an ellipse to ensure smooth chest contours. The periosteum of the rib portion to be resected is stripped, and a high-speed burr creates the osteotomy.

Patients with symptomatic thoracic disk herniations may be amenable to treatment with endoscopic transthoracic decompressions. Patient selection is a critical issue because patients rarely have true radicular or myelopathic symptoms. Patients with diffuse midthoracic back pain and diagnostic imaging showing evidence of multiple degenerative segments with or without herniations are not good candidates for either open or endoscopic diskectomy.

Comparable endoscopic techniques have been described for vertebral corpectomies or osteotomies. The spine is exposed by bluntly dissecting the pleura and ligating only those segmental vessels in the surgical field. A combination of pituitary rongeurs, curets, Cobb elevators, and high-speed burrs are used as they would be with the chest open. The corpectomy reconstruction can

Table 5	Advantages and Disadvantages of Endoscopy
Advantages
Less postoperative pain
Alleviates the physiologic concerns of healing associated with large incisions into the thoracic, peritoneal, or retroperitoneal cavities
Improved visualization of the target tissues
Improved cosmetic result with smaller incisions
Reduced recovery time and hospital stay
Disadvantages
Steep learning curve
Cost
Limitations in tactile feedback
Increased working distance from 4 to 30 cm
Two-dimensional video visualization
Triangulation
Limited depth perception
Necessity for specialized instruments
Adverse effect on ability to deal with certain complications (such as brisk arterial bleeding)
As experience is gained, disadvantages much less limiting

be completed by negotiating allograft struts or mesh cages into the defect after inserting them into the chest through an enlarged portal.

Techniques for endoscopic transthoracic spinal instrumentation continue to evolve with the development of new implants capable of stabilization and correction. Threaded cylindrical interbody fusion cages, in widespread use in the treatment of deformities of the lumbar spine, are now being used to treat deformities of the thoracic spine in the coronal or oblique plane. Such thoracic cage application may be technically less demanding, but the consequences of malpositioning are significant. The fusion rates for patients with single thoracic cages have yet to be evaluated. Existing posterior or anterior rod and screw implant systems have been modified for application in an endoscopic fashion.

Increasingly, open and endoscopic approaches are being combined for instrumentation. In such procedures, one of the portals is enlarged to a 5-cm incision, which allows the use of more standard surgical instruments and significantly simplifies implant introduction.

In the postoperative period, most patients are extubated immediately. A chest tube is maintained at water seal and removed 1 to 2 days postoperatively. An intensive care unit stay is not usually needed. Aggressive respiratory care is required to prevent "down lung" atelectasis and pneumonia.

Complications of thoracoscopic surgery are essentially the same as with an open approach. As in any spinal cord level procedure, spinal cord injury or ischemia is possible. Dural laceration may be noted. Intercostal neuralgia is common (21% of patients), but it is usually transient. Endoscopic releases may be less complete than open releases. Also, trocar or instrument injury to the lung, diaphragm, heart, great vessels, thoracic duct, azygos vein, esophagus, segmental arteries, sympathetic chain, and splanchnic nerves is possible.

One series compared video-assisted thoracoscopic surgery to open thoracotomy in a sheep model. In this series, histologic, biomechanical, and radiographic outcomes were comparable to those of open surgery. However, endoscopic procedures were associated with protracted learning periods, long surgical times, increased blood loss, and increased animal morbidity. Others report that, with increased surgeon experience with these procedures, tissue damage, blood loss, postoperative pain, intensive care unit and hospital stays are reduced and that respiratory and shoulder function are less affected.

Lumbar Spine

Several methods have been described to reduce the exposure needed for posterior decompression surgery. The most common is use of a surgical microscope. Microdiskectomy is the most commonly performed minimally invasive approach to partial disk removal (see chapter 44).

A newer endoscopic diskectomy technique uses a tubular working cannula. The fiberoptic image bundle is housed in a sidewall of the cannula. Standard instruments, such as pituitary or Kerrison rongeurs, are inserted under direct vision. This technique has also been used to treat cervical disk herniations (via laminoforaminotomy) and for microdecompression of lateral recess lumbar spinal stenosis. The benefits of this technique over the more traditional microdiskectomy have not yet been established. For most spine surgeons, microdiskectomy remains the safer technique.

The role of posterior endoscopic and minimally invasive techniques in the treatment of metastatic disease, fractures, and infections is evolving. Although the anterior approach to metastatic disease is favored overall, the use of an endoscope to assist posterolateral decompression may obviate the need for a second anterior surgery in patients undergoing posterior stabilization.

The medial branch of the dorsal primary ramus can be injured when a midline approach is carried beyond the facets and over the transverse processes. To minimize this type of injury, several newer techniques have been developed that use a muscle-splitting approach in the interval between the multifidus medially and the longissimus laterally. This approach is similar to that described by Wiltse for far lateral diskectomy. Exploiting this plane, endoscopic, fluoroscopic, or navigation system assistance allows for transpedicular instrumentation through smaller incisions. Several variations, including

interbody fusion techniques, have been described and are marketed with specialized instruments by the various implant manufacturers. Long-term results of fusions with these implants are not yet available.

Interestingly, much of the current interest in percutaneous pedicle screw technology comes from the increased use of anterior lumbar interbody cages, themselves part of the vanguard of minimally invasive spine surgery. Increasingly, the late instability of fusion constructs resulting from the use of these threaded fusion cages in motion segments with preserved disk height has been described. Additionally, posterior stabilization has been recommended. Translaminar facet screws represent another method of achieving posterior fixation through small incisions with minimal tissue stripping.

Most truly endoscopic lumbar spine procedures are anterior. Unlike the posterior approach, there are several critical anatomic structures that must be avoided when approaching the spine anteriorly, including the inferior epigastric artery and vein, which lie deep to the surface of the rectus muscle. Placement of endoscopic ports through these structures is associated with postoperative hematoma formation. The ureters run obliquely from the retroperitoneal space into the abdomen. The left ureter runs obliquely in the mesentery deep to the sigmoid and is not usually seen. The right ureter runs obliquely over the right iliac into the pelvis and may occasionally be injured. The ureter will sometimes course in midline directly over the L5-S1 disk space and may be directly damaged by surgical exposures. Overretraction of the psoas muscle may injure the lumbar plexus. Injury to the lumbar sympathetic chain, just anterior to the L5-S1 disk, may result in retrograde ejaculation.

Contraindications to anterior spinal endoscopic surgery include peritoneal or pelvic infections, prior open anterior spine surgery, or prior lower abdominal surgery (such as colon resection or hysterectomy). Endometriosis also causes adhesions that can limit anterior spinal endoscopy.

Anterior spinal endoscopy can be performed with or without insufflation. Insufflation involves the use of carbon dioxide to inflate the abdominal cavity to more completely visualize surrounding anatomic structures. Insufflated surgery is a direct extension of conventional laparoscopic surgery. It gives direct access to L5-S1, L4-5, and occasionally to L3-4. The advantages of insufflation include organ retraction, more rapid exposure, increased working space, and decreased bleeding. However, special instruments are required, including expensive trocars with diaphragms. Additionally, air may leak during the procedure. Moreover, carbon dioxide insufflation of the peritoneal cavity increases mean arterial pressure and decreases venous return. Carbon dioxide absorption may lead to hypercapnia and decreased diaphragmatic excursion. Carbon dioxide embolism from open veins has also been reported.

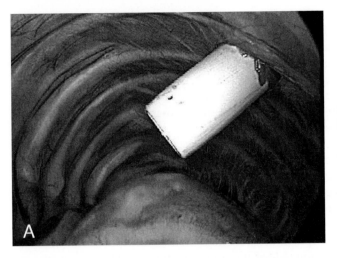
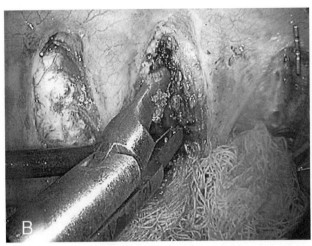

Figure 2 **A,** Photograph of the introduction of a working portal during thoracoscopy. **B,** Photograph of the initial thoracoscopic approach to the disk space.

With a gasless approach, the anatomic approach remains the same, but the working space is created by lifting the anterior abdominal wall with a fan retractor and hydraulic arm (Laparolift, Origin Medsystems, Menlo Park, CA). This technique decreases costs because conventional instruments are used. However, gasless surgery takes longer and is technically more difficult to perform. Moreover, lateral vision is limited with the use of this technique. A combined approach using insufflation for the initial spine exposure to place retractors and Steinmann pins and the subsequent conversion to a gasless/Laparolift procedure falls in the midrange in terms of cost and ease of use.

Operating room positioning of the patient is critical for these procedures. Drains including a Foley catheter and nasogastric tube are placed. The patient is supine with one or both arms tucked at the side or overhead (for fluoroscopic control). Steep Trendelenburg positioning is often required; therefore, a special shoulder harness or foot stirrups may also be needed. Fluoroscopy and endoscopy monitors must be in the direct line of sight of spine and endoscopic surgeons. The preparation materials and drape must allow for bone graft harvest and conversion to an open procedure, if necessary.

The actual approach to the spine may be transperitoneal or retroperitoneal. In transperitoneal endoscopy, the procedure begins with placement of the first (umbilical) portal. Once in place, the peritoneum is insufflated to 15 mm with carbon dioxide. Secondary ports are then placed under visual guidance, including a 17-mm suprapubic working portal. A superficial incision in the midline peritoneum from the sacral promontory to vascular bifurcation is made, exposing the spine. Blunt dissection in the retroperitoneal space is used to identify the middle sacral artery and the several medial branches of the iliac veins, which are clipped. More blunt dissection will expose the disk spaces, the levels of which are con-

firmed on fluoroscopy (Figure 2).

The retroperitoneal approach uses a potential space behind the peritoneal sac. Advantages of this approach include improved spinal access from T12 to S1. In that the peritoneum contains the bowel loops, retraction is facilitated. Additionally, conventional instruments may be used and conversion from a pure percutaneous endoscopic to an endoscopically assisted anterior approach may be performed if increased difficulty is encountered.

In retroperitoneal approaches, a left lateral decubitus positioning of the patient allows abdominal contents to fall freely forward. A skin incision is made, the internal and external obliques are identified, and fibers are spread bluntly. This exposes the transversalis fascia, which is also incised. A finger may be used to bluntly dissect in the retroperitoneal space along the twelfth rib to the transverse process of T12 or L1. The potential space may be increased by inserting an insufflating balloon or a gasless technique with a Laparolift or insufflated technique may be used. The blunt dissection is carried posteriorly to the psoas fibers until the disk space is identified.

Titanium cage or bone dowel implantation, which is among the most commonly performed lumbar endoscopic techniques, is typically used for anterior column fusion in patients with disk-related pain (Figure 3). Advantages include avoidance of extensor muscle stripping, more rigid anterior fusion, and lower pseudarthrosis rates from grafting under compression. Reports of failure of these implants as stand-alone devices have dimmed the initial enthusiasm.

The implementation of endoscopic approaches to the anterior spine has fostered a renewed interest in decreasing the morbidity of traditional open anterior procedures. Various mini-open anterior paramedian muscle-sparing approaches to the lumbar spine have been recently described. Proponents argue that this cosmeti-

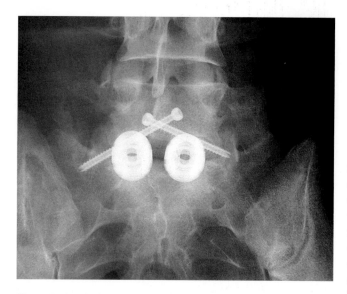

Figure 3 Postoperative AP radiograph of a patient who underwent endoscopic transperitoneal titanium BAK cage (SpineTech, Minneapolis, MN) placement followed by open posterior translaminar facet screw instrumentation.

cally acceptable approach allows better tactile feedback and overall safety than endoscopic techniques. In several centers, the initial enthusiasm for endoscopic techniques has gradually given way to a reversion toward open surgery, but with far more attention given to cosmetics and the minimization of soft-tissue injury.

Summary

Most minimally invasive spine surgery involves a change in approach, not a change in the surgical procedure itself. Therefore, the indications for surgical intervention should not be relaxed merely because these procedures may be performed endoscopically. As in any spine surgery, careful patient selection is paramount in predicting successful outcomes. Few long-term data are available for any of these endoscopic spine surgery techniques. Although many of these procedures are promising, significant advantages over previous techniques have yet to be demonstrated.

The advantages of endoscopic spinal surgery (improved surgical visualization through magnification and lighting, decreased perioperative morbidity, and shortened hospital stays) must be counterbalanced with the steep learning curve for this procedure. Initial experience with endoscopic spinal surgery may be associated with higher complication rates and longer operating times. A less efficacious technique should not be used merely because it is endoscopic.

Endoscopic spine surgery techniques are also both personnel and equipment intensive. Unlike open procedures, a second surgeon may be needed for an endoscopic procedure (to perform a second approach). Specialized and usually disposable instruments are also required for endoscopic spine surgery. Although these

additional costs may be recouped with earlier patient discharge, the potential benefits of a minimal approach are not going to be realized by every surgeon. Because endoscopic approaches limit visualization with a limited field width, decreased three-dimensional perspective, and a loss of tactile sense, surgeons should be prepared for immediate conversion to an open procedure if necessary.

Endoscopic procedures will likely be performed more commonly in the future. Current indications for endoscopic spine surgery include minimally invasive access to the intervertebral disk (both anteriorly and posteriorly), débridement of tumor and infection, releases for deformity, and anterior interbody fusions. Placement of spinal instrumentation anteriorly remains under evaluation. All of these procedures are at risk for achieving overzealous acceptance before independent, randomized studies are done to demonstrate comparable outcomes and risk profiles with accepted techniques.

Annotated Bibliography

Percutaneous Disk Procedures

Biyani A, Andersson GB, Chaudhary H, An HS: Intradiscal electrothermal therapy: A treatment option in patients with internal disc disruption. *Spine* 2003;28:S8-S14.

This review of the histologic, biomechanical, and clinical results of IDET suggests that although the mode of effect is not understood, IDET may be beneficial in some patients. In those who did not have improvement of symptoms, little procedural risk was encountered.

Cohen SP, Larkin T, Abdi S, Chang A, Stojanovic M: Risk factors for failure and complications of intradiscal electrothermal therapy: A pilot study. *Spine* 2003;28:1142-1147.

In this retrospective review of 79 patients undergoing IDET, 48% of patients reported more than 50% pain relief at 6-month follow-up. In this series, there was a 10% complication rate, but most of the complications were transient and self-limited. Obesity was a risk factor for failure of the procedure.

Freedman BA, Cohen SP, Kuklo TR, Lehman RA, Larkin P, Giuliani JR: Intradiscal electrothermal therapy (IDET) for chronic low back pain in active-duty soldiers: 2-year follow-up. *Spine J* 2003;3:502-509.

In this consecutive case series assessing the use of IDET in the management of chronic discogenic low back pain in 36 soldiers, 50% or greater pain reduction was reported by 47% of patients at 6-month follow-up and 16% at 2-year follow-up. The authors also reported that 20 of 31 soldiers (65%) had a persistent decrease in their analog pain scores. Additionally, 7 of 31 soldiers (23%) went on to undergo spinal surgery within 24 months of undergoing IDET. The authors noted that their reasonable early results diminished with time and that up to

20% of patients reported worsening of baseline symptoms at final follow-up. They concluded that IDET should not be used as a substitute for spinal fusion in the treatment of chronic discogenic low back pain in active-duty soldiers.

Lieberman IH, Dudeney S, Reinhardt MK, Bell G: Initial outcome and efficacy of "kyphoplasty" in the treatment of painful osteoporotic vertebral compression fractures. *Spine* 2001;26:1631-1638.

This is a prospective study of kyphoplasty procedures that were performed in 30 patients. The results demonstrate excellent outcomes and low complications.

Lindsay R, Silverman SL, Cooper C, et al: Risk of new vertebral fracture in the year following a fracture. *JAMA* 2001;285:320-323.

This article reviews the clinical consequences of vertebral compression fractures and largely dispels the notion that these injuries follow a benign, self-limited course.

Muramatsu K, Hachiya Y, Morita C: Postoperative magnetic resonance imaging of lumbar disc herniation: Comparison of microendoscopic discectomy and Love's method. *Spine* 2001;26:1599-1605.

The authors of this study compared postoperative MRI studies and found that the effect of microendoscopic diskectomy on the cauda equina was comparable to that of open diskectomy. Furthermore, the postoperative images of the route of entry failed to show that microendoscopic diskectomy is appreciably less invasive with respect to the paravertebral muscles.

Phillips FM, Ho E, Campbell-Hupp M, McNally T, Todd Wetzel F, Gupta P: Early radiographic and clinical results of balloon kyphoplasty for the treatment of osteoporotic vertebral compression fractures. *Spine* 2003;28:2260-2265.

This is an outcomes report of 29 patients who underwent kyphoplasty in 37 separate sessions; a total of 61 vertebral compression fractures were treated. In 30 of the 52 fractures that were considered reducible, a mean 14.2° of correction was noted. Significant pain relief was noted with minimal complications.

Saal JA, Saal JS: Intradiscal electrothermal treatment for chronic discogenic low back pain: Prospective outcome study with a minimum 2-year follow-up. *Spine* 2002;27:966-973.

This 2-year follow-up study of the original designer series demonstrated that the statistically significant improvement in pain scores and SF-36 quality of life scores that was previously reported increased between the 1- and 2-year observation points.

Schick U, Döhnert J, Richter A, König A, Vitzthum HE: Microendoscopic lumbar discectomy versus open sur-

gery: An intraoperative EMG study. *Eur Spine J* 2002; 11:20-26.

This electromyographic study demonstrated that less mechanical irritation of the nerve root occurred with endoscopic approaches than with traditional open surgery.

Spruit M, Jacobs WC: Pain and function after intradiscal electrothermal treatment (IDET) for symptomatic lumbar disc degeneration. *Eur Spine J* 2002;11:589-593.

This small series of prospectively evaluated patients failed to show significant improvement of patient symptoms after undergoing IDET.

Yeung AT, Tsou PM: Posterolateral endoscopic excision for lumbar disc herniation: Surgical technique, outcome, and complications in 307 consecutive cases. *Spine* 2002; 27:722-731.

In this retrospective review of 1-year outcomes in 307 consecutive patients with lumbar disk herniation who underwent posterolateral endoscopic diskectomy, the response rate to the questionnaire was 91%, and 90.7% of those patients reported being satisfied with their surgical outcomes. The combined major and minor complication rate was 3.5%.

Endoscopic and Mini-Open Procedures

Anand N, Regan JJ: Video-assisted thoracoscopic surgery for thoracic disc disease: Classification and outcome study of 100 consecutive cases with a 2-year minimum follow-up period. *Spine* 2002;27:871-879.

In this retrospective review of prospectively collected 4-year follow-up data in 100 consecutive patients who underwent video-assisted thoracoscopic surgery, no permanent complications or spinal cord injuries were reported. The average percentage of improvement in Oswestry scores was most significant in grade 4 patients (myelopathy, 60%), followed by grade 3A patients (axial and thoracic radicular pain, 37%), grade 3B patients (axial with leg pain, 28%), and grade 1 patients (pure axial, 24%). The authors concluded that the procedure was associated with significant clinical improvement in most treated patients.

Escobar E, Transfeldt E, Garvey T, Ogilvie J, Graber J, Schultz L: Video-assisted versus open anterior lumbar spine fusion surgery: A comparison of four techniques and complications in 135 patients. *Spine* 2003;28:729-732.

This is a retrospective report comparing the outcomes of anterior lumbar interbody fusion in 135 patients using one of the following four approaches: transperitoneal endoscopy with insufflation, retroperitoneal endoscopic surgery, mini-open surgery, or traditional open approaches. The incidence of complications for video-assisted techniques was found to be consistent with that reported in the medical literature, but it was higher than that for open techniques. The authors note that they no longer use video-assisted techniques as a result of these findings.

Khoo LT, Beisse R, Potulski M: Thoracoscopic-assisted treatment of thoracic and lumbar fractures: A series of 371 consecutive cases. *Neurosurgery* 2002;51(5 suppl): 104-117.

In this report of 371 patients with thoracic and thoracolumbar spine fractures who were treated with thoracoscopic assistance, the severe complication rate was low (1.3%), with only one instance of each of the following reported: aortic injury, splenic contusion, neurologic deterioration, cerebrospinal fluid leak, and severe wound infection.

Pellisé F, Puig O, Rivas A, Bagó J, Villanueva C: Low fusion rate after L5-S1 laparoscopic anterior lumbar interbody fusion using twin stand-alone carbon fiber cages. *Spine* 2002;27:1665-1669.

This study reported prospective data on 12 patients undergoing twin, stand-alone anterior cage placement. Although significant improvements in visual analog scores, Prolo scores, and Waddell Disability Index scores were noted, the overall CT scan fusion rate at 2-year follow-up was 16.6% and was deemed unacceptably low.

Classic Bibliography

Do HM: Magnetic resonance imaging in the evaluation of patients for percutaneous vertebroplasty. *Topics in MRI* 2000;14:235-244.

Grados F, Depriester C, Cayrolle G, et al: Long-term observations of vertebral osteoporotic fractures treated by percutaneous vertebroplasty. *Rheumatology (Oxford)* 2000;39:1410-1414.

McLain RF: Endoscopically assisted decompression for metastatic thoracic neoplasms. *Spine* 1998;23:1130-1135.

Silverman SL: The clinical consequences of vertebral compression fractures. *Bone* 1993;13:S27-S31.

Section 7

Rehabilitation

Section Editors:
Mitchell Freedman, DO
Tom G. Mayer, MD

Chapter 51

Spinal Cord Injury

Kevin C. O'Connor, MD

Eric K. Mayer, MD

Mitchel B. Harris, MD

Introduction

Over the past two decades, advances in spinal cord medicine have come about at an unprecedented pace. To stay abreast of these advances, it is helpful to review characteristics of the population affected by spinal cord injury (SCI), their prognosis, testing procedures, and major medical and rehabilitation sequelae that are standards of care.

Epidemiology

The annual incidence of SCI in the United States, not including fatalities at the site of injury, is approximately 40 cases per million population, or approximately 11,000 new cases per year. The number of Americans with SCI has been estimated to be between 183,000 and 230,000. SCI primarily affects young adults with an average age of injury of 32.1 years; 55% of all SCIs occur in people between the ages of 16 to 30 years, during the most productive working/earning years. The average age of injury has been increasing since the 1970s, mirroring the increase in the median age of the general population. The fastest growing cohort with SCI is patients older than age 60 years, who now represent 10% of new SCI patients. There remains a 4:1 male to female ratio that has largely remained unchanged since the 1960s.

A significant trend has been observed in the racial distribution of patients with SCI. Since 1990, African-Americans and Hispanics have become disproportionately affected with new SCIs. Percentages of new SCIs have risen for African-Americans from 5.7% in 1974 to 27.6% in 1990, and for Hispanics from 5.7% to 7.7%. During the same time period, the percentage of Caucasians with new SCIs has decreased from 77.5% to 59.1% (Figure 1).

Motor vehicle crashes still account for the largest percentage of SCIs at a current rate of 38.5%, followed by acts of violence (mostly gunshot wounds), falls, and sports-related injuries (Figure 2). The proportion of injuries from falls and acts of violence has increased steadily.

Over the past 20 years, tetraplegia has become less common and paraplegia more common. Approximately one half of all traumatic SCIs in the United States are cervical lesions, and one third are thoracic. The most common neurologic level of injury is C5, followed by C4, and then C6. The most common level of paraplegia is T12. There has also been a trend toward an increased number of incomplete lesions (Figure 3).

Causes of Death

Overall, 85% of SCI patients who survive the first 24 hours after injury are still alive 10 years later. The most common cause of death is diseases of the respiratory system, with most of these resulting from pneumonia. The second leading cause of death following SCI is nonischemic heart disease. Deaths resulting from external causes such as subsequent unintentional injuries and suicides and homicides (but not including multiple injuries sustained during the original accident) are the third leading cause of death. The majority of these deaths are the result of suicide. The fourth leading cause of death is infectious and parasitic diseases (usually septicemia associated with decubitus ulcers, urinary tract or respiratory infections). Mortality rates are significantly higher during the first year after injury than during subsequent years.

Classification

In 1969, Frankel and associates described a five-grade system for classifying traumatic SCI, divided between complete and incomplete injuries. The amount of preserved motor or sensory function determined the specific Frankel classification. The Frankel classification was replaced in 1992 by the American Spinal Injury Association (ASIA) Impairment Scale, which was revised in 1996, and again in 2000. These standards subsequently became known as the International Standards for Neurologic and Functional Classification of Spinal Cord Injury. The ASIA standards have gained widespread acceptance as the preferred classification system for SCI. The initial neurologic examination serves as a baseline

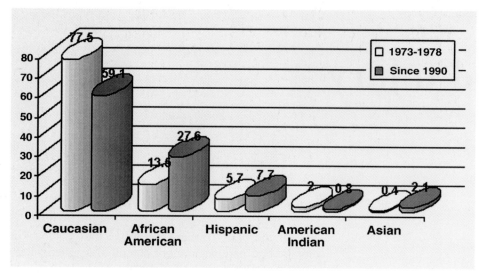

Figure 1 Racial distribution of SCI.

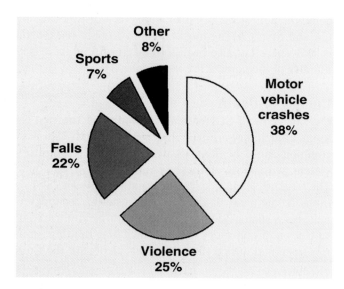

Figure 2 Etiology of SCI since 1990.

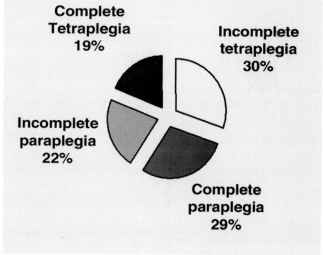

Figure 3 Current percentage of injuries by ASIA classification (since 1991).

for evaluation over the first hours to days after injury; however, neurologic status can change over the first few days and is influenced by resuscitative procedures. The period from 72 hours to 1 week after injury is the earliest time period after injury when detailed neurologic evaluations can reliably be performed to predict neurologic recovery.

The ASIA sensory examination consists of 28 key dermatomes, each separately tested for pinprick/dull (with a safety pin) and light touch (with cotton) sensation on both sides of the body. A three-point scale from 0 to 2 is used, with the face serving as the normal reference point. A score of 0 represents absent sensation, including inability to distinguish the sharp and dull edge of the pin; a score of 1 represents impaired sensation, including hyperesthesia; and a score of 2 is given when the pin or cotton is felt in the same manner as when tested on the face. The sensory level is the most caudal dermatome to have intact (2/2) sensation for both pinprick and light touch on both sides of the body.

The ASIA motor examination consists of testing 10 key muscles (5 in the upper limb and 5 in the lower limb) on each side of the body (Table 1). The patient is supine during testing and strength is graded on a six-point scale from 0 to 5. The motor level is defined as the lowest key muscle that has a grade of at least 3, provided that the segments above that level are graded as 5. Grade 4 is not considered normal, as it previously was, unless the examiner judges that certain factors inhibited full effort, including pain, positioning, disuse, or hypertonicity. In patients in whom there is no key muscle for a segment that has intact sensory dermatomes (C2-C4, T2-L1, and S2-S5), the sensory level defines the motor level.

Table 1 | Key Muscle Groups Involved in ASIA Motor Examination

Root Level	Muscle Group	Root Level	Muscle Group
C5	Elbow flexors	L2	Hip flexors
C6	Wrist extensors	L3	Knee extensors
C7	Elbow extensors	L4	Ankle dorsiflexors
C8	Long finger flexors	L5	Long toe extensor
T1	Small finger abductors	S1	Ankle plantar flexors

Table 2 | ASIA Impairment Scale

A = Complete. No motor or sensory function is preserved in the sacral segments S4-S5.

B = Incomplete. Sensory but no motor function preserved below the neurologic level and includes the sacral segments S4-S5.

C = Incomplete. Motor function is preserved below the neurologic level, and more than half of the key muscles below the neurologic level have a muscle grade less than 3.

D = Incomplete. Motor function is preserved below the neurologic level, and at least half of the key muscles below the neurologic level have a muscle grade greater than or equal to 3.

E = Normal. Sensory and motor functions are normal.

A is a complete injury, while B through E represent incomplete injuries. For an individual to receive a grade of C or D, the injury must be incomplete and have either voluntary anal contraction or sparing of motor function more than three levels below the motor level

The skeletal level of injury is defined as the spinal level where, by radiographic examination, the greatest vertebral damage is found. The neurologic level of injury is the most caudal level at which both motor and sensory modalities are intact on both sides of the body. Because of a poor correlation between vertebral injury and function, the neurologic level of injury is preferred. Because these levels can be different from side to side, up to four levels (right C6 sensory, left C8 sensory, right C5 motor, left C8 motor) may be needed to present a clearer picture of the patient's status.

Tetraplegia, previously called quadriplegia, is defined as impairment or loss of motor or sensory function in the cervical segments of the spinal cord caused by damage of the neural elements within the spinal cord. Tetraplegia results in impairment of function of the arms as well as the trunk and legs. Paraplegia refers to impairment of motor or sensory function in the thoracic, lumbar, or sacral segments of the spinal cord secondary to damage of the neural elements within the spinal cord. Paraplegia results in impairment of the trunk and legs, depending on the level of injury, but the arms are spared. Plexus injury or injury to the peripheral nerves outside the neural canal are not included. The terms quadriparesis and paraparesis are discouraged because they imprecisely describe incomplete lesions.

Complete injury is defined as the absence of sensory or motor function in the lowest sacral segments, and incomplete injury is defined as preservation of motor or sensory sensation below the neurologic level of injury that includes the lowest sacral segments, also known as sacral sparing. Sacral sparing is tested by light touch and pinprick at the anal mucocutaneous junction (S4-5 dermatome) on both sides, as well as by testing for voluntary anal contraction and deep anal sensation. If any of these sensations is present, even if impaired, the patient has an incomplete injury. The zone of partial preservation refers to those dermatomes and myotomes caudal to the neurologic level that remain partially innervated and is used only in complete injuries. The ASIA Impairment Scale describes five levels of SCI severity (Table 2).

Spinal Cord Injury Syndromes
Central Cord Syndrome

The most common of the incomplete syndromes is central cord syndrome, which is characterized by motor weakness of the upper extremities greater than the lower extremities, in association with sacral sparing. Central cord syndrome most frequently occurs in older patients with cervical spondylosis and a hyperextension injury, but can occur in any age group or with any mechanism. The mechanism of injury involves compression of the cord during hyperextension, caused by an inward bulging of the ligamentum flavum on an already narrowed canal.

Central cord syndrome has a typical pattern of recovery that begins with the lower extremities, followed by bowel and bladder function, proximal upper extremities, and hand function. The prognosis is dependent on the patient's age, with those younger than age 50 years having a much better prognosis for independence than older patients. However, for patients with ASIA D tetraplegia, the prognosis for recovery of independent ambulation is excellent, even for those older than age 50 years.

Brown-Séquard Syndrome

Brown-Séquard syndrome involves hemisection of the spinal cord and accounts for 2% to 4% of all traumatic SCIs. Neurologically, there is an ipsilateral loss of position, light touch, vibration, and motor loss, and a contralateral loss of pain and temperature below the level of the lesion. Neuroanatomically, this is explained by the crossing of the spinothalamic tracts at the spinal cord level and the crossing of the corticospinal and dorsal columns at the medulla.

Overall, patients with Brown-Séquard syndrome have the best prognosis for functional outcome and potential for ambulation. Approximately 75% to 90% of patients ambulate independently upon discharge from rehabilitation; patients are more likely to ambulate when the upper limb is weaker than the lower limb on the affected side.

Anterior Cord Syndrome

Anterior cord syndrome is associated with lesions that affect the anterior two thirds of the spinal cord but preserve the dorsal columns. Although anterior cord syndrome can be associated with direct injury to the anterior cord, it is most commonly caused by lesions of the anterior spinal artery, which supplies the anterior two thirds of the spinal cord and can be injured through thrombosis or embolism. There is inconsistent and variable loss of motor strength and pinprick sensation with preservation of light touch, deep pressure, and proprioception. Prognosis is poor with less than a 20% chance of motor recovery.

Conus Medullaris and Cauda Equina Syndromes

The conus medullaris is the terminal segment of the spinal cord. The segment above it is termed the epiconus and it consists of spinal cord segments L4 to S1. Lesions of the epiconus cause upper motor neuron dysfunction of the lower lumbar and sacral segments. Recovery is similar to that of other upper motor neuron SCIs. Lesions of the conus medullaris affect the S2-S5 segments and there is a combination of upper and lower motor neuron deficits because the cauda equina is often injured simultaneously. Frequently the lower motor neuron deficits predominate. With conus medullaris injuries, recovery is limited.

Lesions below the L1 vertebral level injure the cauda equina, producing motor weakness and atrophy of the lower extremities with bowel and bladder involvement and areflexia. Cauda equina injuries have a better prognosis for recovery than other SCIs, because the roots are histologically peripheral nerves and regeneration can occur. Often, traumatic SCI will cause a combination of conus and cauda equina injuries.

Acute Management of Spinal Cord Injury

Acute intervention after SCI may be surgical or nonsurgical. Nonsurgical intervention consists of pharmacologic and realignment techniques. The role of surgical intervention for acute SCIs is still widely debated; however, there exists a significant body of information identifying the benefit of urgent surgical intervention in animal SCI models. Human clinical trials and retrospective analysis have been unable to show a statistical improvement in neurologic outcome related to surgical intervention. According to one recent study, subacute and late decompressive procedures have a major role in the treatment of incomplete SCI.

When the trauma patient is initially assessed at the scene of injury, if there is any suspicion of SCI, additional attention is given to maintaining maximal oxygenation and normalization of blood pressure. These crucial early interventions help to protect the fragile spinal cord blood perfusion. Generally these interventions include nasal cannula administration of oxygen and vasopressors to maintain an optimal blood pressure. Crystalloids are initially administered; however, if adequate pressures cannot be maintained in the SCI patient, pressors (dopamine) should be quickly added to resuscitation efforts. Blood pressure should be maintained at a systolic pressure between 80 and 100 mm Hg to minimize the proliferation of secondary insults to the spinal cord from hypoxemia.

The importance of maintaining adequate spinal cord perfusion following injury is widely accepted though largely unproven. There exists a hypothetical watershed region of partial injury within the cord tissue that has the potential for functional recovery if perfusion is maintained and further trauma avoided. Healthy cord tissue demonstrates autoregulation of blood flow capable of maintaining perfusion through a wide range of systemic blood pressure. This autoregulatory function can be lost following injury, leaving the watershed region vulnerable to fluctuations in systemic blood pressure. Maintenance of mean arterial pressure above 85 mm Hg has been recommended for at least 7 days following injury. Initial efforts at volume expansion using crystalloid or colloid may be insufficient, and require subsequent administration of dopamine or neosynephrine.

Mortality in the acute phase of SCI is frequently secondary to pulmonary failure and shock. Shock is initially managed by the Advanced Trauma Life Support protocol of crystalloid resuscitation, until it is clear that supplementary pressors are required to maintain adequate blood pressure. Early and aggressive pulmonary support is essential in the acute stages after injury. Pneumonia and atelectasis are difficult to avoid and represent the most common early complications. The frequency and severity of these occurrences is related to the level of the SCI, as it relates to the remaining innervation of the respiratory muscles. In the patient with acute SCI, respiratory support is often required.

The loss of sympathetic tone, found with lesions above the T6 level, leads to unopposed vagal input. This imbalanced neural activity can cause increased bronchial secretions and ultimately lead to mucus plug formation. Mucus plugs, an impaired cough reflex, and compromised respiratory muscles all can cause early respiratory arrest in the patient with acute SCI.

High-dose steroids are administered in the patient with acute SCI. Intravenous administration of the glucocorticoid methylprednisolone in high doses (loading dose 30 mg/kg bolus over 15 minutes followed by

5.4 mg/kg hr) is recommended, with the length of time of administration dependent on the time of presentation. If administration of the steroid is initiated within 3 hours of the SCI, administration for 23 hours is recommended, whereas if steroid administration is initiated between 3 to 8 hours after SCI, the steroid should be continued for 48 hours. The original clinical trials did not recommend the use of methylprednisolone if the patient presents after 12 hours from the time of injury. Additionally, the study cohort did not include cord injuries caused by ballistic/penetrating trauma or those with nerve root injury. The studies supporting this protocol have come under increasing scrutiny over the past few years.

Shortcomings of the Second National Acute Spinal Cord Injury Study (NASCIS II) include lack of data regarding the functional significance of apparently incremental improvements in neurologic scores, failure to present raw study data, and absence of a clearly defined initial study hypothesis. Follow-up post hoc subgroup analysis suggests that placebo administration greater than 8 hours following injury achieved an equivalent improvement in motor score in patients who had methylprednisolone administered within 8 hours of injury. NASCIS II has also been criticized for lacking functional outcome measures. Currently the use of high-dose steroids in the treatment of SCI is an off-label use of this drug and has not been approved for this indication by the Food and Drug Administration. High-dose steroid treatment also has been associated with an increased incidence of gastrointestinal bleeding as well as an increased rate of infection.

The glucocorticoids are stabilizing agents that have been shown to affect the neural membranes, preventing uncontrolled intracellular calcium influx. Additional stated positive effects include decreasing the lysosomal enzyme effects and reducing secondary swelling and inflammation.

A second nonsurgical intervention is early indirect reduction of the spinal canal via cranial tong traction. The increasing availability of MRI has dampened some of the enthusiasm for rapid closed reduction techniques, as MRI has identified the presence of associated herniated intervertebral disks. Closed reduction of the traumatic deformity is directed toward restoration of the spinal column to its premorbid alignment and reestablishment of the diameter of the bony spinal canal. This reduction maneuver is applicable to cervical spine injuries only. Additionally, before any significant amount of traction (> 10 lb) can be applied through the tongs, special effort must be made to rule out the possibility of an associated occult craniocervical injury. For patients with distractive injuries of the cervical spine, craniocervical dissociations, or fracture-dislocations associated with ankylosing spondylitis, application of a holding device such as a halo is recommended in the urgent setting. These injuries pose the risk of significant neurologic deterioration if undiagnosed or untreated.

Indirect reduction is infrequently performed in the acute setting for the treatment of a thoracolumbar or lumbar injury in the presence of a spinal cord, conus, or cauda equina injury. Some physicians advocate early open reduction and stabilization of thoracolumbar fracture-dislocations with accompanying neural deficits. Keeping in mind that most SCI models show irreversible cord pathophysiology within 6 to 8 hours, advocates of early decompression, realignment, and stabilization stress the importance of acute intervention. Such intervention, however, often is not possible because of ground transportation of patients and hospital referral networks.

Medical Complications of Spinal Cord Injury
Cardiac
The most important postinjury treatment issue is cardiovascular sequelae. These are often subdivided into direct complications resulting from the injury itself (for example, hypotension, bradycardia, and autonomic dysreflexia) after spinal shock has resolved and indirect complications resulting from sequelae of immobilization and the relatively sedentary lifestyle postinjury (for example, deep venous thrombosis [DVT], pulmonary embolism, and coronary artery disease).

Autonomic dysreflexia is characterized by a sudden sympathetic discharge causing an exaggerated increase in blood pressure, often with bradycardia, in response to a noxious stimulus originating below the injury. This syndrome usually occurs in 48% to 85% of patients with SCI above the T6 level. Associated symptoms include headache, mydriasis, piloerection, nasal congestion, flushing, and sweating. The patient can also experience no symptoms at all, with silent blood pressure elevation. The most common cause of autonomic dysreflexia is bladder distention, followed by fecal impaction, pressure ulcers, ingrown toenails, fractures, and abdominal emergencies. Treatment includes putting the patient in a sitting position, removal of precipitating stimuli, and if the cause cannot be found, use of antihypertensive agents (such as nifedipine, nitrates, and angiotensin-converting enzyme inhibitors).

Deep Venous Thrombosis
DVT has been reported in 15% to 80% of SCI patients and usually develops during the first 2 weeks after injury. Residual motor function in the lower extremities and the level of SCI contribute to the overall incidence. The estimated incidence of pulmonary embolism is 2% to 16%. All patients should receive prophylaxis for DVT unless otherwise contraindicated. If prophylaxis is delayed more than 72 hours, tests to exclude the presence of clots should be done. Anticoagulant prophylaxis

with either low-molecular-weight heparin or adjusted dose unfractionated heparin should be initiated, unless contraindicated, within 72 hours of injury. Vena cava filter placement is recommended in SCI patients for whom anticoagulant prophylaxis has failed or who have anticoagulation contraindications. Filters should also be considered for SCI patients with high-level tetraplegia, or for those with thrombosis of the inferior vena cava despite the use of anticoagulants. Anticoagulant prophylaxis should continue for patients who are categorized as motor incomplete on the ASIA impairment scale while they are hospitalized and for 8 to 12 weeks in motor complete patients, depending on risk factors. Patients with chronic SCI remain at increased risk for DVT, and reinstitution of prophylactic measures should be considered for patients with chronic SCI who are immobilized and on bed rest for a prolonged period, or for those who are to undergo surgical procedures.

Pulmonary

Pulmonary complications after SCI remain the leading cause of death in patients with tetraplegia and paraplegia. Pneumonia accounts for 18.9% of deaths in the first year after injury. The problems of pulmonary management can be classified into three main categories: secretion management, atelectasis (and its sequelae), and hypoventilation. At least two of the following treatments should be available to patients: deep pulmonary suctioning, chest physiotherapy, assisted cough methods (for example, quad cough), mechanical insufflation-exsufflation, abdominal binders, frequent position changes, incentive spirometry or resistive devices, and positive pressure ventilation.

Bladder

The bladder is usually affected in one of two ways after injury. A spastic bladder, or upper motor neuron bladder, fills with urine and a reflex automatically triggers the bladder to empty. A flaccid bladder, or lower motor neuron bladder, results when the reflexes of the bladder muscles are slowed or absent. A flaccid bladder can become overdistended or stretched. Although the upper tracts are at risk in both conditions, they are at greater risk in a spastic bladder. Bladder sphincter dyssynergia occurs when the sphincter muscles do not relax when the bladder contracts, which may also place the upper tracts at risk for injury. This may occur with upper motor neuron dysfunction. To treat the neurogenic bladder, SCI patients are placed on a bladder management program, which will allow acceptable bladder emptying with convenience and help to avoid bladder accidents and infection, and long-term upper tract damage secondary to reflux. Common treatment options include clean intermittent catheterization, an indwelling catheter, and for men, an external condom catheter.

Individuals with SCI are at a high risk for urinary tract infection; complications caused by such infections are the most common cause of SCI morbidity. Other complications include bladder and renal calculi, renal failure, and bladder carcinoma. Individuals with SCI should have annual urologic evaluations including functional studies.

Bowel

Similar to the neurogenic bladder, the neurogenic bowel may be either spastic or flaccid. Patients are placed on a bowel program with predictable, regular, timely, and thorough evacuation of the bowels without the occurrence of incontinence or complications. Pharmacologic agents are not always needed for long-term use but can be an effective adjunctive tool to facilitate the bowel program. A common starting routine for patients with a neurogenic bowel includes a stool softener three times daily, a laxative at bedtime, and a suppository in the morning after breakfast. A bowel routine after eating makes use of the gastrocolic reflex. If a patient usually has a bowel movement in the evening, then the laxative can be given at noon and an enema or suppository in the evening after dinner. It is difficult for patients with a true lower motor neuron bowel to achieve continence and a bulk laxative may be needed to limit loose stool formation with diarrhea.

Skin

Pressure ulcers are a daily concern for patients with SCI. It is estimated that up to 80% of individuals with SCI will have a pressure sore during their lifetime, and 30% will have more than one pressure sore. Education in pressure ulcer etiology (including pressure and shear), use of appropriate equipment to help decrease ulcers, and weight shifts, while seated and in bed is necessary. The treatment of pressure sores may include dressings, bed rest, and surgery. All factors that contributed to pressure ulcer development must be eliminated or minimized. Treatment can be very costly in terms of lost wages and additional medical expenses.

Neuromusculoskeletal

After SCI, many changes occur in bone metabolism. An imbalance between bone formation and bone resorption rapidly develops, resulting in bone loss and osteoporosis. Within the first 4 to 6 months, 25% or more of bone mass is lost. By 16 months, bone mass homeostasis is reached with bone mass at 50% to 70% of normal and near the fracture threshold. Fractures are very common in patients with SCI. Data from the Model SCI Systems show that 14% of patients with SCI will have had a fracture within 5 years after injury. This percentage increases to 28% after 10 years, and 39% after 15 years. The frequency of fractures increases with age and completeness of injury, and is higher in women than men. Most fractures are in the lower extremities and result from falls; fractures can also occur with routine activities of daily living and range-of-motion exercises. Treatment of fractures in nonambulatory patients with SCI is somewhat controversial. Circumferential plaster casts or traction can cause skin breakdown, and surgical intervention for femoral shaft and distal femur fractures is associated with a high complication rate because of bone quality, risk of osteomyelitis, and recurrent bacteremia. Surgical intervention may be indicated when nonsurgical management fails to control rotational deformity, if vascular supply is jeopardized, or in proximal femur fractures with severe spasticity. Often fractures are treated with soft splints without bed rest, and a wheelchair is used to provide functional positioning for healing.

Heterotopic ossification is the formation of true bone at ectopic sites and occurs in up to 50% of adults with SCI. Ankylosis occurs in approximately 5% of patients. Most commonly, heterotopic ossification develops between 1 to 4 months after injury and 90% develops around the hip, followed by the knee and elbow. Description of the diagnosis and treatment of this condition can be found in chapter 53.

Spasticity is a common sequelae of upper motor neuron SCI. It may enhance function and maintain muscle bulk, but when poorly controlled, spasticity may lead to impaired function, pain, and decreased quality of life. A full discussion of spasticity is found in chapter 52.

Prognosis After Spinal Cord Injury

Recovery of motor function has been documented for at least 2 years after injury and changes in neurologic status may continue after 2 years. Recovery from SCI depends on the initial strength of the muscles, and most importantly, on whether the injury is complete or incomplete. Vertebral displacement less than 30% and age younger than 30 years at the time of injury are factors associated with improved recovery. No correlation has been found between degree of vertebral wedging, type of fracture, or etiology of injuries. In evaluating changes after SCI, MRI is the best modality to show intramedullary detail such as hematoma and edema. A hemorrhage found with acute MRI correlates with the poorest prognosis, followed by contusion and edema. A normal MRI scan correlates with the best prognosis. Although MRI may augment the physical examination, it alone is not as accurate a predictor of SCI recovery as the physical examination.

Ninety percent of patients with complete tetraplegia will recover one root level of function. The initial strength of the muscle is a significant predictor of achieving antigravity strength and the rate of strength recovery. In patients with no initial motor strength, there is an improved prognosis of recovering antigravity strength the faster the recovery begins. According to the literature, muscles with grade 1 and 2 strength at 30 days have a 97% chance of recovery to 3/5 strength at 1 year. In comparison, in the first muscle below the neurologic level of injury with 0/5 strength at 1 month, only 57% recover to at least 1/5 strength, and only 27% recover to 3/5 or more strength at 1 year. Most upper extremity recovery occurs during the first 6 months, with the greatest rate of change during the first 3 months.

Upper extremity recovery in patients with incomplete tetraplegia is approximately twice as great as for those with complete tetraplegia. For patients who are initially sensory incomplete, the prognosis for motor recovery is much more favorable in those with pinprick sparing than in those in whom light touch sensation alone is spared.

For patients with complete paraplegia, 76% do not show a change in neurologic level of injury from 1 month to 1 year after injury. Even without a change in neurologic level, patients with incomplete paraplegia have the best prognosis for lower extremity and functional recovery. Overall, 80% of patients with incomplete paraplegia regain strength to grade 3 or more in hip flexors and knee extensors at 1 year. The absence of any motor function at 1 month after injury is not an absolute indicator of poor motor recovery.

Most of the recovery after SCI is spontaneous, but it may be enhanced by several factors. Active exercise can promote motor recovery whereas immobilization may impede motor recovery. Using body weight-supported and interactive locomotor training, ambulation recovery may be enhanced in patients with incomplete SCI. Serotonergic and neuroadrenergic drugs may enhance locomotor recovery, whereas drugs with gamma-aminobutyric acid may impede ambulation.

Functional Outcomes
C1 through C4 Tetraplegia
Patients with C1 and C2 lesions may have functional phrenic nerves. In these patients, implanted phrenic nerve pacemakers can be used, and pacing of the diaphragms may be simultaneous or alternating. If secretions are not a problem, tracheostomies may be plugged or discontinued.

Patients with C3 lesions have impaired breathing and are often ventilator-dependent. They can shrug their shoulders and have neck motion, which may permit the operation of specially adapted power wheelchairs and equipment (such as tape recorders, computers, telephones, page turners, automatic door openers, and other environmental control units). Adaptive devices include mouth (sip and puff) and voice activation controls, or chin, head, eyebrow, or eye blink controls. Patients with

C4 lesions may not require respiratory equipment beyond the initial acute care stage, but may have the same functional equipment needs as ventilator-dependent patients.

In addition to powered wheelchairs, patients with C1-C4 tetraplegia require assistance with all personal care, turning, and transfer functions. Headrests, troughs or a lapboard (for the upper extremities), and lifts may be necessary. Bed surfaces with two or more segments that are alternately inflated and deflated may be indicated for patients who do not have assistance for turning. Power recliners allow independent seated weight shifts. Patients with partial C5 function may benefit from adaptive equipment to enable feeding, writing, and typing.

C5 Tetraplegia

Patients with C5 tetraplegia have functional deltoid and/or bicep musculature. They can internally rotate and abduct the shoulder, which causes forearm pronation by gravity. They can externally rotate the shoulder and cause supination and wrist extension and can flex the elbow. C5 tetraplegia patients require assistance to perform bathing and lower body dressing functions, for bowel and bladder care, and for transfers. With the use of adaptive equipment, C5 tetraplegia patients can feed themselves, perform oral facial hygienic and upper body dressing activities, operate some equipment (such as computers, tape recorders, telephones), and participate in leisure activities. They can propel manual wheelchairs short distances on level surfaces. Powered wheelchairs are needed for community distances and outdoor terrain.

C6 Tetraplegia

Patients with C6 tetraplegia have musculature that permits most shoulder motion, elbow bending, and active wrist extension. Tenodesis orthoses support tenodesis training early in recovery. Wrist-driven flexor hinge splints permit pinching strength that is needed for catheterization and work skills. Short opponens orthoses with utensil slots, writing splints, Velcro handles, and cuffs permit feeding, writing, and oral facial hygiene. C6 tetraplegia patients can perform upper body dressing without assistance; may seldom perform lower body dressing without assistance; may seldom catheterize themselves and perform their bowel program with assistive devices; can perform some transfers independently with a transfer board; can turn independently with the use of side rails; and can relieve pressure by leaning forward, alternating sides, or possibly by push-ups. Water mattresses can lower pressure sufficiently to eliminate the need for turning during the night. They can propel a manual wheelchair short distances on level terrain, operate power wheelchairs, and may drive a specialized van.

C7 to C8 Tetraplegia

Patients with C7 tetraplegia have functional triceps, can bend and straighten their elbows, and also may have enhanced finger extension and wrist flexion. As a result, these patients have enhanced grasp strength, which permits enhanced transfer, mobility, and activity skills. They can turn and perform most transfers independently; can propel a manual wheelchair on rough terrain and slopes, and may therefore not need a powered wheelchair; can drive a specialized van; and can perform most daily activities such as cooking and light housework, and therefore may occasionally live independently. They may, however, require assistance for bowel care and bathing. C8 tetraplegia patients have flexor digitorum profundus function, which permits all arm movement, with some hand weakness. They can propel a manual wheelchair for community distances, including in and out of a car and over curbs, and may even become wheelchair independent.

Ambulation After Spinal Cord Injury

Up to 90% of SCI patients who are initially sensory incomplete and motor complete, with preserved pinprick sensation, will have sufficient motor recovery to walk at the time of discharge from rehabilitation. Motor incomplete patients have a better prognosis for ambulation than sensory incomplete patients. Patients who are able to walk in the community have at least fair hip flexor strength bilaterally and fair strength in at least one knee extensor, so that the maximum bracing needed is one long leg and one short leg orthosis. The Waters Ambulatory Motor Index as well as the ASIA Lower Extremity Motor Score have been found to correlate and the determinants between motor power and walking ability still were applicable. The Lower Extremity Motor Score is determined by adding of the muscle grades of the 10 key muscles. All patients with incomplete injuries who have a lower extremity motor score of greater than or equal to 20 at 1 month will progress to ambulation by 1 year postinjury (Table 3).

Tendon Transfer Surgery

The basic principle of upper extremity muscle transfers is to use functioning proximal musculature to control distal parts, with minimal risk of loss of function. Arthrodesis may be performed in conjunction with tendon transfers to stabilize a joint. Wrist fusion is generally contraindicated in patients with tetraplegia because loss of wrist extension interferes with manual wheelchair propulsion and transfers. Upper extremity surgery is usually not performed before the patient has completed the rehabilitation program.

At the C5 level, patients have functional use of the deltoids and elbow flexors. At this level, the most helpful procedures are transfer of the brachioradialis to the

Table 3 | Lower Extremity Motor Score and Ambulation

Lower Extremity Motor Score at 1 Month	Percentage Ambulatory at 1 Year
Incomplete Tetraplegia	
1-9	21
10-19	63
> 20	100
Complete Paraplegia	
1-9	45
Incomplete Paraplegia	
0	33
1-9	70
10-19	100

extensor carpi radialis brevis to restore wrist extension (C6 level) and transfer of the deltoid to the triceps to provide elbow extension (C7 level).

Upper extremity reconstructive surgery, or functional neuromuscular stimulation of the upper extremity, or both surgery and stimulation can improve function at the C6 level. Stimulation can be provided by external, percutaneous, or implanted electrodes, by shoulder motion using an external system, by key and palmar grip and release, or by a bionic glove, an electrical stimulator garment that provides controlled grasp and hand opening.

To restore lateral or key grip in patients without a natural tenodesis, flexor pollicis longus (FPL) tenodesis is surgically created by securing the proximal end of the tendon to the distal radius. To preserve thumb interphalangeal joint flexion, a screw is inserted through the distal tip of the thumb and placed across the interphalangeal joint. When possible, transfer of an active muscle to the FPL will also provide lateral pinch to the finger flexors and will provide better function. To provide finger flexion in the C6 patient, tendon transfer to the flexor digitorum profundus provides grasp and a firm surface for lateral pinch. The flexor carpi radialis, pronator teres, and extensor carpi radialis longus have all been used for lateral pinch and finger flexors.

Patients with C7 tetraplegia lack finger and thumb flexion and intrinsic hand musculature. Transfer of the brachioradialis to the FPL can achieve restoration of thumb flexion. Restoration of finger flexion can be achieved through transfer of the extensor carpi radialis longus, flexor carpi ulnaris, or pronator teres to the flexor digitorum profundus.

Annotated Bibliography

Burns AS, Ditunno JF: Establishing prognosis and maximizing functional outcomes after spinal cord injury: A review of current and future directions in rehabilitation management. *Spine* 2001;26(suppl 24):S137-S145.

This article reviews the medical literature to provide a framework for predicting neurorecovery and functional outcomes after SCI based on injury severity. The authors conclude that within 72 hours to 1 month after SCI, it is possible to predict with reasonable accuracy the magnitude of expected recovery based on physical examination (and use of the ASIA scale). Future directions for improving functional outcomes through the use of novel interventions such as pharmaceutical treatment, functional neuromuscular stimulation, standard protocols to limit secondary injury, and functional training methods (such as body weight support) to maximize activity-dependent neuroplasticity are also addressed.

Fehlings MG, Sekhon LH, Tator C: The role and timing of decompression in acute spinal cord injury: What do we know? What should we do? *Spine* 2001;26(suppl 24): S101-S110.

This article reviews the role of surgical reduction and decompression, particularly early surgery. A review of the current evidence available in the literature suggests that there is no standard of care regarding the role and timing of surgical decompression. The authors conclude that there are insufficient data to support overall treatment standards or guidelines for this topic. The existence of biologic evidence from experimental studies in animals is noted, which shows that early decompression may improve neurologic recovery after SCI; however, it is concluded that the relevant time frame in humans remains unclear.

Hurlbert RJ: The role of steroids in acute spinal cord injury: An evidence-based analysis. *Spine* 2001;26(suppl 24):S39-S46.

This is a literature review of methylprednisolone protocol that attempts to evaluate the role of steroids in nonpenetrating (blunt) SCIs. From an evidence-based approach, the authors conclude that methylprednisolone cannot be recommended for routine use in acute nonpenetrating SCIs and that prolonged administration (48 hours) of high-dose steroids is not without risk and may be harmful to the patient. Until more evidence is forthcoming, methylprednisolone should be considered to have investigational (unproven) status only.

Kirshblum S, Campagnolo D, DeLisa J: *Spinal Cord Medicine*. Philadelphia, PA, Williams and Wilkins, 2002.

This comprehensive resource of SCI medicine encompasses traumatic and nontraumatic disorders affecting the spinal cord. All aspects of the spinal cord including anatomy, epidemiology, classification, treatment and complications for acute SCI, comprehensive rehabilitation topics, and aging with SCI are reviewed. Various nontraumatic disorders of the spinal cord including motor neuron disorders, multiple sclerosis, and postpolio syndrome are also covered.

National Spinal Cord Injury Statistical Center: Spinal Cord Injury: Facts and Figures at a Glance, University of Alabama at Birmingham, Birmingham, AL. Available at: www.spinalcord.uab.edu. Accessed May 2001.

The National Spinal Cord Injury Database has been in existence since 1973 and includes data from an estimated 13% of new SCI patients in the United States. Since its inception, 25 federally funded Model SCI Care Systems have contributed data to the National SCI Database. As of July 2004, the database contained information on 22,992 patients who sustained traumatic SCI.

Papadopoulos SM, Selden NR, Quint DJ, Patel N, Gillespie B, Grube S: Immediate spinal cord decompression for cervical spinal cord injury: Feasibility and outcome. *J Trauma* 2002;52:323-332.

Ninety-one consecutive patients with acute, traumatic cervical SCI (1990-1997) were prospectively studied to determine the effect of immediate surgical spinal cord decompression on neurologic outcome. The authors concluded that immediate spinal column stabilization and spinal cord decompression, based on MRI, may significantly improve neurologic outcomes.

Sekhon LH, Fehlings MG: Epidemiology, demographics, and pathophysiology of acute spinal cord injury. *Spine* 2001;26(suppl 24):S2-S12.

This review examines the epidemiology, demographics, and pathophysiology of acute SCI. The authors also discuss future goals of increasing understanding of both primary and secondary mechanisms of injury, the roles of calcium, free radicals, sodium, excitatory amino acids, vascular mediators, and apoptosis.

Winslow C, Bode RK, Felton D, Chen D, Meyer PR Jr: Impact of respiratory complications on length of stay and hospital costs in acute cervical spine injury. *Chest* 2002;121:1548-1554.

This article attempts to determine if respiratory complications experienced during the initial acute-care hospitalization in patients with acute traumatic cervical spinal injury are more important determinants of the length of stay and total hospital costs than level of injury. A retrospective analysis of an inception cohort (413 patients) for the 5-year period from 1993 to 1997 was performed. The results showed that both mean length of stay and hospital costs increased monotonically with the number of respiratory complications experienced. The authors concluded that the number of respiratory complications experienced during the initial acute-care hospitalization for cervical spine injury is a more important determinant of length of stay and hospital costs than level of injury.

Classic Bibliography

American Spinal Injury Association: *International Standards for Neurological Classification of Spinal Cord Injury, revised 2002.* Chicago, IL, American Spinal Injury Association, 2002.

Barbeau H, Ladouceur M, Norman K, Pepin A, Leroux A: Walking after spinal cord injury: Evaluation, treatment, and functional recovery. *Arch Phys Med Rehabil* 1999;80:225-235.

Bracken MB, Shepard MJ, Collins WF, et al: A randomized, controlled trial of methylprednisolone or naloxone in the treatment of acute spinal cord injury: Results of the Second National Acute Spinal Cord Injury Study. *N Engl J Med* 1990;322:1405-1411.

Bracken MB, Shepard MJ, Collins WR Jr, et al: Methylprednisolone or naloxone treatment after acute spinal cord injury: One-year follow-up data: Results of the second National Acute Spinal Cord Injury Study. *J Neurosurg* 1992;76:23-31.

Bracken MB, Shepard MJ, Holford TR, et al: Administration of methylprednisolone for 24 or 48 hours or tirilazad mesylate for 48 hours in the treatment of acute spinal cord injury: Results of the Third National Acute Spinal Cord Injury Randomized Controlled Trial. National Acute Spinal Cord Injury Study. JAMA 1997;277:1597-1604.

Brunette DD, Rackswold GL: Neurologic recovery following rapid spinal realignment for complete cervical spinal cord injury. *J Trauma* 1987;27:445-447.

Cotler HB, Miller LS, DeLucia FA, Cotler JM, Dayne SH: Closed reduction of cervical spine dislocations. *Clin Orthop* 1987;214:185-199.

Delamarter RB, Sherman JE, Carr JB: Cauda equina syndrome: Neurologic recovery following immediate, early, or late decompression. *Spine* 1991;16:1022-1029.

Dolan EJ, Tator CH, Endrenyi L: The value of decompression for acute experimental spinal cord compression injury. *J Neurosurg* 1980;53:749-755.

Frisbie JH: Fractures after myelopathy. *J Spinal Cord Med* 1997;20:66-69.

Galandiuk S, Raque G, Appel S, Polk HC Jr: The two-edged sword of large-dose steroids for spinal cord trauma. *Ann Surg* 1993;218:419-425.

George ER, Scholten DJ, Buechler CM, Jordan-Tibbs J, Mattice C, Albrecht RM: Failure of methylprednisolone to improve the outcome of spinal cord injuries. *Am Surg* 1995;61:659-663.

Green D: Prevention of thromboembolism after spinal cord injury. *Semin Thromb Hemost* 1991;17:347-350.

Guha A, Tator CH, Endrenyi L, Piper I: Decompression of the spinal cord improves recovery after acute experimental spinal cord compression injury. *Paraplegia* 1987;25:324-339.

Merli GJ, Crabbe S, Doyle L: Mechanical plus pharmacological prophylaxis and deep vein thrombosis in acute spinal cord injury. *Paraplegia* 1992;30:558-562.

Moberg EA: The present state of surgical rehabilitation for the upper limb in tetraplegia. *Paraplegia* 1987;25: 351-356.

Nesathurai S: Steroids and spinal cord injury: Revisiting the NASCIS II and NASCIS III Trials. *J Trauma* 1998; 45:1088-1093.

Parsons KC, Lammerts DP: Rehabilitation in spinal cord disorders: 1. Epidemiology, prevention, and system care of spinal cord disorders. *Arch Phys Med Rehabil* 1991;72(suppl):S293-S294.

Staas WE, Formal CS, Freedman MK, et al: Spinal cord injury and spinal cord injury medicine, in DeLisa JA (ed): *Rehabilitation Medicine Principles and Practice*, ed 3. Philadelphia, PA, Lippincott Raven, 1998, pp 1259-1292.

Stover SL, Fine PR: The epidemiology and economics of spinal cord injury. *Paraplegia* 1987;25:225-228.

Tarlov IM, Klinger H: Spinal cord compression studies: II. Time limits for recovery after acute compression in dogs. *AMA Arch Neurol Psychiatry* 1954;71:271-290.

Tator CH, Duncan EG, Edmond VE, Lapczak LI, Andrews DE: Complications and costs of management of acute spinal cord injury. *Paraplegia* 1993;31:700-714.

Vaccaro AR, An HS, Betz RR: The management of acute spinal trauma: Prehospital and in-hospital emergency care. *Instr Course Lect* 1997;46:113-125.

Vaccaro AR, Daugherty RJ, Sheehan TP, et al: Neurologic outcome of early versus late surgery for cervical spinal cord injury. *Spine* 1997;22:2609-2613.

Waters RL, Adkins RH, Yakura JS: Motor and sensory recovery following complete tetraplegia. *Arch Phys Med Rehabil* 1993;74:242-247.

Chapter 52

Miscellaneous Neurologic Diseases

Guy W. Fried, MD

Multiple Sclerosis

Multiple sclerosis (MS) is an inflammatory demyelinating disease of the central nervous system that causes multiple focal lesions. The focal lesions and their neurologic effects are progressive and difficult to predict. MS is twice as common in women than in men, is diagnosed at an average age of 30 years, and is 10 times more prevalent in northern geographic areas such as the United States and Canada than in Asia and Africa. MS is characterized by recurrent episodes of inflammation of the myelin and it can affect any area in the central nervous system. The inflammation and immune response destroy the myelin, cause plaque formation, and disrupt nerve conduction. The development and progression of MS usually follows a set pattern according to the history of exacerbations and remissions. Patients may suffer exacerbations following physical and emotional stressors; for example, the stress of a surgical procedure. Good prognostic indicators for MS include having no motor findings at the time of presentation, resolution of early flare-ups, an age younger than 30 years at onset, and having limited cerebellar and pyramidal findings after 5 years.

Because of the complexity of its symptoms, the differential diagnosis of MS is broad. MS may appear as a single subtle symptom or as a more significant constellation of symptoms. The differential diagnosis includes central nervous system tumors, cerebrovascular accident, anterior horn cell disease, myasthenia gravis, and collagen vascular diseases, as well as the secondary effects of Lyme disease and human immunodeficiency virus (HIV). Currently, MRI is the most accurate tool to diagnose MS, with positive findings in 72% to 95% of patients. White matter plaques are a characteristic finding. Gadolinium contrast can help distinguish old from new lesions. Lumbar puncture may also be useful because spinal fluid characteristics may show increased gamma globulin in 60% of patients with definite MS. The oligoclonal band may be seen in the gamma globulin region on gel electrophoresis.

Pain and dysesthesias can often be a prominent feature of MS. More than half of the patients with MS have a history of an acute or chronic pain disorder. These symptoms are best treated with anticonvulsant or tricyclic antidepressant medications. When a patient has pain, evaluation for correctable causes such as carpal tunnel syndrome, cervical myelopathy, and mechanical back pain is important.

Spasticity is a velocity-dependent increase in resistance to a passive stretch. Potential complications include reduced joint range of motion and contracture, poor hygiene, predisposition to decubitus, pain, and an impaired ability to use volitional motor power, resulting in functional impairment. Spasticity can be beneficial in some instances. Spasticity of the knee extensors can assist with stability during transfers and ambulation. The Modified Ashworth Scale is a frequently used rating system for spasticity (Table 1).

If spasticity interferes with function, treatment may be considered. Before treatment is initiated, however, an increase in spasticity should be investigated for an underlying cause. Any noxious stimulation such as bladder distension, bowel impaction, or an ingrown toenail may increase a patient's spasticity. The initial treatment for spasticity is usually oral medications such as baclofen, benzodiazepines, tizanidine, and dantrolene sodium; however, these medications can have a sedating effect and may contribute to fatigue. Other treatments include botulinum toxin serotypes A and B, which are given as an intramuscular injection that binds at receptor sites inhibiting the release of acetylcholine. According to a 2001 study, botulinum toxin injections can be quite useful in diminishing focal spasticity, and do not have any cognitive or fatigue-related adverse effects. However, the injections potentially can lead to temporary weakness and the cost per injection can begin at several hundred dollars. Intrathecal baclofen also can be useful in controlling severe lower extremity spasticity. A surgically implanted pump allows precise titration to deliver varying doses of baclofen to correspond with the need for spasticity control throughout the day. The in-

TABLE 1 | Modified Ashworth Scale

Scale	Description
0	No increase in muscle tone
1	Slight increase in muscle tone, manifested as a catch-and-release or by minimal resistance at the end of range of motion
1+	Slight increase in muscle tone, manifested by a catch, followed by minimal resistance throughout the remainder (less than half) of the range of motion
2	More marked increase in muscle tone throughout most of the range of motion, but the affected limb is easily moved
3	Considerable increase in muscle tone; passive range of motion difficult
4	Affected limb is rigid

(Reproduced with permission from Black-Schaefer R: Stroke (Young), in Frontera W, Silver J (eds): Essentials of Physical Medicine. Philadelphia, PA, Hanley and Belfus, 2002, pp 784-792.)

trathecal baclofen may allow the patient to take fewer oral medications and reduce the overall side effect profile.

Orthotic treatment to support ankle and foot positioning as well as supportive management for impaired functional abilities tend to be the primary rehabilitative focus. Orthotic treatment may or may not be necessary because of the variable presentation of MS. The patient's degree of sensation, tone, and muscle strength, especially at the knee and ankle, must be considered. Orthoses are typically made of metal, plastic, or a combination of these materials. The molded plastic ankle-foot orthosis (AFO), which immobilizes the ankle in gait, is the most commonly used. Plastic AFOs are lighter and more easily concealed, which frequently leads to better patient acceptance. Fluctuating edema is better accommodated in a metal orthosis because it does not closely approximate the skin and therefore allows the limb more flexibility. A limb with poor sensation is also better suited to a metal orthosis because it can be manufactured with a soft leather shoe or inner lining to avoid skin breakdown. A metal AFO also can allow more adjustments for ankle joint control.

The location of the spasticity and how well it is controlled may determine the necessity of surgical procedures. The goal of surgical orthopaedic intervention is to improve function and correct deformity. The split anterior tibial tendon transfer procedure is used to reduce excessive inversion of the foot. The tendon of the tibialis anterior is surgically split, allowing a portion to be attached to the cuneiform and cuboid bones to generate an eversion force. MS will also frequently lead to an equinovarus foot, which interferes with ambulation and may require surgery. Knee flexion contractures can also occur with severe spasticity. Orthopaedic hamstring

lengthening procedures followed by postoperative casting can allow better range of motion. Hip flexion contracture can accompany knee flexion contractures. Iliopsoas tenotomy may be useful if standard range-of-motion techniques fail.

Parkinson's Disease

Parkinson's disease is a chronic, degenerative, central nervous system movement disorder characterized by resting tremor and bradykinesia. Dementia may also develop in about 10% to 15% of patients. In Parkinson's disease, the site of pathology is the basal ganglia and extrapyramidal motor system that is responsible for controlling upright posture, muscle tone, coordination, and the initiation of automatic movements in the face and body. There is also a deficiency of dopamine, which allows acetylcholine to become predominant and precipitate tremor. The classic tremor occurs at rest and is abolished by movement; therefore, the disease is not initially disabling. The major motor disability is bradykinesia and akinesia as evidenced by difficulty initiating movements and decreased associated motions. Clinical observation will show a patient having moderate difficulty rising from a chair, often needing to use their arms to push off. The patient will assume a forward-flexed standing posture and will walk with a slow, moderately wide-based gait with short steps. Patients may exhibit a festinating gait, appearing to be falling forward as they start off slowly and then move faster. The patients show poor postural reflexes in which they do not reorient their balance to environmental changes. Cogwheeling, which represents a basal ganglia disorder of tone, is elicited by passive flexion and extension of a muscle, allowing the examiner to feel repetitive stops during range-of-motion testing. Patients with Parkinson's disease may also have a hypokinetic dysarthria, which presents as limited intonation and affect. Deficits in posture, balance, and tone may lead to frozen joints and falls that create most of the injuries (such as fractures) requiring orthopaedic intervention. Postural instability, bradykinesia, and rigidity are the major predictors of falls. Patients with Parkinson's disease can improve their ability to move with exercises emphasizing range of motion, balance, gait, and fine motor dexterity; gains can be lost if regular exercise is stopped. Maintenance exercises are also useful for management of rigidity and bradykinesia.

The mainstay treatment of symptoms of Parkinson's disease is medication. Centrally acting anticholinergic medications can decrease tremors and saliva production. Amantadine potentiates the action of dopamine and may help with akinesia and rigidity. Levodopa has been found to be effective at improving bradykinesia tremor and rigidity when added to carbidopa. The combination of levodopa and carbidopa allows more medication to enter the circulatory system and cross the blood-brain barrier. It has been noted that a low protein diet allows for more consistent results with levodopa. Levodopa has also been noted to improve the hypokinetic dysarthria, allowing for faster and more natural lip movement and thereby improving speech intelligibility.

Peripheral Polyneuropathy

Peripheral polyneuropathy is a common condition in orthopaedic patients. The lower motor neurons of the peripheral nervous system may be damaged in a variety of diseases. Patients often will have abnormal sensation that may be described as dull, prickling, numbing, or the feeling of pins and needles. In addition, autonomic nervous system involvement may produce gastroparesis, postural hypotension, and problems with regulation of heart rate. It is important to start with a detailed history and physical examination evaluating weakness, atrophy, areflexia, and sensory loss. Physical assessment determines whether involvement is in a focal region of the body associated with an entrapment site such as carpal tunnel syndrome or whether it is a diffuse peripheral condition. Electrodiagnostics can provide an added benefit in helping to clarify the nerve disease process. Needle electromyography and nerve conduction velocity studies can help determine whether the neuropathic process is predominantly axonal, demyelinating, or a combination of both. These studies can also determine whether the findings involve primarily motor or sensory nerves, and whether they are symmetric versus multifocal. A careful family history of primary family members can evaluate for inherited neuropathies, which can appear without a readily apparent clinical etiology.

Diabetes is the most common cause of peripheral neuropathy. It affects multiple organ systems, including the peripheral nervous system. The incidence of peripheral neuropathy in diabetic patients depends largely on how it is defined. If it is defined by patient symptoms, about half of the individuals are affected. If electrodiagnostic characteristics are considered, the incidence increases to 90%. Peripheral neuropathy is also associated with end stage renal disease. Studies indicate that at the time dialysis is initiated, as many as 65% of the patients have a peripheral neuropathy; axonal damage is more common than demyelination. The specific etiology is unclear but it appears to be related to toxin buildup because hemodialysis, peritoneal dialysis, and renal transplantation have led to an improvement in symptoms and electrodiagnostic study results. Chronic alcohol ingestion leads to a similar type of peripheral neuropathy affecting the axons and leading to significant demyelination. Abstinence from alcohol may improve symptoms. Pernicious anemia is frequently caused by a deficiency of gastric intrinsic factor leading to a malabsorption of vitamin B_{12} from the ileum. In patients with pernicious anemia, an axonal peripheral neuropathy is common

with dysesthesias. The peripheral neuropathy can be reversible if vitamin B_{12} is given early in the disease process.

Paraproteinemias including multiple myeloma, amyloidosis, lymphoma, Waldenström's macroglobulinemia, chronic lymphocytic leukemia, and nonmalignant gammopathy may also lead to a neuropathy. Frequently this is a diffuse distal symmetrical problem. Multiple myeloma most commonly occurs in patients between 40 and 70 years of age. A distal sensorimotor involvement will present in about 5% of the patients with multiple myeloma. Radicular pain may occur with or without vertebral fractures. Many demyelinating neuropathies with a diffuse symmetric pattern are inherited; for example, Charcot-Marie-Tooth disease that presents with a progressive symmetric distal muscular atrophy.

HIV is commonly associated with peripheral polyneuropathy. Fifty percent of patients with acquired immunodeficiency syndrome show symptoms of a peripheral polyneuropathy. The HIV infection may produce a neuropathy, which is clinically indistinguishable from Guillain-Barré syndrome. The presentation of the demyelinative neuropathy occurs early in the HIV infection and may in fact be the presenting symptom. Guillain-Barré syndrome is the most common disease producing an acute generalized paralysis from an inflammatory demyelinating polyneuropathy. Patients present with distal paresthesias and then a generalized weakness that progresses. Cranial nerve involvement is not uncommon, with the facial nerve being affected in up to one half of the patients. Early mortality in Guillain-Barré syndrome is related to respiratory failure, and up to 30% of patients may require mechanical ventilation. Autonomic nervous system involvement will result in difficulties regulating blood pressure, heart rate, and body temperature as well as bowel and bladder function. Overall, about 16% of patients with Guillain-Barré syndrome will be left with a degree of permanent disability. Electromyogram studies of the amplitude of the compound of motor action potential have a strong predictive value for ambulation. Children have a much greater potential for recovery.

With all the neuropathies a thorough patient history and physical examination followed by a search for reversible causes are critical. Musculoskeletal treatment emphasizes maintaining basic health status by monitoring autonomic functions including blood pressure, temperature, and breathing. Musculoskeletal supports include a conditioning endurance program. Musculoskeletal weakness can be addressed through range-of-motion activities and orthotic devices such as a lightweight plastic AFO to maintain function. Surgical treatment consisting of Achilles tendon lengthening, split anterior tibial tendon transfer, and plantar fascial release may prevent later problems. Before performing surgical procedures, it should be determined whether the underlying process is progressive, such as Charcot-Marie-Tooth disease, whether there are reversible factors as in vitamin B_{12} deficiency, or ominous factors such as HIV infection.

Postpolio Syndrome

Postpolio syndrome occurs in patients with a history of acute polio. It has been estimated that 25% to 60% of the patients who had acute polio may experience latent effects of the disease. The characteristics of postpolio syndrome include musculoskeletal pain, fatigue, new muscle weakness or atrophy, respiratory impairment, cold intolerance, and a decline in the ability to perform activities of daily living. The specific cause of postpolio syndrome is unknown; the etiology has been attributed to pathophysiologic and functional causes. Pathophysiologic causes include chronic poliovirus infection, death of the remaining motor neurons with aging, premature aging, damage to the remaining motor neurons caused by increased demands or secondary insults, and an immune-mediated syndrome. Functional etiologies for postpolio syndrome include greater energy expenditure as a result of weight gain and muscle weakness caused by disuse or overuse.

A mild conditioning program for patients with postpolio syndrome may be beneficial while avoiding any overuse or excessive fatigue that can be detrimental. Most orthopaedic needs are based on joint, muscle, or back pain. Many patients require revision of orthotic devices such as braces, canes, and crutches or new orthotic devices to treat new symptoms. Common issues include genu recurvatum, knee pain, back pain, degenerative arthritis, or arthralgia. Surgery for scoliosis or fractures may also be necessary to treat new conditions.

Annotated Bibliography

Multiple Sclerosis

Frohman EM: Multiple sclerosis. *Med Clin North Am* 2003;87:867-897.

MS is the most common disabling neurologic disease of young people. It affects up to 450,000 people in the United States. Substantial advances have been made in diagnosis and treatment over the past decade. This excellent review article helps in the formation of initial diagnostic and treatment plans.

Jin YP, de Pedro-Cuesta J, Huang YH, Soderstrom M: Predicting multiple sclerosis at optic neuritis onset. *Mult Scler* 2003;9:135-141.

This prospective study examines patients who develop definite MS at the onset of optic neuritis. Correlations made with MRI and oligoclonal bands in cerebrospinal fluid aid in the diagnosis. The study indicated a strong correlation between optic neuritis leading to definite MS in patients with brain and spinal cord lesions.

Joy JE, Johnston RB (eds): *Multiple Sclerosis: Current Status and Strategies for the Future.* Washington, DC, National Academy Press, 2001, pp 29-69.

This review article is an excellent overview that highlights the pathophysiology, diagnosis, prognosis, and treatment of multiple sclerosis.

Keenan MA, Esquenazi A, Mayer NH: The use of laboratory gait analysis for surgical decision making in persons with upper motor neuron syndromes. *Phys Med Rehabil State Art Rev* 2002;16:249-261.

A description of laboratory gait analysis and its use in identifying muscle groups causing spasticity is presented. The use of this information for presurgical planning is discussed.

Rammohan KW: Axonal injury in multiple sclerosis. *Curr Neurol Neurosci Rep* 2003;3:231-237.

The pathophysiology and pathogenesis of MS are discussed. Axonal injury is recognized as an early occurrence in the inflammatory lesions of MS. Neurologic functional impairment correlates best with axonal damage.

Shapiro RT: Pharmacologic options for the management of multiple sclerosis symptoms. *Neurorehabil Neural Repair* 2002;16:223-231.

This article reviews pharmacologic management of MS. Immunomodulatory drugs that control the underlying disease process but do not cure MS are reviewed. The article emphasizes that optimal disease treatment requires a multidisciplinary approach combining medication, rehabilitation, and patient education.

Yablon SA: Botulinum neurotoxin intramuscular chemodenervation: Role in the management of spastic hypertonia and related motor disorders. *Phys Med Rehabil Clin N Am* 2001;12:833-874.

Botulinum neurotoxin intramuscular chemodenervation use is an important therapeutic tool in focal spasticity management. Botulinum toxin injections have been shown to be effective and safe. Techniques, dosage, targeted muscles, and functional goals are discussed in this review article.

Parkinson's Disease

Samii A, Nutt JG, Ransom BR: Parkinson's disease. *Lancet* 2004;363:1783-1793.

Parkinson's disease is the most common serious movement disorder in the world, affecting about 1% of adults older than 60 years. This review article covers diagnosis, treatment, and pathogenesis.

Peripheral Polyneuropathy

Cannon A, Fernandez Castaner M, Conget I, Carreras G, Castell C, Tresserras R: Type 1 diabetes mellitus in Catalonia: Chronic complications and metabolic control ten years after onset. *Med Sci Monit* 2004;10:CR185-CR190.

This review article confirms that diabetic microvascular complications including polyneuropathy and retinopathy were already present 10 years after the onset of diabetes.

Postpolio Syndrome

Jubelt B: Post-polio syndrome. *Curr Treat Options Neurol* 2004;6:87-93.

Postpolio syndrome describes the late manifestations that occur in patients 30 to 40 years after acute poliomyelitis, such as new weakness, muscle pain, joint pain, peripheral nerve compression, fatigue, and cold intolerance. This review article discusses the diagnosis and treatment plan.

Classic Bibliography

Cheng Q, Jiang GX, Press R, et al: Clinical epidemiology of Guillain-Barre syndrome in adults in Sweden in 1996-97: A prospective study. *Eur J Neurol* 2000;7:685-692.

LaBan MM, Martin T, Pechur J, Sarnacki S: Physical and occupational therapy in the in the treatment of patient with multiple sclerosis. *Phys Med Rehabil Clin N Am* 1998;9:603-614.

McDeavitt JT, Graziani V, Kowalske KJ, Hays RM: Neuromuscular disease: Rehabilitation and electrodiagnosis: 2. Nerve disease. *Arch Phys Med Rehabil* 1995;76:S10-S20.

Meythaler JM, DeVivo MJ, Braswell WC: Rehabilitation outcomes of patients who have developed Guillain-Barré syndrome. *Am J Phys Med Rehabil* 1997;76:411-419.

Miller RG, Peterson GW, Daube JR, Albers JW: Prognostic value of electrodiagnosis in Guillain-Barré syndrome. *Muscle Nerve* 1988;11:769-774.

Chapter 53

Traumatic Brain Injury and Stroke

Barbara J. Browne, MD

Jeanne G. Doherty, MD

Epidemiology

Traumatic brain injury is defined as any insult to the brain caused by an external force, causing temporary or permanent impairments in physical function, cognitive ability, and/or disturbance of behavioral and emotional function. These impairments may cause total or partial functional disability and psychosocial maladjustment. Two million brain injuries occur in the United States each year. Approximately 50,000 patients die from acute brain injury.

Leading causes of traumatic brain injury include motor vehicle crashes (50%), falls (21%), gunshot wounds (12%), and recreational injuries (10%). Alcohol is a factor in approximately 60% of injuries across all age groups.

Approximately 750,000 Americans suffer strokes each year; nearly one third of these patients die. Those who survive experience significant levels of disability, with hemiparesis as the most common impairment. Only 10% of stroke survivors experience a full recovery. Another 10% fail to improve. The remaining 80% have varying degrees of neurologic impairment that will improve with rehabilitative intervention.

Mechanism of Injury

There are primary and secondary mechanisms of injury in traumatic brain injury. Primary injury occurs immediately at the time of impact and is associated with acceleration-deceleration and rotational forces. Secondary injury is the neurochemical and physiologic sequelae of the primary brain insult, which occurs over hours to days after the initial injury.

Primary injury includes skull fracture, intracranial hemorrhage, cortical contusion, diffuse axonal injury (a significant injury to the white matter of the brain), and penetrating injury. The two basic types of skull fractures are those of the cranial vault and the basilar skull. Fractures of the occipital condyles also may occur. Intracranial hemorrhages include epidural and subdural hematomas and intracerebral and subarachnoid hemorrhages.

Although skull fractures increase the risk of seizure and intracranial hematoma, there is no correlation between the severity of the skull fracture and the severity of the neurologic injuries. A cranial vault fracture may be linear or stellate, and depressed or nondepressed. A depressed skull fracture initially may be missed secondary to few or no neurologic symptoms. The mortality rate in individuals with a depressed skull fracture is 11%. Approximately 11% of patients with a depressed skull fracture will be left with permanent neurologic deficits. Depressed skull fractures can be further subdivided into simple or closed (15%) and compound or open (85%). A simple fracture is not associated with a laceration. There is no evidence to suggest that surgical elevation of a simple, depressed skull fracture reduces the incidence of seizures or improves neurologic deficits unless there is a skull fragment compressing the cerebral hemisphere. A compound, depressed skull fracture is associated with a scalp laceration. These types of skull fractures should be explored and surgically elevated to reduce the risk of central nervous system infection. A basilar skull fracture increases the risk of meningitis with a dural tear, pneumocephalus, cerebrospinal fluid fistula, and cranial nerve injury.

Secondary injuries include the effects of intracranial pressure, cerebral edema, and hydrocephalus, which may cause cerebral ischemia and hypoxia of brain tissue. They may also include brain herniation syndromes, which can cause significant damage to the brainstem.

The two major mechanisms causing stroke are ischemia (80%) and hemorrhage (20%). These two groups can be further subdivided by location and cause. Ischemic stroke has three main mechanisms: thrombosis, embolism, and systemic hypoperfusion. Each of these mechanisms can result from various underlying pathologic conditions. Hemorrhages are most commonly associated with uncontrolled hypertension, aneurysms, and arteriovenous malformations.

Types of Deficits

Stroke and brain injury can cause mobility and self-care deficits and behavioral, emotional, and cognitive dysfunction. Certain generalizations regarding types of deficits can be made based on the anatomic location of injury in the brain. Injuries involving the cerebral hemispheres can result in contralateral paralysis, sensory changes, and visual field losses. Paralysis of the arm tends to be more pronounced with middle cerebral artery lesions, whereas lower limb weakness is most pronounced with anterior cerebral artery lesions. Frontal lobe injury often causes impairments of insight, judgment, logical reasoning, problem solving, memory, and higher level executive functioning. It may also cause apathy, withdrawal from social interaction, emotional swings, impulsiveness, and confabulation. Parietal lobe injuries often cause agnosia (inability to recognize sensory stimuli), apraxia (inability to perform purposeful movement despite adequate motor ability), aphasia, visual-spatial disorders, and hemispatial neglect. Injury to the dominant hemisphere can cause language and speech disorders. Nondominant hemispheric injury may cause deficits such as anosognosia (loss of awareness of one's own deficits) and constructional apraxia (inability to reproduce drawings or assemble and build structures despite adequate motor ability). Emotional dysfunction such as depression and indifference may occur. Temporal lobe injury may cause disturbances in behavior, memory, and cognition. Dominant hemisphere injury may cause fluent aphasia, alexia, and agraphia (inability to express thoughts in writing). Anxiety, depression, rage, and fear also may occur. Occipital lobe injury may cause visual impairment or occipital blindness (acting sighted despite blindness). Brainstem stroke generally spares cognitive and language function but often shows diverse symptoms. Impairments can involve both ipsilateral and contralateral functions, cranial nerve dysfunction, ataxia, vertigo, and dysphagia.

In the early period after a stroke, the affected limbs are often flaccid with an absence of deep tendon reflexes. Over several weeks, a progression from flaccidity to spasticity to normal tone may occur. Motor return frequently begins as a synergistic contraction of multiple limb muscles rather than isolated action. Flexor activity predominates in the upper limb. A common pattern is scapular retraction and depression, shoulder adduction with internal rotation, forearm pronation, and flexion at the elbow, wrist, and fingers. Extensor overactivity is predominant in the lower limb with adduction and internal rotation at the hip, extension at the knee, and plantar flexion at the ankle with supination at the foot. The entire recovery process is variable and may halt at any stage. Early motor recovery is usually seen in proximal muscles before distal or isolated muscle movement. Maximal neurologic and functional recovery has been shown to occur within 12 weeks for most patients undergoing standard inpatient rehabilitation.

Complications

Spasticity

Spasticity is discussed in detail in chapter 52.

Contractures

A contracture is defined as a fixed loss of passive joint range of motion (ROM) secondary to pathology of connective tissue, tendons, ligaments, muscles, joint capsule, and/or cartilage. Contractures occur in up to 84% of patients and can be classified as arthrogenic, soft-tissue, or myogenic. Arthrogenic contractures are caused by pathology of the intrinsic joint components, and cause restriction of ROM in all planes. Soft-tissue contractures result in shortening of tendons, ligaments, and skin, causing restriction of movement in one plane. Myogenic contractures can be further classified as intrinsic or extrinsic. Intrinsic myogenic contractures are caused by a primary disorder of muscle fibers, such as muscular dystrophy. In extrinsic myogenic contractures the muscle itself is histologically normal. Such contractures are secondary to muscles being placed in a shortened position for extended periods of time such as occurs in brain injury. Factors that contribute to the occurrence of contractures include spasticity, immobility, prolonged bed rest, weakness, improper positioning, pain, and heterotopic ossification (HO). Muscles such as the iliopsoas, gastrocnemius, hamstrings, biceps, and tensor fascia lata that cross two joints are at greatest risk of contracture. Common locations in the lower extremity for contractures include ankle plantar flexors, hip flexors, and knee flexors. Common locations for contractures in the upper extremity are elbow flexors/supinators and shoulder adductors/internal rotators.

The most important aspect of treatment of contractures is prevention. Early mobilization, daily ROM exercises, stretching, and the use of splints and orthotic devices are essential for preventing contractures. Proper positioning in bed and the wheelchair must also be addressed. To avoid knee and hip flexion contractures in bed, pillows should not be placed under the knees, and lying in the prone position also can be helpful. To avoid extreme shoulder adduction and internal rotation, pillows should be placed to keep the shoulder in a partially abducted and externally rotated position. Elbows should not be positioned in flexion and supination. Resting night splints and bivalved casting can be used as a preventive measure. Ankle plantar flexion contractures are common but preventable. In bed, the use of ankle-foot orthoses ideally placed at 90° can help to prevent these contractures. In addition, there are many wheelchair modifications that can be used to alter a patient's position and assist in preventing contractures. To encourage normal lordosis of the lumbar spine and kyphosis of the thoracic spine, the pelvis should be placed in a slightly anterior tilted position. Armrests and lapboards are used to prevent shoulder contractures. Reclining the back support 10° and placing lateral trunk supports assists in trunk stabilization and proper alignment. Extensions or hip blocks placed laterally keep the pelvis in a symmetrical position and align the lower extremities. Leg straps prevent adduction of the lower extremities. Footrest height can be adjusted to properly position the ankle, knee, and hip. Despite all efforts to prevent contractures they may still develop. If so, treatment measures should be initiated immediately. Treatment includes physical, medical, and surgical intervention. A significant aspect of physical intervention is an aggressive stretching program with sustained stretching techniques. To correctly stretch a joint, it is positioned at the limit of ROM and sustained in that position. Caution should be used with patients who have significant osteoporosis so that fractures are avoided. Before stretching, the use of therapeutic heat including ultrasound can be very beneficial. Patients with impaired sensation should be monitored closely. Serial casting applied to a prestretched limb is a common treatment method for joint contracture. The joint is held at its initial limit of ROM. Casts are periodically removed and new casts placed after increasing joint ROM by 5° to 10°, the new limit of ROM. The skin must be monitored for breakdown. Dynamic splints, which have movable parts to counter contracting forces, are an alternative to serial casting. Medical treatment includes maximizing treatment of spasticity and pain with modalities and medication (see chapter 52). Surgical intervention is reserved for patients who are refractory to conservative treatment. Options include joint manipulation, tendon release, tendon lengthening, and joint capsule release. Complications that can occur following tendon lengthening include reduction of muscle strength and altered ROM. There is also a tendency for tendon shortening to recur. Postoperative therapy is a key component to ensure the most favorable outcome.

Skin Conditions

Skin breakdown and pressure ulcers are preventable complications following traumatic brain injury and stroke. Risk factors include impaired cognition, decreased mobility in bed, diaphoresis, incontinence, infection, diabetes, malnutrition, anemia, muscle atrophy, and impaired sensation. Spasticity and joint contractures are significant contributing factors. The common mechanisms for skin involvement include pressure, shear, maceration, and friction. Preventive treatment includes proper positioning, timely turning in bed, weight shifts in the wheelchair, minimizing excessive perspiration and urinary and fecal incontinence, proper transfer techniques, adequate nutrition, treatment of medical conditions such as diabetes and anemia, and appropriate treatment of spasticity and joint contractures.

Shoulder Pain

Up to 85% of people with hemiplegia experience shoulder pain. Shoulder spasticity and subluxation are among the most frequent causes of pain. Additional factors include adhesive capsulitis, impingement syndrome with rotator cuff injury, complex regional pain syndrome type 1 (CRPS 1), and brachial plexopathy. Effective treatments to reduce spasticity-related muscle imbalance include electromyogram biofeedback with relaxation exercises, botulinum toxin, and phenol blocks. Shoulder subluxation has been implicated as a contributing factor in pain, limited ROM, and function. The use of arm slings can reduce pain and subluxation in some patients and may also improve gait stability by limiting detrimental displacement of the body's center of gravity seen in the hemiparetic gait. However, sling use can also result in increased flexor tone that may lead to contracture formation, and may promote disuse of the extremity. Wheelchair lap trays or arm boards provide support but may also overcorrect the subluxation and lead to impingement syndromes. Corticosteroid injections can be an effective treatment for adhesive capsulitis. Other useful adjuncts include transcutaneous electrical nerve stimulation to reduce subluxation and pain. Current trials of percutaneous intramuscular stimulation show promise for enhanced efficacy. Pain that is thought to originate centrally or related to CRPS 1 may respond to gabapentin, tricyclic antidepressants, oral steroids, or stellate ganglion blocks.

Systemic Complications

Dysphagia resulting in aspiration pneumonia occurs in 20% of stroke survivors and up to 45% of traumatic brain injury survivors. A video fluoroscopic swallow study provides additional sensitivity and identifies most cases of dysphagia with aspiration. Factors that increase the risk of aspiration pneumonia include nasogastric feeding, tracheostomy, lethargy, emesis, and reflux. Specialized diets often involve thickened liquids with soft or pureed solids. Patients believed to be at high risk for aspiration should have enteral feedings. A gastrostomy or jejunostomy tube is inserted if prolonged enteral feeding is anticipated. Malnutrition is a possible complication of dysphagia.

Urinary dysfunction is often seen following stroke and brain injury. Complications include urinary tract infection, neurogenic bladder, and less frequently, nephrolithiasis and urethral stricture.

Esophagitis, gastritis, ulcers, gastrointestinal hemorrhage, pancreatitis, diarrhea, and constipation may also develop. An abnormal liver function test result is a common finding after brain injury. It may be drug induced or related to trauma and often is influenced by some premorbid factor.

TABLE 1 | Brooker Classification Scale for Heterotopic Ossification of the Hip

Class	Description
I	Islands of bone with soft tissue
II	Bone spurs from the pelvis or proximal femur, leaving at least 1 cm between bone surfaces
III	Bone spurs from the pelvis or proximal femur, reducing the space between opposing surfaces to less than 1 cm
IV	Bone ankylosis of the hip

(Reproduced with permission from Blount PJ, Bockenek WL: Heterotopic ossification, in Frontera W, Silver J (eds): Essentials of Physical Medicine. Philadelphia, PA, Hanley and Belfus, 2002, pp 569-574.)

Atelectasis, pneumonia, deep venous thrombosis (DVT), pulmonary embolism, and pneumothorax are possible complications after stroke and traumatic brain injury. The more severely affected patients will require ventilator support and many will require a tracheostomy. Cardiovascular complications include hypertension, arrhythmias, cardiomyopathy, myocardial infarction, and endocarditis.

DVT has been reported in up to 70% of unprotected stroke patients and in approximately 20% of patients after traumatic brain injury. Risk factors include bed rest, hemiplegia, flaccidity, older age, obesity, history of malignancy, and previous thrombosis. An additional risk factor in the posttraumatic brain-injured population is lower extremity fracture. The risk of DVT appears lowest in patients capable of ambulating a distance of more than 100 feet. Differential diagnosis includes cellulites, fracture, tumor, CRPS, and HO. A full discussion of treatment of DVT is found in chapter 51, Spinal Cord Injury.

Seizure Disorder

A seizure occurs in 5% to 25% of stroke survivors. The highest rates follow hemorrhagic, cortical, and embolic strokes. Seizure disorder following traumatic brain injury occurs in 1.5% of patients with mild injuries, 2.9% with moderate injuries, and 17% of those with severe injuries. These posttraumatic seizures can be classified as immediate (occurring within hours of the injury), early (first detected within the first week of injury), and late (occurring more than 1 week after injury). It is estimated that 12% to 15% of new onset seizures following a traumatic brain injury occur 10 to 30 years after the acute injury. Risk factors for posttraumatic seizures include depressed skull fractures, prolonged posttraumatic amnesia, missile injuries with penetration and retained metal fragments, loss of consciousness for more than 24 hours, focal neurologic signs on initial examination, intracerebral hemorrhage, diffuse brain contusion, cortical injury with subcortical extension, advanced age, and rec-

reational drug use. Previously there has been controversy over the need for prophylactic treatment of posttraumatic seizures. It has been shown that prophylactic treatment is not indicated for more than 1 week after traumatic brain injury unless there is documented seizure activity following injury, a history of seizure disorder, or multiple risk factors. A seizure occurring 2 weeks or more after stroke probably represents scar formation and is usually treated with long-term prophylaxis.

Heterotopic Ossification

HO is a musculoskeletal complication that may occur following traumatic brain injury and less frequently after stroke. HO is described as new bone formation in nonskeletal tissue, located periarticularly. HO is not specific to traumatic brain injury and stroke; it also can develop following a spinal cord injury, burn, fracture, total joint arthroplasty, or trauma to muscle or joints. HO is defined as neurogenic when it occurs secondary to traumatic brain, stroke, or spinal cord injury. The reported incidence of HO after traumatic brain injury varies depending on the study and ranges from 11% to 75%. There is an increased incidence to 76% in patients with severe traumatic brain injury. Approximately 20% to 30% of patients have clinically significant loss of ROM from HO and 10% to 15% have complete ankylosis. The Brooker classification system has been used to describe HO of the hip (Table 1).

Risk factors for developing HO subsequent to traumatic brain injury include the presence of fractures, especially those of the long bones; prolonged coma (more than 2 weeks); spasticity; and decreased ROM. HO usually develops within 1 to 6 months of injury but it may develop as early as 2 weeks or as late as 12 months after injury. The clinical presentation of HO is variable. Most commonly it presents initially as decreased joint ROM or increased spasticity. A patient may also present with a low-grade fever, erythema, pain, swelling, or tenderness. Less frequently HO may present with a nerve compression, vascular compression, or lymphedema. It is most frequently found at the hips, then the shoulders and elbows, then the knees. In the hip, HO can form inferomedially, anterolaterally, or posteriorly. In the knee it is usually found anteromedially, in the shoulder it usually forms inferomedially, and in the elbow it forms along the medial collateral ligament. Alternative diagnoses include DVT, cellulitis, CRPS, septic joint, hematoma, or tumor. The gold standard for diagnosing HO is the three-phase radionuclide bone scan. Phase I and II of the bone scan can detect the condition as early as 2 to 3 weeks after the onset and phase III may be positive in 4 to 8 weeks. The bone scan usually normalizes 7 to 12 months from the time of initial diagnosis. Although its sensitivity is high, the disadvantage of using the bone scan for diagnosing HO is its lack of specificity. Serum alkaline phosphatase is another test used in the diagnosis of HO, with elevated levels associated with clinically significant HO. Normal levels range from 38 to 126 IU. Serum alkaline phosphatase levels begin rising to the upper limits of normal within the first 2 weeks and may begin to exceed normal values within the first 3 weeks from the initial onset of HO; peak levels are reached at approximately 10 weeks and elevation may persist for up to 6 months. Serum alkaline phosphatase levels parallel the clinical course of HO. Elevated serum alkaline phosphatase levels also are not specific. Levels may be elevated in clinical findings such as hepatic dysfunction or fractures. If there is a suspicion of HO based on elevated serum alkaline phosphatase levels, a three-phase bone scan should be performed for confirmation.

Treatment of HO includes physical therapy, medication, and surgical intervention. Physical therapy includes early aggressive ROM exercises, stretching, and joint mobilization. There is no evidence to suggest that this intervention increases the formation of HO because of an inflammatory response. At times, manipulation under anesthesia is necessary for active ROM of a joint that has not responded to conservative physical therapy. Medication options for treatment of HO include etidronate disodium and nonsteroidal anti-inflammatory drugs (NSAIDs). Etidronate disodium is a biphosphonate that limits ossification by blocking the formation of hydroxyapatite crystals. The prophylactic oral dose is 20 mg/kg/day for 2 weeks, then 10 mg/kg/day for 10 weeks. The treatment oral dose is 20 mg/kg/day for 6 months or 20 mg/kg/day for 3 months, then 10 mg/kg/day for 3 months. Adverse effects of etidronate disodium include nausea, vomiting, diarrhea, and abdominal discomfort; it can also contribute to osteoporosis and impaired fracture healing. NSAIDs reduce bone formation by inhibiting prostaglandin synthetase. They have been shown to be effective in preventing HO following total hip arthroplasty and HO resection. Indomethacin is the NSAID most often used for treatment. NSAIDs have not been proven specifically to decrease the incidence of neurogenic HO.

Indications for surgical intervention for HO include impaired positioning, which causes difficulty with sitting, lying, hygiene, ambulation, and activities of daily living; and ankylosed joints, which cause skin breakdown, profound pain, and progressive nerve compression. Some studies have indicated that patients with good neuromuscular control in general have the best postoperative functional outcome. Those with a poor neurologic recovery and persistent spasticity have a higher incidence of recurrence and less functional improvement in the limb. The surgery may be a wedge or complete resection. It is essential to defer the surgery until the bone formation is mature, at least 18 to 24 months from the initial diagnosis, to limit excessive bleeding. Cautious dissection, ade-

quate hemostasis, neurovascular bundle isolation, and adequate bone mass exposure are other measures to reduce morbidity. Postoperative complications include hemorrhage, sepsis, and recurrence of HO. Postoperative prophylaxis to prevent recurrence includes medications such as etidronate disodium or NSAIDs. Also, low dose radiation of 600 to 750 rads may be an option. There have been some studies exploring the use of a postoperative continuous passive ROM machine. Therapy for ROM begins when pain and swelling have subsided, usually 10 to 14 days postoperatively.

Fractures

There are certain complications such as fractures and nerve injuries that occur specifically after traumatic brain injury. Fractures occur in approximately 34% of patients; 11% are estimated to be occult fractures. Common types include those of the pelvis, hip, knee, shoulder, and cervical spine fractures and dislocations. Screening diagnostic studies including radiographs of the cervical and thoracic spine, pelvis, hips, and long bones should be obtained in comatose patients, especially those with high velocity injuries. Bone scan should also be considered as a screening study. Treatment of these fractures should include early fixation because of the strong possibility that these patients may eventually become agitated and confused. Delayed treatment of these fractures may become more difficult because of the increased risk for the development of hypertonicity and spasticity. Early stabilization is associated with fewer pulmonary complications, decreased use of pain medications, fewer joint contractures, decreased mortality, and shortened hospital stays. It also allows for earlier mobilization and thus facilitates earlier rehabilitation.

Nerve Injury

Peripheral nerve injuries occur in approximately 34% of patients with severe traumatic brain injuries; 11% are occult injuries. Causes include direct trauma, improper positioning, postoperative complications, and HO. Cranial nerve injuries may also occur and are associated with the direct trauma.

Assessment

There are multiple assessment tools used to measure both severity of brain injury and function after injury. The Glasgow Coma Scale is the gold standard for measuring severity of injury in the acute stage. One score totaling from 3 to 15 is obtained based upon eye opening, verbal response, and best motor response (Table 2). Injury is classified as severe if the score is 3 to 8, moderate from 9 to 12, and mild from 13 to 15. Loss of consciousness for more than 6 hours is indicative of a severe injury. Posttraumatic amnesia is memory loss following in-

TABLE 2 | Glasgow Coma Scale

Scale	Eye Opening	Verbal Response	Motor Response
6			Obeys commands
5		Oriented	Localizes to pain
4	Spontaneous	Confused	Withdraws from pain
3	To speech	Inappropriate	Flexor posturing
2	To pain	Incomprehensible	Extensor posturing
1	No response	No response	No response

(Reproduced with permission from Burke DT: Traumatic brain injury, in Frontera W, Silver J (eds): Essentials of Physical Medicine. Philadelphia, PA, Hanley and Belfus, 2002, pp 806-812.)

jury. A brain injury is mild if it lasts less than 1 hour after initial injury and severe if it persists for more than 24 hours.

Outcome Measures

Although there are a variety of assessment tools used in patients with brain injury, many do not have outcome predictive value. Among the tools used to predict outcome are the Glasgow Outcome Scale, Disability Rating Scale, Functional Independence Measures, Functional Assessment Measures, and Galveston Orientation Assessment Test.

Several general characteristics can predict a good outcome in the brain-injured patient: limited trauma, posttraumatic amnesia for less than 4 weeks, loss of consciousness for less than 2 weeks, Glasgow Coma Scale score greater than 5, age younger than 60 years, strong support system, more highly educated, and premorbid higher intelligence. A poorer outcome is predicted with recurrent injury, a mass lesion, anoxia, elevated intracranial pressure, hypotension, history of alcohol or drug use, premorbid disability, violent etiology, poor work history, and premorbid psychiatric history.

Rehabilitative Intervention

Effective rehabilitation of the multiple impairments arising from stroke and brain injury requires a team approach. Traditional team members include a physician, nurse, psychologist, and physical, occupational, speech, and recreational therapists. Experienced case management is crucial for overall coordination, communication, and successful discharge. Any restrictions such as weight bearing or ROM must be identified before beginning rehabilitation. Conventional approaches include ROM exercises, mobilization activities, and teaching compensatory skills. Newer promising treatments of stroke and brain injury are focused on central nervous system recovery using periods of intensive active motor training. Theoretical explanations for success of these newer treatments include avoiding learned nonuse of the affected side and brain reorganization. Other promising treatments include treadmill gait training with body-weight support, which can promote balance and gait efficiency, and neuromuscular electrical stimulation.

Annotated Bibliography

Epidemiology

Petrilli S, Durufle A, Nicolas B, Pinel JF, Kerdoncuff V, Gallien P: Prognostic factors in the recovery of the ability to walk after stroke. *J Stroke Cerebrovasc Dis* 2002; 11:330-335.

This article presents a prospective study of 93 stroke patients; factors predictive of future ambulation are identified.

Complications

Blount PJ, Bockenek WL: Heterotopic ossification, in Frontera W, Silver J (eds): *Essentials of Physical Medicine*. Philadelphia, PA, Hanley and Belfus, 2002, pp 569-574.

A comprehensive description of HO including definition, diagnosis, and treatment is presented in this chapter.

Brashear A, Gordon MF, Elovic E, et al: Intramuscular injection of botulinum toxin for the treatment of wrist and finger spasticity after a stroke. *N Engl J Med* 2002; 347:395-400.

This article discusses a randomized, blinded, and controlled study that demonstrates the effectiveness of botulinum toxin to reduce spasticity and improve ROM.

Farmer SE, James M: Contractures in orthopedic and neurological conditions: A review of causes and treatment. *Disabil Rehabil* 2001;23:549-558.

This article reviews the scientific literature from 1966 to 2000 on the development and treatment of contractures in neurologic and orthopaedic conditions. Information is presented on predisposing factors, muscle physiology, and the effectiveness of various treatment modalities for contractures.

Gardner MJ, Ong BC, Liporace F, Koval KJ: Orthopedic issues after cerebrovascular accident. *Am J Orthop* 2002;31:559-568.

A review of the most common orthopaedic problems and deformities experienced after stroke is presented. Muscle spasticity, contractures, and HO are discussed along with methods of prevention and surgical intervention.

Melamed E, Robinson D, Halperin N, Wallach N, Keren O, Groswasser Z: Brain injury-related heterotopic bone formation: Treatment strategy and results. *Am J Phys Med Rehabil* 2002;81:670-674.

In this study, the results of 12 excisions of HO in 9 patients were assessed. Functional improvement was noted in all patients 1 year after intervention. There was no evidence of recurrence. Recommendations were made regarding indications for excision of HO.

Assessment

Burke DT: Traumatic brain injury, in Frontera W, Silver J (eds): *Essentials of Physical Medicine*, Philadelphia, PA, Hanley and Belfus, 2002, pp 806-812.

This chapter presents an overview of a number of functional assessment tools used for patients with posttraumatic brain injury.

Rehabilitative Intervention

Chae J: Neuromuscular electrical stimulation for motor relearning in hemiparesis. *Phys Med Rehabil Clin N Am* 2003;14:S93-S109.

This article examines the types of neuromuscular electrical stimulation technologies being used and their clinical usefulness in aiding upper limb functional recovery after hemiparesis.

Hesse S, Werner C, Frankenberg S, Bardeleben A: Treadmill training with partial body weight support after stroke. *Phys Med Rehabil Clin N Am* 2003;14:S111-S123.

This article explores treadmill training with body-weight support as a means to enhance gait recovery after stroke. Technical aspects of using a treadmill gait-trainer are covered.

Snels IA, Dekker JH, van der Lee JH, Lankhorst GJ, Beckerman H, Bouter LM: Treating patients with hemiplegic shoulder pain. *Am J Phys Med Rehabil* 2002;81:150-160.

A literature review of 14 studies is presented, exploring the causes and treatment of hemiplegic patients with shoulder pain.

Taub E, Uswatte G, Morris DM: Improved motor recovery after stroke and massive cortical reorganization following Constraint-Induced Movement therapy. *Phys Med Rehabil Clin N Am* 2003;14(suppl 1):S77-S91.

This article reviews newer theories on brain plasticity and the effects of learned nonuse. The potential for greater motor recovery in both acute and chronic hemiparesis using more intense periods of active use of paretic limbs is explored. Potential efficacy with other impairments such as dystonia, aphasia, and phantom pain are addressed.

Yu D, Chae J: Neuromuscular stimulation for treating shoulder dysfunction in hemiplegia. *Crit Rev Phys Med Rehabil* 2002;14:1-23.

A review of several randomized controlled trials of neuromuscular stimulation to treat shoulder subluxation and pain in hemiplegic patients is presented. Potential causes of shoulder pain are reviewed.

Classic Bibliography

Bonyke C, Boake C: Principles of brain injury rehabilitation, in Braddom R, Buschbacher R, Dumitru D, et al (eds): *Physical Medicine and Rehabilitation*. Philadelphia, PA, WB Saunders, 1996, pp 1027-1052.

Garland DE: A clinical perspective on common forms of acquired heterotopic ossification. *Clin Orthop* 1991;263:13-29.

Garland D, Keenan MA: Orthopedic strategies in the management of the adult head injured patient. *Phys Ther* 1983;63:2004-2009.

Garland DE, Rhoades ME: Orthopedic management of brain-injured adults: Part II. *Clin Orthop* 1978;131:111-122.

Ippolito E, Formisano R, Farsetti P, Caterini R, Penta F: Excision for the treatment of periarticular ossification of the knee in patients who have a traumatic brain injury. *J Bone Joint Surg Am* 1999;81:783-789.

Langhorne P, Stott DJ, Robertson L, et al: Medical complications after stroke: A multicenter study. *Stroke* 2000;31:1223-1229.

Woo BH, Nesathural S (eds): *The Rehabilitation of People With Traumatic Brain Injury*. Boston, MA, Blackwell Science Inc, 2000, pp 13-17, 35-43, 95-99.

Chapter 54

Limb Amputation and Prosthetic Rehabilitation

Michael C. Munin, MD

Gary F. Galang, MD

Incidence and Etiology

The most recent (1993) National Health and Human Services data show that there are about 1.5 million amputees in the United States, with 50,000 new amputations occurring each year. About 5% of amputations are tumor related, 15% result from trauma, and the remaining approximately 80% are vascular in etiology, with diabetes-related ischemic vascular disease as the major cause. In the United States there was a 27% increase in the overall rate of dysvascular amputations from 1988 to 1996, with a large part of the increase occurring in geriatric and minority populations. Traumatic and cancer-related amputations decreased by one half within the same period. The average age for patients with amputation resulting from vascular etiologies is between age 51 to 69 years, whereas the average patient age for trauma-related amputations is 21 to 30 years. The overall male to female ratio is approximately 2:1.

Most adult limb amputations occur in the lower extremity (80%); partial foot amputations comprise 50% and transtibial and transfemoral amputations about 25% each. Upper extremity amputations account for the remaining 20% of all amputations, with most resulting from work-related injuries involving the dominant arm in healthy younger patients. The most common upper limb amputations are at the transradial level (57%), followed by transhumeral amputations (23%).

Congenital abnormalities are the most common cause of limb deficiencies for patients younger than age 10 years. Causes of congenital amputation include intrapartum exposure to drugs and radiation (10%) and genetic deficits (20%); the etiology of the remaining 70% is unknown. Congenital upper limb absence is usually seen at the level of the transverse upper third of the left radius.

Limb salvage or reconstruction has recently become an increasingly viable alternative to amputation for patients with a traumatic or oncologic etiology. A recent multicenter study comparing surgical reconstruction with limb amputation after major trauma (type IIIB, IIIC tibial fractures) reported that the outcomes for patients who underwent reconstruction were not significantly different from those who underwent amputation. However, reconstruction was associated with a higher risk of complications, additional surgeries, and rehospitalization.

Surgical Technique and Functional Outcomes
Bone

In general, ambulation and prosthetic control are optimized with the preservation of the knee joint and maintenance of a longer residual bone length, which provides better pressure distribution that minimizes skin breakdown with prosthetic wear. A longer residual bone length also provides a longer torque arm, improving control and decreasing the metabolic demands of prosthetic ambulation. In geriatric dysvascular amputees, 90% of transtibial amputees will successfully use a prosthesis compared with 25% or fewer of transfemoral amputees. Postoperative surgical wound healing is relatively higher at the transfemoral level (70% to 98%) compared with the transtibial level (30% to 90%) in dysvascular patients. This finding suggests that the transfemoral level may be more suitable for geriatric patients with fewer activity demands. Younger patients can have excellent outcomes at the transfemoral level with appropriate prosthetic prescriptions and training.

At the transtibial level, the ideal surgical margin is at the musculocutaneous junction of the gastrocnemius muscle. Longer bone lengths provide less soft-tissue padding and poorer blood supply for the myocutaneous flap. Furthermore, because of the height requirements of the foot and ankle assembly, longer bone lengths may preclude the addition of important components such as a vertical shock pylon and rotator unit. The recommended transtibial residual limb length is 12.5 cm to 17.5 cm or approximately 2.5 cm of bone length per 30 cm of body height. A residual limb length that measures 33% to 50% of the intact tibial length from the medial tibial plateau to the medial malleolus is also recommended. In transfemoral amputations, a 5-cm stump length measured from the greater trochanter is fitted as a hip disarticulation. A transfemoral residual bone length between 50% to 75% of the intact femur measured from the greater trochanter to the lateral femoral condyle is considered optimal.

Beveling the cut cortical bone at the site of amputation is recommended regardless of surgical level. Ideally, a 45° angle may prevent pressure on the anterior skin flap. In transtibial amputations, sectioning the fibula 1.2 cm shorter than the tibia is also recommended. Complete removal of the fibula and adjacent muscle bulk was previously performed for short residual limbs; however, this practice is not currently recommended because retention of the fibular head is important for anchoring the total contact socket within the residual limb.

Soft Tissue

Adequate padding and coverage to the distal bone is achieved by muscle stabilization techniques and skin flaps with the goal of attaining a muscular, cylindrical, residual limb to provide ideal prosthetic fitting. Muscle stabilization through myoplasty and tension myodesis not only provides more soft-tissue coverage but also acts as a replacement insertion that facilitates muscle contraction and movement. In tension myodesis, transected muscle groups are sutured to bone under physiologic tension. In myoplasty, the muscle is sutured into soft-tissue fascia or opposing muscle groups. In younger more active patients who need firmer stabilization, a myodesis is preferred. In transfemoral amputations, it has been reported that the absence of adductor magnus myodesis results in a loss of 70% of hip adduction power. Furthermore, myodesis prevents the anterolateral drift of the distal femur caused by muscular imbalance from the hip abductors that are unaffected by the transfemoral amputation. Both procedures are relatively contraindicated in ischemic limbs because they may further compromise the already marginal blood supply.

The type of skin and soft-tissue flaps are determined by the vascular supply of the distal limb. In transtibial amputations, blood supply in the posterior and medial aspects of the leg is more abundant than in the anterolateral region. In ischemic limbs, a long posterior myocutaneous flap and a short or even absent anterior flap is recommended. A posterior flap that measures 1 cm more than the diameter of the leg at the level of the bone division is recommended. To preserve all intact vascular connections between muscle and skin, dissection along tissue planes is avoided and myocutaneous flaps are used. Occasionally, to provide more coverage, a vascular graft can be taken from the other leg.

The fish mouth or guillotine transtibial amputation is indicated for patients with ischemic limbs or those who require delayed primary wound closure. The procedure uses equal length anterior and posterior flaps; how-

ever, soft-tissue coverage is less than attained in posterior flap closures.

Nerve

Careful attention should be given to the treatment of the transected nerves in an attempt to prevent symptomatic neuroma formation to minimize future pain. Careful traction followed by transection allows the nerve to recoil within the soft tissues of the residual limb. Silicone capping, grafting with an epidural nerve sheath, or a venous graft may prevent disorganized nerve regeneration and sprouting. However, most techniques currently in use do not eliminate neuroma formation and more studies are required to determine the best long-term outcomes.

Preoperative Consultation

Optimal care begins before surgery. When amputation is considered, patient consultation with a physiatrist, physical therapist, prosthetist, and a functioning amputee is necessary to facilitate a smoother transition into prosthetic training. The physiatrist coordinates all the efforts of the rehabilitative team, provides input on the recommended surgical level of amputation and limb length, informs the patient about the anticipated postoperative rehabilitation protocol and outcomes, and explains potential problems. The physical therapist can initiate preprosthetic training before surgery by educating the patient on conditioning and range-of-motion exercises for the affected extremity. The prosthetist can provide valuable input on the latest advances in rehabilitation technology, concentrating on limitations so as not to create false expectations. A functioning amputee provides the patient with psychological reassurance that a health professional may not be able to convey.

Immediate Postoperative Treatment
Wound Protection and Coverage

Wound protection and edema control can be achieved simultaneously with a postoperative compressive dressing such as an elastic stockinette (stump shrinkers) or elastic bandages. Elastic bandages require proper application to avoid proximal constriction from a tourniquet effect. An elastic stockinette tends to be easier to apply and provides reasonable control of edema. Some patients may experience pain as the stockinette is pulled across the incision line and function better with elastic bandages. A nonremovable plaster cast can be placed immediately after the amputation for protection; however, this technique prevents wound inspection and can result in pistoning and skin breakdown when residual limb edema subsides. A removable rigid dressing made of thermoplastic provides wound coverage and edema control and allows wound inspection and dressing changes. It can be fabricated to resemble a socket to improve residual limb shape or it can be formed into a bivalve or clamshell design. This approach can be used for patients who need protection from falling and accidental contact while waiting for the residual limb to mature.

Range of Motion

A range-of-motion and contracture prevention protocol is integral in the early postoperative course. Lying prone, bedside range-of-motion exercises, and early mobilization can prevent knee flexion and hip abduction/external rotation contractures that are seen in lower extremity amputees. It has been shown that early contracture was independently associated with the inability to complete an inpatient prosthetic rehabilitation program soon after amputation surgery.

Postamputation Pain

The treatment of pain has important functional and prognostic implications. Pain is present in up to 70% of amputees immediately after surgery and in 50% after 5 years. Along with ambulation distance, pain is the most important amputation-specific determinant of health-related quality of life. Pain is experienced as hyperalgesia (a stronger or earlier withdrawal response to noxious stimuli) or allodynia (the sensation of pain from nonnoxious stimuli). Phantom limb pain is defined as the nociceptive sensation of the amputated limb.

Generally, postamputation pain can be attributed to local and biomechanical factors affecting the residual limb or to the changes to the peripheral and central nervous systems caused by the amputation. Local factors include ischemia, infection, wound dehiscence, and skeletal abnormalities (such as ectopic bone formation, excess fibular length, and inadequate tibial beveling). Neuropathic pain is often manifested as residual limb pain secondary to a neuroma, pain in the missing limb (phantom limb pain), or sympathetically driven pain.

The treatment of neuropathic pain after amputation does not produce perfect results and often requires a multidisciplinary approach. Pain management protocols include pharmacologic agents, mechanical, surgical, and physical modalities (exercise), psychological counseling, and behavioral approaches including imagery techniques.

The antiepileptics, tricyclic antidepressants, and opioids are the most commonly used oral medications for postamputation neuropathic pain. Gabapentin, an antiepileptic agent with both gamma-aminobutyric acid and glutamate antagonist properties, is shown to decrease neuropathic pain and is relatively well tolerated. Desipramine, a tricyclic antidepressant, could also be considered a first-line drug. The role of opioids in the treatment of neuropathic pain is controversial but remains clearly indicated in acute postamputation pain. Other medications that are used in neuropathic pain disorders

include α-2 agonists (clonidine), N-methyl D-aspartate receptor antagonists (amantidine, dextromethorphan), anti-inflammatory agents, magnesium sulfate, or cannabinoids.

Preoperative analgesia with intrathecal anesthetics or opioids has been beneficial in patients with longstanding preamputation pain. This regimen is initiated preoperatively and continued for up to 3 days after amputation before converting to an oral regimen. Neuroma excision with the combination of funiculectomy, epineural sleeve suture ligation, or silicone capping is being performed but long-term outcome studies are not yet available. Local neurolysis with phenol/glycerin has provided relief in patients for whom neuroma excision has been unsuccessful. Ultrasound for identification and guidance during neurolysis also has been used with moderate success. Cortical, thalamic, and dorsal column stimulators implanted to stimulate neuroinhibitory pathways can provide neuromodulation of neuropathic pain but not nociceptive pain. Intrathecal pumps that infuse clonidine, anesthetics, or opioids have been implanted in patients with intractable pain.

Mechanical stimulation by gentle residual limb tapping and the application of transcutaneous electrical or vibratory stimulation have been the usual physical modalities for treating postamputation pain. The use of transcutaneous nerve stimulation has had moderate success and can be applied directly to the site of pain, on the contralateral limb, or even auricularly. Prosthetic wear and early mobilization promotes afferent signals that increase cortical reorganization and may relieve neuropathic pain in many patients.

Prosthetic Training

Prior research has supported both immediate prosthetic training and delayed prosthetic fitting. Vascular transtibial amputees treated with a rigid intrasurgical plaster cast followed by early postoperative prosthetic limb fitting have been compared with those referred to an amputee clinic for fitting several weeks after hospital discharge. A significant decrease in the number of total hospitalization days was noted in the group who had early prosthetic limb fitting, implying increased cost effectiveness with this approach. In another study, outcomes for patients with immediate prosthetic transtibial fitting were examined and no significant variation was found in terms of local necrosis or infection. In a more recent study, a 68% success rate in early prosthetic fitting was reported despite strict inclusion criteria that only admitted patients who it was believed would benefit from this approach. Based on this data, a postoperative delay of about 3 weeks before beginning prosthetic rehabilitation was recommended, although some patients will require a preprosthetic rehabilitation program.

Early functional training includes donning and maintenance of the prosthetic device, residual limb desensitization, strengthening, gradual and monitored increased prosthetic wear, and gait retraining. Strengthening of the quadriceps, glutei, and hamstring muscles must be done as these muscle groups compensate for the loss of the ankle and/or knee. The duration of prosthetic wear should be gradual, beginning with 30-minute intervals two times a day and increasing to several hours at a time with frequent skin checks. Gait training is started with parallel bars to facilitate weight acceptance on the residual limb. Weight bearing is gradually increased on the prosthetic limb. Gait retraining is initiated using a step to gait pattern leading to a step through gait pattern. It is important to achieve a smooth gait pattern with equal step-lengths to avoid gait deviations that increase metabolic energy expenditure. The early establishment of an energy-efficient walking pattern has considerable long-term implications that affect function and independence.

Prosthetic Components and Prescription

The technology involved in the development of prosthetic components has evolved significantly in the past decade. The incorporation of titanium, carbon fiber, and other metal alloys has increased the rigidity and tensile strength of the components without adding weight. The use of silicone liners and sockets composed of flexible plastics along with suction suspension has generally increased comfort and decreased skin breakdown. Polycentric and multiaxial joints and terminal devices with pneumatic, hydraulic, and computer-driven controls have contributed to a smoother and more energy-efficient gait pattern. The goal of prosthetic wear has gone beyond community ambulation to educational, vocational, and recreational activities as well.

Partial Foot Amputation

The amputation of a single toe, except for the big toe, results in minimal loss of function. Toe spacers are inserted to fill the void and to prevent further deformities (varus or valgus) in the remaining toes. The amputation of the first ray significantly affects push-off; therefore, a long steel shank and a rocker bottom is usually provided as compensation. For transmetatarsal amputations, a custom molded insole with a toe filler is recommended.

Proximally, the Lisfranc amputation is a transmetatarsal disarticulation whereas a Chopart amputation is a disarticulation at the midtarsal joint through the talonavicular and calcaneocuboid joints. Both of these procedures may result in a significant equinovarus deformity with anterior weight bearing through the scar line, predisposing to skin breakdown over time. Early postoperative rigid dressing and Achilles tendon lengthening

are done to prevent the equinus deformity. For this level of amputation, a special shoe or a slipper-like prosthesis or a combination of both is provided. A ground-reacting ankle-foot orthosis with anterior and posterior shells is prescribed in a muscularly imbalanced and pressure-sensitive foot to provide maximal control.

The Boyd amputation excises all the tarsal bones except the calcaneus. Because of resultant residual limb problems, it is not a popular procedure and is used primarily for the pediatric congenital amputee. The Syme's amputation is an ankle disarticulation with a heel flap attached securely to the distal tibia to provide weight bearing on the residual limb. Cosmetic concerns may limit acceptance of this procedure because the distal residual limb has a bulbous shape. The Syme's prosthesis extends to the proximal tibia but has a removable medial wall to allow the bulbous distal limb to enter the socket. The foot component is similar to that used in a transtibial amputation but with a lower profile to accommodate the residual limb.

Transtibial Components
Foot and Ankle Assembly

The solid ankle cushioned heel exemplifies the earlier foot assemblies. It consists mainly of a semirigid wooden keel surrounded by a resilient material concentrated at the heel. At heel strike, energy is absorbed with the compression of the heel assembly and a plantar flexion moment is simulated. A stable base of support is provided by the keel, which hyperextends at the metatarsophalangeal line at heel-off. During the swing phase, the unloaded toe region reverts to its neutral position. The use of this design is limited to home ambulators or those patients with limited insurance coverage.

Dynamic response feet store energy at heel strike and transmit the forces to the keel during heel-off, providing recoil. Examples include the Seattle (Model and Instruments Works, Inc, Seattle, WA), the Carbon Copy II (Ohio Willow Wood Co, Mt. Sterling, OH), the Quantum (Hosmer Dorrance Corp, Campbell, CA), and the Flex (Ossur North America, Aliso Viejo, CA) foot designs. Because they provide a better spring for running and jumping, these prosthetic foot designs are recommended for more active individuals.

Articulated foot assemblies provide motion at the anatomic location of the ankle, better accommodate uneven surfaces, and absorb torsional forces reducing torque to the limb by the socket. Designs are either single axis, which provide dorsiflexion and plantar flexion, or multiaxis, which provide motion in the dorsiflexion-plantar flexion and inversion-eversion planes. The College Park (College Park Industries, Frasier, MI), Luxon (Otto Bock North America, Minneapolis, MN), and Endolite (Endolite North America, Centerville, OH) designs are common examples of multiaxis foot assemblies.

Heel height adjustability is a feature developed to address cosmetic issues in patients who use footwear of varying heel heights. This option is often incorporated into the foot assembly. The Century 22 (Otto Bock North America) foot offers manual adjustment of varying heel heights from 35 to 50 mm.

Occasionally, a torque absorber is placed between the shank and the foot assembly to absorb torsional forces as the prosthesis twists around the residual limb during ambulation. This modification is recommended for patients with skin conditions or for those who participate in sport activities or vocations that require significant foot rotation.

Pylon
The pylon is the interphase between the foot assembly and the socket and is classified as having an endoskeletal or exoskeletal design. Endoskeletal pylons consist of a rigid and unyielding central support surrounded by a polyurethane, soft cosmetic cover to allow for a more natural appearance. Substitution of isolated components (socket, shank, and foot) is also possible without discarding the entire prosthesis. This situation is ideal in early prosthetic rehabilitation when a temporary or intermediate prosthesis is provided or in the pediatric population to allow for limb growth. Recent improvements in material construction using titanium and carbon fiber have significantly increased the weight limit for these pylons to as much as 350 lb.

Exoskeletal or crustacean shanks are solid blocks of hard plastic or wood molded to resemble the intact limb and hollowed in the middle to reduce weight. The exterior surfaces are laminated to provide waterproofing. Although more rigid and stronger than the endoskeletal pylon designs, they are heavier and revisions often entail discarding the entire prosthesis. Their use is limited to relatively obese patients or people such as farmers or outdoorsmen who are constantly exposed to environments that could corrode the more intricate components of the endoskeletal pylon.

Recent designs have also incorporated the pylon with the foot assembly. The Re-Flex Vertical Shock pylon (Ossur North America) integrates a foot with a vertical shock-absorbing pylon that returns energy both in the vertical and sagittal planes.

Socket
The socket acts as an interphase between the residual limb and the prosthesis and applies weight-supporting forces to the residual limb. In socket fabrication, pressure-tolerant areas are built up for more contact and pressure-sensitive areas are relieved to minimize contact. Pressure-tolerant areas include the patellar ten-

don, the pretibial muscles, the gastrocnemius/gastrocnemius-soleus complex muscles, the popliteal fossa, the lateral flat aspect of the fibula, and the medial tibial flare. The pressure-sensitive areas include the tibial crest, tubercles, condyles, the fibular head, the distal tibia and fibula, and the hamstring tendons.

The patellar tendon-bearing socket is the most frequently used. Although it is designed to put substantial weight on the patellar tendon, its intimate contact with the entire residual limb provides even distribution of pressure with minimal distal end bearing. The trim line extends anteriorly to the lower patella level, mediolaterally to the femoral condyles, and posteriorly below the level of the hamstring tendon insertions.

For shorter residual limbs and those with mediolateral instability, a patellar tendon supracondylar socket is more appropriately prescribed. A supracondylar socket extends above the medial and lateral femoral condyles using the bony ridges to suspend the prosthesis. It provides better mediolateral knee support and is appropriate for shorter residual limbs. A supracondylar/suprapatellar suspension uses the same design but extends the anterior trim line to envelop the patella for added support. This particular feature also helps counteract genu recurvatum forces.

Suspension Systems
Mechanical suspension devices are external devices that are attached to anchor on bony prominences to provide stabilization. They are indicated early after amputation when there is significant volume fluctuation along the residual limb secondary to edema. They also are useful in older amputees with poor hand dexterity and poor residual limb bulk and tone. Examples include: (1) A suprapatellar suspension strap that is fastened to the medial and lateral socket walls passing over the superior border of the patella. This device offers some resistance to knee hyperextension forces and is relatively easy to put on and take off; however, it is prone to mild pistoning and is not indicated for short, painful residual limbs with mediolateral instability. (2) A thigh corset secured to the socket by sidebars and a knee joint assembly is useful to take weight off of the residual limb and to provide better rotational stability. (3) Anteriorly, a fork strap can be attached to a waist or pelvic belt to add stability in the anteroposterior plane and to help suspend the prosthesis, especially in knee flexion. It is indicated for shorter residual limbs and for obese patients who cannot use a suprapatellar strap. (4) Over-the-knee sleeves are fabricated from a flexible material such as neoprene, which extends from the proximal end of the prosthesis to the distal thigh.

Atmospheric or suction types of suspension are generally preferred over mechanical types to minimize pistoning and shearing forces. However, they require adequate hand and visual function to apply. Furthermore, suction suspensions may provide undue stress to a healing surgical wound, thus promoting delayed wound healing or wound dehiscence; they are typically withheld early in the postoperative period until volume fluctuations have stabilized. One example is a prefabricated, closed-end silicone elastomer liner that is flexible enough to adapt to the irregular surfaces in the residual limb and to promote an airtight environment to achieve suspension. This device is rolled proximally up and over the knee and is secured to the socket by means of a shuttle lock mechanism, which consists of a pin at the distal end of the liner and a locking mechanism located at the bottom of the socket. Early in the postamputation period when the residual limb volume fluctuates significantly, the pin and shuttle lock mechanism can be deferred in lieu of a supracondylar strap. The Iceross (Ossur North America) and Alpha (Ohio Willow Wood) liners are examples of silicone liners. Another example is the Vacuum Assisted Socket System (Otto Bock North America), which consists of a silicone liner, a suspension sleeve, and an air evacuation pump that creates an elevated vacuum of 15 mm Hg between the liner and the socket wall. This design controls volume fluctuation and promotes a more secure and intimate fit between the residual limb and socket.

Transfemoral Components
Socket Design
The two main transfemoral socket designs are termed quadrilateral and ischial containment. The quadrilateral socket has its posterior border under the ischial tuberosity and buttocks for weight bearing, with the anterior border providing a posteriorly directed force to control the femur. Therefore, it is narrow anteroposteriorly and wide mediolaterally. An ischial containment socket should contain the ischial tuberosity and apply counter pressure from the lateral wall of the socket. It is narrow mediolaterally and wider anteroposteriorly. Quadrilateral socket designs are useful for obese patients, whereas more active patients may benefit from the ischial containment design that maintains the femur in adduction, allowing the gluteal musculature to generate maximal tension at an ideal resting length. Material construction can be either rigid (wood, plastic laminates), flexible, or a combination of both (Scandinavian or Icelandic-Swedish-New York sockets). The outer hard socket can be windowed posteriorly and anteriorly to allow improved comfort with sitting. In this situation, a flexible inner liner is used in contact with the skin.

Suspension Device
The transfemoral suspension devices can either be mechanical or atmospheric. A pelvic belt and hip joint offers maximal stabilization and is best suited to those with short residual limbs, significant mediolateral stabil-ity, or lack of rotational control. Less restrictive suspension would include a Silesian belt or total elastic suspension belt, which is composed of neoprene with reinforced elastic bands running at oblique angles posteriorly and anteriorly around the waist. A silicone liner with a distal pin and shuttle lock similar to that found in transtibial devices can be used. This component adds length and in combination with the knee unit may cause an uneven knee axis (prosthetic thigh longer than intact thigh), leading to cosmetic and biomechanical deficits. A suction suspension is ideal for patients with mature residual limbs. Surface tension, negative pressure, and muscle contractions suspend the prosthesis from the limb without the need for a waist belt. Suction is generated by placing the residual limb into the socket with a nylon pull sock or using a lubricating lotion, then expelling air with a one-way valve.

Knee Assembly
Knee assemblies consist of a joint or bolt that allows flexion and extension, an extension stop that limits hyperextension, and a friction device that provides smoother motion along the assembly. General classifications are based on axis and control, either on swing or stance phase.

A single axis knee assembly acts as a hinged joint and is preferred for its simplicity, reliability, minimal maintenance, and cost. It is also ideal for children because growth entails frequent changes in prosthetic components. A polycentric or multiaxis knee is more physiologic and uses multiple bar linkages along the bolt to allow a shifting mechanical axis during flexion and extension. This feature provides more stability while allowing for improved performance at higher walking speeds.

Control is provided either at the stance or swing phase. Stance phase control is provided for patients with knee instability who cannot control knee flexion. A manual locking knee is used to maximize stability; however, this eliminates knee motion throughout the gait cycle and is recommended for limited household ambulators. Stance phase weight-activated control is used for those with slightly better overall knee stability who need support during upright activities.

The presence and type of swing phase control is determined by the patient's ability to vary cadence. A constant friction device is used for elderly patients who walk at a constant speed. This unit has a split bushing and clamp around the knee bolt, which provides constant friction throughout the swing phase. The amount of friction is controlled by a friction adjusting screw that tightens or loosens the bushing. For active patients who want to vary walking speeds and run, hydraulic or pneumatic swing phase control devices are used. Hydraulic and pneumatic mechanisms adjust resistance to changes

Table 1 | The Centers for Medicare and Medicaid Services Functional Levels of Ambulation

Level	Amputee and Prosthetic Characteristics
K0	Patient cannot transfer independently
	Prosthesis will not enhance quality of life or mobility
K1	Patient has the ability or potential to use a prosthesis for transfers or ambulation on level surfaces with a fixed cadence
	Patient has limited or unlimited household ambulation
	A solid ankle cushioned heel foot or a single axis foot; a manual locking, single axis or polycentric knee unit (with or without stance phase weight-activated control); or any socket or suspension design is allowed
K2	Patient has the ability to traverse low-level environmental barriers such as curbs, stairs, or uneven surfaces with a constant cadence
	All K1 prosthetic components are allowed with the addition of flexible keels or multiaxial feet, rotators, and torque absorbers
K3	Patient has the ability or potential for ambulation with variable cadences
	Patient can traverse most environmental barriers
	May have vocational, therapeutic, or exercise activity that demands prosthetic use beyond simple locomotion
	All K1 and K2 prosthetic components are allowed with the addition of hydraulic/pneumatic knees and dynamic or shock absorbing pylons
K4	Patients have the ability or potential for prosthetic use that exceeds basic ambulation
	Patients exhibit high impact and energy levels typical of the growing child, active adult, or athlete
	All existing prosthetic components are allowed in this functional level

in the rate of motion and this improves knee control and provides a smoother gait pattern.

The C-Leg

In 1999, a microprocessor knee unit called the C-Leg (Otto Bock North America) was introduced in the United States. This knee unit uses force sensors in the pylon that detect knee angles and loading forces at the foot and ankle that are then sampled by onboard microprocessors 50 times per second. The C-Leg was reported to allow patients to have a significant reduction in oxygen consumption during slower speed ambulation and to achieve a wider range of cadences compared with a conventionally controlled hydraulic single axis knee. However, randomized trials comparing this technology to multiaxis hydraulic knee designs are needed to determine optimal patient selection.

Knee Disarticulation

Knee disarticulations involve the removal of the tibia and fibula at the knee with suturing of the patellar ten-

don to the cruciate ligaments. This procedure is done on patients with traumatic injuries and very short residual tibiae above the tubercle, or on elderly dysvascular patients without prosthetic potential who need to bear weight on the residual limb for transfers. The knee disarticulation prosthesis consists of a modified quadrilateral transfemoral socket with some ischial weight bearing and a four-bar linkage polycentric knee that may result in uneven knee axes.

Functional Levels

The Centers for Medicare and Medicaid Services have identified functional levels of ambulation with corresponding components deemed appropriate for each level of activity (Table 1). This classification system is only applicable to patients with single lower extremity amputation. It is also possible for a classification to be upgraded if initial expectations are exceeded.

Common Gait Abnormalities in Lower Limb Prosthetic Rehabilitation

Transtibial Deviations

Excessive knee flexion during heel strike could be caused by a foot placed in dorsiflexion, an excessively stiff heel cushion, anterior translation of the socket in relation to the pylon, or a residual limb flexion contracture. Insufficient knee flexion can be caused by plantar flexion of the foot, an excessively soft heel cushion, posterior displacement of the socket in relation to the pylon, or weak quadriceps on the residual limb.

Lateral thrust occurs when the pylon is placed medially, creating a varus moment. The patient usually reports concomitant pain and pressure on the medial femoral condyle and lateral distal tibia. Medial thrust is an analogous problem with the pylon placed laterally, causing a valgus moment. Patients often report pain on the lateral femoral condyle and medial distal tibia. These deviations are corrected by repositioning the pylon to the socket in the coronal plane.

Transfemoral Deviations

Lateral trunk bending is a trunk lean to the prosthetic side during the stance phase. It occurs because of an abducted socket, a hip abduction contracture, insufficient lateral support of the prosthetic socket, a short prosthesis, or weak ipsilateral hip abductors.

Circumduction is a curvilinear motion of the prosthesis during the swing phase and is caused by a functionally longer prosthetic limb length, which creates difficulty in clearance. Common causes include an ill-fitting socket that pistons or does not fully accommodate the residual limb, a manual locking knee, a device that causes excessive knee friction, or a foot in plantar flexion.

Table 2 | Metabolic Cost of Ambulation Per Level and Nature of Amputation

Amputation Level	Metabolic Cost
Syme's	Increased 15%
Traumatic transtibial	Increased 25%
Vascular transtibial	Increased 40%
Traumatic transfemoral	Increased 68%
Vascular transfemoral	Increased 100%

(Data from Czerniecki JM: Rehabilitation in limb deficiency: Gait and motion analysis. Arch Phys Med Rehabil 1996;77:S3-S8.)

Vaulting is described as excessive plantar flexion of the intact foot during the prosthetic swing phase and occurs because of a functionally longer prosthetic limb length for reasons similar to those that create a circumduction moment.

Medial or lateral heel whip is often caused by rotational malalignment of the knee apparatus in comparison to the tibial components. A knee unit placed in excessive external rotation leads to a medial whip; a knee unit placed in excessive internal rotation results in a lateral whip.

Long-Term Prosthetic Rehabilitation Issues
Metabolic Requirements
The metabolic requirements of ambulation increase proportionally with decreased length of the amputated limb, the number of amputated joints, and the number of amputated limbs. Furthermore, vascular amputees have higher metabolic requirements than their traumatic counterparts. Amputees, however, offset the increased metabolic demands by choosing a slower self-selected walking pace. Patients should not be denied prosthetic fitting and training on the basis of cardiopulmonary limitations unless these limitations are profound. The metabolic cost of ambulation based on the level and nature of amputation is shown in Table 2.

Functional Outcomes and Work Reintegration
The long-term survival rate for patients after dysvascular lower extremity amputation is 50% to 70% at 2 years, and 30% to 40% at 5 years with a postoperative mortality rate of 10% to 30%. Heart disease is the most common cause of death (51%), followed by carcinomatosis (14%) and cerebrovascular accidents (6%). The risk of contralateral limb amputation reaches 15% to 20% in 2 years after the initial amputation and the reamputation rate of the ipsilateral limb in a transtibial dysvascular patient ranges from 4% to 30%.

Traumatic amputees show more favorable outcomes. In a 2001 study, a 9% acute admission mortality rate with only a 3.5% 10-year mortality rate was found. Further-more, 95% of the survivors wore prostheses and averaged 80 hours of use per week. An earlier study involving younger amputees showed a 79% job reintegration rate. Age at the time of amputation, comfort of the prosthesis, education level, and lowering of the physical demands in the workplace were positive predictors for return to work. Pain did not appear to be associated with return to work but was directly associated with work-related satisfaction.

Upper Limb Amputation and Prosthetic Components
Levels of Amputation
The transradial amputation is the most common and preferred upper extremity amputation. The residual limb length can be classified as either long (55% to 90%), medium (35% to 54%), or short (0 to 34%) based on the length of the intact forearm measured from the medial epicondyle to the distal ulna or radius. Because of component weight and length considerations, the long transradial residual limb provides the longest lever arm most suitable for a body-powered prosthesis. A medium length transradial residual length provides enough clearance for externally powered prosthetic components. The short transradial limb is difficult to suspend and may promote deficits in elbow strength and range of motion. Elbow disarticulations may pose cosmetic concerns because of limited options in externally-powered elbow units available for this amputation level.

Transhumeral amputations are also classified by residual limb length (short, medium, and long), but the prosthetic options and rehabilitative interventions are similar at each level. Shoulder disarticulations and forequarter amputations are reserved for tumor excision surgeries because of the difficulty in providing a prosthesis with adequate suspension.

Prosthetic Control
Upper extremity prosthetic control is usually either body powered, externally powered, or a combination of both. Body-powered control is provided by the intact movements of the residual limb that connects to cables to flex and extend the elbow or open and close the terminal device. The movements include scapular abduction; chest expansion; shoulder depression, flexion and abduction; and elbow flexion. Myoelectric controls use the electrical activity generated by muscle contractions to control the flow of energy from a battery to a motor controlling the terminal device or elbow unit. Comparative studies between myoelectric and body-powered hands showed no significant difference in terms of performance that could limit application of this technology to specialized situations.

Prosthetic Components

The terminal device attempts to approximate the complex functions of the hand and is available in different designs based on the user's preference. The devices can either be hooks that provide lateral pinch or hands that provide a three-jaw chuck pinch. They can be passive or purely cosmetic, body powered, or externally powered. Body-powered designs are either voluntary opening or voluntary closing; the selection depends on the patient's anticipated use (for example, an amputee who plans to work in a factory would benefit from a voluntary closing terminal device, which would not get caught in the assembly line). Terminal devices cannot provide the sensory feedback and dexterity of an intact hand. Myoelectric-powered hands allow for a proportional grasp. Slip control systems have microprocessors that maintain constant pressure on the object to prevent slippage.

Wrist designs can be manually or externally controlled, and most provide passive supination and pronation with a friction lock to control rotation when lifting heavier objects. Quick disconnect wrists allow for easy interchange of terminal devices. Elbow mechanisms are either internal or external and can also be passive, body powered, or externally powered. Body-powered designs are controlled with mechanical cables through movements of the residual limb or can be manually locked by the contralateral hand, chin, or the ipsilateral shoulder. Electrical elbows are operated by electrical switches or myoelectric impulses.

Prosthetic socket design also has progressed with the development of lightweight and durable materials. Flexible thermoplastics provide better fit and comfort and are used in the internal layer, which comes in close contact with the residual limb. Carbon fiber has replaced wood or laminated plastics in the external layer. Mechanical suspension devices usually consist of harness systems that anchor across the shoulders. Fabric liners as well as silicone suction suspension systems are also available for the upper extremity prostheses.

Annotated Bibliography

Incidence and Etiology

Bosse M, MacKenzie EJ, Kellam JF, et al: An analysis of outcomes of reconstruction or amputation after leg threatening injuries. *N Engl J Med* 2002;347:1924-1931.

Limb salvage has replaced amputation as the primary surgical treatment in severe limb trauma. This prospective cohort study examines the long-term outcomes of significant lower extremity injury (grade III tibial or ankle fractures, severe dysvascular and soft-tissue injury) treated either with amputation or limb salvage. The functional outcomes are similar between the two treatment options; however, longer hospital stays, increased number of complications, and more surgeries were found in the limb-salvage group.

Dillingham TR, Pezzin LE, MacKenzie EJ: Limb amputation and limb deficiency: Epidemiology and recent trends in the United States. *South Med J* 2002;95:875-883.

This study provides a comprehensive perspective on the epidemiology of limb amputations in the United States using linear regression techniques on data from 1988 to 1996. Dysvascular amputations have increased to 27%, accounting for 82% of all limb loss. Rates of trauma and cancer-related amputations have declined by one half and the incidence of congenital deficiencies has remained stable.

Immediate Postoperative Treatment

Bone M, Critchley P, Buggy DJ: Gabapentin in postamputation phantom limb pain: A randomized, double-blind, placebo-controlled, cross-over study. *Reg Anesth Pain Med* 2002;27:481-486.

This study used a randomized, double blind, placebo-controlled crossover methodology. Subjects with severe phantom limb pain were enrolled in a 6-week course of gabapentin therapy titrated by increments of 300 mg to a maximum of 2,400 mg per day versus the control group. Significant improvement in terms of pain intensity was found in patients treated with gabapentin as compared with those given the placebo. However, no differences were noticed in terms of rescue medication (codeine/paracetamol) required, sleep disturbance, or function as measured by the Barthel index.

Ernberg LA, Adler RS, Lane J: Ultrasound in detection and treatment of painful stump neuroma. *Skeletal Radiol* 2003;32:306-309.

The use of ultrasound has shown considerable success in the assessment of amputation stump neuromas. This study investigates the usefulness of ultrasound guided localization for steroid injection of amputation stump neuromas.

Munin MC, Espejo-De Guzman MC, Boninger ML, Fitzgerald SG, Penrod LE, Singh J: Predictive factors for successful early prosthetic ambulation among lower-limb amputees. *J Rehabil Res Dev* 2001;38:379-384.

In an effort to predict successful outcomes with early prosthetic rehabilitation, demographic and medical factors were analyzed in a group of lower extremity amputees admitted to an inpatient rehabilitation facility. Sixty-eight percent of the patients met criteria for successful ambulation at time of discharge. The absence of lower extremity contractures and longer length of inpatient rehabilitation stay were significantly related to successful prosthetic ambulation.

van der Schans CP, Geertzen JH, Schoppen T, Dijkstra PU: Phantom pain and health-related quality of life in lower limb amputees. *J Pain Symptom Manage* 2002;24:429-436.

This study analyzed the determinants of health-related quality of life in a population of 437 lower extremity amputees using the RAND-36 Item Health Survey (Dutch Language Version) questionnaire. In general, the most important amputation-specific determinants of health-related quality of life were walking distance and stump pain. Amputees with phantom limb pain had poorer quality of life than those with only phantom limb sensation.

Prosthetic Components and Prescription

Carnesale PG: Amputation of the lower extremity, in Canale ST (ed): *Campbell's Operative Orthopedics*. Philadelphia, PA, Mosby, 2003, pp 575-595.

This chapter examines the different levels of lower extremity amputations including their indications, techniques, and postoperative treatment. Noticeable differences occur in approaches taken in the nonischemic and ischemic lower extremity.

Schmaltz T, Blumentritt S, Tsukishiro K, Kocher L, Dietl H: Energy efficiency of trans-femoral amputees walking on computer-controlled prosthetic knee joint: C-LEG. Otto Bock Website. Available at: http://www.ottobockus.com/products/lower_limb_prosthetics/c-leg_energy.pdf. Accessed June, 2004.

This online article reviews a study of the energy expenditure needed for walking by six transfemoral amputees using several prosthetic devices including the C-Leg with electronic controls.

Long-Term Prosthetic Rehabilitation Issues

Schoppen T, Boonstra A, Groothoff JW, deVries J, Goeken LN, Eisma WH: Employment status, job characteristics and work-related health experience of people with a lower limb amputation in the Netherlands. *Arch Phys Med Rehabil* 2001;82:239-245.

This study examined the occupational status of lower limb amputees in the Netherlands and compared the health experience of working and nonworking amputees. Patients who stopped working because of the amputation had a worse health experience compared with those who continued to work. Patients who later returned to work, reported problems (such as finding a suitable job or obtaining workplace modifications) stemming from the long delay between the amputation and the return to work.

Classic Bibliography

Carabelli RA, Kellerman WC: Phantom limb pain: Relief by application of TENS to contralateral extremity. *Arch Phys Med Rehabil* 1985;66:466-467.

Czerniecki JM: Rehabilitation in limb deficiency: 1. Gait and motion analysis. *Arch Phys Med Rehabil* 1996; 77(suppl 3):S3-S8.

Edelstein JE, Berger N: Performance comparison among children fitted with myoelectric and body-powered hands. *Arch Phys Med Rehabil* 1993;74:376-380.

Esquenazi A: Upper limb amputee rehabilitation and prosthetic restoration, in Braddom RL (ed): *Physical Medicine and Rehabilitation*. Philadelphia, PA, WB Saunders, 2000, pp 263-278.

Gottschalk F: Transfemoral amputation: Biomechanics and surgery. *Clin Orthop* 1999;361:15-22.

Kane TJ III, Pollak EW: The rigid versus soft postoperative dressing controversy: A controlled study in vascular below-knee amputees. *Am Surg* 1980;46:244-247.

Leonard EI, McAnelly RD, Lomba M, Faulkner VW: Lower limb prosthesis, in Braddom RL (ed): *Physical Medicine and Rehabilitation*. Philadelphia, PA, WB Saunders, 2000, pp 279-311.

Leonard JA, Meier RH: Upper and lower extremity prosthesis, in DeLisa JA, Gans BM (eds): *Rehabilitation Medicine: Principles and Practice*. Philadelphia, PA, Lippincott-Raven, 1998, pp 669-697.

Pezzin LE, Dillingham TR, MacKenzie EJ: Rehabilitation and the long-term outcomes of persons with trauma-related amputations. *Arch Phys Med Rehabil* 2000;81:292-300.

Pinzur MS, Littooy F, Osterman H, Wafer D: Early postsurgical prosthetic limb fitting in dysvascular below-knee amputees with a pre-fabricated temporary limb. *Orthopedics* 1988;11:1051-1053.

Yuksel F, Kislaoglu E, Durak N, Ucar C, Karacaoglu E: Prevention of painful neuromas by epineural ligatures, flaps and grafts. *Br J Plast Surg* 1997;50:282-185.

Chapter 55

Musculoskeletal Rehabilitation

Tom G. Mayer, MD

Joel Press, MD

Levels of Care

Nonsurgical care for patients with injuries to the spine and extremities can be classified into three distinct levels of treatment. Timing of the care is dependent on the diagnosis and anticipated healing time from the inciting event.

Primary Care

Primary care is usually provided during an acute stage of an injury with pain control as the primary focus; avoidance of deconditioning is also a consideration. The duration of the period of primary care depends on the type of injury and can range from 10 to 14 days in patients with mild sprains, strains, and lacerations and from 8 to 12 weeks in patients with complex fractures and dislocations. Treatment modalities include thermal (heat/cold) applications, pain medication and muscle relaxants, immobilization, bed rest, traction, and injection methods.

Secondary Care

Secondary care is usually appropriate in the postacute phase of an injury with the goal of providing reactivation to prevent long-term physical deconditioning and psychosocial changes that could extend beyond the normal healing period. This phase can begin when an injury has undergone sufficient partial healing and/or stabilization (through surgery, bracing, casting, or tissue healing) to permit progressive motion and strengthening exercises. Active joint mobilization and strengthening of the involved para-articular muscles are the primary modalities; treatment may be assisted with bracing, manipulation, thermal modalities, medication, and injections. In most patients, secondary care is the last component of musculoskeletal rehabilitation and is administered after an injury is treated nonsurgically or with surgery during the acute stage of injury.

Tertiary Care

Tertiary care is the final phase of musculoskeletal rehabilitation and is needed for only a small percentage of patients who have chronic disabling musculoskeletal pain that does not respond to early surgical and/or nonsurgical intervention. Because this group of patients is often characterized by a complex mix of physical deconditioning, psychosocial and socioeconomic barriers to recovery, and some resistance to care, a multidisciplinary approach is usually needed. Some patients require a functional restoration approach, which includes intensive physical training along with a cognitive behavioral disability management program aimed at increased productivity. Measurement of function, narcotic detoxification, psychotropic medication, and infrequent injections to relieve pain may be components of this approach. At the other extreme, palliative pain management usually involves a more passive role for the patient with an emphasis on pain-relieving injections and long-term use of opiates accompanied by a psychosocial focus on deemphasizing the pain experience. Neuroablative procedures and devices such as drug pumps and spinal cord stimulation also may be used. Chronicity of symptoms is usually established by 6 months after injury; however, more functionally-based programs may be appropriate within 3 to 4 months of symptom onset if significant psychosocial or treatment resistance is evident.

Primary Rehabilitation

The two main objectives of primary rehabilitation are to control pain and to prepare the musculoskeletal system for proper healing from injury. Pain control can be accomplished through the use of medications, physical modalities, injections, and occasionally bracing or relative immobilization (fracture management). No single pain medication is effective for all injuries. With any medication, knowledge of the mechanism of action, side effect profile, and interactions with other medications is essential for proper use. Acetaminophen (less than 4 mg/day) is an excellent first-line analgesic medication for pain because of its low cost. Serious adverse effects are rare except for liver toxicity, which may occur with prolonged use at a high dosage; particularly in association with substantial alcohol intake. Comparisons of effectiveness with nonsteroidal anti-inflammatory drugs (NSAIDs) are inconsistent. NSAIDs, all of which are analgesic, antipyretic, and anti-inflammatory, show no significant differences among the various available compounds. Some patients reported a marked preference and variation in efficacy of different NSAIDs, thus warranting a trial of a second or third class of medication if one class provides no pain relief. An adequate trial of NSAIDs may be 2 to 3 weeks. Several rare, serious adverse effects including clinical hepatitis, aplastic anemia, and agranulocytosis can occur. Gastrointestinal adverse effects are the most common and occur in approximately 25% of patients taking NSAIDs, whereas silent endoscopically demonstrated lesions occur in as many as 60% of patients. The overall risk for serious gastrointestinal bleeding in patients treated with NSAIDs is 1 per 1,000 patients, with the risk significantly greater in patients older than 65 years.

Other medications used for acute pain symptoms with muscle spasms are muscle relaxants. These medications are centrally acting drugs, which produce nonspecific sedation that accounts for their muscle relaxation effect. Although peripherally acting muscle relaxants exist (such as dantrolene sodium), these medications are not used for musculoskeletal disorders because of potential severe adverse effects. Muscle relaxants have been found to be more effective than a placebo in the relief of symptoms of acute musculoskeletal disorders. Oral corticosteroids also may be useful as a strong anti-inflammatory agent for patients with radicular symptoms in the cervical and/or lumbar region. Short-term use (7 to 10 days) or corticosteroids taken at a high dosage (30 to 40 mg prednisone or equivalent) have not been associated with major adverse effects. Opioid analgesics, on occasion, can be used for acute pain symptoms. Opioid analgesics act primarily by binding opiate receptors in the central nervous system and can be associated with tolerance, toxicity, addiction, and illicit use with long-term administration. Even short-term use of these medications should be undertaken with caution because of an association of adverse effects including demotivation, early reactive hyperalgesia, and early dependency problems in a select group of patients. Although more potent than NSAIDs and acetaminophen, in two of three clinical trials, narcotic analgesics were found to be no more effective than these medications in relieving pain. The dosage schedule should be defined and use limited to patients whose pain is unresponsive to alternative medications.

Physical agents including ultrasound, electrical stimulation, and heat and cold have been used to promote tissue healing, increase circulation, decrease inflammation, and reduce pain. Although physical agents are frequently used for symptomatic relief, these passive modalities do not appear to have any effect on clinical outcomes. It is essential to understand indications and contraindications of specific modalities when prescribing these agents. In general, short-term use (1 to 3 weeks) of physical modalities may be appropriate for an acute musculoskeletal problem or a flare-up of a chronic condition. No single modality has been shown to be superior to others for relief of musculoskeletal pain. Prolonged use of these passive modalities should be discouraged. Newer treatments such as vertebral axial decompression and continuous passive motion have been purported to alleviate acute and chronic pain. Until clinical studies confirm these findings, use of these treatments should be viewed as another physical modality and treated accordingly.

Injections of a variety of medications in various anatomic locations can be an adjunct to treating acute painful musculoskeletal conditions. Epidural injections have been shown to be effective in reducing radicular pain; however, the results in some controlled, prospective studies are variable. The benefit of facet joint and sacroiliac injections is controversial. They may provide some short-term pain relief that serves as an adjunct to other treatments (for example, manipulation, mobilization, and exercise) by facilitating joint movement in otherwise hypomobile joints or segments. Trigger point injections may provide some temporary relief for tight, painful muscle spasms to allow earlier activation of the musculoskeletal system. Multiple, repeat injections without concomitant activation of the patient is probably of little benefit.

Secondary Rehabilitation

Secondary rehabilitation focuses on restoring function to the musculoskeletal system once initial pain symptoms have subsided and tissue healing has been initiated. No single component of musculoskeletal rehabilitation is effective for every disorder; most disorders require multiple components to provide a comprehensive program. Understanding the roles and skills of chiropractors, physical therapists, and other health care providers is critical to avoid overuse and abuse of any one treatment. Cornerstones of restoring function are activation of the patient to prevent the sequelae of immobility and exercise to restore muscle flexibility, muscle balance, and coordination. Initially, exercises are emphasized in nonpainful ranges and planes of motion. Manual treatments and mobilization of restricted joints and soft tissues, either by chiropractors, osteopaths, therapists, or physicians, are often initiated before beginning focused strengthening programs. Injections for pain control (for example, local corticosteroids and epidural injections) may play some role in this phase of rehabilitation if the injections are used as an adjunct to increasing the patient's active participation in therapy or exercise. Exercise programs for musculoskeletal rehabilitation should focus not only on mobility and absolute muscle strength but also on muscle balance (agonist and antagonist strength ratios), kinetic chain issues (proximal and distal segment interplay with an injured segment), and muscle endurance or ability to function without fatiguing. Exercise programs should focus on strengthening weaker structures, with minimal aggravation of pain symptoms. Nonspecific exercise programs for nonspecific diagnoses yield nonspecific and often unsuccessful results.

Repetitive flexion-biased exercises for a patient with a typical posterolateral disk herniation may increase symptoms. Exercises that emphasize centralization of pain symptoms to the lumbar spine in patients with low back and leg symptoms may prove useful. The benefit of determining the directional preference and proper plane for flexion for each patient with back pain before initiating exercise treatment has been well documented. A recent study of patients with acute low back pain has shown that a classification-based exercise program improved disability and returns to work status in the exercise group compared with a control group followed for 1 year. Aerobic conditioning has been shown to be beneficial in terms of improving aerobic capacity, muscle strength, and flexibility in patients with nonactive to moderately active rheumatoid arthritis and osteoarthritis of the hip and/or knee. Short periods of immobilization immediately after surgery may be required for adequate tissue healing. However, during the postoperative period, and especially following anterior cruciate ligament reconstruction, early rehabilitation to prevent loss of range of motion and muscle strength has been shown to improve functional outcome.

Physical conditioning programs, called work conditioning or work hardening programs, attempt to improve work status and function; however, there is no evidence of their efficacy for acute back pain. Emphasis should be placed on use of programs that focus on return to work. Patients should participate in restoration programs that simulate the activities of daily living that they need to perform, and emphasize improvement in function. Programs that emphasize pain relief alone and that use short-term passive modalities are not effective. If no improvement is seen in a 4- to 6-week period with physical conditioning or work hardening programs, other options such as tertiary rehabilitation should be considered.

Tertiary Rehabilitation
Multidisciplinary Assessment
Because the diagnosis in patients with chronic pain or disability may be multifactorial, the involvement of many health professionals is often required. Before instituting a tertiary rehabilitation program, a multidisciplinary assessment of the patient's treatment options

should take place. This assessment should include all appropriate imaging tests, supportive electrodiagnostic tests, and diagnostic injection procedures as needed. Electromyography, nerve conduction velocity tests, MRI, CT, myelography, diskography, selective nerve root block, peripheral nerve block, and sympathetic block tests may be included. Careful surgical decision-making and discussions with the patient and family about surgical options should then take place. If the patient agrees to surgery, it should proceed with appropriate postoperative secondary care. Tertiary rehabilitation is the last resort when all reasonable surgical interventions have been exhausted or the patient is unwilling to elect additional surgery.

As a prelude to the tertiary rehabilitation process, special assessment of physical and functional capacity and psychosocial status is needed. From a physical perspective, patients have usually already undergone many weeks or months of physical therapy guided by a variety of health professionals and limited by resistance, fear, and inhibition of function (often termed fear-avoidance). During tertiary rehabilitation, the quantification of physical function by objective measures may help to guide the treatment approach by setting parameters for exercise, by providing feedback on progress to the patient, and by leading to better assessment of permanent impairment. Measurements of the mobility and strength around the injured joint(s) or spinal region(s), aerobic capacity, and the functional capacity of performing various activities of daily living (such as lifting, gripping, climbing) are important. Such tests are often termed physical or functional capacity evaluations and may involve goniometers, inclinometers, or three-dimensional digitizers to measure mobility; isometric, isoinertial, or isokinetic strength testing devices; bicycle or treadmill ergometers; and a variety of lifting protocols and devices. In unmotivated patients or those with chronic pain, measurements of functional capacities may not reflect their true physiologic functional abilities.

Psychosocial assessment is also an essential prerequisite for planning tertiary rehabilitation. Traditionally, clinicians have searched for causes of pain, seeking a physical basis for pain complaints that, once identified, could be eliminated or blocked. When no organic basis was identified, a psychological cause was assumed, hence the term psychogenic pain. However, the concept of a simple dichotomy, that pain is physical or psychological, is inadequate. It is more accurate and clinically effective to identify a variety of psychosocioeconomic barriers to recovery or risk factors creating entitlement, resistance, or fear-avoidance. A variety of simple validated questionnaires have been developed that can be used to assess pain, disability, health status, and depression (Table 1). A psychiatric diagnosis can be made using the Structured Clinical Interview for the *Diagnostic and Statistical Manual of Mental Health Disorders*,

TABLE 1	Questionnaires Available for Patient Physical and Psychological Assessment

Pain Drawing Questionnaire
Oswestry Low Back Pain Disability Questionnaire
Roland-Morris Disability Questionnaire
Medical Outcomes Study 36-Item Short Form
Million Disability Questionnaire

fourth edition. Significant psychopathology has been noted in chronic pain patients. A psychological interview conducted by a clinical psychologist who considers identified risk factors for ongoing disability may be useful. Personality changes may be manifested by anger, hostility, noncompliance, and resistance to the efforts of the therapeutic team. Minor head injuries, organic brain dysfunction, and a history of alcohol or drug use can produce cognitive errors and dysfunctions, which could create clinical management problems and make the patient refractory to education.

Finally, it is imperative that the orthopaedic surgeon is aware of the influence of the disability system, which may create a variety of incentives and disincentives to expected behaviors in treatment. Knowledge of the patient's involvement with the workers' compensation system (state or federal) and the key factors associated with this system is needed for proper assessment. It should be determined if the patient is receiving current temporary total disability benefits, impairment or disability benefits, vocational rehabilitation benefits, or is approaching a variety of financial and medical end points (termed maximum medical improvement or permanent and stationary status). The case manager, adjustor, or attorney for the injured worker may be a valuable resource for information about case status. Other financial benefits from private short- or long-term disability insurers, federal disability systems (Supplemental Security or Social Security Disability benefits), or from a variety of third parties (such as auto or product liability insurance) may affect patient motivation and behavior.

Functional Restoration Approaches

Functional restoration approaches to tertiary rehabilitation are oriented toward recovery from disability as well as pain control. The physical and psychological components of disability are known to be a source of much of the disability and it is believed that regaining greater physical capacity, particularly in the injured "weak link," combined with multimodal disability management will ultimately reduce pain perception. A temporary increase in pain during treatment is considered acceptable. Such programs have increased in popularity over the past 2 decades, with multiple outcome studies available in the lit-

erature. These programs use the measurement of physical and functional capacity to guide the rehabilitation approach quantitatively, limiting the amount of exercise so that patients neither exert excessive efforts nor do so little that their time is wasted. Quantification removes some of the subjectivity inherent in allowing patients to remain in treatment who are giving only a negligible effort while claiming they are "doing their best." A supportive psychological and case management program must provide education about pain control and stress management techniques, provide treatment to resolve the disability, reintegrate the patient into the work force, become involved in school or training as needed, and help in case settlement efforts. Modalities that may enhance mobility or help to control pain, such as intra-articular injections, transcutaneous electrical nerve stimulation, and anti-inflammatory or psychotropic medications may prove to be valuable adjuncts to such programs. Objectively documented outcomes that show return to productivity are the measure of success. Outcome measures for functional restoration programs include work status (for example, return to work and work retention), future healthcare system use (for example, additional surgery to the injured area, persistent healthcare-seeking behavior, number of visits to new providers), recurrent injury after work return (for example, new claims and lost time) and case closure (workers' compensation and third-party claims). Repeated use of pain or disability questionnaires may be useful, but should become the primary outcome measure only if the patient has no outstanding disability issues.

Palliative Pain Management

Many pain management specialists and pain clinics focus on palliation of pain rather than restoration of function. Efforts usually are focused on helping the patient reduce stress and tension while accepting a relatively nonfunctional lifestyle. Multidisciplinary assessment may result in recommendations for procedures that may not be beneficial to functional recovery, but which may ameliorate pain. These may include a variety of neuro-ablative procedures, radiofrequency neurotomies in the spine, spinal cord stimulation, or the use of intrathecal drug pumps. Treatment programs generally focus on psychological interventions, with only minimal physical rehabilitation. Although the physical component of functionally-oriented rehabilitation usually has greater intensity and more elements of supervision than secondary care options, physical components in palliative pain management rely more on elements of primary care (manipulation, acupuncture, massage, and thermal modalities) or very light exercise (aqua therapy, light stretching). Contributing to the limited physical aspects of these programs is a tendency to rely on narcotics as an active component of pain control, with acceptance of long-term narcotic use as a permanent component of the patient's medical care. Although psychotropic drugs and NSAIDs may also be used, the type of narcotic and dosage tends to determine much about the patient's ultimate physical and psychological well-being. The regular use of continuous release narcotics (for example, methadone, meperidine hydrochloride, hydromorphone hydrochloride), or narcotic pumps is a rapidly growing trend. Psychologic therapies focus on stress management and learning techniques to cope with inactivity and lack of societal productivity, even in younger individuals. Federal disability benefits (Supplemental Security or Social Security Disability benefits) provide a safety value for those with preretirement disabilities, with the number of patients receiving such payments increasing from four million to nine million in the United States over the past 20 years. These benefits have increased from $40 billion to $100 billion over the same time period, now accounting for 5% of the US federal budget. Outcome measurement may be problematic, because the patient's self-assessment of pain and health status may be markedly influenced by the treatment team and requirements for continued narcotic use.

Summary

Primary rehabilitation focuses on control of painful symptoms and prevention of sequelae of extensive immobility. Secondary rehabilitation stresses early reactivation of the patient with emphasis on stabilizing the injured area while improving flexibility, strength, endurance, and coordination skills. Tertiary care is reserved for patients with chronic disabling musculoskeletal pain that require a more comprehensive and often multidisciplinary approach to improve function even if some pain symptoms persist. Palliative care is provided when functional progress is no longer deemed feasible.

Annotated Bibliography

General

McGill SM: *Low Back Disorders: Evidence-Based Prevention and Rehabilitation.* Human Kinetics, Champaign, IL, 2002.

This book includes information on epidemiologic studies on low back disorders, relevant functional anatomy and normal and injury mechanics of the lumbar spine, scientifically based approaches to back pain prevention at work, and low back rehabilitation.

Primary Rehabilitation

Fritz JM, Delitto A, Erhard RE: Comparison of classification-based physical therapy with therapy based on clinical practice guidelines for patients with acute low back pain. *Spine* 2003;28:1363-1371.

Seventy-eight patients randomly received therapy based on a classification system or clinical practice guidelines. For patients with acute, work-related low back pain, the use of a classification-based approach resulted in improvement in disability and return-to-work status after 4 weeks as compared with therapy based on clinical guidelines.

Secondary Rehabilitation

Mayer T, Polatin P, Smith B, et al: Spine rehabilitation: Secondary and tertiary nonoperative care. *Spine J* 2003; 3(suppl 3):28S-36S.

This Contemporary Concepts Review presents a position statement of the North American Spine Society Board and summarizes aspects of secondary and tertiary rehabilitation specific to spinal disorders in greater detail.

van Tulder MW, Malmivaara A, Esmail R, Koes BW: Exercise therapy for low back pain, in The Cochrane Library (Update Software on CD-ROM), Issue 3, 2003.

Thirty-nine randomized controlled trials were identified. Exercise therapy was shown to be more effective than the usual care given by general practitioners and equally effective as conventional physiotherapy for chronic low back pain. Exercises may be helpful for patients with chronic low back pain to facilitate earlier return to normal daily activities and work.

Tertiary Rehabilitation

Anagnostis C, Mayer T, Gatchel R, Proctor TJ: The Million Visual Analog Scale: Its utility for predicting tertiary rehabilitation outcomes. *Spine* 2003;28:1051-1060.

When a validated disability outcome questionnaire is given to a group of patients with chronic disabling spinal disorders before and after tertiary rehabilitation, excellent predictive value for socioeconomic outcomes (work status, health system usage, recurrent injury 1 year after treatment) is identified, particularly in patients who report high levels of disability immediately after treatment.

Dersh J, Gatchel RJ, Polatin P: Chronic spinal disorders and psychopathology: Research findings and theoretical considerations. *Spine J* 2001;1:88-94.

This prospective study of the prevalence of psychopathology in a large sample of chronically disabled patients with work-related spinal disorders uses a validated clinician-administered instrument for psychiatric diagnosis. The Structured Clinical Interview for the *Diagnostic and Statistical Manual of Mental Disorders*, fourth edition was used.

Jouset N, Fanello S, Bontoux L, et al: Effects of functional restoration versus 3 hours per week of physical therapy: A randomized controlled study. *Spine* 2004;29: 487-494.

A functional restoration multidisciplinary approach featuring physical training and disability management proved better than therapy alone in a randomized controlled trial assessed by quantifiable outcomes.

Proctor TJ, Mayer TG, Gatchel RJ, McGeary DD: Unremitting health-care-utilization outcomes of tertiary rehabilitation of chronic musculoskeletal disorders. *J Bone Joint Surg Am* 2004;86:62-69.

Comparison of patients who persistently seek health care after tertiary rehabilitation with those who do not reveals that persistent healthcare seekers demonstrate poor outcomes in work-related injuries that lead to higher societal costs and decreased worker productivity.

Schonstein E, Kenny D, Keating J, Koes B, Herbert RD: Physical conditioning programs for workers with back and neck pain: A Cochrane systematic review. *Spine* 2003;28:E391-E395.

A meta-analysis by the Cochrane collaboration of randomized trials of chronic back pain in work-related injuries demonstrates that physical conditioning programs that incorporate a cognitive behavioral approach reduce work loss.

Classic Bibliography

Bendix AE, Bendix T, Haestrup C, Busch E: A prospective, randomized 5-year follow-up study of functional restoration in chronic low back pain patients. *Eur Spine J* 1998;7:111-119.

Hazard RG, Fenwick JW, Kalisch SM, et al: Functional restoration with behavioral support: A one-year prospective study of patients with chronic low-back pain. *Spine* 1989;14:157-161.

Jordan KD, Mayer TG, Gatchel RJ: Should extended disability be an exclusion criterion for tertiary rehabilitation? Socioeconomic outcomes of early versus late functional restoration in compensation spinal disorders. *Spine* 1998;23:2110-2117.

Mayer T, Gatchel R, Polatin P: *Occupational Musculoskeletal Disorders: Function, Outcomes and Evidence*. Lippincott Williams & Wilkins, Philadelphia, PA, 1999.

Mayer T, Gatchel R, Polatin P, Evans T: Outcomes comparison of treatment for chronic disabling work-related upper extremity disorders and spinal disorders. *J Occup Environ Med* 1999;41:761-770.

Mayer T, McMahon MJ, Gatchel RJ, Sparks B, Wright A, Pegues P: Socioeconomic outcomes of combined spine surgery and functional restoration in workers' compensation spinal disorders with matched controls. *Spine* 1998;23:598-606.

Mayer TG, Gatchel RJ, Mayer H, Kishino N, Keeley J, Mooney V: A prospective two-year study of functional restoration in industrial low back injury: An objective assessment procedure. *JAMA* 1987; 258:1763-1767.

Mazanec D: Medication use in sports rehabilitation, in Kibler WB, Herring SA, Press JM (eds): *Functional Rehabilitation of Sports and Musculoskeletal Injuries*. Gaithersburg, MD, Aspen, 1998, pp 71-79.

O'Sullivan PB, Phyty GD, Twomey LT, Allison GT: Evaluation of specific stabilizing exercise in the treatment of chronic low back pain with radiologic diagnosis of spondylolysis or spondylolisthesis. *Spine* 1997;22: 2959-2967.

Section 8

Pediatrics

Section Editor:
Randall T. Loder, MD

Chapter 56

Genetic Diseases and Skeletal Dysplasias

William G. Mackenzie, MD

R. Tracy Ballock, MD

Introduction

The recent advances in the fields of human and mouse genetics and molecular biology have led to rapid progress in understanding the etiology and pathogenesis of many human skeletal dysplasias and other genetic diseases affecting the skeleton. Some of these new findings relate to the diagnosis and treatment of children with inherited disorders affecting the skeleton.

Trisomy 21 (Down Syndrome)

Duplication of a portion of the long arm of chromosome 21 occurs once every 800 to 1,000 live births and results in the disorder known as Down syndrome. The most common chromosomal abnormality in humans, Down syndrome can be diagnosed prenatally by amniocentesis. Postnatal diagnosis can be made by recognition of the characteristic facies (upward slanting eyes, epicanthal folds, and a flattened profile) as well as the single transverse flexion crease in the palm (simian crease). Although mental retardation is usually associated with Down syndrome, the degree of mental deficiency is variable. Other abnormalities may include congenital heart disease, duodenal atresia, hypothyroidism, and hearing loss.

Children with Down syndrome may develop musculoskeletal problems as a result of the increased ligamentous laxity that occurs with this condition. Approximately 10% of patients will exhibit asymptomatic atlantoaxial instability. Therefore, it is recommended that children with Down syndrome have screening flexion-extension radiographs of the cervical spine obtained before athletic participation. Spinal cord compression is rare, and surgical intervention is reserved for children who exhibit symptoms of myelopathy (Figure 1).

In addition to C1-C2 instability, children with Down syndrome also may develop hip instability. Unlike typical hip dysplasia in which the shallow acetabulum allows progressive migration of the femoral head out of the socket, in children with Down syndrome the hip may dislocate out of an acetabulum that may be only mildly dysplastic. This is possible because of the degree of ligamentous laxity present. Brace treatment for 6 to 8

months to achieve stability has been recommended for children younger than 6 years. Surgical intervention for this type of hip dislocation has a high failure rate and has not been shown to improve outcomes.

Other musculoskeletal disorders occurring in children with Down syndrome are also the result of excess ligamentous laxity and joint instability. Patellofemoral subluxation and dislocation may develop in the absence of symptoms. Soft-tissue reconstruction alone is frequently unsuccessful in preventing recurrent instability. Pes planovalgus and hallux valgus are also common and usually respond to shoe wear modifications.

Turner's Syndrome

In 1 of every 3,000 live births, a single X chromosome (XO) is present instead of the normal XX or XY combination, resulting in Turner's syndrome. Patients are phenotypically females with short stature, a webbed neck,

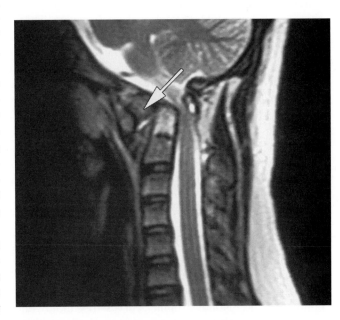

Figure 1 MRI showing spinal cord compression in a 12-year-old girl with Down syndrome. An os odontoideum (*arrow*) has become lodged between the ring of C1 and the dens. The patient had hyperreflexia but was otherwise neurologically intact.

Table 1 | Diagnostic Criteria for Neurofibromatosis 1

Six or more café-au-lait spots whose greatest diameter is 5 mm in pre-pubertal and 15 mm in postpubertal patients

Two or more neurofibromas of any type or one plexiform neurofibroma

Axillary freckling

Optic glioma

Two or more Lisch nodules (iris hamartomas)

A distinctive osseous lesion

A first-degree relative with neurofibromatosis 1

and a low hairline. Girls with Turner's syndrome do not pass through puberty or develop secondary sexual characteristics because of the lack of sex steroid hormones. Cubitus varus is a common finding in Turner's syndrome but rarely requires treatment. Scoliosis may also develop and management is similar to that for idiopathic curves.

Neurofibromatosis

Neurofibromatosis (NF) is divided into two distinct clinical entities, NF1 and NF2. NF1 is the most common single gene disorder, occurring once in every 3,000 births, and it results from a mutation in the gene encoding a protein now known as neurofibromin. Neurofibromin helps regulate cell growth through modulation of the Ras signaling pathway. The diagnosis of NF1 relies on identification of up to six clinical criteria (Table 1). Common clinical findings include café-au-lait macules, axillary freckles, Lisch nodules of the iris, and neurofibromas. Malignant transformation of a neurofibroma to a neurofibrosarcoma results if a somatic mutation occurs in the remaining normal copy of the gene. Therefore, neurofibromas that enlarge suddenly or become painful should be managed as potential sarcomas.

The typical bone lesion in neurofibromatosis is an anterolateral bowing deformity of the tibia that may progress to pseudarthrosis (Figure 2). Prophylactic bracing with a total contact orthosis is recommended to diminish the likelihood of pseudarthrosis formation. Once a pseudarthrosis is established, bone grafting with intramedullary fixation is the initial treatment. For persistent pseudarthroses, either a vascularized bone graft or bone transport by distraction osteogenesis may be required for healing. Although amputation and prosthetic fitting for recalcitrant pseudarthrosis may result in improved lower extremity function over these salvage techniques, this is not commonly performed.

Scoliosis occurs commonly in children with neurofibromatosis, and it is classified as either dystrophic or nondystrophic. Nondystrophic curves resemble idiopathic scoliosis and are managed in a similar fashion. Dystrophic curves are short and sharp, occurring over four to six spinal levels, and represent 80% of scoliosis

in children age 6 years or younger. Nondystrophic scoliosis in younger children can modulate into the dystrophic type over several years. Radiographic features of dystrophic scoliosis include scalloping of the vertebral end plates, foraminal enlargement, and penciling of the ribs. These dystrophic curves are notoriously resistant to brace treatment and will progress if not treated by early anterior and posterior fusion. Preoperative MRI is essential to identify areas of dural ectasia and intraspinal neurofibromas.

Hereditary Multiple Exostosis

Hereditary multiple exostosis (HME) is an autosomal dominant disorder with a prevalence of 1 in 50,000 patients. Bony projections with cartilage caps develop near the ends of multiple long bones (Figure 3). These exostoses continue to grow until skeletal maturity is reached, and they may cause partial growth inhibition in the adjacent physis, resulting in limb deformity, limb-length discrepancy, and occasionally subluxation of an adjacent joint. Although initially a benign lesion, the risk of transformation to a malignant chondrosarcoma or osteosarcoma has been estimated at 0.5% to 3%, which is higher than the general population risk.

HME is caused by mutations in *EXT1* or *EXT2*, members of a newly described family of putative tumor suppressor genes that encode glycosyltransferases. EXT1 and EXT2 proteins have been localized by immunohistochemical techniques to the Golgi apparatus of the cell, where they form a protein complex that is responsible for the biosynthesis of heparan sulfate glycosaminoglycans. The consequence of the disease-causing mutations is loss of heparan sulfate on the cell surface, where the molecule frequently functions as a coreceptor for peptide growth factors to increase binding affinity.

Although *EXT* genes are ubiquitously expressed, the disease appears to only result in aberrant proliferation of growth plate chondrocytes. Histologically, abnormal cytoskeletal inclusions consisting of actin and α-actinin are found in chondrocytes comprising the cartilage cap. The relationship between this observation and the aberrant chondrocyte proliferation is unclear, however. Recently it has been demonstrated that the *Drosophila EXT1* homolog *tout-velu* is necessary for the diffusion of the hedgehog protein in the developing wing tissue of the fly by affecting the transduction of the hedgehog signal across adjacent cells. Therefore, *EXT* mutations may also affect the function of the Indian hedgehog protein in the growth plate, whose role is to modulate the rate at which chondrocytes stop proliferating and differentiate into hypertrophic cells.

Current genetic observations indicate that HME may not be a true chondrodysplasia, but rather a neoplastic condition. According to the Knudsen "two-hit"

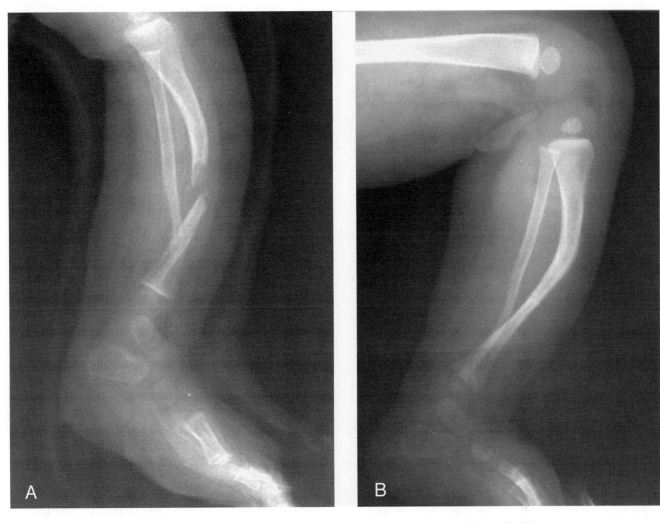

Figure 2 Radiograph showing anterolateral bowing in a child with neurofibromatosis, which progressed to congenital pseudarthrosis of the tibia.

model of tumor suppressor gene inactivation in cancer, both copies of the gene must be inactivated to abolish the normal tumor suppressor activity. In hereditary cancer, the first hit usually consists of a germline mutation, whereas the second hit is the inactivation of the remaining wild-type copy through a somatic mutation. This model has recently been applied to patients with HME. An inherited haploinsufficiency (malfunction of one of the two working copies of a gene within the cell) combined with a subsequent loss of function in the remaining copy of the gene through a somatic mutation is required for osteochondroma formation. The growth dysregulation that ensues then predisposes the cell to further genetic alterations, resulting in chondrosarcoma in a small percentage of patients.

Skeletal Dysplasias

Achondroplasia and Related Disorders

Several chondrodysplasia phenotypes result from mutations in the fibroblast growth factor receptor 3 gene, in-

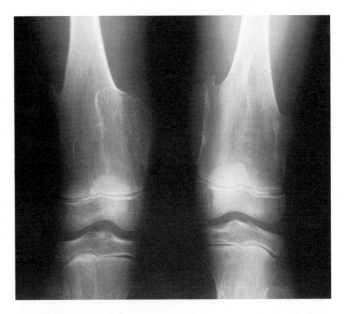

Figure 3 Typical radiographic appearance of multiple osteochondromas around the knees in a patient with hereditary multiple exostosis.

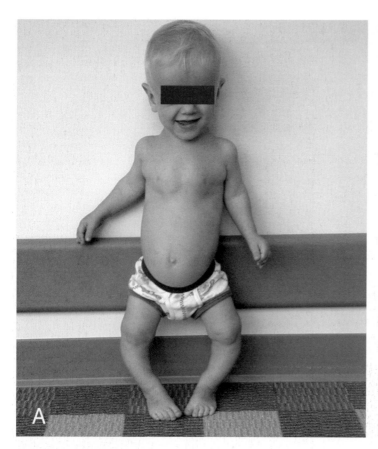

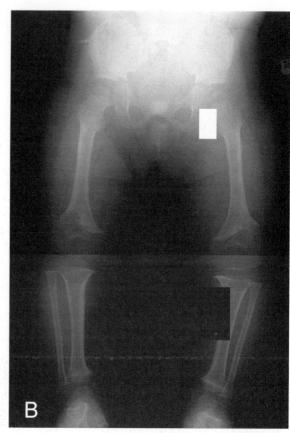

Figure 4 Typical clinical **(A)** and radiographic **(B)** findings in a child with achondroplasia.

cluding achondroplasia, hypochondroplasia, thanatophoric dysplasia, and severe achondroplasia with developmental delay and acanthosis nigricans dysplasia. These disorders are closely related and represent a continuum of severity.

Achondroplasia

Achondroplasia, the most common form of dwarfism, is an autosomal dominant disorder that is caused by a single nucleotide substitution. More than 90% of instances of achondroplasia result from a sporadic mutation. The specific mutation in achondroplasia converts either guanine to arginine or guanine to cysteine at position 380 in the transmembrane domain of the protein, resulting in a glycine to arginine substitution. This single amino acid substitution not only causes stabilization of the fibroblast growth factor receptor protein and its accumulation on the cell surface, but also results in uncontrolled, prolonged ligand-dependent activation of the receptor. The result of this sustained fibroblast growth factor receptor activity is growth retardation in the proliferative zone of the growth plate, leading to decreased bone length. The most profound effect on the skeleton is in the areas of greatest endochondral growth (humerus and femur), resulting in the characteristic rhizomelia. The rhizomelic pattern of shortening in children with

achondroplasia involves the proximal limb bones, including the humerus and femur, whereas children with other disorders have mesomelia (shortening of the forearm and leg) and acromelia (shortening of the hands and feet). The diagnosis is often made prenatally by ultrasound; if not identified prenatally, this disorder is identified at birth by the presence of rhizomelic shortening, a trunk of normal length, macrocephaly, frontal bossing, a depressed nasal bridge, and trident hands (Figure 4). Elbow flexion contractures are the result of bowing of the distal humerus and posterior radial head subluxation/dislocation. Classic radiographic findings include shortening of the long bones, progressive narrowing of the interpedicular distance through the lumbar spine, squared iliac wings, horizontal acetabula, and narrow sacrosciatic notches.

Foramen magnum and upper cervical stenosis is a life-threatening disorder that affects these children at birth and in early life. Cervicomedullary cord compression can result in hypotonia, delayed development, weakness, and apnea. The central apnea can be complicated by obstructive components, including abnormal nasopharyngeal development and enlarged tonsils and adenoids. Routine perinatal screening with MRI is controversial. Symptomatic children are typically assessed with MRI and a sleep study. Surgical management in-

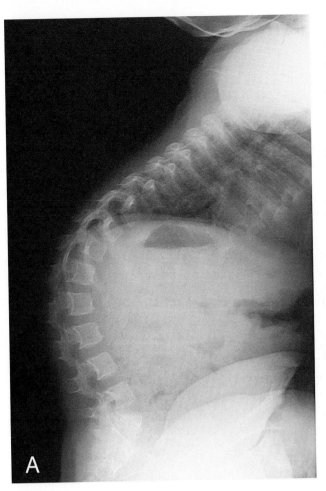
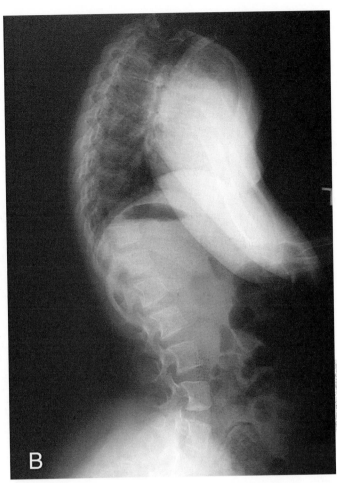

Figure 5 A and **B** Radiographs showing spontaneous correction of thoracolumbar kyphosis.

cludes decompression and occasionally shunting for hydrocephalus. Unlike other forms of skeletal dysplasias, cervical instability is rare.

Thoracolumbar kyphosis occurs commonly in infants. It is thought to be secondary to truncal hypotonia and weakness and an enlarged head. Avoidance of propped sitting is advocated. The kyphosis typically resolves as children achieve independent ambulation (later than in children of average stature with achondroplasia who typically have a mean walking age range of 18 to 24 months) (Figure 5).

Bracing is reserved for those children with severe progressive kyphosis and wedging of the apical vertebra. Anterior and posterior spinal fusion is indicated in older children with persistent severe kyphosis, but it is rarely required. Lumbar spinal stenosis is common (30% of children are symptomatic in the second decade), and it is caused by interpedicular narrowing, short pedicles, disk bulging, and hyperlordosis. In older patients, the stenosis is aggravated by degenerative changes. Lumbosacral decompression is recommended for patients with symptomatic spinal stenosis. Spinal fusion is required in addition to decompression in patients with thoracolumbar kyphosis and those with significant degenerative changes. Scoliosis is unusual in this patient population.

Genu varum is typical in over 90% of patients with achondroplasia. The deformity may occur at multiple levels, including the distal femur, the proximal and distal tibia, and through the lateral ligaments of the knee. Realignment osteotomies are recommended for patients with progressive, symptomatic genu varum. Correction of the associated internal tibial torsion is done concurrently.

Short stature in achondroplasia is moderately severe and can result in functional limitations. Teenagers with achondroplasia have concerns about their body image. Adult studies indicate that function and self-image in patients with achondroplasia are similar to those of average-statured adults. Growth hormone has been advocated in growing children, but its use is controversial because the improvement in final height is variable. Extended limb lengthening to increase stature has been used commonly in Europe, but is more controversial in North America. Long-term effects on the adjacent articular surfaces have not been well studied.

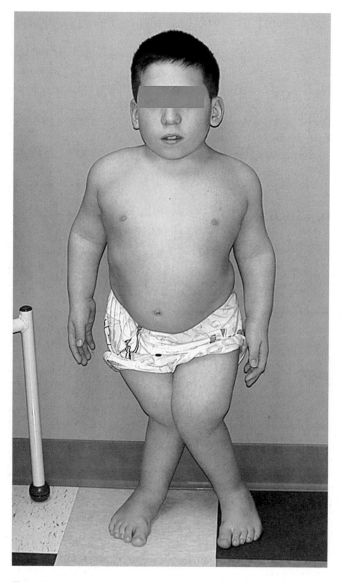

Figure 6 Photograph showing typical clinical appearance of a child with spondyloepiphyseal dysplasia congenita.

Hypochondroplasia

Hypochondroplasia is an autosomal dominant disorder with clinical features and radiographic findings similar to those associated with achondroplasia, but to a milder degree. The diagnosis is rarely apparent before age 2 years and typically results from investigation of short stature. Musculoskeletal problems that present for management in hypochondroplasia include lumbar spinal stenosis, genu varum, and short stature. Management of hypochondroplasia is the same as for the disorders associated with achondroplasia.

Thanatophoric Dysplasia

Thanatophoric dysplasia is a severe, usually lethal disorder resulting from mutations in the fibroblast growth factor receptor 3. Clinical features of this dysplasia include rhizomelic shortening, macrocephaly, platyspondyly, and severe restrictive lung disease resulting from a small thoracic cavity.

Severe Achondroplasia With Developmental Delay and Acanthosis Nigricans Dysplasia

Children with severe achondroplasia with developmental delay and acanthosis nigricans dysplasia exhibit extreme short stature, developmental delay, acanthosis nigricans, and genu varum.

Dysplasias Secondary to Type II Collagen Abnormalities

This spectrum of disorders includes spondyloepiphyseal dysplasia congenita, spondyloepimetaphyseal dysplasia, and Kniest dysplasia.

Spondyloepiphyseal Dysplasia

Spondyloepiphyseal dysplasias are characterized by short stature secondary to a short trunk and short limbs. Many different types of this disorder exist, with the most common type being the congenita form. This is caused by mutations in *COL2A1* (collagen type II α 1 chain). This gene encodes type II collagen, which is found primarily in cartilage and in the vitreous humor, locations consistent with the phenotype of spondyloepiphyseal dysplasia congenita and other disorders such as Kniest dysplasia and type I Stickler's syndrome. Radiographic changes include abnormal spinal development with odontoid hypoplasia and platyspondyly, abnormal formation of the long bone epiphyses with variable metaphyseal involvement, and generalized delay in epiphyseal ossification. The diagnosis is made at birth. Patients have marked short stature with a very short trunk and often a barrel-shaped chest (Figure 6). Lumbar lordosis is typical, and progressive kyphoscoliosis occurs. Retinal detachment, severe myopia, and sensorineural hearing loss are common in childhood and adult life.

Atlantoaxial instability resulting from odontoid hypoplasia and ligamentous laxity must be evaluated early in life and monitored on a regular basis with flexion-extension lateral C-spine radiographs and/or MRI. Surgical management is indicated in patients with significant instability or cervical myelopathy. Progressive kyphoscoliosis in the growing child can be managed with a brace; however, with progression, surgical management is usually required. Lower extremity malalignment is common in these children. Coxa vara, genu valgum, valgus alignment of the distal tibia, and planovalgus foot deformities are typical. These deformities can result in significant gait abnormalities consisting of increased lumbar lordosis, a waddling gait, and a crouch gait with the knees knocking together. The coxa vara is often progressive and is difficult to assess radiographically because of the delayed capital femoral ossification (Figure 7).

When considering realignment of the lower extremities, deformity at the hip, knee, and ankle must be considered and managed together. Abnormal epiphyseal development typically results in early osteoarthritis of the weight-bearing joints, and most young adults require total joint arthroplasty. There is no evidence that realignment osteotomies will delay the need for joint arthroplasty.

An uncommon tarda form of spondyloepiphyseal dysplasia is milder and presents later in the first decade of life. This form has X-linked inheritance and is caused by a mutation in the *SEDL* gene, which is thought to be involved in vesicle transport from the endoplasmic reticulum to the Golgi apparatus. Patients with this type of spondyloepiphyseal dysplasia present with deformities that are milder but similar to those of patients with spondyloepiphyseal dysplasia congenita. In this patient population, the upper cervical spine must be assessed, scoliosis may develop, and osteoarthritis frequently occurs in later life.

Kniest Dysplasia

Kniest dysplasia is an autosomal dominant disorder caused by mutations in *COL2A1*. The trunk is disproportionately shorter than the limbs in patients with Kniest dysplasia, and the face is flattened with midface hypoplasia. Myopia, retinal detachment, deafness, joint contractures, limb malalignment, and kyphoscoliosis can occur throughout life in this patient population. The radiographic features include dumbbell-shaped long bones with broad metaphyses and irregular dysplastic epiphyses. Joint stiffness and pain typically result from deterioration of the articular cartilage.

Metaphyseal Chondrodysplasia

Although many forms of metaphyseal dysplasia have been described, metaphyseal involvement with short stature and bowing of the legs is a common feature to all. The most common Schmid type is autosomal dominant and is caused by a type X collagen mutation (*COL110A1*). This type is the mildest in this group, with patients typically exhibiting moderate short stature, a waddling gait, and genu varum. The diagnosis is usually made in early childhood. The radiographic features resemble those seen in patients with rickets and include metaphyseal irregularity and flaring with widening of the physes.

The Jansen type is a rare autosomal dominant disorder caused by a mutation in the parathyroid hormone receptor gene that regulates the differentiation of growth plate chondrocytes. Severe short stature with deformity is typical, and some affected children have hypercalcemia, hypercalciuria, and hyperphosphaturia.

The McKusick type is an autosomal recessive disorder (also called cartilage-hair hypoplasia) caused by a

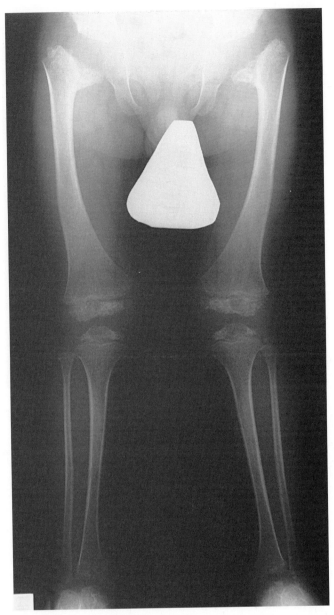

Figure 7 Radiograph showing coxa vara in a child with spondyloepiphyseal dysplasia congenita.

mutation of *RMRP*, a nuclear gene (RNA component of mitochondrial RNA processing endoribonuclease). Patients with this disorder have fine, sparse body hair and significant complications, including impaired cellular immunity, anemia, Hirschsprung's disease, and malignancy. Patients with metaphyseal chondrodysplasia may need surgical management of short stature and limb malalignment (Figure 8).

Pseudoachondroplasia

Pseudoachondroplasia is an autosomal dominant disorder caused by a mutation in the gene encoding for cartilage oligomeric matrix protein (COMP). COMP is an extracellular calcium-binding glycoprotein belonging to

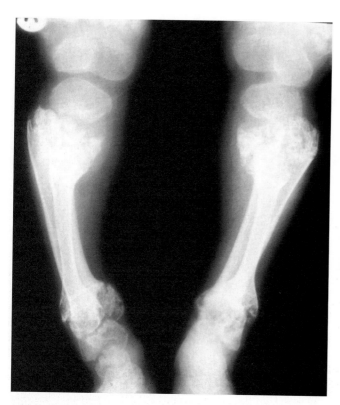

Figure 8 Radiographic appearance of the knees of a patient with Jansen metaphyseal chondrodysplasia.

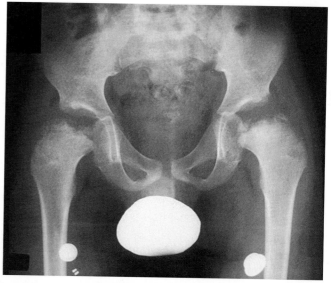

Figure 9 Radiographic appearance of the hips of a patient with multiple epiphyseal dysplasia.

the thrombospondin family, and it is involved in chondrocyte migration and proliferation. The COMP molecule is composed of five flexible arms with large globular domains at the end of each arm, resembling a bouquet of flowers. Mutations affecting the type III repeat region or C-terminal domain of the protein result in decreased calcium binding caused by a structural change in the protein. Approximately 30% of patients have an in-frame deletion mutation, resulting in four aspartic acid residues instead of five at amino acids 469 through 473 of the protein. It is interesting to note that mutations in the *COMP* gene have also been discovered in patients with multiple epiphyseal dysplasia. This suggests that pseudoachondroplasia and multiple epiphyseal dysplasia, although originally described as distinct disorders, are now recognized as part of a disease spectrum.

Children with pseudoachondroplasia have a short trunk and short limb dysplasia that is not usually diagnosed until early childhood. Atlantoaxial instability is common. Generalized ligamentous laxity is present, and this is particularly noticeable in the hands (the fingers are short and hypermobile). Radiographic features include shortening of the long bones with irregular, expanded metaphyses and small fragmented epiphyses. Evidence of platyspondyly can be observed with unique anterior projections. Genu valgum, genu varum, or windswept deformities of the lower extremities can also

be observed. Limb alignment procedures are indicated for patients with severe progressive deformities that interfere with function, but there is a high rate of recurrence because of ligamentous laxity and abnormal bone growth. Early arthritis resulting in hip arthroplasty occurs in about one third of patients with this disorder by the fourth decade of life.

Multiple Epiphyseal Dysplasia

Multiple epiphyseal dysplasia (MED) describes a spectrum of autosomal dominant disorders characterized by epiphyseal dysplastic changes resulting in mild to moderate short stature, genu valgum, and early onset osteoarthritis. Short, hyperextensible fingers are present in patients with severe involvement. The diagnosis is usually made in midchildhood, with reports of pain and joint stiffness in patients with short stature. Radiographs demonstrate delayed epiphyseal ossification with subsequent irregular development of the epiphyses. The spine is usually not affected. The clinical phenotypes are variable, ranging from mild epiphyseal abnormalities in the hips that can lead to a misdiagnosis of bilateral Legg-Calvé-Perthes disease to severe widespread epiphyseal dysplasia with joint contractures, osteoarthritis, and short stature.

In the hips of children with MED, capital femoral ossification is delayed with subsequent fragmented ossification, and it eventually coalesces to form an intact but small ossific nucleus. Although the radiographic appearance in the fragmented stage appears similar to that seen in patients with Legg-Calvé-Perthes disease, the typical stages of sclerosis, collapse, fragmentation, and reossification are not apparent (Figure 9). Osteonecrosis can occur in the hips of patients with MED, thereby complicating the radiographic appearance. Management in this circumstance is similar to the containment methods used for patients with Legg-Calvé-Perthes disease. Painful, stiff joints are managed by avoidance of activities that result in significant joint stress, administration of nonsteroidal anti-inflammatory drugs, and aquatic and physical therapy. The typical genu valgum can be managed by staple hemiepiphysiodesis or osteotomy. Progressive osteoarthritis usually results in total joint arthroplasty.

Three separate genetic loci have been linked to MED. As noted previously, mutations causing all clinical forms of MED have been identified in the gene encoding COMP. The phenotype of the mild pseudoachondroplasia patients overlaps with those of MED. Other mutations have been identified in *COL9A2*, which encodes the α 2 chain of type IX collagen. Type IX collagen is a nonfibrillar heterotrimeric molecule with three chains encoded by three different genes. It is a structural component of hyaline cartilage, intervertebral disks, and the vitreous body of the eye. Type IX collagen decorates the surface of type II collagen molecules to which it is covalently cross-linked. Its function is postulated to involve mediating the interaction of type II collagen with other extracellular matrix components in cartilage.

The phenotype of the *COL9A2* mutants seems to be milder without hip involvement compared with the more severe disease caused by mutations in *COMP*. All mutations in *COL9A2* described to date result in splicing errors that eliminate exon 3, and hence delete 12 amino acids from the N-terminal portion of the molecule. This may affect the structure and function of the molecule in mediating interactions between type II collagen molecules and other extracellular matrix components.

Recently, an unclassified form of MED has been linked to *COL9A3* in a four-generation family with autosomal dominant disease. This is the first disease-causing mutation to be identified in *COL9A3*, which encodes another of the three α chains of type IX collagen. The phenotype of the *COL9A3* mutants overlaps significantly with *COL9A2* mutants, but it differs by the presence of hip involvement.

Ellis-van Creveld Syndrome

Ellis-van Creveld syndrome is an autosomal recessive disorder characterized by postaxial hand polydactyly, short stature with mesoacromelic shortening, sparse, thin hair, and dysplastic nails and teeth. Severe congenital heart disease is seen in approximately 60% of children with this disorder. The diagnosis is typically made at birth. The radiographic features include the postaxial polydactyly, fusion of the capitate and hamate, and medial spikes projecting from the iliac bones. Children with Ellis-van Creveld syndrome develop severe genu val-

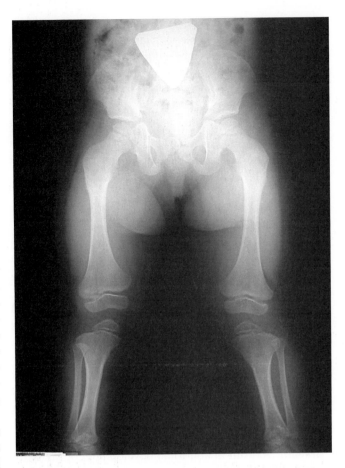

Figure 10 Radiograph showing genu valgum in a patient with Ellis-van Creveld syndrome.

gum resulting from characteristic deficiency of the anterolateral tibial epiphyses (Figure 10). Realignment typically requires femoral and tibial osteotomies.

Ellis-van Creveld syndrome has recently been linked to a new gene named *EVC*, which encodes a protein that has no homology to known proteins. It is expressed at higher levels in the distal limb than the proximal limb in human embryonic tissue, and it is also expressed in the developing vertebral bodies, ribs, heart, kidneys, and lungs. Although the structure of the *EVC* gene product includes both putative nuclear localization signals and a transmembrane domain, its function is currently unknown.

Dyschondrosteosis (Leri-Weill Syndrome)

Dyschondrosteosis (Leri-Weill syndrome) is a common dominant disorder resulting in mild short stature, mesomelic shortening, and Madelung's deformity. The radiographic features are typical of Madelung's deformity, with bowing of the radius and dorsal dislocation of the ulna. Mutations in the short stature homeobox (*SHOX*) gene have recently been implicated as the cause of dyschondrosteosis. Located at the very tip of the short arms of both sex chromosomes, the *SHOX* gene encodes a homeobox-containing DNA transcription factor. *SHOX* defects also appear to be associated with growth failure in Turner's syndrome, although it is not clear why female patients with Turner's syndrome do not develop dyschondrosteosis.

Disorders Caused by Abnormalities in Genes Important in Normal Skeletal Development

This spectrum of disorders includes cleidocranial dysostosis and nail-patella syndrome.

Cleidocranial Dysostosis

Cleidocranial dysostosis is an autosomal dominant disorder with subtle clinical features consisting of a broad forehead, delayed closure of the anterior fontanel, increased ability to appose the shoulders, shortening of the middle phalanges of the third through fifth fingers, delayed eruption of the permanent dentition, and mild short stature. The diagnosis can be made at birth but is often delayed. Radiographic features include multiple wormian bones in the skull, with delayed closure of the sutures and anterior fontanel. The clavicles are small and absent, and there is widening of the symphysis pubis. The disorder is caused by a mutation of core binding factor α1 (*CBFA1*). *CBFA1* is a gene that is important in the induction of osteoblast differentiation. The clinical features result in abnormal development of the anterior midline skeleton. Coxa vara can occur, and if symptomatic or progressive, it can be corrected with a proximal femoral osteotomy.

Nail-Patella Syndrome

Nail-patella syndrome or osteoonychodysplasia is an autosomal dominant disorder characterized by aplasia or hypoplasia of the patellae and dysplastic nails, with the thumbnails being most commonly involved. Mutations of the Lim homeobox transcription factor 1β (*LMX1B*) gene cause this syndrome. *LMX1B* is involved in determining normal dorsoventral patterning in the developing limb bud, and it is expressed in the eyes and kidneys. Up to 30% of affected individuals develop renal failure by the fourth decade of life. Glaucoma is another complication associated with this disorder. The radiographic features include small or absent patellae and iliac horns. Posterior dislocation of the radial head limits elbow extension. Knee deformity and patellar malalignment may require soft-tissue releases and realignment osteotomies.

Disorders Caused by Abnormalities in Genes That Play a Role in the Processing of Proteins

This spectrum of disorders includes diastrophic dysplasia and a large group of lysosomal storage diseases called mucopolysaccharidoses.

Diastrophic Dysplasia

Diastrophic dysplasia is an autosomal recessive disorder characterized by marked short stature and progressive deformity. The diagnosis can be made prenatally by ultrasound and by findings at birth, including a cleft palate, tracheomalacia, hitchhiker thumbs, and bilateral equinocavovarus or skewfoot deformities. Cervical kyphosis is typically present in the perinatal period and in later childhood, joint contractures develop, and kyphoscoliosis is common. Cauliflower ear deformities resulting from cystic swelling in the cartilage of the ear commonly develop after birth.

Mutations in the diastrophic dysplasia sulfate transporter gene have been identified as causing diastrophic dysplasia. The diastrophic dysplasia sulfate transporter gene is ubiquitously expressed and encodes a protein that facilitates the transport of sulfate across the cell membrane. The disease primarily affects cartilage because of the importance of negatively charged sulfate groups in the function of proteoglycan molecules, which is to maintain the hydration and compressive strength of cartilage. One in 70 Finnish citizens are carriers of a mutant diastrophic dysplasia sulfate transporter gene.

Cervical kyphosis often resolves spontaneously. Progressive deformity and/or spinal cord compression requires surgical management. Kyphoscoliosis can also occur in the thoracolumbar spine; if progressive, it typically requires anterior and posterior spinal fusion. Early hip development is normal, but most children with this disorder develop hip flexion contractures with epiphyseal irregularity. End stage osteoarthritis is managed with total joint arthroplasty. Patients with diastrophic dysplasia often have flexion contractures of the knees, valgus alignment, and patellar dislocation. Surgical realignment of the knees can be difficult in these patients. Congenital foot deformities include the equinocavovarus feet or skew feet. The traditional surgical management results in rigid deformities with a high rate of recurrence, of which recurrent equinus is the most common. Supramalleolar osteotomies are often needed for realignment.

Mucopolysaccharidoses

The mucopolysaccharidoses consist of a large group of lysosomal storage diseases. Abnormal function of lysosomal enzymes results in the intracellular accumulation of partially degraded compounds. The mucopolysaccharidoses are subdivided by the enzymatic deficiency and the accumulation of these partially degraded compounds (Table 2). The subtypes are inherited in an autosomal recessive manner, with the exception of Hunter's syndrome, which is a sex-linked recessive disorder.

The clinical features vary depending on the severity of the subtype. Corneal clouding, deafness, hepatosplenomegaly, and cardiovascular abnormality all are present in Hurler's syndrome, and children with this dis-

Table 2 | Mucopolysaccharidoses Subtypes

Subtype	Cause	Prognosis
Type I H (Hurler's syndrome)	Alpha-L-iduronidase deficiency	Type I H: Death in the first decade of life
Type I HS (Hurler-Scheie syndrome)		Type I HS: Death in third decade of life
Type I S (Scheie's syndrome)		Type I S: Good survival
Type II (Hunter's syndrome)	Sulpho-iduronate-sulphatase deficiency	Death in second decade of life
Type III (Sanfilippo's syndrome)	Multiple enzyme deficiency	Death in second decade of life
Type IV (Morquio's syndrome)	Type A (galactosamine-6-sulfate-sulphatase deficiency)	More severe involvement in patients with type IV A than in those with type IV B; survival into adulthood is possible
	Type B (beta-galactosidase deficiency)	
Type VI (Maroteaux-Lamy syndrome)	Arylsulphatase B deficiency	Poor survival with severe form
Type VII (Sly's syndrome)	Beta-glycuronidase deficiency	Poor survival

order usually die in the first decade of life. Morquio syndrome, in contrast, has a much better prognosis, and there is only mild corneal clouding with deafness, no hepatosplenomegaly, and only mild cardiovascular abnormalities. Biochemical analysis of the urine can lead to the diagnosis of the specific mucopolysaccharidoses. Specific enzyme activity known to be abnormal can be detected in skin fibroblast culture and prenatally using chorion villous sampling. All of the subtypes lead to short stature; patients with Morquio syndrome are the most severely affected. Although there are common radiographic findings among this group of disorders, it is not possible to differentiate the various types based on radiographic features alone. The skull is enlarged with a thick calvarium. The ribs are broader anteriorly than posteriorly. The vertebral bodies are ovoid when immature, but in time they develop platyspondyly. In patients with Morquio syndrome, an anterior beak develops at the thoracolumbar junction (Figure 11). Kyphoscoliosis is common. Epiphyseal ossification is delayed, and marked deformity of the joints can develop. The second through fifth metacarpals are narrowed at their proximal ends and the phalanges are bullet-shaped.

Atlantoaxial instability resulting from odontoid hypoplasia and ligamentous laxity is very common, particularly in patients with Morquio syndrome. Soft-tissue deposition in this area also results in further narrowing of the spinal canal. Children with this disorder must be very carefully evaluated for clinical signs of cervical myelopathy and for any evidence of atlantoaxial instability. Treatment is by surgical stabilization of this area and decompression if required. Thoracolumbar kyphosis with anterior wedging is commonly seen in patients with Morquio's syndrome. Bracing may be required; if it is progressive, anterior and posterior fusion is indicated. Severe hip deformity is common in this patient population, and proximal femoral and periacetabular osteotomies are typically used to realign the hip. Genu valgum can be secondary to distal femoral or proximal tibial valgus. If severe and interfering with function, realign-

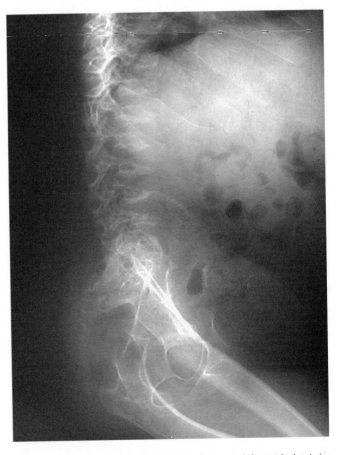

Figure 11 Radiograph showing the presence of characteristic vertebral anterior beaking in a patient with Morquio syndrome.

ment can be achieved by osteotomies or staple hemiepiphysiodesis in the growing child.

Bone marrow transplantation has been used successfully to treat patients with Hurler's syndrome and other mucopolysaccharidoses. Although there has been improvement in the coarse facies and hepatosplenomegaly, the neurologic abnormalities and skeletal deformities persist. Extensive research in the areas of gene therapy and enzyme replacement is ongoing.

Annotated Bibliography

General Reference

Flynn M, Pauli R: Double heterozygosity in bone growth disorders: Four new observations and review. *Am J Med Genet* 2003;121A:193-208.

This article reviews the complex progeny with double heterozygosity and reports that matings between individuals with short stature are common.

Unger S: A genetic approach to the diagnosis of skeletal dysplasia. *Clin Orthop* 2002;401:32-38.

The author recommends that molecular investigation of a skeletal dysplasia should be undertaken only after a limited differential diagnosis is established.

Trisomy 21 (Down Syndrome)

Doyle JS, Lauerman WC, Wood KB, Krause DR: Complications and long-term outcomes of upper cervical spine arthrodesis in patients with Down syndrome. *Spine* 1996;21:1223-1231.

In this outcome study of patients with Down syndrome who underwent upper cervical spine arthrodesis, 11 of 15 patients (73%) had 23 major complications, including nonunion, loss of reduction, neurologic deterioration, late subaxial instability, infection, and wound dehiscence.

Winell J, Burke SW: Sports participation of children with Down syndrome. *Orthop Clin North Am* 2003;34:439-443.

The authors report that patients with Down syndrome can actively participate in athletic activities if their orthopaedic problems are appropriately managed.

Turner's Syndrome

Batch J: Turner syndrome in childhood and adolescence. *Best Pract Res Clin Endocrinol Metab* 2002;16:465-482.

The authors provide a review of the clinical features of patients with Turner's syndrome and discuss management issues.

Ogata T: SHOX haploinsufficency and its modifying factors. *J Pediatr Endocrinol Metab* 2002;15:1289-1294.

This article describes the clinical findings and pathophysiology of SHOX mutations in patients with Turner's syndrome.

Neurofibromatosis

Durrani AA, Crawford AH, Choudry SN, Saifuddin A, Morley TR: Modulation of spinal deformities in patients with neurofibromatosis type I. *Spine* 2000;25:69-75.

In this review of 91 patients with neurofibromatosis and spinal deformity, the authors report that nondystrophic curves may modulate into dystrophic curves, particularly before age 7 years.

Karol LA, Haideri NF, Halliday SE, Smitherman TB, Johnston CE II: Gait analysis and muscle strength in children with congenital pseudarthrosis of the tibia: The effect of treatment. *J Pediatr Orthop* 1998;18:381-386.

The authors of this study report that patients with healed congenital pseudarthrosis of the tibia demonstrated muscle weakness and inefficient gait compared with patients who were treated by amputation.

Parisini P, Di Silvestri M, Greggi T, Paderni S, Cervellati S, Savini R: Surgical correction of dystrophic spinal curves in neurofibromatosis: A review of 56 patients. *Spine* 1999;24:2247-2253.

In this study of patients with neurofibromatosis who underwent surgical correction of dystrophic spinal curves, the authors report that the failure incidence of posterior instrumentation and fusion alone was 53% of patients, and for combined anterior fusion and posterior fusion it was 23%.

Hereditary Multiple Exostosis

Duncan G, McCormick C, Tufaro F: The link between heparan sulfate and hereditary bone disease: Finding a function for the EXT family of putative tumor suppressor proteins. *J Clin Invest* 2001;108:511-516.

The authors of this article review the biology of EXT proteins in vivo and explore the possible roles of these proteins in normal bone development and the formation of exostoses.

Koziel L, Kunath M, Kelly OG, Vortkamp A: Ext1-dependent heparan sulfate regulates the range of Ihh signaling during endochonral ossification. *Dev Cell* 2004;6:801-813.

Exostosin 1 is necessary for the synthesis of heparan sulfate chains of proteoglycans. These regulate the signaling of several growth factors. The authors also found that the loss of tout velu in Drosophila inhibits Hedgehog movement.

Skeletal Dysplasias

Aldegheri R, Dall'Oca C: Limb lengthening in short statured patients. *J Pediatr Orthop B* 2001;10:238-247.

In this article, the authors provide a good review of limb lengthening for stature.

Cooper S, Flaitz C, Johnston D, Lee B, Hecht J: A natural history of cleidocranial dysplasia. *Am J Med Genet* 2001;104:1-6.

This is a review of orthopaedic and other abnormalities observed in patients with cleidocranial dysplasia. The authors also provide management recommendations.

Dalvie S, Skinner J, Vellodi A, Noorden M: Mobile thoracolumbar gibbus in Morquio Type A: The cause of paraparesis and its management. *J Pediatr Orthop B* 2001;10:328-330.

In this article, the authors report that supine spine MRI may underestimate spinal stenosis and cord compression because of mobility of the thoracolumbar kyphosis in patients with Morquio syndrome.

Gomez P, Garcia O, Ginebreda M, Gairi T, Vilarrubius G: Lumbar canal stenosis in achondroplasia: Prevention and correction of lumbosacral lordosis. *An Esp Pediatr* 2001;54:126-131.

The authors of this article report that femoral lengthening improves lumbar hyperlordosis and reduces the symptoms of lumbar spinal stenosis.

Helenius I, Remes V, Tallroth K, Peltonen J, Possa M, Paavilainen T: Total hip arthroplasty in diastrophic dysplasia. *J Bone Joint Surg Am* 2003;85-A:441-447.

The authors of this article report that the rate of implant survival is good and that Harris hip scores increased significantly in patients with diastrophic dysplasia who underwent total hip arthroplasty.

Kitoh H, Kitakoji T, Kurita K, Katoh M, Takamine Y: Deformities of the elbow in achondroplasia. *J Bone Joint Surg Br* 2002;84:680-683.

The authors of this article report that posterior bowing of the distal humerus (primarily) and posterior dislocation of the radial head result in loss of elbow extension.

Morgan K, Rehman M, Schwartz R: Morquio's syndrome and its anaesthetic considerations. *Paediatr Anaesth* 2002;12:641-644.

The authors of this article provide a review of anesthetic care for children with Morquio syndrome.

Munns C, Glass I, LaBrom R, et al: Histopathological analysis of Leri-Weill dyschondrosteosis: Disordered growth plate. *Hand Surg* 2001;6:13-23.

The authors of this article report that the zone of dyschondrosteosis is characterized by marked disruption of the normal physeal arrangement.

Remes V, Marttinen E, Poussa M, Helenius I, Peltonen J: Cervical spine in patients with diastrophic dysplasia: Radiographic findings in 122 patients. *Pediatr Radiol* 2002;32:621-628.

The authors of this article report that the most common alignment of the cervical spine in adulthood is cervical lordosis and that degenerative changes are common. As the prevalence of spina bifida occulta is high, the authors recommend that care be taken during the surgical approach for patients with diastrophic dysplasia.

Remes V, Poussa M, Peltonen J: Scoliosis in patients with diastrophic dysplasia: A new classification. *Spine* 2001;26:1689-1697.

The authors of this article report that scoliosis is common among patients with diastrophic dysplasia; types include early progressive in 10% of patients, idiopathic-like in 50%, and mild nonprogressive in 40%.

Stanley G, McLoughlin S, Beals RK: Observations on the cause of bowlegs in achondroplasia. *J Pediatr Orthop* 2002;22:112-116.

The authors of this study report that tibia vara increased during growth in patients with achondroplasia and that younger children with this disorder tended to have proximal tibial varus and older children tended to have distal tibial varus. Increased fibular length was thought to play a role.

Classic Bibliography

Bailey JA II: Orthopaedic aspects of achondroplasia. *J Bone Joint Surg Am* 1970;52:1285-1301.

Bethem D, Winter RB, Lutter I, et al: Spinal disorders of dwarfism: Review of the literature and report of eighty cases. *J Bone Joint Surg Am* 1981;63:1412-1425.

Fairbank T: Dysplasia epiphysealis multiplex. *Br J Surg* 1947;34:325.

Hastbacka J, Superti-furga A, Wilcox WR, Rimoin DL, Cohn DH, Lander ES: Sulfate transport in chondrodysplasia. *Ann N Y Acad Sci* 1996;785:131-136.

Kopits SE: Orthopaedic complications of dwarfism. *Clin Orthop* 1976;114:153-179.

Mackenzie WG, Bassett GS, Mandell GA, Scott CI Jr: Avascular necrosis of the hip in multiple epiphyseal dysplasia. *J Pediatr Orthop* 1989;9:666-671.

Peltonen JL, Hoikka V, Poussa M, Paavilainen T, Kaitila I: Cementless hip arthroplasty in diastrophic dysplasia. *J Arthroplasty* 1992;7(suppl):369-376.

Poussa M, Merikano J, Ryoppy S, Marttinen E, Kaitila I: The spine in diastrophic dysplasia. *Spine* 1991;16:881-887.

Remes V, Marttinen E, Poussa M, et al: Cervical kyphosis in diastrophic dysplasia. *Spine* 1999;24:1990-1995.

Ribbing S: Studien uber Hereditaire multiple Epiphysenstorungen. *Acta Radiol* 1937;1(suppl):34.

Ryoeppy S, Poussa M, Merikanto J, Marttinen E, Kaitila I: Foot deformities in diastrophic dysplasia: An analysis of 102 patients. *J Bone Joint Surg Br* 1992;74:441-444.

Chapter 57

Neuromuscular Disorders in Children

John F. Sarwark, MD

Arash Aminian, MD

David E. Westberry, MD

Jon R. Davids, MD

Lori A. Karol, MD

Myelomeningocele

Myelomeningocele (spina bifida, myelodysplasia) is the most common major birth defect, with an incidence in the United States ranging from 0.6 per 1,000 to 0.9 per 1,000 births. This neural tube defect results from embryologic failure of closure of neural crests during the neurulation phase of the spine in the third to fourth week after fertilization. The failure results in a cerebrospinal fluid-filled swelling of dura and arachnoid with spinal nerve roots contained in the sac. In 85% to 95% of patients, the disorder is caused by dietary deficiency of folate. Daily supplementation of 0.4 mg (400 µg) of folic acid before conception and during the pregnancy reduces the risk of neural tube defects significantly.

Prenatal diagnosis via enzyme elevation of maternal serum α-fetal protein has an accuracy rate of 60% to 95% for screening neural tube defects. An improved ultrasonographic technique for prenatal diagnosis also has allowed informed prenatal assessment for possible elective termination. Cesarean section is the preferred method of delivery when the diagnosis is known because it avoids trauma to the large myelomeningocele and its neural elements. Fetal sac closure surgery has been postulated to improve neurologic outcome. In one study of 59 patients, intrauterine myelomeningocele repair reduced the incidence of hindbrain herniation (4% versus 50%) and the incidence of shunt-dependent hydrocephalus (58% versus 92%). Functional level was unchanged. Currently, multicenter prospective studies to assess risk and benefits of intrauterine myelomeningocele repair continue.

Latex allergy, sensitivity, or anaphylaxis affects 20% to 70% of patients with myelomeningocele. The etiology is proposed as a result of multiple exposures to latex. Therefore, routine precautions, including latex-free environments, should be taken to limit latex exposure.

Orthopaedic Considerations

The goal of orthopaedic treatment is to maximize function; ambulation is one main goal. Ambulation ability is related to the level of the last intact motor root, which often correlates with the last intact laminar arch (Table 1). Ambulation is generally predicted by age 2 years. A child with myelomeningocele who is not a community ambulator by the age of 6 years is not likely to reach this goal.

Serial, well-documented orthopaedic and neurologic examinations are key components in detecting and avoiding progressive deterioration caused by neurologic loss. Major areas of concern include loss of motor function and rapid progression of scoliosis. Common causes of increasing spasticity and loss of function include hydrocephalus, shunt malfunction, tethered cord, syringomyelia, and posterior fossa compression from Arnold-Chiari malformation.

Hip Deformities

Hip flexion contracture in children with myelomeningocele is caused by muscle imbalance (weak extensors/strong flexors), spasticity as seen in tethered cord patients, or habitual sitting posture. During the first 2 years of life, hip flexion contracture decreases except in high thoracic-level patients. Surgery is usually not indicated in patients younger than 2 years of age. In patients with high thoracic lesions, flexion contracture of 30° to 40° may be tolerated. Greater than 30° to 40° of contracture will result in impairment of standing ability, short stride length, and increased lumbar lordosis. In patients with low lumbar motor deficit, hip flexion contracture of more than 20° causes decreased walking ability as a result of anterior pelvic tilt, decreased velocity, and increased demand of the upper extremities.

Treatment of hip subluxation in patients with myelomeningocele depends on their functional level and the physical demand on the hip. Gait symmetry often corresponds more to the absence of hip contractures and less to the presence of hip dislocation. Therefore, hip reduction is unnecessary in the low-demand hip. Management of most hips focuses on contracture release and/or realignment osteotomies to prevent bracing difficulties and spinal deformities except where significant asymmetry is present. In children with community

Table 1 | Motor Level and Functional Status: Myelomeningocele

Group	Lesion Level	Muscle Involvement	Function	Ambulation
1	Thoracic/high lumbar	No quadriceps function	Sitter Possible household ambulator with RGO	Some degree until age 13 years with HKAFO, RGO 95% to 99% wheelchair dependent as adults
2	Low lumbar	Quadriceps and medial hamstring function, no gluteus medius, maximus	Household/community ambulator with KAFO or AFO	Require AFO and crutches, 79% community ambulators as adults, wheelchair for long distances; significant difference between L3 and L4 level, medial hamstring needed for community ambulation
3	Sacral	Quadriceps and gluteus medius function	Community ambulator with AFO, UCBL, or none	94% retain walking ability as adults
	High sacral	No gastrosoleus strength	Community ambulator with AFO, UCBL, or none	Walk without support but require AFO, have gluteus lurch and excessive pelvic obliquity and rotation during gait
	Low sacral	Good gastrocnemius-soleus strength, normal gluteus medius, maximus		Walk without AFO, gait close to normal

RGO = reciprocating gait orthosis; UCBL = University of California/Berkley Lab (orthosis); KAFO = knee-ankle-foot orthosis; AFO = ankle-foot orthosis; HKAFO = hip-knee-ankle-foot orthosis

ambulation skills, the instability is addressed aggressively with a goal of achieving concentric reduction and acetabular coverage for the high functioning child.

Knee Contractures and Torsional Deformities

Knee flexion contractures and extension contractures are the most common knee deformity in children. Studies have shown that increased knee flexion during gait has a high energy cost. Correction of knee flexion contracture of 20° or more is indicated. In some patients, hamstring lengthening is insufficient and a posterior capsulotomy of the knee may be required. Supracondylar extension osteotomy of the distal femur is recommended in older ambulatory children with fixed flexion deformity of 20° or more after failed radical knee flexor release.

Knee extension contractures are much less common than flexion contractures. Treatment with serial casting to achieve 90° of flexion is successful in most patients. If nonsurgical treatment fails, V-Y lengthening of the quadriceps is favored.

Moderate and severe torsional deformities impede walking and place abnormal stress on the knee. A study of 25 patients with lumbosacral myelomeningocele showed that increased external tibial torsion increased clinical valgus knee stress. A thigh-foot angle greater than 20° significantly increased this stress and supramalleolar tibial/fibular osteotomy is indicated.

Internal tibial torsion is not an acquired deformity in a child younger than 5 years of age with spina bifida. It is present at birth and may lead to a significant in-toeing gait. In patients age 5 years or younger, treatment is observation; orthotic devices may be used. If the condition persists in a child older than 5 years of age, an external supramalleolar tibial/fibular derotation osteotomy is indicated.

Foot Deformities

The goal of treatment is to achieve a supple, braceable, and plantigrade foot. Approximately 30% of children with myelomeningocele have a rigid clubfoot at birth. Initial treatment includes serial casting, but correction is rarely achieved by nonsurgical treatment. Comprehensive posteromedial lateral release is indicated at or before walking age.

Acquired equinus deformity occurs more frequently in children with high lumbar and thoracic-level lesions. Prevention is attempted by bracing and physical therapy. Heel cord resection is indicated to achieve a plantigrade and braceable foot. In patients with mild deformities who are high functioning, Achilles tendon resection can be performed. With severe deformity, a radical posterior release including capsulotomy is required.

Coronal plane malalignments include valgus deformity of the ankle or the hindfoot and are commonly seen in patients with L4-5 level deformity; this condition can lead to difficulty with brace fitting and pressure sores over the medial malleolus. Radiographs help determine the location of the deformity. Ankles in mild valgus are treated with percutaneous screw hemiepiphysiodesis. In severe deformities and in older children, supramalleolar closing wedge osteotomy is indicated. For hindfoot valgus, a medial sliding osteotomy of the calcaneus with displacement of 50% of the width of the fragment is recommended.

Scoliosis

Scoliosis is related to the degree of motor paralysis. Paralytic spinal deformities are expected in 5% of patients with sacral level function, 25% at L5, 60% at L4, 70% at L3, 80% at L2, and more than 90% at L1 and higher. Congenital lumbar kyphosis is a severe spinal deformity occurring in 10% to 15% of patients. This deformity does not respond to bracing. Indications are variable among surgeons. Lumbar kyphosis may have deleterious effects on pulmonary function (because of abdominal compression and thoracic hypokyphosis) and sitting balance, and can progress to skin ulcerations because of the prominent gibbus. Newer approaches to surgical management, including vertebral subtraction or decancellation procedures with instrumentation in young patients, and kyphectomy in the older patient with instrumentation, are complex and carry significant risks for morbidity and mortality.

Physical examination of patients with spinal deformity includes assessment of pelvic obliquity, joint contractures, and leg length inequality as potential reversible causes of spinal deformity. Clinical findings of tethered cord syndrome must be considered in the assessment. Treatment with an orthotic device is advised for moderate scoliotic curves. Studies have shown the greatest curve progression before the age of 15 years, and average curve progression of 5° per year for curves greater than 40°. Intraspinal pathology such as tethering of the spinal cord and syringomyelia contribute to curve progression. Although most curves progress, bracing has a beneficial temporary effect of delaying definitive spinal fusion until adult sitting height is achieved and also supports the trunk in a functional position for those patients with imbalance and hypotonia. Patients who use spinal orthotic devices may find independent gait reduced because of increased energy expenditure and balance disturbances. In wheelchair-dependent patients, increasing spinal deformity may compromise sitting balance and lead to pressure sores. Prevention of sitting imbalance is correlated with prevention of an unbalanced spine to curvature of less than 40° and pelvic obliquity to less than 25°.

Indications for spinal fusion and instrumentation in scoliosis are progression of curve greater than 50°, poor sitting balance, and pulmonary compromise not controlled by bracing. In a study of 29 patients with severe thoracolumbar and lumbar scoliosis, combined anterior and posterior instrumentation gave the best correction of the deformity and pelvic obliquity, and reduced the rate of pseudarthrosis. Surgical complications include wound infection (6% to 15%), fixation failure (15%), and pseudarthrosis (7% to 28%). Patients have an improved sitting balance after surgery, but ambulation may be more difficult.

Cerebral Palsy

Epidemiology

The cerebral palsies (CPs) are the most common causes of physical disability in children. They can be defined as a heterogeneous group of upper motor neuron impairment syndromes caused by chronic brain abnormalities. Causes are multifactorial and include antenatal and postnatal insults to the developing brain. The incidence ranges from 1 to 3 per 1,000 live births. The rate of CP in children weighing less than 1,500 g at birth is 70 times higher compared with those weighing 2,500 g or more. The incidence and prevalence of CP has remained constant over the past 40 years. Improved obstetrical care has resulted in fewer neonatal insults, but improved neonatal care has resulted in the decreased mortality of more preterm infants. Although the cerebral lesion is nonprogressive, musculoskeletal deformities and impairment can be progressive in the growing child.

Major types of CP are described as spastic, dystonic, ataxic, and hypotonic. The spastic variety is the most common, with mixed varieties now being increasingly diagnosed. The clinical spectrum of CP ranges from very minor impairment as seen in a patient with mild hemiplegia with minimal gait deviations to significant cognitive deficits and motor functional limitations as seen in children with severe total body involvement. Patients with severe CP often have comorbidities such as seizures, recurrent pneumonias, and difficulty eating, often requiring feeding tubes.

Care of a child with CP involves a multidisciplinary approach with emphasis on early intervention therapies, tone management, use of orthotic devices, and musculoskeletal surgery. Input from orthopaedists, physical and occupational therapists, neurologists, neurosurgeons, pediatricians, and orthotists are required to maximize the function and activities of daily living of a child with CP. Treatment is focused during the early years of growth on tone management, prevention of contractures, aids for walking, and multilevel bony and soft-tissue surgery to improve gait.

Literature on the treatment of adult CP patients is limited. A recent survey showed that many adults with CP continue to have spasticity and pain-related issues, which contribute to the deteriorating ability to ambulate. Independent walking and other forms of supported ambulation are often lost upon reaching adulthood. Care of adult CP patients is limited by lack of adult health and rehabilitation services.

Outcomes Assessment

With the recent focus on evidence-based medicine and the development of best practice guidelines, greater attention has been focused on the assessment of outcomes in multiple domains (technical, functional, patient and family satisfaction, and cost). Recent studies of CP patients have had variable success using measurement instruments such as the Child Health Questionnaire and Pediatric Outcomes Data Collection Instrument and in attempting to assess outcomes of treatment. A single study found considerable variability in the reliability and validity of these different instruments for patients with CP.

Bone Mineral Density

Multiple factors may adversely affect bone mineral density in children with CP. Impaired weight bearing and short-term immobilization after orthopaedic surgery contribute to low bone mineral density. Poor nutrition, low calcium intake, and anticonvulsants play a negative role as well. A recent controlled clinical trial showed that pamidronate is a safe and effective agent to increase bone mineral density in children with CP.

Treatment Modalities

Botulinum Toxin

Botulinum toxin A is a protein polypeptide chain that irreversibly binds to the cholinergic terminals at the neuromuscular junction and effectively inhibits release of acetylcholine from the synaptic vesicles. The toxin can be injected locally into spastic muscles, causing a rapid onset of weakness that may last for 3 to 6 months. The most common locations benefiting from botulinum toxin A injection are spastic ankle plantar flexors, posterior tibialis, hamstrings, hip adductors, and wrist flexors. The benefits of repeated injections are still unclear. Risks of repeat injections include lessening of the positive effect of the toxin as well as possible antibody formation. A 2000 study of repeat botulinum A toxin injections into calf muscles of patients with spastic equinus showed similar effects after the first and second injections, with a decrease in the duration of response after the third and fourth injections. The long-term benefits of botulinum toxin have yet to be determined.

Baclofen

Baclofen is a γ-aminobutyric acid agonist that acts peripherally and centrally at the spinal cord level to impede the release of excitatory neurotransmitters that cause spasticity. Large doses of oral baclofen are required to detect changes in spasticity, often with the unwanted side effect of sedation. Intrathecal baclofen allows for larger doses to reach the target tissues in the spinal cord. A synchronized implantable infusion pump is now available. Complications, which may be life

threatening, occur in approximately 20% of patients and are primarily related to breakage of the catheter, catheter dislodgment, infection, and skin breakdown at the insertion site. Development of scoliosis in patients with baclofen pumps remains an important concern. Most pumps are implanted in patients with severe spasticity that interferes with function and positioning. A long-term review of this device showed benefits in terms of decreased pain and spasm relief, better sleep, independence, and improved ease of care.

Physical Therapy

Physical therapy is the mainstay of nonsurgical treatment in children with motor dysfunction. Critical periods for intensive therapy include the early ambulatory years and the immediate postsurgical rehabilitation phase. Debate continues regarding the method, indications, and value of therapies offered to patients. Currently, precise objective and collaborative goal setting has been emphasized. However, a recent randomized controlled study failed to show any long-term benefit in intensive, goal-directed therapies versus the traditional forms of therapy.

Recent emphasis has been placed on the weakness seen in spastic muscles. A retrospective analysis failed to show a true relationship between the degree of spasticity and strength of the muscle. There was a trend toward increased spasticity and less strength in distal muscle groups compared with proximal muscle groups.

Orthotic Devices

Ankle-foot orthoses (AFOs) are commonly prescribed to improve gait and stability, prevent deformity, and to protect surgically-treated limbs. In patients with spastic diplegia, solid AFOs have been shown to improve ankle kinetics, whereas floor reaction AFOs are effective in correcting crouch type gait secondary to ankle plantar weakness. AFOs may be used initially to prevent equinus contractures, and are often used to prevent recurrence of deformity after botulinum toxin injection and casting during treatment of dynamic or mild myostatic deformities of the ankle plantar flexors. The AFOs must extend to just below the knee and have a rigid ankle, leaf spring, or hinged design to prevent equinus deformity. Supramalleolar designs are ineffective at preventing equinus. Prevention of equinus has been shown to improve walking speed and stride length for most children. The efficacy of AFOs to help in overcoming functional limitations and preventing contractures is yet to be established.

Alternative Therapies

Electrical Stimulation

Threshold electrical stimulation is based on low-intensity, long-duration electrical transcutaneous stimulation of select muscle groups. It is theorized that electrical stimulation promotes local blood flow, increasing the size of atrophic muscles and perhaps their function. Early studies show improved motor performance and lower incidence of falls after 3 months of treatment. However, two recent randomized trials failed to show any benefit in motor or ambulatory function in children with CP.

Hyperbaric Oxygen Therapy

Evidence for the effectiveness of hyperbaric oxygen therapy treatment in children with CP is largely anecdotal. Known risks include oxygen toxicity (tremors or seizures), barotrauma (tympanic membrane rupture), myopia, and pneumothorax. A randomized multicenter trial showed that hyperbaric oxygen therapy had no greater effect on patients compared with breathing slightly pressurized air.

Horseback Riding

The postulated effects of hippotherapy involve the movement of the horse's hind legs and pelvis to produce a three-dimensional input to the patient. Ambulatory pelvic motion is therefore mimicked while riding horseback. Potential benefits include improvement in overall gross motor function, walking, running, and jumping. Using the Gross Motor Function Measure, a single study of children with CP showed minimal improvement after 18 weeks of hippotherapy.

Neurosurgery

Selective dorsal rhizotomy (SDR) selectively sections dorsal rootlets from L1 to S2. Heightened responses to afferent impulses from muscle spindles are interrupted with an end result of decreased spasticity. Concerns remain regarding the effects of SDR on muscle strength. Original indications for SDR were limited to ambulatory patients with diplegia. Short-term results have shown reduced spasticity and improved function when SDR is followed by intensive physical therapy. There is a lack of consensus in the literature regarding patient indications, surgical techniques, surgical approach, and determination of which rootlets to section. Complications, although rare, include bowel or bladder incontinence, dysesthesia, dural leaks, and risk of musculoskeletal deformities including hip subluxation and spondylolysis, spondylolisthesis, and scoliosis. A meta-analysis of three randomized clinical trials showed functional improvement and reduced spasticity in carefully selected CP patients after SDR and physical therapy when compared with physical therapy alone. Other studies have shown the need for additional orthopaedic procedures in a significant percentage of patients who have undergone SDR.

Gait Analysis

Gait analysis continues to evolve as a diagnostic and research tool. Using computers, cameras, reflective markers, in-floor force plates, dynamic electromyography, and pedobarographs, movement in multiple planes can be captured and analyzed. Preoperative assessment of ambulatory patients provides information across multiple joints and lends direction to appropriate procedures such as muscle tendon lengthening and rotational osteotomies.

A recent longitudinal study using gait analysis evaluated the natural progression of gait in children with CP. Gait function was shown to deteriorate over a 4-year span with respect to temporal/stride measures, passive range of motion, and kinematic parameters. This deterioration was not seen in a similar cohort who had undergone orthopaedic intervention.

The application of quantitative gait analysis in clinical decision making is in evolution. Current controversies are focused on the reliability and variability of data collection and interpretation between centers. Technologic advances in motion analysis and greater experience with the clinical applications of the data will increase the use of gait analysis.

Management of Specific Musculoskeletal Complications

Spine

Spinal deformity is more commonly seen in severely affected CP patients with quadriplegia. The typical long C-shaped thoracolumbar curve is resistant to bracing and often progresses relentlessly. The spinal deformity leads to difficulty with seating systems and unequal balance secondary to pelvic obliquity. Associated comorbidities are commonly present and the decision to pursue surgical correction must be done cautiously. Often, these patients have significant comorbidities such as seizure disorder, poor nutritional status, and respiratory compromise. Aggressive preoperative and postoperative care is required. Current techniques use segmental fixation with Galveston fixation to the pelvis. Severe curves may require an additional anterior procedure to achieve adequate correction. A recent review of skeletally immature patients (with open triradiate cartilage) with neuromuscular scoliosis following posterior spinal fusion to the pelvis revealed minimal evidence of subsequent progression of the deformity caused by anterior overgrowth, also known as the crankshaft phenomenon.

Hip

Hip subluxation secondary to spastic hip adductors and flexors may become evident in children between the ages of 2 to 4 years and is typically seen in children with severe spasticity. AP radiographs of the pelvis should be obtained at regular intervals to monitor for subluxation.

Typical findings include acetabular dysplasia (usually superior or posterosuperior), increased femoral anteversion, and increased femoral neck-shaft angle. Soft-tissue release of the adductors shows a failure rate of 40%. Osteotomies of the proximal femur (varus-producing) in addition to acetabular osteotomies improve the coverage and stability of the developing hip and are typically done after age 4 years. Combined procedures may carry an increased risk of proximal femoral osteonecrosis.

Untreated hip dislocation in the older child or young adult remains a difficult diagnostic and therapeutic challenge. Recent studies show that not all dislocated hips are painful and not all painful hips are dislocated. Determining the degree of pain from a dislocated hip remains difficult. Long-term benefits of salvage operations such as proximal femoral resection or hemiarthroplasty are yet to be determined. For patients with unilateral hip dislocation and the absence of spinal deformity, hip fusion may be an alternative procedure, with a recent review showing diminished pain and postural improvement following hip fusion in a series of older patients with CP.

Knee

Spastic hamstring muscles increase knee flexion during the stance phase of gait. Untreated knee flexion contractures and worsening crouch gait can lead to increased loads across the patellofemoral joint, resulting in pain and late arthritis. Decreased dynamic range and poor transition from stance to swing secondary to rectus femoris spasticity are commonly seen. Treatment consists of medial hamstring lengthening with concomitant posterior transfer of the rectus tendon. Knee flexion contractures following hamstring lengthening can be addressed using serial stretch casting during the postoperative period. Lateral hamstring release is reserved for the older patient with resistant knee flexion contractures or for patients with previous medial hamstring release. Risks of lateral hamstring lengthening include excessive weakness leading to knee hyperextension during the stance phase. Extension osteotomy can be performed at the level of the distal femur for resistant contractures.

Ankle

Equinus is the most common deformity in CP and causes adverse effects during standing and gait. For children younger than 3 years of age, developmental therapy and orthotic devices are used. From ages 3 to 6 years, a combination treatment with serial casting, botulinum toxin, and orthotic devices is recommended. Definitive muscle-tendon surgery is preferably delayed until at least age 6 years for persistent equinus deformity to minimize risk of recurrence. Surgical options vary depending on the degree of deformity and contracture. Selective gastrocnemius-soleus complex recession is performed more commonly. Nonselective Achilles tendon lengthening is reserved for more severe myostatic deformities. There is greater risk of overlengthening with Achilles tendon lengthening, which can result in disruption of the ankle plantar flexion-knee extension couple, leading to a crouch gait pattern.

Foot

Planovalgus and hallux valgus deformities are common in patients with CP. In nonambulatory patients, a shoeable plantigrade foot is the goal of treatment. In ambulatory patients, treatment is directed toward correction of skeletal lever arm deficiency to maximize ankle plantar flexion function and to facilitate bracing. Surgical treatment involves posterior calf muscle lengthening and skeletal realignment by calcaneal lengthening and/or subtalar arthrodesis. Hallux valgus deformities often require metatarsophalangeal fusion in patients with CP to prevent recurrence.

Equinovarus foot deformity is seen in the setting of a spastic posterior tibialis tendon. For flexible deformities, surgical considerations include posterior calf lengthening, intramuscular or Z-lengthening of the posterior tibial tendon, or split posterior or anterior tibial tendon transfers. A recent long-term follow-up survey showed a failure rate in 75% of patients with low-level ambulatory diplegia and quadriplegia undergoing these procedures before age 8 years.

Transverse Plane

In some ambulatory patients with CP, increased femoral anteversion fails to resolve with growth, resulting in lever deficiency at the level of the hip. Assessing the degree of pathologic femoral anteversion requires some combination of clinical examination, two-dimensional CT, and gait analysis. Compensatory actions during the gait cycle include internal rotation of the hip and external rotation of the pelvis to restore the lever arm. Correction of these deviations can be achieved following correction of the increased anteversion by derotational osteotomy of the femur. This procedure can be performed proximally by an intertrochanteric or subtrochanteric osteotomy, or distally above the metaphyseal flare. A prospective study comparing both methods showed excellent clinical results with either technique. If this condition is not corrected by the teenage years, patients may develop compensatory increased external tibial torsion. In such cases, the transverse plane malalignment may need to be corrected at both the femoral and tibial levels. Tibial rotation osteotomy is best performed at the supramalleolar level to minimize the risk of compartment syndrome and neurologic injury. Simultaneous procedures will necessitate an aggressive postoperative physical therapy regimen to enable the patient to return to their preoperative functional level.

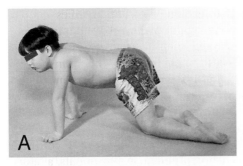
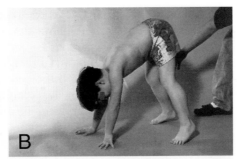
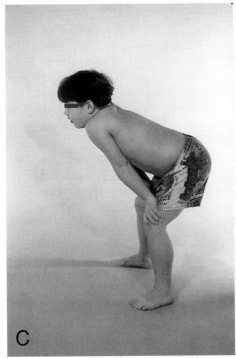
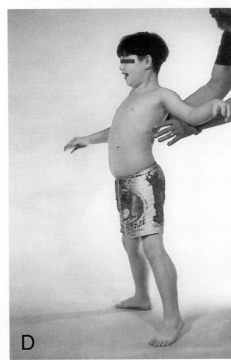

Figure 1 Patient with Duchenne muscular dystrophy show the Gowers' maneuver. **A,** The prone position. **B,** The bear position. **C,** Moving the hands up the thighs to help upright the trunk and augment knee extension. **D,** The upright position. *(Reproduced from Sussman M: Duchenne muscular dystrophy. J Am Acad Orthop Surg 2002;10:138-151.)*

Muscular Dystrophy

The mutation that causes Duchenne muscular dystrophy is a point deletion of a segment of the dystrophin gene, located at Xp21 on the X chromosome. This produces a frame shift resulting in all messenger RNA distal to the deletion coding for a nonsense protein. Thus, formation of the dystrophin protein is absent. Dystrophin is critical to the stability of the cell membrane. Becker muscular dystrophy resembles Duchenne muscular dystrophy in that it is also inherited in an X-linked recessive manner. A less significant mutation in the dystrophin gene does not result in a frame shift, and therefore allows production of smaller amounts of an inferior dystrophin. The onset of weakness in patients with Becker muscular dystrophy is delayed usually until the second decade, and life expectancy is longer. This difference in the mutation results in a significant difference in disease severity such that the amount and quality of dystrophin produces a spectrum of disease.

Duchenne muscular dystrophy can be diagnosed using DNA analysis in at least two thirds of patients.

Duchenne muscular dystrophy should be suspected in boys whose laboratory values show extremely high levels of serum creatine phosphokinase (measuring 10 to 200 times normal), which leaks across the defective cell membrane into the serum. The diagnosis is definitively made by absent dystrophin staining of muscle biopsy specimens in patients who do not have discoverable mutations.

Because of the relatively common presentation of the clumsy child, diagnosis of Duchenne muscular dystrophy is often missed for up to 2 years following presentation. Early diagnosis is extremely important to families because of the possibility of genetic counseling for future offspring. Clinical features seen in young boys with Duchenne muscular dystrophy are a waddling gait, toe walking, falling, and difficulty climbing stairs. Walking is usually delayed until age 18 to 24 months. Unlike in patients with spinal muscular atrophy, deep tendon reflexes are present. Gowers' sign is positive, as the child uses the hands to "walk up" the legs when rising from the floor because of proximal muscle weakness

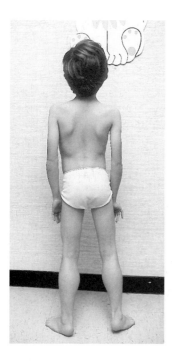

Figure 2 Physical findings in patients with Duchenne muscular dystrophy. A 5-year-old boy with Duchenne muscular dystrophy and marked pseudohypertrophy of the calves. *(Reproduced from Sussman M: Duchenne muscular dystrophy. J Am Acad Orthop Surg 2002;10:138-151.)*

(Figure 1). Documentation of the Gowers' sign should be mandatory in all boys evaluated for weakness or gait disturbances. Calf pseudohypertrophy develops as muscle is replaced by fibroadipose tissue (Figure 2). Gait is wide-based, and lumbar lordosis is increased.

Research is underway in gene therapy using adenovirus vectors in animal models to import the normal dystrophin gene. The production of an immune response to introduction of the gene and reaction to the viral vectors are complications of this therapy. Stem cell and myoblast transplant are also under investigation.

Corticosteroids have been shown to acutely improve muscular strength, and to slow progressive weakening in intermediate follow-up. Ambulation may be prolonged and the deterioration of pulmonary function slowed with corticosteroid therapy. The preferred steroid and mode of administration is debated. Although positive effects on skeletal muscle have been shown, side effects such as obesity and osteopenia are of concern.

Advances in pulmonary care have resulted in longer life spans. A recent study revealed that patients who use nighttime ventilation have up to 50% survival at age 25 years.

Orthopaedic Manifestations

Hip abductor and hamstring releases, Achilles tendon lengthening or release with posterior tibialis tenotomy or transfer may prolong ambulation in those patients whose ability to walk is deteriorating. Timing of the surgery is very important because those children who have already become nonambulatory will not regain the ability to walk after surgery. In a recent study, 42% of boys who underwent multilevel releases with posterior tibia-

lis tendon transfer to prolong ambulation would choose to have the surgery again. Willingness to use knee-ankle-foot orthoses and compliance with postoperative physical therapy must be evaluated preoperatively. Isolated foot surgery consisting of posterior tibialis tendon transfer (combined with Achilles tendon lengthening and toe flexor tenotomy) corrected equinovarus, allowed patients to continue to wear shoes, and had high patient and family satisfaction.

Scoliosis is a major problem in the nonambulatory patient with Duchenne muscular dystrophy. Shortly after transitioning to wheelchair use, up to 95% of patients develop scoliosis, which is progressive in almost all patients. Bracing is contraindicated because it does not prevent progression, and may delay surgery until a time when the pulmonary status of the child precludes safe surgery. Forced vital capacity has been found to decrease 4% yearly, and an additional 4% for each 10° of thoracic deformity. Treatment is early posterior spinal fusion, recommended after a curve reaches 20° to 30° of magnitude in boys without significant cardiomyopathy, and whose preoperative pulmonary function tests reveal forced vital capacity of at least 35% of normal levels. Most authors recommend fusion with segmental instrumentation from the upper thoracic spine to the sacrum or pelvis, although there are reports of maintenance of correction following fusion to L5 in patients with minimal (< 10°) preoperative pelvic obliquity, especially with the use of pedicle screw fixation distally. Outcomes studies suggest improved quality of life in boys who have undergone spinal fusion compared with their peers who have not had surgery.

Fractures are more prevalent in patients with Duchenne muscular dystrophy, occurring in up to 21% of affected boys. Frequent falls, combined with osteopenia, lead to the increased frequency. Loss of mobility occurs in up to 20% of ambulatory boys with Duchenne muscular dystrophy as a result of fractures.

Spinal Muscular Atrophy

Spinal muscular atrophy represents a group of diseases characterized by progressive symmetric muscular weakness caused by the loss of anterior horn cells. Spinal muscular atrophy is inherited as an autosomal recessive trait. A mutation in the survival motor neuron gene on chromosome 5q can be detected in 94% of patients. The survival motor neuron gene is critical to RNA metabolism and is a mediator of apoptosis (programmed cell death). Spinal muscular atrophy can be diagnosed using DNA analysis or by muscle biopsy. Muscle enzyme levels are usually normal. Prenatal diagnosis is possible.

Subtypes of spinal muscular atrophy are distinguished by the age of onset and clinical severity. Type I, known as Werdnig-Hoffmann or acute infantile spinal muscular atrophy, is a lethal condition presenting in patients 6 months of age or younger. The babies exhibit little or no movement of their extremities, with characteristic tongue fasciculations and absent deep tendon reflexes. Most die of respiratory infections before the age of 2 years. Longer survival is possible with tracheostomy or noninvasive ventilation. Orthopaedic treatment is limited to splinting of fractures that may occur at birth.

Patients with type II or chronic infantile spinal muscular atrophy, present between 6 and 12 months of age. These babies have muscle weakness that is more advanced in the legs than in the arms. They achieve head control, and most can sit, but they cannot walk. Survival into adulthood is common.

Type III spinal muscular atrophy is known as Kugelberg-Welander syndrome and has an age of onset between 2 and 15 years, when proximal muscle weakness becomes noticeable. Patients ambulate as children, but become wheelchair users in adulthood.

Orthopaedic Manifestations

Currently there is no effective medical treatment for spinal muscular atrophy. Orthopaedic treatment is needed for scoliosis, which is widespread in patients with type II and III. Soft orthotic devices can delay but not prevent surgery in children younger than 10 years of age. Posterior spinal fusion is recommended for most progressive curves, with fusion to the pelvis in nonambulatory patients.

Hip dislocation and subluxation occur in 62% of hips in patients with type II spinal muscular atrophy, and less frequently in type III patients. Although open reduction of the hip can be performed, even with concomitant pelvic osteotomy, redislocation frequently occurs because of the inherent muscle weakness. Long-term studies show that nearly all hip dislocations in patients with spinal muscular atrophy remain painless; surgery should be avoided in nonambulatory patients.

Friedreich's Ataxia

Friedreich's ataxia is characterized by involvement of the cerebellum and the spinal cord pathways. Clinically, patients present with the classic triad of ataxia, loss of deep tendon reflexes, and an extensor Babinski response. Associated medical conditions include hypertrophic cardiomyopathy, and in some patients, diabetes mellitus. The average age of onset is 12 years, and death occurs on average 25 years after diagnosis because of cardiac deterioration.

Friedreich's ataxia is inherited in an autosomal recessive fashion. The disease is caused by the presence of an expanded guanine-adenosine-adenosine trinucleotide repeat in both copies of the frataxin gene on chromosome 9. The normal number of repeats is less than 33, whereas patients with Friedreich's ataxia have 66 to

1,500 abnormal guanine-adenosine-adenosine repeats. The number of added repeats may correlate with the severity of disease or age of onset. Frataxin is a mitochondrial protein, involved in iron metabolism and oxidative stress. Knowledge of the role of frataxin has led to the initiation of treatment with antioxidants such as Coenzyme Q, which has been shown in preliminary studies to decrease the rate of cardiac deterioration but not the ataxia.

Orthopaedic Manifestations

Patients with Friedreich's ataxia often present for the evaluation of frequently falling and have cavus or cavovarus feet. Surgery to prolong ambulation is performed in selected patients when the position of the foot exacerbates the instability during gait. Scoliosis occurs in more than 80% of patients. Curve types vary between idiopathic-looking curves to long, sweeping thoracolumbar curves. Increased thoracic kyphosis is common. Progression is linked to early age at diagnosis and to curve magnitude. Bracing is ineffective at preventing progression, and may interfere with mobility. Curves that stabilize at less than 40° at skeletal maturity rarely progress. Surgery is indicated for curves of 60° or greater. Posterior spinal fusion from the upper thoracic to the lower lumbar spine is effective.

Charcot-Marie-Tooth Disease

Charcot-Marie-Tooth disease is a clinically and genetically heterogeneous group of hereditary motor sensorineuropathies. Traditionally, Charcot-Marie-Tooth disease has been divided into demyelinating forms that slow nerve conduction velocity (Charcot-Marie-Tooth types 1, 3, and 4), and axonal forms that decrease the compound muscle action potential (Charcot-Marie-Tooth type 2). Overlap between these two forms exists. To date, 10 genes causing various forms of Charcot-Marie-Tooth disease have been identified. These genes are expressed either by Schwann cells and/or accompanying neurons. The most common mutation involves overexpression of the peripheral myelin protein 22 gene on chromosome 17, producing autosomal dominant Charcot-Marie-Tooth disease type 1A. Other genes commonly disturbed include the myelin protein zero gene, and connexin 32, which is present in the x-linked Charcot-Marie-Tooth disease.

In most patients the disease manifests during the second decade of life. Cavovarus foot deformity is frequently the presenting symptom. Physical examination is notable for lower limb areflexia, calf atrophy, an increased longitudinal arch, and clawing of the toes.

Orthopaedic Manifestations

The first line of treatment of mild cavus and cavovarus is the use of orthotic devices. AFOs can improve gait in patients with flexible deformities. Patients with Charcot-Marie-Tooth disease frequently have significant foot drop during swing phase, and this is improved by use of AFOs.

Surgical treatment of the cavovarus foot deformity is based on the flexibility of the deformity. In patients with mild flexible hindfoot varus, plantar fascia release and first metatarsal dorsal closing wedge osteotomy, with or without transfer of the peroneus longus to peroneus brevis, can improve the deformity. The posterior tibialis tendon can be transferred to the dorsum of the midfoot to improve swing phase foot drop. When the hindfoot is rigid, calcaneal osteotomy is necessary. After correction of the hindfoot deformity is achieved, metatarsal osteotomies to align the forefoot may be performed. Alternatively, midfoot dorsal closing wedge osteotomy improves cavovarus by correcting midfoot and forefoot equinus. In severe cases, triple arthrodesis is necessary to obtain and maintain correction. Clawing of the toes may be improved with transfer of the toe extensors to the metatarsal necks. Although initial results following cavovarus surgery are usually satisfactory, progression of the neurologic disease often leads to recurrence of deformity.

Hip dysplasia is also associated with Charcot-Marie-Tooth disease. Ambulatory patients may report symptoms during adolescence. Symptomatic acetabular dysplasia can be treated by pelvic osteotomies. Patients with hereditary motor sensorineuropathies are more prone to sciatic nerve palsy after pelvic surgery.

Scoliosis occurs more frequently in patients with Charcot-Marie-Tooth disease. Left thoracic and kyphotic curves distinguish the radiographic appearance of many of these curves from idiopathic scoliosis. Although bracing rarely is effective, surgical correction can be performed without an increase in complications.

Annotated Bibliography

Myelomeningocele

Gabrieli AP, Vankoski S, Dias L, et al: Gait analysis in low lumbar myelomeningocele patients with unilateral hip dislocation or subluxation. *J Pediatr Orthop* 2003;23: 330-334.

Gait symmetry using motion analysis of 20 patients with low lumbar myelomeningocele with unilateral hip dislocation or subluxation and no scoliosis corresponded to the absence of hip contractures and had no relation to the presence of hip dislocation. The authors concluded that reduction of the hip is unnecessary.

Farmer DL, von Koch CS, Peacock WJ, et al: In utero repair of myelomeningocele: Experimental pathophysiology, initial clinical experience, and outcomes. *Arch Surg* 2003;138:872-878.

Fetoscopic repair of neural tube defects before 22 weeks' gestation is physiologically and technically feasible. Surgical repair of 13 patients showed one third were spared the need for a shunt at 1 year of age, but improvement in neurologic function was unclear.

Nolden MT, Sarwark JF, Vora A, Grayhack JJ: A kyphectomy technique with reduced perioperative morbidity for myelomeningocele kyphosis. *Spine* 2002;27: 1807-1813.

Evaluation of 11 patients with myelomeningocele and lumbar kyphosis showed subtraction vertebrectomy with posterior instrumentation to be a safe and efficacious technique for correction and stabilization of myelomeningocele kyphosis in young patients.

Scoliosis

Berven S, Bradford DS: Neuromuscular scoliosis: Causes of deformity and principles for evaluation and management. *Semin Neurol* 2002;22:167-178.

In a review of the literature, outcomes in patients with neuromuscular deformity who were treated with a combined anterior and posterior fusion showed improvement of the major curve of up to 60%, more effective correction of pelvic obliquity, and a decreased pseudarthrosis rate.

Trivedi J, Thomson JD, Slakey JB, Banta JV, Jones PW: Clinical and radiographic predictors of scoliosis in myelomeningocele. *J Bone Joint Surg Am* 2002;84-A:1389-1394.

In a retrospective review of patients with myelomeningocele over a 5-year period with an average follow-up of 9.4 years, curves of less than 20° often resolved. Clinical motor level, ambulatory status, and last intact laminar arch were predictive factors for development of scoliosis.

Cerebral Palsy

Anderson C, Mattsson E: Adults with cerebral palsy: A survey describing problems, needs, and resources, with special emphasis on locomotion. *Dev Med Child Neurol* 2001;43:76-82.

This article presents a report of a survey of adult CP patients discussing natural history and progression. Of those polled, 77% had difficulty with spasticity, 18% had full disability pension, 35% reported decreased walking ability, and 18% had pain every day.

Bell KJ, Ounpuu S, DeLuca PA, Romness MJ: Natural progression of gait in children with cerebral palsy. *J Pediatr Orthop* 2002;22:677-682.

Using clinical measures and gait analysis, gait function in patients with CP decreased longitudinally compared with the group who had orthopaedic intervention.

Bower E, Michell D, Burnett M, Campbell M, McLellan D: Randomized control trial of physiotherapy in 56 children with cerebral palsy followed for 18 months. *Dev Med Child Neurol* 2001;43:4-15.

Patients in aim and goal directed therapy showed no advantage in acquisition of gross motor function or performance compared with patients undergoing more traditional forms of therapy.

Flynn JM, Miller F: Management of hip disorders in patients with cerebral palsy. *J Am Acad Orthop Surg* 2002; 10:198-209.

This review article discusses surgical options for hip disorders in CP. Childhood and adult hip pathology with treatment options are discussed.

Graham K, Selber P: Musculoskeletal aspects of cerebral palsy. *J Bone Joint Surg Br* 2003;85:157-166.

A comprehensive review of the role of the orthopaedic surgeon in the management of CP is detailed. The etiology, natural history, pathophysiology, and surgical strategies are discussed.

Henderson RC, Lark RK, Kecskemethy HH, Miller F, Harcke HT, Bachrach SJ: Bisphosphonates to treat osteopenia in children with quadriplegic cerebral palsy: A randomized, placebo-controlled clinical trial. *J Pediatr* 2002;141:644-651.

This small clinical trial demonstrated increased bone mineral density following administration of bisphosphonates in nonambulatory children with CP.

McLaughlin J, Bjornson K, Temkin N, et al: Selective dorsal rhizotomy: Meta-analysis of three randomized controlled trials. *Dev Med Child Neurol* 2002;44:17-25.

A consistent reduction in spasticity in seen following selective dorsal rhizotomy (SDR). With respect to functional outcome, the difference between SDR alone and SDR with physical therapy was minimal.

Pirpiris M, Trivett A, Baker J, Rodda G, Nattrass R, Graham H: Femoral derotation osteotomy in spastic diplegia. *J Bone Joint Surg Br* 2003;85:265-272.

Proximal and distal femoral derotation osteotomy was found to be equally effective for correction of increased femoral anteversion and intoeing gait. Distal osteotomy may provide faster rehabilitation and a decrease in surgical complications.

Rosenbaum PL, Walter SD, Hanna SE, et al: Prognosis for gross motor function in cerebral palsy: Creation of motor development curves. *JAMA* 2002;288:1357-1363.

Evidence-based prognostication concerning gross motor progress in children with CP is discussed. Patterns of gross motor development are illustrated relating to the severity of motor impairment.

Ross S, Engsberg J: Relation between spasticity and strength in individuals with spastic diplegic cerebral palsy. *Dev Med Child Neurol* 2002;44:148-157.

No relationship between strength and spasticity in patients with CP was identified.

Saraph V, Zwick EB, Zwick G, Steinwender C, Steinwender G, Linhart W: Multilevel surgery in spastic diplegia: Evaluation by physical examination and gait analysis in 25 children. *J Pediatr Orthop* 2002;22:150-157.

Clinical, kinematic, and kinetic improvements are shown following multilevel bony and soft-tissue procedures in ambulatory CP patients.

Smucker JD, Miller F: Crankshaft effect after posterior spinal fusion and unit rod instrumentation in children with cerebral palsy. *J Pediatr Orthop* 2001;21:108-112.

In skeletally immature children with cerebral palsy, posterior spinal fusion alone with unit rod instrumentation was successful in maintaining correction of neuromuscular scoliosis. Crankshaft deformity was not identified in this series of 50 patients treated with isolated posterior procedures.

Sterba J, Rogers B, France A, Vokes D: Horseback riding in children with cerebral palsy: Effect on gross motor function. *Dev Med Child Neurol* 2002;44:301-308.

A small clinical trial evaluated the effect of recreational horseback riding therapy on Gross Motor Function Measure scores. An increase of 7.6% in these scores was seen after 18 weeks of horseback riding therapy and returned to control levels 6 weeks following therapy. A minimal increase in walking, running, and jumping ability was seen after horseback riding therapy.

Vitale MG, Levy DE, Moskowitz AJ, et al: Capturing quality of life in pediatric orthopaedics: Two recent measures compared. *J Pediatr Orthop* 2001;21:629-635.

Cross-sectional application of Child Health Questionnaire and Pediatric Outcomes Data Collection Instrument among varying diagnoses. The instruments were able to distinguish physical from psychosocial health problems.

Muscular Dystrophy

Bentley G, Haddad F, Bull TM, et al: Treatment of scoliosis in muscular dystrophy using modified Luque and Harrington-Luque instrumentation. *J Bone Joint Surg Br* 2001;83:22-28.

Sixty-four patients with Duchenne muscular dystrophy and 33 patients with spinal muscular atrophy had posterior spinal fusion with sublaminar wiring. Fusion to the pelvis is recommended.

Chan KG, Galasko CS, Delaney C: Hip subluxation and dislocation in Duchenne muscular dystrophy. *J Pediatr Orthop B* 2001;10:219-225.

Nineteen of 54 boys had subluxated or dislocated hips, usually related to pelvic tilt.

Connolly AM, Schierbecker J, Renna R, et al: High dose weekly oral prednisone improves strength in boys with Duchenne muscular dystrophy. *Neuromuscul Disord* 2002;12:917-925.

Improvement in muscle strength was seen up to 2 years following twice weekly prednisone therapy with fewer side effects than daily administration.

Eagle M, Baudouin SV, Chandler C, et al: Survival in Duchenne muscular dystrophy: Improvements in life expectancy since 1967 and the impact of home nocturnal ventilation. *Neuromuscul Disord* 2002;12:926-929.

Using nighttime noninvasive ventilation, survival averaged 50% at 25 years of age in boys without severe cardiomyopathy.

McDonald DG, Kinali M, Gallagher AC, et al: Fracture prevalence in Duchenne muscular dystrophy. *Dev Med Child Neurol* 2002;44:695-698.

Twenty-one percent of boys with Duchenne muscular dystrophy sustained fractures; 48% of the fractures occurred in ambulatory patients as a result of falls, and 20% of boys ceased walking because of the fracture.

Scher DM, Mubarak SJ: Surgical prevention of foot deformity in patients with Duchenne muscular dystrophy. *J Pediatr Orthop* 2002;22:384-391.

Plantigrade shoeable feet were maintained after tibialis posterior transfer, Achilles tendon lengthening, and toe flexor releases.

Sengupta DK, Mehdian SH, McConnell JR, et al: Pelvic or lumbar fixation for the surgical management of scoliosis in Duchenne muscular dystrophy. *Spine* 2002;27:2072-2079.

Increasing pelvic tilt was not seen at 3.5-year follow-up after posterior spinal fusion with pedicle screw fixation to L5 for mild curves.

Sussman M: Duchenne muscular dystrophy. *J Am Acad Orthop Surg* 2002;10:138-151.

A detailed review of current treatment and research on Duchenne muscular dystrophy is presented.

Spinal Muscular Atrophy

Bach JR, Baird JS, Plosky D, et al: Spinal muscular atrophy type 1: Management and outcomes. *Pediatr Pulmonol* 2002;34:16-22.

Although tracheostomy prolonged survival in patients with type 1 spinal muscular atrophy, noninvasive ventilation preserved speech.

Sporer SM, Smith BG: Hip dislocation in patients with spinal muscular atrophy. *J Pediatr Orthop* 2003;23:10-14.

Thirty-nine of 41 patients with spinal muscular atrophy and hip dislocations were pain free at 18-year follow-up.

Freidreich's Ataxia

Lynch DR, Farmer JM, Balcer LJ, et al: Friedreich ataxia: Effects of genetic understanding on clinical evaluation and therapy. *Arch Neurol* 2002;59:743-747.

Molecular genetic research has led to the discovery of mutations in the frataxin gene. The link between genotype and phenotype has been studied. Treatment is under investigation based on frataxin's role in cellular responses to oxidative stress.

Charcot-Marie-Tooth Disease

Berger P, Young P, Suter U, et al: Molecular cell biology of Charcot-Marie-Tooth disease. *Neurogenetics* 2002;4:1-15.

The specific mutations in 10 genes linked with subtypes of Charcot-Marie-Tooth disease are discussed.

Sammarco GJ, Taylor R: Cavovarus foot treated with combined calcaneus and metatarsal osteotomies. *Foot Ankle Int* 2001;22:19-30.

Fifteen feet affected by Charcot-Marie-Tooth disease underwent combined calcaneal and metatarsal osteotomies with improvements in foot scores and radiographs.

Classic Bibliography

Beaty JH, Canale ST: Orthopaedic aspects of myelomeningocele. *J Bone Joint Surg Am* 1990;72:626-630.

Botto LD, Moore CA, Khoury MJ, Erickson JD: Medical progress: Neural tube defects. *N Engl J Med* 1999;341:1509-1519.

Brinker MR, Rosenfield SR, Feiwell E, Granger SP, Mitchell DC, Rice JC: Myelomeningocele at the sacral level: Long term outcomes in adults. *J Bone Joint Surg Am* 1994;76:1293-1300.

Daher YH, Lonstein JE, Winter RB, et al: Spinal deformities in patients with Charcot-Marie-Tooth disease: A review of 12 patients. *Clin Orthop* 1986;202:219-222.

Damiano DL, Abel MF: Functional outcomes of strength training in spastic cerebral palsy. *Arch Phys Med Rehabil* 1998;79:119-125.

Delp SL, Zajac FE: Force and moment generating capacity of the lower extremity muscles before and after tendon lengthening. *Clin Orthop* 1992;284:247-259.

DeLuca PA, Davis RB, Ounpuu S, Rose S, Sirkin R: Alterations in surgical decision making in patients with cerebral palsy based on three-dimensional gait analysis. *J Pediatr Orthop* 1997;17:608-614.

Drennan JC: Current concepts in myelomeningocele. *Instr Course Lect* 1999;48:543-550.

Galasko CS, Delaney C, Morris P: Spinal stabilization in Duchenne muscular dystrophy. *J Bone Joint Surg Br* 1992;74:210-214.

Greene WB: Treatment of hip and knee problems in myelomeningocele. *Instr Course Lect* 1999;48:563-574.

Hensinger RN, MacEwen GD: Spinal deformity associated with heritable neurological conditions: Spinal muscular atrophy, Friedreich's ataxia, familial dysautonomia, and Charcot-Marie-Tooth disease. *J Bone Joint Surg Am* 1976;58:13-24.

Hoffman EP, Kunkel LM: Dystrophin abnormalities in Duchenne/Becker muscular dystrophy. *Neuron* 1989;2: 1019-1029.

Koman LA, Mooney JF III, Smith BP, Walker F, Leon JM: Botulinum toxin type A neuromuscular blockade in the treatment of lower extremity spasticity in cerebral palsy: A randomized, doubled-blind, placebo-controlled trial: BOTOX Study Group. *J Pediatr Orthop* 2000;20: 108-115.

Kunkel LM: Analysis of deletions in DNA in patients with Becker and Duchenne muscular dystrophy. *Nature* 1986;322:73-77.

Labelle H, Tohme S, Duhaime M, et al: Natural history of scoliosis in Friedreich's ataxia. *J Bone Joint Surg Am* 1986;68:564-572.

Lieber RL: Skeletal muscle adaptability: I. Review of basic properties. *Dev Med Child Neurol* 1986;28:390-396.

Lim R, Dias L, Vankoski S, Moore C, Marinello M, Sarwark J: Valgus knee stress in lumbosacral meylomeningocele: A gait analysis evaluation. *J Pediatr Orthop* 1998;18:428-433.

Mazar J, Menelaus MB, Dickens DR, Doig WG: Efficacy of surgical management for scoliosis in myelomeningocele: Correction of deformity and alteration of functional status. *J Pediatr Orthop* 1986;6:568-575.

Muller EB, Nordwall A: Brace treatment of scoliosis in children with myelomeningocele. *Spine* 1994;19:151-155.

Mubarak SJ, Morin WD, Leach J: Spinal fusion in Duchenne muscular dystrophy: Fixation and fusion to the sacropelvis? *J Pediatr Orthop* 1993;13:752-757.

Mubarak SJ, Wenger DR, Valencia F: One-stage correction of the spastic dislocated hip: Use of pericapsular acetabuloplasty to improve coverage. *J Bone Joint Surg Am* 1992;74:1347-1357.

Ounpuu S, Muik E, Davis RB III, Gage JR, Deluca PL: Rectus femoris surgery in children with cerebral palsy:

Part I. The effect of rectus femoris transfer location on knee motion. *J Pediatr Orthop* 1993;13:325-330.

Ounpuu S, Muik E, Davis RB III, Gage JR, Deluca PL: Rectus femoris surgery in children with cerebral palsy. Part II: A comparison between the effect of transfer and release of the distal rectus femoris on knee motion. *J Pediatr Orthop* 1993;13:331-335.

Perry J: Determinants of muscle function in the spastic lower extremity. *Clin Orthop* 1993;288:10-26.

Read L, Galasko CS: Delay in diagnosing Duchenne muscular dystrophy in orthopaedic clinics. *J Bone Joint Surg Br* 1986;68:481-482.

Reimers J: Functional changes in the antagonists after lengthening of the agonists in cerebral palsy. *Clin Orthop* 1990;253:30-37.

Rose SA, Deluca PA, Davis RB III, Ounpuu S, Gage JR: Kinematic and kinetic evaluation of the ankle after lengthening of the gastrocnemius fascia in children with cerebral palsy. *J Pediatr Orthop* 1993;13:727-732.

Skaggs DL, Rethlefsen SA, Kay RM, Dennis SW, Reynolds RA, Tolo VT: Variability in gait analysis interpretation. *J Pediatr Orthop* 2000;20:759-764.

Smith AD, Koreska J, Moseley CF: Progression of scoliosis in Duchenne muscular dystrophy. *J Bone Joint Surg Am* 1989;71:1066-1074.

Strauss DJ, Shavelle RM, Anderson TW: Life expectancy of children with cerebral palsy. *Pediatr Neurol* 1998;18:143-149.

Sutherland DH, Davids JR: Common gait abnormalities of the knee in cerebral palsy. *Clin Orthop* 1993;288:139-147.

Talipan N, Bruner JP, Hernandez-Schulman M, et al: Effects of intrauterine myelomeningocele repair on central nervous system structure and function. *Pediatr Neurosurg* 1999;31:183-188.

Walker JL, Nelson KR, Heavilon JA, et al: Hip abnormalities in children with Charcot-Marie-Tooth disease. *J Pediatr Orthop* 1994;14:54-59.

Wetmore RS, Drennan JC: Long-term results of triple arthrodesis in Charcot-Marie-Tooth disease. *J Bone Joint Surg Am* 1989;71:417-422.

Williams JJ, Graham GP, Dunne KB, Menelaus MB: Late knee problems in myelomeningocele. *J Pediatr Orthop* 1993;13:701-703.

Chapter 58

Pediatric Hematology

Michael T. Busch, MD

Tim Schrader, MD

Gary M. Lourie, MD

Hemophilia

Hemophilia is a group of genetic bleeding disorders that affects about 20,000 Americans. Hemophilia is inherited in about two thirds of patients; the condition results from spontaneous genetic mutations in one third of patients. The most common deficiencies involve factor VIII (classic hemophilia or hemophilia A) and factor IX (Christmas disease or hemophilia B). Because the genes for these deficiencies are carried on the X chromosome, they are usually recessive disorders affecting males. Females, who are genetic carriers of the disease, can have mild deficiencies and may become symptomatic after trauma or surgery. von Willebrand's disease is a deficiency or abnormality of von Willebrand's factor, a large protein that is responsible for the adherence of platelets to damaged endothelium and acts as a carrier protein for the factor VIII molecule. von Willebrand's disease can be inherited in either an autosomal dominant or recessive manner, and it affects almost an equal number of males and females. Other less common clotting factor deficiencies and disorders of platelets may need to be considered when evaluating patients for spontaneous musculoskeletal bleeding that is spontaneous or occurs after trauma or surgery.

The hallmark symptom of severe hemophilia (factor levels ≤ 1% of normal) is spontaneous bleeding. In these patients, bleeding occurs without any recognizable trauma. Recurrent hemarthrosis, or repeated bleeding into the joints, usually begins after a child starts to walk. In children, the ankles and elbows are more commonly affected than the knees and shoulders. Orthopaedic surgeons may encounter these frequently undiagnosed disorders in patients who experience excessive intraoperative, postoperative, or posttraumatic bleeding. Preoperative screening histories should query for frequent gum bleeding, epistaxis, excessive bruising, and menorrhagia. A family history should also be obtained. Because mild deficiencies may not result in significant symptoms, a screening history should be obtained for all patients before surgery, particularly those undergoing more demanding procedures such as spinal fusion. The possibility of an undiagnosed coagulopathy should be considered in patients with compartment syndrome after relative minor injuries and when excessive bleeding is encountered during or after surgery.

Although several substances in blood produce an inflammatory reaction from the synovium, iron is thought to be the primary stimulant. In response to the inflammation, the synovium develops villi that are highly vascular and friable (Figure 1). These villi are then prone to spontaneous hemorrhage with normal activity or minor trauma. Once inflamed, the synovium also releases chondrolytic substances and other factors that alter the normal homeostasis between osteoblasts and osteoclasts, resulting in chondrolysis, periarticular osteopenia, and cyst formation.

Hemophilic arthropathy can develop in patients as young as 3 years of age. Synovitis must be treated early and aggressively to prevent hemophilic arthropathy. This involves medical treatment, including varying degrees of a combination of prolonged factor replacement, physical therapy, and activity modifications. If these measures are not enough to control bleeding, inflamed synovium may become so thick and abundant that control can only be gained from a synovectomy (Figure 2, A).

Prophylaxis

By infusing exogenous clotting factor concentrates on a regular basis (typically two to three times per week), the trough concentrations can be kept above 1% (patients typically bleed when levels are below 1%). Although primary prophylaxis is a good strategy to prevent joint bleeding, there are numerous issues related to cost and difficulty of ongoing administration.

Demand Therapy

The common approach is to treat hemarthroses as they occur. The first dose administered after a joint bleed should elevate the deficient clotting factor level to 80% of normal. This decays to 5% in 48 hours (the half-life for factor VIII is 12 hours), and an additional 40% dose

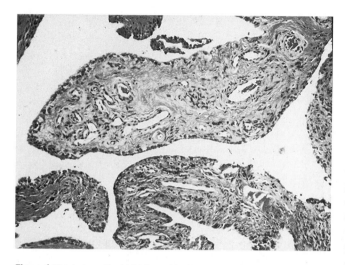

Figure 1 Histologic section of the hemosiderotic synovitis that results from recurrent hemarthrosis in a patient with severe hemophilia. Note the highly vascular villi with little supporting collagen, making this area highly prone to bleeding with minor trauma or even normal joint motion.

is given on the second and third days after a bleed so that levels remain above 5% for 5 days. Rest, ice, compression, and elevation are instituted immediately to reduce the severity of the bleed. As swelling resolves and motion returns, the child gradually resumes activities.

If a joint bleeds more than three times in 6 months, it becomes prone to developing a chronic synovitis. Secondary prophylaxis is instituted for 3 months. If bleeding stops and the synovitis resolves, the options are to continue secondary prophylaxis indefinitely or to resume demand therapy. If the bleeding continues on prophylaxis or if the synovitis fails to resolve after 3 months, the synovitis is considered recalcitrant to medical management and a synovectomy becomes necessary. The primary indications for synovectomy are persistent synovitis or bleeding despite 3 months of prophylaxis and resumption of joint bleeding within 1 year of successful prophylaxis.

Synovectomy is therefore a means of "rescuing" the joint from chronic synovitis, and it is a key treatment modality for the successful use of demand therapy. The primary objective when performing a synovectomy in these joints is to remove most of the friable villous layer of the synovium. Perioperative hemostasis is provided by factor administration, allowing the synovium to heal. The resultant synovial lining is smoother and less prone to repetitive injury.

Radionuclide Synovectomy

By injecting a radioactive pharmaceutical agent into an affected joint, the hypertrophic synovium is ablated, restoring a smoother and less friable surface. In the United States, the most commonly used substance is P32 chromic phosphate. This substance releases primarily β radiation, which only penetrates a few millimeters into

tissue. Although there is still some theoretic risk of subsequent malignant transformation after radionuclide synovectomy, only one associated instance has been reported in a child with hemophilia, and there are no reports of growth disturbances.

The procedure is typically done as an outpatient procedure in the radiology suite, and local anesthesia is usually adequate. An arthrogram is always done to confirm intra-articular placement of the needle tip and to look for venous extravasation (which usually occurs in joints acutely inflamed by a bleed just before the procedure and is a contraindication to proceeding). The dosage varies depending on the joint and the size of the patient. Steroids are simultaneously injected to reduce the inflammatory response that can accompany the treatment. A small-gauge needle is used to minimize leakage up the needle track, and pressure is applied afterward. Follow-up liver and spleen scans are used to look for systemic leakage, but the results of these tests are rarely positive. Patient activities are reduced for 2 weeks, and physical therapy is not usually needed. Radionuclide synovectomy generally reduces the frequency of bleeds by 50% of patients with hemophilia. Radionuclide synovectomy is ideally suited for patients with hemophilia who have developed an inhibitor, which is an immunoglobulin G-mediated antibody response to the clotting factor.

Arthroscopic Synovectomy

Arthroscopic synovectomy offers some advantages over radionuclide synovectomy in that the diseased synovium is physically removed and lesions of articular cartilage can be débrided simultaneously (Figure 2, *B*). This procedure can be done on an outpatient basis using a continuous infusion pump to fully correct the deficient clotting factor before surgery and through the fourth postoperative day. Infusion is then continued every other day for at least 6 to 12 weeks. The most common complication, loss of motion, is associated with preexisting arthritis (significant lost motion already present or radiographic changes of joint space narrowing) or early postoperative bleeding. Arthroscopic synovectomy requires compliance with a rigorous preoperative and postoperative regimen of factor replacement and physical therapy; therefore, a committed family and experienced multidisciplinary team are keys to success. Joints in children as young as 3 years can be arthroscopically treated, and early intervention significantly improves outcomes. Overall, an 80% reduction in hemarthroses can be expected, and virtually all patients should experience improvement.

Although the direct costs of radionuclide synovectomy are less than those of arthroscopic synovectomy, radionuclide synovectomy carries a higher rate of repeat procedures, and arthroscopic synovectomy may be more

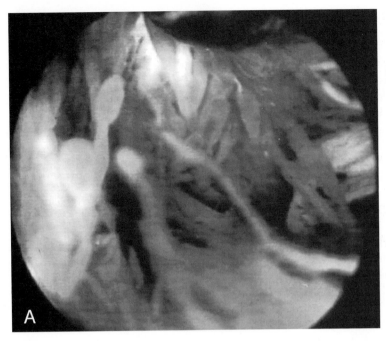 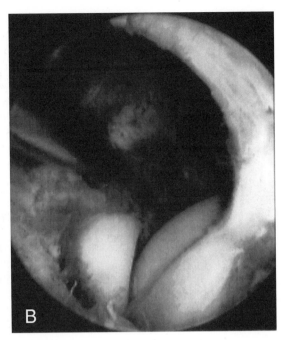

Figure 2 A, Arthroscopic view of the anterior compartment in the elbow of an 8-year-old boy with hemophilic (hemosiderotic) synovitis. Note the vascular villi produced by this proliferative synovitis. **B,** Arthroscopic view of the same region of the anterior elbow compartment seen near the completion of an arthroscopic synovectomy. Note that most of the villi have been removed, but the capsule remains intact. *(Reproduced with permission from Dunn AL, Busch MT, Wyly JB, Sullivan KM, Abshire TC: Arthroscopic synovectomy for hemophilic joint disease in a pediatric population. J Pediatr Orthop 2004;24:414-426.)*

effective, especially in more severely affected joints. Arthroscopic synovectomy also avoids the long-term risks of radiation exposure. Regardless of the type of synovectomy, the key to success is early intervention. Most patients with severe hemophilia who are managed with on-demand therapy protocols will develop a "target joint" by adolescence, and an early "synovectomy rescue" is essential to minimize the risk of premature arthritis.

Sickle Cell Disease

Normal hemoglobin is composed of α and β chains. The gene for β globulin is located on chromosome 11, and a single substitution of valine for glutamic acid at the sixth amino acid position causes an abnormally functioning hemoglobin (the gene for hemoglobin S) to be produced. Heterogeneous individuals have sickle cell trait, and homozygous individuals have sickle cell disease. Other abnormalities can occur in the α and β globulin chains and cause sickle cell disorders, including sickle cell β thalassemia, sickle cell hemoglobin D, and sickle cell hemoglobin E.

Sickle cell trait is common in western Africa, where it provides some protection against malaria. In the United States, about 10% of the African-American population carries the hemoglobin S gene, and 1 in 600 has sickle cell disease. Sickle cell disease primarily affects blacks, but it can occur in other ethnic groups.

Heterozygous individuals have a normal gene for hemoglobin A and a gene for hemoglobin S. Carriers are typically asymptomatic because hemoglobin A still accounts for about 55% to 60% of an individual's total hemoglobin. Only rarely do individuals with sickle cell trait display symptoms. Homozygous individuals with two genes for hemoglobin S, however, have no hemoglobin A, and every organ and tissue in the body can be adversely affected.

As oxygen tension decreases, the hemoglobin S molecules polymerize within the red cells and lead to alteration in red cell shape, membrane changes, cellular dehydration, decreased deformability, and shorter life span of the red cells. Tissues with low oxygen tension and end vessel flow are particularly vulnerable. Musculoskeletal symptoms account for 80% of all hospital admissions.

In infancy, individuals with sickle cell disease are protected by fetal hemoglobin (hemoglobin F). In infants age 4 to 6 months with sickle cell disease, the amount of hemoglobin F begins to decrease and symptoms can occur. Dactylitis (hand-foot syndrome) typically presents between the ages of 6 months and 4 years. This condition is characterized by swelling and tenderness in the hands or feet, and occurs in about 70% of all individuals with sickle cell disease. Dactylitis is thought to represent a vaso-occlusive episode. Treatment consists of analgesia, oxygen, and hydration, with symptoms typically lasting 3 to 7 days. Osteomyelitis must remain in the differential diagnosis, and aspiration can be used to aid in determining the proper treatment. Dactylitis is rare after age 6 years, when hematopoietic marrow disappears in the digits. Forty percent of individuals can have recurrent dactylitis.

The incidence of sickle cell crises in patients with sickle cell disease is around 0.8 episodes per year. Hydroxyurea has been shown to decrease the number of painful episodes in adults, and a multicenter trial of hydroxyurea in children is currently underway.

Although individuals with sickle cell disease are more prone to infection, the incidence of osteomyelitis remains quite low (< 1% per year), and bone infarcts are 50 times more common. Nonetheless, differentiating between osteomyelitis and bone infarcts can be difficult because their signs and symptoms are quite similar. Pain, swelling, redness, warmth, stiffness, and elevated laboratory parameters are common. Erythrocyte sedimentation rates are unreliable in patients with sickle cell disease because of the altered red cells. Blood cultures should be included in routine work-up, and bone aspiration should be done in patients with suspected sickle cell disease. Several imaging modalities have been studied to help differentiate between infection and infarct, including bone scans and MRI. Ultrasonography may be less expensive and equally effective. A recent report has identified serum procalcitonin concentration as a negative predictor of serious musculoskeletal infection. Common pathogens include *Staphylococcus aureus*, *Salmonella*, and *Streptococcus pneumoniae*. Treatment consists of antibiotics, hydration, oxygenation, and surgical drainage of abscesses. Reactive arthritis and septic arthritis can also occur.

Bone marrow hyperplasia can cause bony changes in patients with sickle cell disease. Osteopenia in the vertebral bodies can lead to bulging of the intervertebral disks, compression fractures, and progressive kyphosis. Long bone growth can be affected, and pathologic fractures can occur. Growth retardation is common in patients with sickle cell disease, with height and weight significantly lower than average at 2 years of age. Skeletal maturity can also be delayed. Osteonecrosis of the femoral and humeral heads commonly occurs, with prevalences of 30% and 6%, respectively. Treatment options include restricted weightbearing, core decompression, polymethylmethacrylate injection, vascularized fibular grafts, hemiresurfacing, and total joint arthroplasty. Joint arthroplasty is complicated by higher rates of infection and loosening.

Thalassemia

The thalassemia syndromes comprise a heterogeneous group of hemolytic anemias that result from mutations that affect globulin synthesis. Normal hemoglobin is composed of α and β chains; therefore, α and β thalassemias can occur. Individuals with thalassemia major are homozygous. There is very low to no hemoglobin A pro-

duction, which results in a severe hemolytic, microcytic, hypochromic anemia. Bone marrow hyperplasia ensues, causing bone fragility, growth retardation, and an increased rate of fractures. Slipped capital femoral epiphysis and early osteoarthritis occur at increased rates. Radiographic findings include widened marrow spaces, thinned cortices, severe osteopenia, and "hair-on-end" appearance of the skull. Extramedullary hematopoiesis in the vertebrae can cause paraparesis by compression of the spinal cord. Increased body iron loads can cause tissue fibrosis, resulting in cardiomyopathy, diabetes mellitus, and adrenal, parathyroid, and thyroid hypofunction. Splenectomy in childhood lessens the transfusion requirements, but it increases the already higher than normal rate of infections. Treatments of individuals with thalassemia include early transfusion therapy (maintaining hemoglobin > 9 g/dL), iron chelation, bone marrow transplantation, splenectomy, and supportive medical management.

Leukemia

Acute leukemia is the most common malignancy in childhood, accounting for nearly one third of instances of cancer in children. Acute lymphocytic leukemia accounts for approximately 80% of these instances. With current therapies, approximately 80% of children with acute lymphocytic leukemia now survive.

Although leukemia is primarily a disease of the bone marrow, any organ can be infiltrated by the malignant cell, and this accounts for the highly variable clinical presentation. The musculoskeletal system is often involved, including pain in the extremities, back pain, osteomyelitis, septic arthritis, or fracture. Twenty percent of patients present with a primary report of limp or extremity pain, and up to 50% of patients have these symptoms as secondary complaints at the time of initial diagnosis. Although long bone pain is the most common symptom, the spine may be involved. This becomes an important consideration in the differential diagnosis of the child presenting with back pain. At the onset of the disease, 10% of children have normal peripheral blood counts, making the diagnosis even more challenging. MRI may be helpful because it is very sensitive to marrow changes caused by infiltration and secondary infarct.

Painful joint swelling and fever are common presenting symptoms of the musculoskeletal manifestations of leukemia. These symptoms may mimic sepsis or acute onset of a juvenile idiopathic arthritis (formerly called juvenile rheumatoid arthritis). Typically, patients with juvenile idiopathic arthritis present with morning stiffness and pain localized to the joints, whereas patients with leukemia more often present with night pain and nonarticular bone pain. The radiographs of patients with juvenile idiopathic arthritis may show joint effusions and mild osteopenia surrounding joints, whereas the radiographic changes suggestive of acute leukemia include diffuse osteopenia, metaphyseal bands, periosteal new bone formation, geographic lytic lesions, sclerosis, mixed sclerosis/lysis, and permeative destruction.

Once considered rare, acute megakaryoblastic leukemia now accounts for about 12% of all instances of acute myeloid leukemia in children. Most instances of acute megakaryoblastic leukemia are difficult to diagnose because of their complex clinical presentation and unusual bone marrow morphologic features. In children, acute megakaryoblastic leukemia is often confused with metastatic solid tumors or myelodysplastic syndrome. These abnormalities (bilaterally symmetric periostitis and osteolytic lesions) differ markedly from those commonly reported in association with pediatric acute leukemias.

Treatment protocols for leukemia often include significant doses of steroids because of their antilymphocytic effects. MRI shows changes consistent with areas of osteonecrosis in approximately 25% of children receiving high-dose steroid regimens. Children younger than 10 years are generally not affected. One third or more of those affected develop symptomatic complications of weight-bearing joints. When these complications do occur, treatment options are limited, and end stage joint disease can develop.

Thrombocytopenia With Absent Radii

Thrombocytopenia with absent radii (TAR) syndrome is an autosomal recessive, rare disorder characterized by congenital hypomegakaryocytic thrombocytopenia and bilateral absence of the radius, with shortening of the ulna and a normal thumb. This syndrome develops between the fourth and eighth weeks of gestation when the radii develop and platelet production begins. Significant complications that can occur in infancy secondary to thrombocytopenia include intracranial hemorrhage, anemia, and frequent occurrences of epistaxis. Characteristic hematologic findings include hypomegakaryocytic thrombocytopenia, periodic leukemoid reactions, and eosinophilia. Mortality in early infancy approaches 40% of patients; however, if the child is able to survive the first 1 to 2 years of life, the thrombocytopenia usually resolves and the musculoskeletal problems become the chief manifestation of TAR.

The upper extremity anomalies include bilateral absence of the radii with radial deviation at the wrist, a shortened and bowed ulna, and normal thumbs. Recently, an anomalous muscle spanning the elbow with its origin on the humeral shaft at the deltoid tubercle and insertion into the hand and carpal bones (termed the brachiocarpalis) has been described and its excision has been recommended to negate the strong radial deviation to the hand.

Lower extremity anomalies occur in up to 80% of patients, and they include severe genu varum, instability, and patellar abnormalities, which has prompted some to rename this syndrome TARK, with the letter K signifying involvement of the knee. Other associated deformities include hip dysplasia, pes valgus, talipes equinovarus, synostosis in the metatarsals, and syndactyly involving the toes.

Management of patients with TAR syndrome includes hematologic support, including platelet transfusions until the patient's condition stabilizes, usually around 2 years of age. Musculoskeletal management includes radiographs for patients with occult hip dysplasia. Varus angulation and internal tibial rotation usually recur after corrective osteotomy, which has prompted some to advocate a more conservative management approach using simple adaptive devices and powered mobility aids. Foot and ankle reconstruction including posteromedial release and/or heel cord lengthening have been recommended. The goals of surgical treatment of the upper extremity deformities are to obtain and maintain correction of the radial deviation. The primary indication for upper extremity surgery correction is persistent wrist contracture and reconstruction of function-limiting thumb deficiency.

Annotated Bibliography

Hemophilia

Butler RB, McClure W, Wulff K: Practice patterns in haemophilia A therapy: A survey of treatment centres in the United States. *Haemophilia* 2003;9:549-554.

This study surveyed 52 hemophilia centers with a total of 4,129 patients receiving treatment. Among patients with severe hemophilia, 49% were receiving on-demand treatment, whereas 44% were receiving some form of prophylaxis (13% primary, 20% secondary, and 11% tertiary). Primary prophylaxis was the most common type in children younger than 5 years, who comprised 25% of this age group. In children age 6 to 18 years, 58% were receiving some type of prophylactic regimen, whereas on-demand treatment was most frequent among adult patients.

Dunn AL, Busch MT, Wyly JB, Abshire TC: Radionuclide synovectomy for hemophilic arthropathy: A comprehensive review of safety and efficacy and recommendation for a standardized treatment protocol. *Thromb Haemost* 2002;87:383-393.

This review article compiles the published experience to date using radionuclide synovectomy for hemophilic joint disease. A suggested treatment protocol is presented.

Dunn AL, Busch MT, Wyly JB, Sullivan KM, Abshire TC: Arthroscopic synovectomy for hemophilic joint disease in a pediatric population. *J Pediatr Orthop* 2004;24: 414-426.

This study provides data on 47 pediatric patients who underwent arthroscopic synovectomy (40 ankles, 22 elbows, 9 knees, and 2 shoulders) for hemophilic joint disease. The median patient age at time of surgery was 10.3 years, and median follow-up was 79 months. The authors report that joints with sufficient follow-up data showed a median bleeding frequency decline of 84% ($P < 0.001$).

Journeycake JM, Miller KL, Anderson AM, Buchanan GR, Finnegan M: Arthroscopic synovectomy in children and adolescents with hemophilia. *J Pediatr Hematol Oncol* 2003;25:726-731.

In this study, 28 arthroscopic synovectomies (11 knees, 12 ankles, and 5 elbows) were done on 26 joints in 20 patients with hemophilia. The authors report that the frequency of hemarthrosis diminished significantly in the first year and was maintained for up to 5 years in all but three joints.

Sickle Cell Disease

Scott LK, Grier LR, Arnold TC, Conrad SA: Serum procalcitonin concentration as a negative predictor of serious bacterial infection in acute sickle cell pain crisis. *Med Sci Monit* 2003;9:CR426-CR431.

In this preliminary study of 24 patients with sickle cell disease, pain crisis, and acute inflammation, procalcitonin levels were measured and levels less than 2 ng/mL were reported to have a good negative predictive value of serious infection.

Skaggs DL, Kim SK, Greene NW, Harris D, Miller JH: Differentiation between bone infarction and acute osteomyelitis in children with sickle-cell disease with use of sequential radionuclide bone-marrow and bone scans. *J Bone Joint Surg Am* 2001;83:1810-1813.

This is a study of 70 patients with sickle cell disease and acute bone pain. The findings suggest that serial radionuclide bone marrow and bone scan scintigraphy can provide some differentiation between osteomyelitis and bone infarction.

Leukemia

States LJ: Imaging of metabolic bone disease and marrow disorders in children. *Radiol Clin North Am* 2001; 39:749-772.

In this study, the author reports that MRI provides detailed information about bone marrow and is gaining an increasingly important role in the management of disorders of bone marrow infiltration.

Thrombocytopenia With Absent Radii

Carter PR, Mills J, Ezaki M: (Abstract) Anatomical description of an anomalous muscle in thrombocytopenia absent radius (TAR) syndrome and discussion of its clinical significance, in *American Society for Surgery of the Hand Meeting Abstracts, Phoenix, AZ, 2002*, p 13. Available at: http://www.assh.org. Accessed October 6, 2004.

The authors of this retrospective review of 16 patients with thrombocytopenia absent radius syndrome show the presence of an anomalous muscle spanning the elbow (termed the brachiocarpalis) and emphasize its contribution to the radial deformity. They recommend excision in patients with progressive radial deviation.

Classic Bibliography

Arnold WD, Hilgartner MW: Hemophilic arthropathy: Current concepts of pathogenesis and management. *J Bone Joint Surg Am* 1977;59:287-305.

Chambers JB, Forsythe DA, Bertrand SL, Iwinski HJ, Steflik DE: Retrospective review of osteoarticular infections in a pediatric sickle cell age group. *J Pediatr Orthop* 2000;20:682-685.

Christensen CP, Ferguson RL: Lower extremity deformities associated with thrombocytopenia in absent radius syndrome. *Clin Orthop* 2000;375:202-206.

Hedberg VA, Lipton JM: Thrombocytopenia with absent radii: A review of 100 cases. *Am J Pediatr Hematol Oncol* 1988;10:51-64.

Heinrich SD, Gallagher D, Warrior R, Phelan K, George VT, MacEwen GD: The prognostic significance of the skeletal manifestations of acute lymphoblastic leukemia of childhood. *J Pediatr Orthop* 1994;14:105-111.

Mattano LA Jr, Sather HN, Trigg ME, Nachman JB: Osteonecrosis as a complication of treating acute lymphoblastic leukemia in children: A report from the Children's Cancer Group. *J Clin Oncol* 2000;18:3262-3272.

McLaurin TM, Bukrey CD, Lovett RJ, Mochel DM: Management of thrombocytopenia-absent radius (TAR) syndrome. *J Pediatr Orthop* 1999;19:289-296.

Schoenecker PL, Cohn AK, Sedgwick WG, Manske PR, Salafsky I, Millar EA: Dysplasia of the knee associated with the syndrome of thrombocytopenia and absent radius. *J Bone Joint Surg Am* 1984;66:421-427.

Chapter 59

Shoulder and Humerus: Pediatrics

Ann Van Heest, MD

Introduction

Familiarity with the spectrum of shoulder disorders seen in children is necessary for the treatment of pediatric upper extremity disorders. For the child whose symptoms prevent normal use of the arm, a complete evaluation should include the shoulder girdle because children often are unable to provide details on the history of their disorder and have difficulty localizing symptoms.

A general classification of pediatric shoulder disorders is based on congenital, developmental, or acquired etiology. Congenital shoulder disorders are present at birth and are the result of abnormal fetal formation and development. Developmental disorders are caused by growth disturbances such as growth plate dysfunction, neuromuscular disorders, systemic disease, or manifestations of a syndromic disorder. Acquired disorders are most commonly secondary to trauma, infection, or tumor. This classification system helps provide a general framework for understanding pediatric shoulder disorders.

Sprengel's Deformity

Sprengel's deformity is the congenital failure of descent of the scapula from the embryonic level opposite the fifth cervical vertebra to its final normal position, with its superior border at the seventh cervical vertebra and with its inferior angle at the level of the sixth rib. In up to 50% of patients, an associated omovertebral bar has been described, consisting of a fibrous, cartilaginous, or bony connection between the superior angle of the scapula and the cervical vertebral spinous process, lamina, or transverse process. Additionally, omoclavicular bars have been described. Other common associated anomalies requiring investigation including scoliosis, spina bifida, rib anomalies, Klippel-Feil syndrome, abnormal musculature, foot deformities, torticollis, facial asymmetry, and pulmonary and kidney disorders. The incidence of these disorders is nearly equal on the right and left sides; bilaterality is reported in 10% to 30% of patients. The condition is slightly more common in girls.

Diagnosis of Sprengel's deformity primarily has been made based on a physical examination; physical characteristics include a webbed neck, a palpable scapula into the cervical region, and a loss of range of motion. Radiographs confirm the diagnosis. Recently, prenatal diagnosis through the use of ultrasound has been described.

Recommended treatment is based on the Cavendish classification. Grade 1 deformity is very mild with level glenohumeral joints and no visible deformity when the patient is dressed; no functional impairment is present and treatment is not warranted. Grade 2 deformity is mild with level glenohumeral joints with a visible lump in the neck when the patient is dressed. If the cosmetic deformity is not acceptable, surgical treatment would include extraperiosteal resection of the scapular prominence including resection of the tethering omovertebral bar if present. Hypertrophic scars are common; therefore, parents need to be aware that the bump will be replaced with a scar. Grade 3 deformity is moderate with 2 to 5 cm of shoulder joint elevation compared with the contralateral side, and grade 4 is a severe deformity with the position of the scapula near the occiput. Surgical treatment involves not only resection of the superior angle of the scapula and the tethering omovertebral bar if present, but also derotation of the scapula and relocation to a more caudal position.

The age at which surgical intervention should be undertaken has been discussed by various authors, and the general agreement is for intervention when the child is at least 3 years of age, which is when the child is old enough to tolerate the extensive nature of the procedure yet young enough to maximize correction through subsequent growth. With caudal repositioning of the scapula, there is a risk of compressive injury to the brachial plexus. This risk is greatest in a child older than 8 years and can be lessened by concomitant clavicular osteotomy.

Surgical techniques described for scapular relocation include: (1) the Woodward procedure, which relocates the scapula by detachment and caudal relocation of the midline origin of the parascapular muscle; (2) the Green procedure, which relocates the scapula by extraperiosteal detachment of scapular muscles at their scapular insertion with reattachment after caudal relocation of the scapula using scapular traction cables; and (3) correction by vertical scapular osteotomy. Concomitant clavicular osteotomy or morcellization is recommended to reduce the incidence of neurovascular injury and to provide anterior release allowing greater correction of the deformity.

The Woodward procedure is the most common surgical technique used for correction of a moderate or severe Sprengel's deformity. A recent report has confirmed previous findings of cosmetic and functional improvement with this procedure. The age of the patient and the presence of an omovertebral bone did not influence the results. Associated cervical spine anomalies were indicative of a negative prognosis.

Pseudarthrosis of the Clavicle

Pseudarthrosis of the clavicle in children usually is present at birth, with parents reporting a prominent bump at the midportion of the clavicle. Physical examination reveals little or no pain on palpation of mobile clavicle segments with a prominence in the midportion. Shoulder range of motion is normal or hypermobile. The prominent bump in the midclavicle often becomes more apparent with loss of infantile adipose tissue. If the child is examined at a later age, asymmetry of the shoulder with drooping of the affected side caused by fragment hypermobility may be present. Difficulties with shoulder function are rare, although the recent literature has reported the occurrence of thoracic outlet symptoms in adolescence.

Radiologic evaluation shows lack of bone continuity in the middle third of the clavicle without evidence of reactive bone. The presence of minimal pain and lack of callus formation distinguishes this condition from a birth fracture. Pseudarthrosis of the clavicle can be distinguished from cleidocraniodysostosis because pseudarthrosis is more commonly unilateral with absence of cranial or pelvic involvement. Associated cervical ribs or elevated first ribs may be present in pseudarthrosis of the clavicle. The lesion is usually on the right side; left-sided occurrence is usually in association with dextrocardia. Bilateral occurrences have been reported.

Most children with congenital pseudarthrosis of the clavicle are asymptomatic and do not require surgical intervention. Surgery to establish union is reserved for children with an unacceptable bump, pain, or shoulder dysfunction. Surgical treatment options include resection of the fibrous pseudarthrosis and sclerotic bone ends with suturing of the bone ends, with bone grafting, and/or internal fixation.

Glenoid Hypoplasia

Normal glenoid ossification occurs through consolidation of the secondary ossification centers of the superior glenoid, inferior glenoid, and base of the coracoid. Failure of normal ossification of the inferior glenoid epiphysis is a rarely diagnosed entity. The patient has limited abduction, mild axillary webbing, and aplasia or hypoplasia of the glenoid. Several cases of familial involvement with variable penetrance have been reported. Lack of ossification of the inferior glenoid appears to cause such minimal disability that this condition is often undiagnosed, and is most commonly seen as an asymptomatic incidental finding or as part of other congenital deficiencies.

Birth Brachial Plexus Palsy

The most common pattern of birth brachial plexus injury involves C5 and C6 neurologic injury with complete or partial paralysis of the shoulder girdle muscles. Weakness of the deltoid, biceps, supraspinatus, and infraspinatus results in an adduction internal rotation deformity caused by the unopposed pull of the pectoralis major, subscapularis, teres major, and latissimus dorsi. Secondary skeletal changes include retroversion of the glenoid, posterior subluxation and medial flattening of the humeral head, and elongation with prominence of the acromion. Early radiographic changes of immature ossification of the epiphysis compared with the contralateral side and scapular winging are shown in Figure 1.

During infancy, treatment of the shoulder dysfunction associated with brachial plexus injury is aimed at prevention of both internal rotation contracture and secondary bone deformity during the neurologic recovery period. Brachial plexus exploration with neurolysis, nerve repair, or nerve grafting may be indicated if biceps function has not returned by 6 months of age. If shoulder muscle weakness persists with external rotation deficiency, anterior release or lengthening of the tight anterior structures (pectoralis major, subscapularis, anterior capsule) is recommended, coupled with augmentation of the deficient posterior structures (latissimus dorsi and teres major to rotator cuff tendon transfer).

Children with a history of upper trunk brachial plexus injury with incomplete return of shoulder external rotation usually should be monitored for development of skeletal changes of the glenohumeral joint. Radiographic evaluation for glenohumeral dysplasia has been described using plain radiographs, ultrasound, MRI, CT (Figure 2), and arthrography. Although the method of radiographic evaluation remains controversial, the necessity of monitoring children for glenohumeral dysplasia is not disputed. The natural history of this disease has been well defined; therefore, progressive flattening of the humeral head, posterior subluxation,

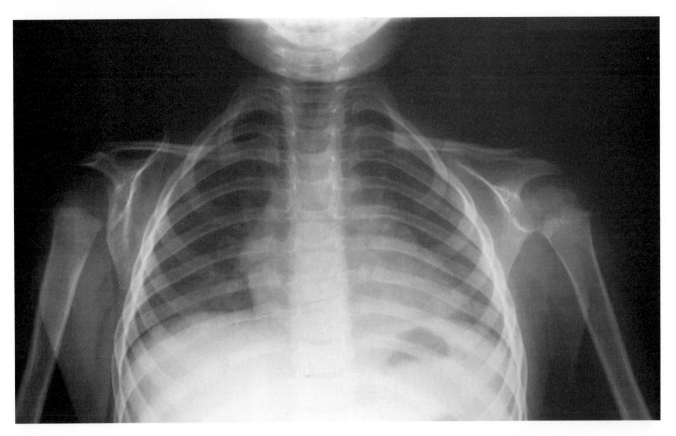

Figure 1 Early radiographic changes associated with glenohumeral dysplasia in a child with upper trunk birth brachial plexus injury are shown. These changes include immature ossification of the epiphysis compared with the contralateral side with scapular winging. Secondary skeletal changes include retroversion of the glenoid, posterior subluxation, medial flattening of the humeral head, and elongation with prominence of the acromion.

eventual dislocation of the joint, and increased retroversion of the glenoid is highly probable. Surgical intervention should be done using tendon transfer surgery before significant glenohumeral dysplasia develops. Recent studies have shown that loss of passive external rotation with the arm in adduction is an early finding on physical examination that glenohumeral dysplasia is developing. If fixed skeletal deformity of the glenohumeral joint exists, a humeral osteotomy with external rotation of the distal fragment is recommended (Figure 3).

Recent studies also have shown that a posterior dislocation can occur in association with birth brachial plexopathy even in infancy (younger than 1 year of age). Whether this condition represents an early manifestation of a severe muscle imbalance or whether the condition occurred acutely at the time of birth is currently unknown. A high index of suspicion for posterior dislocation is essential in the evaluation of an infant with brachial plexus injury at birth. If diagnosed, an open reduction may be necessary.

Clavicle Fractures

A recent study that prospectively screened newborn infants for clavicle fractures reported the incidence of 5 frac-

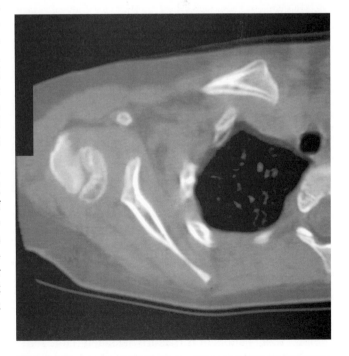

Figure 2 A CT scan more effectively evaluates glenohumeral dysplasia. Radiographic measurements should include glenoid version and the percent of humeral head coverage.

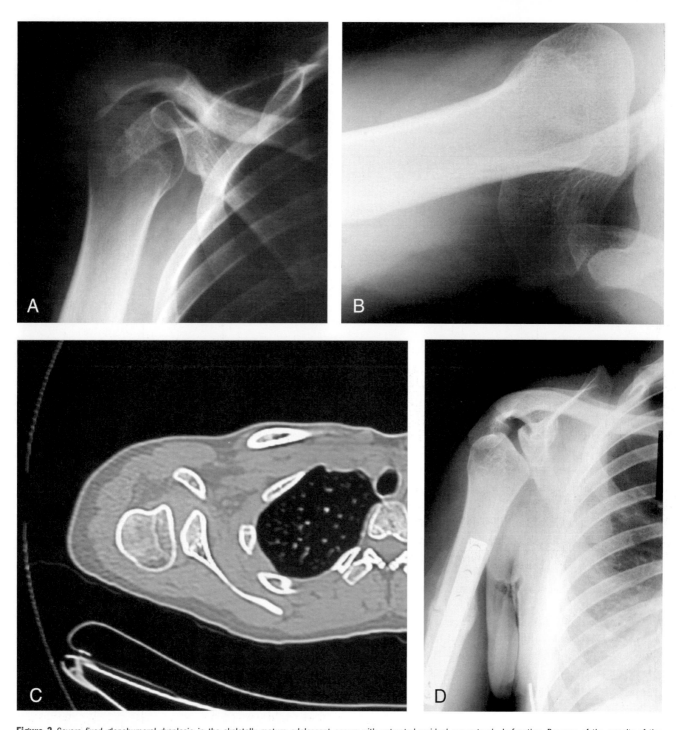

Figure 3 Severe fixed glenohumeral dysplasia in the skeletally mature adolescent occurs with untreated residual upper trunk dysfunction. Because of the severity of the dysplasia and loss of passive joint motion, a humeral rotation osteotomy was necessary for treatment. **A** and **B**, Preoperative radiographs. **C**, CT scan. **D**, Postoperative radiograph.

tures per 1,000 live births. The fractures occurred equally on the right and left side and occurred equally in males and females. All fractures occurred during vaginal deliveries. No clavicle fractures occurred with breech presentation. Risk factors for fracture included large birth weight, shoulder dystocia, mechanically assisted delivery, and prolonged gestational age. One in 11 newborns with a clavicle fracture had an associated brachial plexus palsy.

During the first decade of life, 88% of clavicle fractures are midshaft and 55% are nondisplaced. A recent report of surgical treatment of clavicle fractures indicated that over a 21-year period, only 15 patients with clavicle fractures required surgical stabilization. Surgical treatment was indicated primarily in the older child with a displaced, unstable fracture pattern. Intramedullary elastic nails or plates and screws are options for internal fixation. However, surgery is very rarely needed for pediatric clavicle fractures.

After an isolated nondisplaced midshaft clavicle fracture, the risks of nonunion, malunion, or neurovascular complications are exceptionally rare; therefore, follow-up beyond the initial diagnostic visit is rarely necessary.

Proximal Humerus and Shaft Fractures

Fractures of the proximal humerus are relatively rare (0.5% of all childhood fractures), compared with the more common distal radius, supracondylar elbow, and forearm shaft fractures. Salter-Harris type I injuries are most common in neonates and children younger than age 5 years; metaphyseal fractures are most common in children 5 to 11 years old; and Salter-Harris type II fractures are most common in those older than 11 years.

Diagnosis of proximal humeral fractures in the newborn may be difficult because these fractures must be distinguished from septic arthritis, brachial plexus injuries, and clavicle fractures in the infant with pseudoparalysis of the arm. Plain films may not be helpful in the diagnosis because the proximal humerus epiphysis does not ossify until after 6 months of age. MRI, ultrasound, or aspiration/arthrogram may be necessary. As the child approaches skeletal maturity, pain with arm dysfunction, a history of a fall on an outstretched hand, or a direct blow to the shoulder region along with positive radiographs confirm the diagnosis.

Fractures of the proximal humerus are usually treated using closed techniques. The need for a closed reduction is determined by the extent of displacement and the remodeling remaining, based on the child's age. General guidelines include up to 70° of angulation in the child younger than 5 years old; 40° to 70° of angulation in the child 5 to 12 years old; and up to 40° of angulation in the child older than 12 years.

When reduction cannot be achieved, or when reduction is lost as the arm is moved down to the side, percutaneous pinning is usually recommended. Open reductions are reserved for special circumstances such as in patients with associated injuries, open injuries, concomitant glenohumeral dislocation, or significant muscle interposition. In patients with open injuries, the use of external fixation has been used with good results.

Septic Arthritis and Osteomyelitis

Septic arthritis of the shoulder joint remains an uncommon and difficult diagnosis that requires a high index of suspicion. The disease usually involves very young infants and has a high prevalence of associated infections. In a recent review of the literature, elevated body temperature was present in 90% of pediatric patients with septic arthritis and was the most constant finding of the physical examination. An increased erythrocyte sedimentation rate (that may rise above 100 mm/hr) and increased white blood cell count also may be seen.

The initial radiographs are frequently normal; ultrasonography supports the diagnosis in some patients by showing an accumulation of fluid inside the joint space. Aspiration of synovial fluid from the affected glenohumeral joint is necessary to evaluate the offending pathogen. In a recent review, false-negative Gram stains occurred in approximately 90% of patients, whereas synovial fluid cultures showed the pathogen in 88% of patients. Blood cultures were positive in 90% of pediatric patients. The most common isolated pathogen was *Staphylococcus aureus*, which accounted for 41% of infections. Gram-negative bacilli, which accounted for about 20% of infections, are more prevalent in the pediatric population, especially in neonates.

Pyogenic shoulder arthritis should be treated with intravenous antibiotics after synovial fluid aspiration and joint irrigation. Irrigation (using a wrist arthroscope) or arthrotomy may be chosen.

The close proximity of the proximal humeral metaphysis to the shoulder joint capsule, as well as the perforating vessels from the physis to the metaphysis of the proximal humerus, necessitate investigation to determine if septic arthritis of the shoulder joint coexists with osteomyelitis of the proximal humerus. About half of affected children have both conditions. Treatment of septic arthritis in these children should include intravenous antibiotics and drilling of the metaphyseal bone of the proximal humerus at the time of joint washout. The presence of persistent pain, swelling, and fever in children who have had an arthrotomy or arthroscopy for septic arthritis of the shoulder may indicate concurrent osteomyelitis.

Certain systemic diseases such as sickle cell disease tend to be more closely associated with the development of osteomyelitis. Tuberculous osteomyelitis of the proximal humerus has been described, with the diagnosis confirmed by tissue biopsy and culture. The presence of *Mycobacterium tuberculosis* is confirmed by its growth at body temperature on the agar in the Löwenstein-Jensen culture medium, or can be seen histologically with caseating granulomas. The importance of tissue diagnosis cannot be overemphasized. A high degree of suspicion in patients from immigrant populations is appropriate, as osteomyelitis is more common in this patient group.

Annotated Bibliography

Sprengel's Deformity

Chinn DH: Prenatal ultrasonographic diagnosis of Sprengel's deformity. *J Ultrasound Med* 2001;20:693-697.

This article describes the use of ultrasound for prenatal diagnosis of Sprengel's deformity.

Khairouni A, Bensahel H, Csukonyi Z, Desgrippes Y, Pennecot GF: Congenital high scapula. *J Pediatr Orthop B* 2002;11:85-88.

This recent review of the Woodward procedure confirms the cosmetic and functional improvements achieved. Seventy-nine percent of patients had good or excellent results.

Pseudarthrosis of the Clavicle

Lorente Molto FJ, Bonete Lluch DJ, Garrido IM: Congenital pseudarthrosis of the clavicle: A proposal for early surgical treatment. *J Pediatr Orthop* 2001;21:689-693.

This article presents a review of six children with congenital pseudarthrosis (ages 18 months to 4 years). The patients were surgically treated with bone graft and internal fixation; healing of the pseudarthrosis was obtained in all patients in 6 to 8 weeks.

Glenoid Hypoplasia

de Bellis U, Guarino A, Castelli F: Glenoid hypoplasia: Description of a clinical case and analysis of the literature. *Chir Organi Mov* 2001;86:305-309.

This article discusses the skeletal changes associated with glenoid hypoplasia and describes a case of unilateral glenoid hypoplasia.

Birth Brachial Plexus Palsy

Hoeksma AF, Ter Steeg AM, Dijkstra P, Nelissen GHH, Beelen A, de Jong BA: Shoulder contracture and osseous deformity in obstetrical brachial plexus injuries. *J Bone Joint Surg Am* 2003;85-A:316-322.

A high prevalence of glenohumeral dysplasia on plain radiographs is associated with internal rotation contracture of the shoulder following birth brachial plexus injury. A loss of passive external rotation of the shoulder was highly associated with osseous deformity of the glenohumeral joint.

Moukoko D, Ezaki M, Wilkes D, Carter P: Posterior shoulder dislocation in infants with neonatal brachial plexus palsy. *J Bone Joint Surg Am* 2004;86A:787-793.

Of 134 patients with neonatal brachial plexus palsy, the diagnosis of posterior shoulder dislocations was made in 11 patients (8%). Diagnosis was made on clinical examination and confirmed by ultrasonography at an average patient age of 6 months (range, 3 to 10 months).

Pearl ML, Edgerton BW, Kon DS, et al: Comparison of arthroscopic findings with magnetic resonance imaging and arthrography in children with glenohumeral deformities secondary to brachial plexus birth palsy. *J Bone Joint Surg Am* 2003;85-A:890-898.

The natural history of brachial plexus injury leading to internal rotation contracture, which subsequently leads to glenohumeral dysplasia, is documented within the first 2 years of life. The glenohumeral dysplasia was evaluated comparatively by MRI, arthrography, and arthroscopy.

Clavicle Fractures

Calder JD, Solan M, Gidwani S, Allen S, Ricketts DM: Management of paediatric clavicle fractures: Is follow-up necessary? An audit of 346 cases. *Ann R Coll Surg Engl* 2002;84:331-333.

This study recommends that there is no need for follow-up of children with isolated, uncomplicated midshaft clavicle fractures; these fracture patients can be discharged after their first assessment in fracture clinic.

Kubiak R, Slongo T: Operative treatment of clavicle fractures in children: a review of 21 years. *J Pediatr Orthop* 2002;22:736-739.

This report on the surgical treatment of clavicle fractures showed that, during a 21-year period, only 15 patients with clavicle fractures required surgical stabilization. Surgery was indicated primarily in the older child with a displaced, unstable fracture pattern. Intramedullary elastic nails were the preferred method of internal fixation.

Septic Arthritis and Osteomyelitis

Forward DP, Hunter JB: Arthroscopic washout of the shoulder for septic arthritis in infants: A new technique. *J Bone Joint Surg Br* 2002;84:1173-1175.

The use of a wrist arthroscope for arthroscopic washout of septic arthritis of the shoulder in three children younger than 3 years of age is described. Full recovery was achieved with a single intervention.

Monach PA, Daily JP, Rodriguez-Herrera G, Solomon DH: Tuberculous osteomyelitis presenting as shoulder pain. *J Rheumatol* 2003;30:851-856.

Tuberculous osteomyelitis of the proximal humerus in children is described, along with a review of the relevant literature.

Classic Bibliography

Bennek J: The use of upper limb external fixation in paediatric trauma. *Injury* 2000;31(suppl 1):21-26.

Cavendish ME: Congenital elevation of the scapula. *J Bone Joint Surg Br* 1972;54:395-408.

Sprengel: Die angeborene Verschieburg des Schulterblattes nach oben. *Arch Klin Chir* 1891;42:545.

Goddard NJ, Fixsen JA: Rotation osteotomy of the humerus for birth injuries of the brachial plexus. *J Bone Joint Surg Br* 1984;66:257-259.

Grogan DP, Love SM, Guider KJ, Ogden JA: Operative treatment of congenital pseudarthrosis of the clavicle. *J Pediatr Orthop* 1991;11:176-180.

Hoffer M, Wickenden R, Roper B: Brachial plexus birth palsies: Results of tendon transfers to the rotator cuff. *J Bone Joint Surg Am* 1978;60:691-695.

Lossos IS, Yossepowitch O, Kandel L, Yardeni D, Arber N: Septic arthritis of the glenohumeral joint: A report of 11 cases and review of the literature. *Medicine (Baltimore)* 1998;77:177-187.

McBride MT, Hennrikus WL, Mologne TS: Newborn clavicle fractures. *Orthopedics* 1998;21:317-320.

Schnall SB, King JD, Marrero G: Congenital pseudarthrosis of the clavicle: A review of the literature and surgical results of six cases. *J Pediatr Orthop* 1988;8:316-321.

Webb LX, Mooney JF: Fractures and dislocations about the shoulder, in Green NE, Swiontkowski MF (eds): *Skeletal Trauma in Children*, ed 2. Philadelphia, PA, WB Saunders, 1998, pp 319-341.

Waters PM, Smith GR, Jaramillo D: Glenohumeral deformity secondary to brachial plexus birth palsy. *J Bone Joint Surg Am* 1998;80:668-677.

Woodward JW: Congenital elevation of the scapula: Correction by release and transplantation of muscle origins. *J Bone Joint Surg Am* 1961;43:219-228.

Chapter 60

Elbow: Pediatrics

John M. Flynn, MD

Roger Cornwall, MD

Pediatric Elbow Fractures

Pediatric elbow fractures are common; however, they are challenging to evaluate and treat even for the experienced orthopaedist. The elbow of a young child is composed predominantly of unossified cartilage. In older children, multiple centers of ossification make evaluation difficult. Associated neurovascular injuries frequently occur and may significantly impact the urgency and method of treatment. In general, the pediatric elbow has a relatively limited remodeling capacity. The elbow physes grow more slowly than those in the proximal humerus and distal radius. As a hinge joint, the elbow has a poor tolerance for coronal plane deformities and has a particular propensity for loss of motion. These factors help to explain the disproportionate number of medical liability claims and the anxiety related to pediatric elbow fracture treatment.

Initial evaluation of a child with an injured elbow should begin with a general examination and a search for other sites of injury. Next, the involved upper extremity should be examined carefully for the point of maximal tenderness in the area with maximum swelling. Any upper extremity deformity or a break in the skin integrity should be noted. Because of the high prevalence of neurovascular injuries, a careful neurovascular examination, including a check of the anterior interosseous nerve, is essential. The carrying angle of the uninjured side should be noted, especially in a child with a supracondylar humerus fracture.

Radiographic evaluation should include the bones and joints above and below the site of injury. The presence of a posterior fat pad is an important sign of a possible occult elbow fracture. Radiographs should be studied closely for signs of a secondary injury.

Supracondylar Fractures

Supracondylar fractures, which represent 60% of elbow fractures in children, are classified based on the extent and direction of the displacement of the distal fragment; 98% are extension injuries. The modified Gartland classification system is used to describe the extent of injury.

Type I fractures are minimally displaced, type II are displaced with an intact posterior cortex, and type III fractures have a completely displaced distal fragment. In posteromedial fractures (occurring in approximately 75% of patients), the radial nerve is at risk, whereas in posterolateral fractures, the brachial artery and median nerve are at risk. About 2% of supracondylar fractures are flexion injuries with disruption of the posterior periosteum. The flexion pattern is considered much more difficult to treat with standard closed pinning techniques. A recent study of 29 flexion-type supracondylar humerus fractures reported 86% good or excellent results with casting for minimally displaced fractures, and with closed reduction and percutaneous pinning for all type II and III flexion injuries.

Treatment

The goal of treatment of a pediatric supracondylar humerus fracture is to restore alignment to a position where there is no varus malalignment and the anterior humeral line intersects the capitellar ossification center. Reduction and stabilization should be done without causing iatrogenic nerve injury or using elbow hyperflexion to a degree that will compromise distal perfusion. The use of a long arm cast for 3 weeks is satisfactory treatment for type I fractures, and for type II fractures in which the anterior humeral line intersects the capitellar ossification center and Baumann's angle is acceptable. Closed reduction and percutaneous pinning is indicated for any fracture that does not meet these conditions. The trend toward pinning most type II and III supracondylar humerus fractures has dramatically reduced the incidence of clinically important malunions. Because the technique of reduction and hyperflexion of the elbow is now avoided, Volkmann's ischemic contracture is rare.

Initial evaluation includes a careful neurologic and vascular examination and AP and lateral radiographs of the distal humerus, with separate views of the entire forearm to check for associated injuries. The urgency of surgery was analyzed in a recent study of 158 well-

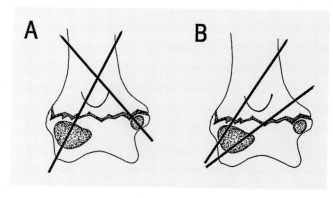

Figure 1 Two pinning techniques for displaced supracondylar humerus fractures are cross pins **(A)** and divergent lateral entry pins **(B)**. These techniques both have been shown to be clinically effective and equally stable to extension varus and valgus testing. The lateral pins do not put the ulnar nerve at risk for injury.

perfused type III fractures. The authors found no correlation between delay to surgery and the complication rate. However, children with a type III supracondylar fracture that will be pinned should be admitted to the hospital and carefully monitored for signs of neurovascular compromise or compartment syndrome.

Before fracture reduction, any entrapped soft tissue should be dislodged by gently milking the brachialis muscle and other soft tissue from the fracture site. The fracture is reduced and held in hyperflexion while percutaneous pins are placed. Recent reports of iatrogenic ulnar nerve injury from the use of a medial pin have focused attention on using only lateral entry pins. Although cadaver models have not shown such a technique to be as biomechanically stable as the use of crossed pins, lateral entry pinning combined with casting has been shown to be clinically effective. In a recent biomechanical study in a synthetic bone model, divergent lateral pins had similar stability to crossed pins on tests of extension and on tests of varus and valgus alignment, but not for axial stress (Figure 1). If there is concern for instability after placing two divergent lateral entry pins, a third lateral pin can be added. The fracture fixation should be tested for stability after pinning by moving the elbow through a range of flexion and extension, and by carefully stressing the fracture in rotation and varus and valgus, before splinting or casting in 70° to 80° of elbow flexion. The percutaneous pins are removed if radiographs show satisfactory callus at 3- to 4-week follow-up.

Neurovascular Compromise

Vascular compromise has been documented in about 10% to 20% of type III extension supracondylar humerus fractures. In these injuries, the brachial artery can sustain an injury ranging from a minor intimal tear to complete arterial disruption. Because there is a rich collateral circulation around the elbow, complete distal ischemia is rare. The absence of a palpable pulse is less important than the integrity of distal perfusion. An initial angiogram is not warranted because the location of the injury is known to be the fracture site. When treating a supracondylar humerus fracture without a palpable pulse, the first step is anatomic closed reduction with percutaneous pinning. Usually, a pulse that can be detected by Doppler ultrasonography will be present shortly after pinning. If this is the case, the fracture should be splinted in 40° to 50° of flexion and the child should be admitted to the hospital for 24 hours of observation. If the hand remains poorly perfused after anatomic reduction and pinning, a vascular consultation is warranted.

Volkmann's ischemic contracture is now a rare complication. A recent study evaluated forearm compartment pressures in supracondylar humerus fractures in 29 children. Pressures in the deep volar compartment were significantly more elevated than in other compartments and fracture reduction did not have an immediate effect on pressures. Most importantly, the investigators found that compartment pressures rose with elbow flexion greater than 90°. Also, deep volar compartment pressures greater than 30 mm often existed without clinical symptoms and without the subsequent development of compartment syndrome. The orthopaedist should be alert for forearm pain after a supracondylar humerus fracture, or for any indication of worsening pain (or analgesic requirements) in a patient after closed reduction and percutaneous pinning.

A neurologic deficit is noted in about 20% of patients with supracondylar humerus fractures. The anterior interosseous nerve is the most common site of nerve injury in extension injuries. In the flexion supracondylar pattern, the ulnar nerve is the most likely to be injured. Most nerve injuries associated with supracondylar humerus fractures will resolve within 6 months. If an iatrogenic ulnar nerve injury is noted after use of a medial pin, some investigators have noted that no intervention is warranted; satisfactory resolution of the injury often occurs. However, most investigators believe that upon recognition, the offending medial pin should be removed and replaced to a safe position.

Malunion

The instability after reduction of severely displaced supracondylar fractures results from failure to obtain good apposition of the distal medial and lateral columns. There is posterior rotation of the distal fragment, then a tilt into varus. Although the deformity may become increasingly apparent as elbow extension is regained, the deformity does not truly worsen over time. Although cubitus varus was considered primarily a cosmetic problem, studies have shown an increased incidence of ulnar neuropathy, late lateral condyle fractures, and postero-

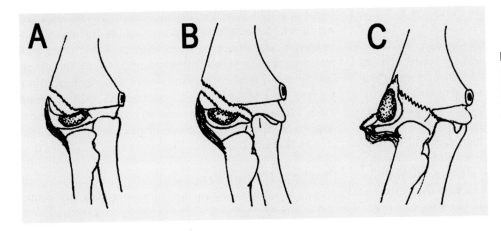

Figure 2 Lateral condyle stages of displacement. **A,** Type I: A fracture in which the fracture line does not completely cross the cartilaginous surface of the distal humerus. **B,** Type II: A complete fracture of the cartilaginous surface without displacement from the joint. **C,** Type III: A complete fracture with displacement of the lateral condylar fragment. *(Adapted with permission from Jakob R, Fowles J, Rang M, et al: Observations concerning fractures of the lateral humeral condyle in children. J Bone Joint Surg Br 1975;57: 430-436.)*

lateral rotatory instability with this condition. Most osteotomy techniques and fixation strategies have been described in small studies. A recent report describes the use of an external fixator to stabilize the fragment after an oblique, incomplete medial opening wedge osteotomy. The complication rate for all techniques tends to be quite high. Currently, there is no clear standard technique for the treatment of cubitus varus after a pediatric supracondylar humerus fracture.

Lateral Condyle Fractures

Because lateral humeral condyle fractures in children involve both the joint and growth cartilage, they are associated with a host of complications including nonunion, malunion, loss of motion, osteonecrosis, and cubitus valgus. The most clinically valuable classification system involves stages of displacement (Figure 2). The oblique radiograph is most helpful in assessing the extent of displacement. A recently published study of the MRI evaluation of lateral condyle fractures with 0 to 3 mm of displacement confirmed previous arthrogram studies and concluded that the stability of the fracture is related to the integrity of the cartilage hinge. Lateral condyle fractures with up to 2 mm of displacement can be treated with casting and close observation. An AP, lateral, and oblique radiograph of the distal humerus with the cast removed should be obtained after about 5 days and again at about 2 weeks to ensure that there is no progressive displacement. If displacement is seen, reduction and pinning is the recommended treatment.

Closed reduction and percutaneous pinning is the preferred treatment for fresh fractures that are only displaced from 2 to 5 mm, are relatively stable, and can be reduced to the anatomic position. Open reduction and internal fixation is usually required in the treatment of lateral condyle fractures. The technique involves a standard lateral approach to the distal humerus with no posterior dissection (the blood supply to the lateral condyle is posterior). An anatomic reduction is ensured both visually and radiographically and two percutaneous Kir-

schner wires are placed to stabilize the fracture. The pins are removed at 4 weeks, followed by 2 additional weeks of casting. Pins left in for longer than 4 weeks are increasingly likely to lead to irritation or infection. A recent study evaluated the rate of healing in 55 patients with lateral condyle fractures. The authors found that radiographic evidence of complete bony healing was not present until 6 weeks after injury, even in children between 1 and 5 years of age.

Lateral condyle fractures are one of the few types of fractures in children in which delayed union or nonunion is not unusual. If open reduction to an anatomic realignment is done more than 3 weeks after injury, osteonecrosis may result if extensive soft-tissue stripping is performed to achieve the reduction. In a recent review of 11 children who had open reduction and internal fixation without soft-tissue stripping, none of the children had osteonecrosis. The authors recommended that nonunions with greater than 1 cm of displacement be fixed without soft-tissue stripping and without restoration to the anatomic position. It was found that despite fixation in a nonanatomic position, overall elbow alignment and range of motion were good. Late lateral condyle nonunion is asymptomatic in some patients, whereas others develop cubitus valgus and a delayed ulnar nerve palsy. Some authors have recommended a supracondylar medial closing wedge osteotomy and transposition of the ulnar nerve for symptomatic patients.

Medial Epicondyle Fractures

Fractures of the medial epicondyle account for 7% to 11% of all pediatric elbow fractures. These fractures result from avulsion of the epicondyle by the flexor-pronator muscles and medial collateral ligament during valgus stress or elbow dislocation. In patients with elbow dislocation where spontaneous or manipulative reduction entraps the medial epicondyle in the joint, the medial epicondyle ossification center may be obscured by the distal humerus or mistaken as the trochlear ossification center. Careful evaluation of radiographs is important whenever a medial elbow injury is suspected in a child.

Treatment recomendations for medial epicondyle fractures are somewhat controversial. Reduction and pin or screw fixation of fractures displaced more than 2 to 5 mm is recommended in three circumstances: if a medial epicondyle is entrapped in the joint; in a fracture with associated ulnar nerve dysfunction; or for displaced fractures in children who place high physical demands on their elbow. The latter group is difficult to define; however, gymnasts and throwing athletes are included. A recent study retrospectively reviewed the results (at more than 30-year follow-up) of 42 patients with medial epicondyle fractures displaced more than 5 mm. Patients treated with cast immobilization had similar functional results to those treated surgically, although radiographic union was much more common in the group treated surgically. Those treated with excision did poorly. Based on these findings, the authors questioned surgical treatment of fractures displaced as much as 15 mm, and did not recommend primary surgical excision.

Medial Condyle Fractures

True medial condyle fractures are rare, accounting for only 1% to 2% of pediatric elbow fractures. Diagnosis may be difficult in the young child, especially before the appearance of the trochlear ossification center. However, the fracture typically involves a metaphyseal bony fragment, clearly differentiating it from a medial epicondyle fracture. Treatment principles for medial condyle fractures are similar to those for lateral condyle fractures. Nondisplaced fractures may be treated with cast immobilization, whereas displaced fractures should undergo closed or open reduction with internal fixation. Arthrography or MRI may be helpful in determining articular displacement and guiding the choice of treatment. A recent study of 21 patients with medial condyle fractures showed that such fractures are associated with a high rate of complications, including delayed or missed diagnosis, osteonecrosis of the trochlea, nonunion, fixation failure, and significant elbow stiffness.

Olecranon Fractures

Olecranon fractures account for approximately 4% to 6% of pediatric elbow fractures and are associated with other elbow fractures in up to 41% of patients. Olecranon fractures in children are similar to those in adults, in that they are usually intra-articular and metaphyseal. However, unlike in adults, many olecranon fractures in children are minimally displaced and suitable for closed immobilization. Fractures with more than 2 mm of articular displacement should be reduced and stabilized with internal fixation. A recent report described a new fixation technique using a pin with a threaded tip and an adjustable locking device at the opposite end. This tech-

nique was biomechanically equivalent to tension band wiring without requiring exposure of the fracture site. A recent review of 39 patients with pediatric olecranon fractures with a mean follow-up of 32 years found encouraging results. Poor results were seen in only three patients, two of whom had associated radial head fractures. The presence of associated injury may be more important than the degree of displacement of the olecranon fracture in determining outcome.

Proximal Radius Fractures

Although not a common injury, fractures of the proximal radius in children result in many complications. In contrast to similar fractures in adults, however, fractures through the neck of the radius are more common than radial head fractures. A variety of treatment algorithms exist for radial neck fractures based on the degree of displacement. Radial neck fractures with less than 3 mm of translation and less than 30° of angulation can be treated with a brief period of immobilization for comfort, followed by early motion. More displaced or angulated fractures should be reduced. Closed reduction is often successful; if it fails, reduction with the use of a percutaneous Kirschner wire manipulation can be done. If these methods of reduction fail, and angulation is greater than 60°, open reduction should be performed. Fixation is usually achieved with the use of Kirschner wires across the fracture but not the joint. A similar algorithm was used to treat 24 patients in a recent study. All of the fractures were reduced to less than 15° of angulation, and all patients had excellent functional and radiographic results at 14- to 25-year follow-up.

Radial head fractures, unlike radial neck fractures, are intra-articular and deserve anatomic alignment. Open reduction is often required to achieve this goal.

Monteggia Fractures

Monteggia lesions include a fracture of the proximal ulna with a radial head dislocation. The ulnar fracture also may be a plastic deformation. A Monteggia fracture should be suspected whenever an "isolated" ulna fracture or radial head dislocation is seen. In a child, closed reduction of the ulna usually reduces the radial head, and the fracture often can be treated with a long arm cast. However, open reduction and internal fixation of the ulna is required when an anatomic reduction of the ulna, radiocapitellar joint, and proximal radioulnar joint cannot be obtained or maintained by closed methods.

Previous reports have discouraged attempted open reduction of a chronic radial head dislocation with or without annular ligament reconstruction because of the high rate of redislocation and other complications. A recent study reviewed 22 patients treated for chronic post-traumatic radial head dislocation. The authors concluded that ulnar osteotomy to correct the malunion

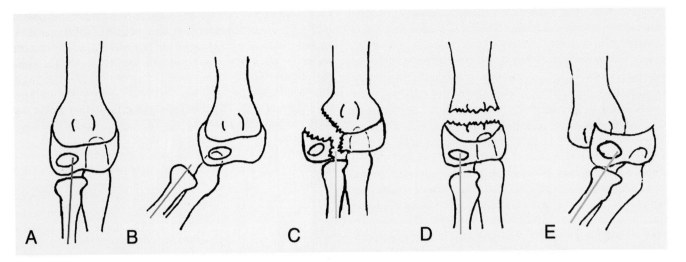

Figure 3 A schematic drawing of the distal humeral proximal radius and ulnar relationship in various pediatric elbow injuries. **A,** Normal elbow. **B,** Elbow dislocation. **C,** Lateral condyle fracture. **D,** Supracondylar fracture. **E,** Distal humeral epiphyseal separation. *(Adapted with permission from Delee JC, Wilkins KE, Rogers LF, Rockwood CA: Fracture-separation of the distal humeral epiphysis. J Bone Joint Surg Am 1980;62:46-51.)*

was essential in treating missed Monteggia fractures, if a normal radial head contour remained. A similar report of 15 patients who underwent open reduction of chronic radial head dislocations and ulnar osteotomies found good to excellent functional results in 12 patients, although most lost some degree of pronation postoperatively.

Transphyseal Distal Humerus Fractures

Displaced fractures through the distal humeral physis can be difficult to diagnose. In the infant, the only sign may be malalignment of the radial and ulnar shafts relative to the distal humerus. This injury is often associated with battered child syndrome (Figure 3). Ultrasound, MRI, arthrography, and stress radiographs can help clarify the diagnosis of a transphyseal fracture. Treatment is similar to that for supracondylar fractures.

Floating Elbow

Ipsilateral fractures of the distal humerus and distal forearm are called pediatric floating elbow. Commensurate with the severity of the trauma is an increased risk of clinically significant swelling, neurovascular compromise, and forearm compartment syndrome. In a recent study of 16 patients with a supracondylar humerus fracture and a displaced distal radius fracture, surgical fixation of both fractures to avoid the high rate of potentially devastating complications (particularly compartment syndrome) was recommended.

Elbow Contractures

Although children are generally less prone to posttraumatic joint stiffness than adults, not all children develop normal or even functional range of motion after elbow injuries. Noninvasive measures such as splinting and physical therapy are successful in many patients. The technique of open capsular release has been used extensively in adults; some authors have reported its use in children. A report on elbow release in 13 adolescent patients with posttraumatic stiffness showed than an average increase of 54° was produced in the flexion extension arc. Only one patient lost motion. Nine patients (69%) achieved at least a 25° to 120° arc of motion. A recent review of 37 patients receiving similar treatment showed only a 25° to 30° improvement in arc of motion; a useful (30° to 130°) arc was achieved only in 46% of patients. After an extended period of observation, surgical release can be a valuable tool in the treatment of stiffness after complex pediatric elbow injuries. The patient and family should be counseled regarding expected improvements in arc of motion.

Annotated Bibliography

Supracondylar Fractures

Battaglia TC, Armstrong DG, Schwend RM: Factors affecting forearm compartment pressures in children with supracondylar fractures of the humerus. *J Pediatr Orthop* 2002;22:431-439.

The authors measured the forearm compartment pressures of 29 children with a type II or III supracondylar humerus fracture. Pressures in the deep volar compartment were significantly elevated compared with the pressure in other compartments. There were also significantly higher pressures closer to the elbow within each compartment. Fracture reduction did not have an immediate effect on pressures. Most importantly, flexion beyond 90° produced significant pressure elevation. The authors also found that pressures greater than 30 mm Hg may exist without clinical evidence of compartment syndrome.

They concluded that to avoid unnecessary elevation of pressures, elbows should not be immobilized in greater than 90° of flexion.

De Boeck H: Flexion-type supracondylar elbow fractures in children. *J Pediatr Orthop* 2001;21:460-463.

Twenty-nine children with a flexion-type supracondylar humerus fracture were reevaluated with an average follow-up of 6.3 years. Seven children with a flexion-type supracondylar humerus fracture were treated in a cast and 22 children with a displaced flexion-type fracture were treated with closed reduction and percutaneous pinning. Good or excellent results were noted in 86.2% of the patients. All patients were satisfied with the end result and had normal use of the elbow. This article reports on a large number of relatively rare flexion-type supracondylar fractures and highlights the good results that can be obtained without an open reduction, even in patients with displaced and unstable fractures.

Koch PP, Exner GU: Supracondylar medial open wedge osteotomy with external fixation for cubitus varus deformity. *J Pediatr Orthop B* 2003;12:116-122.

The authors describe a technique in which an anteromedial approach and a medial opening wedge osteotomy with external fixation are used to treat cubitus varus in children after a malunion and following a supracondylar humerus fracture. The mean valgus correction was 21.75°. At 2-year follow-up, three of the four children had symmetric elbow alignment and one had slight residual varus deformity. The authors concluded that this is a good technique for treating cubitus varus deformity allowing correction of both valgus and flexion.

Lee ST, Mahar AT, Meisen D, Newton PO: Displaced pediatric supracondylar humerus fractures: Biomechanical analysis of percutaneous pinning techniques. *J Pediatr Orthop* 2002;22:440-443.

This biomechanical study of different supracondylar pinning techniques used a pediatric synthetic bone model. The authors concluded that divergent lateral pins had similar stability compared with cross pins in extension, varus, and valgus testing. In axial testing, cross pins were more stable. Divergent lateral pins also had statistically greater stability than parallel lateral pins under varus and valgus loading.

Leet AI, Frisancho J, Ebramzadeh, E: Delayed treatment of type 3 supracondylar humerus fractures in children. *J Pediatr Orthop* 2002;22:203-207.

A retrospective review of 158 patients with well-profused type III supracondylar humerus fractures showed no correlation between an increase in time to surgical intervention and the complication rate. The average time from injury to surgical treatment was 21.3 hours.

O'Driscoll SW, Spinner RJ, McKee MD, et al: Tardy posterolateral rotatory instability of the elbow due to cubitus varus. *J Bone Joint Surg Am* 2001;83:1358-1369.

The authors report on 25 instances of cubitus varus deformity (average 15°) subsequent to a pediatric distal humeral fracture or congenital anomaly in 24 patients who developed posterolateral rotatory instability of the elbow two to three decades afterward. Surgery was performed on 22 limbs, and only 3 limbs had persistent instability at 3-year follow-up. The authors propose that the repetitive external rotation torque on the ulna, resulting from the medial displacment of the mechanical axis, the olecranon, and the triceps line of pull, can stretch the lateral collateral ligament complex and lead to posterolateral rotatory instability in patients with cubitus varus deformity. Surgical correction can relieve symptoms of instability.

Skaggs DL, Cluck MW, Mostofi A, Flynn JM, Kay RM: Lateral-entry pin fixation in the management of supracondylar fractures in children. *J Bone Joint Surg Am* 2004;86:702-707.

The authors reported on 124 consecutive Gartland types II and III supracondylar humerus fractures treated with two or three lateral entry pins. The only complication reported was a pin tract infection. There was no loss of reduction, cubitus varus, hyperextension, loss of motion, or iatrogenic nerve palsies, and no additional surgeries. The authors concluded that the most important technical points for assuring fixation with lateral-entry pins were: separating the pins at the fracture site; engaging the medial and lateral columns proximal to the fracture and sufficient bone in both the proximal segment and the distal fragment; and using three pins to provide additional stability when necessary.

Lateral Condyle Fractures

Cardona JI, Riddle E, Kumar SJ: Displaced fractures of the lateral humeral condyle: Criteria for implant removal. *J Pediatr Orthop* 2002;22:194-197.

The authors reviewed 55 lateral condylar fractures treated at their institution over a 10-year period, with special attention to the rate of healing of the fracture. They concluded that in 50 patients, the fracture was clinically and radiographically healed at 6 weeks. Four patients showed radiographic healing at 5 weeks and one patient at 4 weeks.

Horn DH, Herman MJ, Crisci K, Pizzutillo PD, MacEwan GD: Fracture of the lateral humeral fracture condyle: Role of the cartilage hinge in fracture stability. *J Pediatr Orthop* 2002;22:8-11.

The authors studied 16 patients with a lateral condyle fracture who had both radiographs and MRI. All unstable fractures had complete fractures on MRI scans. Ten of the 12 patients with radiographically stable injuries had incomplete fractures on MRI scans. The authors concluded that the stability of the lateral humeral condyle fractures is related to the integrity of the cartilage hinge.

Wattenbarger JM, Gerardi J, Johnston CE: Late open reduction internal fixation of lateral condyle fractures. *J Pediatr Orthop* 2002;22:394-398.

The authors reviewed the records of 11 children who had a malunion or nonunion of a lateral condyle fracture treated more than 3 weeks after injury and found no patients with osteonecrosis. In fractures with greater than 1 cm of displacement, the fragment position was minimally improved by surgical treatment, but final alignment and range of motion were good. The authors concluded that the risk of osteonecrosis with open reduction of lateral condyle fractures at greater than 3 weeks is reduced if no tissue is stripped off the fracture fragment posteriorly. Even children without an anatomic reduction had functional arms and little or no pain.

Medial Epicondyle Fractures

Farsetti P, Potenza V, Caterini R, Ippolito E: Long-term results of treatment of fractures of the medial humeral epicondyle in children. *J Bone Joint Surg Am* 2001;83-A: 1299-1305.

The authors retrospectively reviewed 42 patients with medial epicondyle fractures that were displaced more than 5 mm. Nineteen patients were treated with cast immobilization without reduction, 17 underwent open reduction and internal fixation, and 6 patients had fragment excision. The functional results at 30-year follow-up were identical for the first two groups, but worse for the excision group. The authors argue that nonsurgical treatment is as effective as open reduction and internal fixation for fractures with displacement of more than 5 mm.

Medial Condyle Fractures

Leet AI, Young C, Hoffer MM: Medial condyle fractures of the humerus in children. *J Pediatr Orthop* 2002;22:2-7.

The authors reviewed a series of 21 children with medial condyle fractures. MRI was used to make the diagnosis or assess displacement in four children. Of the nine patients with displaced fractures that were treated surgically, four had complications, including two patients who lost reduction and required revision with open reduction and internal fixation. Of the 12 patients who were treated in a cast, 2 developed nonunions and 1 developed osteonecrosis of the trochlea. Almost half of the children had some impairment in range of motion.

Olecranon Fractures

Caterini R, Farsetti P, D'Arrigo C, Ippolito E: Fractures of the olecranon in children: Long-term follow-up of 39 cases. *J Pediatr Orthop B* 2002;11:320-328.

Thirty-nine patients with olecranon fractures in childhood were followed at a mean of 32 years. Thirty-four patients had good results and three had poor results. All had minimally displaced olecranon fractures and other associated fractures. Arthritis was rare. The authors concluded that associated injuries may be a stronger predictor of outcome than the degree of displacement in patients with olecranon fractures.

Gicquel P, Maximin MC, Boutemy P, et al: Biomechanical analysis of olecranon fracture fixation in children. *J Pediatr Orthop* 2002;22:17-21.

The authors describe a novel fixation technique for olecranon fractures in children. A pin with a threaded tip is inserted antegrade across the fracture site, without opening the fracture. A locking device is placed proximally on the pin to provide compression. A biomechanical analysis found this technique as strong as tension band wiring. The authors recommended this new technique over tension band wiring because it obviates the need to expose the fracture site.

Proximal Radius Fractures

Malmvik J, Herbertsson P, Josefsson PO, Hasserius R, Besjakov J, Karlsson MK: Fracture of the radial head and neck of Mason types II and III during growth: A 14-25 year follow-up. *J Pediatr Orthop B* 2003;12:63-83.

Twenty-four patients with angulated radial head and neck fractures during childhood were evaluated at a mean follow-up of 19 years. Two patients ultimately required radial head excision. Of the remainder, all but three patients had received closed treatment. All patients had less than 15° of angulation after primary treatment. Nineteen patients had no pain at follow-up, although elbow flexion was typically limited compared with the uninjured side.

Waters PM, Stewart SL: Radial neck fracture nonunion in children. *J Pediatr Orthop* 2001;21:570-576.

The authors describe nine children with radial neck nonunions; eight had associated elbow injuries. Eight children underwent open reduction and fixation, and one had repeated closed reduction attempts with percutaneous fixation. In each case, fixation failed and led to loss of reduction. Four patients were pain free, but all had restriction of motion. Secondary open repair of the nonunion did not guarantee good functional outcome.

Monteggia Fractures

Horii E, Nakamura R, Koh S, Inagaki H, Yajima H, Nakao E: Surgical treatment for chronic radial head dislocation. *J Bone Joint Surg Am* 2002;84-A:1183-1188.

The authors reviewed 22 patients treated for chronic posttraumatic radial head dislocation. Thirteen patients underwent open reduction without ulnar osteotomy, and seven had redislocation of the radial head. In a subsequent group of nine patients who had an ulnar osteotomy, the radial heads of two patients were subluxated at follow-up. Both patients had radial head abnormalities preoperatively. The authors concluded that ulnar osteotomy to correct malunion is essential in treating missed Monteggia fractures if a normal radial head contour remains.

Kim HT, Park BG, Suh JT, Yoo CI: Chronic radial head dislocation in children: Part 2. Results of open treatment and factors affecting final outcome. *J Pediatr Orthop* 2002;22:591-597.

The authors describe 15 cases (14 patients) of open reduction and reconstruction of chronic radial head dislocations, 12 of which were posttraumatic. Results were classified as excellent in 10 elbows, good in 2, fair in 2, and poor in 1. One patient developed a radioulnar synostosis, and 10 lost some degree of pronation postoperatively. All radial heads in the posttraumatic patients remained reduced at follow-up. The authors argue that the results of their series should encourage attempts at reducing chronically dislocated radial heads, especially in posttraumatic patients.

Floating Elbow

Ring D, Waters PM, Hotchkiss RN, Kasser JR: Pediatric floating elbow. *J Pediatr Orthop* 2001;21:456-459.

The authors reviewed a series of 16 patients with pediatric floating elbow injuries. All but one patient's supracondylar humerus fracture was treated with pin fixation. In 10 patients, the distal forearm fractures were treated with closed reduction and cast immobilization. Of these 10 patients, 2 developed compartment syndrome with 1 patient having a subsequent Volkmann ischemic contracture. An additional 4 of these 10 patients required cast removal because of excessive swelling and impending compartment syndrome. The remaining six patients were treated with pin fixation of their distal forearm fractures, and were not placed in circumferential casts. None developed compartment syndrome. The authors recommended surgical treatment of all fractures in this injury pattern to avoid the high rate of potentially devastating complications associated with cast immobilization.

Elbow Contractures

Bae DS, Waters PM: Surgical treatment of posttraumatic elbow contracture in adolescents. *J Pediatr Orthop* 2001; 21:580-584.

The authors describe 13 adolescents who had elbow capsular release for posttraumatic stiffness. An average increase of 54° was achieved in the flexion-extension arc. Nine patients (69%) achieved at least a 25° to 120° arc of motion; one patient lost motion. The authors expressed enthusiasm for surgical release of elbow contractures in adolescents.

Stans AA, Maritz NG, O'Driscoll SW, Morrey BF: Operative treatment of elbow contracture in patients 21-years of age or younger. *J Bone Joint Surg Am* 2002;84-A:382-387.

The authors describe surgical elbow releases in 37 patients younger than 21 years of age. Twenty-eight elbow contractures were posttraumatic. An average increase of only 25° to 30° of motion was obtained in the flexion-extension arc, regardless of the etiology of the contracture. Fewer than half of the patients achieved a flexion extension arc of greater than 30° to 130°. The authors warn of the limited gains that can be expected from elbow releases in children compared with those in adults.

Classic Bibliography

Archibeck MJ, Scott SM, Peters CL: Brachialis muscle entrapment in displaced supracondylar humerus fractures: A technique of closed reduction and report of initial results. *J Pediatr Orthop* 1997;17:298-302.

Bernstein SM, McKeever P, Bernstein L: Percutaneous reduction of displaced radial neck fractures in children. *J Pediatr Orthop* 1993;13:85-88.

Cramer KE, Green NE, Devito DP: Incidence of anterior interosseous nerve palsy in supracondylar humerus fractures in children. *J Pediatr Orthop* 1993;13:502-505.

Culp RW, Ostermann AL, Davidson RS, Skirven T, Bora FW Jr: Neural injuries associated with supracondylar fractures of the humerus in children. *J Bone Joint Surg Am* 1990;72:1211-1215.

Flynn JC: Nonunion of slightly displaced fractures of the lateral humeral condyle in children: An update. *J Pediatr Orthop* 1989;9:691-696.

Foster DE, Sullivan JA, Gross RH: Lateral humeral condylar fractures in children. *J Pediatr Orthop* 1985;5: 16-22.

Fowles JV, Slimane N, Kassab MT: Elbow dislocation with avulsion of the medial humeral epicondyle. *J Bone Joint Surg Br* 1990;72:102-104.

France J, Strong M: Deformity and function in supracondylar fractures of the humerus in children variously treated by closed reduction and splinting, traction, and percutaneous pinning. *J Pediatr Orthop* 1992;12:494-498.

Gaddy BC, Strecker WB, Schoenecker PL: Surgical treatment of displaced olecranon fractures in children. *J Pediatr Orthop* 1997;17:321-324.

Garbuz DS, Leitch K, Wright JG: The treatment of supracondylar fractures in children with an absent radial pulse. *J Pediatr Orthop* 1996;16:594-596.

Keenan WN, Clegg J: Variation of Baumann's angle with age, sex and side: Implications for its use in radiological monitoring of supracondylar fracture of the humerus in children. *J Pediatr Orthop* 1996;16:97-98.

Kissoon N, Gapin R, Gayle M, Chacon D, Brown T: Evaluation of the role of comparison radiographs in the diagnosis of traumatic elbow injuries. *J Pediatr Orthop* 1995;15:449-453.

Lincoln TL, Mubarek SJ: Isolated traumatic radial head dislocation. *J Pediatr Orthop* 1994;14:454-457.

Pirone AM, Graham HK, Krajbich JI: Management of displaced extension-type supracondylar fractures of the humerus in children. *J Bone Joint Surg Am* 1988;70:641-650.

Roye DP Jr, Bini SA, Infosino A: Late surgical treatment of lateral condylar fractures in children. *J Pediatr Orthop* 1991;11:195-199.

Sabharwal S, Tredwell SJ, Beauchamp RD, et al: Management of pulseless pink hand in pediatric supracondylar fractures of the humerus. *J Pediatr Orthop* 1997;17: 303-310.

Williamson DM, Coates CJ, Miller RK, Cole WG: Normal characteristics of the Baumann (humerocapitellar) angle: An aid in assessment of supracondylar fractures. *J Pediatr Orthop* 1992;12:636-639.

Zionts LE, McKellop HA, Hathaway R: Torsional strength of pin configuration used to fix supracondylar fractures of the humerus in children. *J Bone Joint Surg Am* 1994;76:253-256.

Chapter 61

Forearm, Wrist, and Hand: Pediatrics

Peter M. Waters, MD

Alexander D. Mih, MD

Cerebral Palsy

Deformities of the forearm, wrist, and hand, limited function, and decreased sensibility are common in patients with cerebral palsy. Limited motor function occurs with poor release and grasp function resulting from flexor spasticity and contractures, combined with the effects of weak extension of the fingers and wrist. Limited pinch from thumb-in-palm deformity occurs because of intrinsic adductor and flexor spasticity and contractures. Discriminatory sensibility is deficient in more than 50% of these children. Poor voluntary control of the upper extremity limits functional placement of the hand in space; many of these children have visual and cognitive abnormalities that further impair hand function. At best, most patients with cerebral palsy have assistive hand function.

Upper extremity classification systems for patients with cerebral palsy have been used to assess function. The House classification of function has nine levels extending from 0 (no use of the extremity) to 8 (complete spontaneous use). In this schema, the nine levels are further classified into four subgroups based on patient function: no use (level 0), passive assist (levels 1 to 3), active assist (levels 4 to 6), and spontaneous use (levels 7 and 8) (Table 1). Because spasticity varies with stress, growth, and central nervous system changes, it may be difficult to accurately define a patient's level of function based on any single observation. Surgical planning and outcome assessment should be based on the level of function determined preoperatively and postoperatively. Surgery will not create a normal hand but will improve assistive function and cosmesis. The goals of surgery need to be realistic and obtainable.

Treatment

In broad terms, treatment options include observation of the patient's growth and development, use of therapy (including splints), consideration of the need for injections (such as phenol or botulinum toxin), and surgical reconstruction of the forearm, wrist, and hand. Botulinum toxin is currently the most common form of neuro-muscular blockade injection. Injections into the pronator, flexor carpi ulnaris, and adductor pollicis muscles are most often performed. Aggressive therapy should be used to stretch agonist muscle-tendon units and strengthen antagonists. Antibody formation to botulinum toxin will limit its effectiveness in certain patients.

In patients with cerebral palsy, surgery improves level of function and cosmesis in the hemiplegic patient, and ease of nursing care in the patient with quadriparesis while lessening the risk of skin breakdown. The best surgical candidates are patients with hemiplegia and good voluntary control, sensibility, and motivation. The principle of surgery is to correct muscle imbalance by lengthening or releasing tight, spastic muscles and augmenting weak, stretched muscles by tendon transfers and tenodesis procedures. Unstable joints need to be stabilized by soft-tissue or arthrodesis procedures to maximize outcome of tendon reconstruction. The patient and family must understand that surgery will not alleviate all functional deficiency or repair all cosmetic defects of the hand. Even the best outcome will still result in deficiencies of function, cosmesis, and sensibility. However, in properly selected patients, surgery will clearly improve function and patient satisfaction.

Forearm hyperpronation significantly limits hand function in patients with hemiplegia. Release or rerouting of the pronator teres through the interosseous membrane is effective in improving function. Transfer of the flexor carpi ulnaris to the dorsal wrist by rerouting around the ulna also has been shown to provide some degree of active supination. By improving voluntary control of forearm rotation, hand function increases.

Wrist and finger flexion deformity is common in patients with hemiplegia. The flexor carpi ulnaris is usually the major deforming force resulting in wrist flexion. Transfer of the flexor carpi ulnaris to the wrist extensors alleviates the deformity and improves wrist extension and finger tenodesis into flexion. Simultaneous musculotendinous lengthening of the finger flexors are necessary if the extrinsic finger flexors are tight in neutral wrist position; otherwise, the patient will develop a disabling clenched fist postoperatively. Z-lengthenings, su-

Table 1 | House Classification for Hand Function in Patients With Cerebral Palsy

Level	Designation	Activity Level
0	Does not use	Does not use
1	Poor passive assist	Uses as stabilizing weight only
2	Fair passive assist	Can hold onto object placed in hand
3	Good passive assist	Can hold onto object and stabilize it for use by other hand
4	Poor active assist	Can actively grasp object and hold it weakly
5	Fair active assist	Can actively grasp object and stabilize it well
6	Good active assist	Can actively grasp object and manipulate it against other hand
7	Spontaneous use, partial	Can perform bimanual activities easily and occasionally uses the hand spontaneously
8	Spontaneous use, complete	Uses hand completely independently without reference to the other hand

(Reproduced with permission from Waters PM, Van Hest A: Spastic hemiplegia of the upper extremity in children. Hand Clin 1998;14:119-134.)

perficialis to profundus flexor tendon transfers, and bony procedures are reserved for patients with severe contractures and limited function (usually found in the patient with quadriparesis).

Thumb-in-palm deformity limits dynamic pinch and grasp and makes hygiene difficult because of severe contractures. Static contractures are corrected with web space Z-plasty and adductor releases. At times, the static contractures include the flexor pollicis longus and brevis; these muscles will need to be appropriately lengthened or released. Dynamic rebalancing is performed with tendon transfers to weak abductors and extensors of the thumb. There are many possible donor muscles including the palmaris longus, flexor carpi radialis, and brachioradialis. The recipient tendons include the extensor pollicis brevis and longus and the abductor pollicis longus. The metacarpophalangeal joint needs to be stable postoperatively. In most patients, stability is achieved by muscle rebalancing. On occasion, a capsulodesis or arthrodesis procedure will be needed.

Some patients with cerebral palsy have disabling swan neck deformities. If the fingers at the proximal interphalangeal joint lock and hyperextend more than 40° and lock, limited grasp and pain may result. Multiple surgical procedures have been advised, including flexor digitorum superficialis tenodesis, intrinsic muscle slide, lateral band rerouting, spiral oblique ligament recon-

struction, and resection of the motor branch of the ulnar nerve. The lateral band rerouting procedure provides both intrinsic and extrinsic rebalancing and is effective in correcting swan neck deformities.

Patients with cerebral palsy who have disabling dynamic spasticity and fixed contractures of the wrist and hand benefit from surgical reconstruction. Often the more severely affected patients (House level 0 through 2) respond best to musculotendinous lengthenings, tenodesis, and joint stabilization procedures. Patients with more functional ability (House levels 3 through 6) improve with dynamic tendon transfers and releases.

Arthrogryposis

Infants with classic arthrogryposis (amyoplasia) often have stiffness and weakness of all joints and muscles of the upper extremity. Elbow extension, forearm pronation, wrist palmar flexion, ulnar deviation, finger flexion, and thumb-in-palm contractures are typical. Absence of biceps antigravity strength is common and limits the ability to place the hand near the face. Adaptive mechanisms are necessary for function. Children with arthrogryposis often have incomplete syndactyly of all web spaces. Contracture of the first web space is usually functionally significant. Patients usually have marked intrinsic muscle weakness.

Treatment

Initial treatment involves passive range-of-motion therapy and nighttime splinting to improve joint motion and digital strength. The condition of many children improves with growth and therapy over the first several years of life. At the elbow, triceps V-Y lengthening and posterior capsulectomy are performed at 18 months to 3 years of age if passive elbow flexion of approximately 90° does not occur. The wrist palmar flexion contracture is treated with both soft-tissue and bony procedures. A flexor carpi ulnaris release with lengthening or transfer to the wrist extensors is performed in conjunction with a dorsal carpal closing wedge osteotomy.

The thumb-in-palm contracture is treated with a Z-plasty syndactyly release. Care must be taken not to overrelease the adductor. Transfers for thumb abduction and extension are predominantly tenodesis procedures because of the limited strength of the donor muscles.

Children with arthrogryposis will have permanent limited motion and strength in their arms and hands. Because of their high level of intelligence, these children often are quite functionally adaptive.

Forearm and Wrist Trauma
Epidemiology and Prevention Updates

In a longitudinal study from New Zealand, it was determined that 51% of boys and 40% of girls will experience a single fracture by 18 years of age. The most common fracture sites, the wrist and forearm, accounted for 24% of all fractures. It was also found that 23% of boys and 16% of girls had more than one fracture before age 18 years. In a population-based study from Wales, it was noted that there was a seasonal variation in forearm and wrist fractures in children and adolescents. The incidence of such fractures markedly increased in spring and summer, as did the severity of fracture. Twenty-three percent of patients with fractures required hospital admission in the spring and summer compared with only 10% of patients who had fractures during the winter months. In a population-based, case control study from Wales, a significant decrease in bone mass (measured by dual-energy x-ray absorptiometry and metacarpal morphometry) was found in children age 9 to 16 years, with wrist and forearm fractures compared with a control group. Postural balance scores were noted to be significantly poorer in patients with high body weight and a history of previous forearm fracture compared with a control group with normal body weight. The increased body mass index and poor balance appear to contribute to the increased risk of forearm fracture in these patients.

Participants in specific sports such as snowboarding, horseback riding, and soccer (goal keeping) were noted to have an increased risk of wrist fractures. In a retrospective review of skiers and snowboarders from Japan, there was an increased incidence of upper limb injuries, particularly elbow dislocations and wrist fractures, in those who participated in snowboarding. In a randomized controlled study of snowboarders in Norway, it was noted that wrist guards significantly lowered the incidence of wrist injuries without increasing the risks for more proximal fractures or dislocations. Because of the increased risk of head and wrist injuries in horseback riding, and the decrease in severity and number of head injuries with the use of protective headgear, it has been proposed that wrist protectors may be of benefit in this sport as well.

Ligamentous laxity correlates with the site of the fracture. Patients with hyperlaxity are more likely to have a supracondylar humerus fracture after a fall, whereas children with less laxity are more likely to sustain distal radius fractures. In a study of distal radius fractures in young soccer goalkeepers, the size of the ball correlated with the risk of a distal radius fracture.

Forearm and Wrist Fractures

Fractures of the forearm are the most common long bone fractures in children, accounting for 45% of all childhood fractures and 62% of upper extremity fractures. Approximately 75% to 84% of these forearm fractures occur in the distal third of the bone; 15% to 18% in the middle third; and less than 5% in the proximal third. Injuries to the distal radioulnar joint or carpal

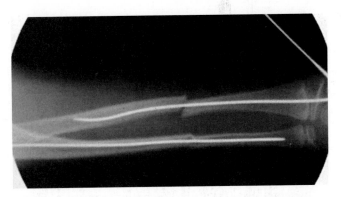

Figure 1 A radiograph showing intramedullary fixation of a diaphyseal radius and ulna fracture. The ulnar pin is inserted proximally and the radial pin is inserted distally.

bones in children are much less common. Scaphoid fracture is the most common carpal bone fracture; however, it accounts for only 0.45% of all upper extremity fractures in children.

Fractures of the Diaphyseal Radius and Ulna

Diaphyseal fractures are classified as plastic deformation, buckle or torus, greenstick or incomplete, and complete. Approximately 50% of diaphyseal fractures are greenstick and most occur in children younger than 8 years of age. The purpose of closed reduction is to correct the malrotation first, then the malangulation.

Complete fractures are more common in preadolescent and adolescent patients and tend to be unstable; these fractures often require internal fixation. There is an increased incidence of loss of reduction. More recently, unstable diaphyseal forearm fractures have been treated with intramedullary fixation. Elastic nails or Kirschner wires can be placed percutaneously after successful closed reduction. The ulnar pin is passed from proximal to distal, while the radial pin is placed from distal to proximal with the entry site proximal to the distal radial physis (Figure 1). Open reduction is indicated for irreducible fractures; unstable fractures, especially in the adolescent patient; displaced segmental fractures; fractures associated with unstable Monteggia, Galeazzi, or supracondylar fractures; refracture; and for patients with a dysvascular limb.

Fractures of the Distal Radius and Ulna
Metaphyseal Fractures

Seventy-five percent to 84% of pediatric forearm fractures involve the distal radius. Most of these radial fractures are metaphyseal and are associated with metaphyseal fractures of the ulna. Nondisplaced metaphyseal torus fractures can be treated with brief immobilization. Studies indicate that removal of the splint at home was more satisfactory for families than return for doctor-supervised removal; the clinical outcome was the same.

Although closed reduction and long arm cast immobilization is indicated for fractures with greater than 10° of malalignment, several studies indicate a high incidence (up to 34%) of loss of reduction. Percutaneous pin fixation avoids the need for rereduction of difficult distal radius fractures but does carry the risks associated with anesthesia, pin placement, possible infection, and limited scarring. Two separate randomized trials of pinning compared with cast immobilization indicated that pinning significantly reduced the risk of loss of reduction requiring remanipulaton; however, long-term clinical outcome was the same for both groups of patients. Pinning is reasonable for fractures with initial angulation greater than 30° and displacement more than 50% of the diameter of the radius. Remodeling of malunited fractures in the flexion/extension plane will occur and, to a lesser extent, remodeling will also occur in the radial deviation/ulnar deviation plane if sufficient gravity remains. Rotational malunion will not remodel.

Percutaneous pinning is clearly indicated for fractures associated with neurovascular compromise and significant soft-tissue swelling, and with concomitant fractures of the elbow (floating elbow) because of the increased risk for development of compartment syndrome in these patients. A smooth Kirschner wire is inserted obliquely from distal to proximal, starting in the radial metaphysis just proximal to the physis. Care must be taken to avoid the radial sensory nerve with insertion. This procedure may be done with a 5- to 10-mm incision and clearing of the pin tract. A second, crossing Kirschner wire can be inserted from between the fourth and fifth dorsal extensor compartments while avoiding the extensor tendons (Figure 2).

Distal Radius Physeal Fractures

Most distal radius physeal fractures are Salter-Harris type II injuries that occur in adolescents. Displacement is typically dorsal with apex volar angulation. An atraumatic closed reduction and long arm cast immobilization is indicated for fractures with greater than 10° of malangulation. The most significant complications are associated with future growth arrest and acute neurovascular compromise. The incidence of associated nerve injuries is approximately 8%. Studies indicate that patients with signs or symptoms of median nerve injury at the time of presentation would be best treated by percutaneous pin fixation rather than cast immobilization to lessen the risk of forearm compartment syndrome, acute carpal tunnel syndrome, or median neuropathy. There is limited evidence of a significant risk of growth arrest with the use of smooth, small diameter pins. The pins should be removed at 3 to 4 weeks postoperatively to lessen the risk of growth arrest.

Long-term follow-up (average, 25.5 years) of 157 patients with distal radius and ulna physeal fractures who were treated with closed reduction showed that 4.4% of

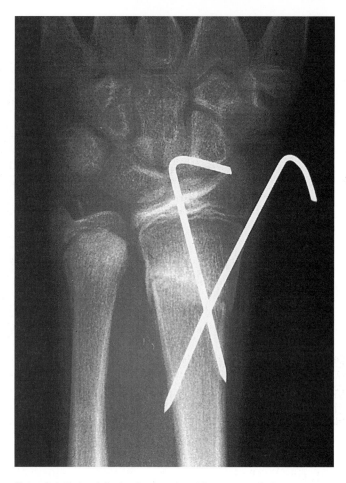

Figure 2 A displaced distal radius metaphyseal fracture treated with percutaneous fixation. Care must be taken to avoid the radial sensory nerve and, if possible, the distal radial physis, with the radial pin. Care must be taken to avoid the extensor tendons with the ulnar pin.

patients with distal radius fractures and 50% of patients with distal ulna fractures had a symptomatic growth discrepancy greater than 1 cm. In addition, 38 asymptomatic patients had growth discrepancies between 2 to 9 mm. Patients with redisplacement or late presentation should not undergo a repeat reduction after 7 days to avoid iatrogenic physeal arrest. Late open reduction should be avoided for the same reason. Because these fractures displace in the plane of motion of the wrist joint and are juxtaphyseal, there is tremendous potential for remodeling of a malunion in the younger adolescent patient. If the malunion does not remodel with growth, a dorsal opening wedge osteotomy with bone graft and internal fixation may be needed for the skeletally mature patient with greater than 10° apex dorsal malangulation. Patients with displaced physeal fractures should be examined for 1 to 2 years after the fracture occurrence to rule out a growth disturbance. If a radial growth arrest occurs, the continued ulnar growth can lead to distal radioulnar joint incongruity, ulnocarpal impaction, and a triangular fibrocartilage tear (Figure 3).

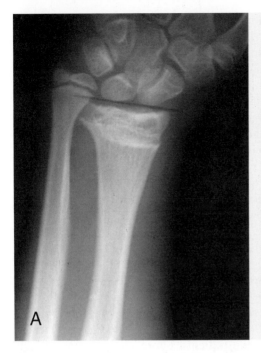
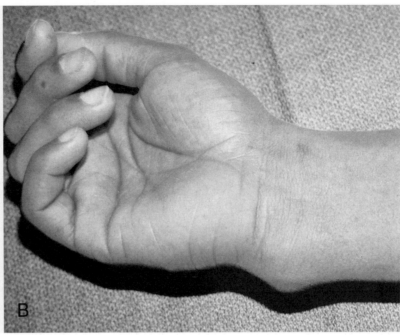

Figure 3 A, Radiograph shows distal radial physeal arrest after repetitive closed reductions of a Salter-Harris type II fracture. Note the ulnar overgrowth with open physis and the radial growth arrest. **B,** Clinical photograph of the patient showing the deformity resulting in ulnar-carpal impaction.

Hand Trauma

Fractures to the pediatric hand account for approximately one quarter of all childhood fractures and have two peak periods of occurrence—in adolescence (from sport-related activities) and in infancy (from crush injuries). Most of these fractures are nondisplaced, nonphyseal injuries that do not have long-term consequences. Physeal injuries account for up to 40% of finger fractures. A Salter-Harris type II fracture of the small finger proximal phalanx is the most common physeal injury. Distal tuft and phalanx fractures are the most common fractures in infants and children up to age 8 years; proximal phalanx fractures of the small finger are most common in the 9- to 12-year age group; and fifth metacarpal neck fractures have the highest incidence in patients age 13 to 16 years. Most pediatric hand fractures heal within 2 to 3 weeks and have excellent functional outcomes regardless of the type of treatment used. Malunions or growth disturbances are rare. However, there is a subset of pediatric hand fractures with comminution, severe displacement, and intra-articular and condylar involvement, which will heal poorly if not recognized and appropriately treated. These fractures account for 12% to 20% of pediatric fractures in most studies.

Problematic Hand Fractures

Phalangeal neck fractures are usually caused by crush injuries. As the child attempts to extract the affected digit, the condyles become entrapped and a fracture occurs in the subcondylar region. The condylar fragment is displaced in extension and often malrotates. The subcondylar fossa is obliterated, blocking interphalangeal flexion. If not properly recognized and treated, complications of malunion and loss of motion occur. The severity of this fracture is often underappreciated in the urgent care setting. Treatment is with either closed reduction and percutaneous pinning or by open reduction and internal fixation. If open reduction is necessary, the collateral ligaments should not be dissected from the distal fragment. This action increases the risk of osteonecrosis. Treatment for a late malunion includes osteotomy, subchondral fossa reconstruction, or remodeling. Remodeling of phalangeal neck malunions rarely occurs because of the significant distance from the physis.

Osteochondral fractures in young children are often challenging to treat. These fractures have a high risk of nonunion, malunion, and osteonecrosis, which is particularly true in crush injuries to the middle phalanx that alter the local blood supply. The fracture is intra-articular, generally displaced, and requires anatomic reduction for a successful outcome. Most often, the fracture needs to be treated aggressively with open reduction. Bone grafts may be necessary to maintain articular congruity and prevent collapse. Even with a well-performed open reduction, complications from osteochondral fractures can occur in young children.

In the adolescent, treatment of intercondylar fractures is similar to that given to adults. Anatomic reduction and pin fixation is necessary to restore the joint surface and to prevent loss of reduction. Open reduction is appropriate for fractures that are not suitable for closed reduction, and can be performed with a volar, midaxial, or dorsal approach. Restoration of an anatomic joint lessens the risk of long-term arthritis, malalignment, and loss of motion.

The major complication of diaphyseal-level phalangeal fractures is malrotation. Frequently, children will refuse to actively move the affected finger in the acute setting, thus preventing accurate assessment of digital alignment. However, possible tenodesis of the wrist enables the physician to assess malrotation and should be performed on all phalangeal and metacarpal fractures regardless of radiographic appearance. If closed treatment is chosen, a solitary finger should never be immobilized; it should be secured to the adjacent digits to prevent subsequent loss of reduction. If the fracture is malrotated and unstable, a reduction pin or screw is necessary for stabilization. Although malrotation is uncommon, it can result in a major complication if it is not discovered until after union takes place. The malrotated digit impairs the function of the adjacent digits secondary to overlap, and can only be corrected with osteotomy.

Scaphoid Fractures

Distal pole scaphoid fractures in the skeletally immature patient heal readily with cast immobilization without risk of nonunion or osteonecrosis. Scaphoid waist fractures are common in the adolescent age group. Recent studies have indicated that both adults and children with clinical pain in the region of the scaphoid and normal radiographs may benefit from MRI, the results of which will alter treatment choices in a high percentage of patients. Waist fractures carry the same risks of nonunion and osteonecrosis in the child as they do in an adult. Open reduction, bone grafting, and internal fixation should be used to treat an established nonunion in a child. The epidemiology of scaphoid fractures continues to change; proximal pole fractures, nonunions, and osteonecrosis now have been described in adolescents. Treatment with distal radial vascularized bone graft has been recommended for these unique complications. The treatment of acute scaphoid fractures, even nondisplaced fractures, with percutaneous screw fixation is controversial. The complication rates in patients with acute scaphoid fractures who were treated with casting compared with those treated with screw fixation have been statistically equivalent.

Flexor Tendon Injuries
Tendon Lacerations

The diagnosis, surgical care, and postoperative rehabilitation of a flexor tendon injury may be more difficult in a child than in an adult. Treatment is especially difficult in a toddler or preschool-age child who offers limited cooperation. The presenting digital cascade and digital excursion with wrist tenodesis serve as the basis for diagnosis of a flexor tendon laceration. If doubt exits, the wound should be explored with the patient under anesthesia. Repair of the tendon lacerations in zones I and II requires meticulous technique with fine sutures. Postoperative cast immobilization for 4 weeks is effective.

No differences have been found in total active motion (TAM) between patients treated with early mobilization protocols and those treated with cast immobilization for 4 weeks. If cast immobilization continues beyond 4 weeks, TAM may decrease by up to 40% by 6 weeks. There was no difference in the results in groups from 0 to 15 years of age.

Two-stage reconstruction of unrecognized zone II lacerations in children has poorer results than in adults, with a higher rate of complications and a mean TAM of only 140°. Better results are achieved with supervised rehabilitation. In a study on uncomplicated flexor pollicis longus tendon laceration repairs, long-term limited motion (> 30°) of the interphalangeal joint occurred in one third of the patients. Short splint immobilization had a negative effect on outcome; however, zone of injury, an early mobilization program, or concurrent digital nerve injury had no significant effect on long-term outcome.

Amputations

The treatment of proximal, complete digital amputations with replantation in children as young as 1 year of age is now standard. In children, the indication for replantation is more liberal than in adult patients and includes cases of multiple digit, thumb, midpalm, hand, and distal forearm amputations, as well as single digit amputations in zones I and II. Crush amputations caused by compression from doors, heavy objects, or bicycle chains have a peak incidence in children 5 years of age, whereas amputations caused by sharp objects occur more commonly in adolescents. Digital survival rates from replantation range from 69% to 89% in pediatric studies. Indications that favor digital survival are amputations resulting from sharp objects, patient body weight greater than 11 kg, more than one vein repaired, bone shortening, interosseous wire fixation, and vein grafting of arteries and veins. Vessel size generally exceeds 0.8 mm in digital replants in children and is not a technical problem for the skilled microvascular surgeon. Index and long finger replants have been more successful than small finger replants in children. A digital survival rate of 95% occurred in children if prompt reperfusion was seen after arterial repair with at least one successful venous anastomosis. Neural recovery rates far exceed those found in adult patients; return of two-point discrimination of less than 5 mm often occurs. Tenolysis may be necessary after tendon repair. Growth arrest or deformity is more common if there is a crush compo-

Table 2 | Classification of Congenital Upper Limb Malformations

I	Failure of formation
	A Transverse arrest
	B Longitudinal arrest
II	Failure of differentiation (separation)
III	Congenital tumorous conditions
IV	Duplication
V	Overgrowth
VI	Undergrowth
VII	Congenital constriction ring syndrome
VIII	Generalized skeletal abnormalities

nent to the amputation. Microvascular toe to thumb transfer is a successful alternative to pollicization as treatment for a failed replant in a young child.

Congenital Upper Extremity Malformations

The prevalence of congenital upper limb anomalies is 2 per 1,000 live births. Forty-six percent of these infants also have another nonhand anomaly; bilateral hand anomalies are found in more than 50% of these patients. Overall, boys are affected more than girls by a ratio of 3:2. Advanced maternal age significantly increases the prevalence of congenital upper extremity malformations.

Recent advances in embryology have greatly improved the understanding of human limb development. Growth factors influence the apical ectodermal ridge and numerous genes influence the zone of polarizing activity and polarity. Genes responsible for specific deformities such as triphalangeal thumb have been identified on specific chromosomes. Modern ultrasound techniques also have increased the rate of prenatal diagnosis of these disorders and may lead to parental consultation before birth.

During embryologic growth, the limb bud appears 26 days after fertilization. The final stage of upper extremity development, separation of the ring and small digits, is completed by day 56. Events occurring at various stages of embryologic growth may have profound effects on the ultimate appearance of the limb.

Classification

The most commonly used classification system is that proposed by the American Society for Surgery of the Hand and the International Federation of Societies for Surgery of the Hand. This system includes eight categories that are based on the proposed etiologic pathways and are found in Table 2.

Trigger Thumb

Trigger thumb is one of the most common malformations in children. Two large studies of consecutive deliv-

eries of more than 12,000 children have not found this condition to be present at birth, supporting the belief that it is not a true congenital condition. The child will have a flexion deformity of the interphalangeal joint that may not be passively correctable. A compensatory hyperextension deformity at the metacarpophalangeal joint may also develop. A palpable nodule at the level of the A1 pulley of the thumb, which appears to be caused by edema within the tendon, will also be present.

Spontaneous resolution occurs in a small number of patients. Nonsurgical treatment has been most popular in Asia where a combination of splinting and passive motion has been shown to allow for correction in up to two thirds of affected patients. When the thumb does not show any sign of spontaneous correction, A1 pulley release is indicated. This procedure may be performed by either transverse incision or a chevron type incision centered over the metacarpophalangeal joint. Longitudinal incisions over this site have been shown to adversely affect range of motion and appearance. Long-term studies of trigger thumb release have found that although recurrence of triggering is extremely rare, approximately 25% of the patients show some limitation in interphalangeal joint motion compared with the unaffected thumb. No long-term functional deficits have been noted with trigger thumb release.

Trigger Finger

Based on large population studies, trigger finger, like trigger thumb, has not been found at birth. Patients with trigger fingers have a higher rate of spontaneous resolution and an earlier age of onset than patients with trigger thumbs. For those digits not showing spontaneous correction, abnormalities are found well beyond the A1 pulley and may include abnormalities of the flexor digitorum sublimis tendon insertion and the A3 pulley. Surgical treatment of a trigger finger requires exploration of the digit well beyond the A1 pulley because almost 50% of patients undergoing simple A1 pulley release will have residual triggering.

Polydactyly

Polydactyly occurs as an isolated disorder, in association with other malformations of the extremities, or as part of a syndrome. It usually occurs sporadically but may be inherited with a mainly autosomal dominant inheritance. Polydactyly is categorized as radial, central, or ulnar with the small finger the most commonly duplicated digit.

Small finger duplication may occur as either a skin tag or a fully developed digit including a fully formed metacarpal bone (Figure 4). The incidence of this disorder has been reported as high as 1 in 300 births in the African American population and 1 in 3,000 in the white population. In the African American population,

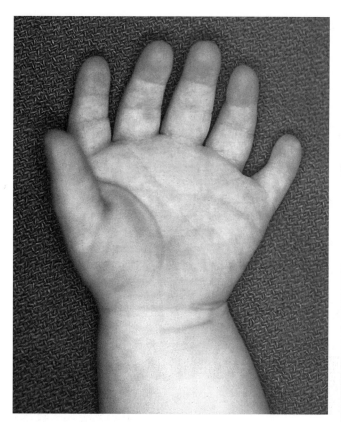

Figure 4 Small finger duplication, complete.

Table 3 | Thumb Duplication

Level	Description
I	Bifid distal phalanx
II	Complete duplication distal phalanx
III	Complete duplication distal phalanx, bifid proximal phalanx
IV	Complete duplication distal and proximal phalanges
V	Complete duplication distal and proximal phalanges, bifid metacarpal
VI	Complete duplication distal, proximal phalanges, and metacarpal
VII	Triphalangeal thumb

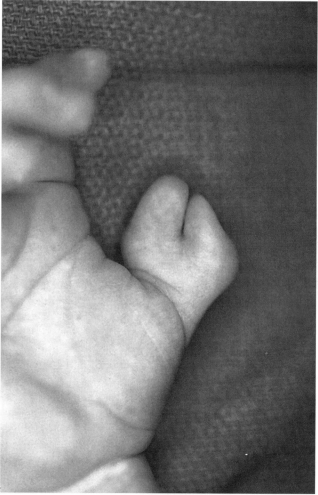

Figure 5 Type IV thumb duplication, converging.

this condition is rarely associated with any other type of malformation, whereas up to 30% of white children with small finger polydactyly will have underlying organ system disorders such as gastrointestinal or genitourinary malformations. Most patients with ulnar polydactyly are treated with either ligation in the nursery or simple excision. One recent study found a 23% complication rate following suture ligation; infection and incomplete removal were the most common complications. Patients with ulnar polydactyly involving neurovascular structures in bone will require more sophisticated reconstruction, which may include transference of hypothenar tendons and collateral ligament reconstruction.

Radial side polydactyly involving the thumb is classified based on the level of duplication (Table 3) and ranges from a bifid distal phalanx to complete duplication of metacarpals (Figure 5). Patients with malformations involving the thumb tips may benefit from a combination type procedure with more proximal duplications treated by excision of the radial digit and reconstruction of the retained ulnar digit. Simple excision produces significant complications of instability and stiffness; formal reconstruction of the duplicated digit including advancement of the thenar tendon and collateral ligament reconstruction should be performed. Because of the difficulty in reconstructing the ulnar collat-

eral ligament, the preferred treatment is preservation of the more ulnar digit, which in most patients is more completely developed. Late deformities have been observed as a result of instability of the interphalangeal joints and eccentric insertions of the flexor and/or extensor tendon. These deformities may have a radial insertion along the retained digit, allowing for a zigzag type of deformity later in life. Although long-term studies show few functional problems with duplicate thumb reconstruction, a large percentage of patients report stiffness and/or instability at the interphalangeal joints.

The triphalangeal thumb falls within the category of thumb duplication and is an autosomal dominant form of an inherited radial abnormality (Figure 6). It may exist in combination with syndactyly. Complications associated with multiple level joint instability have led some physicians to recommend ablation of this digit when it is part of a radial side polydactyly. When seen in isolation, the triphalangeal thumb is best treated by deletion of the middle phalanx and temporary pin fixation of the resulting interphalangeal joint.

Central polydactyly is a rare condition involving duplication of the index, long, or ring digits. These digits often show incomplete duplication with frequent overlapping of the duplicated digits. Most patients are best treated by deletion of these digits, which are often underdeveloped.

Radial Head Dislocation

Congenital radial head dislocation is often asymptomatic and may go undiagnosed until radiographs have been obtained for an injury. True congenital dislocations may have a late diagnosis because of the frequency of bilateral involvement. Recent reports have suggested that open reduction and ligament repair or reconstruction may successfully reduce the radial head. Longer term studies are needed to determine if the bony changes that include capitellar undergrowth, radial head enlargement, and bowing may be prevented by open reduction. Radial head reduction has not been as successful in patients with either radial or ulnar dysplasia and in patients older than 5 years of age at the time of surgery.

In patients who are not evaluated until secondary bone changes have occurred, open reduction has not been recommended. Radial head resection at adolescence remains a mainstay of treatment and has been shown to improve range of motion. Regrowth of the proximal radius has been reported after radial head resection and may cause secondary impingement and loss of motion.

Longitudinal Epiphyseal Bracket (Delta Phalanx)

Delta phalanx may be found in isolation or within a digit affected by other disorders such as syndactyly (Figure 7). In this condition the epiphyseal plate is oriented both transversely and longitudinally, forming a "C" shape. This abnormal epiphyseal plate may cause a significant deviation in digits that are operated on for other conditions, and may be undetected at the time of initial surgery. Studies have shown that this condition

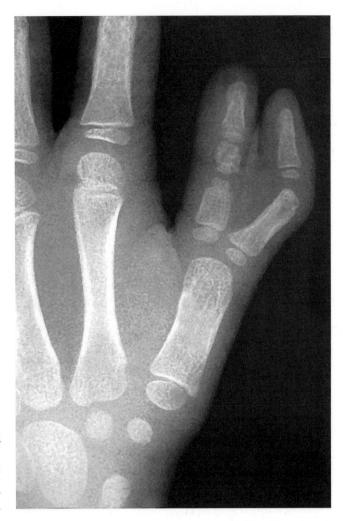

Figure 6 Duplicate thumb, triphalangeal ulnar component.

may not be readily apparent until 18 months of age. In patients with a deviation caused by this abnormal epiphyseal plate, a portion of the plate should be removed and replaced by fat or other material. This technique has been shown to successfully stop the abnormal deviation of the digit. In patients in whom treatment is delayed, treatment may require reversed wedge osteotomy as a method to both correct deformity and arrest the abnormal epiphyseal growth.

Constriction Ring Syndrome

Constriction ring syndrome has been reported in up to 1 in 10,000 births. Although the etiology of this disorder is not completely known, a similar disorder has been produced in laboratory animals by creating a vascular insult late in limb development. In these experiments, the loss of the epidermal layer causes coalescence of digits much like that seen in an untreated burn. Involvement of the digits ranges from mild skin dimpling to complete absence of digits. Acral syndactyly is noted with coalescence of digits at the tip combined with separation at

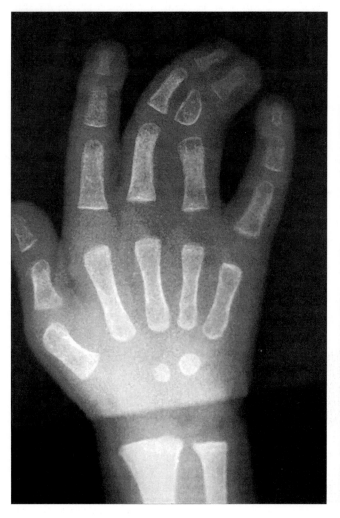

Figure 7 Ring finger delta phalanx.

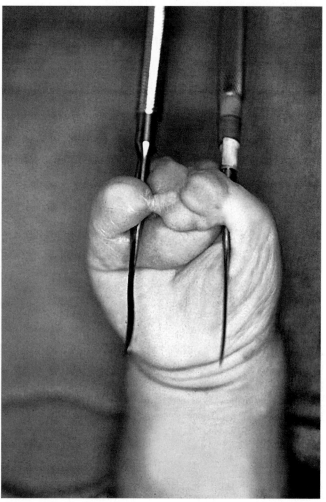

Figure 8 Constriction ring syndrome with web base separation.

the level of the web space (Figure 8). The underlying structures are usually normal to the level of the digital absence; separation of digits may be easily performed as the proper level of the web is already established. Circumferential rings may best be released by performing surgery on one half of the circumference at a time. On rare occasion, this disorder may occur with significant compromise to the digit distal to the site of the constriction ring and will require release of the ring during the first few days of life. In most patients with ring release, a deep fibrous layer must be excised in addition to Z-plasty, which is usually performed at the skin level.

Camptodactyly

Camptodactyly is an isolated congenital flexion deformity of the proximal interphalangeal joint. The patients may present with a broad spectrum of deformity and involvement. The digits have abnormalities of numerous structures including skin, fascia, tendon sheaths, flexor digitorum sublimis tendons, lumbrical and interosseous muscles, bony surfaces, and the central extensor mecha-

nism. Camptodactyly has a bimodal type of distribution, with type I presenting in infancy and type II presenting in adolescence. In type III, the condition is found as part of a syndrome.

Most type I patients improve with stretching and splinting. Patients with type II camptodactyly may improve with splinting and may have significant residual flexion deformity, as do type III patients. Surgery for this disorder must be undertaken with caution because significant residual flexion deformity is usually noted. Most authors recommend reserving surgical release for contractures greater than 60°.

Syndactyly

Syndactyly is the most common congenital hand deformity occurring in approximately 1 in 2,200 births. It may be inherited with an autosomal dominant pattern in up to 40% of patients. Although numerous syndromes include syndactyly, the most common are Apert's syndrome and Poland's syndrome. Syndactyly may be complete or incomplete based on the distal extent of the

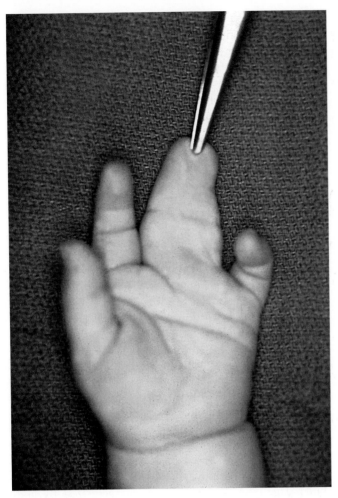

Figure 9 Complete syndactyly of the third and fourth fingers.

web (Figure 9). Syndactyly is also classified as either simple or complex based on any component of shared bone or nail. The geometry of most syndactylous digits usually requires the use of skin graft for separation. A full-thickness graft harvested from either the upper extremity or the groin provides adequate coverage. Recent reports have promoted the separation of syndactylous fingers without grafting by the aggressive defatting of skin flaps. Border digits may require early release because of the disparate length of the ring and small finger or the thumb and index finger. Complications of syndactyly release include infection, web creep, and unrecognized bony anomaly. Web creep is seen in patients undergoing surgery before 16 months of age. The unrecognized bony anomaly of a delta phalanx also may be undetected on radiographs until 18 months of age. These two factors may indicate that delaying surgery until 18 months may be advisable.

Madelung's Deformity

Madelung's deformity is a growth disturbance involving the palmar and ulnar aspects of the distal radius at the epiphyseal plate. A physeal bar has been found that bridges the distal metaphysis of the radius to the epiphysis along the volar aspect of the radius at the lunate facet. Hypertrophy of palmar ligaments (including the radiotriquetral and the short radiolunate ligaments, and an anomalous volar ligament) has been identified. It appears that the physeal bar impedes the normal development of the distal radius causing its palmar and ulnar deformity. The hypertrophied ligament also appears to contribute to the deformity.

Radiographic findings include dorsal bowing of the radius, ulnar tilting of the radius, and radial tilting of the ulna. There is palmar tilting of the distal articular surface of the radius and a triangular appearance of the epiphysis. A fixed pronation deformity of the distal radius is usually present.

Madelung's deformity may occur as an isolated condition or as part of a generalized dysplastic disorder associated with Leri-Weill syndrome (dyschondrosteosis), a condition whose inheritance is autosomal dominant. Deletions or mutations in the *SHOX* (short stature homeobox–containing) gene have now been well documented in those patients.

During the first few years of life, the ulnar portion of the epiphysis fails to ossify, leading to a severely angulated distal articular surface. The carpus then tends to shift toward the ulna with the lunate often overlapping the ulnar head. Patients may seek treatment during the preadolescent years because of the deformity. Pain is rarely a symptom.

Numerous surgical approaches have been described. It appears that the palmar approach to release the hypertrophied ligament combined with either epiphysiolysis or osteotomy may offer the best treatment for correcting this deformity. After epiphyseal plate closure, procedures to correct the deformity should include correction of the articular surface angular deformity combined with ulnar shortening. Salvage type procedures include radiolunate arthrodesis combined with distal ulnar resection.

Synostosis of the Proximal Radius and Ulna

Failure of the proximal radius and ulna to separate leads to a fixed forearm position because of synostosis. Most cases of synostosis are bilateral and may frequently occur in association with other organ system abnormalities. In most patients the disease is characterized by a forearm that is in slight to moderate pronation; minimal treatment may be required for this condition. In patients with significant supination of the forearm, a rotational osteotomy is recommended so that both palms may be positioned for keyboard use. Repositioning of the forearm in patients with congenital radioulnar synostosis may be performed using an osteotomy through the level of synostosis or with a two-level os-

Table 4 | Thumb Hypoplasia

Type I	Mild underdevelopment
Type II	Thenar hypoplasia, abduction contracture, metacarpophalangeal laxity
Type III	Thenar hypoplasia, abduction contracture, metacarpophalangeal instability, extrinsic tendon hypoplasia or absence, metacarpal underdevelopment
A	Stable carpometacarpal joint
B	Unstable carpometacarpal joint
Type IV	Pouce flottant
Type V	Complete absence of thumb

teotomy (one osteotomy performed at the distal third of the radius and one at the proximal third of the ulna). Attempts to separate the synostosis have been successful in a limited number of patients; the use of either a pedicled or free tissue transfer to prevent reformation of the synostosis is required.

Transverse Forearm Deficiency

Most patients with transverse failure of formation have a unilateral, short below-elbow deficiency. Other levels of failure of formation include transcarpal, distal forearm, and transhumeral. Most children will have excellent adaptation to this deficiency with few functional deficits.

The use of a passive prosthesis is usually attempted in patients with a short below-elbow deficiency. In some patients, the forearm portion is quite short and there may be difficulty with prosthetic fitting. In addition, soft-tissue coverage may be inadequate to allow for prosthetic placement. Prosthetic fitting usually begins at 4 to 6 months of age and includes a passive prosthesis to allow for two-handed activity. Many children resist the use of a prosthesis because of its lack of sensory feedback. More proximal levels of deficiency are rarely treated with prosthetic usage.

Longitudinal Deficiency of the Radius

Radial ray deficiency is a condition occurring in 1 in 25,000 births. Radial ray deficiencies include complete or partial absence of the radius and radial digits—most commonly the thumb. Radial deficiencies are usually bilateral. Radial ray deficiency has been categorized as type I, short distal radius; type II, underdevelopment of the entire radius; type III, partial absence of radius; and type IV, complete absence of radius (the most common deficiency). Treatment includes passive stretching with either serial casting or static progressive splinting until 6 months of age at which time centralization or radialization is performed. Alternatively, soft-tissue distraction using external fixation also may be used to provide some level of correction before bony stabilization. Centralization is usually performed in patients who will ulti-

mately undergo pollicization to avoid placement of a pin through the index metacarpal.

A recent long-term assessment of the functional outcome after centralization for radial dysplasia showed that despite surgical intervention, hand function remained markedly abnormal, whereas upper extremity disability was mild. Improvement of wrist alignment and increased forearm length was not found to correlate with improved upper extremity function. Significant radial angulation and limited range of motion and grip strength were all findings in this long-term follow-up study.

Thumb Hypoplasia

Thumb hypoplasia includes the spectrum of deformities from a slightly small thumb to complete thumb absence. Blauth type I thumbs usually appear small but require no reconstruction. Type II deformities have absent or underdeveloped thenar muscles; opponensplasty is required. Type III hypoplastic thumbs are characterized by underdevelopment of the metacarpal bones, absence of extrinsic tendons, and thenar hypoplasia. Type IIIA thumbs show a stable carpometacarpal joint and type IIIB thumbs an unstable carpometacarpal joint, often with a deficient metacarpal. Type IIIA thumbs require significant reconstructive effort including opponensplasty, metacarpophalangeal joint stabilization, and web space deepening. Type IIIB thumbs may best be treated by ablation and pollicization using the index finger as is recommended for the type IV deficiency (pouce flottant). The type V deficiency is characterized by complete absence of the thumb (Table 4). Studies of the long-term outcome following hypoplastic thumb reconstruction did not find any benefit from early reconstruction. More than 30% of patients undergoing pollicization will require opponensplasty. Pollicization is best performed when the patient is 2 to 3 years old because of the increased size of the digital vessels.

Longitudinal Deficiency of the Ulna

Ulnar longitudinal deficiency is one fourth as common as radial ray deficiency and occurs in approximately 1 in 100,000 births. The ulna may show partial or complete deficiency with varying levels of digital deletions. The elbow deformity ranges from joint hypoplasia to complete radiohumeral synostosis. Unilateral involvement is most common and this condition is frequently associated with other musculoskeletal abnormalities such as scoliosis and fibular deficiency. Surgical treatment of patients with ulnar radial deficiency usually focuses on the hand. Up to three fourths of hands have first web abnormalities. Syndactyly is frequently found in the digits that are present, and also requires separation. One study found that slightly fewer than 50% of patients with ulnar ray deficiency also displayed some element of thenar hypoplasia.

Annotated Bibliography

Forearm and Wrist Trauma

Boyd KT, Brownson P, Hunter JB: Distal radial fractures in young goalkeepers: A case for an appropriately sized soccer ball. *Br J Sports Med* 2001;35:409-411.

In a prospective, clinic-based study of young goalkeepers, it was shown that the size of the ball had a direct effect on the risk of a distal radius fracture.

Cannata G, DeMaio F, Mancini F, Ippolito E: Physeal fractures of the distal radius and ulna: Long-term prognosis. *J Orthop Trauma* 2003;17:172-179.

One hundred sixty-three fractures of the distal radius and ulna physes in 157 patients were reviewed at an average follow-up of 25.5 years (14 to 46 years). Seventy-seven were isolated fractures of the distal radius, 54 were associated with ulnar styloid fractures, and 26 were associated with ulnar metaphyseal fractures. Eighteen were Salter-Harris type I fractures and 139 were type II fractures. Symptomatic growth discrepancy of greater than 1 cm at skeletal maturity occurred in 4.4% of the distal radius physeal fractures and 50% of distal ulnar physeal fractures.

Jones IE, Williams SM, Dow N, Goulding A: How many children remain fracture-free during growth?: A longitudinal study of children and adolescents participating in the Dunedin Multidisciplinary Health and Development Study. *Osteoporos Int* 2002;13:990-995.

Results of a longitudinal study of 601 people from New Zealand showed that approximately half (60% girls, 50% boys) of the children in the study did not have a fracture throughout their growth period. More than one fracture occurred in 119 children (16% girls, 23% boys). The forearm was the most common site of fracture (24%).

Ronning R, Ronning I, Gerner T, Engebretsen L: The efficacy of wrist protectors in preventing snowboarding injuries. *Am J Sports Med* 2001;29:581-585.

Results of a randomized, prospective study of 5,029 snowboarders in Norway is presented. A significant decrease in injury rate was found with the use of wrist protectors. Beginners and those using rental equipment were at highest risk for wrist injury.

Wareham K, Johansen A, Stone MD, Saunders J, Jones S, Lyons RA: Seasonal variation in the incidence of wrist and forearm fractures and its consequences. *Injury* 2003;34:219-222.

A longitudinal study from Wales showed a seasonal variation in the incidence of wrist and forearm fractures in children younger than 15 years of age. The incidence in the three winter months (5.7/1,000 per year) was half the incidence for fractures the rest of the year (10.7/1,000 per year). The fractures that occurred during the nonwinter months were more severe with 23% of patients with forearm and wrist fractures requiring hospitalization during the spring, summer, and fall compared with only 10% requiring hospitalization when fractures occurred during the winter.

Waters PM, Bae D, Montgomery K: The surgical management of post-traumatic distal radial physeal growth arrest in adolescents. *J Pediatr Orthop* 2002;22:717-724.

The authors present a case study of patients with distal radial physeal arrests with consequential ulnar overgrowth resulting in complications with ulnar-carpal impaction, distal radial-ulnar joint incongruity, and triangular fibrocartilage tears. Surgical planning and treatment options are outlined for corrective osteotomies and soft-tissue repairs.

Hand Trauma

Mahabir RC, Kazemi AR, Cannon WG, et al: Pediatric hand fractures: A review. *Pediatr Emerg Care* 2001;17:153-156.

The incidence and epidemiology of hand fractures in children are discussed.

Rajesh A, Basu AK, Vaidhyanath R, Finlay D: Hand fractures: A study of their site and type in childhood. *Clin Radiol* 2001;56:667-669.

Radiographs of 280 children with hand fractures were reviewed and categorized by site of the injury and age of the patient. Distal tuft fractures were the most common in the 0- to 4-year age group; distal phalanx fractures occurred most frequently in the 5- to 8-year age group; fractures of the proximal phalanx of the small finger were most common in the 9- to 12-year age group; and fractures of the small finger metacarpal occurred most frequently in the 13- to 16-year old age group.

Congenital Upper Extremity Malformations

Giele H, Giele C, Bover C, et al: The incidence and epidemiology of congenital upper limb anomalies: A total population study. *J Hand Surg [Am]* 2001;26:628-634.

A homogeneous population study found congenital upper extremity anomalies in approximately 2 per 1,000 live births with nearly 50% of those affected having some other anomaly. Failure of separation and duplications were the most common malformations and increased in number with advanced maternal age.

Goldfarb CA, Klepps SJ, Dailey LA, et al: Functional outcome after centralization for radius dysplasia. *J Hand Surg [Am]* 2002;27:118-124.

This long-term review of patients undergoing centralization found residual radial angulation of 36°, wrist arc of motion of 31°, and an average ulnar length that was 54% of that found in the uninvolved contralateral ulna. Surgery resulted in improvement in wrist alignment but with less benefit to functional improvement than previously believed.

Greuse M, Coessens BC: Congenital syndactyly: Defatting facilitates closure without skin graft. *J Hand Surg [Am]* 2001;26:589-594.

The authors performed syndactyly separation with the use of graft by performing extensive defatting. Skin graft was required for complex cases and reoperation was performed in 2 of 16 patients.

Kemnitz S, De SL: Pre-axial polydactyly: Outcome of the surgical treatment. *J Pediatr Orthop B* 2002;11:79-84.

This retrospective study of patients who underwent reconstruction of preaxial polydactyly found high levels of patient satisfaction. Functional outcome was affected by joint stability.

Keswani SG, Johnson MP, Adzick NS, et al: In utero limb salvage: Fetoscopic release of amniotic bands for threatened limb amputation. *J Pediatr Surg* 2003;38:848-851.

The use of fetoscopic laser surgery to release constriction rings at the level of the wrist improved extremity blood flow in utero.

McAdams TR, Moneim MS, Omer GE Jr: Long-term follow-up of surgical release of the A (1) pulley in childhood trigger thumb. *J Pediatr Orthop* 2002;22:41-43.

The authors report on the results of long-term follow-up on patients undergoing trigger thumb release. Patients with a transverse incision had better appearance. Twenty-three percent of these patients had incomplete interphalangeal joint motion, and 17% had metacarpophalangeal hyperextension.

Moon WN, Suh SW, Kim IC: Trigger digits in children. *J Hand Surg [Br]* 2001;26:11-12.

In this study of more than 7,000 newborn infants, no instances of trigger thumb or trigger finger were found. Trigger fingers developed earlier in life than trigger thumb and had a higher spontaneous recovery rate.

Murase T, Tada K, Yoshida T, et al: Derotational osteotomy at the shafts of the radius and ulna for congenital radioulnar synostosis. *J Hand Surg [Am]* 2003;28:133-137.

The authors describe a two-level osteotomy with the radius osteotomy at the distal third and the ulnar osteotomy at the proximal third. Pronation deformity was corrected by manual derotation.

Rayan GM, Frey B: Ulnar polydactyly. *Plast Reconstr Surg* 2001;107:1449-1454.

This study reviews the various types of ulnar polydactyly and their treatments. Most patients (71%) had soft-tissue tags that were treated by ligation. African American patients were most likely to have soft-tissue duplications only, whereas white patients were more likely to have digits with bony elements.

Schmidt-Rohlfing B, Schwobel B, Pauschert R, et al: Madelung deformity: Clinical features, therapy and results. *J Pediatr Orthop B* 2001;10:344-348.

This long-term retrospective review found that most patients with Madelung's deformity are female (77%), with a positive family history in 13% of those affected. Despite surgery, almost all patients had limited range of motion.

Classic Bibliography

Bayne LG, Klug MS: Long-term review of the surgical treatment of radial deficiencies. *J Hand Surg [Am]* 1987; 12:169-179.

Benson LS, Waters PM, Kamil NI, Simmons BP, Upton J III: Camptodactly: Classification and results of nonoperative treatment. *J Pediatr Orthop* 1994;14:814-819.

Buck-Gramcko D: Pollicization of the index finger: Method and results in aplasia and hypoplasia of the thumb. *J Bone Joint Surg Am* 1971;53:1605-1617.

Carter PR, Ezaki M: Madelung's deformity: Surgical correction through the anterior approach. *Hand Clin* 2000;16:713-721.

Cole RJ, Manske PR: Classification of ulnar deficiency according to the thumb and first web. *J Hand Surg [Am]* 1997;22:479-488.

Fitoussi F, Mazda K, Frajman JM, Jehanno P, Pennecot GF: Repair of the flexor pollicus longus tendon in children. *J Bone Joint Surg Br* 2000;82:1177-1180.

Gibbons CL, Woods DA, Pailthorpe C, et al: The management of isolated distal radius fractures in children. *J Pediatr Orthop* 1994;14:207-210.

Horii E, Nakamura R, Sakuma M, Miura T: Duplicated thumb bifurcation at the metacarpophalangeal joint level: Factors affecting surgical outcome. *J Hand Surg [Am]* 1997;22:671-679.

Hung L, Cheng JC, Bundoc R, et al: Thumb duplication at the metacarpophalangeal joint: Management and a new classification. *Clin Orthop* 1996;323:31-41.

James MA, McCarroll HR, Manske PR: The spectrum of radial longitudinal deficiency: A modified classification. *J Hand Surg [Am]* 1999;24:1145-1155.

Mani GV, Hui PW, Cheng JC: Translation of the radius as a predictor of outcome in distal radial fractures of children. *J Bone Joint Surg Br* 1993;75:808-811.

Manske PR, Halikis MN: Surgical classification of central deficiency according to the thumb web. *J Hand Surg [Am]* 1995;20:687-697.

Manske PR, Rotman MB, Dailey LA: Long-term functional results after pollicization for the congenitally deficient thumb. *J Hand Surg [Am]* 1992;17:1064-1072.

McCarroll HR: Congenital anomalies: A 25 year overview. *J Hand Surg [Am]* 2000;25:1007-1037.

McCarty E, Mencio G, Green N: Anaesthesia and analgesia for the ambulatory management of fractures in children. *J Am Acad Orthop Surg* 1999;7:81-91.

Mintzer CM, Waters PM: Surgical treatment of pediatric scaphoid nonunions of the scaphoid. *J Pediatr Orthop* 1999;19:329-337.

Johnson KJ, Haigh SF, Symonds KE: MRI in the management of scaphoid fractures in skeletally immature patients. *Pediatr Radiol* 2000;30:685-688.

O'Connell SJ, Moore MM, Strickland JW, et al: Results of zone I and zone II flexor tendon repairs in children. *J Hand Surg [Am]* 1994;19:48-52.

Ogino T, Kato H: Clinical and experimental studies on teratogenic mechanisms of congenital absence of digits in longitudinal deficiencies. *Cong Anom* 1993;33:187-196.

Proctor MT, Moore DJ, Paterson JM: Redisplacement after manipulation of distal radial fractures in children. *J Bone Joint Surg Br* 1993;75:453-454.

Shoemaker S, Comstock C, Mubarak S, et al: Intramedullary kirschner wire fixation of open or unstable forearm fractures in children. *J Pediatr Orthop* 1999;19:329-337.

Smith PJ, Grobbelaar AO: Camptodactyly: A unifying theory and approach to surgical treatment. *J Hand Surg [Am]* 1998;23:14-19.

Vransky P, Bourdelat D, Al Faour A: Flexible intramedullary pinning technique in the treatment of pediatric fractures. *J Pediatr Orthop* 2000;20:23-27.

Waters PM, Kolettis GJ, Schwend R: Acute median neuropathy following physeal fractures of the distal radius. *J Pediatr Orthop* 1994;14:173-177.

Chapter 62

Hip, Pelvis, and Femur: Pediatrics

Keith R. Gabriel, MD

Eric J. Wall, MD

Developmental Dysplasia of the Hip

Incidence

Most newborn screening studies, usually based on physical examination techniques, suggest that some degree of hip instability can be detected in 1 in 100 to 1 in 250 babies. Actual dislocated or dislocatable hips are much less frequent, being found in 1 to 1.5 of 1,000 live births. Late presentation of developmental dysplasia of the hip (DDH) is found in approximately 4 per 10,000 children.

Etiology

There is no single cause of DDH. The basic structures of the human hip joint are well formed by the 11th fetal week. Subsequent development of the hip requires a continuous synergistic molding and growth of the immature femoral head and the acetabulum. Any process or event that interrupts this interaction can result in structural abnormality and instability. Those hips that dislocate early during the course of fetal development will have extreme anatomic abnormalities, and are called teratologic dislocations.

The risk of DDH has been found to be 34% in identical twins, but only 3% in fraternal twins. The frequency in siblings is approximately 6% to 7%. If one parent and one sibling have DDH, the risk to subsequent infants rises to 36%. The genetic influence may also be seen in comparisons of different ethnic groups, with high rates among Lappish and very low rates among Bantus.

Infants who have been in the breech position during the third trimester and/or perinatally have a higher risk of DDH, as high as 20% for those in the frank breech position. An increased incidence is also found with conditions typically associated with intrauterine crowding, such as oligohydramnios, congenital recurvatum or dislocation of the knee, and congenital muscular torticollis. Postnatally, a high incidence of DDH is found in those societies where infants are customarily strapped or swaddled with the thighs adducted.

DDH is associated with certain neuromuscular conditions and genetic syndromes, especially those in which decreased or abnormal fetal movement is a feature, such as arthrogryposis and spina bifida. Treatment of these hips depends as much on the nature of the overall disorder as on the dislocated hip itself. Although ligamentous laxity has been suggested as a risk factor, DDH is not especially associated with genetic conditions such as the Marfan, Ehlers-Danlos, or Down syndromes, in which generalized joint laxity is a prominent feature.

In infants who are otherwise normal, the most important risk factors for DDH are female gender, family history, and breech positioning. In addition to routine screening, some types of imaging studies are often recommended for these infants.

Diagnosis

Physical Examination

For newborns and neonates, the mainstay of physical diagnosis has been the palpable sensation of the hip sliding out of or into the acetabulum. Barlow's test is a provocative maneuver in which the examiner attempts to subluxate or dislocate the hip by pressing gently downward on the flexed, adducted thigh. Ortolani's test is a reduction maneuver performed by abducting the flexed hip while lifting gently forward under the greater trochanter. Palpable luxation or reduction of the joint constitutes a positive test. Most high-pitched "clicks" are transmitted from the greater trochanteric or knee areas, and are inconsequential.

Between 3 and 6 months of age, the soft tissues tighten sufficiently that a reduced hip does not dislocate with Barlow's test and a dislocated hip cannot be reduced with Ortolani's test. Hip abduction in flexion will be limited on the affected side, and the thigh will be foreshortened. In unilateral cases, the shortening is conveniently demonstrated by the Galeazzi (or Allis) test, in which the infant is positioned supine with the hips and knees flexed so that the relative height of the knees can be assessed.

After these children begin to stand, a flexion contracture usually develops at the affected hip. Increased lumbar lordosis and pelvic obliquity are seen. The pa-

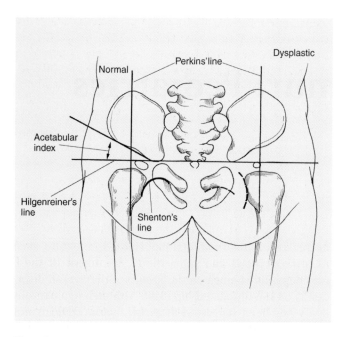

Figure 1 Standard reference lines and angles used to interpret pelvic radiographs in DDH. The femoral ossific nucleus normally is located in the lower, inner quadrant formed by the intersection of Hilgenreiner's (horizontal) and Perkins' (vertical) lines. Shenton's line is a continuous arc along the inferior border of the femoral neck and superior margin of the obturator foramen, which is disrupted when the femoral head is dislocated. The acetabular index measures the inclination of the acetabulum. Normal values for a newborn are less than 30° (average 27.5°). *(Reproduced with permission from Guille J, Pizzutillo P, MacEwen G: Developmental dysplasia of the hip from birth to six months. J Am Acad Orthop Surg 2000;8:232-242.)*

tients walk with gluteus medius insufficiency because of the high position of the greater trochanter. In unilateral cases, the limb-length inequality may either contribute to a limp, or may be compensated by toe-walking on the affected side. Once again, limitation of hip abduction in flexion is a useful finding in all age groups.

Lesser degrees of dysplasia may include a functionally stable but anatomically insufficient hip. These situations are ordinarily clinically silent in younger children. The abnormality may be discovered incidentally, but more often presents in later life as hip pain or degenerative arthritis.

Imaging: Ultrasound, Radiography, CT, MRI, and Arthrography

Ultrasound allows visualization of cartilaginous and soft-tissue structures before femoral head ossification. The static acetabular morphology, as described by Graf, is based on two angles measured in the coronal plane. A reference line common to both angles is first established along the lateral wall of the ilium superior to the acetabulum. The α angle is subtended by this iliac line and a line tangential to the bony roof of the acetabulum. The β angle is subtended by the iliac line and a line tangential through the cartilaginous labrum. In general, a normal, mature infant hip should have an α angle of greater than 60° and a β angle of less than 55°. The per-

centage of coverage of the femoral head can also be assessed. In dynamic ultrasound assessment, the position of the femoral head with respect to the posterior bony wall of the acetabulum is monitored as the hip is stressed with a modified Barlow's test.

The use of ultrasound in the routine screening of all newborns is neither cost effective nor practical. The procedure is so sensitive that routine use has resulted in overdiagnosis, above the expected incidence of DDH. The presence or severity of ultrasound abnormalities in infants who have otherwise normal hip examinations does not correlate with ultimate outcome. Routine ultrasound screening of newborns has not been shown to reduce the prevalence of late-diagnosed dysplasia.

Ultrasound evaluation at 3 to 4 weeks after birth is useful as an adjunct in those patients having equivocal findings on initial nursery examination, and for those in high-risk groups. Ultrasound can be used to check hip stability and document reduction during treatment or at the completion of treatment. The greatest advantage is that serial examinations can be done without exposing the infant to ionizing radiation.

Femoral head ossification usually begins by age 6 months, and plain radiographs then become the primary imaging modality for DDH. Radiography also remains useful to evaluate the distorted anatomy of teratologic dislocations. Traditionally, several lines are projected across the visible ossified portions of the pelvis and proximal femur to assist in interpretation of the plain films. Hilgenreiner's, Perkins', and Shenton's lines are commonly used, as illustrated in Figure 1, to determine the alignment of the proximal femur to the pelvis. The acetabular index provides information about the contour of the acetabulum itself.

CT, MRI, and arthrography do not play a significant role in the primary diagnosis of DDH. Each modality has specific uses in treatment. CT is currently the study of choice for assessing hip reduction in a spica cast after closed or open treatment. Limited use of CT directly through the acetabulum requires a minimum of radiation exposure. Sedation is seldom needed, as the patient is immobilized in the cast and spiral acquisition techniques for CT have decreased the time required for these studies. A method of hip reduction and spica cast application with the infant in the MRI scanner has been investigated, but is not yet feasible in most areas. Both CT and MRI data can be presented as three-dimensional images, and software is available to manipulate these images when planning various osteotomies. Arthrography is unparalleled for showing dynamically the soft-tissue impediments to reduction, and is useful to confirm position and stability in closed or open procedures. However, it is an invasive study that requires sedation or anesthesia.

Screening

All babies should be screened for hip dysplasia. However, the scope, timing, and methodology of neonatal screening for DDH are areas of current controversy. Hips dislocated at birth should be treated, with the exception of certain teratologic situations. However, 75% to 90% of hips found to be subluxatable at birth will spontaneously stabilize within a few weeks. A reasonable protocol is to reexamine all hips having questionable nursery examinations, and infants with recognized risk factors for dysplasia, at 2 to 3 weeks after birth. Hips with persistent laxity at that point should be treated. Ultrasound may be used at week 3 or 4 as an adjunct in questionable or high-risk situations. Hips that are stable at the 3-week examination but show dysplastic anatomy on ultrasound should be reassessed in 2 to 3 months. If the dysplasia persists, treatment is indicated.

Treatment

The fundamental goals of treatment are the same regardless of patient age. Concentric reduction should be obtained and maintained, with a minimum of risk to the blood supply of the capital femoral epiphysis. The later DDH is diagnosed, more complex interventions are needed and the risk of complications increases.

Abduction Splinting

Infants whose hips are subluxatable, reduced but dislocatable, or dislocated but reducible can usually be treated by splinting the hips in flexion and gentle abduction. Most of these infants will be younger than 6 months of age, although occasionally the hips of a slightly older infant remain Ortolani positive. Sometimes abduction splinting is used to achieve reduction of a dislocated hip in infancy. This procedure must be done with care to avoid forced positioning, and the attempt should be abandoned if not successful within 2 to 3 weeks.

The most popular abduction splint used in the United States is the Pavlik harness, although it has some limitations and potential problems. It is an active device, in that normal muscle function is required; it is not effective in patients with paralysis or spasticity. If the anterior straps hold the hips hyperflexed, femoral nerve palsy or inferior hip dislocation can occur. The persistent use of the Pavlik harness with the hip in a posteriorly subluxated position will result in a failure of development of the posterior wall of the acetabulum, sometimes called Pavlik disease. Prolonged prone positioning of the infant wearing the harness should be avoided, because the combined effect of the harness and the weight of the torso forces the hips into maximal abduction, increasing the risk of ischemic necrosis.

Good results are also obtained with other abduction splints such as the von Rosen splint or various Plastazote orthoses. It is critical that forced or extreme abduction be avoided. Regardless of the splint chosen, concentric reduction must be verified within 2 to 3 weeks of initiation of treatment. If reduction is not confirmed within that period, the splinting device should be abandoned and another method of treatment chosen. When successful, the abduction splint should be worn on a full-time basis until the hip is stable, and part-time wear is recommended until acetabular remodeling is confirmed.

Closed Reduction

Most infants older than age 6 months, those whose hips are not reducible with a simple Ortolani maneuver, and those in whom splinting in abduction fails will need a more formal closed or open reduction of the hip. Closed methods are preferred up to about age 2 years, but the reduction must be obtained and maintained without excessive force. Forcible maneuvers and forced rigid immobilization carry a high risk of ischemic necrosis.

The use of traction before closed reduction of the hip has become less common. The goal of traction is to gently and gradually stretch the soft tissues surrounding the hip, so that closed reduction can be achieved without undue force. However, comparison studies have shown that adductor tenotomy and immobilization in the human position (hips flexed 100°, abducted 45° and neutrally rotated) can achieve comparably low rates of ischemic necrosis.

Closed reduction should be done under general anesthesia, with an arthrogram used to verify positioning. A concentric reduction must be obtained, with no more than 5 mm of contrast pooling medially between the femoral head and the acetabulum, and with no soft-tissue interposition. With the hips flexed, a safe zone of abduction should be assessed: an arc of stable positioning between redislocation (toward adduction) and the limit of comfortable, unforced abduction. If the safe zone is unacceptably narrow, an adjunctive procedure such as percutaneous adductor tenotomy may be indicated to release soft-tissue tension and increase the range of available abduction. The infant is then immobilized in a spica cast in the human position (hip flexion of about 100° and abduction of about 45°) for 3 to 4 months. Part-time abduction bracing should be continued until acetabular remodeling is complete. It is not unusual for infants treated by closed reduction to achieve stable hips, but to require a secondary acetabular or femoral procedure to correct residual deformity.

Open Reduction

Failure to obtain a concentric closed reduction of the hip is an indication for open reduction in all age groups. Any hip in which extreme positioning is required to maintain reduction should also be treated by open reduction. In general, children older than 2 years of age will require open reduction.

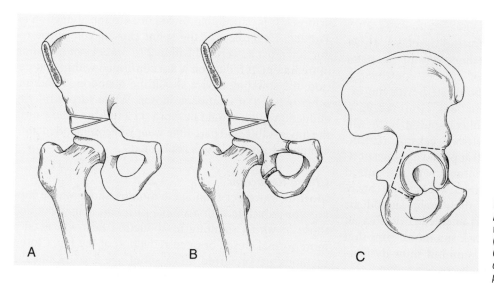

Figure 2 Redirectional osteotomies. **A,** Single innominate (Salter). **B,** Triple innominate (Steel). **C,** Bernese pericapsular (Ganz). *(Reproduced with permission from Gillingham B, Sanches A, Wenger D: Pelvic osteotomies for the treatment of hip dysplasia in children and young adults. J Am Acad Orthop Surg 1999;7:325-337.)*

Anteromedial and medial approaches have most often been recommended for younger children (2 years old or younger). All approaches include division of the origin of the adductor longus. One anteromedial variation then proceeds between the pectineus medially and the femoral neurovascular bundle laterally. Division of the psoas tendon allows direct access to the anteromedial hip capsule. With exception of an inverted labrum, obstacles to reduction can be easily visualized and removed. However, there is no opportunity to perform capsulorrhaphy or osteotomy through this exposure. A potential disadvantage is that the medial femoral circumflex artery is in the field of deep dissection, which some believe increases the risk of ischemic necrosis.

Alternatively, after division of the origin of the adductor brevis, the pectineus may be retracted laterally and the deep dissection can then proceed either anterior or posterior to the adductor brevis. These two variations are conceptually less direct than the anteromedial approach, and are not well suited for high dislocations. Other indications and limitations are similar.

The most commonly used anterior approach for open hip reduction is that of Smith-Peterson, generally modified by using a bikini incision parallel to the groin flexion crease. Dissection is deepened between the tensor fascia femoris and the sartorius, mobilizing the origins of the tensor fascia femoris from the iliac wing. Division of the origins of the rectus femoris then gives access to the anterior, superior, and lateral hip capsule. A separate tenotomy, either percutaneous or open, of the adductor longus is recommended. All of the impediments to reduction can be addressed via this approach. If an inverted labrum is identified, it can be released by making several radial cuts in the tight area. The labrum should not be excised.

This approach is suitable for all age groups. The dissection preserves the medial femoral circumflex vessels.

Capsulorrhaphy and pelvic osteotomy can be performed through this approach. Postoperative immobilization is in the functional position, with approximately 15° of flexion, 15° of abduction, and neutral rotation.

Femoral shortening at the time of open reduction has taken the place of preoperative traction for reducing soft-tissue tension around the hip. This procedure is virtually always necessary for children older than age 2 years, but should be considered in each patient. A separate lateral approach is necessary. The hip is reduced, a subtrochanteric osteotomy of the femur is performed, and the soft tissues are allowed to retract. The resulting overlapped segment of proximal femur is resected, and the femur is internally fixed with a plate and screws. Varus and rotation can be adjusted through this osteotomy as needed for hip stability. It is important to avoid excessive retroversion of the femur, especially if concomitant pelvic osteotomy is done, as this increases the risk of posterior redislocation of the hip.

In older children, the acetabulum will be more severely dysplastic. Anterolateral coverage will be insufficient. It is frequently necessary to consider concomitant pelvic osteotomy at the time of open reduction to ensure stability of the hip. The Salter innominate osteotomy will redirect the acetabulum to restore approximately 25° of lateral coverage and 10° of anterior coverage (Figure 2). As indicated previously, combined pelvic and femoral osteotomy must be done carefully to avoid posterior instability of the joint.

Upper Age Limits

Beyond a certain age, surgical treatment is unlikely to produce a stable, mobile, pain-free joint for the long term. Despite obvious gait abnormalities, bilateral pain-free dislocations probably should not be reduced after age 6 or 7 years. Unilateral dislocations are generally more problematic, because of limb-length inequality and pelvic obliquity. Therefore, reduction of unilateral dislocations is considered until adolescence.

Complications

Redislocation

Redislocation after closed reduction can usually be treated by repeat closed reduction or open reduction with no deleterious effect on long-term outcome. Redislocation following open reduction is usually attributable to some flaw in the initial procedure. Inadequate inferior capsular release, inadequate capsulorrhaphy, and posterior instability from combined pelvic and femoral osteotomies are common errors. Repeat surgery is almost always necessary to correct the problem, and results are generally worse than with primary open reduction.

Ischemic Necrosis

Ischemic necrosis of the femoral head is seen with all forms of treatment. Causes include extrinsic compression of the vasculature supplying the capital femoral epiphysis, and excessive direct pressure on the cartilaginous head. Excessive or forceful abduction, previous failed closed treatment, and repeat surgery are associated with increased rates of ischemic necrosis. The question of whether ossification of the femoral head before treatment might affect ischemic necrosis rates is not fully resolved.

The diagnosis of ischemic necrosis is based on radiographic findings that include failure of appearance or growth of the ossific nucleus 1 year after reduction, broadening of the femoral neck 1 year after reduction, increased density and then fragmentation of the ossified femoral head, or residual deformity of the femoral head and neck after ossification. Classifications of ischemic necrosis separate partial involvement from complete necrosis, which causes progressive femoral head and neck deformity. Treatment depends on degree of severity.

Late Dysplasia

In a growing child, the mechanically stable hip that is reduced but dysplastic may be monitored with serial radiographs. Failure of improvement with growth is an indication for intervention, as is symptomatic dysplasia in the adolescent. Analysis of the late dysplastic hip is facilitated by CT or MRI studies with three-dimensional reconstruction. Femoral, pelvic, or concomitant osteotomy may be required, according to the location of the major deformity. Pelvic osteotomies are grouped into reconstructive and salvage types.

If it is possible to concentrically and congruently reduce a dysplastic hip, a reconstructive osteotomy may be indicated to improve coverage of the femoral head with the native articular cartilage of the acetabulum. Several

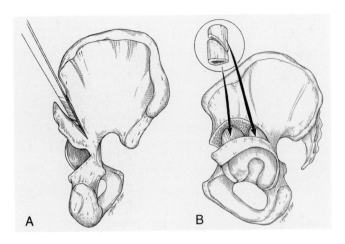

Figure 3 Reshaping osteotomy of Dega, which preserves the sciatic notch and a variable portion of the inner table of the ileum. *(Reproduced with permission from Vitale MG, Skaggs DL: Developmental dysplasia of the hip from six months to four years of age.* J Am Acad Orthop Surg 2001;9:401-411.*)*

osteotomies that reorient the acetabulum without changing its shape have been described, and the choice, in large measure, depends on patient age (Figure 2). The single innominate osteotomy (Salter) depends on flexibility of the symphysis pubis to allow sufficient rotation of the acetabular segment. In older children this flexibility is lost, and triple osteotomy (Steel or Tonnis) is preferred so that the acetabular segment of the pelvis can be rotated without violating the triradiate growth potential. After closure of the triradiate cartilage, the periacetabular osteotomy (Bernese) is appropriate.

If the intrinsic shape of the acetabulum must be altered to improve congruence, reshaping osteotomies such as the Pemberton or the Dega should be considered. These osteotomies require an open triradiate cartilage to allow hinging through the acetabulum itself. The inner and outer tables of the ileum are divided in the Pemberton, whereas only the outer table is cut in the Dega (Figure 3). Both proceed into the posterior limb of the triradiate, and preserve the posterior wall of the ischium at the sciatic notch.

Salvage osteotomies increase the surface area available for weight bearing, and depend on fibrocartilaginous metaplasia of the interposed hip capsule to form an articulating surface. The Chiari innominate osteotomy and various shelf acetabular augmentations are available (Figure 4).

Developmental Coxa Vara

Developmental coxa vara has an estimated incidence of 1 in 25,000 live births. Males and females are affected with equal frequency, there is no predilection for the right or left side, and the condition is bilateral in approximately 50% of patients.

The underlying defect of this condition is unknown. The most widely accepted theory regarding the progres-

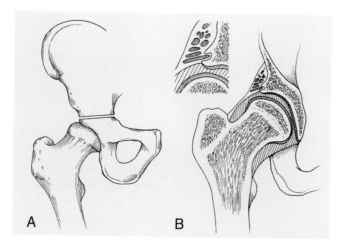

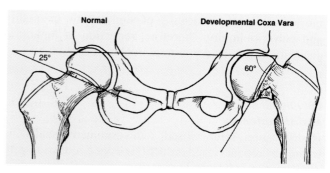

Figure 5 Hilgenreiner's physeal angle is created by a line through the triradiate cartilage and its intersection with a line through the physis. The normal angle is about 25°. *(Reproduced with permission from Beals RK: Coxa vara in childhood: Evaluation and management. J Am Acad Orthop Surg 1998;6:93-99.)*

Figure 4 Salvage procedures. **A,** Chiari. **B,** Shelf slotted acetabular augmentation. *(Reproduced with permission from Gillingham B, Sanchez A, Wenger D: Pelvic osteotomies for the treatment of hip dysplasia in children and young adults. J Am Acad Orthop Surg 1999;7:325-337.)*

sive deformity is that there exists an unspecified primary ossification defect in the inferior femoral neck. Physiologic stresses of weight bearing cause fatigue failure of the local dystrophic bone, resulting in the progressive varus displacement. MRI and some biopsy specimens support this theory.

Patients usually have a progressive but painless gait abnormality during early childhood. The coxa vara creates a high-riding position of the greater trochanter (decrease or reversal of the articulotrochanteric distance) and therefore the hip abductors are functionally weakened. The children walk with a waddling, Trendelenburg pattern. Those with unilateral involvement have an additional component of limb-length inequality, whereas those with bilateral coxa vara have increased lumbar lordosis.

The high-riding greater trochanter is prominent on physical examination. Hip range of motion is restricted in all planes. The loss of abduction is a direct manifestation of the coxa vara. Loss of internal rotation is attributed to a progressive loss of femoral anteversion as the femoral neck displaces. A hip flexion contracture is often present. The lower extremity length discrepancy in patients with unilateral deformity is generally mild.

The radiographic indicator of developmental coxa vara is a triangular metaphyseal fragment in the inferior femoral neck, delineated by an inverted Y-shaped radiolucency. There is a decrease in the femoral neck-shaft angle, sometimes to values below 90°. The position of the physeal plate is measured by Hilgenreiner's physeal angle, determined on the AP view as the angle between Hilgenreiner's line and the plane of the proximal femoral physis. A normal Hilgenreiner's angle should be less than 25° (Figure 5). Spontaneous healing may occur when Hilgenreiner's angle remains less than 45°. A Hilgenreiner's angle of greater than 60° (increasingly

more vertical) is associated with progression of the coxa vara, stress fracture and nonunion of the femoral neck, and early degenerative arthritis of the hip. The overall radiographic appearance of the hip is similar in some skeletal dysplasias, so screening radiographs of other areas should be obtained for every patient on initial presentation.

Nonsurgical treatments have been unsuccessful. Surgical derotational valgus-producing osteotomy of the proximal femur is indicated when Hilgenreiner's physeal angle is greater than 60°, the physeal angle is greater than 45° and the deformity is progressing, the femoral neck-shaft angle is less than 90°, or the patient develops a significant Trendelenburg gait. Surgical goals include overcorrection of the femoral neck-shaft angle to about 160°, restoration of Hilgenreiner's angle to about 25°, and normalization of femoral rotation. Supplemental bone grafting of the inferior femoral neck defect at the time of corrective osteotomy is not necessary. There are differing opinions regarding the best patient age for surgery. In general, corrective osteotomy should be performed as soon as the criteria for intervention are apparent.

If adequate correction into valgus has been achieved, the triangular defect in the inferior femoral neck closes by 6 months postoperatively. Premature closure of the proximal femoral physis occurs by 24 months in most surgically treated hips, even though the physeal plate is not violated during surgery. The patient must therefore be monitored for subsequent limb-length inequality. If premature closure of the proximal femoral physis is recognized, apophyseodesis or advancement of the greater trochanter should be considered. Recurrence of varus is unusual if adequate valgus has been achieved at surgery.

Slipped Capital Femoral Epiphysis

Slipped capital femoral epiphysis (SCFE) is one of the most common hip disorders in the pubertal child. The diagnosis can be delayed because 15% of patients have knee pain instead of hip pain, and those patients with hip pain are often initially believed to have a pulled groin muscle. Historically, the condition and its treatment have been fraught with frequent complications such as chondrolysis, osteonecrosis, slip progression, intra-articular pin penetration, hip stiffness, and degenerative arthritis. Currently, with early diagnosis and single cannulated screw fixation, the outcome is usually excellent in stable SCFE with minimal or moderate displacement. Osteonecrosis, which is usually seen only in unstable SCFE, and severe slip displacement can lead to early hip degeneration.

Etiology

The etiology of SCFE is unknown, but it is probably a mechanical problem of increased sheer stress across a capital femoral growth plate weakened either by rapid growth, or by a condition such as pelvic radiation, hypothyroidism, renal failure, or growth hormone treatment. Most children with SCFE are above the 95th percentile for weight and are obese; these factors place increased stress across the growth plate. Growth plates show physiologic weakness during periods of rapid growth such as the pubertal growth spurt. Endocrine consultation or endocrine screening laboratories are not indicated unless the patient has atypical endocrine findings. Children with SCFE who are younger than 10 years of age or 16 years and older, or whose weight is below the 50th percentile have a high incidence of atypical SCFE and may require further workup. No specific genetic component has been identified with SCFE.

Epidemiology

The prevalence of SCFE in the United States ranges between 2 to 10 cases per 100,000 children. Male children outnumber females with the disease by a 3:2 ratio, and the mean age for diagnosis is about 13.5 years for boys and 12 years for girls, which corresponds with the age at which the adolescent growth spurt occurs. Fifty percent of children with SCFE are above the 95th percentile for weight according to age. There is an increased incidence of SCFE during the summer and fall months and it reportedly is bilateral in 17% to 50% of patients. Approximately half the children who have bilateral hip involvement are identified at the time of initial presentation. Therefore, both hips should be examined and bilateral radiographs obtained for every patient with a unilateral presentation of SCFE.

Diagnosis

Studies show that approximately 85% of children have a history of hip or proximal thigh pain and 15% have only knee pain. Therefore, in any adolescent with knee pain, range of motion should be assessed on the ipsilateral hip. The patient with SCFE will usually have a paradox-

ical limp. When the patient bears weight on the painful lower extremity, they will lean over that extremity during the stance phase of gait. This unusual limp pattern helps localize the cause of pain to the hip. Conversely, patients tend to lean away from the involved side if the pain emanates from below the hip. Patients with SCFE tend to externally rotate their lower extremity while walking.

The hallmark of the clinical examination is that as the examiner flexes the hip of a patient with SCFE, the patient's leg will externally rotate obligatorily. There is usually complete loss of internal rotation, and any attempt at testing hip internal rotation causes pain. The diagnosis of SCFE is confirmed with AP and frog-lateral hip radiographs. The earliest radiographic sign of SCFE can be growth plate widening or lucency (termed epiphysiolysis) and patients with chronic slips may develop a radiodense blush sign on the metaphyseal side of the capital femoral growth plate. On the AP radiograph of a normal hip, a line drawn up along the superior border of the femoral neck (Klein's line) should project over the lateral edge of the femoral head. In a child with SCFE the femoral head may not project over this line (Figure 6). Patients who have the earliest stage of SCFE may have normal radiographs (preslip). MRI can help diagnose a preslip condition by showing metaphyseal high signal next to the growth plate and growth plate widening.

Classification

In the most useful classification for SCFE, the condition is either stable or unstable. Stable slips are defined by the mode of clinical presentation. If a patient can walk into the examiner's office, with or without crutches, they have a stable slip. With an unstable slip, the patient has difficulty with ambulation and usually presents on a gurney or in a wheelchair. This classification helps with prognosis in that the most feared complication of SCFE, osteonecrosis of the femoral head, is usually only seen with unstable slips. Increased SCFE displacement and increased angle of the slip relative to normal anatomy correlate with less favorable outcomes than mild slips.

Treatment

The most popular treatment of SCFE is single screw fixation across the capital femoral growth plate performed in situ (without reduction) in stable slips. Although single screw fixation seems to be the gold standard for most slips, recent articles have shown slip progression after single screw fixation. Single screw fixation using modern fluoroscopic techniques that avoid persistent joint penetration have virtually eliminated the risk of chondrolysis (cartilage deterioration and hip stiffness) that was previously a common complication of SCFE pinning. The success and simplicity of single cannulated

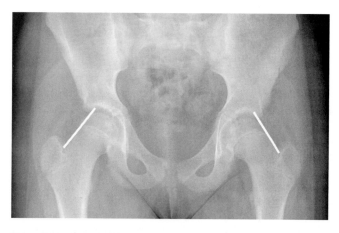

Figure 6 AP radiograph of the pelvis shows that on the left hip the lateral epiphysis does not cross a line drawn along the superior edge of femoral neck (Klein's line). This is consistent with a subtle SCFE on the left hip. The right femoral epiphysis does cross this line and is normal.

screw fixation has decreased the popularity of alternative treatments of stable SCFE such as bone peg epiphysiodesis, hip spica casting, and femoral neck osteotomy.

Technique of Cannulated Screw Fixation

Patients with SCFE are usually pinned on a fracture table that allows clear AP and lateral views of the hip. Because obesity can impair visualization of the hip with SCFE, it is imperative to confirm visualization of the hip joint surface on the AP and lateral radiographic views before commencing the procedure. A radiolucent standard operating room table can also be used instead of the fracture table by rotating the hip between AP and frog-lateral views; however, this is indicated only for stable hips. After the patient is on the table, AP and lateral guidelines can be drawn on the skin surface to mark the entry position. Large cannulated screws are the most popular for fixation, which is usually performed in situ. An adequate number of screw threads should be placed into the center of the epiphysis to facilitate a stable fixation without joint penetration. After fixation is achieved, the hip is rotated under live fluoroscopy to ascertain that the pin is not penetrating the hip joint. Pins that are not placed centrally in the femoral head can inadvertently penetrate the joint despite two orthogonal radiographic views showing no joint penetration. Postoperatively, patients with stable slips are allowed to bear weight as tolerated or limited weight bearing is instituted for 6 to 8 weeks.

Controversies

Although a few recent studies have shown progressive slippage after single screw fixation, the procedure remains the current gold standard because it provides the least risk of inadvertent hip joint penetration and chon-

drolysis. Single pin fixation is also recommended for unstable slips, although some authors have stated a need for two screws. Because unstable SCFE has a high rate of osteonecrosis, some authors recommend early reduction and arthrotomy to reduce possible compression on the extracapsular epiphyseal vessels. Traditionally, reduction was believed to increase the risk of osteonecrosis, hence the emphasis on in situ fixation. Frequently, spontaneous reduction occurs when patients are placed on the fracture table because of the weight of the proximal thigh and femur. One recent study reported an increased risk of osteonecrosis associated with reduction; however, another recent study found no such increase and concluded that spontaneous and gentle reduction is safe. Prophylactic pinning of the unslipped opposite hip, for which the risk of future slip is 25% or less, is also controversial. After one hip has slipped, patients and their families are much more attuned to the condition and will seek treatment early when pain or limp develop in the opposite hip. Most pediatric orthopaedists choose not to perform prophylactic pinning, but recommend that patients return to the office at the first sign of pain or limp in the opposite hip. Because up to 57% of opposite hip slips are asymptomatic and current fixation methods have low complication rates, recent decision analysis reviews tend to support prophylactic pinning of the unslipped opposite hip.

Legg-Calvé-Perthes Disease

Idiopathic osteonecrosis of the femoral head in children is termed Legg-Calvé-Perthes disease. Its specific cause is unknown, but it likely involves a temporary interruption of the blood supply to some portion of the femoral head that can extend to the adjacent capital femoral growth plate and the metaphysis. The condition tends to run its initial course over a period of 3 to 5 years. In the short term most patients recover good hip function; however, long-term studies show that by the fifth or sixth decade of life approximately 50% of patients with prior Legg-Calvé-Perthes disease will develop degenerative arthritis of the hip. Children who experience onset of this disease before the age of 6 years, and those who have healing with good hip joint congruence at maturity have the best long-term results. The main goals of treatment in Legg-Calvé-Perthes disease are to keep the femoral head contained within the acetabulum and to maintain motion. Treatment can range from observation to physical therapy, casting, and femoral or pelvic osteotomy. However, the effect of treatment at altering the natural history of Legg-Calvé-Perthes disease remains controversial.

Epidemiology

Legg-Calvé-Perthes disease most commonly occurs in children age 4 to 10 years, but it has been described in children age 2 years to teens. It is distinguished from adult osteonecrosis of the hip primarily because of its much better healing and revascularization potential. The male to female ratio of occurrence is 5:1. The condition tends to be bilateral in about 10% of children; however, it usually does not present at the same time in both hips. The differential diagnosis for simultaneous bilateral hip osteonecrosis includes Meyer's dysplasia, spondyloepiphyseal dysplasia, multiple epiphyseal dysplasia, sickle cell disease, Gaucher's disease, and hypothyroidism.

Etiology

The etiology of Legg-Calvé-Perthes disease is unknown. Thrombosis caused by abnormalities in the clotting cascade have been recently investigated as the primary etiology with an initial study showing that approximately 75% of children with this disease have abnormal clotting factors. Although the rate of clotting factor abnormalities is small, more recent studies have not validated the high rate of inherited thrombosis and thrombophilia in patients or animals with Legg-Calvé-Perthes disease. Animal models have shown that multiple episodes of infarction are necessary to create changes that simulate the human Legg-Calvé-Perthes disease. As a group, children with this disease tend to be of shorter stature, have a delay in bone maturation of approximately 2 years, have a high rate of attention deficit disorder, and have high rates of exposure to secondhand smoke. However, no systemic causes have been identified in children with Legg-Calvé-Perthes disease. Approximately 2% of children with transient synovitis of the hip will develop Legg-Calvé-Perthes disease; however this scenario probably results from an initial misdiagnosis and is not a cause of the disease.

Stages/Pathogenesis

The stages of Legg-Calvé-Perthes disease are based on radiographs. During the initial stage the infarction occurs, and radiographs may remain occult for the first 3 to 6 months after this initial ischemic event. Most patients present to a physician after radiographic alterations in the femoral head have been noted. In the fragmentation stage, the femoral head appears to fragment or dissolve, either partially or totally. This indicator typically occurs during revascularization as the infarcted bone is resorbed, leaving behind a lucent zone in the femoral head. The third phase, termed reossification, occurs when new bone appears. In the healing stage the femoral head reossifies back to normal bone density; however, residual femoral head and neck deformity including shortening (coxa breva), widening (coxa magna), and flattening may exist.

If the capital femoral growth plate is involved in the process, there can be tilting of the femoral neck (coxa valga) and relative overgrowth of the greater trochanter. This four-stage process typically evolves over 3 to 5 years and tends to proceed more quickly in younger children than in older children.

Clinical Presentation

The typical child with Legg-Calvé-Perthes disease has a painless limp. The patient may report intermittent hip, thigh, or even knee pain that is typically not severe and does not necessitate use of a crutch. The patient may have a Trendelenburg gait in which body weight is shifted over the affected hip during the stance phase of gait. This gait pattern (shifting weight away from the affected side during the stance phase of gait) helps to identify the hip as the source of the patient's pain. On clinical examination, the patient usually exhibits joint stiffness that is most apparent with loss of hip internal rotation and hip abduction. Limb-length discrepancy and leg muscle atrophy are late findings that can occur in patients with more severe hip involvement. On clinical presentation, the differential diagnosis will include septic arthritis, transient synovitis, proximal femoral osteomyelitis, SCFE, and hip dysplasia. Infectious etiologies can usually be ruled out through the clinical history and laboratory studies including erythrocyte sedimentation rate and C-reactive protein levels. DDH and SCFE are usually identified on the radiographs. Transient synovitis of the hip usually improves with anti-inflammatory medications within 1 week and is typically completely resolved within 4 weeks of presentation, versus the longer time course of Legg-Calvé-Perthes disease.

Radiographic Findings

The earliest radiographic finding in Legg-Calvé-Perthes disease is an apparent joint space widening caused by failure of the involved femoral ossific nucleus to grow after the ischemic event.

Irregularity and increased density of the femoral head ossification center are also early findings. A subchondral lucent line (crescent sign) can appear in the femoral head, and forms the basis for the Salter-Thompson classification system. A crescent sign involving less than half the femoral head is class A, and if it involves more than half the femoral head it is class B. The extent of fragmentation of the ossific nucleus forms the basis of the Catterall and Herring lateral pillar classifications. In the Catterall classification stages 1 and 2, fragmentation involves less than half the femoral head, and in stages 3 and 4 it involves more than half the femoral head. The Herring lateral pillar classification is based on an AP hip radiograph obtained approximately at the start of the fragmentation phase (Figure 7). Only the lateral third of the ossific nucleus is evaluated on this view. A lateral pillar that maintains its full height is classified as group A. A lateral pillar that partially collapses but maintains greater than 50% of

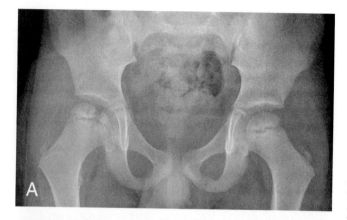

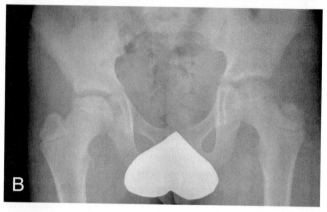

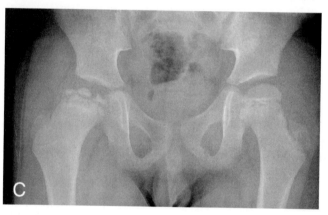

Figure 7 Lateral pillar classification. **A,** Herring group A, right hip with no loss of height in the lateral third of the epiphysis compared with the normal left hip. **B,** Less than 50% collapse of the lateral pillar is shown in the right hip, rendering it a Herring group B hip. **C,** A Herring group C hip with greater than 50% collapse of the lateral pillar.

its height is group B, and a lateral pillar that maintains less than 50% of its height is group C. The increasing grade within each classification system tends to correlate with a poorer prognosis.

Hinge abduction, in which a bump deformity of the lateral femoral head prevents it from rotating under the acetabulum, is considered a poor prognostic sign. Hinge abduction can be seen on arthrogram taken with the patient under anesthesia, or can be inferred by comparing an AP hip radiograph obtained in neutral abduction

with one obtained during maximum hip abduction. The patient's knees should be pointed forward during filming. Failure of the lateral corner of the femoral head to slip under the edge of the acetabulum in the maximum abduction film is evidence of hinge abduction.

Because radiographic changes may not be apparent for 3 to 6 months after the onset of the disease, bone scans and MRI have been investigated to provide an earlier diagnosis, but their clinical value is not clearly established. Although rarely necessary, gadolinium-enhanced MRI has been shown to correlate well with bone scan results in providing an early diagnosis of Legg-Calvé-Perthes disease. MRI without gadolinium enhancement was found to be poor for the evaluation of femoral head necrosis.

Prognosis

The long-term prognosis of Legg-Calvé-Perthes disease is improved with younger age of onset, especially with an onset in patients younger than 6 years, and also with less residual hip joint deformity at skeletal maturity. A recent study suggests that the percentage of physeal involvement on MRI scan may correlate better with long-term prognosis than the percentage of femoral head involvement. The Stulberg classification is the gold standard for rating the residual femoral head deformity and joint congruence at skeletal maturity; however, a recent study has questioned the interobserver and intraobserver reliability of this five-tier grading scale. Lateral epiphyseal calcification and hip subluxation over 4 mm have been recognized as risk factors for poor prognosis. Although most patients with Legg-Calvé-Perthes disease do well during adolescence and early adult life, by age 50 or 60 years 50% of patients develop disabling degenerative arthritis. A recent study indicates that contrary to the popular belief that girls with Legg-Calvé-Perthes disease have a poorer prognosis, the outcomes for boys and girls with the disease are essentially equal.

Treatment

Initial treatment of Legg-Calvé-Perthes disease is typically rest, activity restrictions, the use of nonsteroidal anti-inflammatory drugs, and physical therapy to regain hip motion. Bracing is no longer preferred because two studies showed no significant effect using this treatment. The goal of all treatments is to maintain motion of the hip and to keep the femoral head contained within the acetabulum. Patients who lose substantial motion, who develop hinge abduction, or who start to subluxate or dislocate the hip joint may require more aggressive treatment. Surgical treatment remains highly controversial, but appears to be best suited for children older than 8 years with moderate femoral head involvement. Preliminary results from a large multicenter trial show that surgical treatment is associated with better outcome in lateral pillar B and B/C border hips in patients who are age 8 years and older at onset. Surgical treatment was not beneficial to lateral pillar A and C hips. Lateral pillar classification alone does not seem to be prognostic; however, taking into account other factors such as age of the patient and "head at risk" signs (such as calcification lateral to the epiphysis, metaphyseal lesions, lateral subluxation of the femoral head, and a horizontal growth plate) improves the prognostic value. Patients who develop severe stiffness or whose femoral heads do not remain contained within the acetabulum may benefit from Petrie casting with or without a soft-tissue release.

Femoral varus osteotomy and acetabular rotational osteotomy can also enhance containment but should only be performed after hip stiffness is resolved preoperatively. Salvage procedures such as a shelf arthroplasty or Chiari osteotomy or valgus femoral neck osteotomy can be considered for severe disease.

Some patients who have had Legg-Calvé-Perthes disease will develop recurrence of pain and locking or catching of the hip during their teenage years. Osteochondritis dissecans or loose fragments of cartilage can develop and are best investigated with MRI or CT scan. The presence of an osteochondritis dissecans lesion in a patient who has had Legg-Calvé-Perthes disease is not an indication for open or arthroscopic removal. Nonsurgical treatment seems to work well; the osteochondritis dissecans lesion can end up in the cotyloid fossa where it will cause minimal complications. Older children with Legg-Calvé-Perthes disease can also develop labral tears that can be treated with open or arthroscopic procedures.

Annotated Bibliography

Developmental Dysplasia of the Hip
Duppe H, Danielsson LG: Screening of neonatal instability and of developmental dislocation of the hip: A survey of 132,601 living newborn infants between 1956 and 1999. *J Bone Joint Surg Br* 2002;84:878-885.

This article helps to illustrate the differences in detection and treatment rates according to the experience of screeners and use of adjunctive ultrasound examinations.

Eberle CF: Plastazote abduction orthosis in the management of neonatal hip instability. *J Pediatr Orthop* 2003; 23:607-616.

One hundred thirteen consecutive newborns with hip instability on physical examination were treated with the Plastazote orthosis; only two required additional treatment and there were no instances of ischemic necrosis.

Grudziak JS, Ward WT: Dega osteotomy for the treatment of congenital dysplasia of the hip. *J Bone Joint Surg Am* 2001;83-A:845-854.

This article explains and removes the confusion surrounding this osteotomy. Results for 22 patients are presented.

Guille J, Pizzutillo P, MacEwen G: Developmental dysplasia of the hip from birth to six months. *J Am Acad Orthop Surg* 2000;8:232-242.

This article reviews diagnosis and management of DDH in children from birth to age 6 months.

Holen KJ, Tegnander A, Bredland T, et al: Universal or selective screening of the neonatal hip using ultrasound?: A prospective, randomized trial of 15,529 newborn infants. *J Bone Joint Surg Br* 2002;84:886-890.

The effect of screening was measured by the rate of late detection of dysplasia in children from age 6 to 11 years. Universal ultrasound screening was not statistically better than universal screening by physical examination, with ultrasound reserved for questionable cases.

Konigsberg DE, Karol LA, Colby S, O'Brien S: Results of medial open reduction of the hip in infants with developmental dislocation of the hip. *J Pediatr Orthop* 2003;23:1-9.

Forty hips in 32 patients were reviewed at an average of 10.3 years after medial open reduction. Satisfactory results were obtained in 75% of patients. The authors endorse the procedure as an option for patients younger than 1 year of age.

Lerman JA, Emans JB, Millis MB, Share J, Zurakowski D, Kasser JR: Early failure of Pavlik harness treatment for developmental hip dysplasia: Clinical and ultrasound predictors. *J Pediatr Orthop* 2001;21:348-353.

In 26 of 137 hips, Pavlik harness treatment failed to achieve or maintain hip reduction. Univariate risk factors for failure were bilaterality, initial clinical examination, and initial ultrasound percent coverage.

Luhmann SJ, Bassett GS, Gordon JE, Schootman M, Schoenecker PL: Reduction of a dislocation of the hip due to developmental dysplasia: Implications for the need for future surgery. *J Bone Joint Surg Am* 2003;85-A:239-243.

Reduction of dislocated hips before the appearance of an ossific nucleus resulted in only a slight increase in ischemic necrosis, but delay more than doubled the need for future surgery. These authors do not recommend a delay.

Sampath JS, Deakin S, Paton RW: Splintage in developmental dysplasia of the hip: How low can we go? *J Pediatr Orthop* 2003;23:352-355.

Subluxatable hips at newborn examination were reexamined. By treating only those hips with persistent instability at 2 weeks, and those with persistent anatomic dysplasia at 9 weeks, the rate of abduction splinting was lowered without adversely affecting outcomes.

Sanchez-Sotelo J, Trousdale RT, Berry DJ, Cabanela ME: Surgical treatment of developmental dysplasia of the hip in adults: I. Nonarthroplasty options. *J Am Acad Orthop Surg* 2002;10:321-333.

An overview of the etiology, biomechanics, and principles of treatment of acetabular dysplasia is presented.

Vitale MG, Skaggs DL: Devlopmental dyplasia of the hip from six months to four years of age. *J Am Acad Orthop Surg* 2001;9:401-411.

This article reviews diagnosis and management of DDH in children from ages 6 months to 4 years.

Weintrob S, Grill F: Current concepts review: Ultrasonography in developmental dysplasia of the hip. *J Bone Joint Surg Am* 2000;82-A:1004-1018.

Methods, techniques, indications, and a critical analysis of screening issues are discussed.

Developmental Coxa Vara

Beals RK: Coxa vara in childhood: Evaluation and management. *J Am Acad Orthop Surg* 1998;6:93-99.

This article presents an excellent and comprehensive review of coxa vara in children.

Burns KA, Stevens PM: Coxa vara: Another option for fixation. *J Pediatr Orthop B* 2001;10:304-310.

The authors reported excellent fixation using a modified veterinary plate for valgus osteotomy in 9 patients (12 hips).

Widmann RF, Hresko MT, Kasser JR, Millis MB: Wagner multiple K-wire osteosynthesis to correct coxa vara in the young child: Experience with a versatile "tailor-made" high angle blade plate. *J Pediatr Orthop B* 2001;10:43-50.

By stacking Kirschner wires, the effect of a high angle blade plate was achieved in patients who were otherwise too small for conventional internal fixation devices.

Slipped Capital Femoral Epiphysis

Futami T, Suzuki S, Seto Y, Kashiwagi N: Sequential magnetic resonance imaging in slipped capital femoral epiphysis: Assessment of preslip in the contralateral hip. *J Pediatr Orthop B* 2001;10:298-303.

MRI showed growth plate widening on T1 images as an early sign of SCFE in patients with a preslip condition.

Kennedy JG, Hresko MT, Kasser JR, et al: Osteonecrosis of the femoral head associated with slipped capital femoral epiphysis. *J Pediatr Orthop* 2001;21:189-193.

Osteonecrosis was found only in unstable SCFE in 4 of 27 patients. The magnitude of slip and the magnitude of reduction in the unstable group was not predictive of a poorer outcome.

Loder RT, Greenfield ML: Clinical characteristics of children with atypical and idiopathic slipped capital femoral epiphysis: Description of the age-weight test and implications for further diagnostic investigation. *J Pediatr Orthop* 2001;21:481-487.

Patients with SCFE who are younger than age 10 years or older than age 16 years and those with weight less than the 50th percentile are more likely to have an atypical (nonidiopathic) cause of SCFE such as renal failure, prior radiation treatment, or endocrine disorder.

Schultz WR, Weinstein JN, Weinstein SL, Smith B: Prophylactic pinning of the contralateral hip in slipped capital femoral epiphysis. *J Bone Joint Surg Am* 2002;84-A:1305-1314.

A decision analysis formula based on probabilities of achieving a good long-term outcome supports prophylactic pinning of the unslipped opposite hip.

Tokmakova KP, Stanton RP, Mason DE: Factors influencing the development of osteonecrosis in patients treated for slipped capital femoral epiphysis. *J Bone Joint Surg Am* 2003;85-A:798-801.

In this study, osteonecrosis was found only with unstable SCFE (21 of 36 hips), and complete or partial reduction of unstable SCFE was associated with a higher rate of osteonecrosis.

Legg-Calvé-Perthes Disease

Gigante C, Frizziero P: and Turra, S: Prognostic value of Catterall and Herring classification in Legg-Calve-Perthes disease: Follow-up to skeletal maturity of 32 patients. *J Pediatr Orthop* 2002;22:345-349.

A small study found that Catterall classification was not prognostic but lateral epiphyseal calcification and epiphyseal subluxation greater than 4 mm were prognostic of poor outcome. Herring classification was only prognostic when combined with patient age.

Herring J, Kim H: Browne R: Abstract: Legg-Calve-Perthes disease: A multicenter trial of five treatment methods. Pediatric Orthopaedic Society of North America Annual Meeting, Amelia Island, Florida, 2003, p26.

Preliminary results of a landmark prospective study on the outcome of Legg-Calvé-Perthes disease at maturity, showed that only lateral pillar B hips and borderline B/C hips of patients age 8 years and older had improved outcome with surgery. Lateral pillar A and lateral pillar B hips in patients younger than 8 years did well without treatment; there was no treatment effect for lateral pillar C hips.

Classic Bibliography

Castelein RM, Sauter AJ, de Vierger M, et al: Natural history of ultrasound hip abnormalities in clinically normal newborns. *J Pediatr Orthop* 1992;12:423-427.

Chiari K: Medial displacement osteotomy of the pelvis. *Clin Orthop* 1974;98:55-71.

de Sanctis N, Rondinella F: Prognostic evaluation of Legg-Calve-Perthes disease by MRI: Part II. Pathomorphogenesis and new classification. *J Pediatr Orthop* 2000;20:463-470.

Ganz R, Klaue K, Vinh TS, Mast JW: A new periacetabular osteotomy for the treatment of hip dysplasias: Technique and preliminary results. *Clin Orthop* 1988;232: 26-36.

Goldberg MJ, Harcke TH, Hirsch A, Lehmann H, Roy DR, Sunshine P: Clinical practice guideline: Early detection of developmental dysplasia of the hip (AC0001). *Pediatrics* 2000;105:896-905.

Graf R: Fundamentals of sonographic diagnosis of infant hip dysplasia. *J Pediatr Orthop* 1984;4:735-740.

Guille JT, Lipton GE, Szoke G, et al: Legg-Calve-Perthes disease in girls. *J Bone Joint Surg Am* 1998;80:1256.

Harcke HT, Kumar SJ: The role of ultrasound in the diagnosis and management of congenital dislocation and dysplasia of the hip. *J Bone Joint Surg Am* 1991;73:622-628.

Herring JA, Neustadt JB, Williams JJ, et al: The lateral pillar classification of Legg-Calvé-Perthes' disease. *J Pediatr Orthop* 1992;12:143-150.

Loder RT, Richards BS, Shapiro PS, Reznick LR, Aronson D: Acute slipped capital femoral epiphysis: The importance of physeal stability. *J Bone Joint Surg Am* 1993; 75:1134-1140.

Malvitz TA, Weinstein SL: Closed reduction for congenital dysplasia of the hip: Functional and radiographic results after an average of thirty years. *J Bone Joint Surg Am* 1994;76:1777-1792.

McAndrew MP, Weinstein SL: A long-term follow-up of Legg-Calve-Perthes disease. *J Bone Joint Surg Am* 1984; 66:860-869.

Meehan PL, Angel D, Nelson JM: The Scottish Rite abduction orthosis for the treatment of Legg-Calve-Perthes disease. *J Bone Joint Surg Am* 1992;74:2.

Neyt JG, Weinstein SL, Spratt KF, et al: Stulberg classification system for evaluation of Legg-Calve-Perthes disease: Intra-rater and inter-rater reliability. *J Bone Joint Surg Am* 1999;81:1209.

Pemberton PA: Pericapsular osteotomy of the ilium for treatment of congenital subluxation and dislocation of the hip. *J Bone Joint Surg Am* 1965;47:65-86.

Reinker KA: Early diagnosis and treatment of hinge abduction in Legg-Calve-Perthes disease. *J Pediatr Orthop* 1996;16:3-9.

Salter RB, Dubos J-P: The first fifteen years' personal experience with innominate osteotomy in the treatment of congenital dislocation and subluxation of the hip. *Clin Orthop* 1974;98:72-103.

Salter RB, Thompson GH: Legg-Calve-Perthes disease: The prognostic significance of the subchondral fracture and a two-group classification of the femoral head involvement. *J Bone Joint Surg Am* 1984;66:479-489.

Schoenecker PL, Strecker WB: Congenital dislocation of the hip in children: Comparison of the effects of femoral shortening and of skeletal traction in treatment. *J Bone Joint Surg Am* 1984;66:21-27.

Staheli LT, Chew DE: Slotted acetabular augmentation in childhood and adolescence. *J Pediatr Orthop* 1992;12: 569-580.

Stulberg SD, Cooperman DR, Wallensten R: The natural history of Legg-Calve-Perthes disease. *J Bone Joint Surg* 1981;63:1095-1108.

Tonnis D, Behrens K, Tscharani F: A midified technique of the triple pelvic osteotomy: Early results. *J Pediatr Orthop* 1981;1:241-249.

Walters R, Simon S: Joint destruction: A sequel of unrecognized pin penetration in patients with slipped capital femoral epiphysis, in *The Hip*. St. Louis, MO, CV Mosby, 1980, p 145.

Weinstein SL, Ponseti IV: Congenital dislocation of the hip: Open reduction through a medial approach. *J Bone Joint Surg Am* 1979;61:119-124.

Chapter 63

Knee and Leg: Pediatrics

Kosmas J. Kayes, MD

David A. Spiegel, MD

Anterior Cruciate Ligament Injuries

Anterior cruciate ligament (ACL) tears in patients with an open physis are on the rise, and optimum treatment still remains controversial. Most of these injuries occur during participation in sports activities. The mechanism is a noncontact, deceleration injury with a valgus stress component or a hyperextension injury. Patients almost always report immediate pain and early onset of knee effusion. Accurate history and physical examination in the child younger than 12 years is often difficult because children are not able to provide a good history. The examination may not confirm the diagnosis with only 50% correlation of physical examination findings with findings on MRI or at time of arthroscopy. Most patients will have a positive Lachman test, but a pivot shift is often difficult to elicit. Effusion and loss of motion will be present.

Imaging should consist of plain radiographs of the knee, including AP, lateral, tunnel, and Merchant views. MRI is the imaging study of choice for evaluation of an ACL tear. Studies have shown that MRI can be just as accurate in adolescents with ACL injuries as in adults. Specificity and sensitivity of clinical examination (done by experienced surgeons) and MRI were shown to correlate well with findings at arthroscopy. However, in children younger than 12 years, MRI findings were significantly lower in both sensitivity and specificity.

In children with open physis at the knee, treatment is still controversial. Modifying sports activity or not participating in pivoting sports until near skeletal maturity are options, but often are not acceptable to the family and patient. Bracing and physical therapy may help but will not eliminate the possibility of recurrent episodes of instability that expose the menisci to injury. Complete tears of the ACL are associated with a higher rate of meniscal injury than partial tears, and patients with recurrent episodes of subluxation are at greater risk to eventually injure the meniscus. A teenager with nearly closed physes, with skeletal age 14 years or older (boys tend to be 2 years behind in skeletal maturity compared with girls of the same chronologic age), and

at Tanner stage 4 to 5 can probably be considered skeletally mature and therefore receive adult treatments. If a child has more than 2 cm of growth remaining, hamstring reconstruction should be considered to lessen the likelihood of injury to the physes. More importantly, careful attention should be paid to fixation to prevent damage to the physis.

Primary repair of the ACL has never been shown to be successful. Extra-articular reconstruction has a high rate of failure (greater than 50%) over time and may need to be revised with an intra-articular method when the child is skeletally mature. Intra-articular reconstruction in the skeletally immature patient carries the risk of growth disturbance. This possibility needs to be weighed against the inevitable risk of further and potentially irreversible risk of meniscal damage. Transepiphyseal techniques that avoid the physis potentially offer the solution but are technically demanding and not well studied to date. The literature has reported instances of injury to the physis in younger children after intra-articular ACL reconstruction but most of these injuries are related to technical error in graft placement or fixation.

Partial tears of the ACL are unusual but do occur in children younger than skeletal age 14 years with a normal Lachman test; tears involving less than 50% of the fibers have been shown to respond well to nonsurgical reconstruction. Many MRI studies have shown partial tears of the ACL, however, no good data exist on which tears to treat surgically and which to treat nonsurgically with rehabilitation.

Meniscal Tears

Meniscal tears in children are still difficult to diagnose, with many children not reporting a significant injury and physical examination being less reproducible, especially in children 12 years of age or younger. MRI can have a higher false-positive rate for diagnosing meniscal tears because of increased vascularity of the meniscus in children; diagnosis is improved with review by a good pediatric skeletal radiologist. Tears of the medial meniscus are more common than lateral meniscal tears if discoid menisci are excluded. ACL tears have a 50% rate of associated meniscal tear.

Meniscal repair should be attempted in children and adolescents to preserve meniscal tissue if possible. Suture repair is still the gold standard, with the vertical mattress inside-out technique shown to be the strongest. Not only will peripheral tears or red-on-white tears heal, but new evidence suggests that tears that extend into the white zone greater than 4 mm from the periphery had a 75% healing rate with stable inside-out repair.

Discoid Meniscus

Discoid menisci occur in 3% to 5% of the population. They are more often lateral, with 25% occurring bilaterally. Discoid menisci are often asymptomatic but can become symptomatic at any age. Symptoms often include pain and popping in the lateral joint line and mechanical symptoms of catching and locking. The discoid meniscus does not have the same strength characteristics as a normal meniscus and can be more prone to tear without significant trauma. Classification by Watanabe consists of three types. In type I, the meniscus covers the entire lateral plateau and is stable. In type II, the meniscus only covers part of the plateau and is stable. Type III discoid menisci (Wrisberg variant) are unstable because of absent meniscotibial attachment posteriorly.

Treatment in asymptomatic patients with no tear is observation. For symptomatic patients, treatment consists of repair or débridement if a tear is present and saucerization of the meniscus. For type III unstable menisci, suture stabilization to the capsule is necessary along with saucerization. Complete meniscectomy should be avoided because the meniscus will not regenerate.

Tibial Eminence Fracture

Avulsion of the tibial eminence occurs with a mechanism similar to an ACL tear. Usually occurring between 8 to 14 years of age, the attachment of the ACL on the tibial eminence is avulsed off, bringing a varying amount of bony fragment with it. Historically, these injuries occurred after a fall from a bicycle, but recently more are reported from mishaps during skiing or while playing football. The mechanism of injury is usually forceful hyperextension or a direct blow to the distal end of the femur with a flexed knee. A high incidence of associated injuries (up to 40%) such as medial collateral ligament (MCL) injuries or meniscal tears has been reported.

Meyers and McKeever classify injuries into three types. Type I is nondisplaced, type II is elevation of the anterior fragment up to 3 mm with the posterior hinge intact, and type III is complete displacement of the avulsed fragment; they occur in approximately 15%, 39%, and 45% of patients with tibial eminence frac-

tures, respectively. Treatment of type I injuries is usually long leg casting with the knee in extension or 10° to 15° flexion for 4 to 6 weeks. Type II lesions can undergo closed reduction with hyperextension of the knee, then long leg casting with close follow-up to check for displacement. If the fragment does not reduce to less than 2 mm of displacement, then the same treatment as for type III lesions should be done. Type III fractures are typically treated with open or arthroscopic reduction of the fragment and fixation to secure the fragment while it heals.

The anterior horn of the medial meniscus or the transverse meniscal ligament may be trapped beneath the fragment in many patients and must be mobilized while the fragment is reduced and then secured. Meniscal entrapment is reported in 26% of type II injuries and more than 90% of type III injuries. Several different methods of fixation have been reported, including use of Steinmann pins, cannulated screws into the fragment stopping short of the physis, or suture technique through fibers of the ACL at its base and then down through the crater, exiting out the anterior tibial epiphysis.

Controversy exists as to whether long-term instability continues, either objectively or subjectively, no matter how well the fragment is reduced. The thought is that some ligaments undergo appreciable interstitial failure before the fracture and that even if the fracture is reduced, the ligament may have residual laxity. Most reports show that even if there is some objective laxity on clinical examination, most patients (84%) return to their previous level of activity. A recent report on a small number of patients demonstrates that residual laxity may not be inevitable because good results with minimal objective or subjective laxity were obtained.

Juvenile Osteochondritis Dissecans

Juvenile osteochondritis dissecans refers to an osteochondritis dissecans lesion that occurs before physeal closure. An avascular portion of the subchondral bone in severe cases can undergo separation from the underlying epiphyseal cancellous bone. The cartilage separates with the subchondral bone, although sometimes there is very little bone remaining on the back side of the cartilage. The severity ranges from minimal involvement that results in a soft cartilage bed to complete separation with production of a loose body. The etiology of this disease is unknown but is highly associated with repetitive microtrauma and/or vascular disruption. Boys are affected twice as often as girls, and most patients are very active in sports, giving credence to the theory of trauma as an etiology. The lateral aspect of the medial femoral condyle is most often involved (75%). The lateral condyle, patella, trochlea, and tibial plateau can also develop lesions but are affected much less often. The posterior aspect of the lateral femoral condyle can have normal variations in ossification that can mimic an osteochondritis dissecans lesion on plain radiographs.

Approximately 50% of patients describe a history of trauma to the knee with reports of ongoing, vague knee pain during athletic activities. The pain often improves with rest. Mechanical symptoms of locking, catching, or popping can occur when the condition is more advanced and loose fragments are present. Patients may have pain with palpation over the condyle that is involved. Effusion may or not be present.

A tunnel view is important, along with an AP and lateral view of the knee, as many lesions are best seen on the tunnel view. MRI can be helpful in making treatment decisions. MRI stage I lesions have articular cartilage thickening but no break in the cartilage. Stage II lesions have a break in the cartilage but no increased signal intensity on T2-weighted images between the bone fragment and the intact subchondral bone. Stage III lesions have the increased signal intensity at this interface, an indication that fluid is present between the fragment and the host bone. This finding is a sign of instability of the fragment. Stage IV lesions are loose bodies. MRI with gadolinium enhancement helps to distinguish between type II and type III lesions

Treatment in skeletally immature patients with a stable lesion depends on the symptoms. Patients with open physes have a better prognosis for healing of the lesions. If the patient is relatively asymptomatic, then activity restriction alone may be enough. However, if symptoms of pain and joint effusion are present, restricted weight bearing and possibly immobilization may be warranted for 6 weeks. Range-of-motion exercises should be performed out of the brace. This treatment plan can result in healing in up to 90% of patients at 3 to 6 months. If symptoms persist or the MRI signal does not change, then drilling of the lesion may be indicated. This procedure helps induce vascular supply into the lesion and facilitates healing. The lesions may be drilled retrograde through a portal while visualizing through the scope or antegrade with fluoroscopic guidance to avoid penetrating intact cartilage.

If the lesion is unstable (type III or IV), surgical intervention is indicated. If subchondral bone is present, the bed can be débrided and drilled and the fragment fixed with pins or screws. Results are variable with fixation. If there is no subchondral bone on the fragment, the piece should be removed and the bed débrided and drilled. Other options include autologous chondrocyte transplantation and osteochondral grafts. If the lesion is smaller than 2.5 cm, débridement of the frayed cartilage, drilling, or microfracture may allow the lesion to heal with fibrocartilage. In larger lesions, fixation of the fragment should be attempted only if there is subchondral bone attached to the cartilage. Lesions on the medial femoral condyle tend to respond the best; lesions of the

trochlea, tibia, and patella do not have as good a response to the same treatment.

With larger lesions, newer techniques of cartilage restoration can be considered. At a mean 5-year follow-up (range, 1 to 10 years) of autologous chondrocyte transplantation, 90% of patients had good results. However, only seven patients in this study were younger than 18 years. Mosaicplasty gave the same results at the same length of follow-up; again, most patients who were treated had adult-onset lesions. The outcome of these procedures in the younger population is still unknown because results are not separated from those found with adult-onset lesions.

Tibial Tubercle Fractures

These fractures are rare and account for approximately 2% of all epiphyseal fractures. The mechanism of injury is usually jumping or landing during some type of sports activity, often basketball or track. The force of the massive quadriceps contraction on takeoff or landing against the acutely flexing knee pulls off the tubercle.

The Watson-Jones classification of these fractures includes type I (the fracture line is between the ossification centers of the tibial tubercle and the epiphysis before closure), type II (the fracture pattern courses between the tibial tubercle and the plateau), and type III (the fracture extends vertically behind the tibial tubercle and through the tibial plateau). A few instances have been reported in which a tubercle avulsion fracture with an accompanying epiphyseal fracture, either Salter-Harris II, III, or IV occurs (making a case for a type IV tibial tubercle fracture pattern). These types of fractures are extremely rare but can have higher potential for compartment syndrome.

Treatment of nondisplaced type I injuries is cast immobilization for 6 weeks with the leg in extension. Displaced type II and III lesions require open reduction and screw fixation for stability. Meniscal injury can also occur in type III fractures. Most injuries occur in older children just before physeal closure and heal well; however, if this injury occurs in younger children, smooth pin fixation should be considered to avoid further damage to the proximal tibial physis. Children may have resultant recurvatum deformity if younger than 11 years at the time of injury.

Distal Femoral Physeal Fractures

These fractures comprise less than 1% of all pediatric fractures and about 5% to 6% of physeal fractures. The undulation of the physis contributes to its stability. The mechanism of injury is usually a football injury or being hit by a motor vehicle. Concomitant ligament injury may occur in up to 50% of patients but often is unrecognized initially. Most injuries are closed, and patients have pain, deformity, inability to bear weight, and knee effusion (if the fracture is intra-articular).

Salter-Harris type II fractures are the most common pattern and are seen in adolescents. The risk of growth arrest is significant (between 19% to 25%) even in this pattern. Salter-Harris type III fractures usually result from a valgus stress and involve the medial condyle. These fractures may be minimally displaced. Salter-Harris type IV is uncommon and Salter-Harris type V is extremely rare, with the diagnosis often made later after deformity occurs from growth disturbance. Infants respond to remodeling and require minimal reduction even with significant displacement. In adolescents, minimal remodeling of varus/valgus can be expected; therefore, reduction needs to be near anatomic.

Treatment of nondisplaced Salter-Harris type I and II fractures consists of cast immobilization with close follow-up. If reduction is required, these injuries are unstable and fixation should be considered. Smooth Steinmann pins crossed in the metaphysis are effective for Salter-Harris type I and II fractures with a small metaphyseal fragment. If the metaphyseal fragment is large enough, cannulated screws can be used transversely through the metaphyseal fragment into the remaining metaphysis, thereby avoiding the physis. Salter-Harris type III and IV fracture patterns require anatomic reduction. If no displacement is present, simple immobilization is adequate; however, most Salter-Harris type III and IV fractures will require open anatomic reduction and fixation. Cannulated screws placed parallel to the physis, which travel transversely across the epiphysis and the metaphysis, are excellent constructs.

Proximal Tibial Physeal Fractures

Proximal tibial physeal fractures are rare injuries occurring in patients age 8 to 15 years. Half of these fractures result from motor vehicle crashes and half from injury during sports participation. They can also be found in the newborn and in patients with arthrogryposis who have undergone aggressive stretching in an attempt to improve range of motion. The mechanism of injury can be a direct force, flexion injury, or abduction with or without hyperextension of the lower leg. An associated MCL injury may be present, especially in Salter-Harris type III fractures.

Salter-Harris type fractures account for 15% of the injuries and about half are nondisplaced. For those that are displaced, the metaphyseal portion typically is displaced medially or posteriorly. Salter-Harris type II fracture patterns (43%) are nondisplaced in up to two thirds of patients. When displacement does occur, the metaphyseal fragment is usually displaced medially. Salter-Harris type III fractures (22%) usually involve the lateral epiphysis, and the MCL is often torn in this pattern. Salter-Harris type IV fractures account for 27% and Salter-Harris type

V account for 3% of these injuries. Type V patterns are not usually not noticed until deformity occurs after the injury.

Treatment of Salter-Harris type I and II patterns is casting for 6 to 8 weeks if nondisplaced and gentle closed reduction, often under general anesthetic, if displaced. Crossed pins should be considered for stability or cannulated screws should be used if the metaphyseal fragment if large enough. Salter-Harris type III and IV patterns require open reduction and internal fixation if any displacement is present. They can be fixed with cannulated screws across the epiphysis for type III and across both metaphysis and epiphysis for type IV. These injuries can cause unrecognized arterial damage and lead to compartment syndrome.

Congenital Dislocation of the Knee

Congenital knee dislocation is a spectrum of deformity from simple positional contractures that correct spontaneously to rigid dislocation of the knee joint requiring surgical intervention. The condition often occurs in children with myelomeningocele, arthrogryposis, or other syndromes such as Larsen's. This deformity is often associated with developmental dysplasia of the hip, clubfoot, and metatarsus adductus. It is extremely important to look for associated hip dysplasia when a knee dislocation is present. The deformity is recognized at birth with a knee that is hyperextended and a foot that is extended toward the patient's head because of a flexed hip. The pathology consists of one or all of the following conditions: contractures of the quadriceps tendon, an absent suprapatellar pouch, tight collateral ligaments, and anterior subluxation of the hamstring tendons.

If the condition results from positioning in utero, often the deformity is mild and the knee is still fairly flexible. The knee will correct spontaneously within a few weeks or can be assisted by gentle range-of-motion therapy to accelerate correction. Serial casting also may be helpful if hip dysplasia is present. A Pavlik harness is applied once knee range of motion increases enough to allow proper fit.

A more severe contracture or true dislocation shows minimal response to stretching and casting. This condition usually is evident within the first 3 months of treatment. Failure to gain 30° of knee flexion by 3 months is an indication for surgery. Surgical treatment is with V-Y quadricepsplasty or Z-lengthening of the tendon, release of the anterior joint capsule, transposition posteriorly of the hamstring tendons, and mobilization of the collateral ligaments. Ninety degrees of knee flexion should be achieved and then the knee should be placed in a cast in 45° to 60° flexion for 3 to 4 weeks.

Congenital Dislocation of the Patella

A true congenital dislocation of the patella is rare. This entity must be distinguished from a recurrent dislocation that occurs later in life. In congenital dislocation of the patella, the patella is hypoplastic or absent, and the femoral trochlea is often flattened. The lateral retinaculum is tight, and the patella is completely dislocated laterally. The patella is often adherent to the iliotibial band and often irreducible over the condyle. Genu valgus is often present, as is a flexion contracture of the knee. Surgical intervention is required and involves extensive lateral retinacular release, often to the greater trochanter, medial plication, and either hamstring tenodesis or transfer of one half of the patellar tendon.

Nail-Patella Syndrome

Nail-patella syndrome is rare, involving a tetrad of orthopaedic manifestations: (1) nail dysplasia; (2) hypoplastic (or absent) and often dislocated patellae; (3) iliac horns; and (4) elbow dysplasia, mostly consisting of radial head dislocation. The syndrome is of autosomal dominant inheritance with great variability in the phenotype. Foot abnormalities may also accompany the diagnosis, as well as upper and lower extremity tendon contractures. The foot deformities include metatarsus adductus, pes planus, equinus, clubfoot, vertical talus, and calcaneovalgus. Many patients have nephropathy and glaucoma.

The orthopaedic implications primarily involve the patellar dislocations. Most patients will require early surgical intervention to stabilize the extensor mechanism and prevent long-term complications. Surgical treatment is with lateral release (extensive), medial plication, and hemipatellar tendon transfer or hamstring tenodesis. The nail problems are usually well tolerated. Surgery for radial head dislocation is usually not needed because patients usually will not have significant complications. The iliac horns are asymptomatic.

Patellar Fracture

Fractures of the patella are uncommon in children younger than 16 years. Diagnosis in the younger patient is difficult and often delayed. The mechanism of injury is by direct impact or contraction of the quadriceps muscle. Osteochondral fractures are more likely in the younger age group, especially after a dislocation event. Avulsion fractures are classified by location. Superior pole avulsion is least common; medial avulsion is often caused by dislocation of the patella and is the most common, followed by inferior pole avulsion. Lateral avulsion must be distinguished from the congenital variant bipartite patella. Often a larger fragment is fractured off than appears on radiographs because of the large cartilaginous portion.

Treatment options vary but generally follow the same guidelines as for adult fractures. Nondisplaced fractures can be treated in a cast. For displacement greater than 3 mm, open reduction and fixation is recommended. Small fracture pieces may be excised and screw fixation of a larger fragment should be considered.

Evaluation of Genu Varum in Infants and Children

Bowing of the lower extremities in infants and children is a common reason for referral to an orthopaedic surgeon. Infantile genu varum is physiologic in most instances. Pathologic causes include infantile Blount's disease, skeletal dysplasias, rachitic syndromes (nutritional or metabolic), posttraumatic or postinfectious deformities, and rarely, focal fibrocartilagenous dysplasia.

Historical features that elevate the index of suspicion for infantile Blount's disease include obesity, early ambulation, race (African American), and rarely, a positive family history. The deformity is localized to the proximal tibia, in contrast to physiologic bowing, where the deformity is usually more evenly distributed throughout the diaphyseal region. A varus thrust also should raise the index of suspicion.

A host of radiographic parameters have been investigated to screen for the development of infantile Blount's disease (Figure 1). The tibial metaphyseal-diaphyseal angle (TMDA) is most frequently used for this purpose. The TMDA has been shown in several studies to be effective (< 5% error) for angles less than 9° (physiologic) or greater than 16° (Blount's); however, a significant percentage of cases may be indeterminate (9° to 16°).

In an attempt to improve the accuracy of radiographic screening, several other measurements have been evaluated for their sensitivity, specificity, and predictive value. Both the percentage of tibial deformity (tibial varus/total limb varus) and the ratio of the femoral metaphyseal-diaphyseal angle to the TMDA may be more sensitive and more specific than the TMDA alone. The epiphyseal-metaphyseal angle (EMA) may also be helpful because patients 1 to 3 years of age with a TMDA of 10° or greater and an EMA of greater than 20° are at increased risk for Blount's disease. Serial radiographs are often required to establish the diagnosis, and a comprehensive approach to screening should include both standardized measurements and knowledge of the sequential radiographic changes described by Langenskiöld.

Blount's Disease

Infantile Blount's disease is a progressive varus deformity of the proximal tibia. The etiology is most likely multifactorial, and the pathophysiology involves a dis-

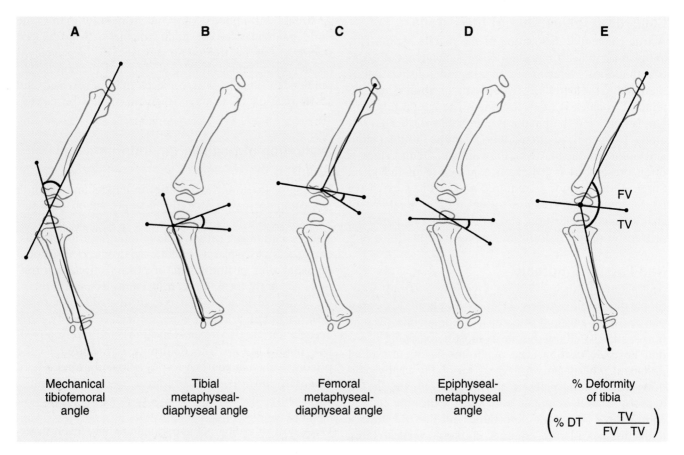

Figure 1 Radiographic indices used in the evaluation of lower extremity bowing in infants and children. **A,** Tibiofemoral angle (mechanical). This is the angle in between a line drawn from the center of the hip to the center of the knee and a line from the center of the knee to the center of the ankle. **B,** TMDA. The TMDA has been used most commonly and is measured as the angle between a line drawn though the most distal aspect of the medial and lateral beaks of the proximal tibia and a line perpendicular to the anatomic axis (most reproducible if drawn along the lateral tibial cortex). **C,** Femoral metaphyseal-diaphyseal angle. This angle is measured in between the anatomic axis of the femur and a line drawn perpendicular to a line parallel to the distal femoral physis. **D,** Epiphyseal-metaphyseal angle. This represents the angle between a line drawn through the proximal tibial physis (parallel to the base of the epiphyseal ossification center) and a line connecting the midpoint of the base of the epiphyseal ossification center with the most distal point on he medial beak of the tibia. **E,** Percent deformity of the tibia ([%DT] = tibial varus [TV]/total limb varus). The %DT is calculated as the degree of tibial varus (angle between the mechanical axis of the tibia and a line parallel to the distal femoral condyles) divided by the total limb varus (tibial varus + femoral varus [FV]). Femoral varus represents the angle between the mechanical axis of the femur and the line parallel to the distal condyles of the femur.

turbance of growth in the posterior and medial regions of the proximal tibia, most likely caused by mechanical overload in a genetically susceptible individual. The sequence of radiographic changes that evolves over the first decade of life has been described by Langenskiöld. Plain radiographs may suggest a depression in the medial tibial plateau in later stages of the disease; however, arthrography (or MRI) often reveals that this region is occupied by unossified cartilage.

The best outcomes are associated with early diagnosis and unloading of the medial joint by either bracing or osteotomy. Although somewhat controversial, a knee-ankle-foot orthosis may be indicated for patients with stage I and II disease who are younger than 3 years. The device should be worn at least during weight-bearing hours, and desirable features include a drop lock and a valgus producing strap.

Valgus osteotomy is indicated for patients with progressive deformity. Overcorrection is essential, and the distal fragment should be translated laterally. An intra-operative arthrogram facilitates visualization of the tibial joint surface. The lowest risk of recurrence is seen in those with Langenskiöld III disease who are younger than 4 years. Unfortunately, recurrence remains common even after a well-executed osteotomy.

Although MRI is not routinely indicated, it may be helpful in documenting the presence, size, and location of a physeal bar in later stages of the disease. Treatment of a physeal bar must be individualized. In addition to angular correction, either a resection of the bar or a lateral hemiepiphysiodesis may be required. Limb lengths should be followed closely, and either lengthening or contralateral epiphysiodesis may be indicated.

Adolescent or late-onset Blount's disease also involves a progressive varus deformity of the proximal tibia and is diagnosed in children older than 8 years. Most patients are obese, and mechanical overload has been implicated. A common radiographic feature is wid-

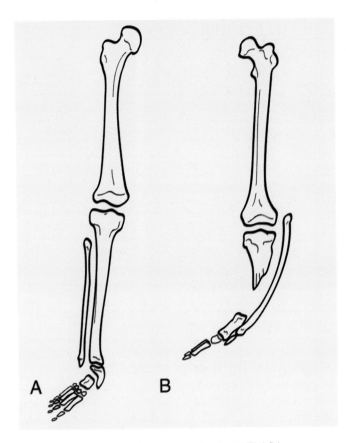

Figure 2 Common osseous anatomy of fibular **(A)** and tibial **(B)** deficiency.

Table 1 | Clinical Findings in the Ipsilateral Extremity That May Be Observed in Patients With Longitudinal Deficiency of the Tibia and Fibula

Fibular Deficiency	Tibial Deficiency
Femur	**Femur**
Shortening	Hypoplasia
External rotation	PFFD
Lateral condylar hypoplasia	
PFFD	
Coxa vara	
Knee	Knee
Absent or attenuated cruciate ligaments	Absent cruciates
Genu valgum	Dysplastic or absent patella
Patellar dysplasia and/or subluxation	
Tibia	**Tibia**
Shortened	Deficient or absent
Anteromedial bowing	
Fibula	**Fibula**
Hypoplastic or absent	Angulation (varus, posterior)
	Proximal instability/dislocation
Ankle	**Ankle**
Valgus	Fibulocalcaneotalar articulation
Ball and socket	
Foot	**Foot**
Equinovalgus	Equinovarus
Tarsal coalition	Tarsal coalition
Longitudinal deficiency (lateral)	Longitudinal deficiency (medial)
Fused metatarsals	

PFFD = proximal femoral focal deficiency

ening and irregularity of the medial proximal tibial physis, which is consistent with a chronic compressive injury. This multiplanar deformity includes varus, procurvatum, and internal torsion. Treatment is by osteotomy or hemiepiphysiodesis, and suggested advantages of external fixation include the ability to address all components of the deformity, to minimize neurovascular complications by enabling a gradual correction, to make adjustments in alignment postoperatively based on standing radiographs, and to enable simultaneous limb lengthening. Hemiepiphysiodesis may be considered for milder deformities in patients with sufficient growth remaining. A coexisting deformity of the distal femur may require either hemiepiphysiodesis or osteotomy.

Longitudinal Deficiency of the Fibula

Given the spectrum of coexisting abnormalities associated with longitudinal deficiency of the fibula (Figure 2 and Table 1), postaxial hypoplasia is a term that has been suggested as more comprehensive in describing this condition. The treatment plan must address limb length inequality, foot and ankle deformity, and coexisting abnormalities such as valgus at the knee and ankle. Growth inhibition varies from 5% to 30% and the fe-

mur contributes to limb shortening in up to 50% of patients.

Classification schemes have traditionally focused on the degree of fibular deficiency and the predicted limb length inequality; however, both the treatment and prognosis also depend on deformity of the foot and ankle. Fibular morphology does not seem to correlate with either the percentage of growth inhibition or the degree of foot deformity; therefore, treatment recommendations should not be based solely on the degree of fibular deficiency. Congenital lower extremity deficiencies are associated with a constant percentage of growth inhibition; thus, the discrepancy at maturity can be estimated at an early age. The position of the foot of the shorter extremity relative to the longer extremity also may be used to estimate the percentage of shortening at skeletal maturity (proximal one third ≥ 26%, middle one third approximately 16% to 25%, distal one third ≤ 15%).

The treatment should be individualized. Patients with a functional (or reconstructable) foot and a milder

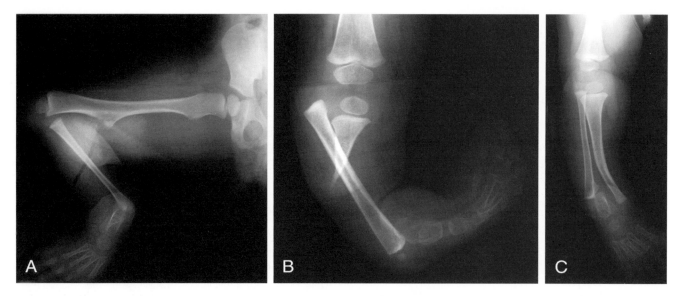

Figure 3 The Kalamchi and Dawe classification for longitudinal deficiency of the tibia. **A,** Type I represents complete absence of the tibia. **B,** Type II deficiencies are associated with absence of the distal tibia. **C,** Type III deficiencies have a distal tibial deficiency (hypoplasia) with a diastasis of the distal tibiofibular articulation.

projected discrepancy may be treated by foot reconstruction and an epiphysiodesis, a single lengthening procedure, or both. A foot with three or more rays can potentially be treated by reconstruction rather than amputation. Those extremities with a nonfunctional foot and/or a large projected limb-length discrepancy (up to 25 cm) are most commonly treated by amputation (Syme or Boyd). In general, most patients with complete absence of the fibula require amputation. The indications for amputation versus limb salvage remain nebulous for the subset of patients with a functional (or reconstructable) foot and a large projected discrepancy. Although a staged reconstruction including two or three lengthening procedures is technically feasible, it remains to be determined whether limb function and patient satisfaction will be enhanced compared with early amputation. The psychosocial impact of multiple reconstructive procedures during childhood and adolescence must also be considered.

Coexisting deformities must also be addressed to maximize outcome. The severity of ankle valgus correlates with the degree of fibular deficiency. There is typically a wedge-shaped distal tibial epiphysis and a tarsal coalition. Milder degrees of ankle valgus may be treated by hemiepiphysiodesis, whereas techniques to restore the lateral buttress in patients with greater deformity include fibular lengthening or distal tibial osteotomy. Valgus deformity at the knee results from hypoplasia of the lateral femoral condyle, and treatment options include a distal femoral osteotomy or distal femoral hemiepiphysiodesis (open versus physeal stapling). Anteromedial bowing of the tibia is common but typically only requires an osteotomy in patients with complete absence of the fibula.

Longitudinal Deficiency of the Tibia

A spectrum of limb abnormalities is seen in patients with partial or complete absence of the tibia. Clinical concerns include instability at the knee and the ankle, an equinovarus foot deformity with or without the loss of medial rays, and limb-length discrepancy. The classification scheme presented by Kalamchi and Dawe is perhaps most practical (Figure 3). The condition occurs sporadically; however, both autosomal dominant and autosomal recessive forms of transmission have been documented. In contrast to fibular deficiencies, associated congenital anomalies in the musculoskeletal system (most often in the hand) and the viscera (congenital heart disease, testicular anomalies) have been reported in patients with tibial deficiencies.

Complete absence of the tibia is usually treated by through knee amputation. A small subset of patients with a strong quadriceps muscle and no knee flexion contracture may be candidates for fibular centralization (Brown procedure). Because a significant subset of these patients may subsequently require an amputation for progressive flexion contracture, most physicians have abandoned this procedure. When the proximal tibia has ossified, stability is achieved by proximal tibiofibular synostosis, and either amputation (Syme or Boyd) or foot salvage is also performed depending on the local anatomy. Two or more limb lengthenings may be required if the foot is retained, and the patient's family must be prepared for the effects on the patient of multiple procedures throughout childhood and adolescence.

The third major type of deformity involves hypoplasia of the distal tibia associated with a diastasis between the distal tibia and fibula, for which the most common treatment has been early Syme or Boyd amputation. Limbs with lesser degrees of anticipated discrepancy and a functional (or reconstructable) foot may be considered for salvage, and the choice of procedure is based on the local anatomy. Options for ankle stabilization include arthrodesis of either the distal tibia or fibula to either the talus or the calcaneus. Talectomy may be required to facilitate closure of the diastasis, and synostosis of the distal tibia to the fibula may be required to maintain stability. An osteotomy of the distal tibia and fibula also may be required to correct angular deformity, and limb-length discrepancy will need to be treated by one or more lengthenings and/or epiphysiodesis.

Congenital Pseudarthrosis of the Tibia and/or Fibula

The etiology of congenital pseudarthrosis of the tibia remains unknown, and the pathophysiology appears to involve a localized deregulation of bone modeling and growth. The condition is associated with neurofibromatosis in approximately 50% of patients; however, only 10% of patients with neurofibromatosis will develop pseudarthrosis of the tibia. In contrast to anterolateral bowing of the tibia, which is associated with a "prepseudarthrosis" or frank pseudarthrosis of the tibia, posteromedial bowing is generally benign and improves with time. However, patients with posteromedial bowing will require either an epiphysiodesis or a limb lengthening to treat limb-length discrepancy.

The goal of treatment is not only to obtain union, but also to prevent progressive deformity/refracture, to treat coexisting limb-length discrepancy and ankle valgus, and to maximize function of the foot and ankle. Follow-up beyond skeletal maturity is required to determine the outcome of a given treatment method. There is evidence to suggest that delaying surgery may increase the chances of achieving union and that results of treatment may be better in patients presenting for surgery at a later age (older than 5 years).

For patients with anterolateral bowing and a prepseudarthrosis, the goal is to prevent or delay fracture by full-time immobilization in a clamshell ankle-foot orthosis or similar device. Prophylactic bypass grafting has not been widely accepted. The primary goal for an established pseudarthrosis is to achieve union. Principles of surgery include resecting all abnormal tissue, providing a stable mechanical environment, and grafting with autogenous bone. The role of electrical stimulation as an adjunct has yet to be determined.

Resection and grafting with intramedullary fixation has been associated with variable rates of union (28% to 80%); concomitant fibular surgery may improve the outcome. In the absence of fibular involvement, osteotomy is usually required to facilitate apposition of the tibial fragments. A coexisting pseudarthrosis of the fibula worsens the prognosis and should be treated by resection and grafting as well. Intramedullary fixation of the fibula should be considered. Ankle valgus may be treated by medial distal tibial hemiepiphysiodesis or distal tibiofibular synostosis because a distal tibial osteotomy may fail to unite.

There has been considerable interest in the use of external fixation and distraction osteogenesis. Following resection of the pathologic tissue, acute shortening and compression at the pseudarthrosis site may be combined with bone transport via a proximal tibial corticotomy. Excellent rates of union have been reported; however, refracture remains a concern. The technique is most appropriate for children older than 5 years. Intramedullary fixation may help to protect against refracture once union has been achieved.

Free vascularized fibular grafting results in union rates of 92% to 95%; however, additional procedures are commonly required for delayed union at the distal transfer site, for refracture or stress fractures, for ankle valgus, and for limb-length discrepancy. Pseudarthrosis may recur above or below the site of transfer. Donor site morbidity (weakness, ankle valgus) remains a concern, and restoring fibular continuity by grafting of the periosteal envelope, or by distal tibiofibular fusion, should be considered. Ipsilateral fibular transfer may be considered in those with no evidence of fibular involvement.

Amputation is most commonly performed for resistant pseudarthroses following multiple attempts to achieve union or when union has been achieved but function is impaired by chronic pain or stiffness. The Syme or Boyd techniques are preferred in children, whereas below-knee amputation may be considered in skeletally mature patients.

Isolated congenital pseudarthrosis of the fibula is extremely rare. The lesion is typically in the distal third, and the goals of treatment are to restore fibular continuity and to prevent or treat ankle valgus. Although observation or splinting may be an option in the absence of a progressive ankle valgus, an attempt to restore fibular continuity by resection, bone grafting, and intramedullary fixation is generally recommended. In younger children, valgus may improve with growth if union is achieved. Arthrodesis of the distal fibula to the distal tibia may be performed as an alternative to resection and grafting or following failed attempts to achieve union at the pseudarthrosis. The procedure will prevent the progression of ankle valgus in older children and adolescents but will not result in correction of valgus. The most common treatment of an established valgus deformity is either distal tibial hemiepiphysiodesis or osteotomy.

Annotated Bibliography

Anterior Cruciate Ligament Injuries

Anderson AF: Transepiphyseal replacement of the anterior cruciate ligament in skeletally immature patients. *J Bone Joint Surg Am* 2003;85-A:1255-1263.

In this small study, skeletally immature patients with ACL tears were treated with transepiphyseal ACL reconstruction, thereby avoiding crossing the physis with the grafts. The technique is demanding but safe and provided effective treatment in this population.

Kocher MS, Micheli LJ, Zurakowski D, Luke A: Partial tears of the anterior cruciate ligament in children and adolescents. *Am J Sports Med* 2002;30:697-703.

Partial ACL tears diagnosed by MRI and arthroscopically confirmed were studied in 45 skeletally mature and 17 skeletally immature patients. Patients who had good outcomes with nonreconstructive treatment were younger than skeletal age 14 years, had normal or near-normal results on the Lachman and pivot shift tests, and had 50% or less predominantly posterolateral tears. Patients not meeting those criteria required reconstructive treatment for a good result.

Meniscal Tears

Noyes FR, Barber-Westin SD: Arthroscopic repair of meniscal tears extending into the avascular zone in patients younger than twenty years of age. *Am J Sports Med* 2002;30:589-600.

In this prospective study, 71 meniscal tears extending into the avascular zone in patients younger than 20 years were examined at an average follow-up of 18 months postoperatively. The repairs were all made with an inside-out vertical divergent suture technique. Seventy-five percent of these patients had good results with no evidence of ongoing symptoms in the tibiofemoral compartment.

Tibial Eminence Fracture

Owens BD, Crane GK, Plante T, Busconi BD: Treatment of type III tibial intercondylar eminence fractures in skeletally immature athletes. *Am J Orthop* 2003;32:103-105.

In this study, 12 patients with type III tibial eminence fractures had good results with absorbable suture repair. These patients had 1 mm or less residual laxity at an average follow-up of 36 months. Five of the 12 patients had associated injuries, including two MCL injuries, two lateral meniscal tears, one medial meniscal tear, and one patellar tendon avulsion.

Shepley RW: Arthroscopic treatment of type III tibial spine fractures using absorbable fixation. *Orthopedics* 2004;27:767-769.

Five patients (average age, 15 years) were treated with absorbable polydioxanone pins for type III tibial spine fractures.

No patient had any objective instability on KT-1000 testing and no functional limitations in high-demand sporting activities.

Juvenile Osteochondritis Dissecans

Peterson L, Minas T, Brittberg M, Lindahl A: Treatment of osteochondritis dissecans of the knee with autologous chondrocyte transplantation. *J Bone Joint Surg Am* 2003;85-A(suppl 2):17-24.

Fifty-eight knees underwent autologous chondrocyte transplantation for osteochondritis dissecans lesions (average of 5.7 cm^2). Mean age at the time of surgery was 26.4 years and mean follow-up was 5.6 years. The population was mixed regarding lesion size, location, and time of onset (skeletally mature versus immature). Ninety-one percent of patients had good or excellent results at follow-up based on clinical evaluation and self-assessment questionnaires.

Nail-Patella Syndrome

Beguiristain JL, De Rada PD, Barriga A: Nail-patella syndrome: Long-term evolution. *J Pediatr Orthop B* 2003;12:13-16.

Eight patients with knee pain caused by patellar instability were reviewed. Five patients were treated surgically and three were not treated.

Evaluation of Genu Varum in Infants and Children

Bowen RE, Dorey FJ, Moseley CF: Relative tibial and femoral varus as a predictor of progression of varus deformities of the lower limbs in young children. *J Pediatr Orthop* 2002;22:105-111.

Progression of varus deformity was evaluated with six radiographic measurements. The percentage of tibial deformity (tibial varus/total limb varus) was more sensitive and more specific than the metaphyseal-diaphyseal angle. All patients with both a deformity of the tibia greater than 50% and a TMDA greater than 16° experienced progression of deformity.

Davids JR, Blackhurst DW, Allen BL Jr: Radiographic evaluation of bowed legs in children. *J Pediatr Orthop* 2001;21:257-263.

The sensitivity, specificity, and positive predictive value of the mechanical axis, the TMDA, and the EMA were evaluated in children 1 to 3 years of age. Those with a TMDA of 10° or greater and an EMA of greater than 20° are at increased risk for Blount's disease.

McCarthy JJ, Betz RR, Kim A, et al: Early radiographic differentiation of infantile tibia vara from physiologic bowing using the femoral-tibial ratio. *J Pediatr Orthop* 2001;21:545-548.

A femoral-tibial ratio (FTR = femoral metaphyseal-diaphyseal angle/tibial metaphyseal-diaphyseal angle) of 0.7 or less or 1.4 or greater was associated with a less than 5% error risk. The FTR had a greater sensitivity and specificity versus the TMDA alone, with less rotational effect.

Blount's Disease

Chotigavanichaya C, Salinas G, Green T, et al: Recurrence of varus deformity after proximal tibial osteotomy in Blount disease: Long-term follow-up. *J Pediatr Orthop* 2002;22:638-641.

The recurrence rate in three groups was evaluated (patient's younger than 4 years [46%], patients older than 4 years with crossed pins [94%], and patients older than 4 years with external fixation [72%]). Early osteotomy and postoperative alignment in valgus decreased the risk of recurrence.

Craig JG, van Holsbeeck M, Zaltz I: The utility of MR in assessing Blount disease. *Skeletal Radiol* 2002;31:208-213.

In patients with infantile Blount's disease, ossification of the medial tibial epiphysis is delayed, and they may have widening and depression of the medial physis, metaphyseal cartilaginous intrusions, edema, lateral physeal widening, femoral osteochondral injury, hypertrophy of the medial meniscus, and focal physeal arrest.

Longitudinal Deficiency of the Fibula

Stanitski DF, Stanitski CL: Fibular hemimelia: A new classification system. *J Pediatr Orthop* 2003;23:30-34.

This classification evaluates fibular morphology (I = nearly normal, II = small fibula, III = absent fibula), tibiotalar joint and distal tibial epiphyseal morphology (H = horizontal, V = valgus, S = spherical), the presence of a tarsal coalition, and the number of rays in the foot.

Longitudinal Deficiency of the Tibia

Alekberov C, Shevtsov VI, Karatosun V, et al: Treatment of tibia vara by the Ilizarov method. *Clin Orthop* 2003; 409:199-208.
Feldman DS, Madan SS, Koval KJ, et al: Correction of tibia vara with six-axis deformity analysis and the Taylor spatial frame. *J Pediatr Orthop* 2003;23:387-391.

In these two studies the advantages of external fixation for the treatment of infantile and adolescent Blount's disease are shown in 91 patients. Multiplanar correction can be achieved gradually, and alignment can be adjusted based on standing radiographs. Limb-length discrepancy can be addressed simultaneously.

Tokmakova K, Riddle EC, Kumar SJ: Type IV congenital deficiency of the tibia. *J Pediatr Orthop* 2003;23:649-653.

Both reconstruction and amputation are considered for this rare deformity, and patients with a functional (or reconstructable) foot and a lesser degree of projected limb-length discrepancy may benefit from reconstruction of the ankle mortise and subsequent limb lengthening.

Congenital Pseudarthrosis of the Tibia and/or Fibula

Johnston CE II: Congenital pseudarthrosis of the tibia: Results of technical variations in the Charnley-Williams procedure. *J Bone Joint Surg Am* 2002;84-A:1799-1810.

Grafting and intramedullary fixation was most successful when concomitant fibular surgery was performed (osteotomy or resection, with or without intramedullary fixation). Outcome did not correlate with the initial radiographic appearance or age at surgery. Fibular involvement correlates with valgus deformity at the ankle.

Kim HW, Weinstein SL: Intramedullary fixation and bone grafting for congenital pseudarthrosis of the tibia. *Clin Orthop* 2002;405:250-257.

Five of 12 pseudarthroses united after one procedure (three refractures), and 4 of the other 7 eventually healed with multiple procedures. A poor prognosis was associated with distal pseudarthroses and concomitant pseudarthrosis of the fibula.

Ng BK: Saleh M: Fibula pseudarthrosis revisited treatment with Ilizarov apparatus: Case report and review of the literature. *J Pediatr Orthop B* 2001;10:234-237.
Yang KY, Lee EH: Isolated congenital pseudarthrosis of the fibula. *J Pediatr Orthop B* 2002;11:298-301.

These two articles review four patients with the rare disorder of pseudarthrosis of the fibula. Treatment priorities are to restore union and to prevent or treat valgus at the ankle.

Classic Bibliography

Achterman C, Kalamchi A: Congenital deficiency of the fibula. *J Bone Joint Surg Br* 1979;61:133-137.

Anderson DJ, Schoeneker PL, Sheridan JJ, et al: Use of an intramedullary rod for the treatment of congenital pseudarthrosis of the tibia. *J Bone Joint Surg Am* 1992; 74:161-168.

Boyd HB: Pathology and natural history of congenital pseudarthrosis of the tibia. *Clin Orthop* 1982;166:5-13.

Feldman MD, Schoenecker PL: Use of the metaphyseal-diaphyseal angle in the evaluation of bowed legs. *J Bone Joint Surg Am* 1993;75:1602-1609.

Greene WB: Infantile Tibia Vara. *J Bone Joint Surg Am* 1993;75:130-143.

Johnston CE II: Infantile Tibia Vara. *Clin Orthop* 1990; 255:13-23.

Jones D, Barnes J, Lloyd-Roberts GC: Congenital aplasia and dysplasia of the tibia with intact fibula: Classification and management. *J Bone Joint Surg Br* 1978;60:31-39.

Kalamchi A, Dawe RV: Congenital deficiency of the tibia. *J Bone Joint Surg Br* 1985;67:581-584.

Schoeneker PL, Capelli AM, Millar EA, et al: Congenital longitudinal deficiency of the tibia. *J Bone Joint Surg Am* 1989;71:278-287.

Chapter 64

Ankle and Foot: Pediatrics

Vincent S. Mosca, MD

William Hennrikus, MD

Clubfoot (Talipes Equinovarus)

Idiopathic clubfoot occurs in approximately 1 of every 1,000 live births, affects males twice as often as females, and is bilateral in approximately 50% of cases. Recent genetic research supports the hypothesis of a multifactorial pattern of inheritance in which genetics plays a central role. Environmental factors, such as maternal smoking and amniocentesis in the first trimester, may modulate the genetic expression of the disorder. Clubfoot can be identified on fetal ultrasound as early as the 12th week of gestation. The sensitivity and specificity are high, making prenatal counseling about treatment and prognosis an appropriate and beneficial activity.

The clubfoot is characterized by four basic deformities: (1) cavus (plantar flexion of the forefoot on the hindfoot, also described as pronation of the forefoot on the hindfoot); (2) adductus of the forefoot on the midfoot/hindfoot; (3) varus (or inversion) of the subtalar joint complex; and (4) equinus of the foot at the ankle. These deformities are not passively correctable. There is a single (occasionally double) posterior ankle skin crease and a deep transverse skin crease across the midfoot. In a clubfoot, the talus is smaller than normal, and the talar neck is deviated in a plantar medial direction. The axes of the anterior and middle facets of the calcaneus create a more acute angle than in the normal foot, with the anterior facet oriented inward. This creates a corresponding varus deformity of the distal end of the calcaneus, resulting in a medial orientation of the calcaneocuboid joint. There also may be varying degrees of medial subluxation at that joint.

A complete physical examination of the child is indicated to rule out a neurogenic or syndromic cause for the deformity. There is no reported increased risk for developmental dysplasia of the hip in children with clubfoot; however, examination of the hips in a newborn is always an important part of the musculoskeletal screening examination. The diagnosis of clubfoot in a newborn can and should be based solely on clinical findings. If radiographs are obtained, either before, during, or after initiation of treatment, they should be taken as stress dorsiflexion AP and lateral views. There is no indication for routine radiographs or ultrasound imaging of the child's hips.

The goal of treatment is a plantigrade foot with good joint mobility that is functional, painless, stable over time, and free of calluses. Initial treatment is nonsurgical. More than 50 years ago, Kite and Ponseti independently proposed significantly different manipulation and casting techniques for clubfoot deformity correction with each reporting extremely high success rates. For unknown reasons, neither technique came into widespread use and the past five decades have been marked by a proliferation of extensive and radical clubfoot surgeries. Short- and intermediate-term follow-up studies on these radical surgical procedures revealed a high percentage of painful, stiff, and deformed feet with the need for additional surgery in 5% to 50% of cases.

The Ponseti method has recently been reintroduced, based on scientific support of the efficacy of this method that was documented in a long-term follow-up study that was published in 1995. That study showed little difference in appearance, comfort, and function in 25- to 45-year-old patients with clubfoot who were treated as infants, compared with age-matched controls.

With the Ponseti method, the clubfoot is manipulated for 1 to 2 minutes before application of an above-knee cast. Cavus is corrected first, by dorsiflexing the first metatarsal against a fulcrum that is the dorsolateral aspect of the head of the talus. In subsequent weekly manipulations and above-knee cast applications, the adductus and varus are corrected by abducting the forefoot against the same fulcrum. Cavus, adductus, and varus are slightly overcorrected and the foot is externally rotated 60° to 70° in relation to the thigh after four to seven casts have been worn. Percutaneous tenotomy of the Achilles tendon is performed in approximately 90% of feet. The final above-knee cast is worn for 3 weeks. The Achilles tendon reforms in a lengthened state during that time. Straight-last shoes externally rotated on an abduction bar are then worn full-time for 3 months and at night for up to 3 years. At least 95% of clubfoot deformities can be corrected without the need for extensive surgery if the treatment is begun soon after birth. To be successful, this method must be studied in detail, mastered, and should not be modified.

Up to 40% of clubfeet will require lateral transfer of the tibialis anterior to the lateral cuneiform between the ages of 2 and 5 years to correct a dynamic muscle imbalance (supination deformity) that is inherent in the clubfoot and not related to the initial method of deformity correction.

Metatarsus Adductus

Metatarsus adductus is characterized by medial deviation of the forefoot on the midfoot with neutral or slight valgus alignment of the hindfoot. An important pathogenic factor may be a developmental abnormality that results in a trapezoid shape of the medial cuneiform with medial orientation of the first metatarsal-medial cuneiform joint. Metatarsus varus refers to a similar deformity in which the metatarsals are adducted as well as supinated. A skewfoot combines adduction and plantar flexion of the forefoot, with moderate to severe valgus deformity of the hindfoot. The literature is inconsistent with these definitions.

Metatarsus adductus can be classified according to the degree of deformity as mild, moderate, or severe using the heel bisector line. A second classification system, based on flexibility, is prognostic. Flexible metatarsus adductus deformities can be easily abducted beyond straight alignment. Partly flexible metatarsus adductus deformities correct to a straight foot alignment with passive abduction, and rigid feet do not straighten manually. Flexible metatarsus adductus, which accounts for 90% to 95% of all deformities, corrects spontaneously in the first 3 to 5 years of life. Partly flexible and rigid feet benefit from serial manipulation and casting in infants younger than 1 year of age. The lateral pressure point is at the calcaneocuboid joint, not the head of the talus as in clubfoot casting. The subtalar joint is held in slight inversion and the ankle in slight plantar flexion to prevent inadvertent eversion of the subtalar joint. Three to four weekly manipulations and long leg cast applications are needed to slightly overcorrect the deformity. A holding device, such as a reverse or straight-last shoe, should be used for several months thereafter to prevent recurrence of deformity. Good results can be expected at long-term follow-up without a need for surgery, even when there is mild to moderate residual deformity. Severe, rigid deformity in the older child may cause pain, callus formation, and shoe-fitting problems for which surgery would be indicated.

Tarsometatarsal capsulotomies and osteotomies at the base of the metatarsals are associated with significant complications. An opening wedge osteotomy of the trapezoid-shaped medial cuneiform offers treatment at the site of the deformity and is associated with few risks or complications. It may be necessary to perform a concurrent closing wedge osteotomy of the cuboid or osteotomies at the base of the lesser metatarsals.

Congenital Vertical Talus

Congential vertical talus is a dorsolateral dislocation of the talonavicular joint associated with extreme plantar flexion of the talus. The foot has a rocker-bottom appearance, and the head of the talus is prominent and palpable on the plantar-medial aspect of the midfoot. The hindfoot is plantar flexed. There is a dorsiflexion contracture of the forefoot on the hindfoot that prevents the creation of a longitudinal arch by passive manipulation. It is reported that the deformity occurs in association with syndromes such as arthrogryposis, myelomeningocele, and sacral agenesis in more than 50% of patients. Congential vertical talus is bilateral in 50% of affected children. The primary differential diagnosis is positional calcaneovalgus deformity, a condition that resolves completely in most patients. It is differentiated clinically by flexibility of the midfoot but a dorsiflexion contracture of the ankle joint. A lateral radiograph of a congenital vertical talus in maximum dorsiflexion shows fixed plantar flexion of the talus. A lateral radiograph in maximum plantar flexion shows an irreducible dislocation of the talonavicular joint and confirms the diagnosis.

Surgery is required for deformity correction in nearly all feet with congenital vertical talus. Preliminary serial plantar flexion casting is used to stretch the dorsal tendons, skin, and neurovascular structures of the foot. Reduction of the talonavicular joint dislocation is desired, but rarely achieved with casting.

In the past, treatment has been surgical reconstruction between ages 6 and 18 months using a single stage circumferential release. Surgical reconstruction through a dorsal approach to the talonavicular joint, with concurrent Achilles tendon lengthening, has more recently been shown to result in excellent and lasting deformity correction, with less scar formation and shorter surgical time. Naviculectomy, by shortening the elongated medial column of the foot, is an effective surgery for correcting recurrent or untreated congenital vertical talus deformity in the older child. This procedure preserves some motion in the resultant pseudo-subtalar joint complex. Subtalar and triple arthrodeses have also been recommended in the older age group, but it is technically challenging to correct severe valgus deformity of the hindfoot with either procedure, and these surgeries lead to stress transfer to adjacent joints. Subtalar arthrodesis has also been associated with progressive overcorrection of the deformity in some feet.

Tarsal Coalition

Tarsal coalition is a fibrous, cartilaginous, or bony connection between two or more tarsal bones that results from a congenital failure of differentiation and segmentation of primitive mesenchyme. It affects at least 1% to 2% of the general population and is most commonly seen as an autosomal dominant condition with nearly full penetrance. Talocalcaneal and calcaneonavicular coalitions occur with about equal frequency, are usually bilateral, and together account for nearly all coalitions. There may be more than one tarsal coalition in the same foot.

Maturation of the coalition coincides with the development of progressive valgus deformity of the hindfoot and restriction of subtalar motion, all of which are more severe in a foot with a talocalcaneal coalition. For an individual with a tarsal coalition who develops pain, the onset of symptoms may coincide with bony transformation of a previously cartilaginous coalition. This generally occurs between 8 and 12 years of age for those children with calcaneonavicular coalitions, and between 12 and 16 years of age for those with talocalcaneal coalitions. The onset of vague, aching, activity-related pain in the sinus tarsi area or along the medial aspect of the hindfoot is often insidious. The peroneal tendons appear to be in spasm and can develop a late contracture. The exact etiology and the anatomic location of the pain and spasm are debated. Examination of the foot reveals stiffness or rigidity of an everted subtalar joint. The hindfoot remains in valgus alignment even with toe standing.

Calcaneonavicular coalitions are best seen on an oblique radiograph of the foot. Talocalcaneal coalitions are best seen on coronal plane images of a CT scan. A CT scan should be obtained for feet with calcaneonavicular coalitions because a talocalcaneal coalition may coexist. MRI is helpful in identifying coalitions that are still in the fibrous stage and not visualized on radiographs or CT scans, but this should not be a first-line study. A bone scan can be helpful in identifying other possible etiologies for a rigid flatfoot with an atypical presentation of pain (osteoid osteoma, infection, fracture).

Treatment is indicated for symptomatic tarsal coalitions. Nonsurgical treatment such as cast immobilization, soft orthotic devices, and anti-inflammatory medications should be used initially. Surgical treatment is indicated if pain recurs after initially successful nonsurgical treatment. Good long-term pain relief can be expected in most patients after resection of calcaneonavicular coalitions with interposition of the extensor digitorum brevis. An osteologic study has shown at least three anatomic variations for calcaneonavicular coalitions. Poor results may correlate with the exact pathologic anatomy of the coalition. The short-term results of resection and soft-tissue interposition for talocalcaneal coalitions have been good, but the results deteriorate rapidly with time and long-term studies are not available. Unsatisfactory results with resection have been reported in feet in which the ratio of the surface area of the coalition to the surface area of the posterior facet was greater than 50% (as determined by CT scan) and in which there was significant valgus deformity of the hindfoot and narrowing of the posterior facet. The independent influence of the size of the coalition was not determined in that or any other study. Some authors recommend resection of a symptomatic talocalcaneal coalition regardless of its size if the foot is not fixed in severe valgus alignment. The presence of a talar beak does not necessarily indicate the presence of degenerative arthrosis and is not, by itself, a contraindication for resection. Documented degenerative arthrosis and persistence or recurrence of pain following coalition resection are considered by some to be indications for triple arthrodesis, though supportive data are lacking. Severe symptomatic valgus deformity of the hindfoot associated with a talocalcaneal coalition can be corrected and pain relieved with a calcaneal osteotomy with or without concurrent resection of the coalition.

Fractures

Intra-articular ankle fractures are uncommon but problematic in children. Four general fracture types are medial malleolar fractures, Tillaux fractures, triplane fractures, and pilon fractures. Controversial aspects in the treatment of these injuries include the indications for a CT scan and how much displacement indicates reduction and fixation. Complications stemming from these injuries center on growth arrest and articular incongruity.

Medial malleolar fractures occur in young children with an average age of injury of 8 years. The mechanism of injury is supination and inversion of the foot resulting in a Salter-Harris type III or IV injury. Three radiographic views of the ankle are recommended: AP (Figure 1), lateral, and oblique. CT is not needed in most instances. Any displacement of a physeal fracture of the medial malleolus requires reduction and possible fixation. These injuries occur in younger children with many years of growth remaining; therefore, anatomic reduction is needed to minimize angular deformity and shortening. Treatment strategies involve closed reduction and pinning or cannulated screw fixation. If open reduction and internal fixation is needed, minimal stripping of the periosteum is recommended to prevent iatrogenic growth arrest (Figure 2). When treating a Salter-Harris type IV injury, the Thurston-Holland fragment can be safely removed to visualize the physis. Visualization of the joint can be accomplished by a small anterior arthrotomy. Fixation should be performed parallel to rather than across the physis. Screws provide compres-

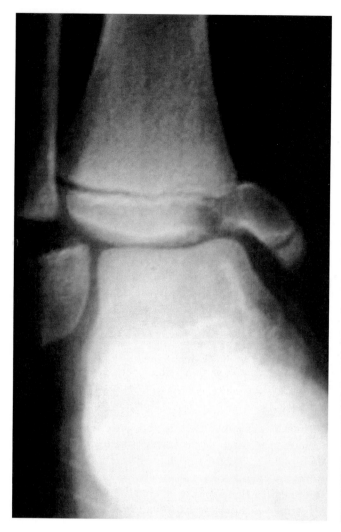

Figure 1 AP radiograph of the ankle showing a displaced medial malleolar physeal fracture and a displaced distal fibular physeal fracture.

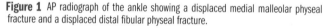

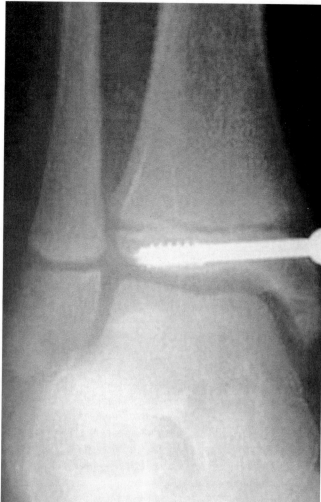

Figure 2 AP radiograph following closed reduction of the fibular fracture and open reduction and internal fixation of the medial malleolar fracture.

sion and may therefore be superior to Kirschner wires. Osteotomy and physeal bar resection may be needed if growth arrest occurs. Long-term follow-up shows that osteoarthritis results in about 10% of these injuries.

Tillaux fractures occur in older children (average age, 13 years). The mechanism of injury is supination and external rotation resulting in the avulsion of the anterior-lateral distal tibial physis by the pull of the anterior-inferior tibia-fibula ligament. The maturing distal tibial physis closes centrally, then medially, then laterally. The open lateral physis is vulnerable to injury in this age group. Three radiographic views are needed. In one third of patients, the Tillaux fracture is only seen on the oblique view. The articular surface displacement needs to be reduced to less than 2 mm to minimize the development of osteoarthritis. Articular congruity is the major concern; physeal arrest is not a concern because the patient is close to skeletal maturity. CT is commonly used and appears to be better than radiographs in determining if the fracture is displaced greater than 2 mm

(Figure 3). Treatment strategies include attempted closed reduction by internal rotation, supination, and direct pressure; percutaneous manipulation with a Steinmann pin; and open reduction and internal fixation using a small anterior arthrotomy. Compression screw fixation can cross the physis because the remaining growth potential is minimal. Long-term follow-up studies are needed.

Triplane fractures occur in children nearing skeletal maturity (average age, 14 years). The mechanism of injury is supination and external rotation. The number of fracture fragments depends on which part of the physis is closed at the time of injury. The fracture occurs in three planes: the coronal plane—the lateral radiograph shows a Salter-Harris type II fracture; transverse plane—epiphysiolysis through the anterior and lateral physis; or sagittal plane—the AP radiograph typically shows a Salter-Harris type III fracture. The extent of the injury is often underappreciated on plain films; therefore, CT is recommended in most cases. CT defines the

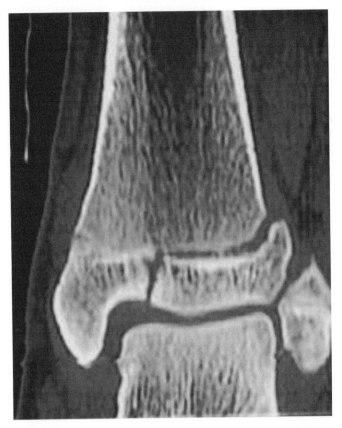

Figure 3 Reformatted CT showing the extent of displacement of a Tillaux fracture.

number of fracture fragments, defines the displacement, and helps in planning surgical incisions. Articular congruity, not physeal arrest, is the major concern with triplane fractures because the patient has almost reached skeletal maturity. The goal of treatment is to restore the articular displacement to less than 2 mm to minimize long-term osteoarthritis. Treatment strategies include closed reduction, closed reduction and fixation, and open reduction and internal fixation. Fixation can cross the physis, and screws are recommended to provide compression. The 2-mm limit of displacement may not be the only factor in long-term outcome. Injury to the distal tibiofibular joint and damage to the articular cartilage at the time of injury may lead to long-term symptoms despite an adequate reduction. Pilon fractures are discussed in chapter 39.

Puncture Wounds

Most puncture wounds of the foot are treated by emergency department and primary care physicians and do not require orthopaedic care. One study defined the natural history of plantar puncture wounds by following 63 patients prospectively. Treatment in the emergency department included surface cleaning alone. Five infections (8%) and two retained foreign bodies (3%) occurred. An infection and/or a retained foreign body are the two most common reasons for a patient with a plantar puncture wound to be referred for orthopaedic care. *Pseudomonas* septic arthritis or osteomyelitis should be suspected in any patient with swelling and foot pain that occurs after stepping on a nail while wearing a sneaker. *Pseudomonas* bacteria commonly grow in the foam rubber in the sole of the sneaker. *Pseudomonas* have an affinity to invade the cartilaginous joint surfaces and physes. Therefore, in infection stemming from a nail puncture wound through a sneaker, open surgical débridement and a course of intravenous antibiotics are recommended. Consultation with an infectious disease specialist should be considered in problematic cases. In patients with suspected retained foreign bodies, radiographs are indicated to detect radiodense objects such as needle fragments and some types of glass; ultrasound can be used to detect radiolucent glass fragments, toothpicks, and splinters. Not all patients require wound exploration and a search for a foreign body. A 3-week period of short leg casting results in the extrusion of radiolucent foreign bodies in some instances. Wound exploration, when deemed necessary, is best done in the operating theater with adequate anesthesia, magnification, and fluoroscopy. A tetanus update is recommended for any patient with a plantar puncture wound.

Apophysitis/Osteochondrosis

Sever's disease (apophysitis of the calcaneus) is a common cause of heel pain in the child and adolescent. Kohler's disease and Freiberg's infraction are less common causes of midfoot pain and metatarsal pain in this age group.

Sever's Disease

Sever's disease is a traction apophysitis at the insertion of the Achilles tendon. The patient reports heel pain that worsens during participation in running sports. Physical examination shows tenderness at the insertion of the Achilles tendon on the calcaneus. In addition, most patients have decreased ankle dorsiflexion compared with the uninvolved side and pain with forced dorsiflexion of the ankle. The pain associated with Sever's disease increases with activity and decreases with rest. Radiographs are normal and rule out conditions such as calcaneal bone cyst or calcaneal stress fracture that can have similar symptoms.

Symptomatic treatment consisting of rest, Achilles tendon stretching, ice, nonsteroidal anti-inflammatory drugs, and modification of running activity is recommended. In addition, a 1-cm heel cushion may be helpful to decrease traction on the apophysis and reduce symptoms. If the pain persists despite the previously outlined treatment, immobilization in a short leg walking cast for 1 to 2 months is recommended. Unfortunately, an undulating course with possible recurrences of pain is common, and patient education about the natural history of Sever's disease is key. The problem abates at skeletal maturity when the apophysis closes. No long-term complications have been reported.

Kohler's Disease

Kohler's disease is osteonecrosis of the tarsal navicular. Radiographs show flattening sclerosis and irregularities. The disorder is more common in boys and is bilateral in about 20% of patients. It is believed that Kohler's disease stems from repetitive microtrauma to the midfoot with weight bearing. A possible genetic predisposition has been suggested. The patient with Kohler's disease limps and bears weight on the lateral side of the foot. Physical examination shows tenderness and occasional swelling at the medial midfoot. Treatment consists of foot support. Rest combined with a soft arch support is recommended for mild symptoms. A short leg walking cast for 1 to 2 months followed by a soft arch support is recommended for more severe symptoms. Casting appears to hasten the resolution of symptoms compared with orthotic devices alone. However, the duration of time for radiographic bone restoration averages 8 months despite the treatment selected. Clinical deformity such as flatfoot does not occur.

Freiberg's Infraction

Freiberg's infraction is osteonecrosis of one of the metatarsal heads. The etiology may involve repetitive microtrauma disrupting the blood supply. The condition occurs most often in adolescent female athletes. The longest metatarsal, usually the second, is typically affected. Radiographs show metatarsal head irregularity, enlargement, flattening, and sclerosis. In patients with advanced etiology, joint space narrowing and osteochondritis dissecans may develop. Patients with Freiberg's infraction report forefoot pain. Physical examination shows local swelling and tenderness over the metatarsal head with occasional stiffness of the metatarsophalangeal joint. Most patients can be treated symptomatically with activity modification, nonsteroidal anti-inflammatory drugs, a metatarsal bar shoe insert, or a change in shoe wear to relieve the weight-bearing stress on the involved metatarsal head. A short leg walking cast followed by a metatarsal bar is sometimes required for more severe cases. Usually, the disease runs its course and the metatarsal head reconstitutes in about 2 years. In the minority of patients in whom conservative care is unsuccessful, surgery is indicated. Surgery should be performed with caution because the reported series are small and without comparison groups. Surgical options include metatarsophalangeal arthrotomy and removal of loose bodies, drilling the metatarsal head, subchondral bone grafting, interposition arthroplasty using the extensor digitorum longus tendon, and dorsiflexion

osteotomy or shortening osteotomy. Metatarsal head resection is not recommended because this procedure may transfer pressure and pain to an adjacent metatarsal head.

Adolescent Bunion

Adolescent bunion is a prominence of the medial aspect of the first metatarsal head associated with a valgus deformity of the hallux. Weight-bearing AP and lateral radiographs of the feet confirm the clinical diagnosis. Normal radiographic angles between the first and second metatarsals (intermetatarsal angle) are from 6° to 10° and between the first metatarsal and the proximal phalanx (hallux valgus angle) are from 10° to 20°. A bunion in an adolescent is present if the intermetatarsal angle exceeds 10° and the hallux valgus angle exceeds 20°. The etiology of adolescent bunion is multifactorial. The patient usually comes for treatment because of the cosmetic deformity and is rarely symptomatic. Physical examination shows abnormal angulation and mobility of the first metatarsocuneiform joint, medial deviation of the first metatarsal, and a congruous first metatarsophalangeal joint. The results of surgery in an adolescent with a bunion are unpredictable with a 50% recurrence rate. Associated pes planus, a tight Achilles tendon, and a long great toe result in the highest recurrence rate. Therefore, surgery should be delayed until skeletal maturity if possible. Suggested treatment options until the patient reaches skeletal maturity include a shoe with a wide, rounded toe box, a total contact insole with a fixed toe separator, and daily exercises combined with a nighttime thermoplastic splint. Surgery may be considered in patients who have exhausted nonsurgical treatment options and still experience pain that interferes with normal activities. No single surgical technique is applicable in all patients. Proximal metatarsal osteotomy should be used with caution if the proximal physis is open; otherwise, growth arrest and shortening may occur. Shortening can result in transfer metatarsalgia.

Annotated Bibliography

Clubfoot (Talipes Equinovarus)

Dietz F: The genetics of idiopathic clubfoot. *Clin Orthop* 2002;401:39-48.

An excellent and comprehensive review of this important aspect of clubfoot is presented.

Herzenberg JE, Radler C, Bor N: Ponseti versus traditional methods of casting for idiopathic clubfoot. *J Pediatr Orthop* 2002;22:517-521.

This is the first report from outside of Iowa comparing the Ponseti method for clubfoot deformity correction with traditional casting followed by extensive posteromedial release surgery. The authors' results with 34 clubfeet treated with the Ponseti method matched the results reported by Ponseti decades ago and recently, and revealed superiority over the traditional method.

Ippolito E, Farsetti P, Caterini R, Tudisco C: Long-term comparative results in patients with congenital clubfoot treated with two different protocols. *J Bone Joint Surg Am* 2003;85-A:1286-1294.

Forty-seven clubfeet treated with extensive posteromedial release (after an average of 16 abduction/pronation casts) were compared with 49 clubfeet treated with an open Achilles Z-lengthening and posterior ankle capsulotomy (after an average of six Ponseti-type supination/abduction casts). Follow-up at 25 years for group one and 19 years for group two showed significantly better results in the second group, although not as good as the results reported by Cooper and Dietz using the traditional Ponseti technique with percutaneous Achilles tenotomy. The authors recommend treating clubfeet according to the method of Ponseti.

Kuo KN, Hennigan SP, Hastings ME: Anterior tibial tendon transfer in residual dynamic clubfoot deformity. *J Pediatr Orthop* 2001;21:35-41.

Forty-two full anterior tibial tendon transfers to the lateral cuneiform were compared with 29 split anterior tibial tendon transfers to the cuboid as treatment of dynamic supination deformity of previously operated clubfeet. There was no significant difference in results between the two techniques.

Pirani S, Zeznik L, Hodges D: Magnetic resonance imaging study of the congenital clubfoot treated with the Ponseti method. *J Pediatr Orthop* 2001;21:719-726.

MRI was performed on infant clubfeet undergoing manipulation and cast treatment according to the Ponseti method at the beginning, middle, and end of treatment. Correction of abnormal relationships between tarsal bones was documented. Additionally, the abnormal shapes of the individual tarsal osteochondral anlages were corrected. This effect can be accounted for by changes in mechanical loading of these fast-growing tissues.

Skelly AC, Holt VL, Mosca VS, Alderman BW: Talipes equinovarus and maternal smoking: A population-based case-control study in Washington state. *Teratology* 2002; 66:91-100.

This article presents an epidemiology study showing an increased risk of having a child with clubfoot if the mother smoked during pregnancy. There was a dose response with increased risk correlated with the number of cigarettes smoked.

Tredwell SJ, Wilson D, Wilmink MA, et al: Review of the effect of early amniocentesis on foot deformity in the neonate. *J Pediatr Orthop* 2001;21:636-641.

Clubfoot was identified in 1.63% of live births in mothers who had undergone early amniocentesis (11 to approximately 12 gestational weeks/day) versus 0.12% in those who underwent midtrimester amniocentesis (15 to approximately 16 ges-

tational weeks/day). The authors hypothesize that decreased amniotic fluid in the early group, during the time of maximum foot growth velocity, leads to decreased fetal movement resulting in joint and limb deformities.

Congenital Vertical Talus

Mazzocca AD, Thomson JD, Deluca PA, Romness MJ: Comparison of the posterior approach versus the dorsal approach in the treatment on congenital vertical talus. *J Pediatr Orthop* 2001;21:212-217.

Twenty-five consecutive congenital vertical tali that were treated with a traditional posterior release operation (average age, 18 months; range, 6 to 67 months) were compared with eight consecutive feet treated with deformity correction via the dorsal approach (average age, 26.5 months; range, 6 to 65 months). The dorsal approach group required 30% less surgical time, had better clinical scores, and fewer complications including no recurrences (versus 32%) and no cases of osteonecrosis of the talus (versus 48%).

Tarsal Coalition

Cooperman DR, Janke BE, Gilmore A, Latimer BM, Brinker MR, Thompson GH: A three-dimensional study of calcaneonavicular tarsal coalitions. *J Pediatr Orthop* 2001;21:648-651.

Thirty-seven presumed calcaneonavicular tarsal coalitions from the Todd Osteological Collection in Cleveland were studied. The anterior facet of the calcaneus was completely spared by the coalition in 8 specimens, partially replaced by the navicular portion of the coalition in 7, and completely replaced by the navicular portion of the coalition in 22. It is hypothesized that this variable coalition anatomy is a potential cause for poor results after resection, particularly if the resection creates joint instability.

Fractures

Barmada A, Gaynor T, Mubarak SJ: Premature physeal closure following distal tibia physeal fractures. *J Pediatr Orthop* 2003;23:733-739.

A residual physeal gap of more than 3 mm following treatment of a distal tibial physeal fracture was associated with high rates of premature physeal closure. The authors suggest that open reduction and removal of entrapped periosteum may be beneficial.

Horn BD, Crisci K, Krug M, et al: Radiologic evaluation of juvenile Tillaux fractures of the distal tibia. *J Pediatr Orthop* 2001;21:162-164.

CT is the preferred imaging modality for detecting more than 2 mm of displacement in juvenile Tillaux fractures.

Leetum DT, Ireland ML: Arthroscopically assisted reduction and fixation of a juvenile Tillaux fracture. *Arthroscopy* 2002;18:427-429.

Arthroscopic visualization assisted with the anatomic reduction of the articular fragment, obviating the need for ankle arthrotomy, is discussed.

Leets M, Davidson D, McCaffrey M: The adolescent pilon fracture: management and outcome. *J Pediatr Orthop* 2001;21:20-26.

Pilon fractures in adolescents result from high-energy trauma and are associated with a high complication rate. Results were good to excellent in only 63% of cases. The authors suggest a new classification system for adolescent pilon fractures.

Marsh JL, Buckwalter J, Gelberman R, et al: Articular fractures: does anatomic reduction really change the result? *J Bone Joint Surg Am* 2002;84-A:1259-1271.

The authors suggest that there is no convincing evidence that improved articular reduction leads to a better outcome or a lower risk of osteoarthritis. Rather, the authors suggest that damage to the articular cartilage at the time of injury is the most important factor in outcome.

Seifert J, Matthes G, Hinz P, et al: Role of MRI in the diagnosis of distal tibia fractures in adolescents. *J Pediatr Orthop* 2003;23:727-732.

The authors report that MRI provided anatomic detail and information about the joint surfaces superior to plain film radiographs.

Apophysitis/Osteochondrosis

Tang SF, Chen CP, Pan JL, et al: The effects of a new foot-toe orthosis in treating painful hallux valgus. *Arch Phys Med Rehabil* 2002;83:1792-1795.

The authors report that using a total contact insole with a fixed toe separator reduced pain and improved the hallux valgus angle without causing skin ulcers or blisters.

Tsirikos AI, Riddle EC, Kruse R: Bilateral Kohler's disease in identical twins. *Clin Orthop* 2003;409:195-198.

Bilateral Kohler's disease in identical twins suggests that a genetic predisposition to the disorder may exist.

Volpon JB, de Carvalo Filho G: Calcaneal apophysitis: A quantitative radiographic evaluation of the secondary ossification center. *Arch Orthop Trauma Surg* 2002;122:338-341.

A radiographic study of patients with Sever's disease compared with normal control patients is presented. The sclerotic aspect of the calcaneus apophysis is a normal finding and should not be used to establish the diagnosis of Sever's disease.

Classic Bibliography

Bleck E: Metatarsus adductus: Classification and relationship to outcomes of treatment. *J Pediatr Orthop* 1983;3:2-9.

Caterini R, Farsetti P, Ippolitio E: Long term follow up of physeal injury to the ankle. *Foot Ankle* 1991;11:372-383.

Clark M, D'Ambrosia R, Ferguson A: Congenital vertical talus: Treatment by open reduction and navicular excision. *J Bone Joint Surg Am* 1977;59:816-824.

Cooper D, Dietz F: Treatment of idiopathic clubfoot: A thirty-year follow-up note. *J Bone Joint Surg Am* 1995; 77:1477-1489.

Coughlin MJ, Bordelon RL, Johnson KA, et al: Evaluation and treatment of juvenile hallux valgus. *Contemp Orthop* 1990;21:169-203.

Duncan RD, Fixsen JA: Congenital convex pes valgus. *J Bone Joint Surg Br* 1999;81:250-254.

Ezra E, Hayek S, Gilai AN, Khermosh O, Wientroub S: Tibialis anterior tendon transfer for residual dynamic supination deformity in treated clubfeet. *J Pediatr Orthop B* 2000;9:207-211.

Farsetti P, Weinstein SL, Ponseti IV: The long-term functional and radiographic outcomes of untreated and nonoperatively treated metatarsus adductus. *J Bone Joint Surg Am* 1994;76:257-265.

Freiberg AH: The so-called infarction of the second metatarsal bone. *J Bone Joint Surg* 1926;8:257.

Grosoia JA: Juvenile hallux valgus: A conservative approach to treatment. *J Bone Joint Surg Am* 1992;74: 1367-1374.

Honein MA, Paulozzi LJ, Moore CA: Family history, maternal smoking, and clubfoot: An indication of a gene-environment interaction. *Am J Epidemiol* 2000; 152:658-665.

Huurman WW, Bhuller GS: Nonoperative treatment of retained radio lucent foreign bodies in lower limbs. *J Pediatr Orthop* 1982;2:506-508.

Ippolitoo E, Ricciardi Pollini PT, Falez F: Kohler's disease of the tarsal navicular: Long-term follow up of 12 cases. *J Pediatr Orthop* 1984;4:416-417.

Katcherian DA: Treatment of Freiberg's disease. *Orthop Clin North Am* 1994;25:69-81.

Kling TF, Bright RW, Hensinger RN: Distal tibial physeal fractures in children that may require open reduction. *J Bone Joint Surg Am* 1984;66:647-657.

Kumar S, Guille J, Lee M, Couto J: Osseous and nonosseous coalition of the middle facet of the talocalcaneal joint. *J Bone Joint Surg Am* 1992;74:529-535.

Laaveg S, Ponseti I: Long-term results of treatment of congenital club foot. *J Bone Joint Surg Am* 1980;62:23-31.

Leonard MA: The inheritance of tarsal coalition and its relationship to spastic flat foot. *J Bone Joint Surg Br* 1974;56:520-526.

McHale KA, Lenhart MK: Treatment of residual club-foot deformity, the "bean-shaped" foot, by open wedge medial cuneiform osteotomy and closing wedge cuboid osteotomy: Clinical review and cadaver correlations. *J Pediatr Orthop* 1991;11:374-381.

Micheli LJ, Ireland ML: Prevention and management of calcaneal apophysitis in children: An overuse syndrome. *J Pediatr Orthop* 1987;7:34-38.

Pennycook A, Makaower R, O'Donnell AM: Puncture wounds of the foot: Can infective complications be avoided? *J R Soc Med* 1994;87:581-583.

Ponseti I: *Congenital Clubfoot.* Oxford, England, Oxford University Press, 1996.

Ponseti IV, Becker JR: Congenital metatarsus adductus: The results of treatment. *J Bone Joint Surg Am* 1966;48: 702-711.

Rebbeck T, Dietz F, Murray J, Buetow K: A single-gene explanation for the probability of having idiopathic talipes equinovarus. *Am J Hum Genet* 1993;53:1051-1063.

Schwab RA, Powers RD: Conservative therapy for plantar puncture wounds. *J Emerg Med* 1995;13:291-295.

Seimon L: Surgical correction of congenital vertical talus under the age of 2 years. *J Pediatr Orthop* 1987;7: 405-411.

Sever JW: Apophysitis of the os calcis. *NY Med J* 1912;95:1025.

Wilde P, Torode I, Dickens D, Cole W: Resection for symptomatic talocalcaneal coalition. *J Bone Joint Surg Br* 1994;76:797-801.

Williams GA, Cowell HR: Kohler's disease of the tarsal navicular. *Clin Orthop* 1981;158:53-58.

Chapter 65

Pediatric Spine Trauma

William C. Warner, Jr, MD

Gregory A. Mencio, MD

Introduction

Cervical spine injuries are uncommon in children and usually are associated with motor vehicle crashes, pedestrian-vehicle accidents, or falls in young children. In older children, sports injuries, diving accidents, and gunshot injuries are the most common causes. An awareness of the unique aspects of the pediatric cervical spine and an understanding of its growth and development are necessary for correct diagnosis and proper treatment. Normal physes may be mistaken for fractures, resulting in overtreatment, and certain fractures that occur through open physes may be undertreated.

The atlas develops from three ossification centers (Figure 1). The posterior arches fuse by 3 to 4 years of age, and the neurocentral synchondrosis between the lateral masses and the body fuse at approximately 7 years of age. The odontoid process is separated from the body of the axis by a synchondrosis, which usually is fused by 6 to 7 years of age. This synchondrosis appears as a "cork in a bottle" on an open mouth odontoid radiograph. The lower cervical vertebrae also are composed of three primary ossification centers, one for the body and two for the neural arches. The neural arches fuse posteriorly by 3 years of age, and the neurocentral synchondrosis fuses with the body between 3 and 6 years of age. The vertebral bodies are wedge-shaped until 7 years of age, and then gradually become rectangular.

Upper cervical spine injuries are more common in children between birth and 8 years of age. After 8 years of age, the injury patterns become more like those in adults, with the lower cervical spine more frequently involved. Factors contributing to the increased frequency of upper cervical spine injuries in the young child include the relatively horizontal facets, the large head size relative to trunk size, muscle weakness, and the increased physiologic motion of the neck in children.

In young children, diagnosis of a cervical spine injury may be difficult; repeated examinations and a high index of suspicion often are needed. Upper cervical spine injuries are frequent in young children with facial trauma (fractures) and head trauma. Any pain or persistent tenderness, paraspinal muscle spasms, limitation of motion, or persistent torticollis should alert the examiner to a possible cervical spine injury. An adequate neurologic examination is difficult in a frightened child, and frequent examinations may be required to reliably determine neurologic status.

Initial radiographs should include cross-table lateral, AP, and odontoid open-mouth views. It is mandatory that the cervicothoracic junction be visible on the plain radiographs. On the lateral radiographs, four lines should be drawn corresponding to the anterior vertebral bodies, the posterior vertebral bodies, the inside of the lamina (spinolaminar line), and the tips of the spinous processes (Figure 2). All four of these lines should follow a smooth, even contour. The articular facets should be parallel and the interspinous ligaments balanced. The retropharyngeal space should be less than 7 mm, and the retrotracheal space should be less than 14 mm in children. An atlanto-dens interval of 4 to 5 mm is normal in young children; in adults and adolescents, this interval should be 3 mm. The atlanto-dens interval is increased in young children because a significant portion of the dens is cartilaginous and not visible on plain radiographs. This situation also gives the appearance of overriding of the atlas on the unossified odontoid on extension lateral radiographic views. Oblique radiographs show details of the facet joints and pedicles and are useful for determining if a fracture or fracture-dislocation is present. Flexion and extension radiographs should be obtained only in an awake and cooperative child under the supervision of a physician; these radiographs may be inappropriate in a very young child or an obtunded patient. Because of the increased physiologic motion in young children, pseudosubluxation of the second cervical vertebra on the third or the third cervical vertebra on the fourth may be present, most commonly in children 1 to 7 years of age. Swischuk's line is helpful in differentiating this phenomenon from true injury. This line is drawn along the posterior arch (spinolaminar line) of C1 to C3 and should pass within 1.5 mm of the posterior arch of C2 (Figure 3).

CT scans with three-dimensional reconstruction views may be helpful in identifying fractures of the upper cer-

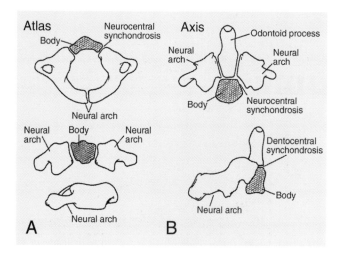

Figure 1 A, Ossification centers of the atlas. **B,** Ossification centers for the axis. *(Reproduced from Copley LA, Dormans JP: Cervical spine disorders in infants and children.* J Am Acad Orthop Surg *1998;6:205.)*

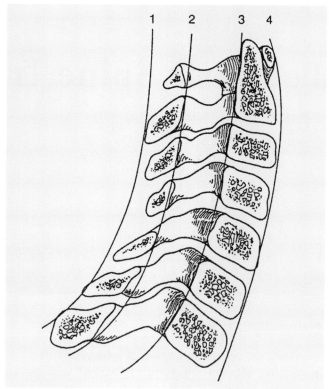

Figure 2 Normal relationships in the lateral aspect of the cervical spine. 1 = spinous processes, 2 = spinolaminar line, 3 = posterior vertebral body line, and 4 = anterior vertebral body line. *(Reproduced from Copley LA, Dormans JP: Cervical spine disorders in infants and children.* J Am Acad Orthop Surg *1998; 6:205.)*

vical spine (base of the skull, C1 or C2 vertebra) and in evaluating atlantoaxial rotatory subluxation. MRI is especially useful for ruling out cervical spine injuries in patients who are obtunded or have a closed head injury and may be difficult to evaluate because of their associated injuries. In a recent study, MRI was able to "clear" the cervical spine in intubated, obtunded, and uncooperative children with suspected cervical spine injuries. MRI also was useful in documenting or ruling out injuries suggested by plain radiographs and CT scans. MRI confirmed the plain radiography diagnosis in 66% of patients and altered the diagnosis in 34%.

Adequate immobilization of the cervical spine is difficult in children. Because commercial cervical collars often do not fit properly, they do not provide adequate immobilization. Sandbags can be placed on each side of the head to prevent motion. Spine boards used for children should be modified to accommodate the large size of the head in relationship to the trunk. An occipital recess or a split mattress technique should be used to prevent unwanted flexion of the cervical spine (Figure 4). A halo ring and vest can be used for immobilization of the cervical spine in children, but an increased complication rate has been reported in children compared with adults. CT scanning can help in pin placement to avoid cranial sutures and thin areas of the skull. Eight to 12 pins with low insertional torques of 1 to 5 inch-lb are used in children. The vest often must be custom fitted to avoid motion in the vest portion while the head is fixed in the halo portion of the orthosis.

Specific Cervical Spine Injuries
Atlanto-Occipital Dislocation

In the past, atlanto-occipital dislocation usually was a fatal injury, but with current emergency medical care

and increased awareness of this injury, more children are surviving atlanto-occipital dislocations. Dislocation of the atlanto-occipital joint is caused by a sudden deceleration injury, such as a motor vehicle or pedestrian-vehicle accident. The child's head is thrown forward on the relatively fixed trunk, causing sudden cranioverte-bral separation. Because the atlanto-occipital joint has little inherent bony stability and most of its stability is provided by its ligamentous attachments, most atlanto-occipital dislocations are unstable and require surgical stabilization. The diagnosis of this condition may be difficult but is suggested by the mechanism of injury and the significant amount of anterior soft-tissue swelling visible on lateral radiographs.

The three most reliable radiographic findings to assist in the diagnosis of atlanto-occipital dislocation are (1) the Wackenheim line, (2) the Powers ratio, and (3) the occipital condylar distance. The Wackenheim line is drawn along the clivus and should intersect tangentially the tip of the odontoid (Figure 5). An anterior or posterior shift of this line indicates an anterior or posterior displacement of the occiput on the atlas. The Powers ratio is determined by drawing a line from the basion to the posterior arch of the atlas and a second line from the opisthion to the anterior arch of the atlas (Figure 6). A ratio of more than 1.0 or less than 0.55 represents a

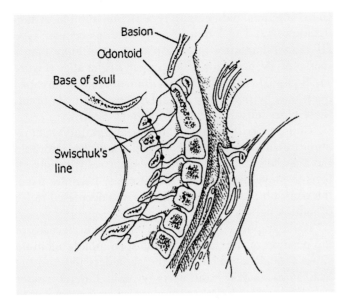

Figure 3 The spinolaminar (Swischuk's) line is used to differentiate pseudosubluxation from true injury. *(Reproduced from Copley LA, Dormans JP: Cervical spine disorders in infants and children. J Am Acad Orthop Surg 1998;6:205.)*

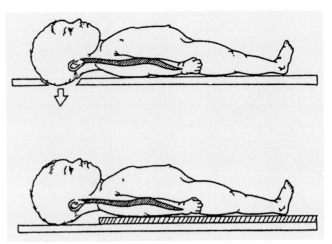

Figure 4 Spine boards used for transportation of young children should be modified to include either an occipital recess (top figure) or a mattress pad (bottom figure) to accommodate the relatively large head. *(Reproduced from Dormans JP: Evaluation of children with suspected cervical spine injury. Instr Course Lect 2002;51:403.)*

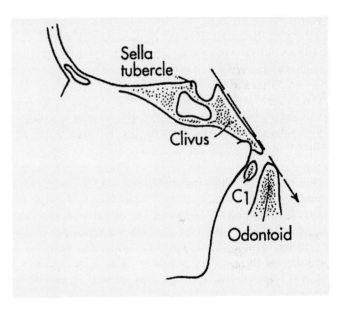

Figure 5 Wackenheim clivus-canal line is drawn along the clivus into the cervical spinal canal and should pass just posterior to the tip of the odontoid. *(Reproduced with permission from Menezes AH, Ryken TC: Craniovertebral junction abnormalities, in Weinstein SL (ed): The Pediatric Spine: Principles and Practice. New York, NY, Raven, 1994.)*

disruption of the atlanto-occipital joint. An occipital condyle facet distance of more than 5 mm from the occipital condyle to the C1 facet also represents a disruption of the atlanto-occipital joint. MRI also is useful for documenting soft-tissue injury associated with atlanto-occipital dislocation.

Atlanto-occipital dislocation should be stabilized surgically with a posterior occiput to C1 or C2 fusion. Because of the instability of this injury, the preoperative use of a halo or traction may be contraindicated.

Fractures of the Ring of C1

Fractures of the ring of C1 are uncommon injuries in both children and adults. The mechanism of injury is an axial load to the head; the force is transmitted through the occipital condyles to the lateral masses of C1. In adults, the ring usually breaks in two places, but in children the open synchondrosis of C1 allows a single fracture of the ring and a greenstick fracture through the synchondrosis. Widening of the lateral masses of more than 7 mm beyond the borders of the axis on an AP radiograph indicates an injury to the transverse ligament. In children, avulsion of the ligament from its attachments is more likely than a true rupture of the transverse ligament. Nonsurgical treatment is recommended for most patients with this injury.

Odontoid Fractures

Odontoid fractures are one of the most common cervical spine fractures in children. Most are associated with head trauma from a motor vehicle crash or a fall from a height, although odontoid fracture can occur with trivial head trauma. In children, this fracture most often occurs

through the synchondrosis of C2 distally at the base of the odontoid and appears on radiographs as a physeal (Salter-Harris type I) injury. The fracture usually is apparent on plain lateral radiographs, which show the anterior displacement of the odontoid. If the fracture through the synchondrosis has spontaneously reduced, it appears as a nondisplaced Salter-Harris type I fracture. CT and MRI may be necessary to fully delineate the injury. Most odontoid fractures in children heal uneventfully and complications are rare. Closed reduction is obtained by extension or slight hyperextension of the neck. At least 50% apposition should be obtained (com-

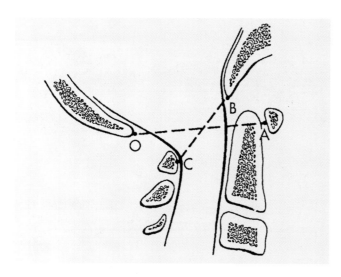

Figure 6 The Powers ratio is determined by drawing a line from the basion (B) to the posterior arch of the atlas (C) and a second line from the opisthion (O) to the anterior arch of the atlas (A). The length of line BC is divided by the length of the line OA. A ratio of more than 1 is diagnostic of anterior atlanto-occipital translation and a ratio of less than 0.55 indicates posterior translation. *(Reproduced with permission from Parfenchuck TA, Bertrand SL, Powers MJ, et al: Posterior occipitoatlantal hypermobiliy in Down syndrome: An analysis of 199 patients. J Pediatr Orthop 1994; 304.)*

plete reduction of the translation is not necessary) before immobilization in a Minerva or halo cast or custom orthosis for 6 to 8 weeks. Manipulation under anesthesia or open reduction and internal fixation rarely are required.

Traumatic Ligamentous Dislocation

Acute rupture of the tranverse ligament is rare, reported to occur in less than 10% of pediatric cervical spine injuries; avulsion of the attachment of the transverse ligament to C1 is more common. The transverse ligament is the primary stabilizer of an intact odontoid against forward displacement. The normal distance from the anterior cortex of the dens to the posterior cortex of the anterior ring of C1 is 4.5 mm in children and a distance of more than this, measured on a lateral radiograph, suggests disruption of the transverse ligament. CT is useful to show avulsion of the transverse ligament from the ring of C1. For acute injuries, reduction in extension is recommended, followed by surgical stabilization of C1 and C2 and immobilization for 8 to 12 weeks in a Minerva cast, halo brace, or cervical orthosis.

Atlantoaxial Rotatory Subluxation

Atlantoaxial rotatory subluxation is a common cause of childhood torticollis and is most often caused by trauma or infection. The most common cause is an upper respiratory infection (Grisel's syndrome), but subluxation can occur after a retropharyngeal abscess, tonsillectomy, pharyngoplasty, or trivial trauma. Atlantoaxial rotatory subluxation is classified into four types: type I, unilateral facet subluxation with an intact transverse ligament

(most common and benign); type II, unilateral facet subluxation with 3 to 5 mm of anterior displacement; type III, bilateral anterior facet displacement of more than 5 mm; type IV, posterior displacement of the atlas (Figure 7). Types III and IV are rare, but neurologic involvement may be present or instantaneous death can occur; these types must be treated with great care.

Children with acute atlantoaxial rotatory subluxation usually report neck pain and headaches and hold the head tilted and rotated to one side, resisting any efforts to move the head. If the deformity becomes fixed, the pain subsides but the torticollis and decreased range of motion persist.

Radiographic evaluation may be difficult because of the position of the head. AP and open-mouth odontoid views should be taken with the shoulders flat and the head in as neutral position as possible. Lateral masses that have rotated forward appear wider and closer to the midline, whereas the opposite lateral mass appears narrower and farther away from the midline. On the lateral view, the lateral facet appears anterior and usually wedge-shaped rather than the normal oval shape. Flexion and extension views can be used to exclude instability. CT scanning is useful to show superimposition of C1 on C2 in a rotated position and to determine the degree and amount of malrotation. Three-dimensional CT scans are helpful to identify rotatory subluxation. MRI is of little value unless neurologic findings are present.

Treatment depends on the duration of symptoms. Many patients probably never receive medical treatment because symptoms are mild and the subluxation reduces spontaneously over a few days. If rotatory subluxation has been present for a week or less, a soft collar, anti-inflammatory drugs, and an exercise program are sufficient. If symptoms persist after a week of this treatment, head halter traction should be initiated, either in the hospital or at home; muscle relaxants and analgesics may be needed. If the subluxation is present for longer than a month, halo traction can be used. If reduction cannot be obtained or maintained, if signs of instability or neurologic deficits are present, or if the deformity has been present for more than 3 months, posterior arthrodesis is recommended to relieve muscle spasms associated with the malrotation and produce normal head appearance.

Hangman's Fracture

Bilateral spondylolisthesis of C2, or hangman's fractures, are caused by forced hyperextension and are most frequent in children younger than the age of 2 years, probably because of the disproportionately large head, poor muscle control, and hypermobility present in this age group. The possibility of child abuse must be considered. Radiographs show a lucency anterior to the pedicles of the axis, usually with some forward subluxation

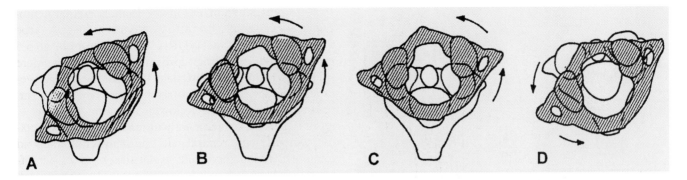

Figure 7 Fielding and Hawkins classification of atlantoaxial rotatory displacement showing four types of rotatory fixation. **A,** Type I, no anterior displacement and odontoid acting as the pivot. **B,** Type II, anterior displacement of 3 to 5 mm and one lateral articular process acting as the pivot. **C,** Type III, anterior displacement of more than 5 mm. **D,** Type IV, posterior displacement. *(Reproduced with permission from Dormans JP: Evaluation of children with suspected cervical spine injury. Instr Course Lect 2002;51:403.)*

of C2 on C3. This injury must be differentiated from a persistent synchondrosis of the axis. Treatment is symptomatic, with immobilization in a Minerva cast, halo, or cervical orthosis for 8 to 12 weeks. If union does not occur, posterior or anterior arthrodesis can be done to stabilize the fracture.

Subaxial Injuries

Fractures and dislocations involving C3 through C7 are rare in children and infants. Because these injuries occur most frequently in older children and adolescents and have fracture patterns similar to those in adults, they generally can be treated as in adults. Atlantoaxial screws and lateral mass plates have been used successfully for fixation of unstable fractures of the cervical spine in children. Image-guided techniques make accurate placement of these implants easier in a child's small vertebrae.

Pediatric Halo Use

Halo vest immobilization is being used with increasing frequency in children with cervical spine injuries. It affords superior immobilization to a rigid cervical collar and is easier to apply and more versatile than a Minerva cast. It permits access for skin and wound care while avoiding the skin problems (maceration, ulceration) typically associated with both hard collars and casts. However, complication rates as high as 68% have been reported with pediatric halo use. The most common problems are pin site infections; however, pin perforation and brain abscesses have also been reported. The thickness of the skull in children is decreased and, in children younger than age 6 years, it has been suggested that CT of the skull to measure calvarial thickness can be helpful in determining optimal sites for pin placement.

In children older than 6 years, the standard adult halo construct using four pins (two anterolaterally, two posterolaterally) inserted at standard torques of 6- to 8-

inch-lb is generally successful. In younger children, more pins (up to 12) placed with lower insertional torques (2- to 4-inch-lb) have been advocated (Figure 8). Standard pediatric halo rings fit most children, but infants and toddlers usually require custom sizing. Although standard pediatric halo vests are available, custom vests or body casts generally provide superior fit and immobilization.

Spinal Cord Injury Without Radiographic Abnormality

The possibility of spinal cord injury without radiographic abnormality (SCIWORA) should be considered in children, particularly in patients younger than 8 years. SCIWORA is defined as spinal cord injury in a patient in whom there is no visible fracture on plain radiographs or CT scan. MRI may be diagnostic in showing spinal cord edema or hemorrhage, soft-tissue or ligamentous injury, or apophyseal end plate or disk disruption, but is completely normal in approximately 25% of patients. SCIWORA is the cause of paralysis in approximately 20% to 30% of children with injuries of the spinal cord. Involvement of the cervical spine has been found to be slightly more common than other levels in most studies.

Potential mechanisms of SCIWORA include hyperextension of the cervical spine, which can cause compression of the spinal cord by the ligamentum flavum followed by flexion, which can cause longitudinal traction; transient subluxation without gross failure; or unrecognized cartilaginous end plate failure (Salter-Harris type I fracture). Ligamentous laxity, hypermobility of the spine, and immature spinal vasculature are thought to be contributing factors. Regardless of the specific mechanism, injury to the spinal cord in this syndrome occurs because of the variable elasticity of the elements of the immature spinal column. Experimentally, it has been shown that the bone, cartilage, and soft tissue in the spinal column can stretch about 2 inches without disruption but that the spinal cord ruptures after a 0.25-

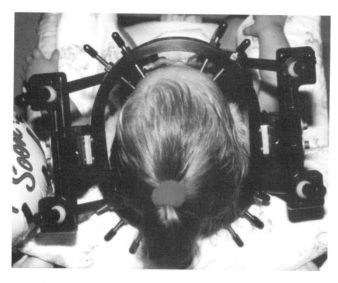

Figure 8 Photograph of a 2-year-old patient showing a halo construct with a total of 10 pins placed with lower insertional torques (2- to 4-inch-lb).

inch displacement. Spinal cord injury occurs when deformation of the musculoskeletal structures of the spinal column exceeds the physiologic limits of the spinal cord.

Neurologic injury may be complete or incomplete. Partial spinal cord syndromes reported in SCIWORA include Brown-Séquard, anterior, and central cord syndromes, as well as mixed patterns of injury. Incomplete neurologic injuries have a good prognosis for recovery, whereas complete injuries carry a dismal prognosis. Approximately 50% of patients have delayed onset of neurologic symptoms or late neurologic deterioration after an initially less severe degree of injury.

SCIWORA may also occur in the thoracolumbar spine in association with high-energy thoracic or abdominal trauma. The mechanisms of injury include vascular insult to the watershed area of the spine associated with profound/prolonged hypotension, distraction mechanism in the seatbelt-restrained patient, or hyperextension mechanism following a crush injury as most often occurs when a child is rolled over by a car while in the prone position, resulting in the spine collapsing into the chest cavity.

Prognosis following SCIWORA is correlated to MRI findings, if any are present, and to the severity of neurologic injury. Children younger than 10 years are more likely to have permanent paralysis than older children, reflecting differences in the types of injuries that occur in these two age groups. SCIWORA in younger children is usually the result of higher-energy trauma such as a motor vehicle crash, whereas in older children the mechanism of injury is more likely to be the result of a lower-energy event such as sports-related trauma or a fall.

Effective treatment requires careful evaluation of the cervical spine to exclude osseous or cartilaginous injury or mechanical instability, and stabilization of the spine to prevent recurrent injury. Immobilization with a rigid cervical collar for 2 to 3 months is usually adequate treatment of SCIWORA. There have been no reports of recurrent spinal cord injury when the cervical spine has been immobilized in this manner. Surgery is occasionally necessary for unstable injury patterns. The prevalence of scoliosis following infantile paralysis is more than 90% for patients with quadriplegia and 50% for patients with paraplegia. Long-term follow-up to monitor for spinal deformity is necessary.

Thoracic and Lumbar Fractures

Thoracic, lumbar, and sacral fractures are relatively uncommon in children. Most of these injuries are caused by motor vehicle crashes or falls. The most common injuries are compression fractures and flexion-distraction injuries. In infants and young children, nonaccidental trauma (child abuse) may be a cause of significant spinal trauma. Avulsion fractures of the spinous processes, fractures of the pars or pedicles, or compression fractures of multiple vertebral bodies are the most common patterns of injury that usually occur from severe shaking or battering. These injuries may be associated with other signs of child abuse, including fractures of the skull, ribs, or long bones and cutaneous lesions. Apophyseal end plate fractures or slipped apophyses are injuries that are unique to older children and teenagers whose symptoms mimic disk herniation.

Compression fractures are caused by a combination of hyperflexion and axial compression. Because the disk in children is stronger than cancellous bone, the vertebral body is the first structure in the spinal column to fail. It is common for children to sustain multiple compression fractures. Compression rarely exceeds more than 20% of the vertebral body. When loss of vertebral body height exceeds 50%, the possibility of injury to the posterior column of the spine should be considered and is best evaluated with CT. Most of these fractures are treated nonsurgically with rest, analgesics, and bracing. Surgical stabilization may be indicated if there is posterior column involvement and instability.

Flexion-distraction injuries (seat belt injuries) occur in the upper lumbar spine in children wearing a lap belt. With sudden deceleration, the belt slides up on the abdomen where it acts as a fulcrum. As the spine rotates around this axis it fails in tension, resulting primarily in disruption of the posterior column with variable patterns of extension into the middle and anterior column. Four patterns of injury have been described. Type A is a bony disruption of the posterior elements extending to a variable degree into the middle column. Type B is an avulsion of the spinous process with facet joint disruption or fracture and extension into the vertebral apophysis. Type C is a disruption of the interspinous ligament with a fracture of the pars interarticularis extending into the body. Type

D is a posterior ligamentous disruption with laminar fracture and disruption of the vertebral apophysis. Because of the transverse plane of orientation of this group of injuries, abnormalities may be missed by thick-section CT and may not be detected even with complementary thin sections, unless sagittal reconstructions are included. A lateral radiograph showing widening of the interspinous space is the most helpful study in diagnosing this fracture, although increased distance between the spinous processes may occasionally be seen on the AP radiograph. MRI may be the single best imaging modality because it can accurately identify soft-tissue and disk injury as well as having predictive value in determining spinal cord and neural injury.

Approximately two thirds of patients have intra-abdominal injuries including ruptures of internal organs and mesenteric tears, which may be life-threatening if not diagnosed and treated appropriately. Neurologic injury is unusual. Lap belt injuries with mostly bony involvement and kyphosis less than 20° can be treated with hyperextension casting. Those with posterior ligamentous disruption and soft-tissue injury require surgical stabilization with compression instrumentation and posterior arthrodesis.

Fracture of the vertebral end plate (slipped vertebral apophysis) usually occurs in teenagers and is characterized by traumatic disruption of the vertebral ring apophysis and disk into the spinal canal. The clinical symptoms are essentially the same as a herniated disk. Patients may have muscle weakness, sensory changes, absent reflexes, and root tension signs. This injury most commonly involves the caudal end plate of L4, but may occur at any level in the lumbar spine. The injuries may be purely cartilaginous with herniation of the apophysis and disk or osseous with fractures of the cortical and cancellous rim of the vertebral body. This injury usually cannot be identified on plain radiographs. CT or MRI is needed to make the diagnosis. Treatment is removal of the bony and cartilaginous fragments and usually requires more extensive exposure (bilateral laminotomies) than simple diskectomy.

Fracture-dislocations of the spine are unstable injuries that usually occur at the thoracolumbar junction and often are associated with neurologic deficits. They are rare injuries in children that require surgical stabilization and fusion. Burst fractures are also rare injuries in children that result from axial compression and typically occur at the thoracolumbar junction or in the lumbar spine. The need for surgical treatment is determined by the stability of the fracture and the presence of neurologic deficits. Nonsurgical treatment is a viable option in neurologically intact children, although most will develop a progressive angular deformity during the first year after the fracture. It has been shown that surgical stabilization prevents kyphotic deformity and decreases the length of hospitalization. Instrumentation should include two levels above and below the fracture. In children with complete neurologic deficits, longer constructs provide better stability and may prevent subsequent paralytic spinal deformity from occurring.

Annotated Bibliography

Specific Cervical Spine Injuries

Flynn JM, Closkey RF, Mahboubi S, Dormans JP: Role of magnetic resonance imaging in the assessment of pediatric cervical spine injuries. *J Pediatr Orthop* 2002;22: 573-577.

In this study of 74 children, MRI confirmed the plain radiography diagnosis in 66% and altered the diagnosis in 34%. MRI is valuable in the evaluation of potential cervical spine injury, especially in obtunded children or those with equivocal plain radiographs.

Kenter K: Worley G, Griffin T, Fitch RD: Pediatric traumatic atlanto-occipital dislocation: Five cases and a review. *J Pediatr Orthop* 2001;21:585-589.

Of five children with traumatic atlanto-occipital dislocation, the three survivors had posterior occipitovertebral fusions. The diagnosis was missed initially in three children. The authors recommend detailed measurements of the initial cervical spine radiographs in pediatric patients at risk for traumatic atlanto-occipital dislocation.

Lustrin ES, Karakas SP, Ortiz AO, et al: Pediatric cervical spine: Normal anatomy, variants, and trauma. *Radiographics* 2003;23:539-560.

Knowledge of the normal embryologic development and anatomy of the cervical spine is important to avoid mistaking synchondroses for fractures and to correctly interpret imaging studies. Familiarity with mechanisms of injury and appropriate imaging modalities also aids in the correct interpretation of radiographs of the pediatric cervical spine.

Thoracic and Lumbar Fractures

Clark P, Letts M: Trauma to the thoracic and lumbar spine in the adolescent. *Can J Surg* 2001;44:337-345.

This article describes thoracolumbar fractures in adolescents. The treatment of these injuries follows many of the same principles as spinal fractures in adults. Nonsurgical treatment is used more frequently because there is less spinal instability and better tolerance of bed rest and spinal immobilization in this population.

Lalonde F, Letts M, Yang JP, Thomas K: An analysis of burst fractures of the spine in adolescents. *Am J Orthop* 2001;30:115-120.

This article describes the results of treatment in 11 children (average age 14.4 years) with burst fractures of the spine; 6 children were treated with posterior spinal fusion and instrumentation. Results showed that (1) mild progressive angular deformity developed at the site of the fracture; (2) spinal instrumentation and fusion prevented kyphotic deformity and decreased the length of hospitalization without contributing to further spinal cord injury; and (3) nonsurgical treatment was a viable option in neurologically intact children, but progressive angular deformity occurred during the first year after the fracture.

Reddy SP, Junewick JJ, Backstrom JW: Distribution of spinal fractures in children: does age, mechanism of injury, or gender play a significant role? *Pediatr Radiol* 2003;33:776-781.

Of the 2,614 pediatric patients referred to a trauma center over a 5-year period, 84 sustained vertebral fracture and 50 had neurologic injury without radiographic abnormality. A total of 164 fractures were identified. The thoracic region (T2-T10) was most commonly injured, accounting for 47 fractures (28.7%), followed by the lumbar region (L2-L5) with 38 fractures (23.2%), the midcervical region with 31 fractures (18.9%), the thoracolumbar junction with 24 fractures (14.6%), the cervicothoracic junction with 13 fractures (7.9%), and the cervicocranium with 11 fractures (6.7%). There was no relationship to gender or mechanism of injury.

Sledge JB, Allred D, Hyman J: Use of magnetic resonance imaging in evaluating injuries to the pediatric thoracolumbar spine. *J Pediatr Orthop* 2001;21:288-293.

This study is a retrospective review of 19 children with thoracolumbar fractures associated with neurologic deficits from three level 1 trauma centers. The authors conclude that MRI is the imaging modality of choice for these fractures because it can accurately classify injury to bones and ligaments and because the cord patterns as determined by MRI have predictive value of neurologic status.

Classic Bibliography

Akbarnia BA: Pediatric spine fractures. *Orthop Clin North Am* 1999;30:521-536.

Banerian KG, Wang AM, Samberg LC, Kerr HH, Wesolowski DP: Association of vertebral end plate fracture with pediatric lumbar intervertebral disk herniation: Value of CT and MR imaging. *Radiology* 1990;177:763-765.

Donahue DJ, Muhlbauer MS, Kaufman RA, Warner WC, Sandford RA: Childhood survival of atlantooccipital dislocation: Underdiagnosis, recognition, treatment, and review of the literature. *Pediatr Neurosurg* 1994;21:105-111.

Dormans JP, Criscitiello AA, Drummond DS, Davidson RS: Complications in children managed with immobilization in a halo vest. *J Bone Joint Surg Am* 1995;77:1370-1373.

Finch GD, Barnes MJ: Major cervical spine injuries in children and adolescents. *J Pediatr Orthop* 1998;18:811-814.

Glass RB, Sivit CJ, Sturm PF, Bulas DI, Eichelberger MR: Lumbar spine injury in a pediatric population: Difficulties with computed tomographic diagnosis. *J Trauma* 1994;37:815-819.

Harris JH, Carson GC, Wagner LK: Radiologic diagnosis of traumatic occipitovertebral dissociation: 1. Normal occipitovertebral relationships on lateral radiographs of supine subjects. *AJR Am J Roentgenol* 1994;162:881-886.

Herzenberg JE, Hensinger RN, Dedrick DK, Phillips WA: Emergency transport and positioning of young children who have an injury of the cervical spine. *J Bone Joint Surg Am* 1989;71:15-22.

Judd DB, Liem LK, Petermann G: Pediatric atlas fracture: a case of fracture through a synchondrosis and review of the literature. *Neurosurgery* 2000;46:991-994.

Mubarak SJ, Camp JF, Vueltich W, et al: Halo application in the infant. *J Pediatr Orthop* 1989;9:612-614.

Odent T, Langlais J, Glorion C, et al: Fractures of the odontoid process: a report of 15 cases in children younger than 6 years. *J Pediatr Orthop* 1999;19:51-54.

Pouliquen JC, Kassis B, Glorion C, Langlais J: Vertebral growth after thoracic or lumbar fracture of the spine in children. *J Pediatr Orthop* 1997;17:115-120.

Subach BR, McLaughlin MR, Albright AL, Pollack IF: Current management of pediatric atlantoaxial rotatory subluxation. *Spine* 1998;23:2174-2179.

Chapter 66

Pediatric Spinal Deformity

Daniel J. Sucato, MD

B. Stephens Richards III, MD

Idiopathic Scoliosis

Idiopathic scoliosis is the most common type of scoliosis and, as its name implies, there is no known definitive etiology for this condition. It is defined as a lateral curvature of the spine with a Cobb angle of 10° or greater and axial plane rotation. The sagittal plane usually demonstrates hypokyphosis in the thoracic spine, junctional kyphosis between two structural curves, and segmental hypolordosis of the lumbar spine when a structural curve is present. Classification of idiopathic scoliosis is usually defined according to the age of the patient at the time of curve development as follows: infantile (from birth to age 3 years), juvenile (from age 3 years to 10 years), and adolescent (from age 10 years to 18 years). The age classifications, although somewhat arbitrary, allow the surgeon to characterize curves and assist in treatment algorithms from the outset.

Infantile Idiopathic Scoliosis

Infantile idiopathic scoliosis is uncommon, and its etiology is not determined. However, patients who present with this presumed diagnosis require more careful evaluation because an underlying cause is more often found with infantile idiopathic scoliosis than juvenile and adolescent scoliosis. A recent multicenter study demonstrated that 21.7% of patients who presented with infantile idiopathic scoliosis measuring greater than or equal to 20° had neural axis abnormalities, and 80% of these patients required neurosurgical intervention. The authors of this study recommended that an MRI scan be obtained at the time of presentation for any patient with presumed infantile idiopathic scoliosis whose curve measures 20° or greater.

Infantile idiopathic scoliosis is the least common type of idiopathic scoliosis. It is more commonly seen in males when compared with juvenile or adolescent idiopathic scoliosis (1:1 male to female ratio), and left curves are more often reported.

Spontaneous correction of infantile idiopathic scoliosis may occur, and can be predicted based on the position of the rib relative to the vertebra and the rib-vertebral angle difference (RVAD) as described by Metha. If the rib overlaps the vertebral body at the apex of the curve (phase 2 rib), the curve is likely to progress, whereas a phase 1 rib pattern (no overlap of the rib) requires measurement of the RVAD to assess for curve progression. A patient with a phase 1 rib and an RVAD greater than 20° has a significant risk for curve progression. Careful observation is warranted in patients with these curves, and treatment with an orthotic device is indicated for those curves that have shown progression or are greater than 30°. For the young patient with a large curve or those patients who do not tolerate an orthotic device, a Risser cast is appropriate to "loosen up" the spine and allow for improved wear of the orthotic device.

Surgical treatment should be delayed as long as possible, primarily because of the concern with creating a small chest and its detrimental effect on pulmonary function. Although there are no definitive indications for surgical treatment, progression despite orthotic treatment or curves greater than 50° are generally accepted indications. A variety of surgical treatment strategies have been described, with the most predictable outcome resulting from an anterior and posterior fusion. Posterior instrumentation is generally recommended, and it is possible in even small patients because of the newer and smaller instrumentations that are currently available. A 5-year follow-up study of 13 patients demonstrated that convex epiphysiodesis combined with a Luque trolley resulted in overall good results, and instrumented growth was 32% of what was expected. Newer instrumentation using dual posterior rods and connectors in the middle of the construct to allow intermittent lengthenings have demonstrated favorable early results. This approach appears to limit the typically high complication rate observed in the traditional growing rod scenario. Longer follow-up is required for these patients.

Juvenile Idiopathic Scoliosis

Juvenile idiopathic scoliosis occurs in patients between the ages of 3 to 10 years; approximately 15% of all patients with idiopathic scoliosis have juvenile idiopathic scoliosis. Females are more commonly affected than males, and this disparity increases with age. As with adolescent idiopathic scoliosis, right thoracic curves are more common.

The natural history of juvenile idiopathic scoliosis is one of steady progression until age 10 years, when curves generally progress fairly rapidly. Unlike infantile idiopathic scoliosis, 95% of all patients with juvenile idiopathic scoliosis have progressive curves, whereas only 5% resolve. The thoracic curves tend to progress more commonly and require fusion more often. Curve patterns may change with extension of the primary curve or a development of secondary structural curves.

As with those with infantile idiopathic scoliosis, patients with juvenile idiopathic scoliosis should have MRI studies to evaluate the neural axis because of a 20% to 25% incidence of abnormalities. These abnormalities often require surgical treatment; therefore, it has been recommended that MRI be done at the time of the initial evaluation.

The nonsurgical treatment of juvenile idiopathic scoliosis is similar to that for adolescent idiopathic scoliosis. Bracing is used to treat patients with curves that have progressed to 30° or for those with curves exceeding 20° that have demonstrated 5° of progression. Surgical management is also similar to that for patients with adolescent idiopathic scoliosis, although the crankshaft phenomenon assumes greater importance in the skeletally immature patient.

Adolescent Idiopathic Scoliosis

Adolescent idiopathic scoliosis is relatively common, with a reported incidence of 2% to 3% for curves between 10° and 20°, and an incidence of 0.3% for curves greater than 30°. There is an equal incidence of smaller curves among males and females, whereas the female to male ratio of curves greater than 30° is 10:1.

The natural history of adolescent idiopathic scoliosis has been well studied, and it is generally accepted that curves progress in two scenarios: (1) continued spine growth and (2) large curve magnitude despite the completion of spine growth. Continued spine growth is assessed using an array of both clinical and radiographic parameters. Clinical parameters include female menarcheal status and height measurements performed at each clinic visit to determine growth velocity. Peak growth velocity is approximately 10 cm per year and occurs just before the onset of menses in females. Radiographic parameters that indicate skeletal immaturity include an open triradiate cartilage, and a Risser grade 0 to 1. Following the completion of growth, curve progression is more likely for patients with thoracic curves exceeding 45° to 50° and thoracolumbar/lumbar curves exceeding 40°, especially when coronal imbalance is

present. The rate of progression in these curves is approximately 1° per year.

Patients with adolescent idiopathic scoliosis should have a complete and organized clinical evaluation to confirm the diagnosis, rule out neural axis abnormalities, and assist in determining treatment. A careful inspection of the skin is necessary to rule out lesions such as café-au-lait spots (neurofibromatosis) and cutaneous manifestations of dysraphism. The extremities, especially the feet, should be inspected to ensure that no deformities (cavovarus feet indicating neural axis abnormalities) are present. Observation of gait (including heel and toe walking) will allow the surgeon to obtain a general sense of the patient's strength and coordination. The neurologic examination should include an assessment of motor function in all muscle groups, a sensory examination, and deep tendon reflexes. Abdominal reflexes that are symmetric confirm a normal neural axis; when abdominal reflexes are asymmetric, the surgeon should obtain an MRI scan. Examination of the patient's back includes an assessment of balance, trunk imbalance, waist asymmetry, pelvic tilt, and limb-length discrepancy. Shoulder height differences are important, especially when deciding whether an upper thoracic curve requires fusion. The Adams forward bend test is performed to analyze axial plane deformity, which is an indication that the curve is structural. Asymmetric forward bending of the patient or tenderness of the spine to palpation may indicate a neural axis abnormality.

Initial radiographic examination should include PA and lateral radiographs of the entire spine (lower cervical spine down to the hips). The PA radiograph should be used to evaluate the spine and determine the Cobb angle for all curves. Skeletal maturity should be assessed using the Risser sign and the maturity of the triradiate cartilage (open or closed). The PA radiograph should always be assessed to ensure that two pedicles are present for each vertebra, no signs of congenital vertebra exist, and that there is no evidence for other abnormalities such as neurofibromatosis (penciling of the ribs, endosteal scalloping, or significantly wedged vertebra). An assessment of spinal balance can be made by dropping a C7 plumb line and comparing it with the center sacral vertical line. Structural characteristics of the proximal thoracic curve include T1 tilt, Cobb angle of greater than 30°, Nash-Moe apical rotation of II or greater, and a transitional vertebra between the upper and middle thoracic curves of T6 or lower. Recently, the clavicle angle (the angle subtended by the intersection of a horizontal line and the line that is tangential to the highest points of each clavicle) has been shown to be the best predictor of postoperative shoulder balance. The lateral radiograph can be used to assess sagittal balance, which is variable, and to ensure that thoracic hypokyphosis is present. The rib heads of the thoracic curve should demonstrate apical lordosis in patients with adolescent idiopathic scoliosis, and its absence should warrant investigation of the neural axis with MRI. A recent study demonstrated that 97% of patients with adolescent idiopathic scoliosis and a normal MRI study had apical lordosis, whereas this sign was absent in 75% of patients with scoliosis and a syringomyelia. The presence of a spondylolysis and/or spondylolisthesis should always be evaluated at the lumbosacral junction and is present in 1% to 2% of patients with adolescent idiopathic scoliosis. Preoperative radiographic assessment should include supine best-effort bend films to the right and left.

MRI should not be used as a screening tool and is indicated when there is an atypical curve pattern, absence of thoracic lordosis, atypical pain, neurologic abnormalities or foot deformities, or extremely rapid curve progression.

The King-Moe classification has been traditionally used for determining curve types in patients with adolescent idiopathic scoliosis. This is a five-part classification that was developed to describe thoracic curve patterns to help guide the surgeon when implanting Harrington instrumentation. As with many orthopaedic classifications, it has fair interobserver and intraobserver reliability. The newer classification system described by Lenke and associates provides a more comprehensive evaluation of both the PA and lateral radiographs and also uses best-effort supine bend films. The following three components are defined in this classification system: curve types (1 through 6), lumbar modifiers (A, B, or C), and thoracic kyphosis (negative, N = normal, or positive). Although more comprehensive, this classification system has 42 possible combinations and therefore introduces more complexity into the curve evaluations. When each of the three components were evaluated individually, the reliability was similar to that of the King-Moe classification. As with any classification system for adolescent idiopathic scoliosis, it should always be used in conjunction with a careful clinical evaluation of the patient.

Nonsurgical treatment includes observation and management with an orthotic device. Observation is indicated for any curve less than 45° in a skeletally mature patient without significant clinical deformity. In the skeletally immature patient, observation of curves less than 25° is warranted. Bracing is used for the skeletally immature patient (Risser grades 0, 1, or 2) with a curve between 30° and 45° or an initial curve between 20° and 25° that has demonstrated 5° of progression. Although numerous braces are available today, the Boston and Charleston braces are most commonly used. The Boston brace can be used to treat all curve patterns. Successful treatment depends on the amount of time the brace is worn, as was reported in a recent study in which a compliance monitor was incorporated into the brace. The Charleston (nighttime) brace has been shown to be effective in treating thoracolumbar/lumbar curves that measure between 25° and 35°.

Surgical Treatment

Generally, the indications for surgical treatment of patients with adolescent idiopathic scoliosis are thoracic curves greater than 45° in the skeletally immature patient or greater than 50° in the skeletally mature patient. Because thoracolumbar/lumbar curves are more likely to progress despite a smaller curve magnitude, surgical intervention is indicated for patients with curves greater than 40° to 45°, especially when there is significant rotation and/or translation. The first goal of surgery is to prevent curve progression with spinal arthrodesis. The second goal of surgery is to safely improve the three-dimensional deformity. Surgical planning depends on the radiographic and clinical deformity present and the skeletal maturity of the patient. Fusion levels depend on the surgical approach used and a careful assessment of the radiographs and clinical deformity. The standard, more traditional posterior approach can be used for all curve patterns, and it is best for double or triple curves. The anterior approach is more commonly used for thoracolumbar/lumbar curve patterns because removal of the disk assists in achieving improvement in coronal plane deformity, and lumbar lordosis can be restored. The anterior approach can also be used for thoracic curve patterns, especially when hypokyphosis is present. In this instance, correction is achieved with convex compression, which produces kyphosis. Use of anterior instrumentation requires close attention to screw length and direction (in the vertebral body) because of the proximity of the aorta to the left side of the spine in patients with right thoracic scoliosis.

For those undergoing posterior instrumentation and fusion, an anterior diskectomy and fusion should also be performed in those who are skeletally immature (Risser grade 0 with open triradiate cartilage) and in those patients who have very large (> 80°) and stiff (< 50% flexibility index) curves.

Advances in spinal instrumentation have improved the correction of scoliotic deformities. Studies have demonstrated improvement and maintenance of deformity when pedicle screws are used in the thoracolumbar/lumbar spine (Figure 1). The use of pedicle screws in the thoracic spine also improves curve correction when compared with hooks, and initial reports demonstrate safe placement (Figure 2). However, anatomic studies demonstrate that it may be challenging to place thoracic pedicle screws, especially on the concavity of the curve, because of the narrow width of the pedicle and the proximity of the aorta laterally and spinal cord medially. Improvement in lateral and posterior translation of the thoracic spine may not be significantly improved when compared with segmental hook and

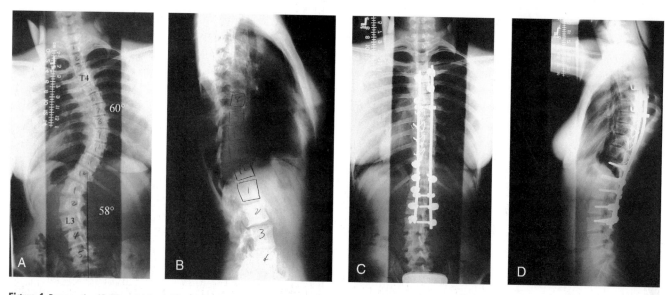

Figure 1 Preoperative AP **(A)** and lateral **(B)** and 3-year postoperative AP **(C)** and lateral **(D)** radiographs of a 14-year-old girl who underwent posterior spinal fusion and instrumentation with a combination of hooks, sublaminar wires, and pedicle screw fixation. Restoration of coronal and sagittal balance is seen in the postoperative radiographs, with excellent correction of the lumbar curve.

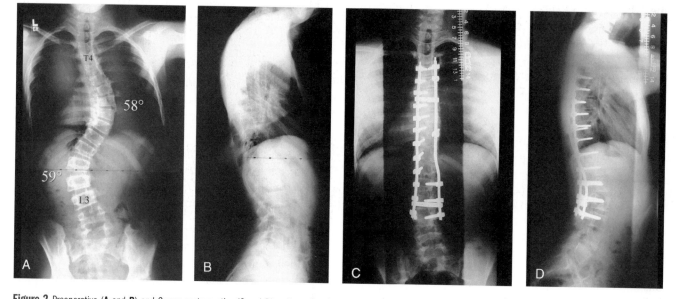

Figure 2 Preoperative **(A and B)** and 2-year postoperative **(C and D)** radiographs of a 14-year-old boy after posterior spinal fusion and instrumentation using pedicle screw fixation alone.

wire fixation; however, the improvement in the ability to correct axial rotation may prove to be its greatest advantage. Confirmation of screw placement is more difficult in the thoracic spine because radiographic visualization is obscured by the ribs and soft tissues. The results of using electromyographic stimulation of screws to confirm intrapedicle placement is not as reliable as lumbar screw stimulation.

The thoracoscopic approach to perform an anterior release appears as effective as open thoracotomy and has minimized the incisions required for anterior access to the spine. A recent study demonstrated that an ante-

rior thoracoscopic release/fusion performed with the patient in the prone position is very effective and better tolerated when compared with a thoracoscopic release with the patient in the lateral position. Thoracoscopic instrumentation for single thoracic curves achieves correction comparable to open anterior or posterior instrumentation (Figure 3). Although less scarring provides excellent cosmetic improvement, the duration of thoracoscopic surgery continues to be significantly longer when compared with more conventional approaches.

Despite recent advancements in spinal instrumentation and techniques, the ultimate goal of surgical treat-

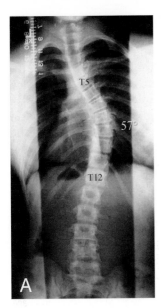
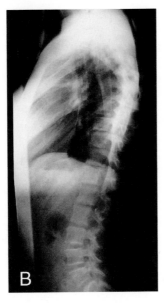
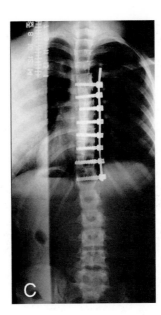
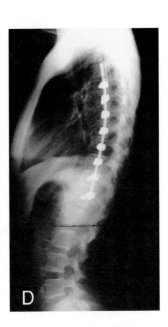

Figure 3 Preoperative (**A** and **B**) and 3-year postoperative (**C** and **D**) radiographs of a 14-year-old girl after a thoracoscopic anterior spinal fusion and instrumentation.

ment is to achieve solid fusion while minimizing complications. Autogenous iliac crest bone continues to be the gold standard to promote fusion in adolescent idiopathic scoliosis. Neurologic monitoring using somatosensory-evoked potentials and/or motor-evoked potentials is now the standard of care. A 50% decrease in amplitude and/or an increase in latency of 10% are generally considered thresholds for concern for neurologic injury when assessing patients using somatosensory-evoked potentials. Critical threshold values for motor-evoked potentials are not as clear and are dependent on the mode of stimulation. The Stagnara wake-up test, which is used when neurologic injury is suspected, is the gold standard for neurologic assessment. Acute complications from the surgical treatment of adolescent idiopathic scoliosis are relatively rare. However, the need for revision following a posterior spinal fusion can be as high as 19%, with revision for late-onset surgical pain from prominent hardware occurring in 8% of patients. Delayed infections can occur up to 3 to 4 years postoperatively and can present as a small draining wound or fluctuance, accompanied by low-grade fevers and a mildly elevated erythrocyte sedimentation rate. Treatment consists of removal of the instrumentation and primary closure, followed by oral administration of antibiotics. Intraoperative cultures usually grow *Staphylococcus epidermidis* or *Propionibacterium acnes*, an organism that requires culture incubation up to 2 weeks.

Scoliosis Research Society-22 Patient Outcome Instrument

This health-related quality-of-life patient questionnaire was developed to correlate patients' perceptions and satisfaction with their scoliotic deformities. Studies have shown this instrument to be simple to use, internally

consistent, and comparable in reliability and validity to the Medical Outcomes Study Short Form-36 Health Survey Questionnaire (SF-36). The Scoliosis Research Society-22 Patient Outcome Instrument (SRS-22) is shorter and more focused on health issues related to scoliosis than is the SF-36. Following surgical treatment for adolescent idiopathic scoliosis, outcomes using the SRS-22 have shown significant improvement from the preoperative status in the domains of pain, general self-image, function from back condition, and level of activity. Improvement in coronal Cobb angle correction does not correlate with improved SRS-22 scores.

One study reported that minimum 20-year follow-up for patients who had posterior surgery with Harrington instrumentation for idiopathic scoliosis demonstrated similar back function when these patients were compared with an age-matched control group from the general population. Those who underwent surgery had a greater likelihood of having back pain (78% versus 58%) and lumbar pain (65% versus 47%). In a 50-year follow-up study of untreated patients compared with a matched control group, the authors reported a greater incidence of shortness of breath (22% versus 15%), which was associated with a Cobb angle of greater than 80°. Despite a greater likelihood of chronic back pain (61% versus 35%), patients with scoliosis were productive and functioning at a high level.

Congenital Spinal Deformities

Congenital vertebral abnormalities lead to a variety of spinal deformities, including scoliosis, kyphosis, or a combination of the two. Its cause remains unknown. Genetic abnormalities or any other traumatic or teratologic type of maternal insults during pregnancy are rarely Kidentified in patients with congenital vertebral abnormalities. Recently, congenital scoliosis has been documented in two monozygotic twins, a finding that contradicts most of the findings in the congenital deformity literature. A potential increase in exposure to chemical fumes and carbon monoxide in mothers of children with congenital spine deformities has also been reported.

Spinal dysraphism, which includes numerous abnormalities such as diastematomyelia, syringomyelia, diplomyelia, Arnold-Chiari malformations, intraspinal tumors, and tethering of the spinal cord, is consistently found in 30% to 40% of patients with congenital spinal deformities. MRI, which best identifies these dysraphic abnormalities, has been recently recommended for all patients with congenital spinal deformity as part of the initial evaluation, even in the absence of clinical findings. The mere presence of a potentially tethering intraspinal lesion may be sufficient reason for prophylactic surgical treatment to address the lesion before the development of any neural dysfunction. This approach, in the absence of neurologic findings, remains controversial.

Congenital Scoliosis

The variety of vertebral anomalies found in congenital scoliosis makes its natural history uncertain. The two basic types, defects of vertebral formation and defects of vertebral segmentation, may occur separately or in combination. In 80% of patients with congenital scoliosis, the anomalies can be classified into one of the two types.

Defects of vertebral formation may be partial or complete. True hemivertebrae result from the complete failure of formation on one side and cause the formation of laterally based wedges consisting of half the vertebral body, a single pedicle, and hemilamina. When present in the thoracic spine, hemivertebrae are usually accompanied by extra ribs. When located at the lumbosacral junction, a significant obliquity between the spine and pelvis can result and is usually accompanied above by a long compensatory scoliosis. This lumbosacral deformity is best treated surgically (usually with hemivertebrectomy) at an early age before the compensatory curve becomes fixed.

Defects of segmentation result in an osseous bridge between two or more vertebrae, either unilaterally or involving the entire segment. The combination of unilateral failure of segmentation and contralateral hemivertebra carries the worst prognosis in congenital scoliosis because it produces the most severe and rapidly progressive deformity. Curves of this kind located in the thoracolumbar spine can be expected to exceed 50° by the age of 2 years. Without treatment, patients with thoracolumbar, midthoracic, or lumbar curves experience severe deformity at an early age. Rib fusions that ac-

company unilateral segmentation defects on the concavity of the curve may adversely affect thoracic growth, resulting in severe limitations in pulmonary function and growth. This rare condition is known as thoracic insufficiency syndrome, which is defined as the inability of the thorax to support normal respiration or lung growth. Left untreated, progressive deterioration occurs and can result in death at an early age. Methods to expand the thoracic cage are being investigated, with the goals being to provide an acute increase in the thoracic volume with stabilization of any flail chest wall defects and to maintain these improvements as the patient grows.

In patients with severe congenital scoliosis, plain radiographs may not provide sufficient information regarding vertebral abnormalities. Should surgical intervention be necessary, a CT scan with reformatted three-dimensional reconstruction provides excellent detail for the understanding of the deformity. These reconstructions are extremely valuable in the preoperative planning for severe deformities. MRI of the spine also must be done for all patients with congenital scoliosis who are undergoing surgical intervention to assess intracanal abnormalities (30% to 40% prevalence). Currently, reformatted images from MRI can provide a clear picture of the canal contents despite the severe three-dimensional deformity associated with some congenital scoliosis patients.

Although bracing has no beneficial effect on congenital curves, it may help to control long flexible compensatory curves below the congenital component. The primary goal of surgical intervention is to stop further progression. Partial correction that can be obtained safely is an added benefit. Even if the curves are relatively small (< 40°), once curve progression has been confirmed, surgical intervention should be undertaken. Surgery should be performed prior to the development of notable deformity, a concept different from that in idiopathic scoliosis. Various surgical approaches are used depending on patient maturity, deformity location, and type of deformity. These approaches include anterior and posterior convex hemiepiphysiodesis, anterior and posterior spinal fusion, posterior fusion with or without instrumentation, hemivertebra excision, and spine osteotomies. Expansion thoracoplasty, a new approach to surgery for congenital scoliosis, is indicated for very young patients who either have or will potentially have thoracic insufficiency syndrome. It consists of lengthening the concave hemithorax with rib distraction by means of a prosthetic rib distractor (Figure 4). This results in increased growth of both the concave and convex sides of the curve, thus allowing additional volume for growth of the underlying lungs. This technique, currently undergoing clinical trials, appears very promising.

In patients with severe congenital spinal deformities, slow gradual correction has recently been reported to be successful in some individuals using preoperative

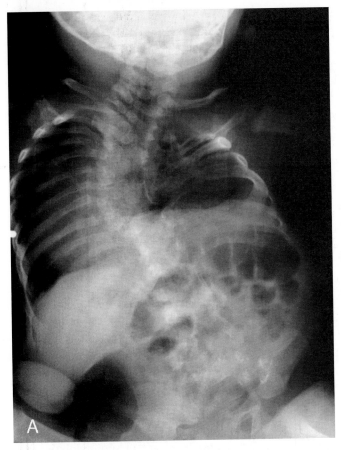 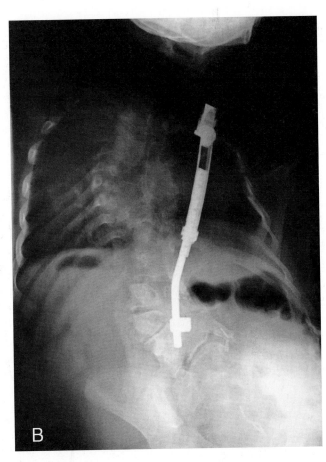

Figure 4 A, Radiograph of a 4-month-old girl with congenital scoliosis, fused ribs, and a unilateral unsegmented bar. **B,** Radiograph of the same patient at age 11 years. After several expansion thoracoplasty procedures, the patient's hemithorax is increased in size beyond that expected with no intervention.

halo traction for 6 to 12 weeks. If this method is used, very close monitoring for any neurologic change (numbness, tingling, and weakness) is essential. When partial correction is obtained or a plateau has been reached, the spine is stabilized by instrumentation and fusion.

Few patients with congenital scoliosis secondary to a hemivertebra need to have the hemivertebra excised. The main indication for hemivertebra excision is a fixed decompensation in a patient in whom adequate alignment cannot be achieved through other procedures (usually involving a hemivertebra of the fourth or fifth lumbar level). Although a combined anterior and posterior resection has been the standard procedure for hemivertebra excision, several recent studies report success with excision through a posterior approach only, with correction maintained using transpedicular instrumentation.

Congenital Kyphosis

Congenital kyphosis represents an abrupt posterior angulation of the spine resulting from a localized congenital malformation of one or more vertebrae. This deformity is caused either by defects of formation (type 1), defects of segmentation (type 2), or a combination of the two. In contrast to congenital scoliosis, failure of segmentation in congenital kyphosis is less common and produces much less deformity than failure of formation. In type 1 kyphosis, there is a partial (or complete) deficiency of the vertebral body, but the posterior elements remain present. With growth, a relentless progression in the kyphosis occurs, leading to anterior impingement on the spinal cord. When this type of deformity is diagnosed, plans for surgical intervention should begin immediately because of the risk of neurologic deficits.

In type 2 kyphosis, the anterior portion of two or more adjacent vertebral bodies are fused, which leads to a deformity that is less progressive, produces less deformity, and has a much lower risk of paraplegia than that seen in patients with type 1 kyphosis.

When imaging congenital kyphosis, MRI will provide the clearest picture of the spinal cord and, in very young patients, the clearest picture of the vertebral bodies. Cord compression may be evident on MRI before any clinical neurologic deficits. Three-dimensional imaging of the spine using CT scan reconstructions is useful for the evaluation of the vertebral anomalies, especially in the older child. Both tests should be obtained before any surgical intervention.

Because nonsurgical treatment has no beneficial effect on congenital kyphosis, the use of an orthotic device is inappropriate. In patients with type 1 kyphosis, surgical intervention should be considered, even in the infant, with the primary goal being prevention of future paraplegia. If the deformity is recognized in patients younger than age 3 to 5 years and before the kyphosis exceeds 50°, simple posterior fusion without instrumentation may be considered. A hyperextension cast is used postoperatively for 4 to 6 months followed by a thoracolumbosacral orthosis for another 6 months. This approach may allow for some growth anteriorly in the abnormal region of the spine, which, over time, may result in progressive improvement in the localized kyphosis. Alternatively, in patients with kyphosis that exceeds 50°, an anterior release with strut graft must accompany the posterior fusion. In the older child or the adult, combined anterior and posterior arthrodesis is mandatory.

Rotatory Dislocation

Segmental spinal dysgenesis, congenital dislocation of the spine, and congenital vertebral displacement of the spine are conditions that create the most severe localized kyphosis of the spine and lead to a neurologic deficit in 50% to 60% of patients. These conditions can be difficult to differentiate from one another. The deformities include severe kyphosis; anterior, posterior, or lateral subluxation of the spine; and scoliosis in association with a severely stenotic spinal canal. The treatment requires combined anterior and posterior spinal fusion because posterior fusion alone is insufficient to achieve solid arthrodesis in patients with these types of congenital instabilities. Exploration and augmentation of the posterior fusion mass should be considered because of a high occurrence of pseudarthrosis. No sudden correction should be attempted in older patients with severe angular kyphosis and progressive neurologic deficit. Function must be favored over cosmetic appearance. Neurosurgical decompression should be used only for patients with a proven recent and progressive neurologic deficit.

Spondylolysis and Spondylolisthesis

Spondylolysis is a defect of one or both of the pars interarticularis in the posterior element of a lower lumbar vertebra. Although it generally results from repetitive stress to the pars interarticularis, it can occur abruptly. Seen in 4% to 6% of the general population, spondylolysis has a predilection in those whose activities involve increased hyperextension of the lumbar spine. The condition primarily affects L5 (in 87% to 95% of patients) and less frequently L4 (in up to 10%) and L3 (in up to 3%). Spondylolisthesis represents a forward slippage of all or part of one vertebra on another and in children is nearly always located between L5 and the sacrum.

Patients usually present with pain localized to the low back that is usually aggravated by extension activities and relieved by rest. Radiation of the pain into the buttocks or posterior thighs is uncommon and a neurologic deficit is rare. Unless the slippage is high grade, the back alignment appears normal and no localized tenderness is present. Hamstring tightness may be present and can lead to a shortened stride length. In patients with a high-grade slip, the buttocks may appear flattened, a step-off may be palpable between the area of the unaffected lumbar spine and loose posterior elements, the torso may appear short, and an olisthetic scoliosis may be present. L5 or S1 nerve root compression symptoms are rare.

Spondylolisthesis is always evident on an upright lateral radiograph of the lumbosacral junction, but spondylolysis may be difficult to visualize. If suspicion of spondylolysis is high, oblique lumbar radiographs should demonstrate sclerosis, elongation, or a distinct defect in the pars interarticularis. If these radiographs are not conclusive, single photon emission CT may demonstrate increased uptake in patients with recent spondylolysis or prefractured stressed regions, but may be normal in patients with established spondylolysis. CT will definitively demonstrate the occult fracture that may not be evident on oblique radiographs. MRI is not needed for diagnosis.

The two most common types of spondylolysis seen in children are isthmic and dysplastic spondylolysis. Isthmic spondylolysis is more common and represents a fatigue fracture of the pars interarticularis. The dysplastic type occurs only at L5-S1 and results from congenital dysplasia of the L5-S1 facet joints. Patients with this type of spondylolysis have an elongated pars interarticularis and are more prone to developing neurologic symptoms and deformity during growth.

Traditionally, radiographic sagittal descriptions of spondylolisthesis have involved the Meyerding classification (grades I through IV) and the slip angle. The Meyerding classification measures the forward translation of L5 on the sacrum. The slip angle measures the sagittal rotation of L5 on the sacrum and reflects the localized kyphosis at this junction, increasing in higher-grade deformities (Meyerding grade IV or spondyloptosis). Pelvic incidence, a newer radiographic measurement that assesses the sacral anatomy and its relationship to the pelvis and spine balance, appears to be more predictive of spondylolisthesis progression. It describes the obliquity of the sacrum to the pelvis and is measured on the lateral radiograph by the angle between the line perpendicular to the middle of the sacral plate and the line joining the middle of the sacral plate to the center of the acetabular axis (femoral heads) (Figure 5). This fixed angle is significantly larger in those patients with higher-grade deformities (when compared with those with low-grade slips and control subjects). Pelvic incidence has a strong correlation with the Meyerding classification; therefore, it may be used early to predict the ultimate severity of spondylolisthesis in early adolescence.

The risk of progression in spondylolisthesis is greatest during the adolescent growth spurt, especially for patients with dysplastic spondylolysis. Findings, such as a vertical, dome-shaped sacrum, a trapezoidal L5, and a kyphotic slip angle increase the risk for progression.

Asymptomatic patients with low-grade spondylolisthesis do not require treatment or activity restrictions. Symptomatic patients will need to be counseled regarding their disorder and temporarily curtail participation in athletic activities. Ultimately, those participating in high-risk sports are five times more likely to have an unfavorable clinical outcome. An acute spondylolysis may heal following the use of a thermoplastic lumbosacral orthosis worn full-time for 6 months, particularly if the spondylolysis is unilateral. If the pars interarticularis defect is chronic, a brace can be used until the child is asymptomatic. Exercises that include hamstring stretching, pelvic tilts, and abdominal strengthening are begun when the patient is pain free. Athletic activities may then be resumed with or without a low-profile antilordotic brace. Should the symptoms recur after a return to higher levels of activity, the following two options need to be discussed: (1) discontinue the activity that produces the symptoms or (2) proceed with surgical treatment to either repair the lytic defect or eliminate movement at the spondylolytic (or spondylolisthetic) segment by a single-level fusion.

Surgical treatment options include repair of a spondylolytic defect, single-level (or two-level) fusions, and reduction of higher-grade spondylolisthesis deformities. The high-grade deformities are uncommon (1% of patients), yet much of the recent literature focuses on the treatment of these deformities. Options that have successfully been described in the recent literature include partial reduction, decompression, and posterior lumbosacral fixation; additional anterior column support; and even in situ posterolateral fusion followed by cast immobilization. Partial (or complete) reduction and instrumentation should be undertaken only by experienced spine surgeons (see chapter 45 for more in-depth information regarding the treatment of adult patients with spondylolisthesis).

Direct repair of spondylolytic defects in patients without spondylolisthesis is usually reserved for those patients with defects at L4 or L3. Defects that occur at L5 can be effectively treated by single-level in situ L5-S1 fusion. If a direct repair is considered, preoperative MRI should be done to rule out adjacent disk pathology. A variety of techniques have been described, including screws across the pars defects, compression wires from transverse process to the spinous process, pedicle screws with wires around the spinous process,

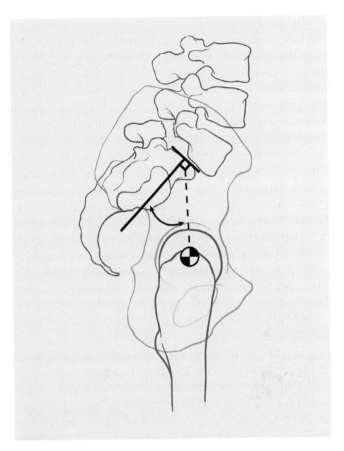

Figure 5 Illustration showing how pelvic incidence in patients with spondylolisthesis is determined by the angle between the line perpendicular to the middle of the sacral plate and the line joining the middle of the sacral plate to the center of the acetabular axis. Pelvic incidence is significantly larger in patients with higher-grade deformities.

and pedicle screws with hooks/rods over the lamina. When a patient with spondylolysis at L5-S1 or low-grade spondylolisthesis requires surgical treatment, a bilateral posterolateral L5-S1 in situ fusion remains the gold standard, and it should be done early in patients with a dysplastic lesion because of the high propensity for progression. Patients with higher-grade spondylolisthesis may require fusion extending to L4. Postoperative brace immobilization may be used for comfort. These treatment options will successfully manage most adolescent patients.

Scheuermann's Kyphosis

Scheuermann's disease represents an exaggerated structural kyphosis involving the thoracic spine. The primary report of poor posture in the adolescent is commonly accompanied by a dull, aching, midscapular, nonradiating discomfort. Physical examination demonstrates an increased, inflexible thoracic kyphosis, which is most evident during forward bending. A compensatory lumbar hyperlordosis is common, but it remains debatable whether this leads to an increased incidence of spondylolysis. Mild scoliosis is present in 15% of patients, but the neurologic examination is almost always normal.

Radiographic features of Scheuermann's disease include kyphosis exceeding 45°, with the apex usually in the middle to lower thoracic spine. If the exaggerated kyphosis is mild, then other accompanying features must be recognized to differentiate Scheuermann's disease from postural kyphosis. These include anterior wedging of three or more adjacent vertebrae in the apical region, end plate irregularities, and narrowing of disk spaces. Schmorl's nodes (herniation of the disk into the vertebral end plate) are occasionally present. Hyperextension lateral radiographs are also helpful in differentiating Scheuermann's disease from postural kyphosis because the apical region in patients with Scheuermann's disease will remain relatively inflexible. Preoperative MRI can be used to rule out disk herniation if necessary.

Nonsurgical treatment consists of exercises and bracing. Although exercises can help alleviate thoracic and lumbar discomfort, they will not result in improvement of the kyphosis. Bracing has been reported to be effective in improving moderate deformity, but lack of patient compliance is a primary limitation.

Surgical indications include large deformities (> 70°), curve progression, persistent pain despite nonsurgical treatment, and, most importantly, genuine cosmetic concerns of the patient. Over the past 15 years, anterior release followed by posterior instrumentation and fusion has been most commonly used. However, recent reports documenting the success of posterior fusion alone, particularly with the use of threaded 4.8-mm compression rods, may obviate the need for additional anterior surgery. Progressive localized kyphosis above or below the fusion can be avoided if the implant extends from the second thoracic vertebra proximally to one level beyond the first lordotic lumbar disk space inferiorly and if the correction is not excessive (> 50%).

Annotated Bibliography

Idiopathic Scoliosis

Asher M, Min Lai S, Burton D, Manna B: The reliability and concurrent validity of the Scoliosis Research Society-22 patient questionnaire for idiopathic scoliosis. *Spine* 2003;28:63-69.

Asher M, Min Lai S, Burton D, Manna B: Scoliosis Research Society-22 patient questionnaire: Responsiveness to change associated with surgical treatment. *Spine* 2003;28:70-73.

These two studies confirm the reliability and validity of the SRS-22 questionnaire when compared with the SF-36. The authors conclude that the SRS-22 is responsive to changes in the postoperative period.

Danielsson A: Back pain and function 23 years after fusion for adolescent idiopathic scoliosis: A case control study. Part II. *Spine* 2003;28:E373-E383.

This is a study of 142 patients who had posterior spinal fusion and instrumentation using Harrington rods at a minimum 20-year follow-up; these patients were compared with 100 age- and sex-matched control subjects. Patients with scoliosis had significantly more degenerative disk changes and lumbar pain than control subjects (65% versus 47%, respectively). However, only 25% of patients who underwent fusion had daily pain, and there were no differences in back function or general health-related quality of life. Patients who underwent fusion also reported pain over their iliac crest incisions when it was made separately.

Dobbs M, Lenke LG, Szymanski DA, et al: Prevalence of neural axis abnormalities in patients with infantile idiopathic scoliosis. *J Bone Joint Surg Am* 2002;84:2230-2234.

This multicenter study analyzed 46 consecutive patients between 1992 and 2000 with infantile idiopathic scoliosis and a curve magnitude greater than or equal to 20°. Ten of the 46 patients (21%) had evidence of neural axis abnormalities on MRI. Eight of these 10 patients had neurosurgical treatment of these abnormalities.

Kuklo TR, Lenke LG, Graham EJ, et al: Correlation of radiographic, clinical, and patient assessment of shoulder balance following fusion versus nonfusion of the proximal thoracic curve in adolescent idiopathic scoliosis. *Spine* 2002;27:2013-2020.

In this retrospective review of 112 patients who underwent surgical treatment for a double thoracic curve pattern, the authors evaluated T1 tilt, clavicle angle, coracoid height difference, trapezius length, first rib-clavicle height difference, shoulder asymmetry as measured by soft-tissue shadows on radiographs, and the translation of the structural curves. They reported that the clavicle angle was the best preoperative predictor of postoperative shoulder balance.

Lenke LG, Betz RR, Harms J, et al: Adolescent idiopathic scoliosis: A new classification to determine extent of spinal arthrodesis. *J Bone Joint Surg Am* 2001;83:1169-1181.

This study introduced the new scoliosis classification, which includes the following three components: curve type, lumbar spine modifier, and a sagittal thoracic modifier. The authors who developed the new system and seven randomly selected surgeons from the Scoliosis Research Society then tested its reliability. The interobserver and intraobserver cap of values for the components of the classification were analyzed and demonstrated good interobserver and intraobserver reliability.

Liljenqvist UR, Allkemper T, Hackenberg L, Link TM, Steinbeck J, Halm HF: Analysis of vertebral morphology in idiopathic scoliosis with use of magnetic resonance imaging and multiplanar reconstruction. *J Bone Joint Surg Am* 2002;84:359-368.

The authors analyzed the morphology of the thoracic pedicles in 307 vertebrae using MRI in multiplanar reconstruction. Maximum intravertebral deformity at the apex of the curve was noted, with transverse endosteal width of the apical pedicles between 2.3 to 3.2 mm on the concavity and 3.9 to 4.4 mm on the convexity.

Merola AA, Haher TR, Brkaric M, et al: A multi-center study of the outcomes of the surgical treatment of adolescent idiopathic scoliosis using the Scoliosis Research Society (SRS) Outcome Instrument. *Spine* 2002;27:2046-2051.

This multicenter study measured outcomes following surgical treatment of adolescent idiopathic scoliosis in 242 patients. Outcome categories included improvement from preoperative pain, general self-image, function from back condition, and level of activity. Overall, the patients were satisfied with the results of surgery. The authors concluded that preoperative pain is typically present in patients with adolescent idiopathic scoliosis, and it improves significantly following surgical treatment.

Newton PO, Betz R, Clements DH, et al: Anterior thoracoscopic instrumentation: A matched comparison to anterior open instrumentation and posterior open instrumentation. *70th Annual Meeting Proceedings*. Rosemont, IL, American Academy of Orthopaedic Surgeons, 2003.

This multicenter study compared three treatment approaches (thoracoscopic, open anterior, and posterior) for patients with right thoracic curves. The radiographic and functional outcomes were similar for the three approaches; however, the patients who had thoracoscopic anterior instrumentation and fusion had longer surgical times.

Ouellet JA, LaPlaza J, Erickson M, Birch JG, Burke S, Browne R: Sagittal plane deformity in the thoracic spine: A clue to the presence of syringomyelia as a cause of scoliosis. *Spine* 2003;28:2147-2151.

Thirty patients with scoliosis and documented evidence of syringomyelia were compared with 54 patients with adolescent idiopathic scoliosis and a normal MRI. The authors analyzed the lateral radiographs for the presence or absence of Dickson apical lordosis. Apical lordosis was seen in 97% of patients with adolescent idiopathic scoliosis and normal MRI scan, whereas only 25% of patients with syringomyelia-associated scoliosis had apical lordosis.

Pratt R, Webb JK, Burwell RG, Cummings SL: Luque trolley and convex epiphysiodesis in the management of infantile and juvenile idiopathic scoliosis. *Spine* 1999;24:1538-1547.

The authors reported 5-year follow-up of patients in whom either a Luque trolley alone or a Luque trolley together with a convex epiphysiodesis was used to treat progressive infantile

or juvenile idiopathic scoliosis. The authors concluded that convex epiphysiodesis together with Luque trolley instrumentation may slow down or improve progressive infantile or juvenile idiopathic curves.

Richards BS: Delayed infections following posterior spinal instrumentation for the treatment of idiopathic scoliosis. *J Bone Joint Surg Am* 1995;77:524-529.

Ten patients (average age, 25 months) with delayed treatment of deep wound infections were observed after undergoing posterior instrumentation for adolescent idiopathic scoliosis. The authors reported that the patients usually had drainage from the wound, fluctuance, and mildly elevated erythrocyte sedimentation rates and were treated using instrumentation removal, primary wound closure, and short-term administration of antibiotics. The authors also discuss the importance of longer culture incubation to identify the infectious organisms.

Richards BS, Sucato DJ, Konigsberg DE, Ouellet JA: Comparison of reliability between the Lenke and King classification systems for adolescent idiopathic scoliosis using radiographs that were not premeasured. *Spine* 2003;28:1148-1157.

Four surgeons analyzed 50 radiographs that had not been premeasured and assigned a classification using both the King and the Lenke classification. The intraobserver and interobserver reliability of the King classification were 83.5% and 68.0%, respectively. These values were similar when only the Lenke curve types were analyzed; however, when the complete classifications were assigned (curve type, lumbar modifier, and thoracic sagittal modifier), there was fair intraobserver and interobserver reliability (65.0% and 55.5%, respectively).

Sucato DJ, Duchene C: The position of the aorta relative to the spine: A comparison of patients with and without idiopathic scoliosis. *J Bone Joint Surg Am* 2003; 85:1461-1469.

Axial T1-weighted MRI scans of the thoracic and lumbar spine were compared for normal control subjects and patients with right idiopathic scoliosis. The aorta was positioned more laterally and posteriorly to the vertebral bodies in patients with idiopathic scoliosis, which was in line with a well-placed vertebral body screw and would be in jeopardy of a laterally misplaced left pedicle screw.

Sucato DJ, Elerson E: A comparison between the prone and lateral position for performing a thoracoscopic anterior release and fusion for pediatric spinal deformity. *Spine* 2003;28:2176-2180.

The technique of an anterior thoracoscopic release using a regular endotracheal tube is described, with ventilation of both lungs with lower tidal volumes. The patient is positioned prone. When compared with patients who underwent this procedure in the lateral position (double lumen endotracheal tube for single-lung ventilation), the anesthesia preparation time and the delay between the anterior and posterior procedure were both shorter and there were fewer respiratory complications (in 0 versus 14.8% of patients).

Suk SI, Kim WJ, Lee SM, Kim JH, Chung ER: Thoracic pedicle screw fixation in spinal deformities: Are they really safe? *Spine* 2001;26:2049-2057.

This study analyzed 462 patients who had 4,604 thoracic screws placed to treat spinal deformity. Neurologic complications directly related to the screws occurred in four patients (0.8%), one of whom had transient paraparesis and three had dural tears. The authors concluded that thoracic pedicle screw fixation is safe when treating spinal deformity.

Weinstein SL, Dolan LA, Spratt KF, Peterson KK, Spoonamore MJ, Ponseti IV: Health and function of patients with untreated idiopathic scoliosis. *JAMA* 2003;289:559-567.

In this prospective natural history study, 117 patients with untreated scoliosis were compared with 62 age- and sex-matched control subjects. The minimum follow-up was 50 years, and multiple parameters were evaluated. The probability of survival was similar between the two groups, however, the incidence of shortness of breath and chronic back pain were greater in patients with scoliosis.

Congenital Spinal Deformities

Basu PS, Elsebaie H, Noordeen MH: Congenital spinal deformity: A comprehensive assessment at presentation. *Spine* 2002;27:2255-2259.

A series of 126 consecutive patients with congenital spinal deformity were assessed for incidence of intraspinal anomaly. This incidence was found in 37% of patients (26% of patients had cardiac defects and 21% had urogenital anomalies). The authors concluded that MRI and echocardiography should be an essential part of the evaluation of patients with congenital spinal deformity.

Campbell RM, Hell-Vocke AK: Growth of the thoracic spine in congenital scoliosis after expansion thoracoplasty. *J Bone Joint Surg Am* 2003;85:409-420.

Expansion thoracoplasty consists of osteotomizing fused ribs on the concavity of the spine followed by expansion of the chest cage using a vertical, expandable prosthetic titanium rib implant. The authors reported that longitudinal growth of the spine was achieved using this technique, likely providing additional volume for growth of the underlying lungs.

Campbell RM, Smith MD, Mayes TC, et al: The characteristics of thoracic insufficiency syndrome associated with fused ribs and congenital scoliosis. *J Bone Joint Surg Am* 2003;85-A:399-408.

This landmark article introduces and defines thoracic insufficiency syndrome, the inability of the thorax to support

normal respiration or lung growth, which is caused by a rare condition of multiple fused ribs and congenital scoliosis.

Kim YJ, Otsuka NY, Flynn JM, et al: Surgical treatment of congenital kyphosis. *Spine* 2001;26:2251-2257.

In this study, 26 patients were retrospectively reviewed. The authors found a low rate of pseudarthrosis even without routine augmentation of the fusion mass if instrumentation was used. They report that although gradual correction of kyphosis occurs with growth in patients younger than 3 years of age with type II and type III deformities after posterior fusion, it appears to be unpredictable.

Klemme WR, Polly DW, Orchowske JR: Hemivertebral excision for congenital scoliosis in very young children. *J Pediatr Orthop* 2001;21:761-764.

Six children (average age, 19 months) underwent anterior-posterior hemivertebra excision. Correction was maintained with plaster immobilization for 3 months. The authors reported that excellent improvements in the curves were obtained and maintained at a minimum 2-year follow-up.

McMaster MJ, Singh H: The surgical management of congenital kyphosis and kyphoscoliosis. *Spine* 2001;26:2146-2154.

In this study, 65 patients with congenital kyphosis or kyphoscoliosis were treated with spine arthrodesis. The authors concluded that all patients with type I or type III congenital kyphosis or kyphoscoliosis should be treated using posterior arthrodesis before age 5 years and before the kyphosis exceeds 50°. If the kyphosis does not reduce to less than 50°, an anterior release and arthrodesis using strut grafting is needed before posterior arthrodesis can be done.

Ruf M, Harms J: Hemivertebra resection by a posterior approach: Innovative operative technique and first results. *Spine* 2002;27:1116-1123.

In this retrospective study, 21 consecutive patients with congenital scoliosis were treated with hemivertebra resection using a posterior approach only with transpedicular instrumentation. Early surgery is recommended to avert severe local deformities, to prevent secondary structural changes, and to avert extensive fusions.

Sink EL, Karol LA, Sanders J, et al: Efficacy of perioperative halo-gravity traction in the treatment of severe scoliosis in children. *J Pediatr Orthop* 2001;21:519-524.

Perioperative halo traction was used in 19 patients, including those with congenital scoliosis. The technique improved balance and frontal and sagittal alignment. No neurologic complications occurred.

Sturm PF, Chung R, Bormze SR: Hemivertebra in monozygotic twins. *Spine* 2001;26:1389-1391.

This is a report on two monozygotic female twins with thoracic hemivertebrae that led to scoliosis.

Suh SW, Sarwark JF, Vora A, et al: Evaluating congenital spine deformities for intraspinal anomalies with magnetic resonance imaging. *J Pediatr Orthop* 2001;21:525-531.

In this study, 41 children with congenital spinal deformities underwent MRI. Evidence of intraspinal anomalies were visible for 31% of the patients, including tethered cord, syringomyelia, and diastematomyelia. The authors recommend MRI as part of the initial evaluation, even in the absence of clinical findings.

Spondylolysis and Spondylolisthesis

Grzegorzewski A, Kumar SJ: In situ posterolateral spine arthrodesis for grades III, IV, and V spondylolisthesis in children and adolescents. *J Pediatr Orthop* 2000;20:506-511.

This study reports on 21 patients who underwent in situ posterolateral L4-S1 fusions to treat severe spondylolisthesis, followed by pantaloon cast for 4 months. The authors report satisfactory results using this technique.

Hanson DS, Bridwell KH, Rhee JM, Lenke LG: Correlation of pelvic incidence with low and high-grade isthmic spondylolisthesis. *Spine* 2002;27:2026-2029.

In this study, pelvic incidence, a fixed angle in an individual, was reported to be significantly higher in patients with low-grade and high-grade isthmic spondylolisthesis when compared with control subjects and correlated significantly with the Meyerding grades of severity.

Lenke LG, Bridwell KH: Evaluation and surgical treatment of high-grade isthmic dysplastic spondylolisthesis. *Instr Course Lect* 2003;52:525-532.

The authors reported that high-grade isthmic dysplastic spondylolisthesis should be treated surgically with appropriate central and foraminal decompressions at the L5-S1 level, followed by lumbosacral fusion. Partial reduction (to improve the slip angle) provides less risk to the L5 nerve root than complete reduction. Anterior and posterior fusion at L5-S1 appears to provide the best long-term results.

Scheuermann's Kyphosis

Johnston CE, Sucato DJ, Elerson E: Correction of adolescent hyperkyphosis with posterior-only threaded rod compression instrumentation. *38th Annual Scoliosis Research Society Meeting Manual.* Quebec, Canada, Scoliosis Research Society, 2003, p 121.

In this study, threaded 4.8-mm posterior compression rods were used to treat 14 patients with thoracic kyphosis (average kyphosis, 78.6° preoperatively). Anterior release was not performed. Correction to 40° was maintained 2.5 years postoperatively. The authors concluded that anterior spinal fusion is not necessary when kyphosis is corrected using this technique.

Papagelopoulos PJ, Klassen RA, Peterson HA, et al: Surgical treatment of Scheuermann's disease with segmental compression instrumentation. *Clin Orthop* 2001; 386:139-149.

Twenty-one patients with kyphotic deformities of 50° or greater underwent posterior compression instrumentation. Seven patients also had anterior release. The authors concluded that the use of the posterior procedure by itself provided significant correction, thereby avoiding the development of any secondary deformity in most patients.

Poolman RW, Been HD, Ubags LH: Clinical outcome and radiographic results after operative treatment of Scheuermann's disease. *Eur Spine J* 2002;11:561-569.

In this study, 23 patients underwent combined anterior and posterior fusion of their kyphotic deformities. On extended follow-up, thoracic kyphosis significantly increased, which was thought to be caused primarily by removal of the posterior implant. This occurred despite solid fusions being shown at the time of implant removal. Use of the SRS-22 questionnaire showed only fair outcomes after surgical intervention, leading the authors to question the indications for surgery.

Stotts AK, Smith JT, Santora SD, et al: Measurement of spinal kyphosis: Implications for the management of Scheuermann's kyphosis. *Spine* 2002;27:2143-2146.

In this study, a broad range of intraobserver and interobserver differences occur in the measurement of thoracic kyphosis in patients with Scheuermann's disease.

Classic Bibliography

Blount WP, Schmidt AC: The Milwaukee brace in the treatment of scoliosis. *J Bone Joint Surg* 1957;39:693.

Cook S, Asher M, Lai S-M, Shobe J: Reoperation after primary posterior instrumentation and fusion for idiopathic scoliosis: Toward defining later operative site pain of unknown cause. *Spine* 2000;25:463-468.

Metha MH: The rib-vertebra angle in the early diagnosis between resolving and progressive infantile scoliosis. *J Bone Joint Surg Br* 1972;54:230-243.

Nachemson AL, Peterson L-E: Effectiveness of treatment with a brace in girls who have adolescent idiopathic scoliosis: A prospective, controlled study based on data from the Brace Study of the Scoliosis Research Society. *J Bone Joint Surg Am* 1995;77:815-822.

Weinstein SL, Ponseti IV: Curve progression in idiopathic scoliosis. *J Bone Joint Surg Am* 1983;65:447-455.

Index

American Academy of Orthopaedic Surgeons